SYS# 1287950

WITHDRAWN

S0-AEH-411

SEX FROM PLATO TO PAGLIA

Advisory Board

David Archard
University of Lancaster

Martha Cornog

John Corvino
Wayne State University

Joseph A. Diorio
Unitec, New Zealand

Ann Garry
California State University, Los Angeles

Christine E. Gudorf
Florida International University

Sarah Hoffman
University of Saskatchewan

Richard T. Hull
State University of New York at Buffalo (Emeritus)

Edward Johnson
University of New Orleans

John Kleinig
John Jay College of Criminal Justice

Timothy F. Murphy
University of Illinois College of Medicine at Chicago

James Lindemann Nelson
Michigan State University

Igor Primoratz
Hebrew University of Jerusalem

J. Martin Stafford

Robert M. Stewart
California State University, Chico

Edward Collins Vacek, S.J.
Weston Jesuit School of Theology

Alan Wertheimer
University of Vermont

SEX FROM PLATO TO PAGLIA
A PHILOSOPHICAL ENCYCLOPEDIA

VOLUME I: A–L

Edited by
ALAN SOBLE

GREENWOOD PRESS
Westport, Connecticut • London

Library of Congress Cataloging-in-Publication Data

Sex from Plato to Paglia : a philosophical encyclopedia / edited by Alan Soble.
    p.   cm.
   Includes bibliographical references and index.
    ISBN 0–313–32686–X (set : alk. paper)—ISBN 0–313–33424–2 (v. 1 : alk. paper)—
ISBN 0–313–33425–0 (v. 2 : alk. paper)
   1. Sex—History—Encyclopedias. 2. Sex—Philosophy—Encyclopedias. I. Soble,
Alan.
HQ12.S423   2006
306.7'03—dc22   2005019218

British Library Cataloguing in Publication Data is available.

Copyright © 2006 by Alan Soble

All rights reserved. No portion of this book may be
reproduced, by any process or technique, without the
express written consent of the publisher.

Library of Congress Catalog Card Number: 2005019218
ISBN: 0–313–32686–X (set)
      0–313–33424–2 (vol. 1)
      0–313–33425–0 (vol. 2)

First published in 2006

Greenwood Press, 88 Post Road West, Westport, CT 06881
An imprint of Greenwood Publishing Group, Inc.
www.greenwood.com

Printed in the United States of America

The paper used in this book complies with the
Permanent Paper Standard issued by the National
Information Standards Organization (Z39.48–1984).

10 9 8 7 6 5 4 3 2 1

For Rachel Soble

Pinball Wizard

Marital continence is so much more difficult than continence out-side marriage, because the spouses grow accustomed to inter-course.... Once they begin to have sexual intercourse as a habit, and a constant inclination is created, a mutual need for inter-course comes into being.

Karol Wojtyła (Pope John Paul II)

[R]estricting sex to a single partner ... reduce[s] its overall fre-quency. Marriage translates a maximum of opportunity into a minimum of desire by continually allowing the release of sexual tension before an ample amount of erotic passion can accumu-late.... Thus marriage seems almost intentionally designed to make sex boring.

Murray Davis

CONTENTS

Preface   xi
Acknowledgments   xix
Introduction   xxi
Abbreviations   xxv
Guide to Related Topics   xxvii

Volume 1: A–L

Abortion   1
Abstinence   7
Activity, Sexual   15
Addiction, Sexual   25
Adultery   30
African Philosophy   38
Animal Sexuality   45
Anscombe, G.E.M. (1919–2001)   50
Aristotle (384–322 BCE)   56
Arts, Sex and the   62
Augustine (Saint) (354–430)   74
Bataille, Georges (1897–1962)   84
Beauty   86
Bestiality   95
Bible, Sex and the   104
Bisexuality   113
Boswell, John (1947–1994)   120
Buddhism   126
Bullough, Vern L. (1928–   )   131
Casual Sex   136
Catholicism, History of   143
Catholicism, Twentieth- and Twenty-First-Century   153
Chinese Philosophy   164
Coercion (by Sexually Aggressive Women)   169
Communication Model   174
Completeness, Sexual   179
Consent   184
Consequentialism   194
Contraception   202
Cybersex   209

Descartes, René (1596–1650)   219
Desire, Sexual   222
Disability   229
Diseases, Sexually Transmitted   235
Dworkin, Andrea (1946–2005)   241
Dysfunction, Sexual   248
Ellis, Albert (1913–)   256
Ellis, Havelock (1859–1939)   261
Ethics, Professional Codes of   268
Ethics, Sexual   273
Ethics, Virtue   279
Evolution   285
Existentialism   292
Fantasy   304
Feminism, French   308
Feminism, History of   315
Feminism, Lesbian   324
Feminism, Liberal   333
Feminism, Men's   342
Fichte, Johann Gottlieb (1762–1814)   347
Firestone, Shulamith (1945–)   353
Flirting   357
Foucault, Michel (1926–1984)   361
Freud, Sigmund (1856–1939)   370
Freudian Left, The   381
Friendship   390
Genital Mutilation   398
Gnosticism   402
Greek Sexuality and Philosophy, Ancient   410
Harassment, Sexual   419
Hegel, G.W.F. (1770–1831)   429
Heidegger, Martin (1889–1976)   435
Herdt, Gilbert (1949–)   439
Heterosexism   442
Hinduism   448
Hobbes, Thomas (1588–1679)   454
Homosexuality, Ethics of   460
Homosexuality and Science   468
Hume, David (1711–1776)   476
Humor   480
Incest   487
Indian Erotology   493
Intersexuality   496
Islam   503
Jainism   510
Jealousy   515
Judaism, History of   521
Judaism, Twentieth- and Twenty-First-Century   533

Kant, Immanuel (1724–1804) 543
Kierkegaard, Søren (1813–1855) 553
Kolnai, Aurel (1900–1973) 563
Lacan, Jacques (1901–1981) 567
Language 574
Law, Sex and the 583
Leibniz, Gottfried (1646–1716) 589
Levinas, Emmanuel (1906–1995) 593
Liberalism 598
Love 606

Volume 2: M–Z

MacKinnon, Catharine (1946–   ) 621
Mandeville, Bernard (1670–1733) 632
Manichaeism 636
Marriage 639
Marriage, Same-Sex 650
Marxism 660
Masturbation 671
Mead, Margaret (1901–1978) 683
Military, Sex and the 684
Money, John (1921–   ) 690
Nagel, Thomas (1937–   ) 698
Natural Law (New) 702
Nietzsche, Friedrich (1844–1900) 711
Nudism 718
Objectification, Sexual 723
Orientation, Sexual 728
Paglia, Camille (1947–   ) 735
Paraphilia 740
Paul (Saint) (5–64?) 748
Pedophilia 755
Personification, Sexual 763
Perversion, Sexual 767
Phenomenology 777
Philosophy of Sex, Overview of 784
Philosophy of Sex, Teaching the 793
Plato (427–347 BCE) 800
Pornography 811
Posner, Richard (1939–   ) 824
Poststructuralism 829
Privacy 839
Prostitution 848
Protestantism, History of 859
Protestantism, Twentieth- and Twenty-First-Century 868
Psychology, Evolutionary 877
Psychology, Twentieth- and Twenty-First-Century 885

Queer Theory   895
Rape   901
Rape, Acquaintance and Date   911
Reproductive Technology   921
Rimmer, Robert (1917–2001)   929
Roman Sexuality and Philosophy, Ancient   933
Rousseau, Jean-Jacques (1712–1778)   939
Russell, Bertrand (1872–1970)   944
Sacher-Masoch, Leopold von (1836–1895)   949
Sade, Marquis de (1740–1814)   952
Sadomasochism   960
Schopenhauer, Arthur (1788–1860)   967
Scruton, Roger (1944–   )   973
Seduction   980
Sex Education   986
Sex Work   997
Sexology   1002
Sexuality, Dimensions of   1010
Sherfey, Mary Jane (1918–1983)   1016
Singer, Irving (1925–   )   1022
Social Constructionism   1026
Spencer, Herbert (1820–1903)   1033
Spinoza, Baruch (1632–1677)   1036
Tantrism   1041
Thomas Aquinas (Saint) (1224/25–1274)   1045
Utopianism   1054
Violence, Sexual   1066
Westermarck, Edward (1862–1939)   1071
Wittgenstein, Ludwig (1889–1951)   1076
Wojtyła, Karol (Pope John Paul II) (1920–2005)   1081

Selected General Bibliography   1091
Editors and Contributors   1095
Name Index   1113
Subject Index   1149

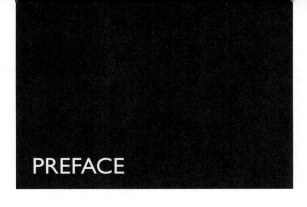

PREFACE

In early 2002, with the encouragement and guidance of Lawrence C. Becker (and, later, Charlotte B. Becker, also an experienced encyclopedist), I undertook this project to assemble an encyclopedia devoted exclusively to a relatively new and quickly growing area in philosophy, the *philosophy of sex*.

The result, *Sex from Plato to Paglia: A Philosophical Encyclopedia*, is a reference tool and resource book directed to undergraduate and graduate students in philosophy, theology, gender studies, psychology, sexology, and the arts and humanities in general, as well as to high school, college, and university teachers (of philosophy of sex courses, and others) and professional researchers and writers, whether independent or affiliated with or housed in an educational institution or think tank. The entries have, with only a few exceptions, been written in such a way that students, faculty persons, and writers in other areas, including the natural and social sciences and the professions, will profit from perusing the encyclopedia, if only out of curiosity. They might be pleasantly surprised and discover that philosophical discussions of sexuality deserve greater attention. The general goal of the encyclopedia is to educate its readers in the fundamental questions, approaches, insights, and conclusions in the continuing and expanding field of the philosophical study of human sexuality and, in the process, to be not only instructive but also thought-provoking and occasionally entertaining.

CONTENT

The encyclopedia is eclectic. It contains entries written in diverse philosophical styles and from various perspectives. Analytic, continental, religious, secular, solemn, curious, liberal, conservative, and feminist pieces cover a wide range of themes in the philosophy of sex, from "Abortion" to "Wojtyła, Karol." The final catalog of contributors and entries is mostly the result of the conscious deliberations of several human brains, but—as editors of large projects and presidents are bound to know—serendipity, too, played a role. Not every possible topic has been covered, but the included entries pick up some of the slack. For example, the intersection of medicine and sex is explored in, among others, these entries: "Diseases, Sexually Transmitted," "Ethics, Professional Codes of," "Intersexuality," "Money, John," "Paraphilia," and "Reproductive Technology."

Sex from Plato to Paglia is composed of 153 entries that break down into these three types: figures, topics/concepts, and history/schools of thought. Fifty entries discuss people who have said something philosophically noteworthy (or more) about sexuality. Most are deceased, from Plato (427–347 BCE) and Aristotle (384–322 BCE) to Michel Foucault (1926–1984), Jacques Lacan (1901–1981), and Robert Rimmer (1917–2001). Eleven, including Albert Ellis (1913–   ), John Money (1921–   ), and Irving Singer (1925–   ), are still alive. Purists will be sure to register the fact that the encyclopedia violates its own title by including entries on figures, topics, and schools that antedate Plato (pre-Platonic philosophy of sex, both Occidental and Oriental); also, some included figures, topics, or history/schools (or a piece of same) fall within a hair space to a decade after the publication of Camille Paglia's (1947–   ) *Sexual Personae* (1990), *Sex, Art, and American Culture* (1992), and *Vamps and Tramps* (1994) (post-Paglian philosophy of sex, both Philadelphian and Opelousan). Philosophers and librarians will also have discriminating opinions about this conundrum—whether the entry "Freudian Left, The" (and others) should be included among figures instead of schools of thought (as the editor did). About 60 entries cover topics or concepts such as abstinence, bestiality, flirting, jealousy, objectification, seduction, and rape, and about 40 entries cover history/schools of thought, such as Catholicism, existentialism, Islam, Jainism, and poststructuralism. Here, too, whether something is a topic or more precisely a school of thought could be puzzling, for example, the entries "Consequentialism," "Nudism," and "Pedophilia." The editor used the following criteria: If the word ended with "ism," or if the word's first letter could, in some context (other than at the beginning of a sentence) exist without too much strain in the upper case, the term was a *good candidate* for the "schools of thought" category. These tests work well for "consequentialism" and "nudism." The editor is not yet convinced that "pedophilia" as a "school of behavior" that has (for some writers) an underlying philosophy—as nudism is both a practice and a philosophy—is properly something other than a topic, despite ancient Greek philosophical pederasty and the more recent exertions of the North American Man-Boy Love Association. Nor are "Heterosexism" and "Sadomasochism" counted as schools of thought, despite the "ism."

STATISTICS

The entries range in length from slightly over 700 words (e.g., "Mead, Margaret") to a hundred or so words over 6,000 (e.g., "Activity, Sexual," "Arts, Sex and the," "Catholicism, History of," "Judaism, History of," and "Masturbation"), including the entry's "References." The average length is roughly 3,500 words per entry. The 153 entries were written by 103 contributors, with 33 contributors writing more than one entry. If we discount the loquacious volume editor's 8 entries, J. Martin Stafford led the pack with 5 entries. Joseph A. Diorio, Christine E. Gudorf, Edward Johnson, and Carol V. Quinn wrote 4 each. Four entries were written by teams of two scholars: Peter B. Anderson and Cindy Struckman-Johnson coauthored "Coercion (by Sexually Aggressive Women)"; Charles M. Culver and Bernard Gert wrote "Paraphilia"; and Jan Steutel and Ben Spiecker cranked out both "Disability" and "Incest."

Most of the authors are philosophers or trained in philosophy. Scholars from other fields also contributed, primarily religious studies and theology, and a handful came from political science, psychology, history, and sociology. Most are inhabitants of the United States, but 21 are from other countries: Canada (4), Finland (4), the United Kingdom (4), Australia (3), Israel (2), Netherlands (2), Denmark (1) and New Zealand (1). American contributors come from 28 states and from Guam (2) and the District of Columbia (2). California (11) beat its nearest competitors, Florida and New York, by 3.

The members of the encyclopedia's advisory board dutifully performed their administrative tasks, which included proposing figures, topics, and schools to be covered in the encyclopedia; suggesting and refining the entry descriptions and thereby the content of the entries; nominating candidate contributors for the entries; volunteering to write entries; reviewing some of the manuscripts; offering general advice about various matters; and providing occasional support and solace to the volume editor. The volume editor takes responsibility, and welcomes both the praise and the blame, for having edited, as editors are wont to do, all the entries.

FORMAT

The entries are arranged alphabetically by title, which was selected by the editor. If the entry is on an individual, his or her birth and death dates (or, in the case of living subjects, only the birth date) are supplied, attached to the title in parentheses. The text of the entry is followed immediately by a "See also" section listing other entries (chosen by the editor) that extend, elaborate, or provide details about the content of the entry. Each entry concludes with two bibliographies. The first, "References," contains works that are referred to or mentioned in the entry's text. The second, "Additional Reading," lists works that are relevant to the content of the entry but not referred to in the text of the entry. The "Additional Reading" items are, to resort to a well-known way of expressing it, "Suggestions for Further Reading." Immediately following "References" is the name of the contributor(s), whose affiliation(s) can be found in the "Editors and Contributors" section at the back of the book.

In the text of the entry, words in boldface type (e.g., **abortion**) are cross-references to other entries in the encyclopedia. Throughout the book, blind entries provide alternative ways of looking up a topic; for instance, users who go to the *E* section to look up "Education" will find the cross-reference "Education, Sex. *See* Sex Education" to lead them to the entry they seek in the *S* section. The first time a deceased person is mentioned in an entry, his or her birth and death dates (the abbreviation "ca." is used to alert the reader to approximate dates) are inserted parenthetically. (Occasionally the year of birth of a still-living person is provided in the text, out of respect for our senior citizens, among whom the editor "self-identifies.") "BCE" and, in a few cases, "CE" are employed instead of "BC" and "AD" for life dates as well as dates of events, appearance of a particular piece of writing, and so on. In the absence of "BCE," assume the date referred to is "CE."

No entry contains any footnotes or endnotes, but the entries do contain in-text citations to material listed in their "References" bibliographies. In-text references are central to the encyclopedia's mission as a research resource, even if they might at times seem to clutter the text. For example, if the entry teaches the reader (and claims) that St. Augustine presented an ingenious but fallacious argument that evil things *cannot* exist, the reader will be told exactly where (in the *Confessions*) Augustine's argument can be located (§7.12), so that the reader is not compelled to page through the entire *book* to find it. The in-text references, then, are meant to make the encyclopedia user-helpful. However, although page references are usually supplied to material in *articles*, sometimes they are not, since in some cases articles are brief and it would not be difficult for readers to find the relevant passage that is paraphrased or discussed. For *quoted* passages, whether from a book or an article, an appropriate reference is given, so that the reader can find it. If a quoted passage contains italicized words, assume that the original was italicized unless advised otherwise.

Note, however, that the in-text references are not always to page numbers in a book or an article. Especially for famous works in the history of philosophy, which exist today in many editions and translations that are paginated differently, it is more convenient for the author and the reader that reference be made not to page number but to, say, chapter number and paragraph number, so that no matter what edition or translation of the work is available, the reader can find the passage that is quoted or referred to. For example, standard marginal numbers are used for anything written by Plato and Aristotle; book, chapter, and section numbers are used for the works of Augustine, Thomas Aquinas, David Hume, and others; "Akademie" numbers are sometimes used for the works of Immanuel Kant; paragraph numbers for G.W.F. Hegel's *Philosophy of Right*; "Remark" letters for Bernard Mandeville's *Fable of the Bees*; and so on. If reference is made to a particular book or article early in a paragraph, and no other, different material is referred to in that paragraph, then the reader should assume that any later in-text references in that paragraph (say, page numbers standing alone) are to that only-named particular book or article. Exceptions to these principles occur in the case of materials referred to that exist on the World Wide Web, which ordinarily have no page or marginal numbers. But these items are almost always brief and, in any event, the reader who accesses a Web page can use his or her browser's search function to find the passage. This procedure is efficient if one searches for a unique word or short string of words.

The "Additional Reading" bibliographies were compiled largely by the volume editor. Every entry, with two exceptions ("Manichaeism" and "Spencer, Herbert"), concludes with an "Additional Reading" list. Many philosophical articles and books on sexuality are valuable sources, yet not all could be discussed or mentioned in the individual entries. The "Additional Reading" lists are meant to alert readers who are interested in the breadth of the philosophical literature, and who wish to pursue matters of special concern more deeply, to this additional material. Also listed are more general philosophical treatises about issues, concepts, and figures that will help readers situate the philosophy of sex within the history of, and current debates in, philosophy. Further, important nonphilosophical articles and books on sexuality, from the humanities and the sciences (some of which are classics in their fields), are significant sources not only for those who wish to evaluate philosophical perspectives on sexuality in the broader context of general human knowledge but also for those who believe, as many scholars do, that knowledge of a wide variety of disciplines is essential to understanding and making progress in the philosophy of sex, which is, and is best approached as, an interdisciplinary field.

The "Additional Reading" bibliography does not include sources discussed, mentioned, or cited in an entry; all these items are listed only in an entry's "References" list. However, occasionally a few sources not referred to in an entry are nevertheless included in its "References" bibliography by virtue of their importance to the content of the entry. Further, an entry's "Additional Reading" list includes not only additional material but also—for the benefit of readers intent on tracking down a particular source or who do not have access to a specific item listed in the "References"—information about reprints and other editions of the sources contained in the "References." This information about reprints and alternative editions has the independent value of providing a historical record of writings in the philosophy of sex.

Readers may notice some repetition in the "References" and "Additional Reading" bibliographies. An item listed in the "References" of one entry may show up in another entry's "References" or in another entry's "Additional Reading." Some items appear in more than one "Additional Reading" list (and may or may not be listed in any entry's "References"). This repetition results from interconnections between the various topics and concepts in the philosophy of sex. It is not to be bemoaned. Rather, the repetition will usefully assist readers in locating relevant material for further research. The essay on the phenomenology of prostitution by Clelia Anderson and Yolanda Estes might be overlooked by readers interested in phenomenological approaches to sexuality, were the essay included only in the bibliographies of the "Prostitution" entry; or it might be missed by those interested in prostitution, were it listed only in the bibliographies of the "Phenomenology" entry. Similarly, Ermanno Bencivegna's "Kant's Sadism," Drucilla Cornell's *The Imaginary Domain: Abortion, Pornography, and Sexual Harassment*, and other "compound" items simply had to be listed several times. The editor suspects that any item listed once could, with justification, have been listed twice, but he wisely eschewed that route. The repetition that does exist will be helpful to those students and scholars—probably most—who read or browse selectively instead of reading universally, that is, digesting the entire encyclopedia.

The encyclopedia's editor is fully responsible for the final selection of the items included in each "Additional Reading" bibliography. The editor, however, received much assistance from the authors of the individual entries, who suggested many items to be included in their entry's "Additional Reading" list and who are therefore responsible (only) for the accuracy of the bibliographic information for the particular items they submitted toward this list. That an item is listed should not necessarily be taken as an endorsement of the book or article or as meaning that either the author of the entry or the editor thinks that the work has merit (although in many cases it does). That is, some items are listed for the sake of completeness and to provide another piece of the intricate historical record. Besides, philosophical tastes vary and change. That which is eminently vacuous in one decade might be eminently sagacious in the next. This could apply to all readers or even only to one reader, who might have "matured"—or "regressed"—as a scholar.

Had space allowed, brief annotations for each item listed could have further enhanced the usefulness of the "Additional Reading" bibliographies. For example, it is obvious why Laura Kipnis's essay "Adultery" is listed for the "Adultery" entry. (Even so, a few words about Kipnis's view of adultery would help the reader.) But its being included for the "Freudian Left" entry may be puzzling. It could be explained easily by appending: "Kipnis coins the term 'surplus monogamy,' deliberately fashioned after Marcuse." Alas, pressing space considerations, as well as time and energy requirements, placed severe limits on what could be accomplished. The reader is encouraged to trust the editor's judgment that good reason exists for the seemingly odd placement of some items. (In a few instances, where it was thought essential, an extremely brief annotation, surrounded by square brackets, has been inserted.)

The following principles were employed by the editor in structuring the items in the bibliographies:

- In the "Additional Reading" lists alone, and never in an entry's "References" bibliography, abbreviations for books are occasionally used, usually when an item has been reprinted in a popular (well-known or much-referred-to) anthology or collection of articles. These books are listed in the "Abbreviations" section found at the front of the book. Sometimes these items are referred to in the "References" as appearing in these collections; there abbreviations are not used, thereby usually (but not always; see the exception, below) signaling that the item's original or primary location of appearance was in fact the anthology itself and not, say, a journal (the item does not appear in the collection as a reprint). This might occur in the "Additional Reading" section of an entry as well, indicating again that the anthology is the original or main location of publication. An exception occurs when a contributor chose to refer in the text of the entry to a reprint of the article in a collection instead of to the original, sometimes on the grounds that the reprint would be more accessible to the reader and sometimes because only the reprint was accessible to the writer. When this happens, it will be made clear in the "Additional Reading" bibliography where the original location of publication, with its earlier date, is provided.

- If an article or essay by an author is included in a book entirely written by that author, the author's name appears only once, as the author of the essay, and not repeated later as author of the whole book. For example,

> Swiss, Charles E. "How to Play Pinball Like a Wizard." In *Games and Other Diversions: A Philosophical Exploration*. Bogalusa, La.: Cheeseworks Enterprises, 2004, 77–93.

In this case, because no other author or editor is provided for *Games and Other Diversions*, the reader should assume that the whole work was authored by Swiss. That is, the formats "In his [or her] *Games* . . ." or "In Charles E. Swiss, *Games* . . ." are not employed. If someone else edited the book, or if the author of the article is in fact the editor of a (this) book that contains essays by other writers, then the editor's name, different or the same, is explicitly provided. In such a case, expect to see:

> Swiss, Charles E. "How to Play Pinball Like a Wizard." In Charles E. Swiss, ed., *Games and Other Diversions: A Philosophical Exploration*. Bogalusa, La.: Cheeseworks Enterprises, 2004, 77–93.

Or if Swiss did not edit the book, it would appear as "In Lucy Butterworth, ed., *Games. . . .*"

- The goal (appreciably achieved but not always) was to supply thoroughly complete bibliographic information. For journal articles, this means full names of author(s); full title of essay; name(s) of translator(s), if any; journal name; volume; issue number (or quarter, season, month); year; and inclusive page numbers. For books, this means full names of all authors or editors ("et al." was used neither for books nor articles; it was deemed by the editor inappropriate for a reference book, which should provide a complete historical record); full name of book, including subtitle, if any; name(s) of translator(s), if any; name of the publisher; place of publication; and year of publication. For an item translated into English, its original date of publication (if available) in its original language is provided after the author's name. Sometimes a year date after the author's name indicates, instead, the year of the item's first edition in English, if a later edition is the one listed in the bibliography. Multiple dates indicate successive editions (for items in any language). And sometimes a year date after the author's name indicates, in particular for ancient texts and classic works, when (roughly) it was written and unleashed onto the world (*perhaps* published, if "published," a relatively modern concept, and grist for the social constructionist mill, even makes sense for these works). The context should successfully disclose what the year date refers to.

The encyclopedia contains other helpful sections. At the end of the front matter is a "Guide to Related Topics," which groups together under a single heading entries having a significant feature in common. A reader who wants to explore ancient thought about sex will find entries of that sort grouped under "Classical Philosophy." Other readers may want to focus on the entries grouped under "Continental Philosophy," "Feminism," "Sexology," and so on. There are twenty-two groupings, from "Analytic Philosophy" to "Theories of

Sexuality." Some entries are listed more than once. "Jealousy," for example, is placed under "Analytic Philosophy," "Ethics," and "Psychology" because the entry discusses in an analytic manner an emotion that has ethical implications.

At the end of the second volume are the "Selected General Bibliography," a section devoted to the authors of the entries and the members of the advisory board, and the indices. The "Selected General Bibliography" lists a number of anthologies and textbooks about the philosophy and theology of sex, works that along with those listed in "Abbreviations" in the first volume might well be said to complete the core literature in the field. This general bibliography also includes helpful treatises in general philosophy, important collections, books, and reference materials from other fields, and (segregated from the rest) the names of journals that exclusively publish studies about sexuality.

Readers curious about the authors of the entries and the members of the encyclopedia's advisory board will find professional and personal information about them in the next section. Their academic positions, affiliations, education, publications, and assorted biographical details were supplied by the persons themselves and only mildly edited by the volume editor. The encyclopedia closes with both a name index and a subject index.

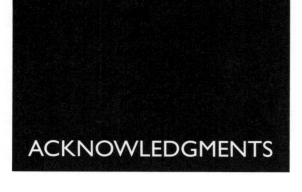

ACKNOWLEDGMENTS

The editor owes some words of thanks to friends and colleagues. From among the contributors to this encyclopedia, these colleagues performed duties above and beyond sending me their entries more or less on time and more or less in good shape: Elizabeth Brake, Keith Burgess-Jackson, David Carr, Carol Steinberg Gould, Mane Hajdin, Raja Halwani, Jeffrey Hershfield, Berel Dov Lerner, Michael P. Levine, Ed Pluth, Lee C. Rice, Lance Byron Richey, and Celia Wolf-Devine. From among the members of the advisory board, these colleagues performed duties above and beyond those required by their burdensome administrative functions: Martha Cornog, Ann Garry, Sarah Hoffman, Richard T. Hull, Edward Johnson, J. Martin Stafford, Robert M. Stewart, and Edward Collins Vacek. From among the contemporary scholars whose work was addressed in entries in the encyclopedia, these writers were especially cooperative in providing generous, witty, or acerbic criticism: Vern L. Bullough, Albert Ellis, John Finnis ("Natural Law, New"), Gilbert Herdt, John Money, Camille Paglia, Roger Scruton, Irving Singer, and Robert C. Solomon ("Communication Model").

Other people who graciously replied to the editor's requests for help or offered it out of the blue include Dirk Baltzly, Steven Barbone, Charlotte Becker, Larry Becker, Aaron Ben-Ze'ev, Charles Bronstein, Ronna Burger, Judy Crane, Russell Dancy, Carrie Delorge, Lara Denis, Laura Drago, Forrai Gábor, Jancy Hoeffel, Rebecca Homiski, Noretta Koertge, Nan Levinson, Peggy Brinkman Matteliano, Elijah Millgram, Seiriol Morgan, Alan Pasch, Sylvia Walsh Perkins, Timothy Perper, Patricia Petersen, Heidi Ravven, Eric Reitan, Marga Ryersbach, Laurie Shrage, Rachel Soble, Edward Stein, Jim Stone, Rosemarie Tong, John Wagner, Yuko Yoshida, Michael Zeleny, and several "I-prefer-to-be-anonymous" reviewers of manuscripts.

To the staff of the Interlibrary Loan Department of the University of New Orleans, I express my gratitude for the stream of books and journal articles they secured for me over the last three years. Finally, a tip of the hat to the personnel at Café Roma (Jefferson Davis Parkway), Rue de la Course (S. Carrollton), the New Orleans East Donut Shoppe ("South Shore Grill"), the Metairie-Causeway Donut Shoppe ("Joe's Cafe"), Z'otz Coffeehouse (Oak Street), Brown's Donut Shop (Read Boulevard), 13 Monaghan (Marigny), Central Perk ("Not Central Park, but Close"), Community Coffee at Riverbend (deceased), Coffee Bean Cafe (a.k.a. "European Coffee House"), and the world-famous house of nunches, the Hoff Street Delicatessen—the only place that survived Katrina.

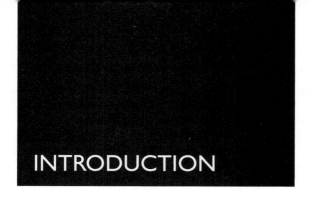

INTRODUCTION

Human sexuality and animal sexuality have been extensively studied by the natural and social sciences. Tens of thousands of books and hundreds of thousands of journal articles, plus a substantial number of excellent reference works (some of which are listed in the "Selected General Bibliography"), attest to the long history of the sexological sciences and to the continuing and irresistible interest among scholars in investigating the variety of sexual desires, sexual behaviors, sexual couplings, and sexual curiosities exhibited by both humans and other animals. This abundant research has seemingly covered every imaginable aspect of sex, from the microscopic to the social, from the mundane to the improbable, from the unspeakably, intimately personal to the public, the political, and the economic. And, of course, the poets, novelists, artists, sculptors, opera writers, musicians, photographers, filmmakers, choreographers, and even the architects and landscapers have illuminated, in their own distinctive, sometimes only implicit, ways the many forms and styles of sexuality. I would not be surprised were a congress of methodical and determined librarians and information historians to discover that of all the topics on which the human mind has pondered, sex is (nearly) the most frequently entertained and dissected.

Indeed, I have heard it said (but have never believed) that men—human males—think about sex once every six to ten seconds. Women, for their part—or so I have been instructed by several authoritative feminists—tend to dwell on food. (In a culture that connives women to be thin, a deliciously fattening but forbidden meal is often in the back of their salivating minds.) Now, what counts, exactly, as "thinking about sex" or "having a thought about sex" (or about food) deserves careful analysis, and this is the sort of thing that *philosophers* do, at least some of them. Consider the question seriously, for it is not far removed from, "What is a *sexual picture*?" and "What is an *obscene image*?"—incomparably difficult questions raised, discussed, and argued over both by philosophers of sex and law and by jurisprudentialists and legal scholars. *Sex from Plato to Paglia* focuses on a slice of all the human thought about sex, the philosophical slice, not the architectural slice nor the choreographical slice and, as such, has its own methods, its own ways of proceeding through the sexual maze, and its own sorts of results.

Moreover, the goals and content of an encyclopedia of the philosophy of sex must, at the beginning, be distinguished from the goals and content of what in popular culture often *passes as* philosophy of sex, by which I mean the stream of lectures and interviews, newspaper columns and books, audio- and videotapes, radio broadcasts, and television programs on sex: from Dr. Ruth's motherly or auntish advice to Dr. Phil's fatherly or uncleish advice, from Rabbi Boteach's fiery encyclicals to Jerry Springer's reconciliatory end-of-the-show monologues. There are differences between popularized philosophy of sex—to be sure, a good deal of it mentions *bona fide* philosophers like Plato (427–347 BCE), St. Augustine (354–430), and Sigmund Freud (1856–1939)—and technical, professional, scholarly, academic philosophy of sex, which also discusses the same catalog of figures.

The central difference may be that whereas pop-culture philosophizing promises a quick fix to ubiquitous problems (indeed, this is its appeal, and it *is* undeniably good for some things), hardcore philosophy promises absolutely no quick fixes at all. What professional philosophy of sex has to offer are "fixes," so to speak, but fixes that take a long time to achieve and require sustained mental attention and deliberation. This is *not* to insist, self-righteously, that (to employ Jeremy Bentham's [1748–1832] metaphor) poetry is always better than pushpin; nor is it to insist (to rely backhandedly on Socrates [469–399 BCE] and John Stuart Mill [1806–1873]) that the unexamined life has absolutely nothing at all going for it—recall the physically gorgeous and ignorantly blissful young heterosexual couple that Alvie (Woody Allen) unabashedly envies in *Annie Hall*. Simply put, philosophy of sex has something to offer to a different group of people, having different needs and interests, who hold a different vision of the valuable or fun life. My own favorites among the entries—an editor can also be a reader—in terms of their value and fun for me, not necessarily the ones that are objectively the best, include: "Augustine (Saint)"; "Descartes, René"; "Desire, Sexual"; "Existentialism"; "Fichte, Johann Gottlieb"; "Hegel, G.W.F."; "Hobbes, Thomas"; "Jealousy"; "Kierkegaard, Søren"; "Mandeville, Bernard"; "Paraphilia"; "Rousseau, Jean-Jacques"; and "Russell, Bertrand." Other readers, having their own equally eccentric standards of value and fun, will construct their own equally compelling lists of favorite entries.

The philosophy of sex provides instruction and practice in clarifying our thought processes, enabling us to progress from an ordinarily quite acceptable, everyday, and usually harmless sloppiness to greater precision in thinking and speaking. It will not offer any psychological consolation. Quite the contrary. Often what is revealed by deep and protracted philosophical thought is hardly the comfort or contentment one might have hoped for, and it is frequently unsettling and upsetting. For what philosophical thought about sexuality tends to reveal, even flaunt, is that the Human Condition cannot be reduced to easy formulas and platitudes, that our sexual existence—our yearnings, desires, motives, actions, and identities—is barely recognized by ourselves and much too complex to be neatly ordered, categorized, and comprehended the way accountants can immaculately sum things up with Power Point in black, white, and red.

For example, sexual jealousy can be painful and difficult to handle, often gaining the better of us. It is not to sell the humanities short by admitting that an attack of severe jealousy is best attended to by psychotherapy, tranquilizers, or several close friends and not by the philosophy of sex. But, again, this is *not* to say that professional, technical, or scholarly philosophy of sex must be arcane, boring, or irrelevant—as the term "academic" often means to those uninitiated to the world of letters. What the philosophy of sex can do will be valuable and interesting in its own right, in the right context. It will help us gain a glimmer of understanding of the existential significance of feeling jealous, inserting it into a larger picture of the meaning of life. It will illuminate how our feeling jealous links up with, even depends on, certain beliefs and attitudes that we possess, ideas we have willy-nilly or, instead, as the result of entrenched social patterns. It will also teach us how to think clearly about exactly what we are experiencing, so that we are able to distinguish jealousy from its various close relatives, such as envy, resentment, and insulted anger, and hence be in a better position to understand and communicate to others the quality and focus of our emotions.

The fear of loss is a ubiquitous human state, but that does not mean we must succumb to it blindly, without any intellectual appreciation of it at all. To take what is for some a less threatening example, consider the practice or phenomenon of "cybersex." Philosophical reflection on cybersex makes us reevaluate the notion of our having a discretely defined body. It forces us to rethink what it means to have "sexual contact" with another person and, derivatively, what forms adultery might, or might not, take in the technologically sophisticated twenty-first century. It also compels us to ask critically why we need or want "actual" or "real" embodied other people when engaging in sex, instead of being happily orgasmic with their virtual representations. The philosophical questions that arise here are in many ways similarly macabre to those that arise about cloning and are equally troublesome and no less pressing.

The philosophy of sex began, in the West, with the ancient Greek philosopher Plato (if not earlier, with Sappho [ca. 610–580 BCE], the pre-Socratics, and the Hebrews), and in the East with ancient religious teachings, including those of Hinduism and Buddhism. Like all subareas in philosophy (ethics, logic, epistemology, and so forth), the philosophy of sex has a history. In the West, for example, it proceeds from Plato to and through—to name just a few figures—Michel Montaigne (1533–1592), David Hume (1711–1776), Immanuel Kant (1724–1804), Søren Kierkegaard (1813–1855), Bertrand Russell (1872–1970), Jean-Paul Sartre (1905–1980), Michel Foucault (1926–1984), and Catharine MacKinnon (1946–   ). That is only *secular* philosophy of sex in the West; the history of the philosophy of sex also has an intertwining theological, religious path, from Plato, again, to and through St. Paul (5–64?), St. Augustine, St. Thomas Aquinas (1224/25–1274), Søren Kierkegaard, and a handful of twentieth-century popes.

It was in the twentieth century that the philosophy of sex blossomed (as did other areas in philosophy, for example, logic, the philosophy of language, and legal philosophy), partially as the result of Thomas Nagel's (1937–   ) pioneering essay "Sexual Perversion," published in the prestigious *Journal of Philosophy* in 1969. "Pioneering" and "prestigious" are used circumspectly, with both trepidation and reluctance, because by the twenty-first century it has become hackneyed, an entrenched professional cliché, to use precisely those words in recounting this revolutionary event. But revolutionary it was, in a genuine sense, for Nagel successfully applied the techniques of (stereotypically) cold analytic philosophy to a rich human phenomenon. Further, he also demonstrated that Anglo-American analytic philosophy had much to learn from the Continental (in this instance, the French) philosophical tradition. After the essay appeared, philosophers increasingly took sexual matters seriously, writing about sexuality unhysterically and without sermonizing, treating sex not as something especially delicate or especially dangerous but as another topic, among other topics of no more or no less importance, about which philosophical thought might fruitfully yield illumination.

There are already in print several reference works in the philosophy of sex. One is Igor Primoratz's *Human Sexuality* (1997), which reprints in a 500-page volume twenty-five of the most important journal articles in the philosophy of sex published during the final thirty years of the twentieth century. *Human Sexuality* is not only historically significant; it is also an indispensable resource for research. (Each article is reprinted as a facsimile, exactly as it appeared when first published, including original font, page numbers, etc.) But the volume is not encyclopedic, nor was it intended to be. Another is Alan Soble's *Sex, Love, and Friendship* (1997), which collects together, in 650 pages, sixty philosophical essays prepared for the Society for the Philosophy of Sex and Love in the period 1977–1992. Like Primoratz's volume, *Sex, Love, and Friendship* is a historically important record and a valuable resource for research but is not encyclopedic. A third is Earl E. Shelp's two-volume, 550-page *Sexuality and Medicine* (1987), whose twenty-eight essays are devoted to the special intersection of sexual ethics and biomedical science. Anyone who has more than a passing interest in the philosophy of sex should obtain copies of, or at least ensure having access to, these three works. The rationale behind *Sex from Plato to Paglia* is that while a great deal of interesting and important philosophical writing has been done on human sexuality, this material remained to be integrated and presented in such a way that a large amount of philosophical thought about sex is succinctly yet accurately and comprehensively summarized. Further, significant advances in the field needed to be distinctly noted and described, and additional lines of research, and questions and issues insufficiently explored or yet to be explored, brought to the attention of those feeling an itch to contribute to the development of the philosophy of sex.

ABBREVIATIONS

The abbreviations listed below are used throughout the entry bibliographies to designate frequently cited works.

HS   Primoratz, Igor, ed. *Human Sexuality*. Aldershot, U.K.: Ashgate, 1997.

P&S1   Baker, Robert B., and Frederick A. Elliston, eds. *Philosophy and Sex*, 1st ed. Buffalo, N.Y.: Prometheus, 1975.

P&S2   Baker, Robert B., and Frederick A. Elliston, eds. *Philosophy and Sex*, 2nd ed. Buffalo, N.Y.: Prometheus, 1984.

P&S3   Baker, Robert B., Kathleen J. Wininger, and Frederick A. Elliston, eds. *Philosophy and Sex*, 3rd ed. Amherst, N.Y.: Prometheus, 1998.

POS1   Soble, Alan, ed. *The Philosophy of Sex: Contemporary Readings*, 1st ed. Totowa, N.J.: Rowman and Littlefield, 1980.

POS2   Soble, Alan, ed. *The Philosophy of Sex: Contemporary Readings*, 2nd ed. Savage, Md.: Rowman and Littlefield, 1991.

POS3   Soble, Alan, ed. *The Philosophy of Sex: Contemporary Readings*, 3rd ed. Lanham, Md.: Rowman and Littlefield, 1997.

POS4   Soble, Alan, ed. *The Philosophy of Sex: Contemporary Readings*, 4th ed. Lanham, Md.: Rowman and Littlefield, 2002.

SLF   Soble, Alan, ed. *Sex, Love, and Friendship: Studies of the Society for the Philosophy of Sex and Love, 1977–1992*. Amsterdam, Holland: Rodopi, 1997.

STW   Stewart, Robert, ed. *Philosophical Perspectives on Sex and Love*. New York: Oxford University Press, 1995.

GUIDE TO RELATED TOPICS

Analytic Philosophy

Abstinence
Activity, Sexual
Adultery
Casual Sex
Completeness, Sexual
Consent
Desire, Sexual
Fantasy
Flirting
Friendship
Harassment, Sexual
Jealousy
Masturbation
Orientation, Sexual
Paraphilia
Perversion, Sexual
Philosophy of Sex, Overview of
Privacy
Seduction

Catholicism, Roman

Abortion
Abstinence
Animal Sexuality
Anscombe, G.E.M.
Augustine (Saint)
Bible, Sex and the
Catholicism, History of
Catholicism, Twentieth- and Twenty-First-
  Century
Completeness, Sexual
Contraception
Natural Law (New)
Paul (Saint)
Thomas Aquinas (Saint)
Wojtyła, Karol (Pope John Paul II)

Classical Philosophy

Aristotle
Augustine (Saint)
Gnosticism
Greek Sexuality and Philosophy, Ancient
Manichaeism
Paul (Saint)
Plato
Roman Sexuality and Philosophy, Ancient

Continental Philosophy

Bataille, Georges
Existentialism
Feminism, French
Fichte, Johann Gottlieb
Foucault, Michel
Freudian Left, The
Hegel, G.W.F.
Heidegger, Martin
Kant, Immanuel
Kierkegaard, Søren
Kolnai, Aurel
Lacan, Jacques
Leibniz, Gottfried
Levinas, Emmanuel
Marxism
Nietzsche, Friedrich
Phenomenology
Poststructuralism
Sade, Marquis de
Schopenhauer, Arthur
Spinoza, Baruch

Ethics

Abortion
Adultery

Animal Sexuality
Bestiality
Bible, Sex and the
Casual Sex
Coercion (by Sexually Aggressive Women)
Consent
Consequentialism
Contraception
Cybersex
Disability
Diseases, Sexually Transmitted
Ethics, Professional Codes of
Ethics, Sexual
Ethics, Virtue
Fantasy
Flirting
Genital Mutilation
Harassment, Sexual
Heterosexism
Hobbes, Thomas
Homosexuality, Ethics of
Humor
Incest
Intersexuality
Jealousy
Kant, Immanuel
Language
Liberalism
Masturbation
Military, Sex and the
Natural Law (New)
Objectification, Sexual
Pedophilia
Personification, Sexual
Philosophy of Sex, Teaching the
Pornography
Privacy
Prostitution
Rape
Rape, Acquaintance and Date
Reproductive Technology
Rimmer, Robert
Russell, Bertrand
Sade, Marquis de
Sadomasochism
Scruton, Roger
Seduction
Sex Education
Sex Work

Sexuality, Dimensions of
Spencer, Herbert
Violence, Sexual
Wojtyła, Karol (Pope John Paul II)

Existentialism

Communication Model
Existentialism
Feminism, French
Kierkegaard, Søren
Nagel, Thomas
Nietzsche, Friedrich
Seduction

Feminism

African Philosophy
Beauty
Bisexuality
Coercion (by Sexually Aggressive Women)
Dworkin, Andrea
Ethics, Sexual
Feminism, French
Feminism, History of
Feminism, Lesbian
Feminism, Liberal
Feminism, Men's
Firestone, Shulamith
Genital Mutilation
Harassment, Sexual
Heterosexism
Language
MacKinnon, Catharine
Mead, Margaret
Objectification, Sexual
Paglia, Camille
Personification, Sexual
Pornography
Prostitution
Sadomasochism
Sherfey, Mary Jane
Social Constructionism
Violence, Sexual

Gay/Lesbian/Bisexual/ Transgendered (GLBT)

Bisexuality
Boswell, John

Diseases, Sexually Transmitted
Dworkin, Andrea
Feminism, French
Feminism, Lesbian
Feminism, Men's
Foucault, Michel
Greek Sexuality and Philosophy, Ancient
Herdt, Gilbert
Heterosexism
Homosexuality, Ethics of
Homosexuality and Science
MacKinnon, Catharine
Marriage, Same-Sex
Mead, Margaret
Military, Sex and the
Orientation, Sexual
Philosophy of Sex, Teaching the
Queer Theory
Roman Sexuality and Philosophy,
    Ancient
Social Constructionism

History

African Philosophy
Beauty
Bible, Sex and the
Boswell, John
Bullough, Vern L.
Catholicism, History of
Catholicism, Twentieth- and Twenty-First-
    Century
Desire, Sexual
Ethics, Professional Codes of
Existentialism
Feminism, History of
Gnosticism
Greek Sexuality and Philosophy,
    Ancient
Incest
Judaism, History of
Judaism, Twentieth- and Twenty-First-
    Century
Love
Manichaeism
Marriage
Philosophy of Sex, Overview of
Poststructuralism
Protestantism, History of

Protestantism, Twentieth- and Twenty-
    First-Century
Psychology, Twentieth- and Twenty-First-
    Century
Roman Sexuality and Philosophy, Ancient
Sexology
Social Constructionism
Utopianism

Legal Philosophy

Arts, Sex and the
Bestiality
Consent
Disability
Diseases, Sexually Transmitted
Dworkin, Andrea
Harassment, Sexual
Humor
Law, Sex and the
Liberalism
MacKinnon, Catharine
Marriage, Same-Sex
Military, Sex and the
Nudism
Paglia, Camille
Pornography
Posner, Richard
Privacy
Prostitution
Rape
Rape, Acquaintance and Date
Sadomasochism
Sex Work

Liberalism

Consent
Consequentialism
Ellis, Albert
Ethics, Sexual
Feminism, Liberal
Hobbes, Thomas
Kant, Immanuel
Law, Sex and the
Liberalism
Nudism
Paglia, Camille
Pornography
Privacy

Prostitution
Rimmer, Robert
Russell, Bertrand
Sadomasochism
Seduction
Sex Work
Singer, Irving

Marxism

Ethics, Sexual
Existentialism
Freudian Left, The
Hegel, G.W.F.
Marxism

Medicine

Addiction, Sexual
Bestiality
Contraception
Disability
Diseases, Sexually Transmitted
Dysfunction, Sexual
Ellis, Albert
Ellis, Havelock
Ethics, Professional Codes of
Firestone, Shulamith
Freud, Sigmund
Genital Mutilation
Homosexuality and Science
Incest
Intersexuality
Money, John
Paraphilia
Pedophilia
Perversion, Sexual
Reproductive Technology
Sexology
Sherfey, Mary Jane

Modern Philosophy

Descartes, René
Hobbes, Thomas
Hume, David
Leibniz, Gottfried
Rousseau, Jean-Jacques
Spinoza, Baruch

Non-Western Philosophy

African Philosophy
Buddhism
Chinese Philosophy
Hinduism
Indian Erotology
Islam
Jainism
Tantrism

Philosophers (Secular)

Aristotle
Bataille, Georges
Boswell, John
Bullough, Vern L.
Descartes, René
Dworkin, Andrea
Ellis, Albert
Ellis, Havelock
Fichte, Johann Gottlieb
Firestone, Shulamith
Foucault, Michel
Freud, Sigmund
Hegel, G.W.F.
Heidegger, Martin
Herdt, Gilbert
Hobbes, Thomas
Hume, David
Kant, Immanuel
Kierkegaard, Søren
Kolnai, Aurel
Lacan, Jacques
Leibniz, Gottfried
Levinas, Emmanuel
MacKinnon, Catharine
Mandeville, Bernard
Mead, Margaret
Money, John
Nagel, Thomas
Nietzsche, Friedrich
Paglia, Camille
Plato
Posner, Richard
Rimmer, Robert
Rousseau, Jean-Jacques
Russell, Bertrand
Sacher-Masoch, Leopold von

Sade, Marquis de
Schopenhauer, Arthur
Scruton, Roger
Sherfey, Mary Jane
Singer, Irving
Spencer, Herbert
Spinoza, Baruch
Westermarck, Edward
Wittgenstein, Ludwig

Philosophers (Theological)

Anscombe, G.E.M.
Augustine (Saint)
Kierkegaard, Søren
Paul (Saint)
Thomas Aquinas (Saint)
Wojtyła, Karol (Pope John Paul II)

Politics

African Philosophy
Arts, Sex and the
Consequentialism
Disability
Diseases, Sexually Transmitted
Dworkin, Andrea
Ellis, Albert
Existentialism
Feminism, Men's
Firestone, Shulamith
Foucault, Michel
Freud, Sigmund
Freudian Left, The
Heterosexism
Law, Sex and the
Liberalism
MacKinnon, Catharine
Mandeville, Bernard
Marriage, Same-Sex
Marxism
Military, Sex and the
Natural Law (New)
Paglia, Camille
Pornography
Privacy
Prostitution
Queer Theory
Rape

Rape, Acquaintance and Date
Scruton, Roger
Sex Education
Sex Work
Sexology
Spencer, Herbert
Utopianism
Violence, Sexual
Wittgenstein, Ludwig

Psychology

Beauty
Completeness, Sexual
Ellis, Albert
Freud, Sigmund
Homosexuality and Science
Humor
Jealousy
Lacan, Jacques
Language
Nagel, Thomas
Plato
Psychology, Evolutionary
Psychology, Twentieth- and Twenty-First-
   Century
Sexology

Religion (Western, Non-Catholic)

Abstinence
Bible, Sex and the
Gnosticism
Islam
Judaism, History of
Judaism, Twentieth- and Twenty-First-
   Century
Manichaeism
Protestantism, History of
Protestantism, Twentieth- and Twenty-
   First-Century

Sexology

Bullough, Vern L.
Dysfunction, Sexual
Ellis, Albert
Ellis, Havelock

Freud, Sigmund
Herdt, Gilbert
Homosexuality and Science
Mead, Margaret
Money, John
Paraphilia
Perversion, Sexual
Psychology, Evolutionary
Psychology, Twentieth- and Twenty-First-
    Century
Sexology
Sherfey, Mary Jane
Singer, Irving
Social Constructionism
Westermarck, Edward

Theories of Sexuality

Animal Sexuality
Aristotle
Communication Model
Completeness, Sexual

Evolution
Freud, Sigmund
Hegel, G.W.F.
Lacan, Jacques
Marxism
Nagel, Thomas
Orientation, Sexual
Philosophy of Sex, Overview of
Plato
Posner, Richard
Psychology, Evolutionary
Psychology, Twentieth- and Twenty-First-
    Century
Queer Theory
Sade, Marquis de
Schopenhauer, Arthur
Sexology
Sherfey, Mary Jane
Social Constructionism
Spencer, Herbert
Thomas Aquinas (Saint)

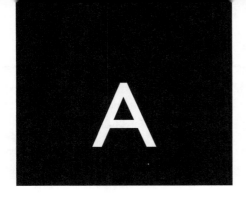

ABORTION. Many believe that one's responsibility to continue a pregnancy is importantly amplified if one is responsible for bringing about its existence in the first place. Just what it takes to count as responsible here is a point on which people diverge—whether voluntary but contracepted intercourse is different from intercourse without the use of **contraception**, and again from intentionally deciding to become pregnant at an *in vitro* fertilization clinic. But a woman who satisfies the relevant criteria, some will say, having in essence invited the fetus into her body, thereby faces a distinct responsibility to sustain and develop this life. For some, indeed, the woman is said thereby to have forfeited a certain dominion: The fetus now has a moral right to the occupation and use of her body (see Wilcox).

Many others regard these claims with deep suspicion. Procreation, we are reminded, especially where abortion is then sought, is usually a low-probability side effect of an activity often pursued for its own reasons; it betrays a retrograde and punitive view of the activity in question to burden its access in this way. The idea of "invitation" is at any rate a red herring. Invitation implies **consent**; use of the body requires contemporaneous consent; and such consent is clearly absent if the woman is seeking to end the pregnancy. More deeply, it is wrong to assume that it ever was present: Giving consent to one's sexual partner to engage in intercourse is not equivalent to giving consent to a fetus to occupy one's body for nine months: Consent just does not travel across parties and activities in quite that way (McDonagh, 60–83).

The issues here are rich ones. What the intersection of abortion and **sexual ethics** really asks us to think about is the important idea of "taking responsibility" for creation; and that idea is nuanced and complex. The voluntariness of heterosexual intercourse can indeed be morally salient, but it is salient to different questions, in different ways, for different reasons.

On one analysis of abortion, it is hard to see how the voluntariness of intercourse could make a moral difference. According to this view, the fetus is a person, and abortion is a gross violation of its right to life. However that life found its way into a woman's body, the life itself is innocent of wrongdoing; hence, killing it is murder (see Pope John Paul II [**Karol Wojtyła** (1920–2005)], 709–11).

This view is of course contested by those who reject fetal personhood. But it is also contested by those who believe that abortion would not count as murder even if the fetus were a person. Assimilating abortion to a violation of the right to life seems to ignore key features of gestation: One who is gestating is providing the fetus with sustenance—donating nourishment, creating blood, delivering oxygen, providing hormonal triggers for development—without which it could not live. Abortion in essence is removal of that assistance. But the right to life, as Judith Jarvis Thomson famously points out, does not include the right to have all assistance needed to maintain that life (55–56). Hence, while ending gestation, at least at early stages, will certainly lead to the fetus's demise, that does not mean that doing so constitutes murder—even, indeed, if that removal is by active means. As Frances Kamm argues (20–41), if the only (safe) way to end the assistance is by active killing, and the killing takes away only that which the person would never have had without your aid (something that cannot be said of a typical street stabbing), there is no wrongful interference. Some killings, in short, exhibit the crucial "formal" feature of letting die: They leave the person, in this case the fetus, no worse off than before he or she encountered the person causing the death.

Many have argued that these arguments, even if sound, do not apply when the pregnancy is the result of voluntary intercourse. In such cases the woman is responsible for introducing the person's need. The woman is not like someone coming upon an accident on the highway who happens to know cardiopulmonary resuscitation. Instead, she is like the person who caused the accident. Her actions introduced a set of vulnerabilities or needs. And we (including pregnant women) have a special duty to lessen vulnerabilities and repair harms we have inflicted on others (see Lee, 115–28; also Werner).

But there is a deep disanalogy between causing the accident and procreating. The fact of causing a crash itself introduces a harm to surrounding drivers: They are in a worse position for having encountered that driver. The simple act of procreating, though, does not worsen the fetus's position, for without procreation the fetus would not exist at all, and the mere fact of being brought into existence is not a bad thing. Creating a human is creating someone who comes with needs, but this is not the same thing as inflicting a need *onto* someone (Silverstein). The woman is (jointly) responsible for creating a life, and it is a life that necessarily includes needs, but that is not the same as her being responsible for the person being needy rather than not needy. The pregnant woman has not made the fetus more vulnerable than it would otherwise have been, for absent her procreative actions, the fetus would not have existed at all.

If the voluntariness of intercourse is morally salient, then, it will not be for the reasons provided by the reparation-based or interference-based arguments. Indeed, if these lessons are correct, the general issue abortion presents is not about wrongful interference at all. It is instead about the far more interesting question of what positive responsibilities, if any, pregnant women have to continue gestational assistance. The more specific question here is whether and how it matters to that issue that the pregnancy results from voluntary intercourse. Let us begin our investigation under the assumption that burgeoning human life is not yet a person, or indeed a creature with interests, but still has a value worthy of respect (Dworkin, 10–15).

Many people admit to moral queasiness when they hear of couples who, knowing full well they would never bring a pregnancy to term, engage in heterosexual intercourse without any regard whatsoever for contraception. Such queasiness is understandable. Imagine a scientist who creates human embryos only for the pleasure of squishing them. What seems morally problematic here is not just the destruction but the attitude displayed toward human life when one's procreative powers are purposefully exercised for such an end. Intentionally bringing about burgeoning human life for frivolous reasons seems to dishonor early life. And if disrespect can be embodied in certain direct intentions, it can also be embodied in callous *disregard* of one's creative potential. If conception is not sought, a scientist experimenting with gametes who fails to take the simplest precautions against egg and sperm joining seems to express an improperly profligate attitude toward human life.

One should not treat one's procreative capacities cavalierly. One should not intentionally start the process without serious (which is not to say unbounded) commitment to support the pregnancy; and one should take at least some precautions to avoid conception when one is not prepared to welcome a new creature into the world. Just how restrictive these norms here should be is, of course, highly contested. Those who value spontaneity in sexual relations and have milder views about the value of burgeoning human life will advance something quite modest—urging, say, good-faith attempts to use contraception control when it is safe, easily obtained, and immediately convenient (see Little). Others (for instance, the Vatican) will advance principles that are stringent indeed—requiring, say, that one not have sex at all until one is prepared to parent. Underlying these (important) differences is commitment to the idea that there are *norms of responsible creation*. To regard things as valuable sometimes enjoins us to create or produce more of them and sometimes, as with people, to take care about the conditions under which we make any.

Notice now, though, that none of this implies one has a special responsibility to gestate if one does get pregnant. Whether strict or modest, the norms of responsible creation are norms about the acts that can lead to procreation. They specify, as it were, the good-faith conditions one should meet for engaging in certain activities. As such, they are commentaries on whether one had any business conducting the activity as one did, not on what responsibilities one faces if it then has certain effects. Indeed, even if the norm is broached—one has sex callously disregarding its potential to lead to new life—that does not itself imply that one now must gestate: It says one should not have had that sort of sex.

A woman who finds herself pregnant after taking poor precautions against conception, now dreading the idea of continued pregnancy, is told, "You should have thought of that earlier!" And indeed she (and her partner) should have; that, after all, is the point of saying one should avoid "negligent" sex. But commitment to this point does not mean that one believes abortion would be unjustified but that contraception is far preferable to even justified abortion. One should try to meet the good-faith criteria of sexual responsibility, but failing to do so does not give one more reason to continue the pregnancy. Indeed, for many, that logic is particularly counterintuitive: That you were sexually irresponsible is no reason at all to bring a child into the world.

This last intuition hints at a very different approach to the ethics of creation. It is an ethic whose concern is with the responsibility involved in bringing a person into the world. Many people have deep convictions about the circumstances in which they feel it right (and wrong) for them to bring a child into existence: Can it be brought into a decent world, an intact family, a society that will respect its agency? These are the sorts of issues that appear in some women's stories of abortion. A woman decides to abort because she knows she could not give up a child for adoption but feels she could not give the child the sort of life, or be the sort of parent, she thinks the child deserves; a woman who would have to give up the child thinks it would be unfair to bring a child into existence already burdened by rejection, however well grounded its reasons; a woman living in a country marked by poverty and gender apartheid wants to abort because she decides it would be wrong for her to bear a daughter whose life, like hers, would be filled with so much injustice and hardship. The normative considerations that can weigh against procreating do not evaporate with the embryo's presence. For those normative considerations are ones that tell against creating persons, and a person, on our current assumption, is just what the fetus as yet is not.

Some have thought that such decisions betray a simple fallacy: Unless the child's life were literally going to be worse than not existing, how can one abort out of concern for the future child? But the worry here is not that one would be imposing a harm on the child by bringing it into existence (as though children who are in the situations mentioned have lives not worth living). The claim is that bringing about a person's life in these circumstances would, more specifically, do violence to a woman's ideals of creating and parenthood. The woman does not want to bring into existence a daughter she cannot **love** and care for; she does not want to bring into existence a person whose life will be marked by disrespect or rejection.

Nor need the claim imply judgment on women who do continue pregnancies in similar circumstances. For the norms in question need not be impersonally authoritative. Like ideals of good parenting, they mark out considerations all should perhaps be sensitive to, but equally reasonable people may adhere to different variations and weightings. Still, they are normative for those who embrace them. Far from expressing mere matters of taste, the ideals one accepts are categorical, issuing imperatives whose authority is not reducible to mere desire. These are, at root, issues about integrity and the importance of maintaining integrity over one's participation in this enterprise, precisely because it is so normatively weighty (Rothman, 80).

What difference, if any, should the voluntariness of intercourse make to our thinking about whether women have positive responsibilities to offer gestational assistance if (or when) we think the fetus is a person? The general question of what positive responsibilities there may be to gestate is here more pressing: On the one hand, what is at stake is nothing less than the life and death of someone with full moral status; on the other hand, the kind of assistance needed to sustain that life is of the most extraordinarily intimate sort. For some, nothing is more obvious than that one who is pregnant from voluntary intercourse has an agent-specific responsibility to nurture this person (Wilcox, 469–75). Over and above what she might owe as a matter of urgent beneficence, if anything, the woman now has a duty to meet the needs of this person that it cannot yet meet itself. After all, it is because of her that this person now exists; the difference between creating widgets and creating persons is that the latter carries positive responsibilities.

For others, nothing is less obvious. Given that creation followed by quick demise does not constitute a setback of interests, the fact that one's activities are causally involved in bringing about this person's existence grounds no special or further responsibility above whatever one owes to the fetus as a matter of urgent beneficence (Boonin-Vail, 302–8). If anything, creating a person does her a favor: Why should this mean one owes her yet more? One might have heightened responsibilities to society here: It is because of an individual's act that a need deserving to be met now exists, and that is a normative burden on the moral community. Especially if that person could reasonably have done more to decrease the risk of that need existing, it is fair to ask the person to be the one who shoulders the burden. But that is a claim that the community, not the person created, has to the individual responsible being the one who does the helping.

What all this asks is how to fill in a picture of how to value persons, given a complex of facts about human beings: Our sexual activities are what bring people into existence—and in a predictably needy state; **sexual activity** has its own honorable place in a flourishing human life; and finally, the assistance required to help this created person is an extraordinarily intimate one.

It is arguable that when pregnancy is not intended, the fact that one's sexual acts are causally related to a person's existence does not ground a separate responsibility to assist. While one should in this case take every precaution against creation occurring, it is no disrespect to the dignity of others to participate in heterosexual activity without a commitment to grant the use of one's body, should the odds go against one and a person comes into existence. But intentional creation seems importantly different. Here one has, metaphorically, called forth the individual. One's sexual acts have arguably created not just a person but a relationship, a relationship that, in Hegelian fashion, predates the relatum's existence. The person comes into the world with a dependent relation already legitimized, grounding a special responsibility to provide for her predictable needs. Such responsibility is not unbounded. It is enormously difficult to predict all that can go wrong with a pregnancy: medical issues, changes in one's life circumstances, the emergence of deep existential understandings of one's own body and life, and other issues that may well emerge that override that responsibility. Still, responsibility exists (again, when or if the fetus is a person) that would need to be overridden if one is decently to decline assistance.

But even where one does have a special responsibility to continue gestational assistance, it gets things badly wrong to construe that responsibility as forfeiting or transferring to the fetus a moral right of occupation and use of one's body. Such a move misunderstands how we should theorize about extraordinary intimate assistances. If I promise you the future sexual use of my body, it would be wrong to say that this grants you a moral right of access to that body, as though you have moral dominion over my body whatever I may say when the time comes around (as in **Saint Paul** [5–64?], 1 Cor. 7:3–5). The body, we might put it, belongs more to the contemporaneous than the past or future self.

This does not mean that our actions cannot normatively encumber our bodies into the future but rather that the way we understand that encumbrance is importantly modulated. The person must take seriously the commitment she has made (the self is, after all, also connected across time); but we can underscore that moral responsibility without reading it as a transfer of moral dominion from one's future self. As always, analyses of abortion's moral status need to pay attention to the unique form of assistance pregnancy actually involves (see Little).

See also Abstinence; Anscombe, G.E.M.; Bible, Sex and the; Consent; Contraception; Ethics, Professional Codes of; Feminism, Liberal; Homosexuality and Science; Manichaeism; Marriage; Privacy; Reproductive Technology; Sex Education; Sexuality, Dimensions of

REFERENCES

Boonin-Vail, David. "A Defense of 'A Defense of Abortion': On the Responsibility Objection to Thomson's Argument." *Ethics* 107:2 (1997), 286–313; Dworkin, Ronald. *Life's Dominion: An Argument about Abortion, Euthanasia, and Individual Freedom.* New York: Knopf, 1993; John Paul II (Pope). "Evangelium Vitae." *Origins* 24:42 (1995), 689–727; Kamm, Frances. *Creation and Abortion: A Study in Moral and Legal Philosophy.* New York: Oxford University Press, 1992; Lee, Patrick. *Abortion and Unborn Human Life.* Washington, D.C.: Catholic University of America, 1996; Little, Margaret Olivia. *Intimate Duties: Re-Thinking Abortion, Law, and Morality.* Oxford, U.K.: Oxford University Press, forthcoming; McDonagh, Eileen. *Breaking the Abortion Deadlock: From Choice to Consent.* New York: Oxford University Press, 1996; Rothman, Barbara Katz. *Recreating Motherhood.* New Brunswick, N.J.: Rutgers University Press, 2000; Silverstein, Harry. "On a Woman's 'Responsibility' for the Fetus." *Social Theory and Practice* 13:1 (1987), 103–19; Thomson, Judith Jarvis. "A Defense of Abortion." *Philosophy and Public Affairs* 1:1 (1971), 47–66; Werner, Richard. "Abortion: The Moral Status of the Unborn." *Social Theory and Practice* 3:2 (1974), 201–22; Wilcox, John T. "Nature as Demonic in Thomson's Defense of Abortion." *The New Scholasticism* 63:4 (1989), 463–84.

Margaret Olivia Little

ADDITIONAL READING

Addelson, Kathryn Pyne. "Moral Revolution." In Julia A. Sherman and Evelyn Torton Beck, eds., *The Prism of Sex.* Madison: University of Wisconsin Press, 1979, 189–227. Reprinted, revised, in Kathryn Pyne Addelson, *Impure Thoughts: Essays on Philosophy, Feminism, and Ethics.* Philadelphia, Pa.: Temple University Press, 1991, 35–61; and Marilyn Pearsall, ed., *Women and Values: Readings in Recent Feminist Philosophy*, 3rd ed. Belmont, Calif.: Wadsworth, 1999, 328–43; Baird, Robert M., and Stuart E. Rosenbaum, eds. *The Ethics of Abortion: Pro-Life vs. Pro-Choice*, rev. ed. Buffalo, N.Y.: Prometheus, 1993; Boonin, David. *A Defense of Abortion*. Cambridge: Cambridge University Press, 2003; Cahill, Lisa Sowle. "Grisez on Sex and Gender: A Feminist Theological Perspective." In Nigel Biggar and Rufus Black, eds., *The Revival of Natural Law: Philosophical, Theological and Ethical Responses to the Finnis-Grisez School*. Aldershot, U.K.: Ashgate, 2000, 242–61; Callahan, Joan C. "The Fetus and Fundamental Rights." *Commonweal* (11 April 1986), 203–7. Reprinted, revised, in Robert M. Baird and Stuart E. Rosenbaum, eds., *The Ethics of Abortion: Pro-Life vs. Pro-Choice*, rev. ed. Buffalo, N.Y.: Prometheus, 1993, 249–62; Callahan, Sidney. "Abortion and the Sexual Agenda." *Commonweal* (25 April 1986), 232–38. Reprinted in Robert M. Baird and Stuart E. Rosenbaum, eds., *The Ethics of Abortion: Pro-Life vs. Pro-Choice*, rev. ed. Buffalo, N.Y.: Prometheus, 1993, 111–21; in Patricia Beattie Jung and Shannon Jung, eds., *Moral Issues and Christian Responses*, 7th ed. Belmont, Calif.: Wadsworth, 2003, 161–72; and POS3 (151–64); POS4 (177–90); Connery, John R. "Abortion: Roman Catholic Perspectives." In Warren T. Reich, ed., *Encyclopedia of Bioethics*, vol. 1. New York: Macmillan, 1978, 9–13; Cornell, Drucilla. *The Imaginary Domain: Abortion, Pornography, and Sexual Harassment*. New York: Routledge, 1995; Davis, N. Ann. "Fiddling Second: Reflections on 'A Defense of Abortion.' " In Alex Byrne, Robert Stalnaker, and Ralph Wedgwood, eds., *Fact and Value: Essays on Ethics and Metaphysics for Judith Jarvis Thomson*. Cambridge, Mass.: MIT Press, 2001, 81–96; Dworkin, Andrea. "Abortion." In *Right-wing Women*. New York: Perigee Books, 1983, 71–105; Dwyer, Susan, and Joel Feinberg, eds. *The Problem of Abortion*, 3rd ed. Belmont, Calif.: Wadsworth, 1997. 1st and 2nd editions, ed. Joel Feinberg, 1973, 1984; Feinberg, Joel, and Barbara Baum Levenbook. (1986) "Abortion." In Tom Regan, ed., *Matters of Life and Death: New Introductory Essays in Moral Philosophy*, 3rd ed. New York: McGraw-Hill, 1993, 195–234; Finnis, John. "The Rights and Wrongs of Abortion: A Reply to Judith Thomson." *Philosophy and Public Affairs* 2:2 (1973), 117–45; Gibson, Susanne. "Abortion." In Ruth Chadwick, ed., *Encyclopedia of Applied Ethics*, vol. 1. San Diego, Calif.: Academic Press, 1998, 1–8; Gilligan, Carol. *In a Different Voice: Psychological Theory and Women's Development*. Cambridge, Mass.: Harvard University Press, 1982; Grisez, Germain. "Is Abortion Always the Wrongful Killing of a Person?" In *The Way of the Lord Jesus*, vol. 2: *Living a Christian Life*. Quincy, Ill.: Franciscan Press, 1993, 488–505; Harrison, Beverly Wildung. *Our Right to Choose: Toward a New Ethic of Abortion*. Boston, Mass.: Beacon Press, 1983; Hursthouse, Rosalind. "Virtue Theory and Abortion." In Daniel Statman, ed., *Virtue Ethics: A Critical Reader*. Washington, D.C.: Georgetown University Press, 1997, 227–44; Kerber, Linda K., Catherine G. Greeno and Eleanor E. Maccoby, Zella Luria, Carol B. Stack, and Carol Gilligan. "On *In a Different Voice*: An Interdisciplinary Forum." *Signs* 11:2 (1986), 304–33; Lasch, Christopher. "Gilligan's Island." In Christopher Lasch, *Women and the Common Life: Love, Marriage, and Feminism*. Edited by Elisabeth Lasch-Quinn. New York: Norton, 1997, 121–36; MacKinnon, Catharine A. "Abortion: On Public and Private." In *Toward a Feminist Theory of the State*. Cambridge, Mass.: Harvard University Press, 1989, 184–94; MacKinnon, Catharine A. (1982) " 'More Than Simply a Magazine': *Playboy*'s Money." In *Feminism Unmodified: Discourses on Life and Law*. Cambridge, Mass.: Harvard University Press, 1987, 134–45; MacKinnon, Catharine A. "Roe v. Wade: A Study in Male Ideology." In Jay L. Garfield and Patricia Hennessey, eds., *Abortion: Moral and Legal Perspectives*. Amherst: University of Massachusetts Press, 1984, 45–54; Mahowald, Mary B. "Concepts of Abortion and Their Relevance to the Abortion Debate." *Southern Journal of Philosophy* 20:2 (1986), 195–207; McMahan, Jeff. *The Ethics of Life: Problems at the Margins of Life*. New York: Oxford University Press, 2002; Mendus, Susan. "Different Voices, Still Lives: Problems in the Ethics of Care." *Journal of Applied Philosophy* 10:1 (1993), 17–27; Mills, Claudia. "What Do Fathers Owe Their Children?" In Alex Byrne, Robert Stalnaker, and Ralph Wedgwood, eds., *Fact and Value: Essays on Ethics and Metaphysics for Judith Jarvis Thomson*. Cambridge, Mass.: MIT Press, 2001, 183–98; Murphy, Timothy F. "Abortion and the Ethics of Genetic Sexual Orientation Research." *Cambridge Quarterly of Healthcare Ethics* 4:4 (1995), 340–50; Nails, Debra. "Social-Scientific Sexism: Gilligan's Mismeasure of Man." *Social Research* 50:3 (1983), 643–64; Nicholson, Susan T. *Abortion and the Roman Catholic Church*. Knoxville, Tenn.: Religious Ethics,

1978; Paden, Roger. "Abortion and Sexual Morality." *Diálogos* 50 (1987), 145–54. Reprinted in SLF (229–36); Perkins, Robert L., ed. *Abortion: Pro and Con*. Cambridge, Mass.: Schenkman, 1974; Pollitt, Katha. "Marooned on Gilligan's Island: Are Women Morally Superior to Men?" In *Reasonable Creatures: Essays on Women and Feminism*. New York: Knopf, 1994, 42–62; Regan, Donald H. "Rewriting *Roe v. Wade*." *Michigan Law Review* 77 (1979), 1569–1646; *Roe v. Wade*. 410 U.S. 113, 93 S.Ct. 705, 35 L.Ed. 2d 147 (1973); Shrage, Laurie. "Fetal Ideologies and Maternal Desires: A Post-Enlightenment Account of Abortion. In *Moral Dilemmas of Feminism: Prostitution, Adultery, and Abortion*. New York: Routledge, 1994, 55–77; Smith, Holly M. "Intercourse and Moral Responsibility for the Fetus." In W. B. Bondeson, H. T. Engelhardt, Jr., S. F. Spicker, and D. H. Winship, eds., *Abortion and the Status of the Fetus*. Dordrecht, Holland: Reidel, 1983, 229–45; Soble, Alan. "More on Abortion and Sexual Morality." In Alan Soble, ed., *Sex, Love, and Friendship*. Amsterdam, Holland: Rodopi, 1997, 239–44; Sommers, Christina Hoff. "Pathological Social Science: Carol Gilligan and the Incredible Shrinking Girl." In Paul R. Gross, Norman Levitt, and Martin W. Lewis, eds., *The Flight from Science and Reason*. New York: New York Academy of Sciences, 1996, 369–81; Sullivan, J. P. "The Ethics and Politics of Abortion." *Philosophy of the Social Sciences* 17:3 (1987), 413–25; Thomson, Judith Jarvis. "A Defense of Abortion." *Philosophy and Public Affairs* 1:1 (1971), 47–66. Reprinted in Robert M. Baird and Stuart E. Rosenbaum, eds., *The Ethics of Abortion: Pro-Life vs. Pro-Choice*, rev. ed. Buffalo, N.Y.: Prometheus, 1993, 197–211; in Thomas A. Mappes and Jane S. Zembaty, eds., *Social Ethics*, 6th ed. New York: McGraw-Hill, 2002, 28–38; in Judith A. Boss, ed., *Analyzing Moral Issues*, 3rd ed. New York: McGraw-Hill, 2005, 91–101; and P&S1 (305–23); P&S2 (210–17); P&S3 (231–45); Wertheimer, Roger. "Understanding the Abortion Argument." *Philosophy and Public Affairs* 1:1 (1971), 67–95; Willis, Ellen. (1979) "Abortion: Is a Woman a Person?" In *Beginning to See the Light*. New York: Knopf, 1981, 205–11. Book reprinted by Wesleyan University Press, 1992. Essay reprinted in Ann Snitow, Christine Stansell, and Sharon Thompson, eds., *Powers of Desire: The Politics of Sexuality*. New York: Monthly Review Press, 1983, 471–76; and POS3 (165–69); POS4 (191–95); Wolf-Devine, Celia. "Abortion and the Feminine Voice." *Public Affairs Quarterly* 3:3 (1989), 81–97. Reprinted in Susan Dwyer and Joel Feinberg, eds., *The Problem of Abortion*, 3rd ed. Belmont, Calif.: Wadsworth, 1997, 160–74; in Louis Pojman and Frances Beckwith, eds., *The Abortion Controversy: 25 Years after Roe v. Wade, a Reader*. Belmont, Calif.: Wadsworth, 1998, 414–29; and Philip E. Devine and Celia Wolf-Devine, eds., *Sex and Gender: A Spectrum of Views*. Belmont, Calif.: Wadsworth, 2003, 163–72.

ABSTINENCE. Although abstinence, celibacy, chastity, and virginity all appear to concern some repudiation of or opposition to **sexual activity**, they are related to each other and to sexual conduct in a variety of complex ways. First, since not all eventual celibates need be virgins, there can be celibacy without virginity. Second, although virginity is arguably terminated by sexual activity, it is not clear that it is terminated by any sort of sexual activity. In an unpleasant Greek myth, a prepubescent Helen is abducted and sodomized by Theseus (Calasso, 122), but it is moot whether she thereby lost her virginity. Third, according to a major tradition of Christian reflection (exemplified by Elizabeth [**G.E.M.**] **Anscombe** [1919–2001]), insofar as chastity signifies a sexual attitude, virtue, or ideal as much if not more than a pattern of behavior, one might be chaste in the absence of celibacy or virginity. Fourth, however, this opens up the interesting possibility (see below) of celibacy without chastity.

In attempting to give sharper definitions to these different notions of abstinence, we might well begin with a fundamental normative question about all abstention from sexual conduct. Given that sexual activity is for most healthy humans a prime source of pleasure, why should engaging in it be regarded as wrong? Indeed, why have some forms of sexual conduct been subject to severe social prohibitions and sanctions?

The most general grounds for sexual prohibition turn on its possible adverse individual or social effects. Such actual or alleged harm may be intrinsic or extrinsic. Although heterosexual intercourse for purposes of pleasure or procreation may be regarded as only contingently harmful (when it is, for example, extramarital, adulterous, or promiscuous), **masturbation**, **bestiality**, and homosexual sodomy have been held to be absolutely wrong in themselves. Moreover, whereas disapproval of extramarital, adulterous, or promiscuous heterosexual intercourse is usually grounded in concerns about unwanted pregnancy, social disruption, and **sexually transmitted diseases**, objections to intrinsically nonprocreative sexual acts are more often grounded in their alleged biological or teleological "unnaturalness." On more extreme views, however, any kind of sexual activity whatsoever may count as intrinsically objectionable, regardless of its legal or procreative status. Such views—of which there is more than a hint in the writings of, among others, **Saint Augustine** (354–430) and **Immanuel Kant** (1724–1804)—may still be with us. In his work on the virtues, for example, Peter Geach (Anscombe's spouse) observes, "Apart from the good of marriage that redeems it, sex is poison" (147). For the most part, however, such past and present hostility to sexuality seems to be based on more than considerations of individual and social utility and to be often religiously motivated.

All the same, it seems possible to make sense of the main varieties of abstinence in terms of individual and social utility without reference to any "other-worldly," religious, or metaphysical considerations. In many cultures, abstinence in the form of virginity has often been valued in or demanded from those outside the married state. This has been and continues to be particularly true of female members of traditional societies, whose virginity is often a key economic counter in the social bargaining for quality spouses and who might incur the direst penalty (death by stoning or fire) for voluntary or even coerced sexual "dishonor." Notoriously, such societies commonly operate a double standard with regard to male and female sexual conduct. Whereas girls who have engaged in or been forced into premarital heterosexual activity are treated as pariahs, and widows may be expected to terminate all sexual and other life on their spouses' funeral pyres, men (married and unmarried) may be covertly if not actively encouraged to seek sexual release with prostitutes or concubines. Still, neither female nor male conformity to socially sanctioned virginity necessarily means adherence to complete sexual abstinence. Although traditional societies take a dim view (officially) of masturbation, homosexual sodomy, and lesbian sex, such activities may nevertheless be consistent with strict conformity to prohibitions of full intercourse, might occur without loss of socially and economically valuable virginity, and might be, for these reasons, at least covertly tolerated. From this viewpoint, the sexual abstinence of virginity appears to be of a different order from celibate and other forms of abstinence.

We might here take note of the "New Virginity" (see Ali and Scelfo) recently invoked in opposition to the "revolution" in sexual attitudes and lifestyles that has gathered momentum in such Western liberal democracies as Great Britain and the United States in the latter part of the twentieth century. This New Virginity is not merely indicative of a physical state of sexual inexperience but signals more general hostility to the alleged sexual decadence of liberal or "permissive" cultural trends. Advocates of the New Virginity, who are often closely associated with conservative or fundamentalist religious groups, reject all forms of unregulated (specifically nonmarital) sexual activity as grave symptoms of contemporary moral decline. From this uncompromising viewpoint, premarital sex is no less reprehensible than **homosexuality**, masturbation, and **pornography**. For most "new virgins," virginity therefore means a state of totally sex-free celibacy outside marriage, an abstinence that excludes not only penetrative intercourse but also alternative, noncoital routes to sexual satisfaction.

Regardless, celibacy seems neither synonymous nor coextensive with virginity. A woman whose hymen is intact, yet who has engaged in alternative noncoital routes to sexual pleasure, might well be a noncelibate virgin; yet after introduction to full sexual activity, she might later abstain from sex and therefore become a nonvirginal celibate. Celibacy is, all the same, a common human condition that is experienced, in one form or another, by most people sometime in their lives. Of course, "celibacy" is prone to narrower or broader, more or less formal, interpretations. First, there is the question of whether celibacy implies sexual abstention as such, since it is often taken to mean little more than forsaking **marriage**. For many people, however, the term is closely associated with religious life and obligation, as in the Roman Catholic requirement that priests be unmarried, and is in this sense taken to involve abstinence. The main purpose of such consecrated abstention is not self-denial for its own sake but the spiritual sublimation or redirection of sexual drives (thought to be otherwise prone to egotistical focus) for the greater glory of the church as Christ's body on earth.

Celibacy might also be observed by lay or secular members of the public for reasons that are neither religious nor moral, and it is not then obvious that such celibacy must exclude all sexual activity. In this less precise sense of "celibacy," individuals might choose to live alone and avoid having sexual relations with others for a variety of reasons relating to social isolation, psychosexual **dysfunction** (including morbid fear of disease or contamination), simple preference for the solitary life, low sexual drive, or other nonmoral or pragmatic considerations. The much loved British comedian Kenneth Williams (1926–1988) seems to have followed a celibate life, in this sense, for some psychologically complex mixture of reasons. In his entertaining and moving posthumous diaries, however, Williams openly admits to regularly practicing homoerotically inspired and sadomasochistic masturbation as part of a generally celibate, but far from sex-free, lifestyle (see *Diaries* throughout, but especially 97–98, 167, 403, 673).

One way of capturing the difference between religious and secular forms of celibate abstention is by reference to the notion of chastity. What mainly seems to distinguish consecrated celibacy from secular celibacy (aesthetically or pragmatically motivated avoidance of sexual relations) is a commitment to abstention as a moral or spiritual ideal of human growth. Whereas some secular (or even religious) celibates might choose the single state from fear of disease or intimacy, or due to a preference for solitary masturbation, the consecrated celibate regards this state precisely as a vehicle for expressing the value or virtue of chastity. But chastity would seem to require the cultivation of certain attitudes toward sexual life—a certain purity of heart or mind—that is not reducible to even complete celibate abstinence. In this light, it is possible to be celibate without being chaste, insofar as one might abstain totally from sex yet cultivate lewd thoughts and desires. Although there is a sense in which Williams might be regarded as celibate, one would be hard put to describe him as chaste: He lusted after the objects of his fantasies.

However, just as it seems possible to have celibacy without chastity, there may also be chastity without celibacy, or circumstances in which one could describe mutual **love** between noncelibate individuals as nonetheless chaste. First, there is a case in which the persons concerned are both married to others and not engaging in sex with each other. The love between Queen Guinevere and Sir Launcelot might be described as chaste so long as it does not lead or tend to physical **adultery**—but as unchaste if it does. Second, the mutual love and sexual activity of persons married to one another might be regarded as chaste when it conforms to certain standards of fidelity and restraint but as unchaste when it does not. Although this point is no longer widely appreciated in the predominantly secular and liberal climate of modern sexual morality, it is recognized in contemporary Catholic and other Christian moral theology, according to which chastity is endorsed as a moral goal for religious celibates and noncelibates alike (see *Catechism of the Catholic Church*, "Vocation to Chastity").

So although virginity, celibacy, and chastity might all involve sexual abstinence, they are conceptually distinct notions and at odds with sexual expression in rather different ways. Roughly, whereas virginity is a state of physical integrity that is terminated only by (perhaps heterosexual) penetrative coitus, celibacy is a particular pattern of human sexual association (or dissociation), and chastity represents a certain ideal of sexual purity. ("New Virginity" and consecrated celibacy might involve all these states and ideals.) However, the more austere conception of chastity as an aspiration to sexual abstinence for its own sake, rather than for any instrumental, pragmatic, or neurotic motive, may well appear the most puzzling of these conditions, not least within the more relaxed sexual ethos of contemporary secular **liberalism**. Indeed, in a live-and-let-live climate in which sexual tastes and inclinations are widely held to be matters of personal preference, it might be said that with the exception of violent or sadistic conduct that harms or injures others, there can be no specifically sexual virtues or vices and therefore that there cannot be any coherent moral (rather than, say, aesthetic or pragmatic) objection to any form of sexuality. It is possible to identify views like this in writers as otherwise diverse as the moral philosopher Bernard Williams (1929–2003; see Magee, 164), revisionist Kantian philosophers (e.g., Thomas Mappes), and progressive educator A. S. Neill (1883–1973) of Summerhill (64).

Perhaps the best way to approach the question whether or if chastity might be a virtue is to ask why some philosophers and theorists have held that the sexual drive, on the face a source of deep human pleasure, is in fact a negative (poisonous) impulse in need of some, if not complete, constraint. Some such dim view of the sexual impulse seems presupposed by any idea that chastity might be a virtue, for although virtues need not be exclusively matters of self-denial or self-control (Carr, "Two Kinds of Virtue"), they are generally concerned with the regulation or proper ordering of potentially wayward passions, appetites, and inclinations. However, if the only moral objection to rampant heterosexual or homosexual promiscuity is that it might harm others through violence or betrayal, and promiscuity does not harm others (since, say, some philanderers consort exclusively with prostitutes on a purely commercial basis), then it is hard to see what specifically moral norms might be invoked (virtue ethically) to regulate this highly gratifying, nonharmful behavior. (Indeed, we could be said to suffer physically harmful or debilitating psychological frustration without it.) How, then, might we make sense of chastity as a moral or sexual virtue?

Much ancient and modern uncertainty or disagreement about the status of chastity rests on recognizing that virtues do not conform to one pattern of psychological structure or organization. Some virtues are straightforwardly concerned with the regulation or control of independently identifiable emotions or appetites that are not inherently objectionable. In this respect, courage and temperance seem concerned with the control or regulation of states of fear and animal appetite, which are in themselves neither negative nor eliminable. No one could be courageous without feeling fear, and it would be absurd to regard as temperate someone who has no appetite for food or drink. In this respect, courage and temperance seem to be virtues of the mean in **Aristotle**'s (384–322 BCE) sense (*Nicomachean Ethics*, bk. 2, sec. 6). They do not require the extinction or elimination of fear and appetite, only that we experience and express them in the right ways. Not all virtues are of this kind. Virtues of truthfulness, fidelity, and honesty, for example, seem straightforwardly opposed to the vices of lying, infidelity, and dishonesty, and such defects cannot be accommodated to virtue in any form, order, or proportion. (**Bertrand Russell** [1872–1970] famously satirized the "Aristotelian" civic leader who always tried to steer a course between partiality and impartiality; 186.) This point, by the way, is unaffected by the consideration (often utilitarian) that it is sometimes morally defensible to kill or tell lies; for this is only to say that it is sometimes defensible to do something *prima facie* wrong to avoid something even worse.

The key question is whether chastity, if it is a virtue, is like temperance or fidelity: Is it more like regulating an inclination or appetite that is not in itself negative or bad, or is it more like extinguishing a tendency, like dishonesty or fidelity, that cannot be reconciled with any virtuous disposition? It is worth noting that despite the temptation to resolve this question quickly in favor of the temperance analogy, sexual appetites are arguably not like appetites for food. They seem no less impossible to deny than inclinations to untruth or infidelity, and although one cannot live without food or drink, one can live without sex. **Thomas Aquinas** (1224/25–1274), for one, regarded sex-free celibacy as not unnatural in this sense, although he added that celibacy without a spiritual reason suggests the vice of insensibility (*Summa contra gentiles*, bk. III, ques. 137). Thus, if one can live (albeit with some struggle and difficulty) without any sexual outlet, and we could identify reasons for regarding any sexual expression as inherently unconducive or inimical to human moral growth (like dishonesty and infidelity), then there would be grounds for regarding chastity— uncompromising sexual abstinence or denial—as a moral virtue. What sort of grounds could these be?

One need not look far in the history of Western (or Eastern) philosophical, religious, and metaphysical reflection to find evidence that all sexual inclination and sexual expression have been regarded in a morally negative way. There is abundant evidence of negative attitudes to sexuality in Western philosophy from its Platonic origins to the present day, and various shades of Christian moral reflection have been deeply informed by sexually negative perspectives. For example, **Saint Paul** (5–64?) advises us that it is good to marry only so that we should not burn (1 Cor. 7:9), and some early church fathers castrated themselves in the light of such stern advice. From whence do these attitudes derive, and might there be any compelling reasons for holding them?

It seems likely that such deep hostility to sexuality derives from a more general antipathy to the material world and to the desires of the flesh that entered ancient Greek and early Christian thought from Middle Eastern religious sources. The ancient Persian religion of Zoroaster had an impact on the postexilic Judaic roots of Christianity; the teachings of the third-century Persian prophet Mani (216–276?) directly influenced the thought of such early church fathers as Augustine; and Eleusian, Orphic, and Pythagorean mysteries appear to have informed Platonic and Neo-Platonist philosophy. These influences also seem to have shaped the mythopoeic character of both authorized and apocryphal Gospel narratives. Despite local differences, such doctrines seem to have agreed in regarding the human soul as a prime site of metaphysical conflict between principles of good (light) and evil (dark), leading to eventual triumph (in the final days) of the light of goodness over the darkness of evil. In identifying goodness with the nonmaterial (spiritual or rational) part of human nature, and evil with the physical or material part, Manichaean and Gnostic dualism regarded the redemption or salvation of the soul as turning on the cultivation of attitudes of denial, contempt for or at least indifference to the desires of the flesh. It is largely in this vein that

Plato (427–347 BCE) saw the task of the philosopher as that of "practicing death" (e.g., *Phaedo*, 64a–67e), and the Pauline epistles characterized the new life in Christ as a matter of the flesh dying to the spirit (e.g., Rom. 8:12–14).

On this view, sexual desires and impulses are morally pernicious particularly because they distract or tempt the soul away from its proper noncorporeal or spiritual concerns with the pursuit of wisdom or knowledge of God (see Paul, Rom. 6:12–13, 19–20, 1 Cor. 7:33–36; Augustine, *Confessions*, bk. 6, chap. 16, bk. 10, chap. 30). It seems to have been largely for this reason that some past Christians practiced extreme sexual self-denial and asceticism, even to the point of sexual self-mutilation. At all events, such early church fathers as Clement of Alexandria (ca. 150–215; see Pagels, 29, citing *Stromata* 3, 57–58; and Friedman, 37, citing *Paidogogus* III, 4, 26) and Augustine (*On Marriage and Concupiscence*, bk. 1, chap. 9) seem to have construed chastity as a matter of strict sex-free celibacy and regarded sex even in the context of marriage as consistent with virtue only if performed for the sake of procreation and not for sensual pleasure. Indeed, in *On the Good of Marriage* Augustine goes beyond this in claiming that "continence from all intercourse [even in marriage] is certainly better than marital intercourse itself which takes place for the sake of begetting children" (chap. 6). This is "the chastity of souls rightly joined together" (chap. 3). That said, the cultivation of Gnostic contempt for or indifference to sexual impulses has sometimes inclined to the opposite extreme of sexual license and indulgence; for if the flesh and bodily desires are of no spiritual or redemptive importance, then indulgence of the appetites may not matter so long as the soul remains spiritually pure. In this respect, early Christians (justly or not) accused some Gnostic sects of extreme sexual permissiveness. Much later, literary figures of pronounced heretical tendencies (e.g., the eighteenth- and nineteenth-century Romantic poets William Blake [1757–1827], George Gordon Lord Byron [1788–1824], and Percy Bysshe Shelley [1792–1822]) may also have regarded sexual license as not incompatible with the achievement of spiritual wisdom. Ironically, it would appear that contemporary perceptions of Christianity as inherently sexually negative derive from its past susceptibility to Gnostic and Manichaean influences.

Whether this is the correct perception of contemporary Christian orthodoxy is another matter. From a philosophical viewpoint, a significant reversal of Platonic, Manichaean, and dualist influences on Christianity was one aim of the Aristotelian reworking of Christian theology by Aquinas in the thirteenth century. The adoption of an antidualist Aristotelian anthropology, and a related reconception of virtue as a reasonable mean between deficiencies and excesses of passion and appetite, opened the way to a more benign view of the place of sexuality in human life and allowed for a more relaxed construal of the virtue of chastity. Thus, although Aquinas regarded sex-free celibacy as a religious and moral ideal, he nevertheless regarded chastity as occupying a mean between excess and defect of **sexual desire** and as therefore not beyond legitimate expression in appropriately regulated contexts. Indeed, although some such conception of chastity has long been apparent in modern Christian theology and church doctrine, it is plainly stated in the modern *Catechism of the Catholic Church* and in the writings of, for example, Anscombe. On this view, chastity is a virtue of sexual temperance that aims to contain sexual impulse and appetite within the bounds of reasonable moderation. Such sexual regulation is likely to be viewed as harsh by contemporary secular liberal standards, insofar as legitimate sexual expression is confined to procreative heterosexual intercourse within marriage, and sodomy, homosexuality, and masturbation are held to be sexually deviant and always impermissible. Still, although Roman Catholic extramarital chastity still remains a matter of uncompromising abstinence, post-Thomist orthodoxy is able to make coherent sense of chastity as a virtue for sexually active marriage partners and hence as a genuine (if exacting) moral ideal for both the faithful married majority and the unmarried or consecrated minority. Moreover, this is not to exclude the possibility of more lenient religious or secular conceptions of chastity as temperance that might rule out only (say) promiscuity, adultery, or pornography, although one should not underestimate the difficulties of this prospect once one drops any biologically functional criterion of sexual propriety (see Carr, "Freud and Sexual Ethics").

See also Activity, Sexual; Adultery; Augustine (Saint); Bible, Sex and the; Casual Sex; Catholicism, History of; Ethics, Sexual; Ethics, Virtue; Gnosticism; Manichaeism; Rousseau, Jean-Jacques; Sex Education; Thomas Aquinas (Saint)

REFERENCES

Ali, Lorraine, and Julie Scelfo. "Choosing Virginity." *Newsweek* (9 December 2002), 61–66; Anscombe, G.E.M. "Contraception and Chastity." *The Human World*, no. 7 (1972), 9–30; Aristotle. (ca. 325 BCE?) *Nicomachean Ethics*. Trans. Terence Irwin. Indianapolis, Ind.: Hackett, 1985; Augustine. (397) *Confessions*. Trans. R. S. Pine-Coffin. Harmondsworth, U.K.: Penguin, 1961; Augustine. (418?–21) *On Marriage and Concupiscence*. Trans. Peter Holmes and Robert Ernest Wallis. In Philip Schaff, ed., *Library of Nicene and Post-Nicene Fathers*, vol. 5. Grand Rapids, Mich.: Eerdmans, 1989, 263–308; Augustine. (401–402) *On the Good of Marriage*. Trans. and ed. Patrick G. Walsh. Oxford, U.K.: Clarendon Press, 2001; Calasso, Roberto. *The Marriage of Cadmus and Harmony*. London: Vintage, 1994; Carr, David. "Freud and Sexual Ethics." *Philosophy* 62:241 (1987), 361–73; Carr, David. "Two Kinds of Virtue." *Proceedings of the Aristotelian Society* 84 (1984–1985), 47–61; *Catechism of the Catholic Church*. London: Geoffrey Chapman, 1994. ("Consecrated Virgins," 992; "Sacrament of Matrimony," 1618–20; "Fidelity," 1646; "Vocation to Chastity," 2337–45); Friedman, David. *A Mind of Its Own: A Cultural History of the Penis*. New York: Free Press, 2002; Geach, Peter T. *The Virtues*. Cambridge: Cambridge University Press, 1977; Magee, Brian. "Conversation with Bernard Williams: Philosophy and Morals." In Brian Magee, ed., *Modern British Philosophy*. London: Secker and Warburg, 1971, 150–65; Mappes, Thomas A. "Sexual Morality and the Concept of Using Another Person." In Thomas A. Mappes and Jane S. Zembaty, eds., *Social Ethics: Morality and Social Policy*, 6th ed. Boston, Mass.: McGraw-Hill, 2002, 170–83; Neill, Alexander S. *Summerhill: A Radical Approach to Education*. London: Gollancz, 1965; Pagels, Elaine. *Adam, Eve, and the Serpent*. New York: Vintage, 1988; Plato. (ca. 378 BCE) *Phaedo*. In *The Last Days of Socrates*. Trans. Hugh Tredennick. (1954) Harmondsworth, U.K.: Penguin, 1977, 99–183; Russell, Bertrand. (1946) *History of Western Philosophy*. London: Routledge, 2000; Thomas Aquinas. (1258–1264) *Summa contra gentiles*, 5 vols. Trans. Anton Pegis. South Bend, Ind.: University of Notre Dame Press, 1975; Williams, Kenneth. *The Kenneth Williams Diaries*. Ed. Russell Davies. London: HarperCollins, 1993.

David Carr

ADDITIONAL READING

Abbott, Elizabeth. *A History of Celibacy*. New York: Scribner's, 2000; Anscombe, G.E.M. (Elizabeth). "Contraception and Chastity." *The Human World*, no. 7 (1972), 9–30. Reprinted in HS (29–50). Reprinted, revised, in Michael D. Bayles, ed., *Ethics and Population*. Cambridge, Mass.: Schenkman, 1976, 134–53; Anscombe, G.E.M. "You Can Have Sex without Children: Christianity and the New Offer." In *Ethics, Religion, and Politics*. Minneapolis: University of Minnesota Press, 1981, 82–96; Baier, Annette. "Good Men's Women: Hume on Chastity and Trust." *Hume Studies* 5 (1979), 1–19; Calderone, Mary S. "The Case for Chastity." In Henry Anatole Grunwald, ed., *Sex in America*. New York: Bantam, 1964, 140–51; Carpenter, Laura M. "The Ambiguity of 'Having Sex': The Subjective Experience of Virginity Loss in the United States." *Journal of Sex Research* 38:2 (2001), 127–39; Carr, David. "Chastity and Adultery." *American Philosophical Quarterly* 23:4 (1986),

363–71; Davis, Murray. *Smut: Erotic Reality/Obscene Ideology*. Chicago, Ill.: University of Chicago Press, 1983; Decter, Midge. (1972) *The New Chastity and Other Arguments against Women's Liberation*. New York: Capricorn, 1974; Deming, Will. (1995) *Paul on Marriage and Celibacy: The Hellenistic Background of 1 Corinthians 7*, 2nd ed. Grand Rapids, Mich.: Eerdmans, 2004; Dworkin, Andrea. "Virginity." In *Intercourse*. New York: Free Press, 1987, 83–119; Foucault, Michel. "The Battle for Chastity." In Philippe Ariès and André Béjin, eds., *Western Sexuality: Practice and Precept in Past and Present Times*. Trans. Anthony Forster. Oxford, U.K.: Blackwell, 1985, 14–25; Geach, Mary. "Marriage: Arguing to a First Principle in Sexual Ethics." In Luke Gormally, ed., *Moral Truth and Moral Tradition: Essays in Honour of Peter Geach and Elizabeth Anscombe*. Dublin, Ire.: Four Courts Press, 1994, 177–93; Hartwig, Michael. *The Poetics of Intimacy and the Problem of Sexual Abstinence*. New York: Peter Lang, 2000; Heid, Stephan. *Celibacy in the Early Church*. Fort Collins, Colo.: Ignatius, 2001; Hume, David. (1739) "Of Chastity and Modesty." In *A Treatise of Human Nature*. Ed. L. A. Selby-Bigge. Oxford, U.K.: Clarendon Press, 1968, bk. III, pt. ii, sec. 12, 570–73; Kant, Immanuel. (ca. 1780) "Duties towards the Body in Respect of Sexual Impulse." In *Lectures on Ethics*. Trans. Louis Infield. Indianapolis, Ind.: Hackett, 1963, 162–71. Reprinted in POS4 (199–205); STW (140–45); Kant, Immanuel. *Lectures on Ethics*. Trans. Peter Heath. Ed. Peter Heath and Jerome B. Schneewind. Cambridge: Cambridge University Press, 1997; Kimmerling, Ben. "Celibacy and Intimacy." In Elizabeth Stuart and Adrian Thatcher, eds., *Christian Perspectives on Sexuality and Gender*. Grand Rapids, Mich.: Eerdmans, 1996, 429–37; Kuefler, Mathew. *The Manly Eunuch: Masculinity, Gender Ambiguity, and Christian Ideology in Late Antiquity*. Chicago, Ill.: University of Chicago Press, 2001; Lea, Henry C. (1867) *History of Sacerdotal Celibacy in the Christian Church*, 4th ed., rev. London: Watts, 1932. New York: Russell and Russell, 1957; Lehrman, Sally. "The Virtues of Promiscuity." *AlterNet* (22 July 2002). <www.alternet.org/story.html?StoryID=13648> [accessed 16 February 2005]; Mappes, Thomas A. (1985) "Sexual Morality and the Concept of Using Another Person." In Thomas A. Mappes and Jane S. Zembaty, eds., *Social Ethics: Morality and Social Policy*, 4th ed. New York: McGraw-Hill, 1992, 203–16. 5th ed., 1997, 163–76. 6th ed., 2002, 170–83. Reprinted in POS4 (207–23); Martin, Christopher F. J. "Are There Virtues and Vices That Belong Specifically to the Sexual Life?" *Acta Philosophica* 4:2 (1995), 205–21; Mead, Rebecca. "Sex and Sensibility: The Histories of Nymphomania and Celibacy." *The New Yorker* (18 September 2000), 146–48; Pheterson, Gail. "The Social Consequences of Unchastity." In Frédérique Delacoste and Priscilla Alexander, eds., *Sex Work: Writings by Women in the Sex Industry*, 2nd ed. San Francisco, Calif.: Cleis Press, 1998, 231–45; Regan, A. "Lust." In *New Catholic Encyclopedia*, vol. 8. New York: McGraw-Hill, 1967, 1081–85; Remez, Lisa. "Oral Sex among Adolescents: Is It Sex or Is It Abstinence?" *Family Planning Perspectives* 32:6 (2000), 298–304; Rhees, Rush. (1963) "Chastity." In *Moral Questions*. Ed. D. Z. Phillips. New York: St. Martin's Press, 1999, 159–63; Russell, Bertrand. *History of Western Philosophy*. London: George Allen and Unwin, 1946. London: Routledge, 2000; Shalit, Wendy. *A Return to Modesty: Discovering the Lost Virtue*. New York: Free Press, 1999; Smullyan, Raymond. "A Query." In *5000 B.C. and Other Philosophical Fantasies*. New York: St. Martin's Press, 1983, 47–50; Stevens-Simon, C. "Virginity: A State of Mind . . . But Not Necessarily of Body." *Journal of School Health* 71 (2001), 87–88; Stubblefield, Anna. "Contraceptive Risk-taking and Norms of Chastity." *Journal of Social Philosophy* 27:3 (1996), 81–100; Tapia, Andres. "Abstinence: The Radical Choice for Sex Education." *Christianity Today* 37:2 (1993), 24–29; Teichman, Jenny. "Intention and Sex." In Cora Diamond and Jenny Teichman, eds., *Intention and Intentionality: Essays in Honour of G.E.M. Anscombe*. Ithaca, N.Y.: Cornell University Press, 1979, 147–61; Thomas Aquinas. (1265–1273) "Abstinence" (2a2ae, ques. 146), "Chastity" (2a2ae, ques. 151). In *Summa theologiae*. 60 vols. Trans. Blackfriars. Cambridge, U.K.: Blackfriars, 1964–1976; Wimbush, Vincent L., and Richard Valantasis, eds. *Asceticism*. New York: Oxford University Press, 1995; Winch, Peter, Bernard Williams, Michael Tanner, and G.E.M. Anscombe. "Discussion of 'Contraception and Chastity.' " In Michael D. Bayles, ed., *Ethics and Population*. Cambridge, Mass.: Schenkman, 1976, 154–63; Woody, Jane D., Robin Russel, Henry J. D'Souza, and Jennifer K. Woody. "Adolescent Non-Coital Sexual Activity: Comparisons of Virgins and Non-Virgins." *Journal of Sex Education and Therapy* 25:4 (2000), 261–68.

ACQUAINTANCE RAPE. *See* Rape, Acquaintance and Date

ACTIVITY, SEXUAL. The sexual activities in which people engage can be examined and understood in many ways: biologically, psychologically, sociologically, anthropologically, economically, philosophically, and theologically. Although certain biological and psychological features of human actions likely *make* some of them sexual actions, what people *believe* is a sexual activity is influenced by social attitudes and norms. Sexologists—biomedical and social scientists—provide information about the types of sexual acts people do; when, how often, with whom, why, and where they do them; and what happens in or to the body and mind before, during, and after. Both theologians and philosophers deliberate and make pronouncements about **sexual ethics**. Philosophers, in addition, make a concerted effort to define (analyze) "sexual act." Of course, everyone is free to define a word, but for philosophers it is often their life's work.

"Sexual activity" is a puzzling concept (Christina agonizes over it). It is difficult to state the conditions that are sufficient and necessary for an act to be sexual, that is, to state (1) what it is that makes an act a sexual act (or in virtue of which it is sexual) rather than some other type of act, and to state (2) what, if absent, would leave us without a sexual act (or is required for an act to be sexual). Defining "sexual act" is important, at least because applying other concepts depends on our being able to identify sexual acts: **Rape** is a forced sexual act or one to which a person does not consent; a married person who engages in a sexual act with someone not his or her spouse commits **adultery**; and in **prostitution** sexual activities are bought and sold. In this way, concepts of *doing* are parasitic on the concept of sexual activity. But the same holds for concepts of *not doing*: **Abstinence**, chastity, and celibacy are in various ways forswearings of sexual activity. If I do not know what a sexual act is, I will not know what to avoid if I plan to be abstinent or remain virginal, and I might without being aware of it engage in forbidden or unwanted sexual acts. Mull over the provocative title of a research report: "Oral Sex among Adolescents: Is It Sex or Is It Abstinence?" (Remez).

It may be, as Alan Goldman urges, that "we all know what sex is, at least in obvious cases, and do not need philosophers to tell us" (270). But the "not obvious" cases are the interesting ones, and about these philosophers might have something illuminating to say. Besides, it is not always obvious how to distinguish obvious cases from those that are not obvious. Philosophers can work on that as well. Simon Blackburn is very confident about a sexual scenario that for other people may be unclear: "[I]n James Joyce's *Ulysses*, Leopold Bloom and Gertie McDowell, eying each other across the beach, use each other's perceived excitement to work themselves to their climaxes. . . . I should have said that Bloom and Gertie had sex together" (91; see **Thomas Nagel** for more about this scenario). But it is not (obvious that it is) obvious that X and Y can be said to have "had sex" while never touching each other. If Blackburn countenances flirting-across-the-beach experiences (i.e., dual **masturbation**) as a case in which two people "had sex," he should be willing to say that two people who chat sexually, using the telephone or while online, to attain sexual pleasure or orgasm through masturbation, are also "having sex." Maybe he is right, but ordinary language does not support him.

A well-known study published in 1999 conducted on college students by two Kinsey Institute researchers found that 60 percent do not think that engaging in oral sex (fellatio, cunnilingus) is "having sex" (Sanders and Reinisch). Other studies have confirmed this finding. Indeed, the figure was about 78 percent for a Canadian student population (Randall and Byers, 91, table 1). If these students do not think that oral sex is "having sex," they would not think that flirting across the beach is "having sex." In fact, they do not: Some 96 to 97 percent of the Canadian students denied that "masturbating to orgasm in each other's presence," telephone chatting, and cyberorgasms are "having sex." (Indeed, only 10 to 14 percent—a dramatically small minority—even think that X's actually touching Y's genitals to the point of orgasm is "having sex.") That such a large percentage refuse to countenance oral sex as "having sex" is at first surprising, even shocking (as is the idea that engaging in oral sex is consistent with abstinence). But postpone judgment. Philosophers and other scholars have no trouble thinking of fellatio and cunnilingus as types of "sexual activity." In their hands that becomes a technical term. "Having sex," by contrast, is an ordinary language expression. Students, as studies have found, reserve it for (voluntary) penis-vagina intercourse and anal intercourse. (They were asked and could answer only about male-female anal intercourse, not about male-male.) Blackburn, employing his own nonordinary language notion of "having sex," claims that "President Clinton['s] standards for having sex with someone were . . . remarkably high" (91). Not at all. When Monica Lewinsky confided to Linda Tripp that she did not "have sex" with President William Clinton, and he denied having "sexual relations with that woman," they were not lying, pulling a disingenuous fast one, or self-deceived. They were merely using the ordinary language notion of "having sex" (and they surely had a right to do so). American and Canadian students agree with those beleaguered lovers, and Aussies, too (Richters and Song).

The finding that 60 to 80 percent do not consider engaging in oral sex to be "having sex" will be shocking if we infer that students thereby deny that fellatio and cunnilingus are *sexual acts*. But the students are not saying that. Even though 78 percent of the Canadian students deny that oral sex is "having sex," about 65 percent still think that if X and Y engage in oral sex, X and Y are "sexual partners," and 98 percent think that X and Y are being "unfaithful" if they are involved in a significant relationship with someone else. (See Randall and Byers, 91, table 2; 92, table 3. For the first two questions, the student subject is X [or Y], while for the last question X [or Y] is the subject's boyfriend or girlfriend; 89.) It is plausible to think that the students would not issue either judgment if they thought that oral sex was not *any* kind of sexual activity, event, or experience. Thus Blackburn would be better off saying that flirting across the beach (as well as talking over the telephone and sending sexually arousing instant or e-mail messages; see Ben-Ze'ev, 4–6) can be a sexual activity, even if it is not "having sex."

Now that we have made a distinction between "having sex" and "sexual activity," where the second is the larger category and includes the first, let us reexamine Goldman's "we all know what sex is." The word "sex" is ambiguous (see Randall and Byers, 87). Does Goldman mean that we all know what "sexual activity" is? (That claim is probably false.) Does he mean that we all know what "having sex" is? (That's true in part.) Or is it something else—**sexual desire**, sexual arousal, sexual pleasure—that we all know? (Maybe we do, maybe not.) Using "sex" ambiguously is common. "If the placement of the clitoris in the female body reflects the divine will, then God wills that sex is not just oriented to procreation, but is at least as, if not more, oriented to pleasure," writes Christine Gudorf (65; see Roth, 434). This claim makes much more sense if "sex" here means "sexual activity," which includes cunnilingus, and not the narrower "having sex," which is not as clitoris-attentive. The feminist legal scholar **Catharine MacKinnon** claims that in our male-dominant society "whatever sexually arouses a man is sex" (*Toward*, 211). Here "sex" seems not to mean either "having sex" or "sexual activity." So what does it mean? When

MacKinnon continues, "[I]nequality is sex . . . humiliation is sex . . . debasement is sex . . . intrusion is sex," we might infer that "is sex" for MacKinnon means "is sexually arousing [for men]." But, if so, the first statement becomes, "[W]hatever sexually arouses a man is sexually arousing [for men]." MacKinnon makes the ambiguity of her use of "sex" more intractable when she writes things like, "Pornography is masturbation material. It is used as sex. It therefore is sex" (*Only Words*, 17). In the terms "**sex education**" and "the philosophy of sex," the wide-ranging ambiguity of "sex" is not a problem but, instead, a virtue, because "sex" allows us to speak about teaching or studying, all at once, the many facets of human sexuality. This is not how MacKinnon uses "sex."

In her marvelous essay "Are We Having Sex Now or What?" Greta Christina wonders about the ontological status of many different acts, including dual masturbation, sado-masochistic encounters, activities between two women, activities among a group of women, and groping, grabbing, rubbing, and roaming while fully clothed. She begins by asking specifically what "having sex" is, but while laying out and discussing these examples, which befuddle her and prevent her from finding a satisfactory answer to the question, the phrase she uses most frequently, by far, is "is sex." That is, she asks, instead, whether these various things are "sex" and, in effect, moves back and forth, with this one word, between asking whether an activity is "having sex" and asking (unbeknownst to her) whether it is a "sexual activity" (and who knows what else). *This* mistake, using the ambiguous "sex," explains why she eventually has to throw up her hands, exasperated. (She ends her essay, after describing a magnificent orgasms-all-around dual masturbation episode, with "I still don't have an answer.") All Christina had to do, to avoid the conclusion that she is trying hard to avoid but sees no way of avoiding—that if something (sadomasochistic events, dual masturbation, and so forth) is not intercourse, then it is not "sex" *at all*—was to say that whatever else they are, these noncoital activities are at least cases of "sexual activity" (which expression she does use once—but only once—in five and a half pages). Then we can negotiate whether to add, which is not prohibited, some of these activities to the "having sex" category. Perhaps at some time we would come to think of solitary masturbation not merely as the sexual act it is now but as a case of *X*'s "having sex" with *X*. (It is doubtful, though, that all sexual activities would turn out to be "having sex.")

One more example: "Whatever else flirting may be, it is not sex," writes John Portmann (227). But that depends on what he means by "sex." Portmann denies that a "dirty" telephone chat is "having sex" (224, 226), and he claims, "The Internet has not given us a new way to *have* sex but rather an absorbing new way to *talk about* sex" (223). It is clear that Portmann equates "sex" and "having sex," so what he asserts about flirting is that it is not "having sex." That is trivial in the ordinary language meaning of "having sex." On his own definition, "sex" ("having sex") "entails skin-to-skin contact" (231). This definition grounds his assertion that flirting is not "sex," for flirting involves no skin-skin contact. (The phenomenon of skin-skin contact may be deployed reductionistically and, perhaps, cynically: "Love as it exists in society is merely the mingling of two fantasies and the contact of two skins," wrote Sébastien-Roch-Nicolas Chamfort [1741–1794], 170.)

Portmann's conclusion, that flirting is not "sex" because it involves no skin-skin contact, is still trivial, for the question should be whether flirting can be a *sexual activity*. Maybe Portmann, even though he uses and defines the expression "having sex," intended to define "sexual activity," instead, as "skin-to-skin contact." If so, flirting is, on his view, neither "having sex" nor a sexual activity. The implication is dubious and, what is worse, his definition is implausible—because sexual acts do not require skin-to-skin contact. Teenagers (and Christina) who "dry hump" while wearing their jeans or shorts are engaging in sexual activity. Hence the notion that flirting is not "sex" (is not a sexual activity) cannot be grounded in or justified by Portmann's definition. And because the ground of that assertion is gone, we are free to go the route of allowing flirting and telephone/Internet chats to count as sexual acts. Further, the weakness of Portmann's definition undermines—takes the support away from—the whole point, the central claim, of his essay, that "chatting is not cheating" (223, 230–34). Hence we are free to agree with Aaron Ben-Ze'ev's reasonable claim that "chatting is sometimes cheating" (199–222; see Collins) and with the Canadian students that masturbation in each other's presence (95 percent), while talking on the telephone (85 percent), and during computer sessions (79 percent) is being "unfaithful" (Randall and Byers). Of course, Ben-Ze'ev and the students are able to arrive at a conclusion opposed to Portmann's because they understand "having sex" and "sexual activity" differently from him. But how *should* we understand these concepts? We would be pleased to have an analysis of "sexual activity" that straightens out this territory.

There are some candidate analyses of "sexual activity," some better than others. Consider an analysis of "sexual activity," (A1), according to which there are *no* sexual activities beyond "having sex," as currently understood. (A1) must be wrong. If an act is sexual if and only if it is "having sex," then penis-vagina and penis-anus intercourse are the only sexual activities. Even if "penis-anus intercourse" is construed broadly enough to include male-male as well as male-female buggery, female-female sexuality is eradicated. Were we to state explicitly the principle deployed here to evaluate the analysis, it might be that any analysis of "sexual activity" entailing that whether two people engage in sexual activity together depends on their sex/gender is false.

The analysis of "sexual activity" in terms of the extension of "having sex" is patently phallocentric. This results from the fact that the students' notion of "having sex" is already phallocentric (see Frye; MacKinnon, *Toward*, 133). Why should it turn out, which seems odd, that "sexual activity," in *addition* to "having sex," gets defined—"hegemonically"—by reference to the male genitalia? When MacKinnon claims that "what is sexual is what gives a man an erection" (*Toward*, 137), she means that in our society sexuality is construed phallocentrically. Missing, for us, is the complementary, "Also, whatever makes a woman lubricate is sexual." But note that the students' notion of "having sex" is not perfectly phallocentric. If it were, they would have included fellatio within "having sex." Both fellatio and cunnilingus were (equally) excluded from that category.

Another possible analysis runs into similar difficulties. (A2) claims that sexual activities are those that are of the reproductive type, plus acts that are the natural biopsychological precursors or concomitants of such acts. On this view, the central case of a sexual activity is penis-vagina intercourse (which is one way of "having sex"), since that is the only act of the reproductive type. The use of contraception (e.g., a condom or intrauterine device) does not, on this view, prevent heterosexual intercourse from being a sexual act. (That would be a strange consequence.) The reason is that contracepted intercourse still has the proper form of a sexual act; it is still of the right type, even if no reproduction will actually occur. After all, many noncontracepted cases of heterosexual intercourse also fail to result in reproduction, and that fact does not change them from being of the reproductive type to some other type. Kissing, mutual masturbation, and oral sex, when engaged in by a male and a female, are all sexual acts, to the extent that they are the natural precursors or concomitants of intercourse.

(A2) also must be wrong. It entails that acts that occur between people who have the same sexual anatomy (e.g., two women) are not sexual, since none are procreative. Like (A1), (A2) succumbs to the principle that whether an act is sexual must not depend on the sex/gender of the persons engaged in it. Further, sexual perversions—such as fondling shoes—could no longer be called *sexual* perversions, because, being nonprocreative, they are not sexual in the first place. Solitary masturbation, too, is (counterintuitively) not a sexual activity. But the main problem is that (A2) denies that male-female anal intercourse is a sexual activity. Heterosexual buggery is neither of reproductive form nor a natural precursor or concomitant of penis-vagina intercourse, yet it is in the current extension of "having sex." But any analysis that entails that a case of "having sex" is not "sexual activity" is false. It is a conceptual truth that what is included in "having sex" will be either equal to or less than what is included in "sexual activity"—no matter how those terms are analyzed. Might (A2) allow that anal intercourse *is* a natural precursor or concomitant of penis-vagina intercourse? That would open the floodgates. (Maybe that is where we should go.) But there is an important question lurking here: the facts that kissing and oral sex are often precursors to heterosexual intercourse, and anal intercourse is not—are these "natural" or the result of social norms and the like? Indeed, some have claimed that the "main event" itself is socially or politically engineered (e.g., Atkinson; Rich).

Other possible analyses of "sexual activity" are superior candidates, but these, too, may be found lacking. Consider this analysis: (A3) Sexual acts are exactly those in which there is contact with a sexual body part (not only the genitals). If so, cunnilingus, fellatio, mutual masturbation, sucking and massaging the breasts, and kissing are sexual acts. On this view, many things that two women can do together count as sexual acts. Further, solitary masturbation counts as a sexual activity, because (A3) does not state that two people must be involved to secure contact with a sexual part. (A3) appears to be better than (A1) and (A2).

Portmann's "skin-to-skin contact" definition, if taken as stating a necessary condition for sexual activity—no skin-skin contact, no sexual act (as in flirting and telephone chatting, on his view)—is a variant of (A3). Portmann's definition does not state, and was not meant to state, a sufficient condition. After all, merely shaking hands is not a sexual act. Similarly, and for the same reason, (A3) had better not be stating a sufficient condition; a gynecologist who examines the genitals of a woman does not automatically perform a sexual act (half of a mutual masturbation), and a man who, to urinate, uses his hand to remove his penis from his pants is not automatically engaged in a sexual act (solitary masturbation).

On the other hand, although dry humping is a counterexample to Portmann's definition, showing that it does not state a necessary condition, dry humping is not a counterexample to (A3), for (A3) does not entail that the contact must be skin-skin. In this sense, Portmann's definition is narrower than (A3), which allows more acts to be sexual—in particular, acts in which contact occurs through, for example, clothing. Thus solitary masturbation through one's pants or pantyhose counts as a sexual act for (A3) but not for Portmann. (A3) did not stumble into this fortuitous situation. "Contact" in that definition must be deliberately articulated in such a way that clothing over a sexual part, or between the toucher and the touched, does not entail that there is no contact—*since* solitary masturbation through one's clothing and dry humping are sexual acts. Moreover, were we to deny that they are sexual activities, we would be in danger of being forced to conclude that cunnilingus with a dental dam and heterosexual intercourse with a condom are not sexual activities. (Both these cases also show that skin-skin contact cannot be necessary.) Of course, were a sexual body part altogether insulated (beyond "jostlability") by an impervious material—a glass or steel bodysuit—there could be no contact and no sexual act.

Nevertheless, (A3) does not state a necessary condition; it cannot dodge counterexamples that were damaging to Portmann's definition: flirting and sexy telephone/Internet chats.

Even though the analysis admits mutual and solitary masturbation into the class of sexual acts, it does not admit dual masturbation—since that type occurs (as does flirting on the beach) at a distance. True, (A3) already has a bloated notion of contact, in allowing contact to happen through things that insulate and isolate sexual body parts and are an obstacle to "direct" or "immediate" contact. But (A3) does not have *carte blanche* to imagine that there *is* contact between two people when they talk in an Internet chatroom. The best thing to say (and which avoids an aura of desperation) is that such acts are sexual *despite* the fact that there is *no* contact, rather than they *are* sexual because there *is* contact.

"Sexual act," according to (A3), depends logically on "sexual body part." To identify sexual acts, we must first catalog sexual body parts; and our understanding of sexual activities could not be any better than our understanding of sexual parts. But can we catalog sexual body parts? Do we clearly understand "sexual body part"? (Portmann's definition is, in one sense, broader than [A3]: *Any* patch of skin will do. It thereby avoids these problems.) The definition of "sexual relations" applied in Clinton's deposition was a body-part definition: "genitalia, anus, groin, breast, inner thigh, or buttocks" (see Toobin, 218). Are the hands, too, sexual body parts? Two people might shake hands, without the act's being sexual. Alternatively, they might press their hands together and experience a rush of sexual pleasure. Sometimes the hands are used nonsexually and sometimes sexually. Hence there is no straightforward answer to the question, "Are the hands sexual body parts?" Whether hands are sexual parts depends on the activity in which they are used. This implies that a body part is sexual by virtue of the sexual nature of the acts in which it is involved. Hence "sexual body part" depends logically on "sexual activity," not the other way around. The point was made above that a gynecological examination is not automatically a sexual act because the genitals are touched, so contact with a sexual body part is not sufficient for an act to be sexual. But we could say, instead, about this case that the genitals are not a sexual body part in the requisite sense to begin with; during a gynecological examination, they are not being treated as sexual body parts.

The fact that on those occasions when holding hands is sexual, the act is accompanied by certain sensations—sexual pleasure—suggests that sexual activity might be profitably analyzed in terms of sexual pleasure. To be precise, as proposed by Robert Gray: (A4) Sexual acts are all and only those acts that produce sexual pleasure; or (equivalently) a necessary and sufficient condition for an act to be sexual is that it produce sexual pleasure. So, as another example, both acts of the reproductive type and acts not of that type are sexual when and only when they produce sexual pleasure. What unites the two types, say, heterosexual fellatio and homosexual (or same-sex) fellatio, is that both can produce pleasure and, we can assume, a qualitatively similar, if not identical, pleasure.

(A4) is a powerful analysis with advantages over the others. Whether an act is sexual does not depend on the sex/gender of its participants but only on whether it produces sexual pleasure. Masturbation, solitary and mutual, can be a sexual act. Further, dual masturbation, too, can be a sexual act, as well as sexy telephone/Internet chatting and flirting ourselves to orgasms on the beach, because producing sexual pleasure does not require contact. And sexual perversions are *sexual* by virtue of producing sexual pleasure. (A4) does not merely entail that these acts can be sexual; it accounts for, explains, the sexual nature of a wide variety of acts.

A similar analysis has been proposed by Deborah Rosen and John Christman, who analyze sexual activity in terms of sexual feelings, not sexual pleasure, where "feelings" is the larger category and includes "pleasure." Their reason for favoring "feelings" is that "many people would claim that pain, or at least a kind of intensity and rapture that connects with tension and conflict, is often closer to the precise nature of the internal 'feel' of their sexual experience" than pleasure (203). If "pleasure" is replaced by "feeling" in the analysis of "sexual activity," it is not clear that what is picked out as a sexual activity changes very much. For the "feelings" analysis to pick out *more* acts as sexual than the "pleasure" analysis (it could not pick out fewer, because "feelings" include "pleasure"), there would have to be acts that consistently gave rise to the "tension and conflict" feelings but never or hardly ever produced pleasure. Are there any such acts? To some extent it might not matter, for where the "sexual pleasure" analysis can be faulted is shared by the "sexual feelings" analysis. According to another variant of (A4), what picks out sexual activities is not pleasure but sexual arousal (see Laumann et al., 176: being "really turned on"). Even if sexual pleasure and sexual arousal largely accompany each other, it is specifically arousal that defines sexual activity (of course—see MacKinnon—both "lubrication" and "erection" are taken as signs of arousal). In this case, whether or how much the sets of acts picked out as sexual by the two analyses diverge depends on the incidence of acts that are sexually arousing but not sexually pleasurable (here Rosen and Christman's observation is relevant; some people might experience a sort of "tension and conflict" sexual arousal) and of acts that are sexually pleasurable but not very, or at all, sexually arousing (that surely happens and is often lamented). Again, divergence might not matter, if what is wrong with (A4) is also a defect of this variation.

A disadvantage of (A4) is that it leaves no conceptual space for sexual acts that fail to produce sexual pleasure (Soble, "Fundamentals," xxxvii–xl; *Philosophy of Sex and Love*, xvii–xlii; *Sexual Investigations*, 127–31). If producing sexual pleasure is partially definitive of "sexual activity," as a necessary feature, then the absence of sexual pleasure *entails* that the act is not sexual. Consider a couple who have lost sexual interest in each other and who engage in routine foreplay and coitus from which they obtain no pleasure. Or consider a Catholic couple that succeeds in fulfilling **Augustine**'s (354–430) wish that in performing the (ideal) marital conjugal act they fulfill its procreative purpose without experiencing sexual pleasure (*On Marriage and Concupiscence*, bk. 1, chap. 9, 170). According to (A4), because these couples experience no pleasure, the coitus they engage in is not a sexual act (nor is it "having sex"). If so, (A4) rules out the *possibility* of "bad sex," for whenever the sexual event is "bad" (not pleasurable), the analysis judges the sexual event not to *be* a sexual act. Hence the category "unpleasurable (i.e., nonmorally bad) sex" is *empty*: "That's a relief. All this bad sex I've been putting up with all my life" [you are hearing the voice of Rodney Dangerfield (1921–2004)] "*wasn't really sex at all*. So I've never *had* any bad sex." Note that the objection to (A4) is not exactly that these couples *are* engaged in a sexual act, one in which they experience no pleasure, and these couples are counterexamples to the analysis. The objection is that (A4) entails that "bad sex" is a contradiction. That implication is counterintuitive, no matter what we say about the activity of the two couples. Both variants of (A4) are vulnerable to this argument: Rosen and Christman's analysis entails that there could not *be* any such thing as "bad sex" in the sense of sexual activity that produced neither pleasure nor a "tension and conflict" feeling, and the other variant entails that there could not *be* any such thing as "bad sex" in the sense of sexual activity that was not sexually arousing. At best, these analyses state a sufficient condition for an act to be sexual but not a necessary condition.

It would, however, also make sense to object to the analysis by claiming that the acts of these couples *are* counterexamples: Coitus is a sexual activity, if anything is, even if the parties are not enjoying it. Or think about another couple: The woman puts up with twenty minutes or so of vaginal intercourse with her husband and derives no pleasure from it.

(He uses a lubricating jelly to make insertion easier and thrusting less painful for her.) Most people, as opposed to a philosopher trying desperately to save his or her cherished position, would say that all six people, even the woman in the last example, engaged in sexual activity. Most people would admit, if honest, that they had, at one time or another, taken part in sexual activity that they did not find arousing or pleasurable. They went through the motions because they were being kind to their partner, or because after a date they feared their partners who refused to leave, or because they were trying to conceive yet also hoped the act would be finished as quickly as possible. Or because they ("erotophobes") utterly dislike sexual activity, with its noxious odors, repulsive fluids, and loss of control, and so do not, by their natures, enjoy it, yet for various reasons must force themselves to engage in bouts of unpleasurable sexual activity. These people have, as frequently and consistently as Dangerfield, "bad sex" for their entire lives, but for a different reason and, unlike Dangerfield, they prefer it that way. (If they do not prefer it that way but wish they could overcome their erotophobia, they have what the American Psychiatric Association diagnoses as "Sexual Aversion Disorder." See DSM-IV, §302.79.) One might say about all these cases that they do not provide counterexamples to (A4), because that these acts are not sexual is not farfetched, exactly because they are zingless and torpid (see Primoratz, 47–49). But that move to defend (A4) only reasserts that if pleasure is absent, the act is not sexual and hence that the set "bad sex" has no members and the phrase is a contradiction.

The weakness of all three versions is that they underestimate the number of sexual acts that occur. This undercounting has dangerous consequences. Suppose I am a social scientist studying patterns of sexual behavior, with the aim of using demographic statistics to understand the incidence of **sexually transmitted diseases**. I want an accurate accounting of how often and with whom people engage in sexual activity. So when I ask you, "How many sexual partners have you had during the last year?" I am not asking with how many people you had a pleasurable, arousing, or satisfactory sexual experience. I do not want you to ignore sexual acts that were disappointing and those partners with whom you had "bad sex." These acts can be just as unsafe as pleasurable experiences. But if you use (A4) in counting your partners, you will be silent about bad experiences. As a result, I might conclude from my survey that all is well in Bogalusa.

What about (A5): trying or intending to produce sexual pleasure (instead of producing it)? On such an analysis, the absence of sexual pleasure does not entail that the act is not sexual, so "bad sex" is logically possible. It is not clear, however, that trying or intending to produce sexual pleasure is sufficient for an act to be sexual. Some ways of trying to produce pleasure might make the act sexual, while other ways of trying might not. Trying to produce sexual pleasure for your partner by rubbing his or her genitals, even if it fails, looks like a sexual act, but trying to produce sexual pleasure by whistling "Dixie" not only will fail but also does not look like a sexual act. (It might be one if your partner has a kinky thing for "Dixie.") Perhaps the particular manner of trying to produce sexual pleasure is a sexual act only if that manner of trying is already a sexual act (say, rubbing the genitals), that is, would be a sexual act if it was not being used to *try* to produce pleasure but *to produce* pleasure. If so, we can know what trying to produce sexual pleasure is only if we know (how?) what acts are sexual. Second, it is also not clear that trying or intending is a necessary condition. One of the couples discussed above is relevant here: The married Catholic pair intending only that she be impregnated, trying only to fertilize her egg, and not concerned with the sexual pleasure of the act, having more important things in mind that they wish to attend to, is still performing a sexual act.

Finally, consider Goldman's proposal that (A6) sexual activity is activity that "tends to fulfill" the desire for the pleasure of physical contact (268). This analysis is more complex than it seems to be at first glance. It has the spirit and content of several previous analyses: As in (A3), sexual activity logically depends on physical contact; as in (A4), sexual activity logically depends on sexual pleasure; as in (A5), sexual activity need not produce pleasure but only "tend to." The new feature is that "sexual activity" logically depends on "sexual desire." Perhaps because (A6) shares certain definitional features with (A3), (A4), and (A5), it also shares their defects. For example, because sexual activity is linked to physical contact, telephone/Internet chatting might not count as sexual activity. But that might turn on whether acts that do not involve physical contact can still "tend to fulfill" the desire for contact, or whether the pleasure of contact can be produced in ways that do not involve contact. Regardless, the distinctive component of Goldman's analysis, that sexual activity is defined in terms of sexual desire, is problematic. If sexual activities are acts that satisfy desire, then if there is no desire, there is no sexual activity. Counterexamples are not hard to imagine. A prostitute usually has no sexual desire for her client. In performing fellatio on him or permitting him coitus, she is not doing something that contributes to satisfying sexual desire, for she has none. She, too, goes through the motions. Yet the fellatio and coitus that she participates in look like sexual acts. That the acts she performs are motivated by a concern for money instead of sexual desire is irrelevant. Perhaps (A6) can be improved—defenders of some of the other analyses may also want to elaborate this suggestion—by focusing not on act-tokens but act-types. That is, "tends to fulfill" can be taken to be about a class of acts, not a single act. Thus it might be possible to argue that the prostitution case is not a counterexample because "tends to fulfill" means that the acts in question, fellatio and coitus (as act-types), usually, in general, or by their nature, do lead to the satisfaction of sexual desire for the performer, even if in particular act-tokens they do not.

Analysis or definition in terms of necessary and sufficient conditions is not always successful. Sometimes none of the proposed conditions can do the job expected of them. This philosophical failure may be only temporary, as when the fault resides in the scientist, not Nature. In any event, analysis is not futile. Much can be learned from the process, even if it does not yield Truth. Working out why things are wrong is as enlightening as working out why things are right.

See also Abstinence; Adultery; Communication Model; Completeness, Sexual; Cybersex; Desire, Sexual; Firestone, Shulamith; Hobbes, Thomas; Homosexuality and Science; Indian Erotology; Judaism, History of; Language; Liberalism; Masturbation; Perversion, Sexual; Philosophy of Sex, Overview of; Prostitution; Rape; Sex Education; Sex Work; Sexuality, Dimensions of; Social Constructionism; Thomas Aquinas (Saint)

REFERENCES

American Psychiatric Association. *Diagnostic and Statistical Manual of Mental Disorders*, 4th ed. Washington, D.C.: Author, 1994; Atkinson, Ti-Grace. (1968) "The Institution of Sexual Intercourse." In *Amazon Odyssey*. New York: Links Books, 1974, 13–23; Augustine. (418?–421) *On Marriage and Concupiscence*. In Marcus Dods, ed., *The Works of Aurelius Augustine, Bishop of Hippo*, vol. 12. Trans. Peter Holmes. Edinburgh, Scot.: T. and T. Clark, 1874, 93–202; Ben-Ze'ev, Aaron. *Love Online: Emotions on the Internet*. Cambridge: Cambridge University Press, 2004; Blackburn, Simon. *Lust: The Seven Deadly Sins*. New York: Oxford University Press/New York Public Library, 2004; Chamfort, Sébastien-Roch-Nicolas. *Products of the Perfected Civilization: Selected Writings of Chamfort*. Trans. by W. S. Merwin. San Francisco, Calif.: North Point Press, 1984; Christina, Greta. (1992) "Are We Having Sex Now or What?" In Alan Soble, ed., *The Philosophy of Sex: Contemporary Readings*, 4th ed. Lanham, Md.: Rowman and Littlefield, 2002, 3–8; Collins, Louise. "Emotional

Adultery: Cybersex and Commitment." *Social Theory and Practice* 25:2 (1999), 243–70; Frye, Marilyn. (1990) "Lesbian 'Sex.'" In *Willful Virgin: Essays in Feminism 1976–1992*. Freedom, Calif.: Crossing Press, 1992, 109–19; Goldman, Alan. "Plain Sex." *Philosophy and Public Affairs* 6:3 (1977), 267–87; Gray, Robert. "Sex and Sexual Perversion." *Journal of Philosophy* 75:4 (1978), 189–99; Gudorf, Christine E. *Body, Sex, and Pleasure: Reconstructing Christian Sexual Ethics*. Cleveland, Ohio: Pilgrim Press, 1994; Laumann, Edward O., John H. Gagnon, Robert T. Michael, and Stuart Michaels. *The Social Organization of Sexuality: Sexual Practices in the United States*. Chicago, Ill.: University of Chicago Press, 1994; MacKinnon, Catharine A. *Only Words*. Cambridge, Mass.: Harvard University Press, 1993; MacKinnon, Catharine A. *Toward a Feminist Theory of the State*. Cambridge, Mass.: Harvard University Press, 1989; Nagel, Thomas. "Sexual Perversion." *Journal of Philosophy* 66:1 (1969), 5–17; Portmann, John. "Chatting Is Not Cheating." In John Portmann, ed., *In Defense of Sin*. New York: Palgrave, 2002, 223–41; Primoratz, Igor. *Ethics and Sex*. London: Routledge, 1999; Randall, Hilary E., and E. Sandra Byers. "What Is Sex? Students' Definitions of Having Sex, Sexual Partner, and Unfaithful Sexual Behaviour." *Canadian Journal of Human Sexuality* 12:2 (2003), 87–96; Remez, Lisa. "Oral Sex among Adolescents: Is It Sex or Is It Abstinence?" *Family Planning Perspectives* 32:6 (2000), 298–304; Rich, Adrienne. "Compulsory Heterosexuality and Lesbian Existence." *Signs* 5:4 (1980), 631–60; Richters, J., and A. Song. "Australian University Students Agree with Clinton's Definition of Sex." *British Medical Journal* 318 (1999), 1011–12; Rosen, Deborah, and John Christman. "Toward a New Model of Sexuality." In Alan Soble, ed., *Sex, Love, and Friendship*. Amsterdam, Holland: Rodopi, 1997, 199–213; Roth, Philip. *Sabbath's Theater*. New York: Vintage, 1996; Sanders, Stephanie, and June Reinisch. "Would You Say You 'Had Sex' If . . . ?" *Journal of the American Medical Association* 281:3 (20 January 1999), 275–77; Soble, Alan. "Analysis." In *Sexual Investigations*. New York: New York University Press, 1996, 111–42; Soble, Alan. "The Fundamentals of the Philosophy of Sex." In Alan Soble, ed., *The Philosophy of Sex: Contemporary Readings*, 4th ed. Lanham, Md.: Rowman and Littlefield, 2002, xvii–xlii; Soble, Alan. *The Philosophy of Sex and Love: An Introduction*. St. Paul, Minn.: Paragon House, 1998; Toobin, Jeffrey. *A Vast Conspiracy: The Real Story of the Sex Scandal That Nearly Brought Down a President*. New York: Simon and Schuster, 2000.

Alan Soble

ADDITIONAL READING

Berk, Richard, Paul R. Abramson, and Paul Okami. "Sexual Activities as Told in Surveys." In Paul R. Abramson and Steven D. Pinkerton, eds., *Sexual Nature Sexual Culture*. Chicago, Ill.: University of Chicago Press, 1995, 371–86; Carpenter, Laura M. "The Ambiguity of 'Having Sex': The Subjective Experience of Virginity Loss in the United States." *Journal of Sex Research* 38:2 (2001), 127–39; Carroll, Mary Ann. "Sexual and Other Activities and the Ideal Life." In Alan Soble, ed., *Sex, Love, and Friendship*. Amsterdam, Holland: Rodopi, 1997, 215–21; Christina, Greta. "Are We Having Sex Now or What?" In David Steinberg, ed., *The Erotic Impulse: Honoring the Sensual Self*. New York: Tarcher, 1992, 24–29. Reprinted in POS3 (3–8); POS4 (3–8). Reprinted, abridged, in *Ms.* (November–December 1995), 60–62; Frye, Marilyn. "Lesbian 'Sex.'" In Jeffner Allen, ed., *Lesbian Philosophies and Cultures*. Albany: State University of New York Press, 1990, 305–15. Reprinted in *Willful Virgin: Essays in Feminism 1976–1992*. Freedom, Calif.: Crossing Press, 1992, 109–19; and Anne Minas, ed., *Gender Basics: Feminist Perspectives on Women and Men*, 1st ed. Belmont, Calif.: Wadsworth, 1993, 328–33; Furbank, P. N. "A Double Life." [Review of *Chamfort*, by Claude Arnaud] *New York Review of Books* (25 June 1992). <www.nybooks.com/articles/2864> [accessed 15 February 2005]; Goldman, Alan. "Plain Sex." *Philosophy and Public Affairs* 6:3 (1977), 267–87. Reprinted in HS (103–23); POS1 (119–38); POS2 (73–92); POS3 (39–55); POS4 (39–55); Gray, Robert. "Sex and Sexual Perversion." *Journal of Philosophy* 75:4 (1978), 189–99. Reprinted in POS1 (158–68); POS3 (57–66); POS4 (57–66); Hamilton, Christopher. "Sex." In *Living Philosophy: Reflections on Life, Meaning and Morality*. Edinburgh, Scot.: Edinburgh University Press, 2001, 125–41; Kaplan, Leonard V., and Beverly I. Moran, eds. *Aftermath: The Clinton Impeachment and the Presidency in the Age of Political Spectacle*. New York: New York University Press, 2001; Michael, Robert T., John H. Gagnon, Edward O. Laumann, and Gina Kolata. *Sex in America: A Definitive Survey*. Boston, Mass.: Little, Brown, 1994; Moore, Gareth. "Sexual Needs and Sexual Pleasures." *International Philosophical Quarterly* 35:2 (1995), 193–204; Nagel, Thomas. "Sexual Perversion." *Journal of Philosophy* 66:1 (1969), 5–17. Reprinted in P&S1 (247–60); P&S2 (268–79); POS1 (76–88). Reprinted, revised, in Thomas Nagel, *Mortal Questions*. Cambridge: Cambridge University Press, 1979, 39–52; in Eugene F. Rogers, Jr., ed., *Theology and Sexuality: Classic and Contemporary Readings*. Oxford, U.K.: Blackwell, 2002, 125–36; and P&S3 (326–36); POS2 (39–51); POS3 (9–20); POS4 (9–20); Pollitt, Katha. "Not Just Bad Sex." *The New Yorker* (4 October 1993), 220–24. Reprinted in *Reasonable Creatures: Essays on Women and Feminism*. New York: Knopf, 1994, 157–68; and Adele M. Stan, ed., *Debating Sexual Correctness: Pornography, Sexual Harassment, Date Rape, and the Politics of Sexual Equality*. New York: Delta, 1995, 161–71; Poovey, Mary. "Sex in America." *Critical Inquiry* 24:2 (1998), 366–92; Radakovich, Anka. "Survey Says: Keeping Score." In *Sexplorations: Journey to the Erogenous Frontier*. New York: Crown, 1997, 185–93; Rich, Adrienne. "Compulsory Heterosexuality and Lesbian Existence." *Signs* 5:4 (1980), 631–60. Reprinted in *Blood, Bread, and Poetry: Selected Prose 1979–1985*. New York: Norton, 1986, 23–75; and Henry Abelove, Michèle Aina Barale, and David M. Halperin, eds., *The Lesbian and Gay Studies Reader*. New York: Routledge, 1993, 227–54; Richardson, Diana. (1993) "Constructing Lesbian Sexualities." In Stevi Jackson and Sue Scott, eds., *Feminism and Sexuality: A Reader*. New York: Columbia University Press, 1996, 267–86; Ross, Stephen David. "The Limits of Sexuality." *Philosophy and Social Criticism* 9:3–4 (1984), 321–36. Reprinted in POS2 (259–75); Soble, Alan. "Sexual Activity." In Alan Soble, ed., *Sex, Love, and Friendship*. Amsterdam, Holland: Rodopi, 1997, 223–27.

ADDICTION, SEXUAL. Sexual addiction is defined as an addiction characterized by a pattern of "out-of-control" **sexual activity**. It is not necessarily defined in terms of the frequency or kind of sexual behavior. Rather, a person's inability to manage his or her life (or "function normally") as a result of sexual behavior is the mark of sexual addiction. The idea that people could be addicted to sexual activity arose in the late 1970s and early 1980s: "[A]ddiction appeared to be everywhere: not only alcohol and drugs, but too much gambling, shopping, working, eating, or having sex" (Groneman, 175). Professional interest in sexual addiction began in 1983 with the publication of psychologist Patrick Carnes's *The Sexual Addiction*. But the claim that the pathological state "sexual addiction" exists has been challenged.

Most people have no problem judging out-of-control alcohol consumption, for example, as both an addiction and unhealthy. Many, however, resist judging out-of-control sexual activity an addiction: The so-called sex addict merely engages in excessive (or gluttonous) sexual activity and, by virtue of bad judgment, ends up having regrettable sex. Further, women who engage in a great deal of sex have often been labeled "nymphos," which is an older version of so-called female sex addiction, but this terminology has often only been a way to disparage female sexuality. (In the past, the charge of nymphomania was often invoked against a female **rape** victim whose "mental illness" led her to fantasize that she had been sexually assaulted; Groneman, 96.)

In Carnes's view, sex addicts are not merely people who are guilt-ridden over their sexual behavior. Nor are they people who engage in scattered episodes of compulsive sexuality (e.g., people going through a "midlife crisis" or are recently divorced). Carnes provides ten "signs" or diagnostic criteria indicating the presence of sexual addiction that distinguish it from other types of regrettable or excessive sexual activity (*Don't Call It Love*,

11–12). Perhaps most crucially, in sexual addiction the life of a person is dominated by sex and, as a result, the rest of his or her life is inadequately governed, organized, and administered. (That is also true for alcohol and narcotics addiction.) The sexual behaviors performed by sex addicts include **masturbation**, engaging in anonymous **casual sex**, viewing **pornography**, going to strip clubs, as well as the illegal activities of visiting prostitutes, engaging in exhibitionism or voyeurism, making indecent phone calls, child molesting, and rape (*Out of the Shadows*, 38 ff.). As a result of these activities, the person suffers severe consequences: being violently injured or raped due to putting oneself routinely in risky or self-destructive situations; experiencing unwanted pregnancies and **abortion**s; contracting **sexually transmitted diseases**, including AIDS (acquired immunodeficiency syndrome); being demoted or losing one's job altogether; being arrested and perhaps either fined or imprisoned for breaking the law; and undergoing financial misfortunes that accompany these consequences or come from squandering one's income on sex. (Again, other addictions come to mind.)

Another sign of sexual addiction is that even though a person suffers these adverse effects, the consequences do not deter the sexual behavior. Most people, should they suffer these kinds of harmful consequences as a result of poor judgment or carelessness with respect to sexual activity, would at least try to avoid engaging again in these behaviors. The sex addict, however, continues to pursue these behaviors (like the narcotics addict), spending inordinate amounts of time seeking or recovering from sexual activity. Further, the sex addict chases sex with an increasing frequency or intensity, because the current level of activity soon fails to satisfy (as in building up tolerance to drugs and alcohol). The addict, obsessed with sex, neglects responsibilities. Relationships with family and friends suffer or are destroyed. By contrast, those who are sexually compulsive only occasionally, are "hypersexual," or engage in sexual activity to some "excess" do not allow sex to become unmanageable and no longer under their control.

Much discussion has focused on one type of sex addiction: **cybersex** addiction. People are using the Internet for sexual satisfaction. In itself, this is not a problem. But the Internet, which makes sexual experiences easily available, permits or encourages potentially self-destructive sexual behavior. One can become as addicted to cybersex as to "real" sexual experiences and suffer similar harmful consequences. Cybersex activities include viewing pornographic images, reading and writing sexually explicit e-mails, sending e-mails or "instant messages" to set up personal sexual encounters, placing advertisements to meet partners, visiting sexually oriented chat rooms, and engaging in online masturbation with another person, perhaps while viewing each other with electronic cameras (Schneider, 36). The appeal of cybersex is its anonymity and convenience and the **fantasy** it provides. It is far less shameful to download pornography from a Web site in the privacy of one's home than to venture into an adult bookstore or strip club. The anonymity of the Internet makes it particularly appealing to women but also dangerous to them. Women cybersex users might ignore normal inhibitions that keep them safe (Carnes, *Out of the Shadows*, 83). Online contacts or relationships can escalate to real-life encounters; meeting men they really do not know is physically and emotionally risky.

If sexual addiction shares so many features with other addictions, why is there reluctance to accept the notion? Carnes answers the question by pointing to the sexism, sexual stereotypes, and expectations about gender and sexual behavior that exist in our society (*Don't Call It Love*, 29). For example, the commonplace, stereotypical expression "boys will be boys" obscures sexual addiction by portraying it as only the normal, even natural, course of events. A male sex addict might very well be praised and admired for his sexual pursuits and conquests; he fulfills the social expectation that, as a "real" man, he will be sexually successful. Our culture also says (falsely; see Ferree) that women cannot be sex addicts, since women, according to a sexist stereotype, are the guardians of morality and are not prone to excessive sexual behavior. Women who do engage in such behavior are "nymphos" or the "happy accidents" eager to satisfy the male's insatiable sexual appetite. The implication seems to be (but this might be disingenuous) that acknowledging sexual addiction as a genuine problem and pathology that afflicts both men and women is fully consistent with feminist philosophical and political concerns about sexist social expectations and stereotypes.

Sexual addiction, according to Carnes and his colleagues, is a pathological condition for which one popular treatment is that used for other addictions: following the Twelve Steps of Alcoholics Anonymous. How has psychiatry addressed the issue? When the American Psychiatric Association's *Diagnostic and Statistical Manual of Mental Disorders* (DSM) was first published (1952), "nymphomania" was classified as "sexual deviation" along with other deviant sexual behavior, including **homosexuality** (7, 38–39, 98, 121; see Groneman, 142–44). In a later edition (1980), nymphomania in women and "Don Juanism" in men were classified as "psychosexual disorders" and characterized by "distress about a pattern of repeated sexual conquests with a succession of individuals who exist only as things to be used" (DSM-III, 283). The revision of the third edition (DSM-III-R, 1987) eliminated "nymphomania" and "Don Juanism," preferring to employ the term "sexual addiction" (296). This inclusion was short-lived, for the fourth edition of DSM (1994) no longer used the expression, because "the concept of sexual addiction is troublesome in that the term *addiction* has a specific meaning associated with physiological processes of withdrawal" and "there is no scientific database to support the concept of excessive sexual behavior as being in the realm of an addiction" (Wise and Schmidt, 1140). Some psychologists claim that according to DSM-IV's definitions and descriptions of a wide variety of mental disorders, patients with sexual addiction can be included within numerous other diagnostic categories (Irons and Schneider).

Since it has eschewed "sexual addiction," how does DSM-IV categorize excessive sexual activity? It is noteworthy that while DSM-IV includes the **sexual dysfunction** "hypoactive sexual desire" (496), there is no category "hyperactive" sexual desire. However, in its catch-all category "Sexual Disorder Not Otherwise Specified," DSM-IV includes a variation of what is found in DSM-III: "Distress about a pattern of repeated sexual relationships involving a succession of lovers who are experienced by the individual only as things to be used" (538). This diagnostic category is rich with allusions (e.g., to the moral philosophy of **Immanuel Kant** [1724–1804]). But the sentence that expresses this diagnosis is awkward. What *is* clear is that this mental disorder, by definition, must be accompanied by psychic distress: no distress, no illness. What the person's distress is *about*, however, is ambiguous. Does a person have a sexual mental disorder if he or she is distressed simply at having a succession of sexual experiences? Then I exhibit mental pathology if I am distressed by my promiscuity, but not if it does not bother me. Or is the disorder constituted by the fact that while being promiscuous I am distressed over the fact that I experience people as "things to be used"? In that case, *removing* my distress at experiencing other people as things is *therapeutic*. This odd implication runs counter to a Kantian moral psychology according to which I *should*, if I am mentally healthy, be bothered by the fact that I experience as mere things the people with whom I have casual sex. Note, too, an intriguing difference between DSM-III and DSM-IV: In DSM-III, the sexual partners of the disordered person "exist" as things to be used, while in DSM-IV they are "experienced" as things to be used. (The wording in the next revision [2000] of DSM remained the same; see DSM-IV-TR, 582.) In a judicious observation, the American Psychiatric Association states, "The whole issue of excessive sexual behavior is worthy of scientific study" (Wise and Schmidt, 1140).

In addition to the rejection of "sex addiction" by the American Psychiatric Association, other scholars have raised doubts about the notion. According to a sociologist and historian of sexology, Janice Irvine, "The rise of sex addiction . . . is best understood in the context of very powerful social influences and the rise of the culture and language of addiction, cultural tensions concerning sexuality, and competing sexual ideologies within feminism, where any troublesome behavior is susceptible to the label of addiction" (441). Further, "sexual addiction" also reflects backlash against the sexual permissiveness of the 1960s and 1970s. Far from being consistent with **feminism**, the notion of sexual addiction was built on conservative "family values," according to which sexual behavior is "healthy" and "normal" only when it takes place within a committed, monogamous, heterosexual relationship. (Note that domestic sexuality may itself involve addiction. Germaine Greer thinks that some women can successfully "bind" their husbands in marriage if the men are "addicted" to a certain type of sexuality that the wives are willing to supply [152]. Men, too, can make their wives dependent on them and reluctant to leave by providing sexual pleasure; see Rubin, 91.)

Sexual addiction, from this sociological perspective, may be seen as a cultural invention, another example of the medicalization of deviance (see Conrad and Schneider). A sexual behavior that was once seen as "sinful" (say, within older Christian theologies of sex) became identified, instead, as a disease or "sickness" (within newer medical discourses of sexuality) and thereby fell within the dominion of the medical establishment. But medicalization of deviance is a two-edged sword. On the one hand, as Irvine suggests, those who engaged in the "sin" of uncontrollable sex themselves had a stake in reclassifying such behavior as "disease," insofar as disease language not only serves to protect the deviant from profoundly negative social judgments but also encourages the tolerance and sympathy usually afforded those with illnesses. On the other hand, being labeled "mentally ill" as a result of desiring or engaging in deviant sexual behavior—the fate of gays and lesbians until 1973–1974, when the American Psychiatric Association eliminated homosexuality *per se* as a diagnostic category from the DSM (Conrad and Schneider, 208–9)—does not usually confirm a person's self-esteem or self-respect.

See also Adultery; Casual Sex; Cybersex; Dysfunction, Sexual; Ethics, Virtue; Foucault, Michel; Paraphilia; Perversion, Sexual; Psychology, Twentieth- and Twenty-First-Century; Sexology; Sherfey, Mary Jane; Social Constructionism

REFERENCES

American Psychiatric Association. *Diagnostic and Statistical Manual of Mental Disorders*, 1st ed. [DSM-I] Washington, D.C.: Author, 1952; American Psychiatric Association. *Diagnostic and Statistical Manual of Mental Disorders*, 3rd ed. [DSM-III] Washington, D.C.: Author, 1980; American Psychiatric Association. *Diagnostic and Statistical Manual of Mental Disorders*, rev. 3rd ed. [DSM-III-R] Washington, D.C.: Author, 1987; American Psychiatric Association. *Diagnostic and Statistical Manual of Mental Disorders*, 4th ed. [DSM-IV] Washington, D.C.: Author, 1994; American Psychiatric Association. *Diagnostic and Statistical Manual of Mental Disorders*, text revision of the 4th ed. [DSM-IV-TR] Washington, D.C.: Author, 2000; Carnes, Patrick J. *Don't Call It Love: Recovery from Sexual Addiction*. New York: Bantam, 1992; Carnes, Patrick J. *Out of the Shadows: Understanding Sexual Addiction*, 3rd ed. Center City, Minn.: Hazelden, 2001; Carnes, Patrick J. *The Sexual Addiction.*

Minneapolis, Minn.: Compcare, 1983; Conrad, Peter, and Joseph W. Schneider. *Deviance and Medicalization: From Badness to Sickness*. St. Louis, Mo.: C. V. Mosby, 1980; Ferree, Marnie C. "Females: The Forgotten Sexual Addicts." In Patrick J. Carnes and Kenneth M. Adams, eds., *Clinical Management of Sex Addiction*. New York: Brunner-Routledge, 2002, 255–69; Greer, Germaine. *The Female Eunuch*. New York: Bantam, 1971; Groneman, Carol. *Nymphomania: A History*. New York: Norton, 2000; Irons, Richard, and Jennifer Schneider. "Differential Diagnosis of Addictive Sexual Disorders Using the DSM-IV." *Sexual Addiction and Compulsivity* 3:1 (1996), 7–21; Irvine, Janice M. "Reinventing Perversion: Sex Addiction and Cultural Anxieties." *Journal of the History of Sexuality* 5:3 (1995), 429–50; Rubin, Lillian B. *Intimate Strangers: Men and Women Together*. New York: Harper and Row, 1983; Schneider, Jennifer. "Effects of Cybersex Addiction on the Family: Results of a Survey." In Al Cooper, ed., *Cybersex: The Dark Side of the Force*. New York: Brunner-Routledge, 2000, 31–58; Wise, Thomas N., and Chester W. Schmidt, Jr. "Paraphilias." In Thomas Widiger, Allen Frances, Harold Pincus, Ruth Ross, Michael First, and Wendy Davis, eds., *DSM-IV Sourcebook*, vol. 2. Washington, D.C.: American Psychiatric Association, 1996, 1133–47.

Carol V. Quinn

ADDITIONAL READING

American Psychiatric Association. *Diagnostic and Statistical Manual of Mental Disorders*, 2nd ed. [DSM-II] Washington, D.C.: Author, 1968; Bergner, Raymond M. "Money's 'Lovemap' Account of the Paraphilias: A Critique and Reformulation." *American Journal of Psychotherapy* 42:2 (1988), 254–59; Blackburn, Simon. "Excess." In *Lust: The Seven Deadly Sins*. New York: Oxford University Press/New York Public Library, 2004, 21–27; Carnes, Patrick J., and Kenneth M. Adams, eds. *Clinical Management of Sex Addiction*. New York: Brunner-Routledge, 2002; Coleman, Eli. "Sexual Compulsivity: Definition, Etiology, and Treatment Considerations." In Eli Coleman, ed., *Chemical Dependency and Intimacy Dysfunction*. New York: Haworth Press, 1988, 189–204; Coleman, Eli. "Treatment of Compulsive Sexual Behavior." In Raymond C. Rosen and Sandra R. Leiblum, eds., *Case Studies in Sex Therapy*. New York: Guilford, 1995, 333–39; Conrad, Peter, and Joseph W. Schneider. *Deviance and Medicalization: From Badness to Sickness*. St. Louis, Mo.: C. V. Mosby, 1980. Expanded ed., Philadelphia, Pa.: Temple University Press, 1992; Cooper, Al, ed. *Sex and the Internet: A Guide Book for Clinicians*. New York: Brunner-Routledge, 2002; Herman, Judith L. "Considering Sex Offenders: A Model of Addiction." *Signs* 13:4 (1988), 695–724; Irons, Richard, and Jennifer P. Schneider. "Differential Diagnosis of Addictive Sexual Disorders Using the DSM-IV." *Sexual Addiction and Compulsivity* 3:1 (1996), 7–21. <www.jenniferschneider.com/articles/diagnos.html> [accessed 28 October 2004]; Kasl, Charlotte. *Women, Sex, and Addiction: A Search for Love and Power*. New York: Harper and Row, 1989; Mele, Alfred R. "Volitional Disorder and Addiction." In Jennifer Radden, ed., *The Philosophy of Psychiatry: A Companion*. New York: Oxford University Press, 2004, 78–88; Morris, Betty. "Addicted to Sex." *Fortune* (10 May 1999), 68–80; Nathan, Sharon G. "Sexual Addiction: A Sex Therapist's Struggles with an Unfamiliar Clinical Entity." In Raymond C. Rosen and Sandra R. Leiblum, eds., *Case Studies in Sex Therapy*. New York: Guilford, 1995, 350–67; Norwood, Robin. *Women Who Love Too Much: When You Keep Wishing and Hoping He'll Change*. Los Angeles, Calif.: Jeremy P. Tarcher, 1985; Peele, Stanton. *Diseasing of America: Addiction Treatment Out of Control*. Lexington, Mass.: Lexington Books, 1989; Schmidt, Chester W., Jr., Raul C. Schiavi, Leslie R. Schover, R. Taylor Segraves, and Thomas N. Wise. "DSM-IV Sexual Disorders: Final Overview." In Thomas Widiger, Allen Frances, Harold Pincus, Ruth Ross, Michael First, Wendy Davis, and Myriam Kline, eds., *DSM-IV Sourcebook*, vol. 4. Washington, D.C.: American Psychiatric Association, 1998, 1087–95; Schmidt, Chester W., Jr., Raul C. Schiavi, Leslie R. Schover, R. Taylor Segraves, and Thomas N. Wise. "Introduction to Section VI: Sexual Disorders." In Thomas Widiger, Allen Frances, Harold Pincus, Ruth Ross, Michael First, and Wendy Davis, eds., *DSM-IV Sourcebook*, vol. 2. Washington, D.C.: American Psychiatric Association, 1996, 1081–89; Schneider, Jennifer, and Robert Weiss. *Cybersex Exposed: Simple Fantasy or Obsession?* Center City, Minn.: Hazelden, 2001; SexHelp. (Web site) "Sex Addiction Q & A." <www.sexhelp.com>

[accessed 3 September 2004]; Verghese, Abraham. "Annals of Addiction: The Pathology of Sex." *The New Yorker* (16 February 1998), 42–49; Weiss, Robert. "Treatment Concerns for Gay Male Sexual Addicts." In Patrick J. Carnes and Kenneth M. Adams, eds., *Clinical Management of Sex Addiction*. New York: Brunner-Routledge, 2002, 331–42.

ADULTERY. According to dictionaries, adultery occurs when a married person voluntarily engages in sexual intercourse with someone other than his or her spouse. Adultery is a topic of great moral interest in most societies and has been studied by many academic disciplines (see Lampe). The central issue is when and why adultery is immoral. Additional issues concern the wisdom of making commitments of sexual exclusivity, how to minimize harm to third parties, the responsibilities of single individuals contemplating or conducting affairs with married persons, and how to respond to the adultery of a spouse, friend, political leaders, religious leaders, or the military.

The dictionary definition of "adultery" is vague and, more interesting, sometimes contested. One vagueness pertains to sexual intercourse. Suppose that a married person engages in "brinkmanship" with an extramarital partner, enjoying myriad sexual activities over a period of weeks but always stopping short of full-blown intercourse. Many people would consider that adultery, prompting a widening of the dictionary definition. In contrast, what if the spouse and the extramarital partner engage in extensive Internet intimacies and fantasies accompanied by **masturbation (cybersex)**? Virtual (cyber) infidelity can be genuine infidelity, but adultery seems to require more by way of bodily conjugations (for discussion, see Ben-Ze'ev; Collins; Maheu and Subotnik; Portmann; Warburton). Again, when President Jimmy Carter confessed in a *Playboy* interview to having "looked on a lot of women with lust" (Scheer, in Richardson, 58), was his "mental adultery" real adultery, morally speaking, as the New Testament would have it?: "You have heard that it was said, 'Do not commit adultery.' But I tell you that anyone who looks at a woman lustfully has already committed adultery with her in his heart" (Matt. 5:27–28). Christian fundamentalists say yes: Lustful looking, or at least lusty desiring, is adultery. Most people, however, say no. **Sexual desire** is not adultery; indeed, it contributes to a healthy sex life, although moral issues arise when **fantasy** turns into intention to pursue an affair. This disagreement illustrates how moral perspectives shape definitions of adultery.

Another vagueness concerns **marriage**. Can we speak of adultery when individuals cheat on their partners within long-term committed relationships that are not (legally) marriages? A plausible answer is yes. Again, do unmarried persons commit adultery when they have an affair with a married person? Perhaps we should say no, although they do "participate in" adultery. There are also technical matters. Does adultery occur when there is an error in the legal paperwork for divorce, so that a new liaison constitutes sex with an extramarital partner? Does adultery occur when a person begins an affair mistakenly believing the spouse is dead (for example, was killed in war)? No doubt these cases are ruled out by the conceptual requirement that the intercourse in adultery must be voluntary, which also excludes **rape** (see Soble, 111–14). But "voluntary" is a slippery notion. In the tradition of Mata Hari (1876–1917), a German spy who allegedly had a sexual liaison with the French minister of war during World War I, the East German spy service, the Stasi, made sexual espionage part of the job of spies serving in brothels (see Wark). If these spies happened to be married, we might say they engaged in adultery for their country, but we might also deny they are paradigmatic adulterers.

Of greater interest, some individuals who attach extremely negative connotations to the word "adultery" define adultery more narrowly (Hunt, 9; Lawson, 39). Thus, a couple might agree that occasional one-night stands, and "mere sex" without emotional involvement, do not count as adultery. For them, adultery implies erotic **love** for another person or involvement in an extended extramarital affair. Or individuals might tell themselves that oral sex does not qualify as adultery. And, conceivably, Thomas Jefferson (1743–1826) might have believed that sexual relations with his slave was not actual adultery. Such conceptual gerrymandering is usually the product of bad faith and self-deception, as is much rationalization about the permissibility of adultery. Yet occasionally it represents good-faith efforts by couples to negotiate the requirements they place on each other to sustain their love or marriage while augmenting their sexual freedom.

Definitions can be useful without stating necessary and sufficient conditions, and greater precision can be added where necessary, as in laws concerning adultery (see Posner and Silbaugh, 103–10). We can employ the dictionary definition of "adultery" while appreciating that key moral issues also arise regarding other sexual infidelities, whether between spouses or between gay, lesbian, or heterosexual couples in committed relationships.

We can group the substantive moral issues into five broad categories. First, the most widely discussed issues are about keeping marital commitments to sexual exclusivity. Are the obligations created by these commitments absolute, in the sense of having no permissible exceptions? Fundamentalist interpretations of the Ten Commandments say the obligations are absolute: "Thou shalt not commit adultery" (Sixth Commandment) and "Thou shalt not covet thy neighbor's wife" (Tenth Commandment). Or are the obligations only *prima facie*, such that they might allow some exceptions when required by other important moral considerations? If so, how many are the permissible exceptions and how strong is the presumption against adultery? Whether the obligations are absolute or *prima facie*, how serious is the wrongdoing in committing adultery, and how much guilt is warranted? If adultery is sometimes permissible, can it also be a positive good in some situations?

Second, is it desirable to make commitments of sexual exclusivity in the first place? In particular, is it wise to make such commitments at a time when people are living far longer than was envisioned when traditional marriage vows were invented? Is it permissible, even prudent, for couples to have "open marriages" in which they give each other permission to have extramarital affairs, perhaps on the condition of telling each other about them? What about "serial monogamy," in which individuals have a series of shorter but monogamous relationships? What is, and what should be, the connection between marriage, love, self-fulfillment, happiness, and other important values in meaningful lives?

Third, when adultery occurs, how should extramarital affairs be pursued to minimize harm? Is deception permissible? At what point, if any, are adulterers obligated to tell their spouses about the affair, even at the risk of ending a good marriage? When and how should extramarital affairs be ended? Fourth, when adultery involves a single person having or planning an affair with a married person, what are the responsibilities of the unmarried person? Is the single person a contemptible home wrecker, or does the primary responsibility and fault belong to the married participant? Fifth, how should we evaluate other people who engage in adultery? If the adulterer is our spouse, should we be willing to forgive, when there is genuine remorse and when children are involved? What are the responsibilities of friends or family who learn about the affair? How should citizens respond to adulterous politicians, and how should members of religious groups react to adultery by their leaders? Is the military justified in banning adultery and punishing adulterers in its ranks?

All these issues have been explored within various ethical frameworks (see, for example, **Edward Westermarck** [1862–1939], 58–73; **Richard Posner** [1939–], 183–86; Primoratz, 78–85). In illustrating some general approaches, I emphasize the first two clusters of issues: keeping and making commitments of sexual exclusivity.

One approach is to apply a general ethical theory. Deontological theories, which emphasize duties and rights, highlight duties to keep promises (in particular wedding vows), to avoid deception, to avoid harming family members, and to meet responsibilities to support and care for one's spouse. Kantians argue that adulterers adopt inconsistent policies of sexual exclusivity and extramarital affairs that cannot be universalized (see Wreen). Utilitarians attend to the consequences of adultery. In some instances, the consequences might be good, enriching the lives of lovers and occasionally even strengthening marriages. Perhaps more often, the consequences are destructive **jealousy**, anger, and hatred, if not unwanted pregnancy and **sexually transmitted diseases**, that destroy otherwise good marriages. Virtue-oriented ethicists highlight desirable features of persons. In their view, adultery usually involves failures to be honest with one's spouse and with oneself and also failures of responsibility and self-control, fidelity and integrity, and caring for one's spouse (see Carr; Putman). In addition, the marital promise of sexual exclusivity might be viewed as a promise to be a certain kind of person, one who is sexually faithful, which involves additional virtues of honesty, loyalty, and self-control (Halwani, "Morality of Adultery," "Virtue Ethics and Adultery"). Note that these approaches seem not to condemn adultery merely because it is sexual, unlike part of **Thomas Aquinas**'s (1224/25–1274) Natural Law rationale for judging adultery sinful: It is the satisfying of sexual desire merely for the sake of sexual pleasure. Further, a man's adultery with another man's wife violates the rights of that man and is a kind of theft (*Summa theologiae*, IaIIae, ques. 73, art. 7).

A second approach skirts disagreements about ethical theories and focuses on lower-level principles. In particular, it relies on everyday moral rules, allowing that different ethical theories justify those rules in different ways. Richard Wasserstrom (1936–) adopts this approach in his classic 1973–1974 essay "Is Adultery Immoral?" He argues that adultery is wrong when it violates widely shared moral rules such as keep your promises, do not deceive, do not harm others, and be fair (which implies not being permitted the rewards of extramarital affairs that are denied to one's partner). These rules are *prima facie*, however, and there are legitimate exceptions to them. Wasserstrom also raises, but leaves unanswered, questions about the wisdom of making promises of sexual exclusivity and of linking sex and love.

A third approach deemphasizes rules and shifts the focus to particularities and context. Whether relying on intuitive judgments or emphasizing that adultery is too complex to be handled by general rules, this approach was favored by Christian ethicist Joseph Fletcher (1905–1991) in *Situation Ethics*: "Is adultery wrong? . . . One can only respond, 'I don't know. Maybe. Give me a case. Describe a real situation'" (142–43). This approach often illuminates adultery by drawing on literature, including plays, memoirs, and novels such as Nathaniel Hawthorne's (1804–1864) *The Scarlet Letter* (1850), Gustave Flaubert's (1821–1880) *Madame Bovary* (1857), Leo Tolstoy's (1828–1910) *Anna Karenina* (1877), Kate Chopin's (1851–1904) *The Awakening* (1899), and D. H. Lawrence's (1895–1930) *Lady Chatterley's Lover* (1928).

Some feminists also adopt a contextual approach and call for appreciating the great variability and vicissitudes of relationships and situations, while insisting that women's rights and well-being be taken into account equitably. Traditionally, women have been punished far more severely than men for committing adultery. Indeed, adultery by males has sometimes been taken for granted, or not even called adultery, but adultery by women has been punished by death. At the other extreme, "wife lending" was practiced for many reasons by the pre–Christian missionary Inuit (see "Do Eskimo Men"). Beyond calling for nonmaleficence and fairness for women, feminists do not agree about adultery. Some underscore the need to protect caring relationships, including marriage and family. Others emphasize the importance of sexually fulfilling relationships that sometimes draw women, as much as men, into extramarital relationships (see Heyn; LeMoncheck). Feminists, among others, also warn of adulterous husbands transmitting HIV (human immunodeficiency virus) to their unsuspecting wives.

A fourth approach, overlapping with care-oriented feminist analyses, shifts the focus to love. The primary marital commitment is "to love, honor, and cherish until death do us part." Accordingly, the central ideal, virtue, and responsibility is faithfulness or constancy in love, in which the requirement of sexual fidelity ("forsaking all others") is supportive. To be sure, the fidelity commitment remains enormously important for many couples. It helps establish a context of the trust, stability, and emotional intimacy that sustains love. It helps protect the love against sexual affairs and potential new loves that could destroy the relationship, as well against disruptive jealousies. And it establishes the powerful symbolism that having sex is quite literally "making love."

What, then, is erotic love? It does not have a simple essence but instead must be understood in light of the moral, religious, and personal values and ideals that couples bring to their relationships. Accordingly, this approach to adultery has many variations. It can be argued that erotic love is a wide array of sex-involving and virtue-structured ways to value a person as singularly important in one's life (Martin, "Adultery and Fidelity," *Love's Virtues*). The relevant virtues guiding and embedded in love typically include deep caring, respect, honesty, fairness, constancy (faithfulness of love), and sexual fidelity (sexual faithfulness). These virtues define relationships in myriad ways, reflecting broader cultural, religious, and personal ideals about relationships and meaningful life that couples embrace.

Some conceptions of love build in a rejection of adultery. That is true of many religious conceptions of love, but even in secular terms some philosophers insist that linking sex and love within sexually exclusive relationships is part of "true love," at least within mainstream Western traditions (see Steinbock). Other philosophers emphasize the great variety of personal ideals and understandings about love, even within marriages (see Barnhart and Barnhart; Higgins on Cicovacki). Affirming the diversity of legitimate ideals, each advancing particular goods, these philosophers might then explore the special goods made possible within sexually exclusive relationships.

Affirming a pluralism of ideals in defining love greatly complicates the ethics of adultery. On the one hand, it affirms the moral autonomy of couples to develop shared understandings about the importance of sexual fidelity in their marriages and loving commitments. It allows that open marriages might contribute to the self-fulfillment of some couples, while appreciating the importance to other couples of foreswearing adultery and even making its absence a condition for the continuance of the relationship. Even so, affirming a plurality of permissible ideals is only a first step in understanding the moral complexities of adultery.

Suppose that couples begin with a shared commitment to sexual exclusivity. Later, they rethink that ideal, perhaps because one partner becomes impotent or sexually uninterested (and therapy fails to help), or perhaps because both desire sexual variety. Respect for their autonomy may permit this revision in light of their shared history and decision making. But suppose only one person goes through a fundamental change of attitude, a change that causes terrible pain to the other spouse. Or suppose one partner falls out of love with the partner, after making a good-faith effort to keep the marriage viable. Or suppose one partner falls deeply in love with another person, contrary to serious attempts not to let that happen. These are hard cases, to which moral philosophy provides no easy answers. Moreover, humility forces us to recognize an important role for luck, in addition to responsible effort, in sustaining initial commitments.

Moral pluralism can recognize a very strong presumption against adultery within relationships based on commitments of sexual exclusivity, while acknowledging limited exceptions in special circumstances. A markedly different emphasis challenges sexual fidelity as even a supportive virtue. Such challenges have come from many quarters, including social critics who renounce marriage as a social institution and sociobiologists who regard promiscuity as natural, a product of human evolution, for both men and women (see Barash and Lipton).

Perhaps the most disarming challenge to conventional views, grounded in the name of love itself, is presented by Richard Taylor (1919–2003) in *Love Affairs*. Taylor celebrates the joys of loving and passionate extramarital affairs: "[T]he joys of illicit and passionate love are overwhelmingly exciting and good" (16). At the same time, he affirms that good marriages are more fulfilling than extramarital affairs and acknowledges that affairs tend to destroy marriages. The task he sets himself is to affirm extramarital love while finding ways to minimize the damage it causes and thereby strengthen marriages. He bases his argument primarily on promoting human happiness. To this end, he develops an elaborate set of rules for pursuing adulterous affairs. Some of the rules apply to the adulterer—for example, to be discrete and to be honest with one's lover. Other rules apply to the spouse; for example, do not spy on or try to entrap one's spouse and try to avoid jealousy. Taylor's approach is useful for open marriages and other relationships based on nontraditional ideals of love. Yet much of his book is directed at marriages in which traditional vows are made, thereby inviting the charge that his perspective on adultery is morally inconsistent, if not subversive. He also reinforces stereotypes of men as naturally promiscuous and women as naturally monogamous, a view that feminists rightly renounce.

Finally, a fifth approach frames the issues in terms of mental health and related notions, such as healthy relationships and psychological maturity. Especially in the United States, the general public's understanding of moral issues is dominated by the therapeutic trend in ethics, that is, the tendency to approach moral issues in terms of mental health. Whether going to professional therapists, reading self-help literature, participating in self-help and mutual aid groups, or watching talk shows, the public apparently heeds psychology and therapy more than philosophy and theology. We might expect therapists to adopt a nonjudgmental stance, either avoiding moral judgments about adultery or conveying a largely tolerant attitude. In fact, therapists often make strong moral pronouncements, albeit in varied directions.

Havelock Ellis (1859–1939) is typical of 1960s thinking that tolerated and even celebrated adultery as a healthy expression of natural desires for sexual variety and freedom (see his posthumous *Sex and Marriage*). Today, however, many therapists oppose adultery when it involves dishonesty and threatens harm to families, as it usually does (see Pittman). A few therapists go further, condemning adultery as "almost always a sign of a conflicted marriage" and narcissistic regression (Strean, xi). In any case, mental health approaches presuppose concealed moral values that need to be made explicit to shed light on adultery (Edwards, 17).

Let us now note some issues concerning third-party responses to adultery. Retaliatory adultery might be pursued with a sense of fair play but might also do further damage to a marriage. Is there any obligation to forgive a wayward spouse who is sincerely contrite? There might be a tug in that direction, especially where relationships remain viable, where marriage is valued for religious or other reasons, or where children are involved (see DeSalvo). Without forgiveness, many relationships cannot improve, but forgiveness itself is morally complex. Although it remains largely the prerogative of individuals who have been wronged, there are obligations in some situations to forgive and in others not to forgive (see Haber).

Controversies about adultery have entered prominently into politics. Does adultery have any relevance to unfitness for public office, beyond crass mudslinging during political campaigns? Psychological and moral studies reveal that character is not all of a piece, suggesting that character flaws in personal life might be irrelevant to leadership in public life (see Doris). Further, a public that made adultery a major issue would deprive itself of leaders such as Thomas Jefferson, Franklin D. Roosevelt (1882–1945), and John F. Kennedy (1917–1963). Most political controversy is not about adultery *per se* but instead about dishonesty and hypocrisy, especially when politicians directly lie to the public. When President William Jefferson Clinton (on January 26, 1998) looked into the camera and denied the allegations about Monica Lewinsky, and when the 1988 front-running democratic candidate Gary Hart lied about his affair with Donna Rice and dared the press to prove otherwise (which it did), questions were raised about their integrity. Certainly, many citizens viewed the recklessness involved in the adulteries of Clinton and Hart as relevant to assessing their character. Perhaps the only feasible thing for politicians to do, at least until the public gains greater clarity about how personal and public life are related, is to refuse to comment on matters of personal privacy.

The gap between private and public life is even less clear regarding adulterous religious leaders. If they are leaders within traditions that strongly forbid adultery, dishonesty about adultery undermines their leadership. Keeping it concealed can make one vulnerable in other ways, even if we set aside the flagrant abuses by the Federal Bureau of Investigation in the surveillance of the adulteries of Martin Luther King, Jr. (1929–1968). The problem of hypocrisy is pronounced when adulterous conservative politicians (such as Newt Gingrich; see Speers) and religious leaders self-righteously defend parochial conceptions of "family values."

Consider, next, the military, which only recently achieved gender integration in the United States. There was a public outcry when Lieutenant Kelly Flynn was disciplined for having an affair with the spouse of another soldier. (The Air Force discharged her in 1997.) Some observers thought she was unfairly singled out, and others objected to the military's interference in a private matter. Yet the U.S. Military's Manual for Courts-Martial explicitly forbids both adultery and extramarital affairs with married persons when there is a threat to "good order and discipline" or to the reputation of the armed forces. This requirement has a point as part of preparedness for combat, although administering the regulation requires wisdom and sensitivity to context (see Davenport; Whitman).

Adultery raises a wide array of moral questions. It can be understood within a plurality of moral frameworks, including ethical theories, general moral rules, religious traditions, attention to contextual nuance, ideals of love, and connections between morality and mental health. A humane understanding of adultery will appreciate the wide diversity of moral ideals and understandings that couples develop to structure their relationships. In this way, adultery is a prism through which to view the moral complexity of human love and sexuality.

See also Abstinence; Activity, Sexual; Aristotle; Bible, Sex and the; Casual Sex; Cybersex; Ellis, Albert; Jealousy; Love; Marriage; Military, Sex and the; Rimmer, Robert; Russell, Bertrand; Sex Education; Thomas Aquinas (Saint); Westermarck, Edward

REFERENCES

Barash, David P., and Judith Eve Lipton. *The Myth of Monogamy: Fidelity and Infidelity in Animals and People*. New York: Henry Holt, 2001; Barnhart, Joseph E., and Mary Ann Barnhart. "Marital Faithfulness and Unfaithfulness." *Journal of Social Philosophy* 4 (April 1973), 10–15; Ben-Ze'ev, Aaron. "Chatting Is Sometimes Cheating." In *Love Online: Emotions on the Internet*. Cambridge: Cambridge University Press, 2004, 199–222; Carr, David. "Chastity and Adultery." *American Philosophical Quarterly* 23:4 (1986), 363–71; Cicovacki, Predrag. "On Love and Fidelity in Marriage." *Journal of Social Philosophy* 24:3 (1993), 92–104; Collins, Louise. "Emotional Adultery: Cybersex and Commitment." *Social Theory and Practice* 25:2 (1999), 243–70; Davenport, Manuel M. "What We Do in Private." *Southwest Philosophy Review* 15:1 (1999), 177–83; DeSalvo, Louise. *Adultery*. Boston, Mass.: Beacon Press, 1999; "Do Eskimo Men Lend Their Wives to Strangers?" (21 January 2003). <www.straightdope.com/mailbag/meskimowifeswap.html> [accessed 20 May 2005]; Doris, John M. *Lack of Character: Personality and Moral Behavior*. New York: Cambridge University Press, 2002; Edwards, Rem B. "Value Dimensions of 'Mental Illness' and 'Mental Health.'" In Rem B. Edwards, ed., *Ethics of Psychiatry*. Amherst, N.Y.: Prometheus, 1997, 17–21; Ellis, Havelock. (1951) *Sex and Marriage*. Westport, Conn.: Greenwood Press, 1977; Fletcher, Joseph. *Situation Ethics*. Philadelphia, Pa.: Westminster Press, 1966; Haber, Joram Graf. *Forgiveness*. Lanham, Md.: Rowman and Littlefield, 1991; Halwani, Raja. "The Morality of Adultery." *Dialogue* 38:2–3 (1996), 43–49; Halwani, Raja. "Virtue Ethics and Adultery." *Journal of Social Philosophy* 29:3 (1998), 5–18; Heyn, Dalma. *The Erotic Silence of the American Wife*. New York: Turtle Bay Books, 1992; Higgins, Kathleen Marie. "How Do I Love Thee? Let's Redefine a Term (A Response to Predrag Cicovacki)." *Journal of Social Philosophy* 24:3 (1993), 105–11; Hunt, Morton. *The Affair*. New York: World Publishing, 1969; Lampe, Philip E., ed. *Adultery in the United States*. Buffalo, N.Y.: Prometheus, 1987; Lawson, Annette. *Adultery: An Analysis of Love and Betrayal*. New York: Basic Books, 1988; LeMoncheck, Linda. *Loose Women, Lecherous Men: A Feminist Philosophy of Sex*. New York: Oxford University Press, 1997; Maheu, Marlene M., and Rona B. Subotnik. *Infidelity on the Internet: Virtual Relationships and Real Betrayal*. Naperville, Ill.: Sourcebooks, 2001; Martin, Mike W. "Adultery and Fidelity." *Journal of Social Philosophy* 25:3 (1994), 76–91; Martin, Mike W. *Love's Virtues*. Lawrence: University Press of Kansas, 1996; Pittman, Frank. *Private Lies: Infidelity and the Betrayal of Intimacy*. New York: Norton, 1989; Portmann, John. "Chatting Is Not Cheating." In John Portmann, ed., *In Defense of Sin*. New York: Palgrave, 2001, 223–41; Posner, Richard A. *Sex and Reason*. Cambridge, Mass.: Harvard University Press, 1992; Posner, Richard A., and Katharine B. Silbaugh. *A Guide to America's Sex Laws*. Chicago, Ill.: University of Chicago Press, 1996; Primoratz, Igor. *Ethics and Sex*. London: Routledge, 1999; Putman, Dan. "Sex and Virtue." *International Journal of Moral and Social Studies* 6:1 (1991), 47–56; Scheer, Robert. "Playboy Interview: Jimmy Carter." *Playboy* (November 1976). Reprinted in Don Richardson, ed., *Conversations with Carter*. London: Lynne Rienner, 1998, 33–58; Soble, Alan. *Sexual Investigations*. New York: New York University Press, 1996; Speers, W. "Newsmakers." *Philadelphia Inquirer* (10 August 1995), F2; Steinbock, Bonnie. "Adultery." *QQ: Report from the Center for Philosophy and Public Policy* 6:1 (1986), 12–14; Strean, Herbert S. *The Extramarital Affair*. Northvale, N.J.: Jason Aronson, 2000; Taylor, Richard. (1982) *Love Affairs: Marriage and Infidelity*. Amherst, N.Y.: Prometheus, 1997; Thomas Aquinas. (1265–1273) *Summa theologiae*. 60 vols. Cambridge, U.K.: Blackfriars, 1964–1976; Warburton, Nigel. "Virtual Fidelity." *Cogito* (November 1996), 193–99; Wark, Wesley K. "Sex, Spies, and Stereotypes." *Los Angeles Times* (27 May 2003), B13; Wasserstrom, Richard A. "Is Adultery Immoral?" *Philosophical Forum* 5 (Summer 1973–1974), 513–28;

Westermarck, Edward. "Adultery and Jealousy." In *The Future of Marriage in Western Civilization*. New York: Macmillan, 1936, 58–79; Whitman, Jeffrey P. "Women, Sex, and the Military." *Public Affairs Quarterly* 12:4 (1998), 447–69; Wreen, Michael J. "What's Really Wrong with Adultery." *International Journal of Applied Philosophy* 3:2 (1986), 45–49.

Mike W. Martin

ADDITIONAL READING

Allan, Graham, and Kaeren Harrison. "Marital Affairs." In Robin Goodwin and Duncan Cramer, eds., *Inappropriate Relationships: The Unconventional, the Disapproved, and the Forbidden*. Mahwah, N.J.: Erlbaum, 2002, 45–63; Bartky, Sandra Lee. "Semper Fidelis? Some Observations on Adultery." *American Philosophical Association Newsletters* [Feminism] 01:2 (Spring 2002), 72–75; Belliotti, Raymond. *Good Sex: Perspectives on Sexual Ethics*. Lawrence: University Press of Kansas, 1993; Boteach, (Rabbi) Shmuel (Schmuley). *Kosher Adultery: Seduce and Sin with Your Partner*. Avon, Mass.: Adams Media, 2002; Broido, Michael. "Killing, Lying, Stealing, and Adultery: A Problem of Interpretation in the Tantras." In Donald S. Lopez, Jr., ed., *Buddhist Hermeneutics*. Honolulu: University of Hawai'i Press, 1988, 71–118; Cicovacki, Predrag. "Can Love Resolve the Problem of Marriage?" In Thomas Magnell, ed., *Explorations of Value*. Amsterdam, Holland: Rodopi, 1997, 221–33; Ellis, Albert. "Adultery: Pros and Cons." In *Sex without Guilt*. New York: Lyle Stuart, 1958, 51–65; English, O. Spurgeon. "Positive Values of the Affair." In Herbert A. Otto, ed., *The New Sexuality*. Palo Alto, Calif.: Science and Behavior Books, 1971, 173–92; Fisher, Helen E. *Anatomy of Love: A Natural History of Mating, Marriage, and Why We Stray*. New York: Ballantine, 1994; Fisher, Helen E. *Anatomy of Love: The Natural History of Monogamy, Adultery, and Divorce*. New York: Norton, 1992; Giroud, Françoise, and Bernard-Henri Lévy. (1993) "On the Pleasures of Fidelity." In *Women and Men: A Philosophical Conversation*. Trans. Richard Miller. Boston, Mass.: Little, Brown, 1995, 137–57; Gould, Terry. *The Lifestyle: A Look at the Erotic Rites of Swingers*. New York: Firefly, 2000; Greeley, Andrew. "Marital Infidelity." *Society* (May–June 1994), 9–13; Halwani, Raja. "Virtue Ethics and Adultery." *Journal of Social Philosophy* 29:3 (1998), 5–18. Reprinted in David Benatar, ed., *Ethics for Everyday*. Boston, Mass.: McGraw-Hill, 2002, 226–40; Kipnis, Laura. "Adultery." *Critical Inquiry* 24:2 (1998), 289–327; Kipnis, Laura. *Against Love: A Polemic*. New York: Pantheon, 2003; Lawson, Annette. *Adultery: An Analysis of Love and Betrayal*. Oxford, U.K.: Blackwell, 1987. New York: Basic Books, 1988; Marquis, Don. "What's Wrong with Adultery?" In David Boonin and Graham Oddie, eds., *What's Wrong? Applied Ethicists and Their Critics*. New York: Oxford University Press, 2005, 231–38; Martin, Mike W. "Adultery and Fidelity." *Journal of Social Philosophy* 25:3 (1994), 76–91. Reprinted in David Benatar, ed., *Ethics for Everyday*. Boston, Mass.: McGraw-Hill, 2002, 212–25; P&S2 (151–64); Martin, Mike W. (1989, 2001) "Marriage and Adultery." In *Everyday Morality: An Introduction to Applied Ethics*, 2nd ed. Belmont, Calif.: Wadsworth, 1995, 230–44; Masters, William H., and Virginia E. Johnson. "Extramarital Sex: Who Gambles—and Why?" In *The Pleasure Bond: A New Look at Sexuality and Commitment*. Boston, Mass.: Little, Brown, 1974, 99–139; McMurtry, John. "Monogamy: A Critique." *The Monist* 56:4 (1972), 587–99. Reprinted in P&S1 (166–77); P&S2 (107–18); Mead, Rebecca. "Love's Labors: Monogamy, Marriage, and Other Menaces." *The New Yorker* (11 August 2003), 80–82; Mendus, Susan. "Marital Faithfulness." *Philosophy* 59 (1984), 243–52. Reprinted in Alan Soble, ed., *Eros, Agape, and Philia: Readings in the Philosophy of Love*. New York: Paragon House, 1989, 235–44; P&S3 (130–38); Neubeck, Gerhard, ed. *Extramarital Relations*. Englewood Cliffs, N.J.: Prentice-Hall, 1969; O'Neill, Nena, and George O'Neill. *Open Marriage: A New Life Style for Couples*. New York: M. Evans, 1972; Primoratz, Igor. "Marriage, Adultery, Jealousy." In *Ethics and Sex*. London: Routledge, 1999, 69–87; Randall, Hilary E., and E. Sandra Byers. "What Is Sex? Students' Definitions of Having Sex, Sexual Partner, and Unfaithful Sexual Behaviour." *Canadian Journal of Human Sexuality* 12:2 (2003), 87–96; Russell, Bertrand. *Marriage and Morals*. London: Allen and Unwin, 1929; Schlabach, Gerald W. "Friendship as Adultery: Social Reality and Sexual Metaphor in Augustine's Doctrine of Original Sin." *Augustinian Studies* 23 (1992), 125–47; Schwartz, Mimi.

"Negotiating Monogamy." In *Thoughts from a Queen-Sized Bed*. Lincoln: University of Nebraska Press, 2002, 26–29; Scruton, Roger. *Sexual Desire: A Moral Philosophy of the Erotic*. New York: Free Press, 1986; Shrage, Laurie. "Interpreting Adultery." In *Moral Dilemmas of Feminism: Prostitution, Adultery, and Abortion*. New York: Routledge, 1994, 31–54; Singer, Peter, ed. "Sexual Morality." In *Ethics*. Oxford, U.K.: Oxford University Press, 1994, Part I.B.iii, 93–112; Steinbock, Bonnie. "Adultery." *QQ: Report from the Center for Philosophy and Public Policy* 6:1 (1986), 12–14. Reprinted in POS2 (187–92); Stern, Lawrence. Review of *Having Love Affairs*, by Richard Taylor. *Ethics* 98:1 (1987), 190–92; Tanner, Tony. *Adultery in the Novel: Contract and Transgression*. Baltimore, Md.: Johns Hopkins University Press, 1979; Taylor, Richard. *Love Affairs: Marriage and Infidelity*. Amherst, N.Y.: Prometheus, 1997. Previously published as *Having Love Affairs*. Buffalo, N.Y.: Prometheus, 1982, 1990; Wasserstrom, Richard A. "Is Adultery Immoral?" *Philosophical Forum* 5 (Summer 1973–1974), 513–28. Reprinted in Richard A. Wasserstrom, ed., *Today's Moral Problems*. New York: Macmillan, 1975, 240–52; and P&S1 (207–21); P&S2 (93–106); P&S3 (139–50); STW (159–67); Westley, Richard. "Justifying Infidelity." *Listening* 10 (1975), 36–44; Wilson, Thomas J. B., with Everett Mayers. *Wife-Swapping: A Complete Eight-Year Survey of Morals in North America*. New York: Counterpoint, 1965; Wreen, Michael J. "What's Really Wrong with Adultery." *International Journal of Applied Philosophy* 3:2 (1986), 45–49. Reprinted in POS2 (179–86).

AFRICAN PHILOSOPHY. A vast number of societies occupy the African continent. Here we focus on one specific ethnic group's construction of sexuality, providing a philosophical analysis of the conceptual scheme of the Igbo of Nigeria and an account of the social implications of that conception and the sorts of practices it permits. In the West, stereotypical myths about black or African sexuality abound. Further, African sexuality has often been addressed on negative grounds, centering on disease and contagion in colonial times (see Jackson), on **bestiality** during the period of the slave trade (see Samuels), on HIV (human immunodeficiency virus) and AIDS (acquired immunodeficiency syndrome) since the 1980s (see Watney), and on **genital mutilation** in the 1990s (see Kouba). The West has frequently represented African sexuality as deviant and perverted (see Blasingame).

Africa, very much part of the modern world, has been influenced by sexual attitudes and norms from three major sources: former colonizers, two world religions (Christianity and **Islam**), and the entertainment industry. In the first half of the twentieth century, the colonization of Africa by European powers (Britain, France, Germany, Belgium, Portugal, Italy, Spain) brought it under the jurisdiction of the sexual mores of those nations. Colonial policies privileged monogamy and nuclear family values as well as a subordinate, invisible identity for women. These were imposed in all the colonies, devaluing some indigenous sexual and marital practices that deviated from European moral schemes and proscribing others that were viewed as morally repugnant. Some of the censured practices included polygyny, woman-woman marriages, women "marrying" men, girl-bride marriages, and infant son marriages. In the process, a pool of "free women" that colonial governments tagged prostitutes was created. But not all the indigenous practices died out. Some, for example, the modern variant of polygamy, were transformed.

Christianity and Islam left imprints on African sexuality. Missionaries castigated local sexual and marital practices that did not conform to the religion's values. Believing, for example, that Igbo marriages were unstable because women possessed sexual autonomy, Christian missionaries condemned the ethical scheme that made such autonomy possible. Christians were especially hostile to the idea that women could have lovers before and during **marriage**. Islamic clerics as well frowned on sexual relations outside marriage. For these religions, sexual relations had to be conducted only within marriage; otherwise, a woman would be deemed a prostitute. The Christian and Muslim emphasis on marriage, and on marital fidelity as upholding the sanctity of marriage, constrained women's sexual autonomy and subverted the indigenous moral scheme that did not include a sexually restrictive role for women. But even after colonial and religious influences permeated African sexual ideas, indigenous sexual practices and attitudes continued until the late 1970s.

The greatest recent influence on African attitudes has been the Western entertainment industry: films, soap operas, **pornography**, and music videos. During the second half of the twentieth century, many sexual practices—kissing, oral sex, anal sex, the use of toys— were introduced to generations of Africans. The idea of **casual sex** without consequences also entered social consciousness and radically reshaped the values of both educated and uneducated Africans.

Unlike the colonials and the religions, which had patriarchal tendencies, many African societies had a mother-centered ideology and possessed a female-affirming worldview. A concrete manifestation of this female affirmation in Igboland was the existence of women's governance and political institutions that secured and consolidated their rights. Consequently, women in Igbo communities were assertive, economically independent, and industrious, and these traits were socially valued. Unlike European women of a similar historical period, Igbo women were far from the passive beings that early British anthropologists in Igboland had assumed them to be. After the 1929 uprising against the British colonial government, studies of Igbo women corrected the erroneous image of them. Even when these women were in polygynous marriages, they reserved the right to have lovers. Their husbands had to abide by clearly defined rules of equity and fairness in their relations with them. Otherwise the polygynous compound would end up in chaos. To avoid the breakdown of family relations, the first wife rather than the husband was in charge of the compound.

Going beyond the various influences of colonialism, religion, and modernity is crucial in understanding Igbo sexual attitudes prior to their assimilation of norms that were designed to instill passivity in women and constrain their sexual autonomy. If one raised the question of the nature of sexuality in, say, the 1950s, the answer would vary depending on the respondent. Some educated men of the time would stress their dominant role as heads of households, underscoring the subordinate sexual role of wives. By contrast, were mature wives to respond, they would speak of having to supplement unsatisfactory spousal sexual relations with sexual relations carried out with men of their choice. A husband's sexual obligations to a number of wives and lovers depleted his sexual energy, leaving unsatisfied wives no option but to take lovers. That wives asserted their right to sexual satisfaction with other men explodes the myth of African men's large sexual appetite and the attendant idea that the duty of their many wives is to minister to their sexual needs. The myth that African men are polygynous by nature has been used to secure the myth of their large sexual drive. But this grounding is questionable, for polygyny as a form of marriage is a social institution that need not at all involve sexual relations between the partners. Besides, Igbo women, too, married wives of their own, and some of these marriages were polygamous.

The Igbo conception of sexuality does not presuppose a Western discursive framework that assigns sexual dominance to men. Within the Igbo cultural scheme, principles that authorized men's sexuality validated women's and wives' sexual needs as well. The principles also permitted the formation of social practices and family organizations that accommodated both women and men. The way women retained sexual agency and were able to exercise it outside their husband's control can be revealed by incorporating women's voices into an account of the nature of Igbo sexuality. The increasing participation of African women in scholarship would uncover a range of formerly concealed practices as well as sexual desires and behaviors rooted in pleasure and not necessarily tied to procreation. It is true that different Igbo societies emphasized the link between sex and procreation during women's childbearing years, but this link did not exist for the duration of a woman's life. The importance of nonprocreative, pleasurable sexual activity is a reflection of the Igbo conception of sexuality that affirms women's autonomy, permitted wives to have lovers, and authenticated practices such as woman-woman marriages.

What happens to a conception of sexuality when women are positively affirmed? How does our understanding of sexuality change when the vagina instead of the penis is perceived as the dominant organ in the heterosexual act? Consider the lyrics of a song that was popular among the young in the 1950s:

> Gbaba lu'm egwu ukwu
> Ikpu na eli amu
> Oke opa kwa anyi a'naa.
>
> Do the hip dance with me [the one in which]
> The vagina devours the penis [and]
> When the cock crows, we'll depart.

Performed in its cultural content, the song/dance is rich with sexual allusions. "Hip" in the first line refers to dance movements that evoke the flexible midbody motions of copulation. The dance movements comprise circular gyrations of the hip and quick forward and backward thrusts of the pelvis. The dance is energetically enacted, and its racy beat incorporates swift short runs and turns. The men and women, keeping pace with the pulsating rhythm of the music, dance in a sexually charged manner. They sing lustily that the penis will be devoured. The imagery of the devouring vagina joins food, sexuality, and dance together in one aesthetic experience. The singers/dancers appreciate that the penis is eaten because it is filling and flavorful. So, too, is copulation. The apparently incongruent assimilation of copulation to consumption is not value neutral: It assigns the values of agency to the vagina and passivity to the penis. (On sexuality as consumption, see **Camille Paglia**, 16.)

The notion that the vagina is a devouring agent comes from the penis's nonvisibility during copulation. The vagina's "engulfing" the penis reverses common Western sexual wisdom by positioning the male in a subordinate position, even though he may be on top of the woman during the act. (About this reversed conception of copulation, see **Andrea Dworkin** [1946–2005], 64–65.) Being on top does not necessarily imply being in a superior psychological or physical position, for severe damage can be done to the male whose penis is enveloped, swallowed, made to disappear. This enveloping act grants the vagina great power. After all, to eat something is to assert one's will over it. However, this consumption does not deny all power and agency to that which is eaten. The penis's frantic activity of withdrawal, being reswallowed, and withdrawing again is a mode of "resistance." This resistance ends only when the man is pushed to the peak of arousal, at which point the penis is compelled to release its seed (as if pulled from it by the vagina), goes limp (and hence becomes even less powerful), and is then expelled. (In the West, these ideas often hint at the male's "castration." **Sigmund Freud** [1856–1939] wrote that "probably no male human being is spared the terrifying shock of threatened castration at the sight of the female genitals" [154].)

The idea of copulation as unidirectional consumption is illustrated by the fact that only men give up something of themselves to complete the act. After the semen's extraction, they are physically and emotionally drained. Ordinarily, eating something involves its demise, but there is no demise in human sexuality (see Shaffer, 188–89) and no fear of death in Igbo consumption, even though the vagina sucks out a vital part of the male. (For a similar conception in Melanesian cultures, see **Gilbert Herdt**.) The owner of the penis relishes the consumption, oblivious to the energy expended in each act. The process of extraction in copulation forces men to replenish themselves so they can function as males. Even when procreation is not the goal of copulation, the exercise still follows the script of extraction and expulsion. The disappearance (symbolic death) and reemergence (symbolic rebirth) of the penis alludes to the drama of life and death.

In both the theoretical and everyday construction of sexuality in the West, the dominant sexual being is (or largely has been) the man, and sexual discourse privileges male anatomy. The penis is represented as the central and dominating copulatory organ; the vagina is merely a sheath for the penetrating penis, a passive receptacle that receives, responds to, and stimulates the invading penis that drives deep into the woman. (See Laqueur for the Western "scientific" notion that the vagina is merely a penis turned inside out.) The question is not raised why the penis, as a sword, always seeks penetration and the needless expenditure of energy. On this model, which privileges the penis, the erect organ is pictured both as one that can harm and as one that can give pleasure. Whatever the preferred description of the penis, as instrument of subjection or pleasure, the focus (glossing Protagoras [ca. 480–410 BCE]) is always on the man as the measure. In this framework, no analogous imageries of the vagina exist. It is an unmentionable part of the female anatomy that exists for the Other, for male enjoyment. If the penis is pictured as a weapon of harm or pain (see Garry), it is an instrument for subduing or terrorizing a woman, designed, at times, to place her under a rapist's will. But even in a loving relationship, the penis is pictured as an instrument for pleasuring primarily the man. Because women are not pictured as desiring subjects, copulation might or might not stimulate them to orgasm; but good women are not, on this model, expected to enjoy sex. Only "fallen women" (nymphomaniacs, prostitutes) were thought to crave sex, and their desires were labeled "pathological." A liberalization of this perspective occurred among young people in the 1960s and among sexologists, who explored female sexuality and the clitoral orgasm (see especially William Masters [1915–2001] and Virginia Johnson).

Igbo culture championed a positive role for the vagina without castrating male libido. Men still played an important role in sexual matters; it is just that the emphasis is different. The positive conception of the vagina derives from its vital role as the birth canal from which all people come, regardless of sex, class, and social status. Every Igbo was duly reminded of this fact. The vagina, due to its important role in the continuation of life and the expansion of families, became the seat of women's power. A cavernous chamber that incubates life and later delivers it into the world, the vagina does so after extracting and preserving the man's seed. The capacity and functionality of the vagina makes it both a desirable and fearful organ. (See Kofman: "[W]oman's genital organs arouse an inseparable blend of horror and pleasure"; 84–85.) Its moist, warm chamber allures and arouses men and powerfully drives them to seek copulation. But it sucks into its mysterious depths that which enters. Its muscular walls rhythmically grip and pull the penis into its recesses and impel the male to an emotional peak. It is fearful also because its concealed inner depths contain the origin of life (see Farber, 156). As owners of this passage, women dictate to men the terms of entrance. Women can make entrance a pleasurable experience through muscular rhythmic contractions, or they can mute or deny that experience by stilling their bodies.

The positive conception of vagina and the recognition of women's sexual autonomy in the Igbo have social ramifications. One notable area is sexual **language**. A richer description of the vagina evolves: They can be "mature and experienced," "taunting" (referring to dexterous pelvic movements during intercourse), "assertive," "firm," "tight," "moist," "warm," "rhythmic," "textured," and "pulsating." A corollary of these linguistic developments is that the penis equally comes up for review. Is it long and big enough? How adequate is its performance? How long can it retain its turgidity? Does it flail about in the vagina? Women declare the criteria for judging penises; their evaluations are required so men can improve their performance. This conception of sexuality arguably accommodates the interests both sexes have in fulfilling sexuality. But the colonial and religious frameworks made no room for women's active, autonomous sexuality and, as a result, Igbo women's views on sexuality were not sufficiently respected postcolonially.

Before the Christian and Islamic influence, the social institutions and practices governing women's sexuality were fundamentally progressive. Marital norms allowed women to control their sexuality. Most Igbo marriages did not make physical paternity an issue. It was marriage, not impregnation, that made one a father. What mattered was the child's birth into a family that had received the legal and moral right to fatherhood from the bride's family. This scheme had three main implications: It detached sexuality from the institution of marriage; it placed wives' sexuality outside the purview of husbands; and it made childbearing a prominent social duty for wives. But this reproductive duty entailed that society ensured that women had the means to perform this task and become mothers regardless of the competence of their husbands.

Consequently, Igbo societies authorized wives to procreate even if their husbands were absent and even if husbands were incapable of fertilizing them. Women could begin a relationship with another man if within a year she was not pregnant. Infidelity, as conventionally defined, was not intelligible within this scheme because marriage did not convey the personhood of a woman to a husband. A different understanding of faithfulness was part of the culture's ethical scheme. Fidelity was not associated with bodies but with loyalty to the lineage. Spouses did not command each other to be chaste; nor did they expect each other not to satisfy their sexual urges with other partners. However, spouses were expected to be loyal to each other's families and to work for their safety. If a husband was unable to perform his sexual duties satisfactorily, the aid of a husband helper (paramour) was promptly elicited. It was both unreasonable and unacceptable to expect a wife to repress her sexuality or her desire for children.

Women in many Igbo communities engaged in two types of transmarital relationships: those sanctioned by the community and those that were not. They were sanctioned—to provide a number of cases—when for professional reasons spouses undertook journeys that kept them away from their conjugal units for months; when a husband had difficulty producing sons and a wife had relations with a man prone to beget sons; when the groom was impotent and a surrogate was solicited to cause impregnation; when pregnancy did not occur within a year of marriage and she returned to her natal home for "medical treatment" that included relations with other men; when a much older husband is unable to satisfy the sexual needs of a younger wife and she solicits the services of a husband helper; when there were ritualized grounds for a bride/wife to accept a lover and she exercised that right; and when a man, who has a desirable physical trait according to the wife or the couple, is brought into their conjugal unit. Nonsanctioned relationships were "abominations," for example, when a wife had relations in a sacred space or with a member of her kin group.

Male scholars have been reluctant to discuss these examples of women's sexual autonomy, but they are common practices in Igbo social life. In traditional Igbo culture, procreation was marriage's *raison d'être*, but that did not entail that only the husband could be the biological father or that a husband could not be the father of children he did not sire. Consequently, Igbo fathers/husbands embraced all the children born within their conjugal unit and were content with the role of caring for the children of both the marriage and the lineage. They nurtured and bonded with them and shaped them to be members of the community.

Many Christian Igbo men and women are disinclined to acknowledge that Igbo culture embraces a principle of sexual autonomy for women. They do not want to endorse what they see as the immoral practices of a bygone, primitive era. With the spread of home-grown Christian evangelism in the late 1980s, a strong push to reign in the sexual autonomy of women occurred. With the rise of this censorious attitude about women's sexuality, respectable Igbo women learned to live on both sides of the divide. Publicly, they affected a posture of the good Christian woman, but privately they conducted extramarital affairs when they chose. As one interviewee confidently asserted, "No one needs to know; after all, there is no meter down there" (personal communication, Lagos, Nigeria, 1981). This subterfuge is troubling; the older conception of female sexual autonomy was candid and healthy. Although the moral scheme that accredited this state of affairs has largely been constrained by the Christian demand for fidelity, it nonetheless provides grounds to critique any coercive ideology that attempts to control women's autonomy and sexuality.

See also Adultery; Bisexuality; Diseases, Sexually Transmitted; Feminism, French; Freud, Sigmund; Genital Mutilation; Herdt, Gilbert; Islam; Kant, Immanuel; Marriage; Protestantism, History of; Psychology, Twentieth- and Twenty-First-Century; Sexology; Sherfey, Mary Jane; Social Constructionism

REFERENCES

Basden, George T. (1938) *Niger Ibos*. New York: Barnes and Noble, 1966; Blasingame, Brenda Marie. "The Roots of Biphobia: Racism and Internalized Heterosexism." In Elizabeth Reba Weise, ed., *Closer to Home: Bisexuality and Feminism*. Seattle, Wash.: Seal Press, 1992, 47–53; Dworkin, Andrea. *Intercourse*. New York: Free Press, 1987; Farber, Leslie. *Lying, Despair, Jealousy, Envy, Sex, Suicide, Drugs, and the Good Life*. New York: Basic Books, 1976; Freud, Sigmund. (1927) "Fetishism." In *The Standard Edition of the Complete Psychological Works of Sigmund Freud*, vol. 21. Trans. James Strachey. London: Hogarth Press, 1953–1974, 152–57; Garry, Ann. "Pornography and Respect for Women." *Social Theory and Practice* 4:4 (1978), 395–421; Green, Margaret M. *Ibo Village Affairs*. London: Frank Cass, 1964; Herdt, Gilbert. *Guardians of the Flutes: Idioms of Masculinity*. New York: McGraw-Hill, 1981; Herdt, Gilbert. *The Sambia: Ritual and Gender in New Guinea*. New York: Holt, Rinehart, and Winston, 1987; Jackson, Lynette A. "'When in the White Man's Town': Zimbabwean *Chibeura*." In Jean Allman, Susan Geiger, and Nakanyike Musisi, eds., *Women in African Colonial Histories*. Bloomington: Indiana University Press, 2002, 191–215; Kofman, Sarah. *The Enigma of Woman: Woman in Freud's Writings*. Trans. Catharine Porter. Ithaca, N.Y.: Cornell University Press, 1985; Kouba, Leonard J. "Female Circumcision in Africa: An Overview." *African Studies Review* 28:1 (1985), 95–110; Laqueur, Thomas. *Making Sex: Body and Gender from the Greeks to Freud*. Cambridge, Mass.: Harvard University Press, 1990; Leith-Ross, Sylvia. (1939) *African Women: A Study of the Ibo of Nigeria*. London: Routledge and Kegan Paul, 1965; Masters, William H., and Virginia E. Johnson. *Human Sexual Response*. Boston, Mass.: Little, Brown, 1966; Paglia, Camille. *Sexual Personae: Art and Decadence from Nefertiti to Emily Dickinson*.

New Haven, Conn.: Yale University Press, 1990; Samuels, Herbert. "Race, Sex, and Myths: Images of African American Men and Women." In Vern L. Bullough and Bonnie Bullough, eds., *Human Sexuality: An Encyclopedia*. New York: Garland, 1994, 507–11; Shaffer, Jerome A. "Sexual Desire." *Journal of Philosophy* 75:4 (1978), 175–89; Thomas, Northcote Whitridge. *Anthropological Report on the Ibo-Speaking Peoples of Nigeria*. London: Harrison and Sons, 1913–1914; Watney, Simon. "Missionary Position: AIDS, Africa, and Race." In Russell Ferguson, Martha Gever, Trinh T. Minh-Ha, and Cornel West, eds., *Out There: Marginalization and Contemporary Culture*. Cambridge, Mass.: MIT Press, 1990, 89–103.

Nkiru Nzegwu

ADDITIONAL READING

AfricaResource. (Web site) <www.africaresource.com> [accessed 12 November 2004]; Basden, George T. *Among the Ibos of Nigeria*. London: Seeley, Service, and Co., 1921; Baum, Robert M. "Homosexuality and the Traditional Religions of the Americas and Africa." In Arlene Swidler, ed., *Homosexuality and World Religions*. Valley Forge, Pa.: Trinity Press, 1993, 1–46; Chernoff, John M. *Exchange Is Not Robbery: More Stories of an African Bar Girl*. Chicago, Ill.: University of Chicago Press, 2005; Chernoff, John M. *Hustling Is Not Stealing: Stories of an African Bar Girl*. Chicago, Ill.: University of Chicago Press, 2004; Douglas, Kelly Brown. "The Black Church and Homosexuality: The Black and White of It." *Union Seminary Quarterly Review* 57:1–2 (2003), 32–45; Douglas, Kelly Brown. *Sexuality and the Black Church: A Womanist Perspective*. Maryknoll, N.Y.: Orbis Books, 1999; Edwards, Allen, and R.E.L. Masters. *The Cradle of Erotica: A Study of Afro-Asian Sexual Expression and an Analysis of Erotic Freedom in Social Relationships*. New York: Julian Press, 1963; Franklin, Clyde W., II. (1984) "Black Male–Black Female Conflict: Individually Caused and Culturally Nurtured." In Michael S. Kimmel and Michael A. Messner, eds., *Men's Lives*, 3rd ed. Needham Heights, Mass.: Allyn and Bacon, 1995, 285–92; Garry, Ann. "Pornography and Respect for Women." *Social Theory and Practice* 4:4 (1978), 395–421. Reprinted in Sharon Bishop and Marjorie Weinzweig, eds., *Philosophy and Women*. Belmont, Calif.: Wadsworth, 1979, 128–39; Garry, Ann. "Sex, Lies, and Pornography." In Hugh LaFollette, ed., *Ethics in Practice: An Anthology*, 2nd ed. Malden, Mass.: Blackwell, 2002, 344–55; Gilman, Sander L. *Difference and Pathology: Stereotypes of Sexuality, Race, and Madness*. Ithaca, N.Y.: Cornell University Press, 1985; Janz, Bruce B. "African Philosophy Resources." <pegasus.cc.ucf.edu/~janzb/afphil> [accessed 8 September 2004]; Kumashiro, Kevin K., ed. *Troubling Intersections of Race and Sexuality: Queer Students of Color and Anti-Oppressive Education*. Lanham, Md.: Rowman and Littlefield, 2001; Lott, Tommy L., and John P. Pittman, eds. *A Companion to African-American Philosophy*. Malden, Mass.: Blackwell, 2003; Marable, Manning. (1993) "The Black Male: Searching beyond Stereotypes." In Michael S. Kimmel and Michael A. Messner, eds., *Men's Lives*, 3rd ed. Needham Heights, Mass.: Allyn and Bacon, 1995, 26–32; Martey, Emmanuel. "Church and Marriage in African Society: A Theological Appraisal." In Elizabeth Stuart and Adrian Thatcher, eds., *Christian Perspectives on Sexuality and Gender*. Grand Rapids, Mich.: Eerdmans, 1996, 199–209; Mba, Nina Emma. *Nigerian Women Mobilized: Women's Political Activities in Southern Nigeria, 1900–1965*. Berkeley, Calif.: Institute of International Studies, 1982; Nzegwu, Nkiru. *Family Matters: Feminist Concepts in African Philosophy of Culture*. Albany: State University of New York Press, 2005; Nzegwu, Nkiru. "Feminism and Africa: Impact and Limits of the Metaphysics of Gender." In Kwasi Wiredu, ed., *A Companion to African Philosophy*. Malden, Mass.: Blackwell, 2003, 560–69; Oniang'o, Clement M. P. "The Foundations of African Philosophy." Lock Haven University of Pennsylvania. <www.lhup.edu/library/InternationalReview/african_phil.htm> [accessed 8 September 2004]; Parks, Carlton W. "African American Lesbian and Gay Identities." In Timothy F. Murphy, ed., *Reader's Guide to Lesbian and Gay Studies*. Chicago, Ill.: Fitzroy Dearborn, 2000, 15–16; Shaffer, Jerome A. "Sexual Desire." *Journal of Philosophy* 75:4 (1978), 175–89. Reprinted in SLF (1–12); Simson, Rennie. "The Afro-American Female: The Historical Context of the Construction of Sexual Identity." In Ann Snitow, Christine Stansell, and Sharon Thompson, eds., *Powers of Desire: The Politics of Sexuality*. New

York: Monthly Review Press, 1983, 229–35; Staples, Robert. (1986) "Stereotypes of Black Male Sexuality: The Facts behind the Myths." In Michael S. Kimmel and Michael A. Messner, eds., *Men's Lives*, 3rd ed. Needham Heights, Mass.: Allyn and Bacon, 1995, 375–80; Wieringa, Saskia, ed. *Subversive Women: Women's Movements in Africa, Asia, Latin America, and the Caribbean*. New Delhi, India: Kali for Women, 1995; Wiredu, Kwasi, ed. *A Companion to African Philosophy*. Malden, Mass.: Blackwell, 2003; Yamauchi, Edwin M. *Africa and the Bible*. Grand Rapids, Mich.: Baker Academic, 2004.

AIDS. *See* Diseases, Sexually Transmitted

ANCIENT GREEK SEXUALITY AND PHILOSOPHY. *See* Greek Sexuality and Philosophy, Ancient

ANCIENT ROMAN SEXUALITY AND PHILOSOPHY. *See* Roman Sexuality and Philosophy, Ancient

ANIMAL SEXUALITY. Can the study of nonhuman animal sexuality reveal anything interesting about human sexuality? At first, this question appears straightforward, but it raises thorny philosophical issues. Are humans *sufficiently* similar to animals to warrant the investigation of animal sexuality for clues to our own? Jared Diamond senses a conundrum here: "It's obvious that humans are unlike all animals. It's also obvious that we're a species of big mammal, down to the minutest details of our anatomy and molecules" (*Third Chimpanzee*, 1). We are very much like, and very much unlike, animals.

But which animals are we talking about? Which are the right or best ones to look at? The Book of Genesis tells us immediately that the sexuality of animals (as an undifferentiated group) and the sexuality of humans have something salient in common: This universally shared sexuality is by nature (God's design) heterosexual, and its purpose is reproduction. St. **Thomas Aquinas** (1224/25–1274) similarly lumps the animals together when explaining the foundations of Natural Law: "There is in man an inclination to things that pertain to him . . . according to that nature which he has in common with other animals: and in virtue of this inclination, those things are said to belong to the natural law, which nature has taught to all animals, such as sexual intercourse, education of offspring and so forth" (*Summa theologiae*, IaIIae, ques. 94, art. 2). Yet Aquinas fine-tunes his account: He selects birds in particular among the animals as providing the right analogy for understanding human sexuality and rejects a mammalian model, because in birds both parents are involved in the rearing of the young (*Summa contra gentiles*, bk. 3, chap. 122). "Zoologists have long known that most mammals are polygamous and most birds are monogamous" (Ridley, 221), but the fact that humans are mammals seems not to have influenced Aquinas. On his view, human infants, unlike dog infants, require the constant contribution of their father, from which "fact" he derives the naturalness for humans—and the morality—of monogamous **marriage**.

Others who have thought about the links between animal and human sexuality look to the primates, especially the great apes, for clues about human sexuality. They cite our close genetic affinity (humans share roughly 98 percent of their genetic material with chimpanzees and bonobos), which resulted from an evolution in which modern humans did not "split off" from the branch of the great apes until relatively recently, about 6 million years ago. Christine Gudorf's "reconstituted" Natural Law theology of human sexuality, for example, relies on primatology, sociobiology, and human female sexual anatomy in arriving at conclusions about God's design that are very different from Aquinas's (62–70). By contrast, some cast their nets far wider into the animal kingdom. The phenomena of sperm choice and sperm competition, for example, may play a significant role in shaping the sexual repertoires of a diverse range of animals—from dung flies through garter snakes to chimpanzees as well as humans. (Sperm competition and sperm choice are postinsemination analogs of Darwinian sexual selection; see Birkhead, ix.)

One area in which humans differ from animals is cognition. Our minds are very unlike and cognitively superior to those of even our closest primate relatives. The impressive performance of the cognitive mind, including **language**, culture, science, and art, are largely absent in the "lower" animals. Insofar as human sexuality has a significant cognitive component, skepticism about our learning anything important about human sexuality from animals seems justified. **Thomas Nagel**, who emphasizes the discontinuity between animals and humans in terms of self-consciousness, analyzes human sexual arousal in sophisticated Gricean terms as involving a mutual recognition of intentions (10–13). The elaborate sexual fantasies of humans are dramatic evidence of Nagel's discontinuity. Data on frequency of partners (Laumann et al., chap. 5) also indicate cognitive dimensions in human sexuality: Humans conform their behavior to social norms—or deliberately resist them. People in the United States of all ages tend to have fewer sexual partners while married than single. The cohort with the largest number of sexual partners, within marriage or outside, is that which came of age during the "sexual revolution" of the 1960s and 1970s. This suggests a large social and historical component in patterns of human sexuality. Humanity has a history in a special way that dogs do not. The question, Are humans more like birds or dogs or chimps? turns out to be a trick. Humans are *sui generis*.

Meredith Small, acknowledging the importance of such examples, asks, "[I]s the layer of culture so thick that we humans approach sexual activity, make mate choices, and accomplish reproduction differently from other animals?" (*Female Choices*, 187). Social constructionists (e.g., Tiefer), who give roughly a yes answer to Small's question, reject explanations of human sexuality that ignore the centrality of social context. By contrast, essentialists, who answer with a rough no, feel no reservation about making cross-species comparisons to study human sexuality (e.g., Wilson; see Stein for the **social constructionism**–essentialism debate). Social constructionists contend that there are no universal facts about human sexuality that exist in the abstract apart from social context. Susan Sperling agrees that "[h]uman gendered behavior involves uniquely human cultural, cognitive, and linguistic characteristics." But she also asserts that primate ethology "may have something to offer by elucidating developmental mechanisms that apply across primate phyla" (including humans) and, at the same time, that this ethology "defin[es] the important differences between human and nonhuman primates" (27). Matters may indeed be this complex.

Another tangle is that human biology itself may explain some differences between human and animal sexuality. Jared Diamond points out that menopause, the preference for sex in private, and the pair-bond are unique to human sexuality. (Also see Hrdy on the significance for human sexuality of concealed ovulation; i.e., estrus is absent in human females; *Woman*, 141–43.) These evolved sexual characteristics depend "on both ecological parameters and the parameters of a species' biology, both of which vary among species"

(Diamond, *Why Is Sex Fun?* 12). Small also mentions the pair-bond as a human achievement, which she explains as the compromise we strike to solve a dilemma many primates face, the conflict between wanting to pass on one's genes to the next generation and the desire for sexual satisfaction (*Female Choices*, chap. 7).

If insights into human sexuality can be gleaned from animals, the most obvious candidates, according to some scholars, are primates. Males and females of many primate species, including bonobos and chimpanzees, experience sexual pleasure, engage in nonreproductive sex, and bear infants that are dependent on their parents (especially mothers) for long stretches of time. Many primates live in social structures that require social skills, and some studies suggest that some primates have the capacity for self-reflection (Smith et al.). Even so, enormous variation exists in primate sexuality. In chimpanzees, aggressive males dominate females and sometimes kill the offspring of rival males. (Is anyone tempted to do a Thomistic extrapolation here?) In bonobos this aggression is rare; females are dominant in bonobo society, and they use sex to cement bonds, share food, and limit male-male competition (by providing almost unlimited access). But in the bonobos, sexual encounters (which include same-sex genital rubbings) average thirteen seconds. Female gorillas live in "harems" controlled by a single male who has exclusive sexual access. Orangutans live solitary lives; males and females come together only to mate. All these primates are our close relatives, yet from such variety no lesson about human sexuality can be learned. Although Frans de Waal claims that humans share female bonding with bonobos and male bonding with chimpanzees, he is doubtful that these similarities run very deep. On his view, "the exact role of sex in human society depends on an evolutionary and cultural history that has been separate from that of our closest relatives for millions of years" (135). Like Small and Diamond, Waal sees the human nuclear family as marking a significant departure.

Sarah Hrdy warns of the pitfalls of using cross-species comparisons to understand human sexuality. Some scholars "looked to the animals not to make unbiased empirical observations but to use nature to confirm their own and their society's preconceptions about how humans should behave" (*Mother Nature*, 10–11). Aquinas's selecting a bird analogy seems to be a case in point. Hrdy accuses Charles Darwin (1809–1882) and **Herbert Spencer** (1820–1903) of letting Victorian notions of the sexually passive female bias their theories of sexual selection. Hrdy's studies of female primates show how evolutionary theory, freed from sexist bias, challenges traditional assumptions about female sexuality even as her cross-species comparisons indicate the imprint on human nature of our primate heritage. She points out, for example, that primate mothers make use of others to assist in the rearing of children (alloparents) and suggests that some human practices, such as employing wet nurses, exemplify the same strategy (91). Aquinas's view that human infants strictly require contributing fathers is looking specious. (Marlene Zuk raises similar methodological concerns, suggesting that "feminism has more to offer biology than biology does feminism" [201] because feminists can alert biologists to gender biases in their theories.)

Whether humans are naturally monogamous (as in Aquinas) or naturally promiscuous is a hot topic, both among scholars and in the popular media. According to mainstream evolutionary biology (perhaps under the spell of myopic preconceptions about humans), males, having millions of sperm easily spread, tend as a result toward promiscuity, while females, having very few eggs and investing nine months in gestation, tend as a result toward monogamy (Ridley, chaps. 6, 7; Symons, 23–25 and chap. 7). Hrdy, however, points out that in some primate species (baboons, macaques) females exhibit an aggressive, promiscuous sexuality that "goes far beyond the necessary minimum for ensuring insemination" and is not linked to the maintenance of the pair-bond (*Woman*, 144). Female chimpanzees during estrus copulate with several different males in their own troop; they might even copulate—which is risky—with males of neighboring troops. As a result of this female promiscuity, male chimpanzees developed large testes capable of producing copious amounts of sperm, for only such males were able to compete successfully and leave offspring (Small, "Sperm Wars," 52–53). In contrast to chimpanzees, the testes of gorillas are small, which resulted from single males' dominating harems of monopolized females. This pattern, a correlation between testes size (in relation to body mass), sperm production, and promiscuity, is exemplified across the primates and in other species, including rodents (Buss, 74–75; Harvey and May; Morton, 102; Ridley, 119–21; Ruse, 215–16; Short). The size of human testes falls between chimpanzees and gorillas, indicating "an average level of sperm competition for a primate" (Birkhead, 80). It would seem to follow that on the promiscuity-monogamy continuum, humans should fall somewhere between chimpanzees and gorillas.

Of course, even if the study of animal sexuality could usefully illuminate the nature of human sexuality, normative questions would not necessarily be resolved. What could animal studies tell us about what is good or bad, right or wrong, in human sexual behavior? Aquinas took his meditations on birds to have clear ethical implications for human sexuality, because his cross-species comparisons were, for him, indicative of a divinely ordained monogamous order. But Aquinas's birds do not have any choice about being monogamous; they are not moral agents. We are. And, in the West at least, we no longer hold so strongly to the Natural Law tradition or other teleological construals of human nature (see Priest). The question whether human beings are naturally monogamous or promiscuous is different from whether human beings ought to be monogamous or promiscuous. The upshot might be that even if we are successful in drawing significant parallels between animal and human sexuality, that would not have much impact on our lives.

Can the study of animal sexuality reveal interesting things about human sexuality? To the extent that human sexuality straddles biology and culture, body and mind, perhaps not. But sex is in this way hardly unique. Consider the human relationship to food. Much about why and when we become hungry, what we eat, how we eat it, how we digest it, turning it into physiologically useful material, and so on, is simply a matter of biology. Yet there is much about humans and food—the variety, even oddness, of what we eat (and refuse to eat), the different utensils we employ to ingest it, with whom we eat (or refuse to eat with), and at what times—that is bound up with individual psychological attitudes and cultural or ethnic practices. Perhaps these influences on our relationship to food will also eventually prove to be a matter of our biology, broadly construed, but this is controversial. In the meantime, we are left with Diamond's conundrum.

See also Augustine (Saint); Bestiality; Casual Sex; Evolution; Marriage; Nagel, Thomas; Psychology, Evolutionary; Sherfey, Mary Jane; Social Constructionism; Spencer, Herbert; Spinoza, Baruch; Thomas Aquinas (Saint)

REFERENCES

Birkhead, Tim. *Promiscuity: An Evolutionary History of Sperm Competition*. Cambridge, Mass.: Harvard University Press, 2000; Buss, David M. *The Evolution of Desire: Strategies of Human Mating*. New York: Basic Books, 1994; Diamond, Jared. *The Third Chimpanzee: The Evolution and Future of the Human Animal*. New York: HarperCollins, 1992; Diamond, Jared. *Why Is Sex Fun? The Evolution of Human Sexuality*. New York: Basic Books, 1997; Gudorf, Christine E. *Body, Sex, and Pleasure: Reconstructing Christian Sexual Ethics*. Cleveland, Ohio: Pilgrim, 1994; Harvey, Paul, and Robert May. "Out for the Sperm Count." *Nature* 337:6207 (1989), 508–9; Hrdy, Sarah Blaffer. *Mother Nature: A History of Mothers, Infants, and Natural Selection*. New York: Pantheon, 1999; Hrdy, Sarah Blaffer. *The Woman That Never Evolved*. Cambridge, Mass.: Harvard University Press, 1981; Laumann, Edward O., John H. Gagnon, Robert T. Michael, and Stuart Michaels. *The Social Organization of Sexuality: Sexual Practices in the United States*. Chicago, Ill.: University of Chicago Press, 1994; Morton, Oliver. "Doing What Comes Naturally: A New School of Psychology Finds Reasons for Your Foolish Heart." *The New Yorker* (3 November 1997), 102–7; Nagel, Thomas. "Sexual Perversion." *Journal of Philosophy* 66:1 (1969), 5–17; Priest, Graham. "Sexual Perversion." *Australasian Journal of Philosophy* 75:3 (1997), 360–72; Ridley, Matt. *The Red Queen: Sex and the Evolution of Human Nature*. New York: Macmillan, 1993; Ruse, Michael. *Darwin and Design: Does Evolution Have a Purpose?* Cambridge, Mass.: Harvard University Press, 2003; Short, Roger. "Sexual Selection and the Descent of Man." In *Proceedings of the Canberra Symposium on Reproduction and Evolution*. Canberra: Australian Academy of Sciences, 1977, 3–19; Small, Meredith F. *Female Choices: Sexual Behavior of Female Primates*. Ithaca, N.Y.: Cornell University Press, 1993; Small, Meredith F. "Sperm Wars." *Discover* 12:7 (July 1991), 48–53; Smith, J. David, Wendy Shields, and David Washburn. "The Comparative Psychology of Uncertainty Monitoring and Metacognition" (with open peer commentary). *Behavioral and Brain Sciences* 26:3 (2003), 317–73; Sperling, Susan. "Baboons with Briefcases: Feminism, Functionalism, and Sociobiology in the Evolution of Primate Gender." *Signs* 17:1 (1991), 1–27; Stein, Edward, ed. (1990) *Forms of Desire: Sexual Orientation and the Social Constructionist Controversy*. New York: Routledge, 1992; Symons, Donald. *The Evolution of Human Sexuality*. Oxford, U.K.: Oxford University Press, 1979; Thomas Aquinas. (1258–1264) *On the Truth of the Catholic Faith. Summa contra gentiles. Book Three: Providence. Part II*. Trans. Vernon J. Bourke. Garden City, N.Y.: Image Books, 1956; Thomas Aquinas. (1265–1273) *Summa theologiae*, 60 vols. Trans. Blackfriars. Cambridge, U.K.: Blackfriars, 1964–1976; Tiefer, Leonore. (1995) *Sex Is Not a Natural Act and Other Essays*, 2nd ed. Boulder, Colo.: Westview, 2004; Waal, Frans B. M. de. *Bonobo: The Forgotten Ape*. Berkeley: University of California Press, 1997; Wilson, Edward O. *Sociobiology: The New Synthesis*. Cambridge, Mass.: Harvard University Press, 1975; Zuk, Marlene. *Sexual Selections: What We Can and Can't Learn about Sex from Animals*. Berkeley: University of California Press, 2002.

Jeffrey Hershfield

ADDITIONAL READING

Archer, John, and Lynda Birke, eds. *Explorations in Animals and Humans*. Wokingham, U.K.: Van Nostrand Reinhold, 1983; Bagemihl, Bruce. *Biological Exuberance: Animal Homosexuality and Natural Diversity*. New York: St. Martin's Press, 1999; Baker, Robin. *The Sperm Wars*. New York: Basic Books, 1996; Barash, David P., and Judith Eve Lipton. *The Myth of Monogamy: Fidelity and Infidelity in Animals and People*. New York: Henry Holt, 2001; Birke, Lynda. *Feminism, Animals and Science: The Naming of the Shrew*. Buckingham, U.K.: Open University Press, 1994; Birkhead, Tim, and Anders Moller, eds. *Sperm Competition and Sexual Selection*. San Diego, Calif.: Academic Press, 1998; Diorio, Joseph A. "Feminist-constructionist Theories of Sexuality and the Definition of Sex Education." *Educational Philosophy and Theory* 21:2 (1989), 23–31; Dixson, Alan F. *Primate Sexuality: Comparative Studies of the Prosimians, Monkeys, Apes, and Human Beings*. New York: Oxford University Press, 1998; Geertz, Clifford. "Sociosexology." [Review of *The Evolution of Human Sexuality*, by Donald Symons] *New York Review of Books* (24 January 1980), 3–4; Haraway, Donna J. "Animal Sociology and a Natural Economy of the Body Politic, Part 1: A Political Physiology of Dominance." *Signs* 4:1 (1978), 21–36; Haraway, Donna J. "Animal Sociology and a Natural Economy of the Body Politic, Part 2: The Past Is the Contested Zone: Human Nature and Theories of Production and Reproduction in Primate Behavior Studies." *Signs* 4:1 (1978), 37–60; Haraway, Donna J. "Investment Strategies for the Evolving Portfolio of Primate Females." In Mary Jacobus, Evelyn Fox Keller, and Sally Shuttleworth, eds., *Body/Politics: Women and the Discourses of Science*. New York: Routledge, 1990, 139–62; Haraway, Donna J. "Monkeys, Aliens, and Women: Love,

Science, and Politics at the Intersection of Feminist Theory and Colonial Discourse." *Women's Studies International Forum* 12:3 (1989), 295–312; Haraway, Donna J. *Primate Visions: Gender, Race, and Nature in the World of Modern Science.* New York: Routledge, 1989; Haraway, Donna J. "Primatology Is Politics by Other Means." In Ruth Bleier, ed., *Feminist Approaches to Science.* New York: Pergamon, 1986, 77–118; Haraway, Donna J. *Simians, Cyborgs, and Women: The Reinvention of Nature.* New York: Routledge, 1991; Harvey, Paul, and M. D. Pagel. *The Comparative Method in Evolutionary Biology.* Oxford, U.K.: Oxford University Press, 1991; Hrdy, Sarah Blaffer. "The Evolution of Human Sexuality: The Latest Word and the Last." *Quarterly Review of Biology* 54:3 (1979), 309–14; Hrdy, Sarah Blaffer. "Female Reproductive Strategies." In Meredith F. Small, ed., *Female Primates: Studies by Women Primatologists.* New York: Alan R. Liss, 1984, 103–9; Jones, Steve. "Go Milk a Fruit Bat!" [Review of *Why Is Sex Fun? The Evolution of Human Sexuality*, by Jared Diamond] *New York Review of Books* (17 July 1997), 39–41; Jung, Patricia Beattie. Review of *Body, Sex, and Pleasure: Reconstructing Christian Sexual Ethics*, by Christine E. Gudorf. *Theological Studies* 56:3 (1995), 603–5; Maple, Terry. "Unusual Sexual Behavior of Nonhuman Primates." In John Money and Herman Musaph, eds., *Handbook of Sexology.* Amsterdam, Holland: Excerpta Medica, 1977, 1167–86; Masson, Jeffrey Moussaieff. *The Pig Who Sang to the Moon: The Emotional World of Farm Animals.* New York: Random House, 2003; Midgley, Mary. *Beast and Man: The Roots of Human Nature.* Hassocks, U.K.: Harvester, 1979; Morell, Virginia. "Called 'Trimates,' Three Bold Women Shaped Their Field." *Science* 260 (16 April 1993), 420–25; Morris, Desmond. *The Naked Ape.* New York: Dell, 1967; Nagel, Thomas. "Sexual Perversion." *Journal of Philosophy* 66:1 (1969), 5–17. Reprinted in P&S1 (247–60); P&S2 (268–79); POS1 (76–88). Reprinted, revised, in Thomas Nagel, *Mortal Questions.* Cambridge: Cambridge University Press, 1979, 39–52; and P&S3 (326–36); POS2 (39–51); POS3 (9–20); POS4 (9–20); STW (105–12); Pavelka, Mary S. McDonald. "Sexual Nature: What Can We Learn from a Cross-Species Perspective?" In Paul R. Abramson and Steven D. Pinkerton, eds., *Sexual Nature Sexual Culture.* Chicago, Ill.: University of Chicago Press, 1995, 17–36; Pope, Stephen J. "Primate Sociality and Natural Law Theory." In Robert W. Sussman and Audrey R. Chapman, eds., *The Origins and Nature of Sociality.* New York: Aldine de Gruyter, 2004, 313–31; Short, Roger. "Sexual Selection and Its Component Parts, Somatic and Genital Selection, as Illustrated by Man and Great Apes." *Advances in the Study of Behavior* 9 (1979), 131–58; Small, Meredith F. "Prime Mates: The Useful Promiscuity of Bonobo Apes." *Nerve* (9 September 1997). By subscription, <www.nerve.com/Dispatches/Small/bonobo> [accessed 30 August 2004]; Small, Meredith F., ed., *Female Primates: Studies by Women Primatologists.* New York: Alan R. Liss, 1984; Sperling, Susan. "Baboons with Briefcases: Feminism, Functionalism, and Sociobiology in the Evolution of Primate Gender." *Signs* 17:1 (1991), 1–27. Reprinted in Barbara Laslett, Sally Gregory Kohlstedt, Helen Longino, and Evelynn Hammonds, eds., *Gender and Scientific Authority.* Chicago, Ill.: University of Chicago Press, 1996, 364–90; Stein, Edward. "Animal Homosexuality." In Timothy F. Murphy, ed., *Reader's Guide to Lesbian and Gay Studies.* Chicago, Ill.: Fitzroy Dearborn, 2000, 46–47; Stein, Edward, ed. *Forms of Desire: Sexual Orientation and the Social Constructionist Controversy.* New York: Garland, 1990. Reprinted, New York: Routledge, 1992; Waal, Frans B. M. de. "Bonobo Sex and Society." *Scientific American* (March 1995), 82–88; Waal, Frans B. M. de. *Peacemaking among Primates.* Cambridge, Mass.: Harvard University Press, 1989; Waal, Frans B. M. de. "Sex as an Alternative to Aggression in the Bonobo." In Paul R. Abramson and Steven D. Pinkerton, eds., *Sexual Nature Sexual Culture.* Chicago, Ill.: University of Chicago Press, 1995, 37–56; Wilson, Edward O. *On Human Nature.* Cambridge, Mass.: Harvard University Press, 1978.

ANSCOMBE, G.E.M. (1919–2001). Gertrude Elizabeth Margaret Anscombe, a native of Limerick, Ireland, was one of the leading Anglo-American philosophers of the twentieth century. In 1937, while she was still in her teens, two momentous events occurred: She entered St. Hugh's College of the University of Oxford, and she converted to

Roman Catholicism. A year after entering St. Hugh's, she met philosophy student Peter Thomas Geach, three years her senior and also a convert to Roman Catholicism. The couple married in 1941, the year of Anscombe's graduation (with First Class Honours). The following year, Anscombe began postgraduate studies in philosophy at Newnham College of the University of Cambridge, where she attended lectures by Ludwig Wittgenstein (1889–1951). She was named Research Fellow (later Fellow) at Somerville College, Oxford, in 1946. During the next year she made weekly visits to Wittgenstein at Cambridge. He died in 1951, having named her one of his three literary executors, along with Georg Henrik von Wright (1916–2003) and Rush Rhees (1905–1989). The three young philosophers were charged with editing, translating, and publishing his philosophical writings, which were voluminous.

Anscombe's English translation of Wittgenstein's *Philosophical Investigations* (from the original German) was published in 1953. This was a monumental event in twentieth-century philosophy. She went on to translate and edit several more of his works, some by herself and some with others. Her monograph *An Introduction to Wittgenstein's Tractatus* was published in 1959. Two years earlier, she had published *Intention*, which her contemporary Donald Davidson (1917–2003) described as "the most important treatment of action since Aristotle" (Dolan). Two of her students, **Thomas Nagel** and **Roger Scruton** (Dolan; and personal communication), have made their own mark in the philosophy of sex. In 1970, three years after being elected Fellow of the British Academy, Anscombe was elected to Wittgenstein's Chair of Philosophy at Cambridge, where she remained until her retirement in 1986. Her *Collected Philosophical Papers* were published in three volumes in 1981. The final publication during her lifetime ("Practical Truth") appeared in 1999, when she was eighty. Anscombe died two years later in Cambridge, survived by her husband of fifty-nine years and their seven children.

Anscombe's philosophical work was subtle, original, and wide-ranging. Throughout her career, she was interested in ethics, both theoretical and applied. Her 1958 essay "Modern Moral Philosophy," which is still read and discussed in graduate seminars, helped revive study of the virtues. (Geach published a book on the topic, *The Virtues*, in 1977.) She coined the expression "**consequentialism**" to describe those normative ethical theories that make the rightness of actions depend solely on their consequences, an extrinsic property of action ("Modern Moral Philosophy," 12). Her own approach to morality, in keeping with the Roman Catholic Natural Law tradition to which she subscribed, was deontological. Certain act-types, she maintained, are intrinsically wrong. For example, it is always wrong to directly (intentionally) kill the innocent, however good the consequences of doing so may be. Anscombe considered U.S. President Harry S. Truman (1884–1972) a murderer (literally) for ordering the bombing of Hiroshima and Nagasaki ("Mr Truman's Degree"). She was also a lifelong opponent of **abortion**, which she considered murder. To put her beliefs into practice, she and her daughters blocked the entrance to an abortion facility in the early 1990s. They were arrested and jailed. John Finnis provided legal counsel.

Anscombe's views on **sexual ethics** are presented most perspicuously in a pair of essays: "You Can Have Sex without Children," from 1968, and the 1972 "Contraception and Chastity" (this has been widely reprinted, but Anscombe considered the former to be "perhaps argued more delicately and problematically"; *Collected Philosophical Papers*, vol. 3, viii). "Chastity," she points out, has both broad and narrow meanings. Narrowly speaking, it refers to **abstinence** from sexual intercourse (i.e., virginity). Broadly speaking, it refers to sexual virtue—the virtue that is distinctive to sex ("Contraception and Chastity," 136). In these essays Anscombe uses the word in the broad sense.

The aim of Anscombe's essays is to show that there is a *logical* difference, and therefore *possibly* a *moral* difference, between so-called safe-period sex (often referred to as "the rhythm method") and the various forms of contraceptive intercourse: those involving "the pill" (birth-control pills), condoms, and intrauterine devices (IUDs), for example. Anscombe's audience is her fellow Catholics. She is not trying to persuade non-Catholics of anything; nor could she, since she argues from distinctively Catholic premises (see *Collected Philosophical Papers*, vol. 3, vii). One way to understand Anscombe's essays is as an attempt to vindicate the Church's long-standing teaching on **contraception**. (Note that the first essay appeared before, and the latter after, Pope Paul VI's [1897–1978] 1968 encyclical *Humanae vitae*.) She is trying to show that the Church's teaching is *coherent*, not that it is true. She *assumes* its truth ("Contraception and Chastity," 137, 146). She is replying to the charge, leveled by Catholics and non-Catholics alike, that the distinction between safe-period sex and contraceptive sex is arbitrary. In her view, it is not.

To understand Anscombe, one must understand the concept of an intrinsically generative act. Some sex acts, considered as physical acts, are intrinsically generative, while others are intrinsically nongenerative. An act can be intrinsically generative even if it does not in fact produce offspring. Anscombe explains this by means of an analogy: "In order to be an intrinsically generative *sort* of act, an act need not *itself* be actually generative; any more than an acorn needs to produce an actual oak tree in order to be an acorn" ("You Can," 85). She then distinguishes between those sex acts that are intrinsically generative *in their intention* and those that are intrinsically *non*generative in their intention. The two distinctions cut across one another, producing four jointly exhaustive and mutually exclusive categories of sex act:

1. *Intrinsically generative both qua physical act and qua intentional act.* This category includes sexual intercourse performed with an intention to procreate but also safe-period intercourse.

2. *Intrinsically generative qua physical act but intrinsically nongenerative qua intentional act.* This category includes the pill and postcoital douching.

3. *Intrinsically generative qua intentional act but intrinsically nongenerative qua physical act.* This category includes artificial insemination.

4. *Intrinsically nongenerative both qua physical act and qua intentional act.* This category includes condoms and IUDs.

It may seem that the rhythm method and the pill are alike, for in both cases there is an intention not to procreate. But this is not the relevant intention. Some intentions are intrinsic to ("embodied in") acts, while others are extrinsic to acts. When a couple uses the pill, their act, considered as an intentional act, is intrinsically nongenerative. But when the same couple has intercourse during the safe period, their act, considered as an intentional act, is intrinsically generative. In the second case, the couple is leaving open the possibility of generation, whereas in the first case—involving the pill—they are not. In the second case, the couple is *evading* pregnancy; in the first case, the couple is *preventing* pregnancy. Jenny Teichman explains:

> [T]he intention to deprive someone of his goods is part of the essence of *fraud* but it is not part of the essence of *telling tall stories* although one may tell tall stories with the intention of depriving someone of his goods. It is part of the essence of *contraceptive sex* that there is an intention to avoid conception but it

is not part of the essence of *safe period sex*, under *that* description, that there is an intention to avoid conception, although one may choose the safe period with the intention of avoiding conception. (154; italics in original)

Anscombe takes it for granted (as part of Catholic teaching) that only marital intercourse is permissible. This of course rules out **homosexuality** as well as **adultery**. She also assumes (again, as part of Catholic teaching) that contraceptive intercourse, even within **marriage**, is impermissible. She is trying to show that safe-period sex is *not contraceptive* and therefore does not fall under the prohibition against contraceptive sex. This does not mean that a married couple may use safe-period sex with the intention never to procreate. This further (extrinsic) intention shows the couple to be unchaste. Moreover, if a couple marries with the *intention* of never procreating, their marriage is "invalid" or "no marriage at all" ("You Can," 90).

One should not infer from Anscombe's discussion that she believed sex to be bad. To the contrary: "[C]opulation, like eating, is of itself a good kind of action, since like eating it preserves human life" ("You Can," 89). We might say that there is a normative presumption in favor of marital sex acts. That presumption, like any other, can be overridden:

[O]ne individual act of eating or copulation can be bad only because there is something special about it that makes it bad: normally intercourse is morally good simply as a part of married life—it is a chaste act, and an act of the virtue of chastity in one who possesses that virtue. ("You Can," 89)

Nor does Anscombe hold the view that a desire for sexual pleasure is bad in itself. Here she criticizes St. **Thomas Aquinas** (1224/25–1274), whose doctrine on that point, she says, is "faulty and confused" ("You Can," 89). "God gave us our sensitive appetite, and its arousal without our calculation is part of the working of our life." But there *is* such a thing as intercourse "purely for pleasure," and it is condemned as such by Christianity.

Some marks of "being purely for pleasure" would be: immoderation in, or preoccupation with sexual pleasures; succumbing to desire against wisdom; insisting against the *serious* reluctance of the other partner (the qualification is needed because of some facts of male and female psychology). In all these cases but the last both parties may be heartily consenting. (90)

The motive of pleasure, for Anscombe, must be integrated into the marital life.

According to Anscombe, then, there is a logical difference between safe-period sex and contraceptive sex, where the latter includes use of the pill, condoms, IUDs, and the like. But not all logical differences are morally significant. There is a logical difference between being right-handed and being left-handed, for example, but nobody thinks that this difference grounds a difference in treatment. Why does Anscombe think that the logical difference she has identified makes a *moral* difference? As Teichman puts it, "The distinction . . . is obvious enough, but it is not always obvious just how and when it applies. Furthermore it is not obvious what the distinction rests on" (154–55). Why must a marital sex act be intrinsically generative both qua physical act and qua intentional act to pass moral muster? Why is the former not enough?

Here, Anscombe falls back on her Catholic Natural Law deontology. There are, according to Natural Law, certain basic goods that must not be chosen against (see Finnis, chap. 4, sect. 2). One of these is human life. To have contraceptive sex is to choose against the basic good of human life, for the sake of which marriage exists. It is to foreclose the *possibility* of conceiving. The act therefore betrays a disrespect for, indeed a defiance of, the moral law.

Anscombe's essays on contraception have not been warmly embraced by her fellow philosophers. Peter Winch (1926–1997) criticized Anscombe's 1972 essay by claiming that there is not, in fact, a logical difference between contraceptive sex and safe-period sex since, if a couple engages in safe-period sex as part of a "method" designed to avoid conception (it is not by accident that it is called the rhythm *method*), the couple is intending not to conceive. Anscombe replied, in effect, that Winch was confused. She reiterated the distinction between intentions that are embodied in acts and what she calls "further" intentions. She illustrated this distinction with the case of "industrial action." There are two ways one might thwart the aims of one's employer. The first is by "working to rule," which means doing one's job but no more than one's job. The second is by sabotaging the works. The intention of these acts—their *further* intention—may be the same, namely, thwarting the aims of one's employer, but the acts themselves, considered as intentional acts, differ. In the first case, one intends to do one's job (but no more). In the second case, one intends not to do one's job.

The analogy to safe-period and contraceptive sex is clear. In both cases, the couple's further intention may be to avoid conception, but only in the case of safe-period sex is one doing one's job, so to speak. In safe-period sex, one performs an act that is intrinsically generative both qua physical act and qua intentional act. In contraceptive sex, one performs an act that is intrinsically nongenerative qua intentional act, even if, as in the case of the pill, it is intrinsically generative qua physical act. This distinction shows, quite clearly, that Anscombe is a deontologist, for a consequentialist would evaluate the two acts solely in terms of their consequences, which, by hypothesis, are the same. A consequentialist would say that there is no intrinsic moral difference between safe-period and contraceptive sex. Anscombe believes that there *is* an intrinsic difference and that it resides in the intention that the act embodies. The distinction between evading and preventing is not *ad hoc*; it is familiar from many other contexts.

Bernard Williams (1929–2003) and Michael Tanner, who were colleagues of Anscombe at Cambridge at the time, criticized her 1972 essay by making the same point as Winch, although in different words. "We conclude that Prof. Anscombe has failed, even within her own kind of argument, to provide any coherent defence of the moral distinction between the pill method and the rhythm method" (Winch et al., 158). Anscombe replied as she had to Winch, by saying, in effect, that they were confused. They confused the intention *embodied* in an act with the *further* intention with which the act is performed—a distinction Anscombe had taken pains to highlight ("Contraception and Chastity," 145). Williams and Tanner went on to make a number of irrelevant (and, it must be said, impertinent) claims, such as that because contraception is "a momentous social and moral issue, involving the welfare and dignity of millions of people" (Winch et al., 159), it cannot be resolved by making careful distinctions between act-types. This assertion must have come as a shock to many philosophers, who believe that careful thought about human action (or any other topic) cannot possibly be in conflict with human welfare and dignity.

Williams and Tanner also chastised Anscombe for being insensitive to homosexuals. They said that "she is blankly ignorant if she believes that there are no homosexual unions in which the sexual act is as expressive of love . . . and as significant in the lives of the people concerned, as acts in a heterosexual union can be" (Winch et al., 160). But these were only passing remarks in Anscombe's essay; they had nothing to do with her central argument about contraception and should not, therefore, have come up in a critique of that essay. Finally, Williams and Tanner take Anscombe to task for "assimilat[ing] homosexual acts to masturbation." But to say that two things have something in common is not to say that they have all or even most things in common. In Anscombe's view, as we have seen, all nonmarital sex is morally impermissible: "[O]utside marriage, sexual acts are simply excluded" ("You Can," 91). Neither a homosexual act nor **masturbation** constitutes marital sex. Anscombe does not *argue* for the proposition that nonmarital sex is morally impermissible. She *assumes* it. It is part of the normative background of her discussion of contraception. To quote her husband Peter Geach, "Apart from the good of marriage that redeems it, sex is poison" (147).

See also Abstinence; Casual Sex; Catholicism, Twentieth- and Twenty-First-Century; Consequentialism; Contraception; Marriage; Marriage, Same-Sex; Natural Law (New); Russell, Bertrand; Thomas Aquinas (Saint); Wojtyła, Karol (Pope John Paul II)

REFERENCES

Anscombe, G.E.M. *The Collected Philosophical Papers of G.E.M. Anscombe.* Vol. 1: *From Parmenides to Wittgenstein.* Vol. 2: *Metaphysics and the Philosophy of Mind.* Vol. 3: *Ethics, Religion and Politics.* Oxford, U.K.: Blackwell, 1981; Anscombe, G.E.M. (1972) "Contraception and Chastity." Revised. In Michael D. Bayles, ed., *Ethics and Population.* Cambridge, Mass.: Schenkman, 1976, 134–53; Anscombe, G.E.M. *Intention.* Ithaca, N.Y.: Cornell University Press, 1957; Anscombe, G.E.M. *An Introduction to Wittgenstein's Tractatus.* London: Hutchinson University Library, 1959; Anscombe, G.E.M. "Modern Moral Philosophy." *Philosophy* 33 (January 1958), 1–19; Anscombe, G.E.M. (1957) "Mr Truman's Degree." In *The Collected Philosophical Papers of G.E.M. Anscombe,* vol. 3. Oxford, U.K.: Blackwell, 1981, 62–71; Anscombe, G.E.M. "Practical Truth." *Logos: A Journal of Catholic Thought and Culture* 2:3 (1999), 68–76; Anscombe, G.E.M. (1968) "You Can Have Sex without Children: Christianity and the New Offer." In *The Collected Philosophical Papers of G.E.M. Anscombe,* vol. 3. Oxford, U.K.: Blackwell, 1981, 82–96; Dolan, John M. "G.E.M. Anscombe: Living the Truth." *First Things: The Journal of Religion, Culture, and Public Life* 113 (May 2001), 11–13. <www.firstthings.com/ftissues/ft0105/opinion/dolan.html> [accessed 11 January 2005]; Finnis, John M. *Natural Law and Natural Rights.* Oxford, U.K.: Clarendon Press, 1980; Geach, Peter. *The Virtues: The Stanton Lectures 1973–74.* Cambridge: Cambridge University Press, 1977; Nagel, Thomas. "Sexual Perversion." *Journal of Philosophy* 66:1 (1969), 5–17; Paul VI (Pope). *"Humanae vitae." Acta Apostolicae Sedis* 60:9 (1968), 481–503; Scruton, Roger. *Sexual Desire: A Moral Philosophy of the Erotic.* New York: Free Press, 1986; Teichman, Jenny. "Intention and Sex." In Cora Diamond and Jenny Teichman, eds., *Intention and Intentionality: Essays in Honour of G.E.M. Anscombe.* Ithaca, N.Y.: Cornell University Press, 1979, 147–61; Winch, Peter, Bernard Williams, Michael Tanner, and G.E.M. Anscombe. (1972) "Discussion of 'Contraception and Chastity.' " Revised. In Michael D. Bayles, ed., *Ethics and Population.* Cambridge, Mass.: Schenkman, 1976, 154–63; Wittgenstein, Ludwig. *Philosophical Investigations.* Trans. G.E.M. Anscombe. New York: Macmillan, 1953.

Keith Burgess-Jackson

ADDITIONAL READING

Anscombe, G.E.M. "Contraception and Chastity." *The Human World,* no. 7 (May 1972), 9–30. Reprinted in HS (29–50). Reprinted, revised, in Michael D. Bayles, ed., *Ethics and Population.* Cambridge, Mass.: Schenkman, 1976, 134–53. <www.uwichill.edu.bb/bnccde/PH19B/conchastity .html> and <www.orthodoxytoday.org/articlesprint/AnscombeChastityP.htm> [accessed 6 October 2004]; Anscombe, G.E.M. "Modern Moral Philosophy." *Philosophy* 33 (January 1958), 1–19. Reprinted in *The Collected Philosophical Papers of G.E.M. Anscombe,* vol. 3: *Ethics, Religion and Politics.* Oxford, U.K.: Blackwell, 1981, 26–42; Anscombe, G.E.M. (1968) "You Can Have Sex without Children: Christianity and the New Offer." In *Renewal of Religious Structures: Proceedings of the Canadian Centenary Theological Congress* (Toronto, Canada, 1968). Reprinted in *The Collected Philosophical Papers of G.E.M. Anscombe*, vol. 3: *Ethics, Religion and Politics*. Oxford, U.K.: Blackwell, 1981, 82–96; Anscombe, G.E.M., and Peter T. Geach. *Three Philosophers*. [Aristotle, Thomas Aquinas, Gottlob Frege] Ithaca, N.Y.: Cornell University Press, 1961; Beis, Richard H. "Contraception and the Logical Structure of the Thomist Natural Law Theory." *Ethics* 75:4 (1965), 277–84; Cohen, Carl. "Sex, Birth Control, and Human Life." *Ethics* 79:4 (1969), 251–63. Reprinted in P&S1 (150–65); P&S2 (185–99); Conant, James. "Nietzsche, Kierkegaard, and Anscombe on Moral Unintelligibility." In D. Z. Phillips, ed., *Religion and Morality*. New York: St. Martin's Press, 1996, 250–98; Diamond, Cora. "Anscombe, G[ertrude] E[lizabeth] M[argaret]." In Lawrence C. Becker and Charlotte B. Becker, eds., *Encyclopedia of Ethics*, 2nd ed., vol. 1. New York: Routledge, 2001, 74–77; Ellis, Anthony. "Casual Sex." *International Journal of Moral and Social Studies* 1:2 (1986), 157–69. Reprinted in HS (125–37); Finnis, John M. "Natural Law and Unnatural Acts." *The Heythrop Journal* 11 (1970), 365–87. Reprinted in HS (5–27); Geach, Mary. "Marriage: Arguing to a First Principle in Sexual Ethics." In Luke Gormally, ed., *Moral Truth and Moral Tradition: Essays in Honour of Peter Geach and Elizabeth Anscombe*. Dublin, Ire.: Four Courts Press, 1994, 177–93; George, Robert P. "Elizabeth Anscombe, R.I.P." *National Review Online: NRO Weekend* (3–4 February 2001). <www.nationalreview.com/weekend/philosophy/philosophy-george020301.shtml> [accessed 15 February 2005]; Grisez, Germain. *Contraception and the Natural Law*. Milwaukee, Wis.: Bruce, 1964; Grisez, Germain, Joseph Boyle, John Finnis, William E. May, and John C. Ford. *The Teaching of "Humanae Vitae": A Defense*. San Francisco, Calif.: Ignatius Press, 1988; Kosnick, Anthony, William Carroll, Agnes Cunningham, Ronald Modras, and James Schulte. *Human Sexuality: New Directions in American Catholic Thought*. New York: Paulist Press, 1977; Kristjansson, Kristjan. "Casual Sex Revisited." *Journal of Social Philosophy* 29:2 (1998), 97–108; Paul VI (Pope). "*Humanae vitae*." *Acta Apostolicae Sedis* 60:9 (1968), 481–503. *Catholic Mind* 66 (September 1968), 35–48. Reprinted in Claudia Carlen, ed., *The Papal Encyclicals 1958–1981*. Raleigh, N.C.: Pierian Press, 1990, 223–36; and P&S1 (131–49); P&S2 (167–84); P&S3 (96–105); Rhees, Rush. (1963) "Chastity." In *Moral Questions*. Ed. D. Z. Phillips. New York: St. Martin's Press, 1999, 159–63; Scruton, Roger. "Sexual Morality and the Liberal Consensus." In *The Philosopher on Dover Beach—Essays*. Manchester, U.K.: Carcanet, 1990, 262–72; Stubblefield, Anna. "Contraceptive Risk-taking and Norms of Chastity." *Journal of Social Philosophy* 27:3 (1996), 81–100; Watt, E. D. "Professor Cohen's Encyclical." *Ethics* 80:3 (1970), 218–21; Winch, Peter, Bernard Williams, Michael Tanner, and G.E.M. Anscombe. "Discussion of 'Contraception and Chastity.'" *The Human World* (November 1972), 41–51. Reprinted, revised, in Michael D. Bayles, ed., *Ethics and Population*. Cambridge, Mass.: Schenkman, 1976, 154–63.

AQUINAS, THOMAS. *See* Thomas Aquinas (Saint)

ARISTOTLE (384–322 BCE). Aristotle, born in the small town of Stagira in northern Greece, can be counted among the two or three greatest and most influential philosophers in history. He studied and taught philosophy and science in Athens for most of his life, first as a student of **Plato** (427–347 BCE) in his school, the Academy, and later as the director of his own school, the Lyceum. A large number of Aristotle's works, none of them originally intended for publication, have been preserved, mostly as derived from the notes for lectures at the Lyceum. Even a relative chronology for Aristotle's works is extremely difficult to provide. Aristotle, perhaps more than Plato, was the true founder of philosophy as a discipline divided into specialized branches with concepts and methods of their own. He was, however, not only a philosopher but also an empirical scientist interested in collecting and organizing all humanly achievable knowledge. Aristotelian concepts, theories, and methods have been strongly influential in many areas of intellectual inquiry for more than 2,000 years.

Aristotle explores issues related to the philosophy of sex in various contexts. In the tenth book of the *Metaphysics* ([ca. 350 BCE?]; X 10, 1058a29–b26), he is interested in the relation between the notion of species and the sexual notions of male and female. He insists that the sexual difference between male and female is not a formal difference. Male and female are contrary attributes that belong to the genus animal as such but do not divide that genus into different species. Aristotle argues that male and female are not essential attributes of animals but instances of another type of belonging-to-something as such: They are attributes, the definitions of which include a reference to their subject. Male and female in animals correspond to odd and even in numbers: Only animals can be male or female, and each animal is one or the other (with minor exceptions, mentioned in Aristotle's biological works; see below). Aristotle also argues that male and female are differences in the matter of the genus animal and each animal species, but not in their forms.

The upshot of the metaphysical analysis is that the male and the female in each species have identical forms and, accordingly, the same essential capacities, but differ only in their material constitution. There are, of course, differences between male and female capacities related to reproduction, but in Aristotle's view, these capacities do not belong to the essence of what it is to be a member of certain animal species. Aristotle has a clear tendency to minimize the difference between the two sexes.

Aristotle's biological works are based on careful empirical research of animal life. The crucial text from the viewpoint of sex is the *Generation of Animals* (*Gen. an.*; ca. 340 BCE?), in which the reproductive capacity, its physiological preconditions, and the sexual behavior of animals are meticulously studied. Aristotle's approach is never purely descriptive even in biological studies. He applies metaphysical notions, for example, the distinction between material, formal, efficient, and final causes, as well as actuality and potentiality. He outlines a general theory of reproduction that proceeds from agreed starting points, based on a large collection of empirical material, and works toward basic theoretical principles.

Aristotle's theory shows a common reproductive pattern underlying differences between animal species in their sexual organs and ways of copulation. It was quite an imaginative and progressive accomplishment in its own time, despite its obvious faults from the viewpoint of modern biology. Aristotle's starting point, based on agreed observation, is that most animals generate as a result of intercourse between the male and the female. Exceptional cases of asexual and spontaneous generation are said to occur among primitive species, but in more developed animals the male and female and their copulation are needed for the reproduction of offspring.

The male and female in each species obviously have different reproductive roles. Aristotle explains these roles with reference to the sexual capacities of the sexes, the outward indications of which are the respective differences in sexual organs. There is surprisingly little difference between the male and female in the process that both sexes undergo in reproduction. Both male and female animals transform the food they eat by concocting (*pettein*) it into blood and further into seed (*sperma*), but the capacity to concoct is stronger in males due to the greater amount of natural heat and a special kind of air, *pneuma*, inserted into male blood during copulation. Aristotle calls the product of the concoction in both sexes seed (*sperma*, in a broad sense). It is semen (*sperma* in a restricted sense, or *gonê*) in males, and its female equivalents are the menses (*katamênia*).

The quantitative difference in concocting capacity turns into a qualitative one when Aristotle interprets the roles of male and female as corresponding to the metaphysical distinction between form and matter. He assumes that the male is the formal cause and the female the material cause of generation. The stronger capacity to concoct makes the male capable of forming and ejaculating seed, whereas being female is defined by the lack of these capacities. The female, however, has an important role of its own in reproduction. Here Aristotle rejects a view according to which the womb is only a container for the embryo, which is exclusively generated by the male. The female has the capacity to receive the form of an animal and to provide the matter for future offspring through the menses. So the embryo gets its form from the semen and its matter from the menses.

Aristotle's theory of generation is also targeted to refute a current view (the so-called pangenesis theory), according to which the seed derived either from one or both parents must contain elements from all the bodily parts. This view was used to explain, for instance, the likeness of offspring to its parents, but Aristotle considers it problematic and unnecessary to assume that the structures of the future animal are fully present in the seed. The seed only has to be capable of becoming an animal or, in Aristotelian terms, be potentially an animal. So the female parent provides the matter for the offspring through the menses, and the potential to become a certain type of animal inherent in the matter is actualized through the formative movement provided by the semen. Likeness to parents is explained (*Gen. an.*, IV, 1–3) by reference to the success of the semen (form) in prevailing over the menses (matter) in conception. In the ideal case, a male child resembling the father is generated, in a bit less ideal case, a male child resembling the mother, but female offspring are generated only when some kind of failure happens in conception.

Aristotle's theory of generation is not just a neutral philosophical theory; it also indicates a strong conviction of the supremacy of the male over the female. Aristotle assumes a hierarchical relation between form and matter, so the ascription of the formal role to the male can be taken to give support to the idea that the male is the more active, governing, and plainly better sex. The female is even called a natural imperfection in the species (*anapheria phusikê*; *Gen. an.*, IV 3, 767b6–12). One could ask why it is the male that is picked up as the formal cause instead of the female. The only supposedly neutral pieces of evidence for this choice are the greater natural heat of the male and the corresponding stronger ability to concoct blood. Aristotle's belief in male supremacy seems to have been more ideological than philosophical.

Aristotle presents plenty of examples of the hierarchical relation between the sexes in the animal world as well as in human societies. There is an extensive list of differences in lives (*bioi*) and habits (*ethê*) in the *History of Animals* (*Hist. an.*; ca. 340 BCE?): The female is, for example, softer in disposition, more mischievous, less simple, more impulsive, and more attentive to the nurturing of the young, whereas the male is more spirited, more savage, more simple, and less cunning (*Hist. an.*, IX 1, 608a1–b18). In the *Politics* (*Pol.*; ca. 330 BCE?), Aristotle suggests that men should hold permanent authority over women in the household, and women should be left out of political offices. The claim for male power is derived from the nature of the female deliberative faculty, which Aristotle famously says to be "without authority" (*akuron*; *Pol.*, I 12, 1260a12). He does not see any crucial moral or intellectual differences between men and women, but unlike Plato in the *Republic* (bk. 5, 451d–457d), he endorses a strict hierarchical and functional division of gender roles. Here, as well as elsewhere, Aristotle's thought reflects mainstream Greek popular morality.

Apart from an innovative theory of generation, Aristotle's biological works provide plenty of perceptive observations of the sexual life of animals. Different types of sexual organs and various methods of intercourse are explored and classified in a detailed way. Aristotle even pays attention to the pleasure experienced by females in intercourse. He observes that the pleasure of intercourse is caused by touch in the same region of the female as the male. The female's pleasure is said to be qualitatively similar to the male's and accompanied by liquid discharge. But this is not the female equivalent of semen, since its occurrence is accidental to conception (*Gen. an.*, I 20, 727b34–37).

Given his keen biological interest in sex, it is a bit surprising that the sexual aspect of **love** is a peripheral topic in Aristotle's works on human psychology and ethics. This negligence is all the more conspicuous when one looks at the careful attention Aristotle gives to **friendship** and love (*philia*) in his ethical treatises. Yet there is much of philosophical interest in Aristotle's scattered remarks on erotic love.

Following common usage, Aristotle refers to sexual appetite, and the pleasure resulting from its satisfaction, by the term *ta aphrodisia*, "the (desire for) the pleasures of Aphrodite" (*Ethica Nicomachea* [*Eth. Nic.*; ca. 325 BCE?], III 10, 1118a32; *Ethica Eudemia* [*Eth. Edu.*; ca. 330 BCE?], III 2, 1230b27). Sexual appetite is understood, in accordance with the Platonic tradition, as structurally analogous to the appetites for eating and drinking. These basic appetites are common to all animals. They are directed to the pleasures of taste and touch and related to the bodily processes of replenishment and dissolution. A pain produced by dissolution initiates an appetite, which is then directed to a pleasure produced by the corresponding replenishment (cf. *Rhetoric* [ca. 350 BCE?], I, 10–11). These types of pains and pleasures are perceived by the senses of touch and taste.

In Aristotle's ethics, the virtue of moderation (*sôphrosunê*) is concerned with the control of the appetites for food, drink, and sex. These appetites are natural and not morally reproachable. Unlike Plato, who considered bodily appetites unreliable and misleading by their essential nature, Aristotle thought that humans are innately disposed to develop correct forms of desires and emotional responses in situations related to bodily pleasures. The term "natural virtue" is used of this disposition (*Eth. Nic.*, VI 13, 1144b3–17). The basic appetites generate moral problems, because without the guidance of reason they are likely to develop in harmful directions. Excessive attention to them is slavish and bestial, because appetites do not belong to us as humans but as animals. The virtue of moderation is concerned with finding the correct mean between excess and deficit in appetites. Aristotle, however, says that "mistaking on the side of deficiency as regards pleasure, and taking less than the proper amount of delight in them, does not occur often, since such insensitivity is not human" (*Eth. Nic.*, III 11, 1119a6–7).

Aristotle's psychology of sex is, however, not quite as simple. **Sexual desire** has a more complex structure than the appetites for food and drink. First, sexual pleasure is connected not only to touch and taste, but it is sight that is the most salient sense in the experience of erotic pleasure (*Eth. Eud.*, III 2, 1230b26). The sight of erotically arousing objects not only initiates the appetite but also is often sufficient to give pleasure; one does not actually have to touch or taste the object of erotic appetite. Second, Aristotle distinguishes two aspects of erotic desire in some contexts: the appetite for intercourse (*epithumia sunousias*), on the one hand, and the desire for receiving affection (*phileisthai*), on the other (*Prior Analytics* [ca. 330 BCE?], II 22, 68a40–b7). The sense of sight might have operated as a mediating factor between these two aspects. Aristotle outlines a kind of expansive process in the development of erotic love. Love typically begins from the sight of an erotically arousing person, but the perception of bodily beauty and the sexual appetite aroused by it are able to expand into a recognition of the beloved's more abstract qualities (e.g., the beauty of his or her character).

Aristotle shows only limited interest in the problems of **sexual ethics** in his preserved works. His view of **marriage** was exceptional in the context of his time. While many

Greek writers regarded marriage merely as a means to produce legitimate children, Aristotle saw much broader prospects for the relationship of husband and wife. Despite the permanent hierarchical division of roles in family, the husband's rule over his wife is defined as political (*Pol.*, I 12, 1259b1–2), not aristocratical (as parents rule over children) or despotical (as masters rule over slaves); that is, the husband's rule over the wife is based on a kind of equality. Aristotle stresses that family life should aim at activities performed together for the common good as well as for mutual affection and delight. Husband and wife may even reach the highest form of friendship, based on virtue, if each partner is good in an appropriate way. Aristotle never explicitly mentions erotic love between husband and wife but clearly recognizes it to be possible. He says that erotic love (*to eran*) is an excess of friendship (*huperbolê philias*)—that is, an intense and exclusive attitude that can be directed at just one person (*Eth. Nic.*, IX 10, 1171a10–13). The intense quality of erotic love apparently allows it to be virtuously realized only between husband and wife, in the relation that Aristotle regarded as the most basic social tie humans are inclined to form (*Eth. Nic.*, VIII 12, 1162a16–19).

Although Aristotle might be exceptional in his views about marital love, his remarks about the violations of marriage are much more mainstream. **Adultery** (*moicheia*) is one of the acts he says is always wrong, but the term he uses means violating the rights of other men to their wives and possibly daughters. Extramarital sex with prostitutes or pederastic lovers is not morally problematic, while sleeping with a married woman is always unjust, given that the adulterer is aware of the status of his partner (*Eth. Nic.*, V 6, 1134a19–22). It is also implied that the man should take pains to find out his partner's marital status, since Aristotle elsewhere argues that ignorance does not relieve a person of his responsibility, if it is in his own power to acquire or maintain the relevant knowledge (*Eth. Nic.*, III 5, 1113b30–33).

Aristotle does not comment much on same-sex relationships. He criticizes Plato for accepting erotic relations, albeit without intercourse, between biological brothers or fathers and their sons in the ideal society of the *Republic* (bk. 3, 403a–c), in which permanent families were abolished (*Pol.*, II 4, 1262a33–39). In Aristotle's view, restrictions against **incest** should be stricter, but he does not seem to consider same-sex erotic relations otherwise morally problematic, even if they involve intercourse.

There is a famous passage (*Eth. Nic.*, VII 5, 1148b15–1149a4) that is often cited as an example of Aristotle's condemnation of same-sex relationships as morally depraved. Aristotle here mentions certain activities that are not naturally pleasurable but may become so as the result of sickness, habit, or innate deformities. These activities extend from cannibalism and cutting the stomachs of pregnant women to more harmless habits such as biting one's nails or eating coal or earth. Among the latter group an item is mentioned that is called *hê tôn aphrodisiôn arresin*. The problematic Greek phrase is plausibly interpreted as meaning the disposition of some men toward passivity in sexual conduct. Aristotle indicates that this disposition is likely to be developed as a result of violent treatment, presumably sexual abuse, in childhood. This disposition does not cover the active role in same-sex relationships, and it is not morally condemned, even though it is regarded as some sort of uncomfortable deviation.

Aristotle's interest in sex as a biologist and natural philosopher resulted in an original and influential theory concerning the roles of the male and female in generation. In his writings on human psychology and ethics, he does not systematically discuss topics related to the philosophy of sex but nevertheless makes interesting remarks on the topic. It was natural in Aristotle's view for humans to seek pleasure in sex. Sexual appetite is not a source of moral anxiety in itself, but it has to be controlled by reason in a virtuous human life. Desire for sex could also be expanded into a higher-level desire for mutual affection and erotic love between virtuous partners. Aristotle does not see particular moral problems of their own in same-sex relationships.

See also Abstinence; Beauty; Ethics, Virtue; Fichte, Johann Gottlieb; Friendship; Greek Sexuality and Philosophy, Ancient; Hegel, G.W.F.; Homosexuality, Ethics of; Judaism, History of; Plato; Thomas Aquinas (Saint)

REFERENCES

Aristotle. *The Complete Works of Aristotle. The Revised Oxford Translation*, vols. 1–2. Ed. Jonathan Barnes. Princeton, N.J.: Princeton University Press, 1984; Deslauriers, Marguerite. "Sex and Essence in Aristotle's Metaphysics and Biology." In Cynthia A. Freeland, ed., *Feminist Interpretations of Aristotle*. University Park: Pennsylvania State University Press, 1998, 138–67; Nussbaum, Martha C. "Platonic Love and Colorado Law: The Relevance of Ancient Greek Sexual Norms to Modern Sexual Controversies." *Virginia Law Review* 80:7 (1994), 1515–1651; Plato. (ca. 375–370 BCE) *The Republic. Cambridge Texts in the History of Political Thought*. Ed. Giovanni R. F. Ferrari. Trans. Tom Griffith. Cambridge: Cambridge University Press, 2000; Price, A. W. *Love and Friendship in Plato and Aristotle*. Oxford, U.K.: Clarendon Press, 1989; Sihvola, Juha. "Aristotle on Sex and Love." In Martha C. Nussbaum and Juha Sihvola, eds., *The Sleep of Reason: Erotic Experience and Sexual Ethics in Ancient Greece and Rome*. Chicago, Ill.: University of Chicago Press, 2002, 200–221.

Juha Sihvola

ADDITIONAL READING

Allen, Prudence. *The Concept of Woman: The Aristotelian Revolution*. Grand Rapids, Mich.: Eerdmans, 1997; Anscombe, G.E.M., and Peter T. Geach. *Three Philosophers*. [Aristotle, Thomas Aquinas, Frege] Ithaca, N.Y.: Cornell University Press, 1961; Aristotle. (ca. 340 BCE?) *De Partibus animalium* I and *De Generatione animalium* I (with passages from II. 1–3). Trans. David M. Balme. Clarendon Aristotle Series. Oxford, U.K.: Clarendon Press, 1992; Baltzly, Dirk. "Peripatetic Perversions: A Neo-Aristotelian Account of the Nature of Sexual Perversion." *The Monist* 85:1 (2003), 3–29; Clark, Elizabeth A. *Clement's Use of Aristotle: The Aristotelian Contribution to Clement of Alexandria's Refutation of Gnosticism*. New York: Mellen Press, 1977; Cole, Eve Browning. "Aristotle." In Timothy F. Murphy, ed., *Reader's Guide to Lesbian and Gay Studies*. Chicago, Ill.: Fitzroy Dearborn, 2000, 53–54; Cooper, John M. "Aristotle on Friendship." In Amélie Rorty, ed., *Essays on Aristotle's Ethics*. Berkeley: University of California Press, 1980, 301–40; Cooper, John M. "Aristotle on Natural Teleology." In Malcolm Schofield and Martha Nussbaum, eds., *Language and Logos: Studies in Ancient Greek Philosophy Presented to G.E.L. Owen*. Cambridge: Cambridge University Press, 1982, 197–222; Dover, Kenneth J. (1978) *Greek Homosexuality*, 2nd ed. London: Duckworth, 1989; Freeland, Cynthia A., ed. *Feminist Interpretations of Aristotle*. University Park: Pennsylvania State University Press, 1998; Furth, Montgomery. "Specific and Individual Forms in Aristotle." In Daniel Devereux and Pierre Pellegrin, eds., *Biologique, logique et métaphysique chez Aristote*. Paris: Editions du CNRS, 1990, 106–110; Gannon, Frank. "Aristotle on Relationships." *The New Yorker* (26 January 2004), 40; Gooch, Paul. "A Mind to Love: Friends and Lovers in Ancient Greek Philosophy." In David Goicoechea, ed., *The Nature and Pursuit of Love: The Philosophy of Irving Singer*. Amherst, N.Y.: Prometheus, 1995, 83–97; Halperin, David. *One Hundred Years of Homosexuality: And Other Essays on Greek Love*. London: Routledge, 1990; Knuuttila, Simo, and Juha Sihvola. "How the Philosophical Analysis of Emotions Was Introduced." In Juha Sihvola and Troels Engberg-Pedersen, eds., *The Emotions in Hellenistic Philosophy*. Dordrecht, Holland: Kluwer, 1998, 1–21; Kraut, Richard. *Aristotle on the Human Good*. Princeton, N.J.: Princeton University Press, 1989; Lloyd, G.E.R. *Science, Folklore, and Ideology: Studies in the Life Sciences in Ancient Greece.*

Cambridge: Cambridge University Press, 1983; MacKinnon, Catharine A. (1999) "Toward a New Theory of Equality." In *Women's Lives, Men's Laws*. Cambridge, Mass.: Harvard University Press, 2005, 44–57; Millgram, Elijah. "Aristotle on Making Other Selves." *Canadian Journal of Philosophy* 17:2 (1987), 361–76; Nussbaum, Martha C. "Eros and the Wise: The Stoic Response to a Cultural Dilemma." *Oxford Studies in Ancient Philosophy* 13 (1995), 231–67; Nussbaum, Martha C. *The Fragility of Goodness: Luck and Ethics in Greek Tragedy and Philosophy*. Cambridge: Cambridge University Press, 1986; Nussbaum, Martha C., and Juha Sihvola, eds. *The Sleep of Reason: Erotic Experience and Sexual Ethics in Ancient Greece and Rome*. Chicago, Ill.: University of Chicago Press, 2002; Okin, Susan Moller. "Aristotle." In *Women in Western Political Thought*. Princeton, N.J.: Princeton University Press, 1979, 73–96; Price, A. W. "Plato, Zeno, and the Object of Love." In Martha C. Nussbaum and Juha Sihvola, eds., *The Sleep of Reason: Erotic Experience and Sexual Ethics in Ancient Greece and Rome*. Chicago, Ill.: University of Chicago Press, 2002, 170–99; Rogers, Kelly. "Aristotle on Loving Another for His Own Sake." *Phronesis* 39:3 (1994), 291–302; Saxonhouse, Arlene. (1985) "Aristotle: Defective Males, Hierarchy, and the Limits of Politics." In Mary Lyndon Shanley and Carole Pateman, eds., *Feminist Interpretation and Political Theory*. University Park: Pennsylvania State University Press, 1991, 32–51; Sherman, Nancy. "Aristotle on Friendship and the Shared Life." *Philosophy and Phenomenological Research* 47:4 (1987), 589–613; Sihvola, Juha. "Emotional Animals: Do Aristotelian Emotions Require Beliefs?" *Apeiron* 29:2 (1996), 105–44; Sihvola, Juha, and Troels Engberg-Pedersen, eds. *The Emotions in Hellenistic Philosophy*. Dordrecht, Holland: Kluwer, 1998; Singer, Irving. "Friendship in Aristotle." In *The Nature of Love*, Vol. 1: *Plato to Luther*, 2nd ed. Chicago, Ill.: University of Chicago Press, 1984, 88–110; Spelman, Elizabeth V. "Aristotle and the Politicization of the Soul." In Sandra Harding and Merrill B. Hintikka, eds., *Discovering Reality: Feminist Perspectives on Epistemology, Metaphysics, Methodology and Philosophy of Science*. Dordrecht, Holland: Reidel, 1983, 17–30; Stanton, Domna C., ed. *Discourses of Sexuality: From Aristotle to AIDS*. Ann Arbor: University of Michigan Press, 1992; Tress, Daryl McGowan. "The Metaphysical Science of Aristotle's *Generation of Animals* and Its Feminist Critics." *Review of Metaphysics* 46:4 (1992), 304–41; Vlastos, Gregory. "The Individual as an Object of Love in Plato." In *Platonic Studies*. Princeton, N.J.: Princeton University Press, 1973, 3–34. Reprinted in Alan Soble, ed., *Eros, Agape, and Philia: Readings in the Philosophy of Love*. New York: Paragon House, 1989, 96–124; Winkler, John J. *The Constraints of Desire: The Anthropology of Sex and Gender in Ancient Greece*. New York: Routledge, 1990; Witt, Charlotte. "Form, Normativity, and Gender in Aristotle: A Feminist Perspective." In Cynthia A. Freeland, ed., *Feminist Interpretations of Aristotle*. University Park: Pennsylvania State University Press, 1998, 118–37.

ARTIFICIAL INSEMINATION. *See* Reproductive Technology

ARTS, SEX AND THE. This entry provides an overview of the principal ways issues about sexuality and philosophy are integrally related to the arts and an explanation for the close connection. "Arts" here refers to literature (fiction, drama, poetry), film, photography, architecture, and the performing arts—ballet but also circus. It includes what is termed "mass art" and so-called high art like opera and, with its shrinking audience, classical music. Exploring in detail the particular philosophical issues raised by sex and any individual art form, or discussing particular philosophical problems about sex, the body, and relationships that are often the focus not only of literature but of all the varieties of the fine and performing arts, is impossible. The specific topic will be the philosophical dimension of the treatment of sexuality by items of art and what that dimension tells us about sex and philosophy in relation to the arts. We will not discuss, say, D. H. Lawrence's (1885–1930) or Simone de Beauvoir's (1908–1986) views on women or the role of sex in relationships, unless they have implications for the philosophical dimensions of sexual representation in literature. Why, for example, is sex so often the central focus of much art? What does this tell us, philosophically, about sex in relation to art? Is there anything about sex and the way it is variously portrayed in the arts that explains the philosophical significance of sexuality, the arts, and the intimate relationship between them? With respect to representational art (film, some painting) and nonrepresentational art (most music, some dance), asking questions like, "Can music, dance, architecture, or landscape be gendered?" (see Brett et al.; Citron; McClary) and "Is ballet for 'sissies'?" may yield something philosophically significant about art and sex.

The interface between philosophy, sex, and the arts might be expected to exist primarily through aesthetics. Certainly, aesthetics and sex cross paths in ways that raise questions for both aesthetics and sexuality (e.g., in painting, of what is the focus on the [female] nude indicative; see Clark). However, the connection between aesthetics and (**sexual**) **ethics** has long been a topic in both these philosophical arenas. Aesthetic Formalism insists that aesthetic and moral judgments about works of art are logically separable and should be kept separate. Though this issue predates Oscar Wilde (1854–1900), he is often associated with it. In the preface to *The Picture of Dorian Gray*, Wilde proclaims, "There is no such thing as a moral or immoral book. Books are well written, or badly written. That is all." Although he is usually regarded as an aesthetic formalist, his work is so entwined with ethical issues that taking Wilde at his word is difficult. His books are morally charged in ways that make it nearly impossible to consider their aesthetic value apart from the moral stance they embody. Wilde's proclaimed aesthetic formalism may have been dictated more by social necessity than the belief that aesthetics and ethics, particularly sexual ethics, can or should be separated either in judgment or in life. The relationship between aesthetics and ethics, and its application in other, new fields like film studies and architectural theory, has become much discussed in philosophy (see Bermúdez and Gardner; Levine et al.; Levinson).

While connections between aesthetics and sexuality in the philosophy of the arts are well established, no less important or omnipresent for philosophy are ethical issues between sex and the arts and, emerging from yet beyond the ethics, fundamental problems in social, legal, and political philosophy, philosophical psychology, and metaphysics and theories of the self. There are, arguably, few areas of philosophy on which questions about sex and the arts do not touch. How television portrays the "nuclear family"; same-sex relationships, including **marriage**; the redevelopment of Times Square; religious attitudes toward sex—all are fodder for philosophizing about sex and the arts. It is primarily in film, literature, and the other arts that sexuality becomes problematized and sexual concerns are identified and portrayed. Everything from growing up to growing old has a sexual component. And it is through the arts that audiences or spectators come to reflect on sexually significant issues in their own lives.

Sex has been and continues to be theorized (some say overtheorized) in relation to the arts, perhaps because sex has been closely involved with the arts from their very inception. But philosophy in relation to sex and the arts has not been much discussed. With some exceptions—**Plato** (427–347 BCE), **Thomas Aquinas** (1224/25–1274), **Immanuel Kant** (1724–1804), and **Arthur Schopenhauer** (1788–1860)—sex has not been regarded as a topic worthy of philosophical inquiry (see Alexander). Philosophically investigating sex, like sex itself, has been largely suppressed and to some degree remains suppressed. By contrast, sex and philosophical issues about sex have long been portrayed and taken up in the arts, whether by Chaucer (ca. 1342–1400) or in cave paintings.

If any explanation seems necessary for the centrality of sex in art and literature—other than the generalizations that we are sexual beings, that from birth we develop psychosexually as well as physically, and that sexuality matters to us, consciously and unconsciously, because it is integral to life and the meanings we construct (all staples of psychoanalytic theory and of contemporary common sense)—then **Sigmund Freud**'s (1856–1939) account of sublimation offers the most well known theoretical account. Sublimation is

> a developmental process by which instinctual energies are discharged in non-instinctual forms of behaviour. The process involves (a) displacement of energy from activities and objects of primary (biological) interest on to those of lesser instinctual interest; (b) transformation of the quality of the emotion accompanying the activity such that it becomes "desexualized." . . . And (c) liberation of the activity from the dictates of instinctual tension. (Rycroft, 176)

Not only is much art and literature concerned with sex, but Freud's theory of sublimation (as well as common sense) maintains in this explanatory scheme that much of art itself is the product of sex (or its lack), along with unconscious desires and fantasies that are themselves irreducibly sexual. There are links between the concern, and at times preoccupation, of the arts with sexual themes and the aetiology of the arts in unconscious processes and feelings of **love** (including narcissism), hate, guilt, aggression, and shame. Even apart from Freud's theory of sublimation and the role repression plays in it, sex as often depicted in the arts is bound up with repressed motives and desires—a realm of consternation and confusion—where people do not clearly understand their own feelings, why they love those they love, why they do not love those they prefer to love. To say that the arts' discourse on love and sex primarily explores their irrationality and the ways in which that occurs, recurs, and is manifest in people's lives is not an inaccurate generalization.

Sublimation is just one part, albeit a central one, of a theme that is nearly ubiquitous in Freud's writing: the conflict between the individual and civilization. He discusses sublimation as a way of dealing with repression in *An Autobiographical Study* (*SE*, vol. 20, 64–65), where he says:

> The artist, like the neurotic, had withdrawn from an unsatisfying reality into this world of imagination; but, unlike the neurotic, he knew how to find a way back from it and once more get a firm foothold in reality. His creations, works of art, were the imaginary satisfactions of unconscious wishes, just as dreams are, and like them, they too were in the nature of compromises, since they too were forced to avoid any open conflict with the forces of repression. But they differed from the asocial, narcissistic products of dreaming in that they were calculated to arouse sympathetic interest in other people and were able to evoke and to satisfy the same unconscious wishful impulses in them too.

And in the *Introductory Lectures on Psycho-Analysis* (Part III; *SE*, vol. 16, 376–77), Freud goes on to say that the artist "earns their gratitude and admiration and he has thus achieved through his *phantasy* what originally he had achieved only *in* his phantasy—honour, power, and the love of women."

Take it or leave it, this is at least an explanation for the predominance of sexual themes in art—a reason why "art mirrors life"—and one that resonates with ordinary experience. To those worried about the apparent universality of Freud's claims about art, sex, and sublimation, it is worth saying that, contrary to received opinion and his own occasional misleading statements, Freud no more thought that *all* art was linked with the sexual than he thought that all dreams were sexual or that parents were responsible for all their children's neuroses. Nevertheless, he is not alone in thinking that sexuality is not only ever present but the most significant and revealing dimension of human nature and human relations, not merely by itself but also in its ramifications in other aspects of life. Freud explicitly affirms the ways sexuality informs character and subjectivity in ways so prevalent and profound as to be constitutive of a person—"identity-conferring," if you will. Many writers and artists who are known for examining the "human condition" would by and large concur.

On Freud's view, what is true of the connection between art, artists, and sublimation is true to a lesser extent about everyone or is manifested in different ways. Work—physical as well as intellectual labor—also involves sublimation, as does being the audience for art: watching films, reading books, listening to music. It is the ways in which sublimation is manifest in works of art that is unique to artists, not the sublimation. This ability to sublimate is an essential feature of being human.

Attempting to explain, perhaps, why sex is difficult to handle artistically, **Thomas Nagel** writes:

> Sex is the source of the most intense pleasure of which humans are capable, and one of the few sources of human ecstasy. It is also the realm of adult life in which the defining and inhibiting structures of civilization are permitted to dissolve, and our deepest presocial, animal, and infantile natures can be fully released and expressed, offering a form of physical and emotional completion that is not available elsewhere. ("Personal Rights," 100)

This view is common. It is, however, terribly wrong in ways that art, as a "reflection of life," not only testifies to but exposes when it is itself not deluded that in sex we are liberated. Sex is precisely a place where "the defining and inhibiting structures of civilization" are expressed, where our infantile natures are as much inhibited as expressed, and where "physical and emotional completion" is in varying degrees more often thwarted than not. If in sex the "inhibiting structures of civilization" disappear and our infantile nature is given free play, psychotherapy and therapists would be largely otiose. Further, the foundations of the artistic exploration of human beings as sexual beings would be missing, as would be the basis for the artistic examination of most of our lives, since they are bound up with sexuality in nearly every way at every turn. The romanticism rampant in literature and film undermines and harms philosophical reflection on sex and art, no matter how satisfying in other ways it may be. But views about sex and repression, like Nagel's, that are naively and hopelessly romantic do so as well. Freud thought that little sex was or could be completely satisfactory, for anyone, and that all sexual partners were, and had to be, ill-matched to some degree ("Universal Tendency"). Not only is Nagel's account of sex as emancipatory a traditional romanticization, but his view of the normal structure of sexual attraction is likewise ultraromantic, and it is this that grounds his understanding of sexual perversion (*Mortal Questions*, 39–52).

The romanticization of sex is itself a form of sublimation. In and of itself, none of this—sublimation, repression, even neurotic activity—is harmful. Indeed, it is necessary. Only when people are in the grips of certain misleading, albeit satisfying, conceptions (cognitive/emotional constructs) about love and sex are they unable to find (relative) satisfaction in them; only then do love and sex become a problem. All the arts, in their sexual representations, exploit, sustain, and construct these misleading conceptions, which is a large part of their attraction, along with their catering to harmless voyeurism and their transient mobilization and satisfaction of certain perverse, sadistic, and violent (but also usually harmless) tendencies in their audiences (see Levine). At the same time, however, art, using the same tools, may attempt to do just the opposite. Sexual representation by art may expose romanticizations and myths and elicit more accurate, or less misleading, conceptions of sex and love. But more often than not, art substitutes one partial truth or misrepresentation with another. Sex in art is controversial, in part, because it has this dual nature. Asserting what it might well elsewhere deny is constitutive of the dialogical and exploratory nature of artistic sexual representation (a feature absent in **pornography**).

Sex in art is often meant to inspire debate and evoke discourse. What usually passes as mere entertainment is also a form of both public discourse and public therapy. (It does not have to be very insightful discourse.) Art may be, as least partially, a result of sublimation or, to use Freud's description of a neurotic symptom as a "substitutive satisfaction"—"a substitute for something else that did not happen" (*Introductory Lectures on Psycho-Analysis* [Part III], *SE*, vol. 16, 280). But sexual representation in art, as in dreams, may also be therapeutic in dealing with repressed fantasies and desires, as a way of temporarily overcoming the need to express them. Particular repressions may be overcome, but repression, and so neurotic activity in general, can never be overcome *tout court*. It is a necessary part of ego protection and hence of living.

Jerome Neu asks whether "a morality of desire and fantasy [exists] alongside the ordinary morality governing action" (177). I assume the question rhetorical, that Neu is asking something more or other than whether *having* certain desires and fantasies is immoral. Sex in art often explores the reality and impact of the manifestations, reverberations, and consequences of desire and **fantasy**, a kind of moral enterprise. The arts, more than any other activity, recognize sex as the driving force that psychoanalysis and common experience have always contended it was. Art and literature both reflect and investigate ways in which sex is implicated even in areas of life that seem to have little to do with sex—for example, mourning and melancholia in relation to narcissism and suicide (see Freud, *Mourning and Melancholia*) and a fascination with horror and horror films *via* the "uncanny" (see Freud, "The Uncanny"; Schneider).

Consider "Cremaster," Matthew Barney's visually stunning, intellectually and artistically challenging exhibition and film series about gender, identity, and the moment a fetus becomes male or female. "Cremaster" examines and portrays these issues in artistic, technical, and intellectual ways that would not have been possible in an earlier epoch. It thereby illustrates that art is, at its most challenging but also at its worst, both a product of and a critical reflection on its era. Art is often a meditation on and engagement with the spirit of an age. Sexuality is always in large part definitive of such a spirit; it is always a central feature of a culture's ethos, including but not limited to its morals and mores. Nagel writes:

> Sex is one of the most difficult subjects to treat artistically, and what appears in the public domain is largely dominated by conventions that change over time but are not very reliable guides to the truth. Sex tends to be treated, for the most part, from a safe distance, however explicitly. Occasionally a brilliant writer like Henry Miller will get closer, but it doesn't happen very often. ("Personal Rights," 101)

True, artistic treatment of sex is "largely dominated by conventions that change over time." But this does not mean that the arts must be unreliable "guides to the truth" about sex. Whatever the "truths" about sex may be, artistic efforts to uncover them can no more avoid convention than they can avoid challenging it. Nagel does not say what the "truth" about sex is that Miller (1891–1980) approaches, nor what makes his writing "brilliant." Nagel, then, is merely revealing his own dated predilections (some might say "boyish") for the graphic: We are all products of an age. The irony in Nagel's assertions about literary and cinematic culture is that his view of sexual reality accepts much of the ordinary, public understanding of sex ("ultraromanticism") that he is here critical of such culture for promoting.

Why Nagel hesitates to congratulate more of the artistic culture, beyond Miller, is unclear. For even if we focus only on literary figures as examples, Dante (1265–1321), Shakespeare (1564–1616), George Eliot (1819–1880), Henry James (1843–1916), Edith Wharton (1862–1937), D. H. Lawrence, D. M. Thomas (1914–1953), Saul Bellow (1915–   ), Iris Murdoch (1919–1999), Philip Roth (1933–   ), and countless others, including some mass art romance novelists like Barbara Cartland (1901–2000), are extraordinarily insightful about the many "truths" (values, facets, salient features) of sexual reality. Whatever their aesthetic value, that their portrayal of sex and love satisfies people explains their broad appeal. The difficulty in compiling a list of artistic figures who portray sexual reality as it is, who get it right, is that the multifaceted and ubiquitous nature of sex requires a vast array of representations and, further, that sex is manifest in so many personal, social, and political issues. And all these in turn must be treated in ways that reflect the changing sensibilities of an age. Miller's and Lawrence's depictions of sex cannot be significant for later generations in the way they were for their contemporaries. (Thank goodness.) The artistic treatment of sex is ample evidence that attitudes about and understandings of sex, for better and for worse, are altered and inexorably continue to change. Clifford Geertz (1923–   ) claimed that cultural patterns as sets of symbols, religious ones in particular, are both models *of* and models *for* reality (93). Much the same can be said for the arts. While visual and literary representations of sex do not themselves denote cultural patterns, they may depict and dissect such patterns. They are caught up and implicated in such modeling in ways that make them constitutive of the models, part of the worldview and ethos of an age.

In an article on moral evolution in America written in the early 1960s, Sidney Ditzion (1908–   ) observed:

> Almost every social reform movement in American history carried a sexual component. The feminists, although mainly devoted to economic, political, and legal aspects of sexual democracy, harbored elements devoted to marriage reform and to the achievement of more satisfying sexual alliances for women. . . . Sex was on the mind of America at all times but found public expression only from the pens and mouths of the most daring citizens. (86)

Ditzion thinks there is a direct link between social reform movements and sexuality and between those movements and the arts. The arts—not all the arts all the time, of course, but some—are directly implicated in social reform. Insofar as the arts incorporate ethical and other philosophical perspectives, philosophical discourse on sex and the arts is also involved in social reform and, through social reform, in personal, political, and legislative changes affecting the sexual. Though the general trend in the link between the arts and social reform has been toward liberalization on sexual matters, the question whether liberalization has been good, sexually, morally, and in other ways, is debatable. Nor has social/sexual reform always been in the direction of liberalization. The arts can be equally instrumental in promoting the personal, social, and political *status quo* or in advancing conservative and reactionary, and at times philosophically informed, agendas. Is Hollywood reactionary or *avant-garde*? With film, as with other art forms, the answers are contested and can be adequately defended, if at all, only in a context that takes philosophical inquiry into sex seriously. Yet it has long been the case that analysis of these issues is done not by professional philosophers but mostly by art historians, cultural and literary theorists, and others. Just about every university department in the humanities and social sciences has been engaged with topics relating to philosophy/sex—except philosophy. This becomes less surprising when one realizes that philosophers have had relatively little to do even with the emotions until, in no small measure due to **feminism**, interest in the affective life burgeoned (see Soble, "Introduction").

Philosophical issues relating directly to sex and art include censorship and free speech, **privacy**, pornography, autonomy, identity, and others, both moral and metaphysical. But indirectly the subjects are virtually endless. A history of sex in the arts is also the history of art's engagement with human nature, with human relationships, with fidelity and infidelity, with interpretations of the problems of life, and with the role, significance, and meaning of sex in different kinds of lives and families. Freud has been criticized frequently for seeing or explaining so many things—some would say everything—in terms of sex. This is a vast oversimplification. But if there is an element of truth in asserting that art, like life, is "all about sex," it is because sex is all about, or all involved in, so many other things. It is implicated, for example, in the centrality, or lack thereof, of emotion to life, and the values and meanings attached to emotion. The visual arts and literature, in particular, along with humanities scholarship, have examined its connections with power, pleasure, and pathology. Insofar as art engages these themes, sexuality is a component. Without art, relatively little would be known about both daily life and civilization. The extent to which the arts engage sex, and have always done so, is evidence of the significance of both sex and the arts. Some aspects of art, like some philosophy, are concerned with improving human understanding. While one can extract philosophical themes from art and literature, there can also be a closer connection. Philosophy, literature, and art sometimes coalesce, so that doing art or writing a novel *is* doing philosophy. Thus, Martha Nussbaum and Iris Murdoch are right in seeing some literature as serious moral philosophy, an indispensable part of the ethical enterprise and a much needed tonic for professional moral philosophy. Similarly, the novels of Fyodor Dostoyevsky (1821–1881), Franz Kafka (1883–1924), and Saul Bellow are serious and profound, even if not systematic, reflections on meaning, fear, and transcendence or spirituality.

To think that issues of censorship, privacy, and the value of sex (especially religious versus secular views) that have always occupied the arts have changed or been transformed in or by contemporary art is mistaken. This is interesting, that the tensions and the subjects of discourse, like the body, remain similar, albeit not the same, despite a level of openness (some would say a lack of taste) about sex in the arts that is prevalent and unprecedented (see McNair; Soble, "The Mainstream"). The philosophical issues underlying sex in the arts remain more or less the same, as does the artist's (some artists) perennial clash with the personal, social, and political *status quo*. Nevertheless, there are new technologies embraced by the arts, new forms of performance art, new art forms (for example, videos and DVDs), and everything that is made possible by computer technology, from sophisticated graphic design and increased powers of digital photography to software-generated musical scores. Writing about the artists in her edited volume *Bad Boys and Sick Girls*, Linda Kauffman describes the artists she discusses as "interpreters of this brave new world" and as analyzing the "larger implications" of innovations in science, medicine, and technology (1–2). "By seizing these new technologies to radicalize artistic practices, they challenge society's most cherished assumptions about the body's integrity and rectitude. . . . Only they can expose the latent and manifest meaning of the world that already invisibly envelops us." For Kauffman, an irreducibly philosophical aspect to such art exists, though she does not call it philosophical. Concern with sexuality, gender, race, and the body is of course nothing new in art and literature, but the specific focus and artistic practices through which they are now examined are often distinctively contemporary. (See, for example, Barney; Brooks; Grosz and Probyn.) Contemporary artistic practices at times reflect postmodern themes and social malaise, but they are also inventive insofar as they incorporate the new technologies and reflect on the world, as artists have always done, morally as well as aesthetically, denying, in effect, that art, morality, and sex can or ever should be separated. It may well be the artists—writers, poets, filmmakers, composers, musicians, architects—rather than philosophers, historians, politicians, and religious leaders, who most meaningfully and most influentially, and often most profoundly, interpret, evaluate, and critically examine our ways of living, the ethos, values, tastes, and notions of right and wrong, dominant in the age.

Our discussion so far has been of a general nature. I now examine one specific case, a work of art that illustrates the contentious nature of sexual representation in contemporary art and its clash with politics and values. The case also illustrates the challenging (difficult to understand) and disturbing nature of sexual representation in contemporary art. It is therefore a good example of the continuing significance—personal, political, cultural, social—and remarkable novelty of sexual representation in contemporary art. If one role of art has been to enlarge and improve traditional understanding of those things that concern us most, then despite the Christian Right and politicians who for various reasons have undermined serious, progressive art in the United States, neither contemporary art nor literature has lost its way.

Bob Flanagan (1952–1996) was a poet, writer, and performance artist who died of cystic fibrosis (CF). Kauffman describes and discusses the significance of a site-specific installation and performance piece, *Visiting Hours*, that he and his partner Sheree Rose exhibited in museums from 1992 to 1995.

> *Visiting Hours* transforms the museum into a pediatric hospital ward, complete with a waiting room filled with toys, medical X-rays of Flanagan's lungs, and video monitors of his naked, bound body. In one chamber, the visitor comes upon Flanagan himself, propped up in a hospital bed, his home away from home. (21)

> Flanagan juxtaposes the pathology of CF with the "pathology" of masochism. He traces his masochistic proclivities back to infancy, when he spent long hours bound in his crib. From infancy forward, he was prodded and probed, X-rayed, transformed into a medical "specimen." . . . With Sheree Rose, his dominant "mistress," Flanagan takes sadomasochism into the art museum. While Robert Mapplethorpe's exposure of the forbidden world of gay sadomasochism was an important precursor, Flanagan and Rose make us realize how little theorizing has been devoted to *heterosexuality*, which for so long has been presumed to be "natural." (21)

> Male heterosexual submissives, moreover, constitute a substantial subculture, unacknowledged because their existence defies too many taboos. Flanagan exposes one of commercial sadomasochism's best-kept secrets: the majority of customers are not sadistic men seeking submissive women. Instead, a growing

number of men are willing to pay hefty sums to be clothed in diapers, put in playpens, suckled with bottles. On the one hand, such playacting permits men to return unashamedly to the pre-oedipal bliss of harmony with the mother. On the other hand, they enjoy being punished, spanked, made to clean house, do dishes. Since these men are often highly successful in public life, their sexual proclivities suggest a strong compulsion to repudiate masculine authority and privilege privately. (21)

Men are not fleeing from masculinity, they are fleeing from adulthood—adult responsibilities, failures, impossible social problems, unhappiness, complex relationships with women *and* with other men. Women are fleeing, too. But where men pay to act out fantasies of babyism privately, women prance down fashion runways in babydoll dresses. How else can one explain the current fashion phenomenon of preteen waifs carrying baby rattles and pushing other fashion models in prams? . . . *Visiting Hours* explores head on what fashion and advertising explore at one or more removes: the fulfillment of childhood wishes *un-idealized* by Madison Avenue. . . . Mike Kelley [another artist Kauffman discusses in the same essay] photographed Sheree Rose, eerily humping a stuffed toy rabbit (appropriately, since she is dominant, she is on top), while Bob, a "bottom," is smeared with excrement, wiping his bottom (22). . . . Signs of infantile existence litter the museum: a port-a-potty, pacifiers, blankets, a crib that seems more like a cage, toys like a Superman doll and Visible Man, which is designed to teach children anatomy, although this one excretes shit, mucus, and sperm. (24)

Neither money, success, fame, nor possessions bring happiness, Freud warned; the only source of satisfaction comes from the fulfillment of *childhood* wishes. *Visiting Hours* evokes scenes of infantile satisfactions (oral and anal, passive and aggressive). Since antipornography activists always argue that pornography must be banned so as not to sully the "impressionable minds" of children, it is particularly interesting how much *Visiting Hours* concentrates on childhood. Childhood, the exhibit implies, is tinged with sexual curiosity. (25)

Flanagan's art audaciously exposes the *process* of gender construction, particularly its weird ridiculousness. Rather than disavowing castration anxiety, Flanagan acts it out—he *performs* it. Rather than fetishizing the female body, he pokes and pierces his own. He was inspired in part by Rudolf Schwarzkogler, who "had himself photographed (supposedly) slicing off pieces of his penis as if it were so much salami." . . . Schwarzkogler's acts, however, are fake, whereas Flanagan's actions are real. He pierces the penis, attaches weights, clothespins, and nails it to a board. His acts are at once too literal for art, too visceral for porn. While Camille Paglia worships the penis and Andrea Dworkin damns it, Flanagan deflates it and them both. (26)

Kauffman discusses how Flanagan and other "transgressive artists" became the focus of the Christian Action Network and Senator Jesse Helms (1921–   ), who harassed these artists and sought, successfully in many cases, to stop the National Endowment for the Arts as well as private groups, publishers, and corporations from funding work like theirs. Predictably and simple-mindedly—if Kauffman's interpretation is anywhere near the truth—they see the work as pornographic and of course quite correctly as critically examining and undermining values fundamentalists and conservatives hold dear. These include a strong antihomosexual bias, an anti-pro-choice stance on **abortion**, and pro-censorship. Kauffman writes, "Literally hundreds of other recent art exhibitions besides Bob Flanagan's demonstrate that experimentation with the body is *the* aesthetic at Century's end" (37). If so, an interesting coalescence about what to focus on has emerged between visual, literary, and performance art.

This is not to say that all or most, or even the best, art in the late twentieth century and early twenty-first century is necessarily concerned with "philosophy of the body" (which includes gender, race, intersexuality, the disabled). But it is indicative of "where the action is." If one wants to study and investigate what is new in philosophy, sex, and the arts, go with the "body." This area deals with gender construction, the "constructedness . . . of all experiences, from birth to death" (Kauffman, 37), technology and science, the self, **beauty**, subjectivity, **objectification**, medicalization, along with more traditional artistic and philosophical concerns like privacy, sex, love, morality, rationality, truth, the emotions, and happiness. Such art remains the subject of censorship and so challenges it. And it must routinely weather the charge that it is obscene and/or pornographic.

If pornography refers to that which is the object, solely or primarily, of prurient or lewd interest, then these charges against creations like Flanagan's truly miss their mark (for most audiences). Kauffman's lucid explanation of his work makes this clear. In connection with the charge of obscenity, it is worth noting that similar accusations were leveled against Gustave Flaubert's (1821–1880) *Madame Bovary*, James Joyce's (1882–1941) *Ulysses*, Lawrence's *Lady Chatterley's Lover*, William Faulkner's (1897–1962) *Sanctuary* and *The Wild Palms*, J. D. Salinger's (1919–   ) *Catcher in the Rye*, Philip Roth's *Portnoy's Complaint*, Mark Twain's (1835–1910) *Huckleberry Finn*, and many other notable literary works and films. (See Bard for a history of film censorship, the extraordinary role religious groups [for example, the Catholic Legion of Decency] played in controlling the content of Hollywood films, and the gradual move toward liberalization.) Many of these novels, now acclaimed as classics and a solid part of the Western canon, explore sexuality—desire, repression, subjectivity—in ways that resonate with shared and formative experience. They are not simply literature; they are also deeply philosophical. Literature and art that approach sexuality philosophically have been far more influential than the academic philosophy that they have now come to influence and be influenced by.

See also Beauty; Completeness, Sexual; Desire, Sexual; Fantasy; Freud, Sigmund; Humor; Lacan, Jacques; Language; Law, Sex and the; Nagel, Thomas; Personification, Sexual; Perversion, Sexual; Philosophy of Sex, Overview of; Pornography; Poststructuralism; Utopianism

REFERENCES

Alexander, W. M. "Philosophers Have Avoided Sex." *Diogenes* 72 (Winter 1970), 56–74; Bard, Geraldine E. "Movies: Sexuality in the Cinema." In Vern L. Bullough and Bonnie Bullough, eds., *Human Sexuality: An Encyclopedia*. New York: Garland, 1994, 403–11; Barney, Matthew. "Cremaster." [Exhibition and film series] Guggenheim Museum, New York (January–May 2003); Bermúdez, José Luis, and Sebastian Gardner, eds. *Art and Morality*. London: Routledge, 2003; Brett, Philip, Elizabeth Wood, and Gary C. Thomas, eds. *Queering the Pitch: The New Gay and Lesbian Musicology*. New York: Routledge, 1994; Brooks, Peter. "Invasions of Privacy: The Body in the Novel." In *Body Work: Objects of Desire in Modern Narrative*. Cambridge, Mass.: Harvard University Press, 1993, 28–53; Citron, Marcia. *Gender and the Musical Canon*. Cambridge: Cambridge University Press, 1993; Clark, Kenneth. (1956) *The Nude: A Study in Ideal Form*. Princeton, N.J.: Princeton University Press, 1972; Ditzion, Sidney. "America, Moral Evolution in." In Albert Ellis and Albert

Abarbanel, eds., *The Encyclopedia of Sexual Behavior*, vol. 1. New York: Hawthorn, 1961, 82–89; Faulkner, William. (1931) *Sanctuary*. New York: Garland, 1987; Faulkner, William. (1939) *The Wild Palms*. New York: Garland, 1986; Flaubert, Gustave. (1881) *Madame Bovary*. Trans. Sylvère Lotringer. New York: Fine Creative Media, 2004; Freud, Sigmund. The following works by Sigmund Freud are in *The Standard Edition [SE] of the Complete Psychological Works of Sigmund Freud*, 24 vols. Trans. and ed. James Strachey. London: Hogarth Press, 1953–1974: (1925–1926) *An Autobiographical Study*. vol. 20, 3–74. (1915–1917) *Introductory Lectures on Psycho-Analysis*. vols. 15, 16. (1915) *Mourning and Melancholia*. vol. 14, 237–60. (1912) "On the Universal Tendency to Debasement in the Sphere of Love." vol. 11, 179–90. (1919) "The Uncanny." vol. 17, 217–56; Geertz, Clifford. "Religion as a Cultural System." In *The Interpretation of Cultures*. New York: Basic Books, 1973, 87–125; Grosz, E. A., and Elspeth Probyn, eds. *Sexy Bodies: The Strange Carnalities of Feminism*. London: Routledge, 1995; Joyce, James. (1922) *Ulysses*. Mineola, N.Y.: Dover, 2002; Kauffman, Linda S. "Contemporary Art Exhibitionists." In Linda S. Kauffman, ed., *Bad Girls and Sick Boys: Fantasies in Contemporary Art and Culture*. Berkeley: University of California Press, 1998, 19–49; Lawrence, D. H. (1928) *Lady Chatterley's Lover*. New York: New American Library, 2003; Levine, Michael. "Depraved Spectators and Impossible Audiences." *Film and Philosophy* [special edition] (2001), 63–71; Levine, Michael, Kristine Miller, and William Taylor, eds. ["Ethics and Architecture" issue.] *Philosophical Forum* 35:2 (2004); Levinson, Jerrold, ed. *Aesthetics and Ethics: Essays at the Intersection*. Cambridge: Cambridge University Press, 1998; McClary, Susan. *Feminine Endings: Music, Gender, and Sexuality*. Minneapolis, Minn.: University of Minnesota Press, 1991; McNair, Brian. " 'Not Some Kind of Kinky Porno Flick': The Return of Porno-Fear?" *Bridge*, no. 11 (August–September 2004), 16–19; Murdoch, Iris. *The Sovereignty of Good*. London: Routledge and Kegan Paul, 1970; Nagel, Thomas. *Mortal Questions*. Cambridge: Cambridge University Press, 1979; Nagel, Thomas. "Personal Rights and Public Space." *Philosophy and Public Affairs* 24:2 (1995), 83–107; Neu, Jerome. "Freud and Perversion." In Jerome Neu, ed., *The Cambridge Companion to Freud*. Cambridge: Cambridge University Press, 1991, 175–208; Nussbaum, Martha C. *Love's Knowledge: Essays on Philosophy and Literature*. New York: Oxford University Press, 1990; Roth, Philip. *Portnoy's Complaint*. New York: Random House, 1969; Rycroft, Charles. (1968) *A Critical Dictionary of Psychoanalysis*, 2nd ed. London: Penguin, 1995; Salinger, J. D. (1951) *The Catcher in the Rye*. Boston, Mass.: Little, Brown, 2001; Schneider, Steven. "Monsters as (Uncanny) Metaphors: Freud, Lakoff, and the Representation of Monstrosity in Cinematic Horror." *Other Voices: The (e)Journal of Cultural Criticism* 1:3 (January 1999). <www.othervoices.org/1.3/sschneider/monsters.html> [accessed 9 August 2004]; Soble, Alan. (1976) "Introduction." In Alan Soble, ed., *Sex, Love, and Friendship*. Amsterdam, Holland: Rodopi, 1997, xli–lii; Soble, Alan. "The Mainstream Has Always Been Pornographic" [Reply to McNair]. *Bridge*, no. 12 (October–November 2004), 33–36; Twain, Mark (Samuel L. Clemens). (1884) *The Adventures of Huckleberry Finn*. West Berlin, N.J.: Townsend Press, 2004; Wilde, Oscar. (1890) *The Picture of Dorian Gray*. London: Penguin, 2003.

Michael P. Levine

ADDITIONAL READING

Alexander, W. M. "Philosophers Have Avoided Sex." *Diogenes* 72 (Winter 1970), 56–74. Reprinted in POS2 (3–19); Barmé, Scot. *Man, Woman, Bangkok: Love, Sex, and Popular Culture in Thailand*. Lanham, Md.: AltaMira, 2002; Beardsmore, R. W. *Art and Morality*. London: Macmillan, 1971; Beauvoir, Simone de. (1949) *The Second Sex*. Trans. Howard M. Parshley. New York: Knopf, 1953; Bersani, Leo. *The Freudian Body: Psychoanalysis and Art*. New York: Columbia University Press, 1986; Bordo, Susan. " 'Material Girl': The Effacements of Postmodern Culture." In *Unbearable Weight: Feminism, Western Culture, and the Body*. Berkeley: University of California Press, 1993, 245–75; Bruce, Lenny. *The Essential Lenny Bruce*. Ed. John Cohen. New York: Random House, 1967; Budd, Malcolm. *Music and the Emotions*. London: Routledge, 1995; Bullough, Vern L. "Art: Painting, Sculpture, and Other Visual Art." In Vern L. Bullough and Bonnie Bullough, eds., *Human Sexuality: An Encyclopedia*. New York: Garland, 1994, 43–50; Bullough, Vern L. "Music and Sex."

In Vern L. Bullough and Bonnie Bullough, eds., *Human Sexuality: An Encyclopedia*. New York: Garland, 1994, 413–15; Butler, Judith. *Gender Trouble: Feminism and the Subversion of Identity*. New York: Routledge, 1990; Carroll, Noël. *A Philosophy of Mass Art*. Oxford, U.K.: Clarendon Press, 1998; Clark, Kenneth. *The Nude: A Study in Ideal Form*. New York: Pantheon, 1956. Princeton, N.J.: Princeton University Press, 1972; Colomina, Beatriz, ed. *Sexuality and Space*. New York: Princeton Architectural Press, 1992; Copjec, Joan. *Imagine There's No Woman: Ethics and Sublimation*. Cambridge, Mass.: MIT Press, 2002; Creekmur, Corey, and Alexander Doty, eds. *Out in Culture: Gay, Lesbian, and Queer Essays on Popular Culture*. Durham, N.C.: Duke University Press, 1995; Dynes, Wayne R., and Stephen Donaldson, eds. *Homosexuality and Homosexuals in the Arts*. New York: Garland, 1992; Ellis, Albert. "Art and Sex." In Albert Ellis and Albert Abarbanel, eds., *The Encyclopedia of Sexual Behavior*, vol. 1. New York: Hawthorn, 1961, 161–79. 2nd ed., New York: Jason Aronson, 1973, 161–79; Gay, Volney P. *Freud on Sublimation: Reconsiderations*. Albany: State University of New York Press, 1992; Gay, Volney P. *Reading Freud: Psychoanalysis, Neurosis, and Religion*. Chico, Calif.: Scholars Press, 1983; Grosz, E. A. *Space, Time, and Perversion: Essays on the Politics of Bodies*. New York: Routledge, 1995; Grosz, E. A. *Volatile Bodies: Toward a Corporeal Feminism*. St. Leonards, New South Wales: Allen and Unwin, 1994; Gurstein, Rochelle. *The Repeal of Reticence: A History of America's Cultural and Legal Struggles over Free Speech, Obscenity, Sexual Liberation, and Modern Art*. New York: Hill and Wang, 1996; Hamilton, Christopher. "Art and Moral Education." In José Luis Bermúdez and Sebastian Gardner, eds., *Art and Morality*. New York: Routledge, 2003, 37–55; Henberg, M. C. "George Eliot's Moral Realism." *Philosophy and Literature* 3:1 (1979), 20–38; Hersey, George L. *The Evolution of Allure: Sexual Selection from the Medici Venus to the Incredible Hulk*. Cambridge, Mass.: MIT Press, 1996; Hess, Thomas B., and Elizabeth C. Baker, eds. *Art and Sexual Politics: Women's Liberation, Women Artists, and Art History*. New York: Macmillan, 1973; Karlen, Arno. "The Arts and Sexuality." In Vern L. Bullough and Bonnie Bullough, eds., *Human Sexuality: An Encyclopedia*. New York: Garland, 1994, 50–53; Kaveny, Cathleen. "What Women Want: 'Buffy,' the Pope, and the New Feminists." *Commonweal* (7 November 2003), 18–38; Levine, Michael P. "Depraved Spectators and Impossible Audiences." In *Film and Philosophy* [special edition] (2001), 63–71; Levine, Michael P. "A Fun Night Out: Horror and Other Pleasures of the Cinema." In Steven Schneider, ed., *The Horror Film and Psychoanalysis: Freud's Worst Nightmares*. Cambridge: Cambridge University Press, 2004, 35–54; Levine, Michael P. "Lucky in Love: Love and Emotion." In Michael P. Levine, ed., *The Analytic Freud: Philosophy and Psychoanalysis*. London: Routledge, 2000, 231–58; Levine, Michael, ed. *The Analytic Freud: Philosophy and Psychoanalysis*. London: Routledge, 2000; Levine, Michael, and Steven Schneider. "Feeling for Buffy—The Girl Next Door." In James B. South, ed., *Buffy the Vampire Slayer and Philosophy*. Chicago, Ill.: Open Court, 2003, 294–308; Macarthur, Sally. "The Power of Sound, the Power of Sex: Alma Schindler-Mahler's *Ansturm*." In *Feminist Aesthetics in Music*. Westport, Conn.: Greenwood Press, 2002, 63–80; Miller, Henry. (1934) *The Tropic of Cancer*. New York: Medusa, 1940; Nagel, Thomas. "Sexual Perversion." *Journal of Philosophy* 66:1 (1969), 5–17. Reprinted in P&S1 (247–60); POS1 (76–88). Reprinted, revised, in Thomas Nagel, *Mortal Questions*. Cambridge: Cambridge University Press, 1979, 39–52; and POS2 (39–51); POS3 (9–20); POS4 (9–20); STW (105–12); Neu, Jerome. "Freud and Perversion." In Jerome Neu, ed., *The Cambridge Companion to Freud*. Cambridge: Cambridge University Press, 1991, 175–208. Reprinted in *A Tear Is an Intellectual Thing: The Meanings of Emotion*. New York: Oxford University Press, 2000, 144–65; STW (87–104). Original publication in Earl E. Shelp, ed., *Sexuality and Medicine*, vol. 1: *Conceptual Roots*. Dordrecht, Holland: Reidel, 1987, 153–84; Ollman, Bertell. *Social and Sexual Revolution: Essays on Marx and Reich*. Boston, Mass.: South End Press, 1979; Paglia, Camille. *Sexual Personae: Art and Decadence from Nefertiti to Emily Dickinson*. New Haven, Conn.: Yale University Press, 1990; Reitz, Charles. *Art, Alienation, and the Humanities: A Critical Engagement with Herbert Marcuse*. Albany: State University of New York Press, 2000; Robinson, Paul. *Opera, Sex, and Other Vital Matters*. Chicago, Ill.: University of Chicago Press, 2002; Roth, Philip. (1969) *Portnoy's Complaint*. [Twenty-fifth Anniversary Edition, with "Afterword"] New York: Vintage, 1994; Salmon, Catherine, and Donald Symons. *Warrior Lovers: Erotic Fiction, Evolution, and*

Female Sexuality. New Haven, Conn.: Yale University Press, 2001; Schjeldahl, Peter. "Nothing On: Sex and the Victorians." *The New Yorker* (30 September 2002), 143–44; Scruton, Roger. *Art and Imagination: A Study in the Philosophy of Mind*. London: Methuen, 1974; Swift, Jonathan. *Jonathan Swift: The Complete Poems*. Ed. Pat Rogers. New Haven, Conn.: Yale University Press, 1983; Wilcox, Rhonda V., and David Lavery, eds. *Fighting the Forces: What's at Stake in* Buffy the Vampire Slayer. Lanham, Md.: Rowman and Littlefield, 2002.

AUGUSTINE (SAINT) (354–430). The teachings of Christian theologian and bishop Augustine on **marriage**, reproduction, and sexuality, although developed in the midst of arcane theological controversies, decisively shaped the later Western tradition to our own time.

Aurelius Augustine was born in Thagaste, a town in the Roman province of Numidia (North Africa). Although his father Patricius (d. 372), a minor Roman official, remained unbaptized during Augustine's youth (*Conf*. 9.9), his mother Monica (d. 387) was an ardent Christian whose fervent hope for his conversion, Augustine later claimed, marked him even as a child (*Conf*. 1.11). Augustine's *Confessions*, from which our knowledge of his early life is derived, probably dates to 397 (O'Donnell, vol. 1, xli). The *Confessions* is unique in ancient literature for its retrospective analysis of a young man's intellectual and spiritual development—although such retrospective analyses must be treated with caution. Augustine's father, despite his somewhat limited resources, attempted to provide his son with the best possible education in grammar and rhetoric (*Conf*. 2.3). This education led to Augustine's early career as a teacher of rhetoric in North Africa and Italy, culminating in his appointment as public orator of Milan (*Conf*. 5.13).

Augustine had not been baptized as an infant. Christians of the first few centuries, anxious that postbaptismal sin might incur divine condemnation, often postponed baptism until the storms of adolescence were safely past. Although Augustine portrays himself as unusually undisciplined and sensual, the peccadilloes he reports seem minor in light of late-ancient custom. Nonetheless, he highlights these incidents to show the devious workings of libido and selfishness in "fallen" humans (*Conf*. 1.10, 1.19, 2.2–2.4, 3.1).

Like many young men marked for higher careers who would in mature adulthood need a wealthy wife of good social standing, Augustine in midadolescence took a concubine (*Conf*. 4.2, 6.11, 6.13). Concubinage was an arrangement sanctioned by Roman law, yet fell short of the economic, social, and other entailments of full matrimony. This unnamed woman, to whom Augustine reports he was faithful throughout their relationship of around fifteen years, bore a son, Adeodatus ("gift from God"), within the first year, but no other children followed. This fact is perhaps significant for interpreting Augustine's later condemnation of **contraception**.

In 384, when Augustine was thirty, his mother arranged a marriage for him with a suitable girl whose assets would assist his rising career. His betrothed, however, was only ten and a half; by Roman law she was ineligible for marriage until she was twelve (*Conf*. 6.13). The concubine of long standing was dismissed, while their gifted son (who died a few years later) remained with Augustine (*Conf*. 6.15). Unable to remain sexually abstinent until his betrothed reached marriage age, Augustine took yet another concubine for the interim (*Conf*. 6.15). His marriage, however, was never celebrated. After his "conversion," he committed himself to a life of perpetual celibacy and chastity.

In the *Confessions* (8.11), Augustine rhetorically describes the tug-of-war that existed within him as "Lady Continence" beckoned him to a life of sexual **abstinence** (but one full of "spiritual children"), while his "toys of toys," his old mistresses, lured him in another direction. He apparently never considered that he could be a *married* Christian; for him, the choice was absolute. A conversion experience, impelled by his reading of Romans 13:13, sealed his decision (*Conf.* 8.12). Renouncing sexual practice (although later plagued by sexual dreams; *Conf.* 10.30), Augustine was baptized at Easter time in 386 by Ambrose (339–397), bishop of Milan (*Conf.* 9.6), whose Platonizing exegesis of the Bible made it more intellectually palatable to Augustine (*Conf.* 5.14, 6.3–6.4). He returned to North Africa in 389–390 and adopted monastic practice. Within a few years Augustine was consecrated as priest and, in 395, as bishop of Hippo Regius. From this relatively insignificant town, he became a major voice in Latin-speaking Christianity.

In the mid-390s, Augustine studied the apostle **Paul**'s (5–64?) Epistle to the Romans, which described the tussle within humans between will and desire. Reading Romans 5–7, Augustine began to contemplate the depths of human sinfulness and its mysterious connection to Adam's disobedience, although some years would lapse before he elaborated a theory of original sin to displace his youthful, perhaps philosophically inspired, optimism that the will and reason could triumph over "lower" human inclinations.

For about nine years during his adolescence and early twenties, Augustine was an "Auditor" in the Manichaean sect (*Conf.* 3.11, 4.1). A dualistic and syncretistic religion of salvation originating in the third century, **Manichaeism** incorporated themes of Persian religion, Hellenistic philosophy, and (at least in North Africa) Christianity. Denying the goodness of creation, including God's ordination of human reproduction, Manichaeism posed a serious challenge to Christianity. (In Roman North Africa, Manichaeism, although outlawed, was favored by elite intellectuals [Brown, *Augustine*, 43].) The Manichaean "Elect," through sexual abstinence and dietary practices, were thought to assist the salvation of the cosmos. The "Auditors" or "Hearers," laypeople who lived in "the world," were subject to milder dietary, vocational, and sexual discipline.

The Manichaean myth of creation taught that the power of Darkness attacked, defeated, and consumed the power of Light in the first round of a protracted battle, dispersing sparks of Light, pieces of divine substance, throughout creation. Humans were created by Darkness who confined the sparks of Light within material bodies. Agents of Darkness tricked Adam into having sexual intercourse with Eve to ensure that the remaining sparks would be increasingly dispersed and encased in "matter" by repeated acts of procreation. So procreation is the invidious trick of the power of Darkness to defeat the forces of Light.

Manichaean "Auditors" (in contrast to the "Elect") might marry but were expected not to reproduce. From Augustine's guarded words and other sources, we gather that *coitus interruptus* was one contraceptive method that Manichaeans employed. In addition, they developed an early form of the "rhythm method," based on a calculation of a woman's fertile and infertile periods (*De mor. Man.* 18.65; *C. Faust.* 22.30). Given ancient ignorance of female fertility cycles, this method could not have been too effective. It is a guess, but only a guess, that Augustine's son was the result of "contraceptive failure." In the subsequent (thirteen to fourteen) years of nonprocreative sexual relations with his concubine, Augustine appears to have mastered contraceptive techniques. The Manichaean denigration of reproduction, however, left its mark on the Christian Augustine: Inverting the Manichaean evaluation, he held that reproduction was a "good," while contraception was an "evil."

The newly baptized Augustine embarked on an anti-Manichaean writing career, attacking their notions of reproduction and sexual practice. Denying Manichaean boasts of continence (*Conf.* 6.7; *De cont.* 26.12; *De mor. eccl. Cath.* 2.1), Augustine insinuates that they consumed human seed to free the divine Light within (*De mor. Man.* 68, 70–72; *De cont.*

27.12; *De nat. boni* 45–47; *De haer.* 46). While Manichaeans disdain motherhood, Augustine alleges, they boast that prostitutes "spare God" by preventing the furthering scattering of Light through reproduction (*C. Sec.* 21).

Thus the Manichaean creation myth served to justify their sexual practices. In one episode, an agent of Light devised a strategy to reunite the scattered sparks: He showed beautiful forms of males and females to the archons ("evil rulers" of the cosmos) to excite them, leading to ejaculations that would release the sparks of the divine fallen among the powers of Darkness. Augustine alludes to this myth at least six times in his anti-Manichaean writings (*C. Fel.* 2.7, 2.22; *C. Faust.* 6.8, 20.6, 22.98; *De nat. boni* 44; also *De haer.* 46.7–8.14). When a Manichaean opponent faulted the indulgent sexual practices of the patriarchs of the Old Testament, Augustine rejoined: *No* acts of the patriarchs could compare to the wickedness of the Manichaean teaching that God's substance, confined in bodies, is subjected to the violent motion of sexual acts and is released in ejaculation (*C. Faust.* 22.98).

Moreover, Augustine labels the Manichaean use of contraceptive measures "adultery," since it strikes at the central purpose of marriage, the production of children (*C. Faust.* 15.7). He counters Manichaean jibes at the polygamy and sexual activities of the Old Testament patriarchs; they were not motivated by lust but solely by the desire to produce children for God, a blessed activity at a time of population scarcity. Augustine also develops his infamous interpretation of the sin of Onan in Genesis 38 as *coitus interruptus*: Onan "spilled his seed upon the ground" so as not to impregnate his dead brother's wife (the practice of "levirate marriage," considered by ancient Hebrews to show a man's devotion to familial continuance). Augustine interprets Onan's behavior as a contraceptive practice rather than as a failure of fraternal charity (*C. Faust.* 22.84). That Pope Pius XI's (1857–1939; pope, 1922–1939) encyclical *Casti connubii* (31 December 1930) championed Augustine's interpretation illustrates the long reach of his influence (see "On Christian Marriage," 55).

Despite Augustine's campaign against Manichaean teachings, late in life he was branded as a "Manichaean" for his view that original sin tainted each developing fetus with guilt: The sex act was somehow, rather obliquely, associated with the process. To Augustine's opponents, his view implied that procreation was evil and that parents brought forth children doomed to the Devil—an interpretation that Augustine hotly disputed.

Augustine also composed in 388–389 a commentary on Genesis to refute Manichaeans who had charged that the book portrayed God anthropomorphically and made God complicit with the evil practices of humans (*De Gen. c. Man.* 1.17.27). Augustine's exposition of Genesis allegorized the story so much that he nearly lost flesh-and-blood characters. Augustine here *denied* that God's command to "reproduce and multiply" meant sexual, as contrasted with spiritual union. Thus the couple was enjoined to bring forth "good works" (*De Gen. c. Man.* 1.19.30, 2.11.15). At this stage, Augustine believed that God did *not* intend that sexual reproduction take place in Eden but allowed it only after the first sin (*De Gen. c. Man.* 1.19.30). Had the original righteousness of Adam and Eve been maintained in the Garden, no sexual union would ever have taken place.

Augustine retreated from this spiritualizing exegesis of Genesis 1–3 sometime early in the opening years of the fifth century. This time the debate centered on ascetic renunciation. By the late fourth century, enthusiasts for asceticism such as Jerome (330/47?–420) were encouraging virgins, as well as the widowed and the married, to honor God through lives of complete sexual abstinence. They should become "eunuchs for the sake of the Kingdom of heaven" (Matt. 19:12), like "the angels in heaven who neither marry nor give in marriage" (Matt. 22:30). Jerome assures renunciants that they will recapture the innocence of Eden and be "brides of Christ" in the afterlife (*Ep.* 22.1).

From early times, to be sure, Christianity had counseled sexual restraint. In 1 Corinthians 7, Paul had argued that because of the impending end of the world, it would be better for all who could control themselves to renounce sexuality and remain, like himself, unmarried. The ascetic movement of the mid- and late fourth century, inspired in part by the model of the Egyptian desert fathers and mothers, embraced sexual abstinence with enthusiasm. Although Jerome differentiated himself from "heretics" who championed asceticism out of hatred for the Creator, the material world, and the body (*Adv. Iov.* 1.3), he came dangerously close, or so his opponents thought, to denigrating marriage. In interpreting the Parable of the Sower, Jerome argued that the 100-fold harvest signaled virgins, the 60-fold widows, and the 30-fold married people (*Epp.* 48.2, 123.9). His treatise *Against Helvidius* (383) argued for the perpetual virginity of Jesus's mother Mary—and also for that of Joseph. He advocated the celibacy of the clergy and raised suspicions about the purity of married clergy (*Adv. Iov.* 1.34).

Jerome's views did not stand unchallenged. Christian opponents, for example, Jovinian, counterargued in the early 390s that married and celibate Christians, once they were baptized, were on a par if they were equally virtuous in other respects. They also cited numerous examples of married biblical characters who were blessed by God (see Jerome, *Adv. Iov.* 1.3, 1.5). Jerome's treatise *Against Jovinian* (392/393) is a rancorous attack on his opponent's "leveling" of marriage and celibacy. Championing celibacy, Jerome announced that professed Christian virgins would enjoy the highest quarters in heaven's "many mansions" (John 14:2; *Adv. Iov.* 2.28).

Augustine entered the fray somewhat belatedly. Attempting to rescue marriage from Jerome's denigration, Augustine composed two treatises in (probably) 401–402, *On the Good of Marriage* and *On Holy Virginity*. In these works Augustine agreed with Jerome that virginity was superior to marriage. But, unlike Jerome, he worried that ascetic renunciation would encourage pride (*De bono con.* 9.9, 26.35; *De sanc. virg.* 1.1). The abstinent who proudly imagine that they are "better" than the Old Testament patriarchs and matriarchs who married and bore children should, instead, fear for their own salvation (*De bono con.* 22.27). To those who "murmur," What would happen to the human race if everybody refrained from intercourse? Augustine replies (with Jerome) that the City of God would then, blessedly, be more quickly filled (*De bono con.* 10.10). Yet neither Jerome nor Augustine thought this scenario likely, given human "weakness." To explain why abstinence is now superior to procreation, even though God seemingly encouraged abundant procreation in the Old Testament, Augustine points to a "mysterious difference in times" (*De bono con.* 15.17).

In these treatises, Augustine argues that God had created male and female with the intention that they would unite for the production of children and for the "mutual companionship" of the sexes (*De bono con.* 1.1–3.3). Although he speculates on the mechanism by which Adam and Eve might have "multiplied" if they had not sinned, he breaks off his discussion with the note that it would be "tedious" to decide which theory was best (*De bono con.* 2.2–3.2)—an endeavor he would later find considerably less "tedious." Augustine argues that although children are one chief blessing of marriage, other blessings obtain as well, even if the couple remains childless. For example, marriage encourages an "order of charity" and provides a sexual outlet that forestalls extramarital **sexual activity**. In addition, marriage establishes a "sacred bond" between the couple that cannot be dissolved except by death (*De bono con.* 3.3, 4.4, 7.7, 15.17). Augustine would elaborate the three "goods" of marriage (reproduction, "fidelity," the "sacramental bond") in later works, for example, *On Marriage and Concupiscence* ([418?–421], *De nupt.* 1.11.10, 1.19.17, 1.23.21).

In *On the Good of Marriage*, Augustine briefly mentions another theme that he later develops: If a couple engages in sexual relations for the purpose of procreating a child, no sin attaches to the act. Marital sex undertaken out of lust, by contrast, constitutes a venial sin, yet God readily forgives such sins if the couple asks forgiveness (*De bono con.* 6.6, 10.11). **Adultery**, or fornication, on the other hand, constitutes mortal sin, which incurs damnation unless the sin is forgiven before the person's death. Those who change "the natural use" of sex into one "contrary to nature" (for example, using "a member" not ordained for the purpose) are strongly condemned (*De bono con.* 10.11–11.12). Augustine develops these themes later in *On Marriage and Concupiscence* (*De nupt.* 1.17.15, 2.35.20). There he condemns the "lustful cruelty" that attempts to secure barrenness or, failing that, procures **abortion**: Couples who engage in such practices do not deserve the title of "married" (*De nupt.* 1.17.15).

About the same time that Augustine composed his treatises on marriage and virginity, he undertook a second, less allegorized, exposition of Genesis. By Book III of *Literal Interpretation of Genesis* (*De Gen. ad litt.* [401–414]), he entertained the hypothesis that Adam and Eve could have had sexual intercourse, unmotivated by lust, in the Garden of Eden, had they not sinned (3.21.33). This thesis he affirms in Book IX: Their sexual organs would have obeyed their wills; they would have conceived children without experiencing bodily passion; and Eve would have given birth without pain (9.3.6, 9.14, 9.10.16–18). Later, during the Pelagian controversy, Augustine develops this affirmation of the essential goodness of marriage and reproduction while simultaneously condemning the evil of "lust."

The Pelagian controversy prompted Augustine to further develop his theology of sexuality and reproduction. The controversy, in its early stages, centered on the degree to which sin disabled the human will and in what God's grace to overcome that disability might consist (Brown, *Augustine*, chaps. 29–31). Pelagius (350?–after 418), a Christian from Britain who took up residence in Rome in the late fourth century, was apparently shocked by the laxity of Roman Christians. He heard that Augustine considered humans so corrupted by sin that they could will nothing good without God's special enabling intervention. In the *Confessions* (10.37), Augustine had prayed to God regarding his seeming inability to practice chastity: "Give what Thou commandest, and command what Thou wilt." To Pelagius, such teaching encouraged sloth and blasphemed against God's creation of good human nature. Pelagius argued that God had created humans with reason and free will (which was not forfeited through sin), had provided them with commandments for right living as well as examples of holy people in the Bible, most especially Jesus. Given these means of assistance, plus the cleansing of baptism, there was no reason why Christians could not scrape off the "rust" of sin and improve their lives. (Pelagius's *Letter to Demetrias* [413] provides a good summary of his teaching.) Pelagius appears as a "behaviorist" *avant le lettre*: Human social conditioning and bad examples, not "nature," were responsible for sin. Pelagius thus denied the notion of original sin that Augustine had progressively elaborated, and he called Christians to a more rigorous morality.

Augustine for years had pondered Paul's description, in his letter to the Romans, on the struggle between will and desire. In the *Confessions*, he had reflected on his own inability to keep chaste and on the propensity of humans from infancy onward toward greed, jealousy, and other forms of sinfulness (*Conf.* 1.7). To Augustine, the sinfulness of humankind seemed increasingly like a "given": Although God had not created the first humans sinful, sin was not, as Pelagius believed, a kind of "rust" that could be scraped off. Something had gone deeply astray very early in human history that rendered humans unable to **love** God and serve his will (*De civ. Dei* 10.30). Augustine dated this defect to the sin of Adam and Eve in the Garden.

In six or more treatises from this period of the Pelagian controversy (ca. 412–418) and in Book XIV (418?) of *City of God* (413–427), Augustine sets forth what Adam and Eve's disobedience in Eden entailed for all later humans (excepting Jesus). Although the first couple had been created with the ability to keep from sinning, with that one act of disobedience they had plunged the whole human race into perdition. Humans were henceforth rendered incapable of willing and doing the good, of loving God above all else. All now must die, rather than enjoy the immortality that would have been the first couple's, had they not sinned. One sign of human disobedience now affects the sexual organs, which the will cannot control; a second indication lies in the shame that humans feel at nakedness and sexual intercourse (*De civ. Dei* 14.17–18, 14.20). Since humans disobeyed God, the genital organs disobey the human will: Both unwanted erections and impotence when sexual relations were desired signal the sexual disorder (*De civ. Dei* 14.16). The "healing" of the now-disordered human person, Augustine believes, comes only from God's action in Jesus. Through God's "prevenient" grace, those whom God elects receive a special ability to respond, to achieve eternal life (albeit not on earth), to will and do the good (at least to a limited degree) with the proper motivation of love for and "delight in" God. Those who do not receive this grace are left in the "mass of perdition" in which the first sin had thrust all humans (see *De corrept. et gratia* 34–38; *De spiritu et litt.* 5; *De dono persev.* 35). Christian baptism does not wash away all the traces of original sin, and death and unruly sexual appetites remain to remind humans of that sin and its punishment.

Book XIV of *City of God* provides a kind of (now) untestable "thought experiment": If Adam and Eve had not sinned, they would have reproduced by sexual means while still in Eden, but their sexual organs would have moved at the command of their wills (as do other body parts), no raging lust would have overtaken them, and defloration and labor pains would have been unknown. Free from sickness, death, weariness, hunger, and thirst, the first humans and their offspring would have enjoyed a "purity of love" (*De civ. Dei* 14.10, 15–16, 22–26). Augustine compares his imaginary Adam to the placid farmer of Virgil's (70–19 BCE) *Georgics* (3.136), preparing his mares to receive the generating seed (*De civ. Dei* 14.23; *Opus imperf.* 5.14).

Try as Augustine might to uphold the goodness of marriage and reproduction, a new generation of Pelagian opponents arose to challenge him. Chief among them was Julian of Eclanum (early fifth century; died after 420), an Italian bishop of good family who argued that Augustine's teaching displayed an ignorance of human biology and blasphemously implied that God had so mismanaged human reproduction that all babies enter the world tainted by original sin. Julian and other Pelagian bishops (who had been condemned in "Tractoria" [418] by Zosimus, the Bishop of Rome [reigned, 417–418], on the grounds that they denied grace and underestimated the ravages of sin) solicited highly placed friends to accuse Augustine of "Manichaeism" in his alleged denigration of human creation (see Augustine, *C. duas ep. Pelag.* 1.3.1; 1.4.2). Augustine defended his views, Julian replied to Augustine, and the battle was joined (see Brown, *Augustine*, chap. 32; Clark, "Vitiated Seeds").

In declaring Augustine ignorant of human biology, Julian mentioned what "everyone" knew, that sexual excitement (spurred by the "vital fire") was necessary for erection to occur, the seeds to "cook," and pregnancy to result (see Augustine, *De nupt.* 2.25.12; *C. Iul.* 3.26.13). In Peter Brown's memorable phrase, the body was a "human Espresso machine" that must bubble up to the right degree of "heat" for erection and impregnation to occur (*Body and Society*, 17). By contrast, Augustine denies that the seed is formed by "lust"; it is formed by God directly (*C. Iul.* 4.12.2). Although Augustine wished to affirm God's blessing of procreation (*C. Iul.* 5.34.8), his claim, to Julian, only further implicated God in the passage of sin from generation to generation. Moreover, Julian (appealing to **Aristotle** [384–322 BCE]) argued that properties acquired "by accident" (the guilt of the first sin) cannot "wander off " from their proper subject (Adam and Eve) to others (see Augustine, *C. Iul.* 5.51.14), and what is given "by nature" to humans at the first creation cannot be changed by one man's act of will (see Augustine, *C. Iul.* 6.16.6; *Opus imperf.* 1.96, 2.94, 3.109.2–3, 3.142.2, 4.120, 5.46, 6.26–27). Furthermore, if parents can transmit sin to their children through their sexual act, they must not have been released from that sin through regenerating baptism. So did Augustine deem the sacrament ineffective? (See Augustine, *C. Iul.* 6.18.7.) Julian found Augustine's teachings irreligious: God's power and goodness are called into question if we believe that the womb of a baptized woman, a "temple of God," becomes the site for the Devil to work his ravages (see Augustine, *C. Iul.* 6.43.14). Are we to think that parents are, in effect, "murderers of their own children"? (See Augustine, *C. Iul.* 5.43.10.) Augustine's zeal to condemn unbaptized infants seemed cruel to Julian (see Augustine, *C. Iul.* 5.43.10).

Following a widely accepted notion of his day, that an essential feature of marriage lay in sexual intercourse, Julian faults Augustine's novel insistence that Joseph and Mary were truly "married" even though they had never—so Christian teachers were affirming—had intercourse (see Clark, " 'Adam's Only Companion' "). Such a view would support the notion that sexless marriage was a higher state (see Augustine, *C. Iul.* 5.46.12, 5.48.12, 5.62.16; *De nupt.* 2.37.22). And in his last attacks on Augustine, Julian rebuts Augustine's notion that shame at nakedness and sexual intercourse, as well as women's pain in labor, result from original sin. In making this argument, Julian appeals to a kind of "comparative anthropology" and animal behavior (see Augustine, *C. Iul.* 4.81.16; *Opus imperf.* 4.43–44, 6.26, 6.29).

Julian also attacks Augustine's interpretation of Paul. For Julian, when Paul wrote that sin arose "through one man" (Rom. 5:12), he could not possibly have meant "through reproduction," for everyone knows that reproduction takes two (see Augustine, *Opus imperf.* 2.56.1, 2.75). Augustine responds that it is not from *woman's* "seed" that generation occurs but from the man's. Since male insemination precedes female conception, Paul is correct in saying "through one man" (*Opus imperf.* 2.83, 3.85.4). For Augustine, the woman receives the already-vitiated seed from the man, conceives, and bears the child (*Opus imperf.* 2.179). The transfer of original sin, as well as the disorderly behavior of the sexual organs, commentators have noted, appears to be a "male problem."

Julian finds Augustine's views to be so antisexual and antiscientific that he mocks his opponent's image of the placid farmer sowing his seed and preparing his mares. Augustine, he suggests, would have liked a world without wombs and penises. As Julian pictures that world, the woman's entire body would have been fecund, and children would have "sweated out" of her pores and joints. The male would have assisted her, not with a penis, but with plowshares and hoes, "harvesting" the "forest" of her unbridled fecundity. Poor woman, Julian laments, scraped over by ploughs and hoes! Only a "Manichaean" (which he declares Augustine to be) would favor that sort of arrangement (see Augustine, *Opus imperf.* 5.15).

The newly discovered letters of Augustine reveal that late in life he slightly relaxed his position. In *Letter* 6*, which Augustine wrote to Atticus, bishop of Constantinople I around 421, he faults his opponents for implying that he condemns marriage and God's blessing on reproduction (6*.3). He now distinguishes a legitimate "conjugal concupiscence" from that raging "concupiscence of the flesh" that prompts illicit relations outside (as well as inside) of marriage (6*.5). Even if we go so far as to posit that there might have been some "concupiscence of the flesh" in Eden, it certainly was not such that the spirit would have had to struggle against the flesh (6*.7–8).

Augustine's praise of the "goods of marriage" rescued that institution from the denigrations of both Manichaeans and zealous ascetics. Nonetheless, his condemnation of contraception and abortion, of sexual practices that could not lead to conception, and of "lust" as a venial sin, marked Western Christian **sexual ethics** for centuries to come.

See also Abstinence; Animal Sexuality; Anscombe, G.E.M.; Beauty; Catholicism, History of; Catholicism, Twentieth- and Twenty-First Century; Desire, Sexual; Gnosticism; Manichaeism; Marriage; Paul (Saint); Thomas Aquinas (Saint); Wojtyła, Karol (Pope John Paul II)

WORKS OF AUGUSTINE

Abbreviations of Augustine's works stand for the following titles (in English): *C. Faust.* = *Against Faustus the Manichean*; *C. Fel.* = *Against Felix the Manichean*; *C. duas ep. Pelag.* = *Against Two Letters of the Pelagians*; *C. Iul.* = *Against Julian the Pelagian*; *C. Sec.* = *Against Secundinus*; *Conf.* = *Confessions*; *De bono con.* = *On the Good of Marriage*; *De civ. Dei* = *On the City of God*; *De cont.* = *On Continence*; *De corrept. et gratia* = *On Correction and Grace*; *De dono persev.* = *On the Gift of Perseverance*; *De Gen. ad litt.* = *On the Literal Interpretation of Genesis*; *De Gen. c. Man.* = *On Genesis against the Manichees*; *De haer.* = *On Heresies*; *De mor. eccl. Cath.* = *On the Morals of the Catholic Church*; *De mor. Man.* = *On the Morals of the Manichees*; *De nat. boni* = *On the Nature of the Good*; *De nupt.* = *On Marriage and Concupiscence*; *De sanc. virg.* = *On Holy Virginity*; *De spir. et litt.* = *On the Spirit and the Letter*; *Ep. Epp.* = *Letter, Letters*; *Opus imperf.* = *The Unfinished Work against Julian of Eclanum*.

Augustine's works cited can be found in (1) *Nicene and Post-Nicene Fathers*, 1st series, vols. 1–5. Ed. Philip Schaff. Grand Rapids, Mich.: Eerdmans, 1978–1979; (2) *Fathers of the Church*, vols. 8, 14, 16, 21, 24, 27, 35, 81, 86. Washington, D.C.: Catholic University of America, 1947–   ; (3) *Works of Saint Augustine: A Translation for the 21st Century*, vols. I/1, I/9, I/23–I/26. Ed. John E. Rotelle. Trans. Edmund Hill. Brooklyn, N.Y.: New City Press, 1990–   ; and (4) Elizabeth A. Clark, ed. *St. Augustine on Marriage and Sexuality*. Washington, D.C.: Catholic University of America, 1996.

REFERENCES

Brown, Peter. (1967) *Augustine of Hippo: A Biography*, rev. ed. London: Faber and Faber, 2000; Brown, Peter. *The Body and Society: Men, Women, and Sexual Renunciation in Early Christianity*. New York: Columbia University Press, 1988; Clark, Elizabeth A. " 'Adam's Only Companion': Augustine and the Early Christian Debate on Marriage." *Recherches Augustiniennes* 21 (1986), 139–62; Clark, Elizabeth A. "Vitiated Seeds and Holy Vessels: Augustine's Manichean Past." In *Ascetic Piety and Women's Faith: Essays on Late Ancient Christianity*. Lewiston, N.Y.: Mellen Press, 1986, 291–349; Jerome. *Against Jovinian* [*Adv. Iov.*]. *Against Helvidius. Letters.* In *Nicene and Post-Nicene Fathers*, 2nd series, vol. 6. Ed. Philip Schaff. Grand Rapids, Mich.: Eerdmans, 1979; Julian of Eclanum. [Writings found in the texts of Augustine referred to in the entry]; O'Donnell, James J. *Augustine's Confessions*, 3 vols. Oxford, U.K.: Clarendon Press, 1992; Pelagius. (413) *Letter to Demetrias*. In *The Letters of Pelagius and His Followers*. Trans. and ed. B. R. Rees. Woodbridge, U.K.: Boyell Press, 1991, 29–70; Pius XI (Pope). "On Christian Marriage" (*Casti connubii*). *Catholic Mind* 29:2 (1931), 21–64; Virgil. (37–29 BCE) *Georgics*. Trans. T. C. Williams. Loeb Classical Library. Cambridge, Mass.: Harvard University Press, 1913.

Elizabeth A. Clark

ADDITIONAL READING

Alexander, W. M. "Sex and Philosophy in Augustine." *Augustinian Studies* 5 (1974), 197–208; Anderson, Gary. "The Garden of Eden and Sexuality in Early Judaism." In Howard Eilberg-Schwartz, ed., *People of the Body*. Albany: State University of New York Press, 1992, 47–68; Augustine. *The Works of Saint Augustine, III/11: Newly Discovered Sermons*. Trans. Edmund Hill. Hyde Park, N.Y.: New City Press, 1997; Babcock, William S. "Augustine's Interpretation of Romans (A.D. 394–396)." *Augustinian Studies* 10 (1979), 55–74; Babcock, William S. "Cupiditas and Caritas: The Early Augustine on Love and Human Fulfillment." In William S. Babcock, ed., *The Ethics of St. Augustine*. Atlanta, Ga.: Scholars Press, 1991, 39–66; Babcock, William S., ed. *The Ethics of St. Augustine*. Atlanta, Ga.: Scholars Press, 1991; Barbone, Stephen. "Augustine." In Timothy F. Murphy, ed., *Reader's Guide to Lesbian and Gay Studies*. Chicago, Ill.: Fitzroy Dearborn, 2000, 63–64; Beatrice, Pier Franco. *Tradux peccati: alle fonti della dottrina agostiniana del peccato originale*. Milano, Italy: Università Cattolica del Sacro Cuore, 1978; BeDuhn, Jason. *The Manichaean Body in Discipline and Ritual*. Baltimore, Md.: Johns Hopkins University Press, 2000; Blackburn, Simon. "The Christian Panic." In *Lust: The Seven Deadly Sins*. New York: Oxford University Press/New York Public Library, 2004, 49–63; Bohlin, Torgny. *Die Theologie des Pelagius und ihre Genesis*. Uppsala, Sweden: A.-B. Lundequistska Bokhandeln; Wiesbaden, Ger.: Otto Harrasowitz, 1957; Bourke, Vernon J. *Joy in Augustine's Ethics*. Villanova, Pa.: Villanova University Press, 1979; Boyarin, Daniel. *Carnal Israel: Reading Sex in Talmudic Culture*. Berkeley: University of California Press, 1993; Brown, Peter. *Augustine and Sexuality*. Berkeley, Calif.: Center for Hermeneutical Studies, 1983; Brown, Peter. "A New Augustine" [Review of *Saint Augustine*, by Garry Wills] *New York Review of Books* (24 June 1999), 45–50; Brown, Peter. *Religion and Society in the Age of St. Augustine*. New York: Harper and Row, 1972; Chadwick, Henry. *Augustine*. Oxford, U.K.: Oxford University Press, 1986; Clark, Elizabeth A. *History, Theory, Text: Historians and the Linguistic Turn*. Cambridge, Mass.: Harvard University Press, 2004; Clark, Elizabeth A. (1979) *Jerome, Chrysostom, and Friends: Essays and Translations*, 2nd ed. New York: Mellen Press, 1982; Clark, Elizabeth A. "Vitiated Seeds and Holy Vessels: Augustine's Manichean Past." In *Ascetic Piety and Women's Faith: Essays on Late Ancient Christianity*. Lewiston, N.Y.: Mellen Press, 1986, 291–349; and Karen L. King, ed., *Images of the Feminine in Gnosticism*. Philadelphia, Pa.: Fortress Press, 1988, 367–401; Clark, Elizabeth A., and Herbert Richardson, eds. *Women and Religion: A Feminist Sourcebook of Christian Thought*, 1st ed. New York: Harper and Row, 1977. Rev. and expanded ed., *Women and Religion: The Original Sourcebook of Women in Christian Thought*. San Francisco, Calif.: HarperCollins, 1996; Coyle, J. Kevin. "The Cologne Mani Codex and Mani's Christian Connections." *Eglise et Thèologie* 10 (1979), 179–93; Dittes, James E. "Continuities between the Life and Thought of Augustine." *Journal for the Scientific Study of Religion* 5:1 (1965), 130–40; Dollimore, Jonathan. *Sexual Dissidence: Augustine to Wilde, Freud to Foucault*. Oxford, U.K.: Clarendon Press, 1991; Fredriksen, Paula. "Paul and Augustine: Conversion Narratives, Orthodox Traditions, and the Retrospective Self." *Journal of Theological Studies* [n.s.] 37 (1986), 3–34; Gardner, Iain, and Samuel N. C. Lieu, eds. *Manichaean Texts from the Roman Empire*. New York: Cambridge University Press, 2004; Hartle, Ann. *The Modern Self in Rousseau's Confessions: A Reply to St. Augustine*. Notre Dame, Ind.: University of Notre Dame Press, 1984; Hugo, John J. *St. Augustine on Nature, Sex, and Marriage*. Chicago, Ill.: Scepter, 1969; Hunter, David G. "Resistance to the Virginal Ideal in Late-Fourth-Century Rome: The Case of Jovinian." *Theological Studies* 48 (1987), 45–64; Kaye, Sharon M., and Paul Thomson. *On Augustine*. Belmont, Calif.: Wadsworth, 2001; Laeuchli, Samuel. "What Did Augustine Confess?" *Journal of the American Academy of Religion* 50:3 (1982), 379–409; Lieu, Samuel N. C. (1985) *Manichaeism in the Later Roman Empire and Medieval China: A Historical Survey*, 2nd ed. Tübingen, Ger.: J.C.B. Mohr, 1992; MacDonald, Scott. "Primal Sin." In Gareth B. Matthews, ed., *The Augustinian Tradition*. Berkeley: University of California Press, 1999, 110–39; Markus, R. A. (1970) *Saeculum: History and Society in the Theology of St. Augustine*, rev. ed. Cambridge: Cambridge University Press, 1988; Merdinger, J. E. *Rome and the African Church in the Time of Augustine*. New Haven, Conn.: Yale University Press, 1997; Miles, Margaret R. *Augustine on the Body*. Missoula, Mont.: Scholars Press, 1979; Miles, Margaret R. *Desire and Delight: A New Reading of Augustine's Confessions*. New York: Crossroad, 1992; Miles, Margaret R. "Infancy, Parenting, and Nourishment in Augustine's *Confessions*." *Journal of the American Academy of Religion* 50:3 (1982), 349–64; Nolan, John Gavin. *Jerome and Jovinian*. Washington, D.C.: Catholic University of America, 1956;

Noonan, John T., Jr. (1965) *Contraception: A History of Its Treatment by the Catholic Theologians and Canonists*, enlarged ed. Cambridge, Mass.: Harvard University Press, 1986; O'Connell, Robert J. *St. Augustine's Confessions: The Odyssey of Soul*. Cambridge, Mass.: Harvard University Press, 1969; O'Donnell, James J. *Augustine: A New Biography*. New York: HarperCollins/Ecco, 2005; O'-Donnell, James J. *Augustine's Confessions*, 3 vols. Oxford: Clarendon Press, 1992. <www.georgetown .edu/faculty/jod/> [accessed 17 November 2004]; Pagels, Elaine. *Adam, Eve, and the Serpent*. New York: Random House, 1988; Parsons, Wilfrid. *A Study of the Vocabulary and Rhetoric of the Letters of St. Augustine*. Washington, D.C.: Catholic University of America, 1923; Plinval, Georges de. "Points de vues rècents sur la thèologie de Pèlage." *Recherches de science religieuse* 46 (1958), 227–36; Power, Kim. *Veiled Desire: Augustine on Women*. New York: Continuum, 1996; Rackett, Michael R. *Sexuality and Sinlessness: The Diversity among Pelagian Theologies of Marriage and Virginity*. Unpublished Ph.D. dissertation. Duke University, 2002; Ranke-Heinemann, Uta. (1988) *Eunuchs for the Kingdom of Heaven: Women, Sexuality, and the Catholic Church*. Trans. Peter Heinegg. New York: Penguin, 1990; Rees, B. R., ed. *The Letters of Pelagius and His Followers*. Trans. B. R. Rees. Woodbridge, U.K.: Boyell Press, 1991; Schlabach, Gerald W. "Friendship as Adultery: Social Reality and Sexual Metaphor in Augustine's Doctrine of Original Sin." *Augustinian Studies* 23 (1992), 125–47; Schmitt, Emile. *Le Mariage chrètien dans l'oeuvre de saint Augustin: Une thèologie baptismale de la vie conjugale*. Paris: Etudes Augustiniennes, 1983; Schott, Robin May. (1988) "Augustine's Views of Women and Sexuality." In *Cognition and Eros: A Critique of the Kantian Paradigm*. University Park: Pennsylvania State University Press, 1993, 43–58; Shaw, Brent. "The Family in Late Antiquity: The Experience of Augustine." *Past and Present* 115 (1987), 3–51; Soble, Alan. "Correcting Some Misconceptions about St. Augustine's Sex Life." *Journal of the History of Sexuality* 11:4 (2002), 545–69. Rev. version, <www.uno.edu/~asoble/pages/augbos.htm> [accessed 17 November 2004]; Solomon, Robert C. " 'I Can't Get It Out of My Mind': (Augustine's Problem)." *Philosophy and Phenomenological Research* 44:3 (1984), 405–12; Warfield, Benjamin Breckinridge. *Studies in Tertullian and Augustine*. Westport, Conn.: Greenwood Press, 1970; Wermelinger, Otto. *Rom und Pelagius: Die theologische Position der Römischen Bishöfe im Pelagienischen Streit in den Jahren 411–432*. Stuttgart, Ger.: Anton Hiersemann, 1975; Wills, Garry. *Saint Augustine*. New York: Viking, 1999.

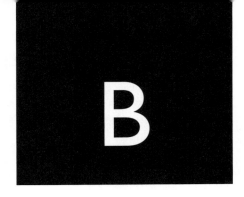

BATAILLE, GEORGES (1897–1962). Georges Bataille, the French writer, pornographer, and philosopher, spent his childhood and school days in Rheims. His childhood was traumatic, as his father, Joseph-Aristide (a postmaster), suffered from advanced syphilis, a fact that influenced Bataille's thought in many ways (see his *Story of the Eye*). Bataille used several pseudonyms for his early clandestine novels (e.g., *Madame Edwarda* [1941]), such as "Lord Auch," "Pierre Angélique," and "Luis Trente." As a young man, Bataille was deeply religious and wanted to be a priest. Instead he became a librarian, in Paris (1922), but religious motives, or countermotives, loom large in his writings. Bataille's lifestyle was, to a certain degree, debauched; he liked to drink, gamble, and visit prostitutes. All this has definite meaning for his novels and philosophy.

Bataille wrote much, but a large part of his work is peculiarly fragmented and has an unfinished feel about it. Some books have an autobiographical character, such as *On Nietzsche*. His ideas are intended to be radically shocking; they invert normally accepted thought about sexuality and eroticism as if to show their soft underbellies (see, especially, *Erotism: Death and Sensuality*). He was involved with French intellectuals and artists of his time and exerted considerable influence over them as well as over the younger generation, including **Michel Foucault** (1926–1984). His thought is far-ranging, and his ideas of eroticism form only a part of it. The philosophers who influenced him were **G.W.F. Hegel** (1770–1831) and **Friedrich Nietzsche** (1844–1900). He was an expert on the **Marquis de Sade** (1740–1814) and **Sigmund Freud** (1856–1939).

Bataille separates **love**, about which he says little, from sexuality and eroticism. This makes his thought disturbing from the view point of Christianity. A key feature is his insistence on a close connection among eroticism, pain, and death. "Pain" here means torture—the meaning of the word should not be taken figuratively or metaphorically. In 1925, Bataille received an authentic photograph (1905) of the Chinese Torture of One Hundred Pieces, in which a young man is tied to a pole and a torturer is cutting him to pieces. Bataille kept this rare picture all his life and used to meditate by looking at it closely. He ultimately decided that the victim was erotically ecstatic or that the expression on his face was of infinite joy. Bataille claimed that this picture, in which eroticism is clearly not connected with love, changed his life. It is also important to see the bridge between the Chinese Torture and the Christian Mystery of the Cross. Bataille was never far from the Christianity that he wanted to subvert.

Bataille was thus able to join the deepest joy and the erotic feelings with the most horrible of pains and torture. But he also sought a connection between sex and death. One way of forging it is through biology (surprising as that might sound). Bataille asks us to think of a single-cell organism, such as an amoeba, which reproduces by dividing into two new amoebae. In doing so, the original organism vanishes, dies, and two new organisms are formed. Here death and reproduction are connected in a manner that cannot fail to entertain the

Hegelian dialectical imagination: The original organism dies yet lives on in its offspring. The next step for Bataille was to draw a distinction between sexuality and eroticism. This is done again through biology: Sexuality is reproductive, and all animals practice it, but eroticism requires human thought, values, **fantasy**, and desire. If love is uninteresting, sex is, too. Love is too soft; sex is too hard. Only eroticism and its fantasies are the proper object of research and subject of fiction.

Bataille's fictional world has been defined as that of a debauchee but not a libertine. This distinction is important. To be a libertine means that someone tries to maximize his or her pleasures by any means. A true libertine, like Sade, might turn to crime or any subversive or perverted act to satisfy desire. He or she might also develop idiosyncratic whims that require satisfaction. A debauchee, by contrast, wants to degrade and ruin himself or herself through (paradoxically) fantasy, desire, and pleasure-seeking. The debauchee seeks waste, excrement, disgust, remorse, and terror, where the deepest satisfactions are supposed to be found. Bataille gazed at the Chinese torture picture (terror), visited brothels (disgust), and gambled (disaster) to satisfy his debauched lust. His philosophy of eroticism reflects these personal experiences and cannot be understood without acknowledging them. His father had syphilis; brothels meant syphilis; Bataille frequented brothels, which he loathed. The interpretation is clear.

Bataille's idea that eroticism is connected with debauched desire, and that debauchery is focused on waste, must be understood theoretically, not only biographically. By doing so its paradoxical nature can be minimized. Why would anyone want pain, disgust, and waste? This is the key question in Bataille's theory of eroticism. How can one enjoy that which is unenjoyable?

Bataille was familiar with the work of sociologist Marcel Mauss (1872–1950) on the potlatch ritual of the American Indians of the Northwest. In this ritual, large quantities of goods are given away or destroyed. Bataille saw here an alternative kind of economic system, one not based on the accumulation of goods and their enjoyment in a rationally maximizing manner. On the contrary, the ritual wasted goods, but this empowered people and gave them enjoyment. Bataille found in this ritual the inspiration for an economics in which waste, exemplified by sperm, menstrual blood, urine, and feces, was the key concept. These materials he connected with the taboos and ritual sacrifices that are, according to cultural anthropology, widespread. Especially important for Bataille were the Aztec sacrificial practices in which thousands of victims were killed in a colorful manner and their flesh eaten. He read this as a sign of a carnal and happy culture. The economy and culture of waste justified, for Bataille, the thesis that eroticism is a debauched activity geared toward loss, humiliation, pain, and death. Behind this philosophy the figure of Sade, whose heroes eat human excrement as a great delicacy, looms large.

Bataille's view of eroticism is both radical (*viz.*, his theory of waste and debauchery) and conservative. It is conservative because his thought is always connected to the Catholic ideas of God and salvation. There is no hope for the salvation of man without God, but God is dead (Bataille accepts Nietzsche's thesis); yet Bataille struggles with the idea of God throughout his writing career. If there is no God, every act is a meaningless symbol of death. We are all promised death, and we reach the abyss in debauchery. In mystical fashion, Bataille announces that the abyss itself is God. So God is dead and death is god.

Bataille says little about **homosexuality**. He might flirt with perverted forms of **incest**, but even this requires corpses. Bataille's basically male model of eroticism emphasizes heterosexual copulation and contact with female prostitutes, which is again connected with the ideas of waste (money), risk (illness), and shame (desiring unworthy persons). For

Bataille, prostitutes are (dead) beasts. His view of women in general seems to be colored by his love for and loathing of female prostitutes. In *Erotism* he designates women as "the privileged objects of desire" and claims that "[n]ot every woman is a potential prostitute, but prostitution is the logical consequence of the feminine attitude" (131). His discussion of religious **prostitution** suggests that he sees commercial prostitution as in some sense divine. The whore, Madam Edwarda, is God.

See also Arts, Sex and the; Beauty; Buddhism; Hegel, G.W.F.; Paglia, Camille; Paraphilia; Perversion, Sexual; Poststructuralism; Sacher-Masoch, Leopold von; Sade, Marquis de; Sado-masochism; Tantrism

REFERENCES

Bataille, Georges. (1957) *Erotism: Death and Sensuality*. Trans. Mary Dalwood. San Francisco, Calif.: City Lights, 1986; Bataille, Georges. *My Mother, Madame Edwarda and the Dead Man*. Trans. Austryn Wainhouse. London: Marion Boyars, 2000; Bataille, Georges. (1945) *On Nietzsche*. Trans. Bruce Boone. New York: Paragon House, 1992; Bataille, Georges. (1928) *Story of the Eye by Lord Auch*. Trans. Joachim Neugroschel. San Francisco, Calif.: City Lights Books, 1987; Mauss, Marcel. (1950) *The Gift: The Form and Reason for Exchange in Archaic Societies*. Trans. W. D. Halls. New York: Norton, 1990.

Timo Airaksinen

ADDITIONAL READING

Bataille, Georges. (1961) *The Tears of Eros*. Trans. Peter Connor. San Francisco, Calif.: City Lights Books, 1989; Bataille, Georges. *Visions of Excess: Selected Writings, 1927–1939*. Trans. Allan Stoekl, with Carl R. Lovitt and Donald M. Leslie. Minneapolis: University of Minnesota Press, 1985; Benjamin, Jessica. "Master and Slave: The Fantasy of Erotic Domination." In Ann Snitow, Christine Stansell, and Sharon Thompson, eds., *Powers of Desire: The Politics of Sexuality*. New York: Monthly Review Press, 1983, 280–99; Bersani, Leo. "Is the Rectum a Grave?" *October*, no. 43 (Winter 1987), 197–222; Ferguson, Frances. "Eugénie, or Sade and the Pornographic Legacy." In *Pornography, the Theory: What Utilitarianism Did to Action*. Chicago, Ill.: University of Chicago Press, 2004, 75–95; Gallop, Jane. *Intersections, a Reading of Sade with Bataille, Blanchot, and Klossowski*. Lincoln: University of Nebraska Press, 1982; Kolnai, Aurel. (1929) *On Disgust*. Ed. Carolyn Korsmeyer and Barry Smith. Chicago, Ill.: Open Court, 2003; Miller, William Ian. *The Anatomy of Disgust*. Cambridge, Mass.: Harvard University Press, 1997; Nussbaum, Martha C. *Hiding from Humanity: Disgust, Shame, and the Law*. Princeton, N.J.: Princeton University Press, 2004; Stoekl, Allan, ed. *On Bataille. Yale French Studies*, no. 78 (1990); Surya, Michel. *Georges Bataille: An Intellectual Biography*. Trans. Krzysztof Fijalkowski and Michael Richardson. London: Verso, 2002.

BEAUTY. Philosophers have tended to think that beauty is much better than sex. This is true whether they hold that beauty is objectively real or a matter of subjective taste. Philosophical discussions of beauty and sex reflect a view of the mind and other "higher" things as superior to the body and "lower" instincts.

Accounts of the relation of beauty to sex fall into three types. The "Ideal" view claims that mere physical beauty is ephemeral: Gorgeous supermodels are air-brushed, and movie stars are not so glamorous in real life. Like Don Juan, we face frustration if our only aim is to seduce beautiful people. It is far better to transform the erotic passion induced by beauty into pursuit of a higher, ideal beauty—whether of art, nature, poetry, or God. **Plato**'s (427–347 BCE) classic statement of this view is his account of *eros* in the *Symposium*. The second, "Deceit," view emphasizes the downside of sexual attraction. The beauty that dazzles our eyes and stirs our longing blinds us to flaws and makes us violate moral limits to obtain it. Beauty misleads—an "ecstasy of the eye, [it] drugs us" (Paglia, 16)—so is a temptation to be avoided. Not surprisingly, we find this view in medieval Christian philosophers but also in the Enlightenment thinker **Immanuel Kant** (1724–1804), who sharply favored reason over natural instincts. A third view, the "Romantic," is more optimistic about the role of beauty in sex. It attracts us to sexual partners but adds something beyond animal lust. It links **sexual desire** to **love**, or even transforms it into love. This view, as stated by the early modern philosophers Edmund Burke (1729–1797) and **David Hume** (1711–1776), differs from the Ideal view by asserting that we can be happy with our human beloved; we do not need an Ideal. Let us examine these views in more detail.

In ancient Athens, Plato extended earlier philosophical criticisms of the anthropomorphic Olympian gods, who often parlayed their ideal beauty into sexual romps. In dialogues featuring his teacher Socrates (469–399 BCE), Plato described a realm of abstract qualities, "Forms" ("Ideas"), where Beauty Itself (or Absolute Beauty) subsisted, along with virtues like Courage, Justice, and Wisdom. The beautiful things of our world, like Helen of Troy, only "participated in" the eternal, immaterial Forms of Beauty. For Plato, the true philosopher longs for these higher realities rather than physical beauty.

Plato's philosophy may seem otherworldly, but human sex and love figured centrally in his thought. We use the term "Platonic love" now for nonsexual friendships between a woman and a man. For Plato, however, love was both sexual and homoerotic, reflecting a norm characteristic of upper-class males (who were nonetheless expected to marry and have children). The *Symposium* ("Drinking Party") defines *eros* as the desire to reproduce in beauty. Married couples reproduce physical offspring, but Platonic lovers seek immortal offspring. An older man desires a young boy with physical beauty, who may reciprocate in loving his partner's inner beauty. Growing together in wisdom, the lovers pursue beauty until they ascend to a vision of the Form of Beauty, which never fades or diminishes (*Symposium*, 211a).

Plato's view of love is "Ideal" because sexual passion inspired by beauty impels lovers to seek higher, better things. A variant of his view appears again in the work of the late classical (or early medieval) philosopher and theologian **Saint Augustine** (354–430), for whom ideal qualities like Beauty do not subsist as Forms but as qualities of God. Augustine, a convert to Christianity, revealed in his *Confessions* shame over his former sexual passions: "I polluted the stream of friendship with the filth of unclean desire and sullied its limpidity with the hell of lust" (§3.1). For Augustine, lust is carnal hunger that can never be satisfied, since only God provides "incorruptible food." Still, all love involves some aspects of the soul and so can be turned in a better direction—by seeking God. Augustine therefore offers a version of the Ideal view: Human desire for things in this world may eventually lead to worship of the ultimate source of everything good and beautiful. (For Augustine on beauty, see *Confessions*, §4.13.)

After the seventeenth-century scientific revolution, philosophers replaced religious accounts of the universe with naturalistic ones. They even used molecular theories of matter to explain human perception and action. British writer Edmund Burke is a typical example. In his book *A Philosophical Enquiry into the Origin of Our Ideas of the Sublime and the Beautiful* (1759), Burke explained our attraction to beauty in physical terms: "[B]eauty is, for the greater part, some quality in bodies, acting mechanically upon the human mind by the intervention of the senses" (146). Qualities that give rise to beauty include being small, smooth, varied, nonangular, delicate, and brightly colored.

Burke distinguished two fundamental human passions, one for self-preservation and one for reproduction (or what he called "the society of the sexes"). On Burke's version of the

Romantic view, the reproductive instinct alone carries men toward women (Burke's discussion is framed in the sexist terms of his time), but this instinct can attach men to particular women in virtue of their beauty. Because beauty is "the object . . . of this mixed passion which we call love" (89), animal lust can be "directed" and "heightened" by beauty into "higher social qualities" in humans—not only love but an individualized love. So sexual desire and love, for Burke, remain distinct (in a way in which, for Plato, they are not), an idea Burke argues for:

> We shall have a strong desire for a woman of no remarkable beauty; whilst the greatest beauty in men, or in other animals, though it causes love, yet excites nothing at all of desire. Which shews that beauty, and the passion caused by beauty, which I call love, is different from desire, though desire may sometimes operate along with it. (128)

An account resembling Burke's was offered by Scottish philosopher David Hume. In his work "Of the Standard of Taste," Hume rejected the idealized beauty of Plato and Augustine. Still, he denied that beauty was merely subjective, because, on his view, there are "standards of taste" that can be agreed on by connoisseurs.

In his *A Treatise of Human Nature* (1739–1740), Hume assumed, with Burke, that the beauty of persons is associated with our sexual desire ("the appetite for generation") for them. But Hume thought our attraction to beauty is also naturally tied to benevolence. He regarded beauty as the mediator in this association of our natural emotions. That is, beauty can be linked at the same time with both sexual desire and benevolence (see Norton, I51–52, I58–59; **Roger Scruton**, 217) so as to generate a new emotion, "love betwixt the sexes." As Hume put it, this love

> is deriv'd from the conjunction of three different impressions or passions, *viz.* The pleasing sensation arising from beauty; the bodily appetite for generation; and a generous kindness or good-will. . . . [T]here arises such a connexion betwixt the sense of beauty, the bodily appetite, and benevolence, that they become in a manner inseparable. (II.ii.11)

Significant contributions to the theory of beauty were made by Kant, who in this area and others wrote critically about Hume. In the *Critique of the Power of Judgment* (1781), Kant argued that beauty is not merely a matter of the consensus of experts with good taste. Yet it is not something ideal, or a property of God, as in Plato and Augustine. Still, the beauty of something is the objective basis for valid human subjective responses to it. Beauty arises when some form of an object pleases our cognitive faculties and stimulates broad enjoyment in a nonutilitarian or nonpragmatic way, that is, without any specific purpose. The person who marvels at the red glow of a sunset is seeing its beauty, unlike the sailor who uses it to forecast good weather.

Since for Kant any response to an object that betrays an ulterior motive—that we want to use it or get something from it—is not a response to beauty, he discounts sexual attraction to potential mates. Sexuality is *always* related to a purpose: our own satisfaction. Hence Kant shared Hume's view of the instincts, but he was more pessimistic than Hume about integrating sex into a moral love. He did not accept the Romantic idea that beauty unites sexual passion with generosity to inspire love. Sexual desire invariably motivates both men and women to treat their partners as mere objects serving their own satisfaction. And "as soon as a person becomes an Object of appetite for another, all motives of moral relationship cease to function" (*Lectures on Ethics*, 163).

Kant can be classified as a "Deceit" theorist because, for him, people who work to make themselves sexually attractive deny their higher human nature and invite partners to do the same. They primp to be beautiful but actually lure others into seeking mere physical satisfaction. As he put it, "[A]ll men and women do their best to make not their human nature but their sex more alluring" (*Lectures*, 164). Beauty neither prompts love, as Hume held, nor launches lovers onto the path to something higher, as Plato believed, since by itself sexual love "is nothing more than appetite" (163). Kant argued that sex can be made moral only within **marriage**, a mutual contract between a man and a woman to use each other's body sexually.

The Deceit view was elaborated by nineteenth-century philosopher **Arthur Schopenhauer** (1788–1860). His essay "On Women" (1851) developed a notoriously misogynist picture of women: "It is only the man whose intellect is clouded by his sexual impulses that could give the name of *the fair sex* to that undersized, narrow-shouldered, broad-hipped, and short-legged race: for the whole beauty of the sex is bound up with this impulse" (441). "On Women" also claims that women are mentally weak, dependent, childlike, and viciously competitive with one another. Since their "primary business" is to attract the men from whom they acquire status and livelihood, women see other women as a threat. And women capture men with their physical beauty, which Schopenhauer sees as a trap for men. Nature endows women with beauty when they are young, but once their beauty serves its purpose, and they give birth, they then lose their beauty (just as some female ants lose their wings after becoming fertile, since wings are now superfluous). It is too late for the man when his woman's true nature is revealed in all its nasty detail, since he is honor-bound to care for wife and children. Schopenhauer's view has surprising echoes in twentieth-century **evolutionary psychology** (see below).

One important twentieth-century philosophical discussion of sex and beauty is in Guy Sircello's (1936–1992) book *Love and Beauty*. Sircello thinks that beauty is an important quality *during* **sexual activity**. It can be exhibited by the physical qualities of the other person, his or her character traits, and our own features. During sexual activity a person might enjoy experiencing another person's gorgeous muscles or admirable generosity and/or his or her own sleek legs. Sircello's emphasis on qualities, including the beauty of character (174), lends a Platonic, idealizing flavor to his thought. When Sircello says that the beautiful features we can enjoy during sex include character and personality, he sounds like the handsome Alcibiades in the *Symposium*, who loved the beauty of Socrates's soul, not his embodiment as a snub-nosed, balding man (*Symp.* 215a–17a). In his book, Sircello wrote openly of his finding beauty in and hence being sexually aroused by other men, students (in particular, those who showed sparks of comprehension and intelligence), and people in paintings (see also Sircello, "Beauty and Sex," 117–18). But some philosophers think the Platonic idea that moral or psychological traits can exhibit beauty is misguided, stretching the concept of beauty past the breaking point. In *The Abuse of Beauty*, art theorist Arthur Danto claims that "it muddles the concept of beauty irreparably if we say that these qualities are another species or order of beauty" (92). Danto is like Burke, who remarked that the association of beauty with virtue "has given rise to an infinite deal of whimsical theory" and involves a "loose and inaccurate way of speaking" (Burke, 146).

Even if Sircello's view is like Plato's, he differs from Plato in holding that we can love "the downright unpleasant and the positively painful" (*Love and Beauty*, 180). It happens at times that a person becomes sexually obsessed with, and perceives as beautiful, unusual features that most consider repellent (as in some fetishes). Consider J. G. Ballard's chilling novel *Crash*, which describes the sex lives of people badly injured in automobile accidents.

Afterward, they come to find scars, wounds, and even body brace equipment arousing. They experience car parts as highly erotic and make love only in cars. When the narrator has sex with the group's charismatic leader, he writes, "I hesitated at finding myself wrestling with this ugly golden creature, made beautiful by its scars and wounds" (*Crash*, 201); "The dark hairs of his pallid forearm, the scar tissue on the knuckles of his ring and index fingers, were now irrigated with a harsh beauty" (198). Sircello would explain that these aesthetic judgments are valid, because the negative qualities of scars and wounds "are only loved for some nonnegative elements of which they are, in part, composed" (*Love and Beauty*, 187). These lovers appreciate certain uniquely shared experiences of crashes along with the drama and strength of endurance that they represent.

During the twentieth century and beyond, scientists, too, examined beauty and sexuality. One influential approach is that of evolutionary psychology, which employs Charles Darwin's (1809–1882) theory of **evolution** by natural selection. For example, according to anthropologist Donald Symons, "[A] scientific, evolution-based account of humans shows extreme differences between men and women" (*Evolution*, 239; but see Geertz). Males achieve reproductive success with multiple matings, so incline toward polygamy or promiscuity; females maximize their chance of having genetic survivors by more monogamous behavior, keeping males around to protect and help rear their offspring.

Symons and other evolutionists argue that beauty is important in sexuality because people look for markers of reproductive fitness in potential mates, and these markers are what we take to be their beauty. The features women find attractive in men, such as height, a V-shaped body, and a strong chin, are indicators of testosterone levels and thus of their suitability as impregnators. Qualities males find attractive in human females include full red lips; smooth, clear skin; and a youthful appearance with high, firm breasts—again, forecasters of fecundity (Etcoff; Symons, "Beauty," "Psychology"). Research by psychologist Devendra Singh has found that having a specific waist-to-hip ratio, a ratio that reflects greater chances of reproducing successfully, makes women seem more desirable to men than women deviating from this ratio. Beauty is not the only trait relevant to sexual attraction, however. Symons cites studies of animal behavior that show that novelty ("fresh features") is itself desirable for rams and bulls. This is often called the "Coolidge Effect" (Bermant; Symons, *Evolution*, 208–13) and would seem to follow from, or be an aspect of, the relatively polygamous/promiscuous nature of males.

Evolutionary psychology can be understood as falling within the Deceit view of beauty. Beauty is not in itself what is desired, even if we think it is, for it is only an outward sign of a less visible physical characteristic, fertility, and it is reproduction that is ultimately desired from sexual activity. Further, even though these markers are generally reliable, they are not infallible. It is to deceive or mislead potential mates that older women apply lipstick or undergo cosmetic surgery to lift breasts and tuck tummies. There are echoes here of Schopenhauer's view, since evolutionary psychology describes an innate biological tension between the needs of men and the needs of women. As a result, "Men and women find it intuitively hard to understand one another" (Symons, *Evolution*, 237). Female beauty may attract male mates and keep them around to help raise children; but the beauty fades and males inevitably wish to stray, perhaps finding a less attractive woman more beautiful just because of her novelty.

Not all social scientists invoke evolution to understand human mating preferences. By contrast, the prominent "sexual script" theory of sexuality articulated by sociologists William Simon and John Gagnon proposes that culture and social conditioning affect sexual desire by providing a variety of scripts or scenarios for arousal and behavior. Such scripts are "far from identical in all social settings or for all individuals in any given setting" (Simon and Gagnon, in Simon, *Postmodern Sexualities*, 44). This theory makes attraction to sheer physical beauty far less important to sexual behavior than other factors. Since, on this view, culture is more important than biology for human sexuality, human sexuality is not a given. Indeed, Simon argued in his later book *Postmodern Sexualities* that sex has no material or biological essence. "Human sexuality is really nothing, at least nothing specific. It is nothing specific in an almost infinite variety of ways. It is almost never the same even when it looks the same. . . . Sexuality is really nothing that is constant" (145).

Although some evolutionists argue that **feminism** profits from taking evolutionary biology seriously with respect to sexual matters, such as **rape** and **sexual harassment** (Buss and Malamuth), many feminists have criticized the field, often because sociobiology and evolutionary psychology claim that differences between the sexes are biologically innate and largely immune from change. Many claims about differences between the sexes are rejected by feminist critics, who contend that the assumptions, hypotheses, and methodologies of evolutionary biology are sexist (Hubbard et al.; Lowe).

A well-known book written in this critical vein is Naomi Wolf's *The Beauty Myth*. Wolf identifies the "beauty myth" as the view that the

> quality called "beauty" objectively and universally exists. Women must want to embody it and men must want to possess women who embody it. . . . None of this is true. Beauty is a currency system like the gold standard. Like any economy, it is determined by politics, and in the modern age in the West it is the last, best belief system that keeps male dominance intact. (12)

Wolf argues that the beauty myth is oppressive to women. Psychologically, the myth makes women feel perpetually inadequate as they measure themselves against media standards of perfection. It narrows female sexuality into a concern for what men find attractive. It injures women's health by prompting them to wear shoes that damage their feet and girdles that cut off circulation and to diet endlessly or restrict food intake to the point of anorexia or bulimia.

Camille Paglia takes a very different approach in her equally well known *Sexual Personae*. She argues, partially on psychoanalytic grounds, that beauty helps attract men to women, who otherwise are threatening due to men's fear of castration, resentment at their mothers, and dread of female embodiment. "Feminism," Paglia asserts, "has been simplistic in arguing that female archetypes were politically motivated falsehoods by men. The historical repugnance to women has a rational basis: disgust is reason's proper response to the grossness of procreative nature" (12). For Paglia—whose thought resembles Schopenhauer's version of the Deceit view—female beauty, as the power that overcomes men's fears, tricks men into being seduced. Hence the *femme fatale* is central in Paglia's book—the woman whose cool, unattainable beauty conceals a hidden threat. In Paglia's Nietzschean vision, male sexuality is inherently superior because it aims at transcendence.

Peg Brand reminds us in *Beauty Matters* (a book devoted to giving women a voice in the discussion of beauty) that in traditional aesthetics "the concept of beauty has been exclusively within the province of male philosophers" (5). Despite their varying views on the relationship between sex and beauty, Kant, Hume, Burke, Schopenhauer, and Plato associated beauty more with women or boys (*objects*) and the sexual desire for it more with men (*subjects*). Consider this passage from Burke:

Observe that part of a beautiful woman where she is perhaps the most beautiful, about the neck and breasts; the smoothness; the softness; the easy and insensible swell; the variety of the surface, which is never for the smallest space the same; the deceitful maze, through which the unsteady eye slides giddily, without knowing where to fix, or whither it is carried. (149)

Schopenhauer, too, wrote as if men were the subjects, women the objects, of desire. He did not discuss whether females are attracted to male beauty or whether they have any sexual desire at all. Paglia reflects these masculine views by focusing (as Plato did) on homoerotic male desire for transcendent Beauty. The modern Deceit views of evolutionary biology have the same pattern in suggesting that females care more about the ability of a male to provide food and protection (resources) than men's physical appearance, while men are almost comically propelled by their gonads into mating frenzies at the sight of attractive females (but see Murstein).

Does a new approach to beauty by other investigators offer alternatives to the traditional three views? Danto speaks of the promise of inquiry into what he labels a "Third Realm," neither of artistic beauty nor natural beauty but of beauty in daily life, a realm that he thinks involves stronger ties to morality. The key notion here is "beautification," which can affect our attitude toward houses and clothing as well as our desires to "prettify" our bodies. Danto defers to feminists who have shown this interest can be harmful to women and deceptive to men; he envisages a scientifically enhanced future of cloning and erectile prostheses, a future that would make beauty less relevant for arousal in men and for reproduction in general. In such a realm, men would be "sexually required only for sexual pleasure—or might even be cloned because of social disorders blamed on testosterone" ("Beauty and Beautification," 81–82). Liberated women in such a world might even be indifferent to male beauty. A holdout for Romanticism might still hope that such humans could still love one another for inner beauty of character.

See also Aristotle; Bataille, Georges; Chinese Philosophy; Dworkin, Andrea; Evolution; Fantasy; Firestone, Shulamith; Genital Mutilation; Greek Sexuality and Philosophy, Ancient; Leibniz, Gottfried; MacKinnon, Catharine; Mandeville, Bernard; Nietzsche, Friedrich; Objectification, Sexual; Paglia, Camille; Philosophy of Sex, Overview of; Pornography; Prostitution; Psychology, Evolutionary; Schopenhauer, Arthur; Social Constructionism; Utopianism

REFERENCES

Augustine. (397) *Confessions*. Trans. F. J. Sheed. Indianapolis, Ind.: Hackett, 1993; Ballard, J. G. (1973) *Crash*. New York: Farrar, Straus and Giroux, 1996; Bermant, Gordon. "Sexual Behavior: Hard Times with the Coolidge Effect." In Michael H. Siegel and H. Philip Zeigler, eds., *Psychological Research: The Inside Story*. New York: Harper and Row, 1976, 76–103; Brand, Peg Zeglin, ed. *Beauty Matters*. Bloomington: Indiana University Press, 2000; Burke, Edmund. (1757, 1759) *A Philosophical Enquiry into the Sublime and Beautiful and Other Pre-Revolutionary Writings*. Ed. David Womersley. London: Penguin, 1998; Buss, David M., and Neil M. Malamuth, eds. *Sex, Power, Conflict: Evolutionary and Feminist Perspectives*. New York: Oxford University Press, 1996; Danto, Arthur C. *The Abuse of Beauty. Aesthetics and the Concept of Art*. [The Paul Carus Lectures, 21] LaSalle, Ill.: Open Court, 2003; Danto, Arthur C. "Beauty and Beautification." In Peg Zeglin Brand, ed., *Beauty Matters*. Bloomington: Indiana University Press, 2000, 65–83; Etcoff, Nancy. *Survival of the Prettiest: The Science of Beauty*. New York: Anchor Books, 2000; Geertz, Clifford. "Sociosexology." [Review, *The Evolution of Human Sexuality*, by Donald Symons] *New York Review of Books* (24 January 1980), 3–4; Hubbard, Ruth, Mary Sue Henifin, and Barbara Fried, eds. *Biological Woman—The Convenient Myth*. Cambridge, Mass.: Schenkman, 1982; Hume, David. (1757) "Of the Standard of

Taste." In *The Philosophical Works of David Hume*, vol. 3. Ed. T. H. Green and T. H. Grose. London: Longman, Green, 1874–1875, 268–84; Hume, David (1739–1740). *A Treatise of Human Nature*. Ed. L. A. Selby-Bigge. Oxford, U.K.: Clarendon Press, 1968; Kant, Immanuel (1781). *Critique of the Power of Judgment*. Trans. Paul Guyer and Eric Matthews. Cambridge: Cambridge University Press, 1990; Kant, Immanuel. (ca. 1780) *Lectures on Ethics*. Trans. Louis Infield. Indianapolis, Ind.: Hackett, 1980; Lowe, Marian. "Sociobiology and Sex Differences." *Signs* 4:1 (1978), 118–25; Murstein, Bernard I. "Physical Attractiveness and Marital Choice." *Journal of Personality and Social Psychology* 22 (1972): 8–12; Norton, David Fate. "Editor's Introduction." In David Hume, *A Treatise of Human Nature*. Ed. David Fate Norton and Mary J. Norton. Oxford, U.K.: Oxford University Press, 2000, I9–I99; Paglia, Camille. *Sexual Personae: Art and Decadence from Nefertiti to Emily Dickinson*. New Haven, Conn.: Yale University Press, 1990; Plato. (ca. 380 BCE) *Symposium*. Trans. Alexander Nehamas and Paul Woodruff. Indianapolis, Ind.: Hackett, 1989; Schopenhauer, Arthur. (1851) "On Women." In *Selections*. Ed. DeWitt H. Parker. New York: Charles Scribner's Sons, 1956, 434–47; Scruton, Roger. *Sexual Desire: A Moral Philosophy of the Erotic*. New York: Free Press, 1986; Simon, William. *Postmodern Sexualities*. New York: Routledge, 1996; Simon, William, and Gagnon, John. "Sexual Scripts. Permanence and Change." *Archives of Sexual Behavior* 15:2 (1986), 97–120. Reprinted in William Simon, *Postmodern Sexualities*. New York: Routledge, 1996, 40–58; Singh, Devendra. "Female Mate Value at a Glance: Relationship of Waist-to-Hip Ratio to Health, Fecundity, and Attractiveness." *Neuroendocrinology Letters* [Special Issue] 23 (2002), 81–91; Sircello, Guy. "Beauty and Sex." In Alan Soble, ed., *The Philosophy of Sex: Contemporary Readings*, 2nd ed. Totowa, N.J.: Rowman and Littlefield, 1991, 117–32; Sircello, Guy. *Love and Beauty*. Princeton, N.J.: Princeton University Press, 1989; Symons, Donald. "Beauty Is in the Adaptations of the Beholder: The Evolutionary Psychology of Human Female Sexual Attractiveness." In Paul R. Abramson and Steven D. Pinkerton, eds., *Sexual Nature Sexual Culture*. Chicago, Ill.: University of Chicago Press, 1995, 80–118; Symons, Donald. *The Evolution of Human Sexuality*. Oxford, U.K.: Oxford University Press, 1979; Symons, Donald. "The Psychology of Human Mate Preference." *Behavioral and Brain Sciences* 12 (1989), 34–35; Wolf, Naomi. *The Beauty Myth: How Images of Beauty Are Used against Women*. New York: Morrow, 1991.

Cynthia Freeland

ADDITIONAL READING

Aertsen, Jan A. "Beauty." In Michael Kelly, ed., *Encyclopedia of Aesthetics*, vol. 1. New York: Oxford University Press, 1998, 237–51; Berscheid, Ellen, and Karen Dion. "Physical Attractiveness and Dating Choice: A Test of the Matching Hypothesis." *Journal of Experimental Social Psychology* 7 (1971), 173–89; Blumstein, Philip, and Pepper Schwartz. *American Couples: Money, Work, Sex*. New York: Morrow, 1983; Bordo, Susan. *Unbearable Weight: Feminism, Western Culture, and the Body*. Berkeley: University of California Press, 1993; Buss, David M. "Men Want Something Else." In *The Evolution of Desire: Strategies of Human Mating*. New York: Basic Books, 1994, 49–72; Buss, David M. "Sex Differences in Human Mate Preferences: Evolutionary Hypotheses Tested in Thirty-seven Cultures." *Behavioral and Brain Sciences* 12:1 (1989), 1–49; Cavell, Stanley. Review of *Love and Beauty*, by Guy Sircello. *Philosophical Review* 101:4 (1992), 953–56; Clifford, Margaret M., and Elaine Walster. "The Effect of Physical Attractiveness on Teacher Expectations." *Sociology of Education* 46 (1973), 248–58; Cogan, Jeanine C., and Joanie M. Erickson, eds. *Lesbians, Levis, and Lipstick: The Meaning of Beauty in Our Lives. Journal of Lesbian Studies* 3:4 (1999). Also New York: Harrington Park Press, 1999; Cosmides, Leda, and John Tooby. "Evolutionary Psychology: A Primer." <www.psych.ucsb.edu/research/cep/primer.html> [accessed 2 February 2005]; Crenshaw, Theresa. *The Alchemy of Love and Lust: How Our Sex Hormones Influence Our Relationships*. New York: Pocket Books, 1997; Darwin, Charles. *The Descent of Man, and Selection in Relation to Sex*. London: John Murray, 1871. Photoreproduction: Princeton, N.J.: Princeton University Press, 1981; Darwin, Charles. (1859) *On the Origin of Species*. Cambridge, Mass.: Harvard University Press, 1964; Dawkins, Richard. *The Blind Watchmaker*. New York: Norton, 1986; Dawkins, Richard.

(1976) *The Selfish Gene*, 2nd ed. New York: Oxford University Press, 1989; Dion, Karen, Ellen Berscheid, and Elaine Walster. "What Is Beautiful Is Good." *Journal of Personality and Social Psychology* 24 (1972), 285–90; Eaton, Marcia M. "Kant and Contextual Beauty." *Journal of Aesthetics and Art Criticism* 57:1 (1999), 11–15. Reprinted in Peg Zeglin Brand, ed., *Beauty Matters*. Bloomington: Indiana University Press, 2000, 27–36; Fisher, Helen. *Anatomy of Love: A Natural History of Mating, Marriage, and Why We Stray*. New York: Fawcett Columbine, 1992; Giroud, Françoise, and Bernard-Henri Lévy. (1993) "On Ugliness as a Basic Injustice." In *Women and Men: A Philosophical Conversation*. Trans. Richard Miller. Boston, Mass.: Little, Brown, 1995, 28–47; Goldman, William, and Philip Lewis. "Beautiful Is Good: Evidence That the Physically Attractive Are More Socially Skillful." *Journal of Experimental Social Psychology* 13:2 (1977), 125–30; Graziano, William G., Lauri A. Jensen-Campbell, Laura J. Shebilske, and Sharon R. Lundgren. "Social Influence, Sex Differences, and Judgments of Beauty: Putting the *Interpersonal* Back in Interpersonal Attraction." *Journal of Personality and Social Psychology* 65:3 (1993), 522–31; Hatfield, Elaine, and Susan Sprecher. *Mirror, Mirror . . . The Importance of Looks in Everyday Life*. Albany: State University of New York Press, 1986; Hersey, George L. *The Evolution of Allure: Sexual Selection from the Medici Venus to the Incredible Hulk*. Cambridge, Mass.: MIT Press, 1996; Irigaray, Luce. (1984) *An Ethics of Sexual Difference*. Trans. Carolyn Burke and Gillian C. Gill. Ithaca, N.Y.: Cornell University Press, 1993; Kant, Immanuel. "Duties towards the Body in Respect of Sexual Impulse." In *Lectures on Ethics*. Trans. Louis Infield. New York: Methuen, 1930. Indianapolis, Ind.: Hackett, 1980, 162–71. Reprinted in POS4 (199–205); STW (140–45); Lakoff, Robin T., and Raquel L. Scherr. *Face Value: The Politics of Beauty*. Boston, Mass.: Routledge and Kegan Paul, 1984; Lambert, Craig. "The Stirring of *Sleeping* Beauty: After Decades in Scholarly Eclipse, Beauty Rears Its Beautiful Head." *Harvard Magazine* (September–October 1999). <www.harvardmagazine.com/issues/so99/beauty.html> [accessed 15 September 2004]; Laqueur, Thomas. *Making Sex: Body and Gender from the Greeks to Freud*. Cambridge, Mass.: Harvard University Press, 1990; McCall, Bruce. "Ethnicity, Genetics, and Cuteness." *The New Yorker* (5 December 1994), 152; McCosker, Anthony. "A Vision of Masochism in the Affective Pain of *Crash*." *Sexualities* 8:1 (2005), 30–48; Miller, Geoffrey. *The Mating Mind: How Sexual Choice Shaped the Evolution of Human Nature*. New York: Doubleday, 2000; Miller, Geoffrey. "Sexual Selection and the Mind: A Talk with Geoffrey Miller." Ed. and publ. John Brockman. *Edge* 41 (26 May 1998). <www.edge.org/3rd_culture/miller/index.html> [accessed 8 October 2004]; Perper, Timothy. "Theories and Observations on Sexual Selection and Female Choice in Human Beings." *Medical Anthropology* 11:4 (1989), 409–54; Nussbaum, Martha C. *The Fragility of Goodness: Luck and Ethics in Greek Tragedy and Philosophy*. Cambridge: Cambridge University Press, 1986; Nussbaum, Martha C. *Love's Knowledge: Essays on Philosophy and Literature*. New York: Oxford University Press, 1990; Paglia, Camille. "Pagan Beauty." *Sexual Personae: Art and Decadence from Nefertiti to Emily Dickinson*. New Haven, Conn.: Yale University Press, 1990, 99–139; Pinker, Steven. *The Blank Slate: The Modern Denial of Human Nature*. New York: Viking, 2002; Pinker, Steven. *How the Mind Works*. New York: Norton, 1997; Pinker, Steven. *The Language Instinct*. New York: Morrow, 1994. New York: HarperCollins, 1995; Plato. (ca. 365 BCE) *Phaedrus*. Trans. Alexander Nehamas and Paul Woodruff. Indianapolis, Ind.: Hackett, 1995; Ramachandran, V. S. "Why Do Gentlemen Prefer Blondes?" *Medical Hypotheses* 48 (1997), 19–20; Ramachandran, V. S., and William Hirstein. "The Science of Art: A Neurological Theory of Aesthetic Experience." *Journal of Consciousness Studies* 6 (June–July 1999), 15–51; Ridley, Matt. *The Origins of Virtue: Human Instincts and the Evolution of Cooperation*. New York: Viking, 1996; Ridley, Matt. "The Uses of Beauty." In *The Red Queen: Sex and the Evolution of Human Nature*. New York: Macmillan, 1993, 277–306; Salmon, Catherine, and Donald Symons. *Warrior Lovers: Erotic Fiction, Evolution, and Female Sexuality*. New Haven, Conn.: Yale University Press, 2001; Santayana, George. (1896) *The Sense of Beauty: Being the Outline of Aesthetic Theory*. New York: Dover, 1955; Schopenhauer, Arthur. (1851) "On Women." In *Parerga and Paralipomena*, vol. 2. Trans. E.F.J. Payne. Oxford, U.K.: Clarendon Press, 1974, 614–27; Singer, Irving. "The Morality of Sex: Contra Kant." *Critical Horizons* 1:2 (2000), 175–91. Reprinted in *Explorations in Love and Sex*. Lanham, Md.: Rowman and Littlefield, 2001, 1–20; and POS4 (259–72); Singh, Devendra.

"Adaptive Significance of Female Physical Attractiveness: Role of Waist-to-Hip Ratio." *Journal of Personality and Social Psychology* 65 (1993), 293–307; Singh, Devendra. "Female Judgment of Male Attractiveness and Desirability for Relationships: Role of Waist-to-Hip Ratio and Financial Status." *Journal of Personality and Social Psychology* 69 (1995), 1089–1101; Singh, Devendra. "Ideal Female Body Shape: Role of Body Weight and Waist-to-Hip Ratio." *International Journal of Eating Disorders* 16 (1994), 283–88; Sircello, Guy. "Beauty and Sex." In D. F. Gustafson and B. L. Tapscott, eds., *Body, Mind, and Method*. Dordrecht, Holland: Reidel, 1979, 225–39. Reprinted in POS2 (117–32); Sircello, Guy. *A New Theory of Beauty*. Princeton, N.J.: Princeton University Press, 1975; Soble, Alan. "Beauty." In *Sexual Investigations*. New York: New York University Press, 1996, 175–213; Soble, Alan. "Love and Value, Yet *Again*." *Essays in Philosophy* 6:1 (2005). <www.humboldt .edu/~essays/soble2rev.html> [accessed 28 January 2005]; Soble, Alan. "Physical Attractiveness and Unfair Discrimination." *International Journal of Applied Philosophy* 1:1 (1982), 37–64; Struckman-Johnson, Cindy, and David Struckman-Johnson. "Men's Reactions to Hypothetical Forceful Advances from Women: The Role of Sexual Standards, Relationship Availability, and the Beauty Bias." *Sex Roles* 37:5–6 (1997), 319–33; Symons, Donald. "On the Use and Misuse of Darwinism in the Study of Human Behavior." In Jerome Barkow, Leda Cosmides, and John Tooby, eds., *The Adapted Mind: Evolutionary Psychology and the Generation of Culture*. New York: Oxford University Press, 1992, 137–59; Travis, Cheryl B., and K. L. Meginnis-Payne. "Beauty Politics and Patriarchy: The Impact on Women's Lives." In Judith Worell, ed., *Encyclopedia of Women and Gender: Sex Similarities and Differences and the Impact of Society on Gender*. San Diego, Calif.: Academic Press, 2001, 189–200; Wilson, Edward O. *Consilience: The Unity of Knowledge*. New York: Vintage, 1999; Wilson, Edward O. *Sociobiology: The New Synthesis*. Cambridge, Mass.: Harvard University Press, 1975. Twenty-fifth Anniversary Edition, 2000.

BEAUVOIR, SIMONE DE. *See* Existentialism

BESTIALITY. Sexual contact between human beings and nonhuman animals is bestiality—or zoophilia, zooerastia, or sodomy. (For how various the kinds of "contact" can be, see Love, 298–303; for a comparison of different dictionary definitions, see Aman.) Though found sometimes in legal or theological works, "sodomy" is confusing and best avoided. The other terms are used variously by different authors, but three elements should be distinguished: (1) *sexual acts* involving human and animal ("bestiality"); (2) *sexual orientation*, where a human prefers or requires an animal as a sexual object for arousal or satisfaction (best called "zooerastia"); and (3) *sexual love* directed to an animal (best called "zoophilia").

"To many persons," Alfred Kinsey (1894–1956) and his colleagues dryly note, "it will seem almost axiomatic that two mating animals should be individuals of the same species" (*Human Male*, 667). In fact, "human contacts with animals of other species have been known since the dawn of history, they are known among all races of people today, and they are not uncommon in our own culture" (669). In Kinsey's sample, animal intercourse resulted in "only a fraction of 1 per cent of the total number of orgasms" (670), but "the entire human male population might have animal contacts as frequently as farm boys do if animals were available to all of them." (About half of all farm boys have "some sort of animal contact"; 671.) The Kinsey report on women acknowledges animal contacts, though in much smaller numbers, and with domestic companions such as dogs more likely partners than livestock (*Human Female*, 505–6, 509).

There are objections to Kinsey's methods but, if anything, incidence is probably underreported. Kinsey notes frequency of animal contacts rising with educational level (*Human*

Male, 671), which suggests knowledge and imagination encourage openness in selecting sex partners and practices. Though "persons other than scientists must evaluate" ultimate judgments (678), Kinsey is tolerant of bestiality because "such activities are biologically and psychologically part of the normal mammalian picture" (677). He suggests that despite its long history of condemnation, particularly among urban populations relatively isolated from animals, "most human sexual activities would become comprehensible to most individuals, if they could know the background of each other individual's behavior" (678). Indeed, "It is not a problem of explaining why individuals of different species should be attracted to each other sexually. The real problem lies in explaining why individuals do not regularly make contacts with species other than their own" (*Human Female*, 504; see **Sigmund Freud** [1856–1939], 145–46).

The majority of human-animal sexual contacts are temporary or experimental. Bestiality, says **Havelock Ellis** (1859–1939), "resembles masturbation and other abnormal manifestations of the sexual impulse which may be practiced merely *faute de mieux* and not as, in the strict sense, perversions of the impulse" (*Studies*, vol. V, 81). The line between bestiality (animal contact) and zooerastia (animal preference) is blurred because choice may be due to practical considerations. As Robert Stoller (1924–1991) notes, "A child may use a pet for masturbation without the animal itself precipitating the excitement but rather functioning to give a special quality of sensation to the genitals" (197). One enthusiast told R.E.L. Masters that "you haven't lived until you've had what they call a 'heat ride,'" because in sexual intercourse with a cow in heat "there is a strong pulsating movement of internal feeling that I have found in very few women" (*Sex-Driven*, 125, 184).

When there is a psychological preference for animal partners, especially if they become necessary for satisfactory sexual experiences, analysts speak of "**perversion**" or "**paraphilia**." The American Psychiatric Association used to list "zoophilia" (zooerastia) as a major paraphilia (a sexual mental disorder), where "the animal is preferred no matter what other forms of sexual outlet are available" (DSM-III, §302.10). Sex with an animal "because of the unavailability of suitable human partners" was viewed as "nonpathological." By 1994, however, "zoophilia" (because it does not occur with sufficient frequency) had been demoted from a major paraphilia to a "Paraphilia Not Otherwise Specified" (DSM-IV, §302.9).

For maverick sexologist Masters, zoophilia involves "a genuine feeling for the animal on the part of the human, and in exceptional cases it may approximate what is called 'erotic love' when humans only are involved." He adds, "Sometimes the term zoophilia is extended to embrace morbid or exaggerated emotional attachments to animals where no sexual intercourse occurs and sexual desires are not consciously present" (*Forbidden*, 64). Such an exaggerated emotional attachment to an animal is called "nonerotic zoophilia" by Ellis, who believes it exemplifies "maternal" more than "erotic" symbolism (*Studies*, vol. V, 77). For true zoophilia, Masters recommends tolerance:

> True zoophiles are encountered with comparative rarity, and their condition is, of course, one calling for psychiatric (or, better, psychoanalytic) intervention— unless they are happy with it, and otherwise well-adjusted, in which case it would be better if society rose to the challenge posed by nature's wealth of variations from the norm and just let them alone. . . . Zooerasts, too, need be of no concern to society. (*Forbidden*, 65)

The American Psychiatric Association is similarly unconcerned, as long as the behavior is not "ego-dystonic" and involves no "functional impairment" (DSM-III, 267–68; DSM-IV, 523).

In Western art and literature, bestiality has had a significant presence. Erwin Haeberle observes that "some of the greatest masterpieces in the history of art are devoted to this subject." Noting the disproportionate presence of women, he suggests that these works "are created largely to satisfy certain male fantasies" (239; cf. Kinsey, *Human Female*, 502–3). Bestiality is rife in world myth. Indian mythology, for example, contains a wide range of instances: A doe drinks water mixed with the semen of a Brahmin ascetic, falls in love with him, and gives birth to his child (Doniger, 43). Cross-cultural psychiatrist George Devereux (1908–1985) finds in bestiality a hidden source of Greek culture's vitality:

> [W]hile it is probable that . . . few Greeks engaged in bestiality, they had many myths about Gods cohabiting, in an animal shape, both with each other (as Poseidon did with Demeter), with human beings (as Zeus did with Leda) and perhaps (like Boreas) even with animals. Now . . . these myths . . . must assuredly be viewed as reflections of a (more or less unconscious) indiscriminateness in the choice of a sexual partner. . . . Greek "homosexuality" is, thus, probably not so much a manifestation of a definitely homosexual partner choice, as of an almost indiscriminate sexual responsiveness . . . and it is, *perhaps*, this which accounts *in part* for that adolescent-like freshness of vision, in love with all of reality, which is one of the characteristic traits of the genius of Greece. (106–7; see Freud, *Three Essays*, 145–46, 149, 191)

Historian of Greek philosophy W.K.C. Guthrie (1906–1981) judges that Devereux "makes out a good case for seeing Greek homosexual behaviour as not a true perversion but an expression of adolescence prolonged into adult life" (393). Does the same logic mean that bestiality is "not a true perversion"?

In rare cases, bestiality has been viewed favorably by a religious or magical sect. In the late nineteenth century, a certain Abbé Boullan (1824–1893) settled in Lyons, France, with members of a splinter group of the Church of Carmel and preached salvation through sexuality. As Francis King reports, "If humanity indulged in sexual activities with angels and other heavenly beings, said Boullan, it was enabled to more rapidly climb the ladder of spiritual evolution that led to the Divine Union. Similarly, copulation with animals speeded up their spiritual evolution—and was therefore meritorious" (181).

Against acceptance stands a long tradition of abhorrence. In Jewish scriptures, and so in the Christian Bible, humans who engage in bestiality are condemned (Lev. 18:23; Deut. 27:21) and sentenced to death (Exod. 22:19) along with their animal partners (Lev. 20:15). Of course, the Bible condemns many things now tolerated. **Homosexuality** receives the same condemnation (Lev. 18:22, 20:13). So does cursing one's parents (Exod. 21:17) and being a disobedient and drunken son (Deut. 21:18–21). Edward Payson Evans (1831–1917) comments:

> It is rather odd that Christian law-givers should have adopted a Jewish code against sexual intercourse with beasts and then enlarged it so as to include the Jews themselves. . . . Nicolaus Boër . . . cites the case of a certain Johannes Alardus or Jean Alard, who kept a Jewess in his house in Paris and had several children by her; he was convicted of sodomy on account of this relation and burned, together with his paramour, "since coition with a Jewess is precisely the same as if a man should copulate with a dog." . . . Damhouder . . . includes Turks and Saracens in the same category, "inasmuch as such persons in the eye of the law and our holy faith differ in no wise from beasts." (152–53)

The logic that undermines visceral racism may also question traditional attitudes toward cross-species sex. Objections to bestiality have traditionally rested on four grounds: disgust, fertility, **consent**, and moral status.

The *disgust objection* is emotionally powerful but logically weak. Tastes vary; natural history and ethnography do not support claims about what is universally disgusting (see Ford and Beach). It may be true, as William Ian Miller argues, that "sexual desire depends on the idea of a prohibited domain of the disgusting. . . . [S]omeone else's tongue in your mouth can be a sign of intimacy *because* it can also be a disgusting assault" (137). But that does not legitimate viewing kisses as disgusting just because they cross species boundaries. Still, many people would be bothered by Paul Goodman's (1911–1972) kissing a dog at a party:

> The dog licked him, and Paul licked him back, and for a full twenty minutes they exchanged kisses. The voices in the room fell silent. . . . The two red tongues touched again and again, and Paul opened his mouth to the dog's tongue. . . . The longing expressed by his open mouth was real, and was disquieting, as of something beyond placation. His affection for the dog was real, too. (Garber, 154–55)

Similarly, many would be disturbed by the hypothetical case posed by Joel Feinberg (1926–2004):

> A passenger with a dog takes an aisle seat at your side. He or she keeps the dog calm at first by petting it in a familiar and normal way, but then petting gives way to hugging, and gradually goes beyond the merely affectionate to the unmistakably erotic, culminating finally with oral contact with the canine genitals. (12)

But they might also be troubled by what their neighbor is eating: if, for example, he picks up a cockroach and pops it in his mouth. Disgust about food, though strong, is plainly culturally relative. *De gustibus non disputandum.* Is there any reason to treat disgust about sex as more morally compelling than disgust about food? *Chacun à son gout?*

Some moral critics argue that disgust has moral import. Robert Bork, for example, believes that what is morally offensive is *ipso facto* harmful: "Knowledge that an activity is taking place is a harm to those who find it profoundly immoral." People will agree, he thinks, for cases they really find immoral. He appeals specifically to the example of bestiality, supposing that people will "agree that it could be prohibited by law, although the only objection to it is moral. . . . Moral outrage is a sufficient ground for prohibitory legislation" (124–25). (But the obstacles to treating offenses as harms are daunting; cf. Feinberg.) **Richard Posner** also suggests that "disgust and other strong emotions in fact supply the sturdiest foundations for moral feelings." Someone who has a radically divergent emotional reaction to situations "inhabits a different moral universe from you, and there is no arguing between universes" (230). Though Posner recognizes that attitudes change over time, that does not make him think we should take feelings less seriously:

> [I]f prostitution, homosexuality, fornication, or any other offense against traditional Christian sexual morality evoked as wide and deep an antipathy as infanticide, gladiatorial contests, or suicide, those offenses would *be* immoral. Period. . . . But since the requisite intensity and unanimity of feeling on these matters no longer exist, their immorality is contestable (as, increasingly, is that

of suicide). . . . [Still,] some fragments of the traditional sexual morality retain their compelling moral authority: the taboos against rape, against certain forms of public nudity, against bigamy, and . . . against bestiality. The challenge for the traditional moralist is to derive the remaining tenets of the traditional morality from these taboos, viewed as unshakable moral intuitions. (232)

But even those who share Posner's convictions about the limited power of philosophical argument to move people away from their prejudices must recognize that this provides no reason not to try to change people's values. **Immanuel Kant** (1724–1804), who views crimes against nature as "so abominable . . . that they are unmentionable" (170–71), worries that "frequent mention would familiarize people with them and the vices might as a result cease to disgust us and come to appear more tolerable." Argument that something should continue to disgust us, however, must rest on some foundation other than the mere current fact of disgust. (Kant's alternative is discussed below.)

Martha Nussbaum attacks disgust as a basis for the legal proscription of homosexuality, concluding that "sodomy laws, the traditional focus of disgust-based lawmaking . . . do not stand up to serious scrutiny" (152). However, she supposes that "sex with animals . . . usually inflicts tremendous pain and indignity on animals, using them as instruments of human whim" (80). Condemning infliction of pain, through deliberate sadism or cruel indifference, does not mean condemning all, or even most, sex with animals. It is unlikely that most of the animal contacts noted by Kinsey involved such pain. While Robert Stoller suggests that "true bestiality (preference for animals)," that is, zooerastia, "frequently is accompanied by sadism," he also finds such cases to be rare. "Very few cases have been reported in which animals are the preferred sex object" (196–97). Cases of *faute de mieux* sex with animals sometimes involve cruelty—but probably not "usually" and certainly not always. Nor is there any reason to believe that sex between humans and animals "usually" inflicts indignity on the animals. Even Diana E. H. Russell, a noted feminist critic of **pornography**, defines erotica (which she approves) as "sexually suggestive or arousing material that is . . . respectful of all human beings and animals portrayed" (3), which suggests that the involvement of animals in a sexual encounter is not intrinsically disrespectful. Michael Ryan describes how he was quickly moved by his dog's apparent discomfort and disaffection to abandon the experiment (178–80).

For those seeking a more rational basis than disgust, the *fertility objection* is an old favorite. Authoritatively formulated by **Saint Thomas Aquinas** (1224/25–1274), it has roots in **Aristotle**'s (384–322 BCE) attempt to found an ethics of virtue on natural teleology. If there is no sense in the idea of a morally compelling natural *telos* (purpose, aim, or end), or in the idea that the purpose of sex is reproduction, the fertility objection must fail (cf. Priest). Aquinas argues (*Summa theologiae*, 2a2ae, ques. 154, art. 11–12) that bestiality is the greatest sin among the unnatural lusts. It is even worse than homosexual **sexual activity**, oral sex, and **masturbation**, which are unnatural because sexual pleasure is sought in ways that exclude reproduction. But if homosexuality, masturbation, and oral sex can be defended, the argument against "unnatural" sexual desires, including the argument against bestiality, is weakened. And so we find:

> Christians have increasingly accepted that masturbation or even nonvaginal heterosexual intercourse, in and of themselves, are not wrong. Bestiality, where it is the casual recourse of the young or of people isolated over long periods of time from other humans, should occasion little concern. It is probably too isolated a phenomenon to justify strong feelings. (Countryman, 244)

Those who view reproduction as the "purpose" of sexuality must also reject contraceptive sex and infertile human sexual contacts (but about infertility see Finnis, 1066–68). We do not condemn sexual activity between partners who are infertile because of menstruation or menopause. Moreover, if infertility is no objection to same-sex relations, why should it stand in the way of cross-species relations? In terms of fertility, why should other-species sex partners be less eligible than other-race or same-sex partners? (Cross-species sex once raised fertility fears not because it was nonreproductive but because it was believed to produce monstrous offspring; cf. D'Emilio and Freedman, 17. Such worry is now *passé*, except perhaps in genetic engineering.)

The *consent objection* claims that human-animal sex may involve coercion or exploitation, because the animal cannot consent. If so, in bestiality as in **pedophilia**, the impossibility of one partner's consent seems to turn sex into **rape**. (Donald Levy, however, suggests that the impossibility of the sheep's consenting means that it makes no "sense to speak of raping a sheep"; 174). Philosophers who reject the consent objection deny that children, or animals, are always incapable of providing consent or a suitable analogue (see Califia). We do not suppose that we should not feed a dog because it cannot consent to eat. Why would masturbating a willing dog be different? Masters's informant (perhaps self-deceptively) insisted that the cow "seems to welcome a continuation of intercourse, which she does not get with a bull" (*Sex-Driven*, 184). Moreover, how can a consent requirement rule out animals for sexual interactions if it does not rule out other uses of them? If we can eat them, or experiment on them, why can we not use them for sexual gratification? As **Edward Westermarck** (1862–1939) was asked during his travels in Morocco (245), "Why should not a man be allowed to do with his animal whatever he likes?"

The *moral status objection* claims that human beings (either in virtue of their species or insofar as they are moral agents) enjoy a special moral status that is incompatible with cross-species sex. Kant argues that masturbation, homosexuality, and bestiality constitute the most degrading human conduct. But Kant's argument is based on the debatable normative assumption that "the end of humanity in respect of sexuality is to preserve the species without debasing the person" (170–71) as well as on the false empirical assumption that such perversions are not found among animals. Like Kant, **Roger Scruton** rejects masturbation, homosexuality, and bestiality. He sees bestiality as "a paradigm of perversion" (292) because it evades the mutual intentionality of sex. Bestiality is based, he thinks, on "a fear of confrontation with the perspective of another" (293), an attempt "to flee from the burden of interpersonality" (27). (For criticism of Scruton's views, see Johnson.)

Peter Singer, well-known defender of animal liberation, points out that "sex with animals does not always involve cruelty" and raises the utilitarian question: Where no damage is done, what exactly is the objection? The fact that we are animals ourselves "does not make sex across the species barrier normal, or natural, whatever those much-misused words may mean, but it does imply that it ceases to be an offense to our status and dignity as human beings" ("Heavy Petting"). Singer's argument acknowledges that neither utilitarians nor deontologists have succeeded in explaining why human moral status is incompatible with animal contact. If petting a dog is acceptable, why not kissing? Neil Levy suggests that Singer is partially correct:

> [T]here is nothing wrong with bestiality, at least from the point of view of morality understood narrowly. Nevertheless, the repugnance that we, most of us, feel with regard to it is not irrational. It . . . reflects the culturally defined conditions of our sense of who we are. This is not to say that we *must* retain the

taboo against bestiality. . . . Whether we want this particular limit to remain in place or not is a decision for all of us to make, individually and collectively. (454)

Such a decision would be uninformed, however, if it did not examine the possibilities for human-animal relations. J. R. Ackerley (1896–1967) dedicates his remarkable memoir to his dog, of whom he says, "peace and contentment reached me in the shape of an animal, an Alsatian bitch" (216). After decades of sexual frustration with human beings, he became passionately attached to this dog, judging that "the fifteen years she lived with me were the happiest of my life" (217). Stuart Hampshire remarks, "Ackerley was the only friend I have had who was in love with a dog and who settled down to live with the handsome creature. 'In love' is the only possible term for the relation between this particular man and this particular dog" (35). The relationship can hardly be described as nonsexual:

> One of my friends . . . asked me whether I had sexual intercourse with her. . . . I said no. In truth, her love and beauty when I kissed her, as I often did, sometimes stirred me physically; but . . . the thought of attempting to console her myself, even with my finger, never seriously entered my head. What little I did for her in her burning heats—slightly more than I admitted in *My Dog Tulip*—worried me in my ignorance of animal psychology, in case, by gratifying her clear desires, which were all addressed to me, I might excite and upset her more than she was already excited and upset. The most I ever did for her was to press my hand against the hot swollen vulva she was always pushing at me at these times, taking her liquids upon my palm. (Ackerley, 217–18)

The stimulation Ackerley derived was plainly erotic: "[L]ooking at her sometimes I used to think that the Ideal Friend . . . should have been an animal-man, the mind of my bitch, for instance, in the body of my sailor" (218).

Unless we settle for disgust and outrage, philosophical critiques of bestiality must answer two questions. First, why should choices be limited if no one is harmed? Second, is not the basis for choice, especially in sexual matters, too mysterious for interference? Both questions are familiar from John Stuart Mill's (1806–1873) defense of liberty. Edward Albee's 2002 play *The Goat* uses bestiality as a symbol of love's unpredictability. Commenting on the love of dogs, Marjorie Garber writes that what matters is

> not to argue about whether dog love is a substitute for human love, but rather to detach the notion of "substitute" from its presumed inferiority to a "real thing." Don't all loves function, in a sense, within a chain of substitutions? For Freud, the original object is the parent, and all nonincestuous loves are then substitutes for the love that has become taboo. For Winnicott . . . the first "not-me" object can be a thumb, a blanket, a teddy bear, or a nursery rhyme. We learn to love by loving, and it is a long, indeed, an interminable process. To distinguish between primary and substitutive loves is to understand little about the complexity of human emotions. (135)

For those who view human sexuality as part of an exclusive moral relationship between (human) persons, animal contact seems degrading and "contrary to nature." Those who see in sex natural inclinations, in the service of individual choice, find personal fulfillment paramount. Despite philosophical tradition, common experience recognizes the reality of friendships with animals (see Gaita; Masson). And if *philia* can flourish between animal and human, perhaps *eros* can as well.

See also Animal Sexuality; Bible, Sex and the; Consequentialism; Friendship; Greek Sexuality and Philosophy, Ancient; Kant, Immanuel; Law, Sex and the; Liberalism; Masturbation; Nudism; Paraphilia; Perversion, Sexual; Privacy; Rape; Scruton, Roger; Sexology

REFERENCES

Ackerley, J. R. *My Father and Myself*. New York: Coward-McCann, 1969; Albee, Edward. *The Goat, or Who Is Sylvia?* New York: Overlook, 2003; Aman, Reinhold. "Offensive Words in Dictionaries: III. Sodomy, Bestiality, Buggery, Bugger, Pederasty." *Maledicta* 9 (1986–1987), 227–46; American Psychiatric Association. *Diagnostic and Statistical Manual of Mental Disorders*, 3rd ed. [DSM-III] Washington, D.C.: Author, 1980; American Psychiatric Association. *Diagnostic and Statistical Manual of Mental Disorders*, 4th ed. [DSM-IV] Washington, D.C.: Author, 1994; Bork, Robert H. *The Tempting of America: The Political Seduction of the Law*. New York: Free Press, 1990; Califia, Pat. "A Thorny Issue Splits a Movement." *Advocate* (30 October 1980), 17–24, 45; Countryman, L. William. *Dirt, Greed, and Sex: Sexual Ethics in the New Testament and Their Implications for Today*. Philadelphia, Pa.: Fortress, 1988; D'Emilio, John, and Estelle B. Freedman. *Intimate Matters: A History of Sexuality in America*. New York: Harper and Row, 1988; Devereux, George. *From Anxiety to Method in the Behavioral Sciences*. The Hague, Holland: Mouton, 1967; Doniger [O'Flaherty], Wendy. *Asceticism and Eroticism in the Mythology of Śiva*. Oxford, U.K.: Oxford University Press, 1973. Paperback reprint, *Śiva: The Erotic Ascetic* (1981); Ellis, Havelock. (1897–1928) *Studies in the Psychology of Sex*. New York: Random House, 1936. (Four, later two, volumes; paginated according to the original seven volumes); Evans, E. P. *The Criminal Prosecution and Capital Punishment of Animals*. London: Heinemann, 1906; Feinberg, Joel. *The Moral Limits of the Criminal Law*, vol. 2: *Offense to Others*. New York: Oxford University Press, 1985; Finnis, John. "Law, Morality, and 'Sexual Orientation.'" *Notre Dame Law Review* 69:5 (1994), 1049–76; Ford, Clellan S., and Frank A. Beach. "Relations between Different Species." In *Patterns of Sexual Behavior*. New York: Harper and Brothers/Paul B. Hoeber, 1952, 144–52; Freud, Sigmund. (1905) *Three Essays on the Theory of Sexuality*. In *The Standard Edition of the Complete Psychological Works of Sigmund Freud*, vol. 7. Trans. and ed. James Strachey. London: Hogarth Press, 1953–1974, 125–245; Gaita, Raimond. *The Philosopher's Dog: Friendships with Animals*. New York: Random House, 2002; Garber, Marjorie. *Dog Love*. New York: Simon and Schuster, 1996; Guthrie, W.K.C. *A History of Greek Philosophy*, vol. 3. Cambridge: Cambridge University Press, 1969; Haeberle, Erwin J. "Sexual Contact with Animals." In *The Sex Atlas*. New York: Continuum, 1981, 239–41; Hampshire, Stuart. "Love Story." *New York Review of Books* (18 January 1990), 34–35; Johnson, Edward. "Inscrutable Desires." *Philosophy of the Social Sciences* 20:2 (1990), 208–21; Kant, Immanuel. (ca. 1780) *Lectures on Ethics*. Trans. Louis Infield. New York: Harper and Row, 1963; King, Francis. *Sexuality, Magic, and Perversion*. Secaucus, N.J.: Citadel Press, 1972; Kinsey, Alfred C., Wardell B. Pomeroy, and Clyde E. Martin. *Sexual Behavior in the Human Male*. Philadelphia, Pa.: Saunders, 1948; Kinsey, Alfred C., Wardell B. Pomeroy, Clyde E. Martin, and Paul H. Gebhard. *Sexual Behavior in the Human Female*. Philadelphia, Pa.: Saunders, 1953; Levy, Donald. "Perversion and the Unnatural as Moral Categories." In Alan Soble, ed., *The Philosophy of Sex: Contemporary Readings*, 1st ed. Totowa, N.J.: Rowman and Littlefield, 1980, 169–89; Levy, Neil. "What (If Anything) Is Wrong with Bestiality?" *Journal of Social Philosophy* 34:3 (2003), 444–56; Love, Brenda. *The Encyclopedia of Unusual Sex Practices*. Fort Lee, N.J.: Barricade Books, 1992; Masson, Jeffrey Moussaieff. *The Pig Who Sang to the Moon: The Emotional World of Farm Animals*. New York: Random House, 2003; Masters, R.E.L. "Bestiality: Human-Animal Sex Contact." In *Sex-Driven People: An Autobiographical Approach to the Problem of the Sex-Dominated Personality*. Los Angeles, Calif.: Sherbourne Press, 1966, 121–209; Masters, R.E.L. "Bestiality: The Sexual Relations of Humans with Beasts." In *Forbidden Sexual Behavior and Morality*. New York: Julian Press, 1962, 5–137; Mill, John Stuart. (1859) *On Liberty*. Ed. Elizabeth Rapaport. Indianapolis, Ind.: Hackett, 1978; Miller, William Ian. *The Anatomy of Disgust*. Cambridge, Mass.: Harvard University Press, 1997; Nussbaum, Martha C. *Hiding from Humanity: Disgust, Shame, and the Law*. Princeton, N.J.: Princeton University Press, 2004; Posner, Richard. *Sex and Reason*. Cambridge, Mass.: Harvard University Press, 1992; Priest,

Graham. "Sexual Perversion." *Australasian Journal of Philosophy* 75:3 (1997), 360–72; Russell, Diana E. H. "Introduction." In *Making Violence Sexy: Feminist Views on Pornography.* New York: Teachers College Press, 1993, 1–20; Ryan, Michael. *Secret Life: An Autobiography.* New York: Pantheon, 1995; Scruton, Roger. *Sexual Desire: A Moral Philosophy of the Erotic.* New York: Free Press, 1986; Singer, Peter. "Heavy Petting." *Nerve* (1 March 2001). <www.nerve.com/Opinions/Singer/heavyPetting/main.asp> [accessed 14 October 2004]. Printed in *Prospect* (April 2001), 12–13; Stoller, Robert J. "Sexual Deviations." In Frank A. Beach, ed., *Human Sexuality in Four Perspectives.* Baltimore, Md.: Johns Hopkins University Press, 1977, 190–214; Thomas Aquinas. (1265–1273) *Summa theologiae*, vol. 43: *Temperance* (2a2ae, ques. 141–54). Cambridge, U.K.: Blackfriars, 1968; Westermarck, Edward. *The Future of Marriage in Western Civilisation.* New York: Macmillan, 1936.

Edward Johnson

ADDITIONAL READING

Ackerley, J. R. *My Dog Tulip: Life with an Alsatian.* New York: Fleet, 1965; Ackerley, J. R. *We Think the World of You.* New York: Obelensky, 1961; Baranzke, Heike. "Does Beast Suffering Count for Kant: A Contextual Examination of §17 in *The Doctrine of Virtue.*" *Essays in Philosophy* 5:2 (2004). <www.humboldt.edu/~essays/baranzke.html> [accessed 15 February 2005]; Belliotti, Raymond. "Bestiality." In *Good Sex: Perspectives on Sexual Ethics.* Lawrence: University Press of Kansas, 1993, 228–33; Braun, Walter. "Sadism and Bestiality." In *The Cruel and the Meek, Aspects of Sadism and Masochism: Being Pages from a Sexologist's Notebook.* Trans. N. Meyer. London: Luxor Press, 1967, 55–59; Cornog, Martha, and Timothy Perper. "Bestiality." In Vern L. Bullough and Bonnie Bullough, eds., *Human Sexuality: An Encyclopedia.* New York: Garland, 1994, 60–63; de River, J. Paul. "Sadistic Bestiality." In *The Sexual Criminal: A Psychoanalytical Study*, 2nd ed. Springfield, Ill.: Charles C. Thomas, 1956, 143–52; Dekkers, Midas. (1992) *Dearest Pet: On Bestiality.* Trans. Paul Vincent. New York: Verso, 1994; Denis, Lara. "Kant on the Wrongness of 'Unnatural' Sex." *History of Philosophy Quarterly* 16:2 (1999), 225–48; Dworkin, Andrea. "Bestiality." In *Woman Hating.* New York: Dutton, 1974, 187–88; Eichler, Barry L. "Bestiality." In Keith Crim, ed., *The Interpreter's Dictionary of the Bible*, supp. vol. Nashville, Tenn.: Abingdon, 1976, 96–97; Evans, E. P. (1906) *The Criminal Prosecution and Capital Punishment of Animals.* London: Faber, 1987; Forberg, Fred Chas. "Of Intercourse with Animals." In *Manual of Classical Erotology (De figuris Veneris).* Trans. Julian Smithson. Manchester, U.K.: Privately printed, 2 vols., 1844. Reprints, New York: Medical Press of New York, 1964, 227–31; and New York: Grove Press, 1966, vol. 2, 168–77; Hentig, Hans von. *Soziologie der zoophilen Neigung.* Stuttgart, Ger.: Enke Verlag, 1962; Jamieson, Dale, ed. *Singer and His Critics.* Oxford, U.K.: Blackwell, 1999; Johnson, Edward. "Inscrutable Desires." *Philosophy of the Social Sciences* 20:2 (1990), 208–21. Reprinted in HS (53–66); Kauffmann-Doig, Federico. "Bestiality or Zooerasty." In *Sexual Behavior in Ancient Peru.* Lima, Peru: Kompaktos, 1979, 51–55; Levy, Donald. "Perversion and the Unnatural as Moral Categories." *Ethics* 90:2 (1980), 191–202. Reprinted, revised, in POS1 (169–89); Lissarrague, François. "The Sexual Life of Satyrs." In David M. Halperin, John J. Winkler, and Froma I. Zeitlin, eds., *Before Sexuality: The Construction of Erotic Experience in the Ancient Greek World.* Princeton, N.J.: Princeton University Press, 1990, 53–81; Malinowski, Bronislaw. *The Sexual Life of Savages in North-Western Melanesia: An Ethnographic Account of Courtship, Marriage, and Family Life among the Natives of the Trobriand Islands, British New Guinea.* London: Routledge and Kegan Paul, 1929; Meyer, Robert G., and Sarah E. Deitsch. *The Clinician's Handbook: Integrated Diagnostics, Assessment, and Intervention in Adult and Adolescent Psychopathology*, 4th ed. Boston, Mass.: Allyn and Bacon, 1995; Midgley, Mary. *Animals and Why They Matter.* Athens: University of Georgia Press, 1984; Midgley, Mary. *Beast and Man: The Roots of Human Nature.* Hassocks, U.K.: Harvester, 1979; Money, John. "Transcultural Sexology: Formicophilia, a Newly Named Paraphilia in a Young Buddhist Male." In *The Adam Principle. Genes, Genitals, Hormones, and Gender: Selected Readings in Sexology.* Buffalo, N.Y.: Prometheus, 1993, 334–40; Nussbaum, Martha C. " 'Secret Sewers of Vice': Disgust, Bodies, and the Law." In Susan A. Bandes, ed., *The Passions of Law.* New York: New

York University Press, 2000, 19–62; Patai, Raphael. "Bestiality." In *Sex and Family in the Bible and the Middle East*. Garden City, N.Y.: Dolphin Books/Doubleday, 1959, 178–80; Posner, Richard A. "Emotion versus Emotionalism in Law." In Susan A. Bandes, ed., *The Passions of Law*. New York: New York University Press, 1999, 309–29; Posner, Richard A., and Katharine B. Silbaugh. "Bestiality." In *A Guide to America's Sex Laws*. Chicago, Ill.: University of Chicago Press, 1996, 207–12; Regan, Tom. *The Case for Animal Rights*. Berkeley: University of California Press, 1983; Reinhardt, James Melvin. *Sex Perversions and Sex Crimes*. Springfield, Ill.: Charles C. Thomas, 1957; Richards, Jeffrey. *Sex, Dissidence and Damnation: Minority Groups in the Middle Ages*. London: Routledge, 1991; Shulman, Alix Kate. "A Story of a Girl and Her Dog." In Ann Snitow, Christine Stansell, and Sharon Thompson, eds., *Powers of Desire: The Politics of Sexuality*. New York: Monthly Review Press, 1983, 410–15; Singer, Peter. (1975, 1990) *Animal Liberation*, 3rd ed. New York: Ecco/Harper-Collins, 2002; Soble, Alan. "Kant and Sexual Perversion." *The Monist* 86:1 (2003), 57–92; Soble, Alan. "Other Animals." In *Sexual Investigations*. New York: New York University Press, 1996, 227–31; Sunstein, Cass R., and Martha C. Nussbaum, eds. *Animal Rights: Current Debates and New Directions*. New York: Oxford University Press, 2004; Taylor, G. Rattray. (1970) *Sex in History*. New York: Harper Torchbook, 1973; Thornhill, Randy, and Craig T. Palmer. *A Natural History of Rape: Biological Bases of Sexual Coercion*. Cambridge, Mass.: MIT Press, 2000; Tiffany, Grace. *Erotic Beasts and Social Monsters: Shakespeare, Jonson, and Comic Androgyny*. Newark: University of Delaware Press, 1995; Zeus. "My Life with Women." *The Onion* (14 April 1999). By subscription, <www.theonion.com> [accessed 9 December 2004].

BIBLE, SEX AND THE. The Bible—the Old and New Testaments—is accorded a certain normative authority within the Christian religious tradition, although how that authority is understood, particularly in relation to current practice, is much debated. Jewish tradition shares a similarly debated commitment to the Old Testament, and is usually supplemented by the Talmud (the "oral Torah") and other ancient materials and commentaries. As one might anticipate about writings deemed to provide a guide for "faith and practice," the Bible makes frequent reference to **sexual activity**. Debates over biblical authority therefore have important implications for **sexual ethics**, especially concerning the extent to which biblical stories and injunctions relating to sex should be interpreted "timelessly," "contextually," or simply as significant records in an evolving history of human spirituality. Biblical materials can be viewed as part of a continuous tradition, although the problems of constructing a coherent account from materials that have multiple authors separated by time, place, and culture must be acknowledged (see Jordan, chap. 1).

Sex and Creation. The two creation stories of Genesis 1 and 2 provide a framework for much subsequent reflection, not only in the Old Testament but also in the New Testament (Mark 10:6; Matt. 19:4). The creation of man and woman "in God's image," the "blessing" that they "be fruitful and multiply," and their being brought together as "one flesh" in a distinctive partnership have usually been taken to center human sexual activity in an ongoing heterosexual framework encompassing reproduction. The narrative, however, is nuanced, and its implications are not always clear.

In the first of these stories, men and women are given a special place within the created order: they, unlike the rest of creation, are made "in the image of God." They are, furthermore, given "dominion" over the rest of creation, although the power to "be fruitful and multiply" is shared with other animals (Gen. 1:22, 28). Each element of this account has occasioned much discussion. Is "image" to be interpreted literally? Does it refer to some variant of rational or moral self-consciousness? Does it speak of creativity? Might it even bespeak a divine gender-duality? Or does it, rather, link with the dominion that is granted and, if so, what, if any, are the constraints on such authority? Is being fruitful and multiplying a command or simply the articulation of a blessing (Daube, "The Duty") and, whichever, does it have implications for such contested contemporary issues as zero-population growth, **contraception**, and family planning? If it is a command, is it a burden placed on each human being or on the man and woman in some representative capacity?

The account given in Chapter 2 of Genesis moves the focus from the place of humans in the created order to the relations between men and women. One might have anticipated, given that "male and female" are both created in God's image, that men and women would be accorded equal status. This is probably intended, although a long tradition of interpretation has understood the term *ezer*, frequently translated as "helpmate" (Gen. 2:18), as implying female subordination. The context provides little support for this; *ezer* is better understood to mean "fellow worker" or "companion." The man is not fulfilled without the woman; she is fashioned from and recognized to be of the same substance; and the unity that the man and woman realize when they become husband and wife constitutes a natural and self-regulating social unit (Gen. 2:18–24). In this context, the bond is not viewed reproductively but as one having intrinsic value for the couple. It is not until the account of rebellion in Chapter 3 that there is any suggestion of subordination and, then, not as a divinely intended feature of gender relationships but as a consequence of refusal to observe divinely intended constraints (cf. Hosea 2:16).

Given this, we might expect the biblical writers to favor a generally heterosexual view of sexuality and one, moreover, that contributes to the perpetuation of those given preeminence within the created order (but see Whitaker). Whether such a positive valuation can or should be taken to have negative implications for other relationships and, even if negative, as warranting moral condemnation are other matters. As with the pain of childbirth, the sweat of labor, and male domination (Gen. 3:16–19), naturally occurring but atypical attractions or senses of the self may be viewed as consequences of a general human alienation from the created order. What is "natural" may therefore have two referents: that which conforms to a pristine order and that which naturally occurs in an order characterized by an alienation from what had been intended for it. The latter order may be burdened with infirmities without those infirmities being objects of moralization (cf. Luke 13:4). This is not to deny that certain willful breaches of that creation nexus might be viewed as wrong and thus subject, at least in theory, to sanctions (although of what kind would be a further issue).

We might think of the biblical writings as constituting an ideal theory (outlined in the first two chapters of Genesis) followed by the development of a nonideal theory that takes account of humans as we find them and that seeks to develop an understanding of sexuality and relationships constrained by a certain perspective on the human condition. This is a world in which polygamy and divorce may occur, even though it was not so "in the beginning." If we view biblical writings as attempts to articulate an ethic for people no longer as they were intended to be, it is reasonable to see that tradition of reflection as evolving, a project to discover or create norms of conduct that will work for those who have to live this mundane life with the significant burdens of alienation (cf. Rom. 8:22–23).

Marriage and Family. Although **marriage** and family life are staples of the biblical social world, and infertility is viewed as a personal and social burden (Gen. 30:1, 2, 22, 23; 1 Sam. 1:4–20; Luke 1:24, 25), it is often difficult to draw strong and direct normative inferences from biblical data for contemporary situations. One cannot, for example, extrapolate from rules relating to the treatment of household slaves that it would therefore be biblically permissible to reinstitute slavery. And so although some form of "marriage" was "ordained" and given public recognition (Gen. 29:27–28; Judg. 14:10, 12; John 2:1–10), it cannot be inferred from the record that the kinds of formalized arrangements with which we are now familiar (along with their various implications for conjugal and property rights and custody) should be seen as being biblically "authorized." At most, there is the view that however nuclear or extended family arrangements are, the joined man and woman constitute a normatively independent unit.

The biblical writers generally evince a strong interest in marital fidelity and the integrity of familial bonds. The marital bond, as understood in Genesis 2, is often treated—in the Old Testament—as a metaphor for the relationship between God and Israel and—in the New Testament—for that between Jesus and the church. The focus is on God's or Jesus's fidelity to those who are "betrothed" to him and therefore on the need for their reciprocal fidelity. **Adultery** and **incest** are thus generally frowned on and sometimes strongly condemned. In Leviticus 18 and 20, the strong injunctions against incest, adultery, homosexual relations, **pedophilia**, **bestiality**, and intercourse during menstruation are linked to the expectation that Israel will echo God's holiness (or separateness). The sanctions levied against prohibited conduct are probably to be understood against a social background in which the political and religious orders are not clearly differentiated and in which the Israelites are under pressure to distinguish their practices from those of neighboring tribes. In many respects, such teachings express what is sometimes referred to as a "garrison ethic," in which the preservation of the whole depends on the cooperation of all.

Even though some wish to reimpose a comparable social order, the one in which we currently live is somewhat closer to that of the New Testament, in which followers comprise a social minority and political power is secular. In the New Testament, many of the proscriptions dealing with sexual behavior are directed to congregational life (with less draconian sanctions than those countenanced by the Old Testament; cf. 1 Cor. 5), and few if any implications can be drawn for what was seen as essentially a separate political order (Rom. 13:1–7). It is a permanent question whether what is unambiguously rejected by New Testament writers is ever intended, even aspirationally, to be enforced in the wider juridicopolitical order.

Patriarchy. There is little doubt that the dominant social relationship of man and woman has been patriarchal, and the biblical writings are frequently seen to mirror, and even to attempt to justify, that tradition (see, for example, 1 Cor. 11; 1 Tim. 2:11–15). Inheritance is patrilineal (cf. Num. 27:1–11). Polygamy (not polyandry) is countenanced, divorce is viewed as a male prerogative, and a bride price is often exacted when the woman passes from her father's possession into the power of the husband. If a virgin is seduced by someone to whom she is not betrothed, her father is owed compensation (cf. Gen. 34:11 f.; cf. Exod. 22:15 ff.; Deut. 22:28 f.). Such rules as there are have a very different background from that outlined in Genesis 1, 2. Nevertheless, a closer and more historical reading, even of passages in which submission is upheld, sometimes (though not always easily; see Titus 2:4–5) point in other directions. Jesus's teachings frequently purport to be an advance on earlier traditions and return to something approximating ideal theory. And **Saint Paul** (5–64?), by likening the subjection of wife to husband to the subjection of the church to the Christ who serves, transforms that relationship into one of mutual service (Eph. 5:21–33). Even so, biblical texts bearing on the relationship of the sexes often lend themselves to multiple interpretations.

Monogamy and Polygamy. In the Old Testament writings, it was not uncommon for a man, even major figures, to have more than one wife or to have a concubine along with a wife (for example, Abraham and Jacob; cf. Judg. 8:30–31; 1 Sam. 1:2; 2 Sam. 3:2–5; 1 Kings 11:1–8; 2 Chron. 13:21). Although it is arguable that the underlying understanding of the writers favored monogamy (cf. Deut. 17:17), alternative relationships did not generally attract condemnation, absent some other factor. Indeed, there are even rules to govern such relationships (Deut. 21:15–17). The Old Testament writers seem more concerned to keep **sexual desire** attached to appropriate relationships than to condemn polygamous ones. Such arguments as there are for monogamy tend to be inferences drawn from the exclusive relationship that Israel's God expects from his betrothed (Isa. 50:1; Jer. 2:1 f.; 3:1 ff.; Ezek. 16:23; Hosea 1–3). This symbolism is replicated in the New Testament (see 1 Cor. 11:3; Eph. 5:22 ff.; although cf. 1 Cor. 7:2).

Adultery and Extramarital Sex. Rather than monogamy, the biblical writers appear to be more concerned with infidelity, as exemplified in adultery (Exod. 20:14; Lev. 20:10; Deut. 5:18; 22:22). Sexual activity, sometimes referred to as "knowing," is generally considered expressive not only of intimacy but also (likely due to the probable nexus of intercourse with children) of an ongoing commitment. The Song of Songs is a paean to sexual pleasure and commitment. The picture is complicated, however, by views about the chattel status of women. The virgin who engages in premarital relationships may violate expectations about the significance of sexuality, but her father also finds the value of his property diminished, and this sometimes appears to be of as much concern as any cheapening of sexual behavior (Exod. 22:15–17). Even **rape** requires a remedy more than punishment, including marriage between rapist and victim (Deut. 22:28–29; although see Gen. 34).

Prostitution, both male and female, is acknowledged and sometimes condemned (Lev. 19:29; 21:9), but condemnation is often associated with a defiling of cultic activity or syncretism rather than with its character as "sex for sale" (Deut. 23:18; Num. 25:1–3; 1 Kings 14:23; 15:12; 22:46; 2 Kings 23:7; cf., however, Prov. 6:26, where recourse to a prostitute is recommended over adultery). Israel's "playing the harlot" is constituted by her religious defection (Judg. 2:17; 8:33; Ezek. 16:41; Hosea). Along with prostitutes and slaves, concubines populate aristocratic circles without too much comment (Gen. 30:1–5; 2 Sam. 16:21–22) and even some protection (Exod. 21:7–11). Rahab the harlot, moreover, is given a special place in the annals of faith (James 2:25; Josh. 2; Heb. 11:31).

Divorce. Divorce attracts considerable attention. Although God is said at one point to "hate divorce" (Mal. 2:16), and priests are forbidden to marry divorcees (Lev. 21:7; cf. 17:2, 5; Lev. 21:13–14), the practice is an established feature of life in ancient Israel (Lev. 21:7, 14; 22:13; Num. 30:10) and governed by various rules. In keeping with patriarchal traditions, divorce appears to have been a male initiative and prerogative (Deut. 21:14; 24:1, 3; Lev. 21:7; Ezra 10:3), permitted, for the most part, for no more important reason than permanent loss of affection. However, rash divorces were discouraged by prohibiting a man from remarrying a woman who had subsequently married someone else (Deut. 24:4; Jer. 3:1; see Daube, "The Return") and limited in only minor ways (Deut. 22:28–29). Women who abandoned their husbands normally suffered significant social consequences (though see Exod. 21:10–11).

Old Testament attitudes to divorce become an issue in the New Testament, where Jesus reaffirms the "sanctity of marriage" as a creation ordinance (Matt. 19:4–6) and claims that the permission was a concession to human weakness. His own position, variously reported, is either that it is not sanctioned at all or at best only in cases of infidelity. As if to reinforce that position, remarriage after divorce is considered a form of adultery (Matt. 5:32b; 19:19; Mark 10:11 f). Adultery was seen as a matter of mental and not simply bodily betrayal (Matt. 5:28).

Virginity and Celibacy. Virginity is valued because intercourse is associated with a certain kind of knowing of another. And thus prostitution, when not viewed as cultic profanation, is generally seen as a corruption of sexual congress not simply, if at all, because it involves the selling of sexual services but more because it detaches sexual activity from ongoing commitment. In the Old Testament, however, female virginity seems to be more closely associated with honor and economics than the idea of commitment (Deut. 22:13–21). A double standard is evident, reflected in the idea that a father is to be compensated if his virgin daughter is seduced but not if his virgin son is (Exod. 22:15–17; Deut. 22:28, 29).

Although eunuchs often held positions of trust in (non-Jewish) courts (2 Kings 9:32, 33; Esther 2:3, 14, 15; Dan. 1:9; Acts 8:27), they were barred from certain religious privileges (Lev. 21:20; Deut. 23:1; 2 Kings 20:18).

In the Old Testament, celibacy is not viewed as a virtue (Judg. 11:37, 39), and though it is later sometimes accorded a strategic value (Matt. 19:10–12; 1 Cor. 7:1, 7, 8, 25, 26, 32–40), it is not considered inherently praiseworthy (cf. 1 Tim. 4:1–3).

Homosexuality. It can hardly be denied that the biblical record accords a certain normative centrality to heterosexual relationships. What is much less clear is whether this centrality reflects derogatorily (and if so, how) on **homosexuality** and whether it has anything clear to say about **bisexuality**, transvestitism (see, though, Deut. 22:5), transgendering, and a whole host of other sexually charged proclivities and arrangements.

The biblical passages taken to express some condemnation of homosexual relationships are less clear in their implications than they are often taken to be. One of the most forthright of these, Leviticus 20:13 (cf. 18:22), which outrightly condemns male homosexual intercourse, does so as an abomination (*to 'evah*), which then raises the difficult question as to how that is to be understood. It occurs in the context of a series of prohibitions designed to preserve the integrity of familial bonds, often visiting violations with garrison-like penalties. Of the offenses delineated, only male homosexual relations are condemned as an abomination, and it is unclear whether the violation is seen as ritual, moral, or both. "Abomination" can be used in each of these ways (Waltke). Some have argued that the condemnation attaches only to anal intercourse, in which there is an inappropriate mixing of bodily fluids (Daube, "Old Testament"; Olyan). Attempts to draw inferences from the condemnation are complicated by the fact that, at least for a later Christian tradition, Levitical rulings have an ambiguous status. Not only are many of the Levitical laws "superseded," but even when not, the penalty structure is usually considered obsolete. Moreover, were one to argue that male homosexual intercourse was still to be condemned, only some other reason could explain the gender-differential condemnation that befalls those who have homosexual relations.

Less clear, but frequently cited, is the story in which two "angels" visit Sodom, supposedly to carry out the foretold destruction of the city (Gen. 19). They are noticed by a current resident of the city, Abraham's nephew Lot, and entreated to accept his hospitality. Before the evening is over, the house is surrounded by local men who demand that the visitors be sent out so that they may "know" them. Lot refuses but tries to mollify the locals by offering his two virgin daughters, to be treated as they please. It is to no avail, and only the miraculous intervention of the angels prevents the house from being stormed. It has been common to interpret the sin of Sodom as an implicit condemnation of (here, at-tempted) male homosexual conduct. But it is not usually seen so by other biblical writers, who see Sodom's downfall in various other failings. That seems reasonable, given that the purpose of the angels' visit was to effect the destruction of Sodom for reasons that existed prior to the incident. Still it might be argued that the homosexual demands of the Sodomites typified the sins of Sodom, an interpretation requiring that we understand the "knowing" (*yada*) demanded by the Sodomites as sexual knowing—likely, though not strictly demanded, by the text. The demand to know them could be grounded in conven-tions of hospitality, especially given Lot's sojourner status (as Bailey argues, 4–8). But even if the knowing is sexual, as suggested, perhaps, by Lot's willingness to offer instead his daughters "who have not known man," it would not be clear that the offense lay in the homosexual conduct per se as in its nonconsensual nature or, possibly, in the fact that the men in question were angels. That Lot gets off scot free for offering his daughters, whereas the men of Sodom are wiped out for demanding "knowing" his guests, suggests that the point of the story is not to condemn homosexual conduct per se. A somewhat similar story in Judges 19 is no more decisive (cf. Stone).

New Testament references to homosexual relations are also susceptible to anachronis-tic interpretations. Jesus appears not to have addressed the issue. But in Paul's letter to the church at Rome, he claims that Gentiles, no less than Jews, are unable to establish their innocence before God. Their consciences witness against them. As a result of their turn-ing away from such evidence of God as they have toward baser creations of their own, God has abandoned them, both men and women, to "degrading passions," lustfully turn-ing from natural intercourse to that which is "against nature" and suffering appropriate consequences as a result (Rom. 1:23–27). The latter has been used (anachronistically) to diminish compassion for gays who have contracted AIDS (acquired immunodeficiency syndrome).

The focus of the passage is unclear. Does it target the development of a gay culture, or is it better read as the abandonment, by those who are "naturally" (heterosexually?) inclined, for "unnatural" (homosexual?) sexual relations, a product of "unrestrained" sexuality such as one might find in bestiality (or pederasty or other forms of sexual satisfaction that lie be-yond the usual boundaries of sexual attraction)? (See Scroggs, 109–18; and the critique in Smith.) Although the biblical writings make no distinction between homosexual inclina-tions (or **orientation**) and homosexual conduct (a concession sometimes made to deal with "natural," or at least deep-seated, inclinations in the devout), it cannot be readily deployed here, since it is the expression of "natural" tendencies that Paul is concerned with and not the tendencies themselves. It is arguable that the focus of Paul's concern is on unrestrained lust rather than the particular form it takes (and therefore on the "natural" inclinations of the parties in question), although there is also a substantial literature to the effect that what Paul has in mind is a departure from the ordering of Genesis 1–2 (see, further, DeYoung, "Meaning of Nature"; Mauser; Ward; Whitaker).

Other Pauline passages do not help much here. In 1 Corinthians 6:9, the exclusion of *malakoi* and (also in 1 Tim. 1:10) *arsenokoitai* from the kingdom of God (along, *inter alia*, with adulterers, drunkards, the greedy, and those who live immoral lives) cannot unam-biguously be translated by the tendentious terms "catamites" and "sodomites." The former might refer to the licentious or (in later Catholic theology) masturbators and the latter to pederasts (Scroggs, 106–8; challenged by Malick) or male prostitutes (John Boswell [1947–1994], 107; Martin; but see DeYoung, "The Source"; Wright). The point is not to deny the Pauline reference but to recognize that it does not provide a stable scaffolding for the social opprobrium that it is used to support. In any case, the context of Paul's remarks is congregational life and not social and legal exclusion.

Bestiality. The condemnation of bestiality (Exod. 22:19; Lev. 18:23; Deut. 27:21) is not explained. Some ground it in the prohibition against the mixing of disparate kinds (cf. Lev. 19:19; Deut. 22:9–11), others in the creation story's assertion that animals do not constitute an appropriate companionship for humans (Gen. 2:19, 20).

Masturbation, Contraception, Sterilization, and Birth Control. Little can be inferred from the biblical writings on the topic of **masturbation**. The use of Onan's sin (Gen. 38:8–10) to condemn male masturbation misconstrues what is really a condemnation of *coitus interruptus* as failing to fulfill the *prima facie* obligations of levirate law, whereby a childless widowed woman might normally expect the brother of her dead husband to take her in as his own wife (Deut. 25:5–10). The later interpretation of *malakos* as masturbators is similarly tendentious, as is the view (associated also with opposition to contraception) that sexual activity is to be both confined to the marital bond and not artificially obstructive of the possibility of a reproductive outcome. At most one might argue that masturbation frequently involves adulterous or other inappropriate fantasies, a view that is given some marginal support by Jesus's teaching on adultery (Matt. 5:28). The lack of a textual basis for this common form of sexual expression perhaps explains nineteenth-century attempts to associate it with various debilitating physical consequences and attempts to Christianize these consequences by seeing them as failures to be a good steward of the "temple of the Holy Spirit" (1 Cor. 6:19–20).

Although attempts at contraception have a long history, reliable contraception is a relatively modern phenomenon and perhaps for this reason does not figure unambiguously as an item of biblical concern. More to the point, though, the Genesis account of sexual expression does not appear to restrict sexual intercourse to that which is reproductively open. Onan's obligation cannot be construed as a general obligation to ensure the reproductive potential of intercourse.

Abortion. **Abortion** is not directly discussed by the biblical writers, although inferences concerning the unborn are drawn from certain passages. The Psalmist, for example, discerns a continuity between his present self and the protective environment of the womb (Ps. 139:13), although it might be questioned whether it is only in the light of the later self that the earlier one is incorporated. Various laws relating to pregnant women might also be invoked. Exodus 21:22–23 is sometimes used to show that a fetus is given a lower status than a developed human life. There is, however, an ancient disagreement over the precise intent of the passage: whether the harm is to the mother or fetus. Even if the latter, some interpreters have taken the passage to refer only to harm done to a "fully formed" fetus. Although much contemporary debate concerns fetal development and the attributes that a fetus must have to qualify for the protections afforded a person, some biblical scholars argue that the status to be accorded a fetus (and humans generally) is not a function of fetal development but of divine investment. People (and fetuses) are said to possess an "alien dignity" (Helmut Thielicke [1908–1986], 286, 287).

Although the biblical writers have a good deal to say about human sexuality, what the implications of their pronouncements might be for issues of sexuality as currently encountered are inherently problematic. The scope of various sexual categories and the social and religious context have changed (and there are shifts even within the writings themselves). Moreover, even if inferences can be drawn for those who accept the theological framework within which the discussion is cast, their wider translation into social policy is much less clear.

See also Abstinence; Adultery; Bestiality; Boswell, John; Bullough, Vern L.; Catholicism, History of; Greek Sexuality and Philosophy, Ancient; Homosexuality, Ethics of; Judaism, History of; Marriage; Paul (Saint); Protestantism, History of; Roman Sexuality and Philosophy, Ancient; Thomas Aquinas (Saint); Wojtyła, Karol (Pope John Paul II)

REFERENCES

Note: A variety of editions of the Bible were used, including the Revised Standard Version, the Jerusalem Bible, and the New International Version, as well as Strong, James. (1890) *The New Strong's Exhaustive Concordance of the Bible*. Nashville, Tenn.: Thomas Nelson, 1990. Bailey, Derrick Sherwin. *Homosexuality and the Western Christian Tradition*. London: Longmans, Green, 1955; Boswell, John. *Christianity, Social Tolerance, and Homosexuality: Gay People in Western Europe from the Beginning of the Christian Era to the Fourteenth Century*. Chicago, Ill.: University of Chicago Press, 1980; Daube, David. (1977) "The Duty of Procreation." In Calum Carmichael, ed., *Biblical Law and Literature: Collected Works of David Daube*, vol. 3. Berkeley, Calif.: Robbins Collection, 2003, 951–70; Daube, David. (1986) "Old Testament Prohibitions of Homosexuality." In Calum Carmichael, ed., *Biblical Law and Literature: Collected Works of David Daube*, vol. 3. Berkeley, Calif.: Robbins Collection, 2003, 949–50; Daube, David. (1992) "The Return of the Divorcee." In Calum Carmichael, ed., *Biblical Law and Literature: Collected Works of David Daube*, vol. 3. Berkeley, Calif.: Robbins Collection, 2003, 937–48; DeYoung, James B. "The Meaning of Nature in Romans 1 and Its Implications for Biblical Proscriptions of Homosexual Behavior." *Journal of the Evangelical Theological Society* 31:1 (1988), 429–41; DeYoung, James B. "The Source and NT Meaning of *arsenokoitai*, with Implications for Christian Ethics and Ministry." *Masters Seminary Journal* 3:2 (1992), 191–215; Jordan, Mark D. *The Ethics of Sex*. Oxford, U.K.: Blackwell, 2002; Malick, David. "The Condemnation of Homosexuality in 1 Corinthians 6:9." *Bibliotheca Sacra* 150:600 (1993), 327–40; Martin, Dale. "Arsenokoités and Malakos: Meanings and Consequences." In Robert L. Brawley, ed., *Biblical Ethics and Homosexuality: Listening to Scripture*. Louisville, Ky.: Westminster John Knox, 1996, 117–36; Mauser, Ulrich W. "Creation and Human Sexuality in the New Testament." In Robert L. Brawley, ed., *Biblical Ethics and Homosexuality: Listening to Scripture*. Louisville, Ky.: Westminster John Knox, 1996, 3–16; Olyan, Saul M. "And with a Man You Shall Not Lie the Lying Down of a Woman: On the Meaning and Significance of Leviticus 18:22 and 20:13." *Journal of the History of Sexuality* 5:2 (1994), 179–206; Scroggs, Robin. *The New Testament and Homosexuality: Contextual Background for Contemporary Debate*. Philadelphia, Pa.: Fortress Press, 1983; Smith, Mark. "Ancient Bisexuality and the Interpretation of Romans 1:26–27." *Journal of the American Academy of Religion* 64:2 (1996), 223–56; Stone, Ken. "Gender and Homosexuality in Judges 19: Subject—Honor, Object—Shame?" *Journal for the Study of the Old Testament* 67 (September 1995), 87–107; Thielicke, Helmut. *The Evangelical Faith*, vol. 1: *Prolegomena: The Relation of Theology to Modern Thought-Forms*. Trans. Geoffrey W. Bromiley. Grand Rapids, Mich.: Eerdmans, 1974; Waltke, Bruce K. "Abomination." In Geoffrey W. Bromiley, ed., *The International Standard Bible Encyclopedia*, 3rd ed., fully rev., vol. 1. Grand Rapids, Mich.: Eerdmans, 1979, 13–14; Ward, Roy. "Why Unnatural? The Tradition behind Romans 1:26–27." *Harvard Theological Review* 90:3 (1997), 263–84; Whitaker, Richard E. "Creation and Human Sexuality." In Choon-Leong Seow, ed., *Homosexuality and Christian Community*. Louisville, Ky.: Westminster John Knox, 1996, 3–13; Wright, David F. "Homosexuals or Prostitutes? The Meaning of *arsenokoitai* (1 Cor. 6:9, 1 Tim. 1:10)." *Vigiliae Christianae* 38 (June 1984), 125–53.

John Kleinig

ADDITIONAL READING

Bailey, Derrick Sherwin. *The Man-Woman Relation in Christian Thought*. London: Longmans, Green, 1959; Balch, David, ed. *Homosexuality, Science, and the "Plain Sense" of Scripture*. Grand Rapids, Mich.: Eerdmans, 2000; Brawley, Robert L., ed. *Biblical Ethics and Homosexuality: Listening to Scripture*. Louisville, Ky.: Westminster John Knox, 1996; Brenner, Athalya, and Carole R.

Fontaine, eds. *A Feminist Companion to Reading the Bible: Approaches, Methods and Strategies.* Sheffield, U.K.: Sheffield Academic Press, 1997; Brewer, David I. "Jesus' Old Testament Basis for Monogamy." In Steve Moyise, ed., *The Old Testament in the New Testament: Essays in Honour of J. L. North.* [*Journal for the Study of the New Testament*, supp. series, no. 189.] Sheffield, U.K.: Sheffield Academic Press, 2000, 75–105; Carr, David M. *The Erotic Word: Sensuality, Spirituality, and the Bible.* Oxford, U.K.: Oxford University Press, 2003; Clark, Elizabeth A. " 'Adam's Only Companion': Augustine and the Early Christian Debate on Marriage." *Recherches Augustiniennes* 21 (1986), 139–62; Countryman, William. *Dirt, Greed, and Sex: Sexual Ethics in the New Testament and Their Implications for Today.* Philadelphia, Pa.: Fortress, 1988; Daube, David. *The Duty of Procreation.* Edinburgh, Scot.: Edinburgh University Press, 1977; Davidson, Richard M. "The Theology of Sexuality in the Beginning: Genesis 1–2." *Andrews University Seminary Studies* 26:1 (1988), 5–24; Davidson, Richard M. "The Theology of Sexuality in the Beginning: Genesis 3." *Andrews University Seminary Studies* 26:2 (1988), 121–32; Davies, Margaret. "On Prostitution." In M. Daniel Carroll R., David J. A. Clines, and Philip R. Davies, eds., *The Bible in Human Society: Essays in Honour of John Rogerson.* [*Journal for the Study of the Old Testament*; supp. series, no. 200.] Sheffield, U.K.: Sheffield Academic Press, 1995, 225–48; Deming, Will. (1995) *Paul on Marriage and Celibacy: The Hellenistic Background of 1 Corinthians 7,* 2nd ed. Grand Rapids, Mich.: Eerdmans, 2004; Eichler, Barry L. "Bestiality." In Keith Crim, ed., *The Interpreter's Dictionary of the Bible,* supp. vol. Nashville, Tenn.: Abingdon, 1976, 96–97; Frymer-Kensky, Tikva. "Virginity in the Bible." In Victor H. Matthews, Bernard M. Levinson, and Tikva Frymer-Kensky, eds., *Gender and Law in the Hebrew Bible and the Ancient Near East.* [*Journal for the Study of the Old Testament*; supp. series, no. 262.] Sheffield, U.K.: Sheffield Academic Press, 1998, 79–96; Gravrock, Mark. "Why Won't Paul Just Say No? Purity and Sex in 1 Corinthians 6." *Word and World* 14:4 (1996), 444–55; Gross, Robert E., and Mona West, eds. *Take Back the Word: A Queer Reading of the Bible.* Cleveland, Ohio: Pilgrim Press, 2000; Helminiak, Daniel A. "The Bible on Homosexuality: Ethically Neutral." In John Corvino, ed., *Same Sex: Debating the Ethics, Science, and Culture of Homosexuality.* Lanham, Md.: Rowman and Littlefield, 1997, 81–92; Helminiak, Daniel A. *What the Bible Really Says about Homosexuality.* San Francisco, Calif.: Alamo Square, 1994; Jung, Patricia Beattie, and Ralph F. Smith. "The Bible and Heterosexism." In *Heterosexism: An Ethical Challenge.* Albany: State University of New York Press, 1993, 61–88; McGrath, R. H. "Sex (in the Bible)." In *New Catholic Encyclopedia,* vol. 13. New York: McGraw-Hill, 1967, 150; Morgan, Douglas N. *Love: Plato, the Bible, and Freud.* Englewood Cliffs, N.J.: Prentice-Hall, 1964; Patai, Raphael. "Bestiality." In *Sex and Family in the Bible and the Middle East.* Garden City, N.Y.: Dolphin/Doubleday, 1959, 178–80; Ringgren, Helmer. "קדשׁ." [qodesh; "holiness"] In G. Johannes Botterweck, Helmer Ringgren, and Heinz-Joseph Fabry, eds., *Theological Dictionary of the Old Testament,* vol. 12. Trans. Douglas W. Stott. Grand Rapids, Mich.: Eerdmans, 2003, 521–45; Schmidt, Thomas E. "Romans 1:26–27 and Biblical Sexuality." In John Corvino, ed., *Same Sex: Debating the Ethics, Science, and Culture of Homosexuality.* Lanham, Md.: Rowman and Littlefield, 1997, 93–104; Seow, Choon-Leong. ed. *Homosexuality and Christian Community.* Louisville, Ky.: Westminster John Knox, 1996; Smith, Carol. "Challenged by the Text: Two Stories of Incest in the Hebrew Bible." In Athalya Brenner and Carole R. Fontaine, eds., *A Feminist Companion to Reading the Bible: Approaches, Methods and Strategies.* Sheffield, U.K.: Sheffield Academic Press, 1997, 114–35; Smith, Carol. "Stories of Incest in the Hebrew Bible: Scholars Challenging Text or Text Challenging Scholars?" *Henoch* 14 (1992), 227–42; Soards, Marion. *Scripture and Homosexuality: Biblical Authority and the Church Today.* Louisville, Ky.: Westminister John Knox, 1995; Thielicke, Helmut. *The Ethics of Sex.* Trans. John W. Doberstein. New York: Harper and Row, 1964; Thomas, Keith. "Rescuing Homosexual History." *New York Review of Books* (4 December 1980), 26–29; Vacek, Edward. "A Christian Homosexuality?" *Commonweal* (5 December 1980), 681–84. Reprinted in POS3 (129–35); POS4 (127–33); Yamauchi, Edwin M. *Africa and the Bible.* Grand Rapids, Mich.: Baker Academic, 2004.

BIRTH CONTROL. *See* Contraception

BISEXUALITY. Bisexuality, heterosexuality, and **homosexuality** are forms of **sexual orientation** or sexual object preference. While the proper characterization of sexual orientation is still debated, commonly proposed criteria include sexual behavior, or the type of person one has sex with; **sexual desire**, or the type of person one is attracted to or finds arousing; **fantasy**, or the content of one's sexual imaginings; and self-identification, or how one labels or thinks of oneself (see De Cecco, "Definition"; Morrow; Shively and De Cecco). Broadly speaking, the sexual orientation of homosexuals is for their own sex/gender, the orientation of heterosexuals is for the other sex/gender, and the orientation of bisexuals is for both. Gary Zinik has usefully distinguished between *simultaneous* bisexuality, in which an individual engages in sexual acts with men and women at the same time (say, a triad); *concurrent* bisexuality, in which an individual carries on distinct sexual relationships with a man and with a woman during the same period of his or her life; and *serial* bisexuality, in which an individual practices serial monogamy, alternating same-sex and other-sex relationships.

The seemingly simple task of estimating the incidence of bisexuality has generated vastly different results, depending on one's analysis of sexual orientation in general and bisexuality in particular. Some theorists explicitly deny that bisexuality even exists. Kenneth Altshuler asserts that bisexuality is only a transition between heterosexuality and homosexuality. For Edmund Bergler, bisexuals are frauds attempting to cover up their homosexual orientation: "The clinical facts . . . are that 'bisexuality' . . . is a blatant misnomer. 'Bisexuality' in adults denotes clearcut homosexuality, with a few *defensive* traces of mechanical heterosexuality retained" (*Counterfeit-Sex*, ix-x; see *Homosexuality: Disease*, 89–108). It is still common for researchers to treat bisexuals and homosexuals as a homogenous group to be contrasted with heterosexuals (see two essays by MacDonald; also Van Wyk and Geist). At the other end of the spectrum, some sexologists postulated that humans were by nature either bisexual or polymorphously sexual. Richard von Krafft-Ebing (1840–1902), for example, claimed that in children "the *psychical* relation to persons of the opposite sex is still absolutely wanting, and the sexual acts during this period exhibit more or less a reflex spinal character" (186), in which the type of object producing or used for sexual pleasure is irrelevant. **Sigmund Freud** (1856–1939), in his *Three Essays*, affirms that basic human psychosexual nature is either bisexual (145, note added in 1915; 147, end of note added in 1920; see also Lang, 156) or "polymorphously perverse" (182, 191; see Herbert Marcuse [1898–1979], 49).

Between these extremes lies a body of empirical research on the incidence of bisexuality inaugurated by Alfred Kinsey's (1894–1956) mid-twentieth-century finding that about 37 percent of males and 13 percent of females engaged in some homosexual activity to orgasm at some time in their lives up to age forty-five (*Human Female*, 487; see *Human Male*, fig. 156 on 625, and 650). More recent studies have found that 22 percent of men and 17 percent of women have had homosexual experiences (Janus and Janus, 69). The National Health and Social Life Survey (NHSLS) found, in face-to-face interviews, that only 7.1 percent of the men and 3.8 percent of the women had some homosexual experience; these figures increased slightly to 9.1 percent and 4.3 percent, respectively, when subjects reported their experiences on a self-administered form placed into a sealed envelope (Laumann et al., 294, 296). The NHSLS data reveal that among individuals with any homosexual sexual experience at all, over 90 percent also had heterosexual experiences (311, table 8.3A; 312). In the NHSLS study, 0.8 percent of the men identified themselves as bisexual, 2 percent identified themselves as gay, 0.5 percent of the women identified themselves as bisexual, and 0.9 percent identified themselves as lesbian (311, table 8.3B;

note that a few pages earlier [297] the figures are slightly different: 1.12, 2.8, 0.78, and 1.4, respectively).

What the data show is that in the United States bisexual behavior is not uncommon—yet bisexual behavior does not correlate with self-attributions of bisexual orientation. The data also illustrate that different rates of bisexuality are found, depending on whether bisexuality is defined in terms of behavior, attraction and/or arousal, self-identification, and so forth. Many theorists prefer criteria based on a person's dispositions for sexual contact rather than behavior, since at least some bisexual behavior (for example, that which occurs in prison) reflects a lack of preferred options instead of deep preferences (Stein, 50). In actual research protocols, however, the dispositional model is often set aside in favor of more easily measurable phenomena such as behavior and fantasies.

Kinsey himself eschewed classifying individuals in discrete categories of heterosexuals or homosexuals (or bisexuals, for that matter):

> Males do not represent two discrete populations of heterosexuals and homosexuals. . . . It is a fundamental of taxonomy that nature rarely deals in discrete categories. Only the human mind invents categories and tries to force facts into separated pigeon-holes. The living world is a continuum in each and every one of its aspects. The sooner we learn this concerning sexual behavior the sooner we shall reach a sound understanding of the realities of sex. (*Human Male*, 639)

Kinsey argued that a seven-point scale (0–6) measuring sexual behavior, sexual attraction, and sexual fantasy toward and with same-sex and other-sex partners best represents the *continuum* of sexual object choice. In the Kinsey system, a "0" person is purely heterosexual; a "6" is purely homosexual. In practice, researchers often just select those who rank as 3's, or perhaps 2's–4's, and label them bisexual (De Cecco, "Sex and More Sex"). The bisexuals, then, are roughly those who have sex more or less equally with men and women. (This group seems to include the people that Bergler says are "bisexual" only by *misnomer*, really being homosexuals.) Some researchers have refined and augmented Kinsey's scale. Michael Storms includes additional scales measuring the intensity of attractions and fantasies. This enables bisexuality to be characterized in terms of *strong* homosexual and heterosexual attractions, which is not possible on Kinsey's scale. Fritz Klein has sought an even more multidimensional approach, adding social preference, affective preference, lifestyle preference, and self-identification (Klein et al.).

How are bisexuality, sex, and gender linked? Since bisexuality is defined in terms of attractions to the same and other sexed/gendered individuals, bisexuality presupposes the everyday view that both sex and gender are dichotomous. But bisexuality also challenges our everyday views, for bisexuals violate the social edict that it is natural (and even right) for women (men) to be exclusively sexually attracted to men (women). Of course, homosexuals already make manifest the point that sex and gender do not determine or always correlate with orientation. But bisexuality is the only sexual orientation in which sex and gender are irrelevant to sexual object choice, so bisexuals exhibit more gender flexibility than heterosexuals and homosexuals, both of which predicate sexual object choice on the specific sex/gender of the other person (Weinberg et al., 288–89). Some bisexuals, however, do retain an attachment to sex/gender categories in the sense that their attractions to men and women are gender-specific: A bisexual woman may be attracted to a man because of his penis and physically intense style of intercourse, and she might be attracted to a woman because of her soft breasts and diffuse eroticism (Weinberg et al., 50–53).

There may also be persons we can call "bisexual" whose erotic desires are directed to others in virtue of their perceived mixing and matching of biological and gender traits. Specific attractions to intersexed or transgendered individuals would fit here. Some bisexuals' attractions, however, appear to be gender "blind"; that is, they are attracted to individuals independently of sex- and gender-linked attributes (Ross and Paul). Their sexual attractions are based on generally *human* traits: the other's character or personality, interests and hobbies, projects and goals. In gender-blind attraction, the gender of one's partner is irrelevant to sexual object choice. The term "bisexuality," then, might not be the most appropriate label for this sexual orientation, since it is clearly outside the tripartite division—bisexuality, homosexuality, heterosexuality—all of whose members presuppose dichotomous sex and gender and classify persons and their acts in terms of sex-specific or gender-specific attraction. People with a gender-blind or "pansexual" orientation are open not only to relations with men and women as traditionally figured in our society but also to relations with individuals who identify themselves as some combination of man/woman or some alternative gender entirely. Pansexuality need not presuppose a strict dichotomy in biological sex but embraces emotional, affective, and sexual relationships with natal males and females as well as intersexed and transexual individuals. From this perspective, puzzles that currently arise in sexual orientation attributions disappear, such as whether a woman "becomes" bisexual if her husband, after sex reassignment surgery, is or identifies as a transexual/transgender woman. Whether pansexualism represents a utopian ideal of freedom from stereotypes or a radical "destabilization" of our binary identity categories—or something else—is up for political debate.

The idea that traditional binary identity categories—male/female, feminine/masculine, heterosexual/homosexual—should be "destabilized" arises from a cluster of poststructuralist views often labeled **queer theory** (Butler, 142–49). A central tenet of queer theory is that sex/gender/sexual orientation and maybe even sexual desire/pleasure are not biologically determined. Nor do they even comprise transhistorical or cross-cultural categories. Further, queer theorists, following **Michel Foucault** (1926–1984), are skeptical of the affirmation of a gay identity as part of the effort to resist homophobia in the dominant culture. Such strategies, it is believed, reinscribe the original binary relations. For this reason, queer theorists and activists have embraced bisexuals and transgender individuals, while many gay and lesbian groups have not. While queer theory and politics has had some success in bringing together groups to fight heterosexism, its goals may be problematic in relation to bisexuality. In its attempt to destabilize "fixed" identities, it leaps over the fact that bisexuality, in contrast to heterosexuality and homosexuality, is an identity that has barely spoken its name, has barely had the opportunity to announce itself as a viable sexual orientation. Bisexuality, constituted in the *space* or gap between heterosexual and homosexual norms, continually gets erased by vested interests on both sides. (It is not erased, however, by the American Psychiatric Association, which classifies psychically distressing or "ego-dystonic" homosexuality, heterosexuality, *and* bisexuality as sexual mental disorders; DSM-IV-TR, 535.)

Bisexuals, like other sexual minorities, face an array of pressures in our society, including prejudicial attitudes, susceptibility to physical attack, and civil rights violations. Bisexuals, of course, do benefit from heterosexual privilege, at least in some contexts, but in other contexts they clearly suffer from both informal and formal discrimination in virtue of their engagement in socially proscribed "homosexual" activities. Bisexuals, like homosexuals, are viewed as deviant *because* they have same-gender attractions. They are subject to dismissal from the U.S. **military** for performing "homosexual" acts or for announcing their sexual orientation; they are forbidden from engaging in **marriage** with their same-gender partner; and in many jurisdictions they have no protection from discrimination in employment and housing.

However, distinctive forms of attitudinal and perhaps even legal discrimination may exist on the basis of the bisexual orientation itself. Both heterosexuals and homosexuals subscribe to stereotypes about bisexuals, stereotypes that often contradict one another but nevertheless persevere. On the one hand, bisexuality simply does not exist—these people are really homosexual. On the other hand, these nonexistent bisexuals bring HIV/AIDS (human immunodeficiency virus/acquired immunodeficiency syndrome) into the heterosexual community. (The topic of bisexuality and HIV/AIDS is fraught with anxiety, blame, fear, and ignorance. Bisexuals have been the scapegoats; regarded as disease vectors lacking any semblance of conscience, they contract HIV from homosexuals and then infect unknowing, virtuous heterosexuals.) They are regarded as weak, indecisive, "sitting on the fence" rather than owning up to an orientation. They are seen as promiscuous, predatory, and untrustworthy in relationships. Naomi Mezey suggests that these stereotypes are not based on the perceived homosexuality of bisexuals but on their transgressing the homosexual/heterosexual divide:

> [T]he paradigm of mutually exclusive heterosexuality and homosexuality ensures that bisexuality retains its currency as the formless receptacle of sexual confusion and fear—fear about the rapid spread of AIDS, about sexual voraciousness, about promiscuity, and unarticulated fear of the taboo and degenerate. Bisexuality serves the function of deviancy so well not because it is thought to include some homosexual behavior, but precisely because it challenges the dual sexual categorization altogether. (103)

Loraine Hutchins and Lani Ka'ahumanu point out that heterosexuality has an interest in denying any morally ambiguous space between heterosexuality and homosexuality: "Heterosexuality *needs* homosexuality, to be reassured that it is different. It also needs the illusion of dichotomy between the orientations to maintain the idea of a fence, a fence that has a right (normal, good) and a wrong (abnormal, evil) side to be on, of fall from" (xxxii). It is not surprising that homosexual communities, as they resist heterosexism and acclaim their own sense of what is right, normal, and good, end up erasing bisexuality or treating bisexuals as morally inferior. For instance, the principle "**feminism** is the theory, lesbianism is the practice" sanctions lesbian chauvinism, thereby disenfranchising bisexual women (see Ault, 117). Another case of privileging is the foundational feminist text, Adrienne Rich's "Compulsory Heterosexuality and Lesbian Existence," which extends lesbian affiliation to many famous women of the past—women whose eroticism, emotional bonds, and **friendship**s may well be regarded more precisely as bisexual.

Although much antipathy to bisexuals involves unconscious tensions and prejudice, some homosexuals are consciously alert to the threat that bisexuals pose for their political strategies aimed at ending discrimination on the basis of sexual orientation. For instance, much gay and lesbian activism is committed to "essentialist" views of gays. It is often argued that homosexuals are a minority group, like African Americans, who cannot choose their membership and therefore deserve the protection of civil rights. The familiar line in this approach is that gays and lesbians are "born that way" so should not be held responsible for their orientation or be deprived on account of it. But can bisexuals plausibly be said to be "born that way," as gays and lesbians are purported to be? (See Van Wyk and Geist.) If not, that would raise problems for the essentialist view of homosexuality and the politics that essentialism generates. Further, it seems odd to think that same-sex object choice is biologically determined for homosexuals but not for bisexuals. If that were true, however, would that mean that civil rights should be extended to gays and lesbians but not bisexuals?

The legalization of **same-sex marriage** is of great political concern to gays, lesbians, and bisexuals. Those bisexuals having partners of the same sex would benefit from receiving the rights already accorded to bisexuals whose partners are of the other sex. The extension of marriage rights to gays is based on the values of individualism and personal freedom, which already ground marital freedom of choice for heterosexuals. Further, the basis of marriage is often perceived to be romantic **love** and eventual commitment, which are at least partly generated through mutually intimate **sexual activity**. However, would the legalization of two-partner gay marriages fully secure bisexuals' civil rights in this area? It might be argued that if bisexuals have a right to full sexual expression in marriage, some bisexuals might form relationships composed of at least three individuals and two different sexes. These relationships might have the same characteristics as heterosexual and homosexual marriages, although the concept and ideal of sexual fidelity would have to be expanded to include all the members of the marriage. The fact that this possibility is rarely considered in public discourse may be a sign of the continued erasure of bisexuality or fear on the part of homosexuals that such a proposal, in opening the door to polygamy, would kill the gay marriage movement. For political reasons, the assumption that romantic unions of more than two individuals are unstable or otherwise objectionable remains unexamined.

In any event, the question of gay marriage brings to light many deeper ethical and political issues concerning homosexual and bisexual sexual expression (see Vernallis). Some gays and bisexuals believe that the gay marriage movement is an attempt to appease heterosexist culture—by displaying gays and lesbians as good citizens who merely want to engage in the long tradition of marriage—and thereby reinforces the demonization of less normative sexual practices (see Rubin on the "sex hierarchy"). Bisexuals disagree over whether to emphasize their capacity for "normal" (lifelong, monogamous) sexual relations or to celebrate nonmonogamy, regarding the ideas of multiple partners, primary and secondary partners, and serial monogamy as distinctively bisexual contributions to sexual thought and freedom. **Margaret Mead** (1901–1978) has explained that while heterosexuals can understand homosexuals as like themselves (namely, as monosexuals but with the reverse sexual object preference), grasping bisexuality may demand a more profound revolution: "Changing traditional attitudes toward homosexuality is in itself a mind-expanding experience for most people. But we shall not really succeed in discarding the strait jacket of our cultural beliefs about sexual choice if we fail to come to terms with the well-documented, normal human capacity to love members of both sexes" (271).

See also Casual Sex; Diseases, Sexually Transmitted; Feminism, French; Feminism, Lesbian; Friendship; Herdt, Gilbert; Heterosexism; Homosexuality and Science; Orientation, Sexual; Psychology, Twentieth- and Twenty-First-Century; Rimmer, Robert; Sexology; Social Constructionism

REFERENCES

Altshuler, Kenneth Z. "On the Question of Bisexuality." *American Journal of Psychotherapy* 38:4 (1956), 484–93; American Psychiatric Association. *Diagnostic and Statistical Manual of Mental Disorders*, text revision of the 4th ed. [DSM-IV-TR] Washington, D.C.: Author, 2000; Ault, Amber. "Hegemonic Discourse in an Oppositional Community: Lesbian Feminists and Bisexuality." *Critical Sociology* 20:3 (1994), 107–22; Bergler, Edmund. (1951) *Counterfeit-Sex: Homosexuality, Impotence, Frigidity*, 2nd ed. New York: Grune and Stratton, 1958; Bergler, Edmund. (1956) "Does 'Bisexuality' Exist?" In *Homosexuality: Disease or Way of Life?* New York: Hill and Wang, 1957,

89–108; Butler, Judith. *Gender Trouble: Feminism and the Subversion of Identity*. New York: Routledge, 1990; De Cecco, John P. "Definition and Meaning of Sexual Orientation." *Journal of Homosexuality* 6:4 (1981), 51–67; De Cecco, John P. "Sex and More Sex: A Critique of the Kinsey Conception of Human Sexuality." In David P. McWhirter, Stephanie A. Sanders, and June M. Reinisch, eds., *Homosexuality/Heterosexuality: Concepts of Sexual Orientation*. New York: Oxford University Press, 1990, 367–86; Freud, Sigmund. (1905) *Three Essays on the Theory of Sexuality*. In *The Standard Edition of the Complete Psychological Works of Sigmund Freud*, vol. 7. Trans. and ed. James Strachey. London: Hogarth Press, 1953–1974, 125–245; Hutchins, Loraine, and Lani Ka'ahumanu, eds. *Bi Any Other Name: Bisexual People Speak Out*. Boston, Mass.: Alyson, 1991; Janus, Samuel S., and Cynthia L. Janus. *The Janus Report on Sexual Behavior*. New York: John Wiley, 1993; Kinsey, Alfred, Wardell Pomeroy, and Clyde Martin. *Sexual Behavior in the Human Male*. Philadelphia, Pa.: Saunders, 1948; Kinsey, Alfred, Wardell Pomeroy, Clyde Martin, and Paul Gebhard. *Sexual Behavior in the Human Female*. Philadelphia, Pa.: Saunders, 1953; Klein, Fritz, Barry Sepekoff, and Timothy Wolf. "Sexual Orientation: A Multi-Variable Dynamic Process." *Journal of Homosexuality* 11:1–2 (1985), 35–50; Krafft-Ebing, Richard von. (1886) *Psychopathia Sexualis: With Especial Reference to the Antipathic Sexual Instinct. A Medico-forensic Study*. Trans. (from the 12th German ed.) Franklin S. Klaf. New York: Stein and Day, 1965; Lang, Theo. *The Difference between a Man and a Woman*. New York: John Day, 1971; Laumann, Edward O., John H. Gagnon, Robert T. Michael, and Stuart Michaels. *The Social Organization of Sexuality: Sexual Practices in the United States*. Chicago, Ill.: University of Chicago Press, 1994; MacDonald, A. P., Jr. "Bisexuality: Some Comments on Research and Theory." *Journal of Homosexuality* 6 (1981), 21–35; MacDonald, A. P., Jr. "A Little Bit of Lavender Goes a Long Way: A Critique of Research on Sexual Orientation." *Journal of Sex Research* 19:1 (1983), 94–100; Marcuse, Herbert. (1955) *Eros and Civilization: A Philosophical Inquiry into Freud*. Boston, Mass.: Beacon Press, 1966; Mead, Margaret. (1975) "Bisexuality: A New Awareness." In Margaret Mead and Rhoda Metraux, *Aspects of the Present*. New York: Morrow, 1980, 269–75; Mezey, Naomi. "Dismantling the Wall: Bisexuality and the Possibility of Sexual Identity Classification Based on Acts." *Berkeley Women's Law Journal* 10 (1995), 99–133; Morrow, Gregory D. "Bisexuality: An Exploratory Review." *Annals of Sex Research* 2 (1989), 283–306; Rich, Adrienne. "Compulsory Heterosexuality and Lesbian Existence." *Signs* 5:4 (1980), 631–60; Ross, Michael, and Jay Paul. "Beyond Gender: The Basis of Sexual Attraction in Bisexual Men and Women." *Psychological Reports* 71:3, pt. 2 (1992), 1283–90; Rubin, Gayle S. "Thinking Sex: Notes for a Radical Theory of the Politics of Sexuality." In Carole S. Vance, ed., *Pleasure and Danger: Exploring Female Sexuality*. London: Routledge and Kegan Paul, 1984, 267–319; Shively, Michael G., and John De Cecco. "Components of Sexual Identity." *Journal of Homosexuality* 3:1 (1977), 41–48; Stein, Edward. *The Mismeasure of Desire: The Science, Theory, and Ethics of Sexual Orientation*. Oxford, U.K.: Oxford University Press, 2001; Storms, Michael D. "Theories of Sexual Orientation." *Journal of Personality and Social Psychology* 38:4 (1980), 783–92; Van Wyk, Paul, and Chrisann Geist. "Biology of Bisexuality: Critique and Observations." *Journal of Homosexuality* 28:3–4 (1995), 357–73; Vernallis, Kayley. "Bisexual Monogamy: Twice the Temptation But Half the Fun?" *Journal of Social Philosophy* 30:3 (1999), 347–68; Weinberg, Martin, Colin Williams, and Douglas Pryor. *Dual Attraction: Understanding Bisexuality*. Oxford, U.K.: Oxford University Press, 1994; Zinik, Gary. "Identity Conflict or Adaptive Flexibility? Bisexuality Reconsidered." *Journal of Homosexuality* 11:1–2 (1985), 7–19.

Kayley Vernallis

ADDITIONAL READING

Alexander, Jonathan, and Karen Yescavage, eds. *Bisexuality and Transgenderism*. Binghamton, N.Y.: Harrington Park/Haworth, 2004; Almaguer, Tomas. "Chicano Men: A Cartography of Homosexual Identity and Behavior." In Henry Abelove, Michèle Aina Barale, and David M. Halperin, eds., *The Lesbian and Gay Studies Reader*. New York: Routledge, 1993, 255–73; Anderlini-D'Onofrio, Serena, ed. *Women and Bisexuality: A Global Perspective*. Binghamton, N.Y.: Harrington Park/Haworth,

2003; Angelides, Steven. *A History of Bisexuality*. Chicago, Ill.: University of Chicago Press, 2001; Atkins, Dawn. *Bisexual Women in the Twenty-First Century*. Binghamton, N.Y.: Harrington Park/Haworth, 2003; Baker, Karin. "Bisexual Feminist Politics: Because Bisexuality Is Not Enough." In Elizabeth Reba Wise, ed., *Closer to Home: Bisexuality and Feminism*. Seattle, Wash.: Seal Press, 1992, 255–67; Bell, Alan P., and Martin S. Weinberg. *Homosexualities: A Study of Diversity among Men and Women*. New York: Simon and Schuster, 1978; Bowie, Malcolm. "Bisexuality." In Elizabeth Wright, ed., *Feminism and Psychoanalysis: A Critical Dictionary*. Oxford, U.K.: Blackwell, 1992, 26–31; Cantarella, Eva. *Bisexuality in the Ancient World*. Trans. Cormac Ó Cuilleanáin. New Haven, Conn.: Yale University Press, 1992; Coleman, Eli. "Bisexuality: Challenging Our Understanding of Human Sexuality and Sexual Orientation." In Earl E. Shelp, ed., *Sexuality and Medicine*, vol. 1: *Conceptual Roots*. Dordrecht, Holland: Reidel, 1987, 225–42; Daumer, Elizabeth. "Queer Ethics, or the Challenge of Bisexuality to Lesbian Ethics." *Hypatia* 7:4 (1992), 91–106; Eadie, Jo. "Activating Bisexuality: Towards a Bi/Sexual Politics." In Joseph Bristow and Angelia Wilson, eds., *Activating Theory: Lesbian, Gay, Bisexual Politics*. London: Lawrence and Wishart, 1993, 139–70; Esterberg, Kristin G. *Lesbian and Bisexual Identities: Constructing Communities, Constructing Selves*. Philadelphia, Pa.: Temple University Press, 1997; Firestein, Beth, ed. *Bisexuality: The Psychology and Politics of an Invisible Minority*. London: Sage, 1996; Fox, Ronald C. "Bisexuality in Perspective: A Review of Theory and Research." In Beth Firestein, ed., *Bisexuality: The Psychology and Politics of an Invisible Minority*. London: Sage, 1996, 3–52; Garber, Marjorie. *Vice Versa: Bisexuality and the Eroticism of Everyday Life*. New York: Simon and Schuster, 1995; Gregory, Deborah. "From Where I Stand: A Case for Feminist Bisexuality." In Sue Cartledge and Joanna Ryan, eds., *Sex and Love: New Thoughts on Old Contradictions*. London: Women's Press, 1983, 141–56; Griffin, Jasper. "The Love That Dared to Speak Its Name." [Review of *Bisexuality in the Ancient World*, by Eva Cantarella] *New York Review of Books* (22 October 1992), 30–32; Gudorf, Christine E. "The Erosion of Sexual Dimorphism: Challenges to Religion and Religious Ethics." *Journal of the American Academy of Religion* 69:4 (2001), 863–91; Haeberle, Erwin, and Rolf Gindorf, eds. *Bisexualities: The Ideology and Practice of Sexual Contact with Both Men and Women*. New York: Continuum, 1998; Hemmings, Clare. *Bisexual Spaces: A Geography of Sexuality and Gender*. New York: Routledge, 2003; Herdt, Gilbert. "Developmental Discontinuities and Sexual Orientation across Cultures." In David P. McWhirter, Stephanie A. Sanders, and June M. Reinisch, eds., *Homosexuality/ Heterosexuality: Concepts of Sexual Orientation*. New York: Oxford University Press, 1990, 208–36; Herdt, Gilbert, ed. *Third Sex, Third Gender: Beyond Sexual Dimorphism in Culture and History*. New York: Zone Books, 1994; Klein, Fritz. *The Bisexual Option: A Concept of One-Hundred Percent Intimacy*. New York: Arbor House, 1978; Klein, Fritz. "The Need to View Sexual Orientation as a Multivariable Dynamic Process: A Theoretical Perspective." In David P. McWhirter, Stephanie A. Sanders, and June M. Reinisch, eds., *Homosexuality/Heterosexuality: Concepts of Sexual Orientation*. New York: Oxford University Press, 1990, 277–82; Mitchell, Juliet. (1974) "Masculinity, Femininity and Bisexuality." In *Psychoanalysis and Feminism: Freud, Reich, Laing, and Women*. New York: Vintage, 1975, 42–52; Money, John. "Androgyne Becomes Bisexual in Sexological Theory: From Plato to Freud and Neuroscience." In *The Adam Principle. Genes, Genitals, Hormones, & Gender: Selected Readings in Sexology*. Buffalo, N.Y.: Prometheus, 1993; Money, John. *Gay, Straight and In-Between: The Sexology of Erotic Orientation*. New York: Oxford University Press, 1988; Money, John. "Prison Is Paradise for Bisexual Machos." In *The Adam Principle. Genes, Genitals, Hormones, & Gender: Selected Readings in Sexology*. Buffalo, N.Y.: Prometheus, 1993, 237–46; Namaste, Ki. "The Everyday Bisexual as Problematic: Research Methods beyond Monosexualism." In Janice Ristock and Catherine Taylor, eds., *Inside the Academy and Out: Lesbian/Gay/ Queer Studies and Social Action*. Toronto, Can.: University of Toronto Press, 1998, 111–36; O'Donovan, Oliver. "Transsexualism and Christian Marriage." *Journal of Religious Ethics* 11:1 (1983), 135–62; Paul, Jay P. "The Bisexual Identity: An Idea without Social Recognition." *Journal of Homosexuality* 9:2–3 (1984), 45–64; Pielke, Robert. "Are Androgyny and Sexuality Compatible?" In Mary Vetterling-Braggin, ed., *"Femininity," "Masculinity," and "Androgyny": A Modern Philosophical Discussion*. Totowa, N.J.: Littlefield, Adams, 1982, 187–96. Reprinted in SLF (101–6); Queen, Carol. "Strangers at Home: Bisexuals in the Queer Movement." *Out/Look*, no. 16 (Spring 1992), 23, 29–33. Reprinted, revised, in John Corvino, ed., *Same Sex: Debating the Ethics, Science, and Culture of Homosexuality*. Lanham, Md.: Rowman and Littlefield, 1997, 258–63; Rado, Sandor. "A Critical Examination of the Concept of Bisexuality." *Psychosomatic Medicine* 2 (1940), 459–67. Reprinted in *Psychoanalysis of Behavior. Collected Papers*, vol 1: *1922–1956*. New York: Grune and Stratton, 1956, 139–50; Raymond, Janice G. *The Transsexual Empire: The Making of the She-male*. Boston, Mass.: Beacon, 1979; Rich, Adrienne. "Compulsory Heterosexuality and Lesbian Existence." *Signs* 5:4 (1980), 631–60. Reprinted in *Blood, Bread, and Poetry: Selected Prose 1979–1985*. New York: Norton, 1986, 23-75; and Henry Abelove, Michèle Aina Barale, and David M. Halperin, eds., *The Lesbian and Gay Studies Reader*. New York: Routledge, 1993, 227–54; Rosenberg, Mila. "Trans/positioning the (Drag?) King of Comedy: Bisexuality and Queer Jewish Space in the Works of Sandra Bernhard." In Jonathan Alexander and Karen Yescavage, eds., *Bisexuality and Transgenderism: InterSEXions of the Others*. New York: Harrington Park Press, 2003, 171–79; Rubin, Gayle S. "Thinking Sex: Notes for a Radical Theory of the Politics of Sexuality." In Carole S. Vance, ed., *Pleasure and Danger: Exploring Female Sexuality*. London: Routledge and Kegan Paul, 1984, 267–319. Reprinted in Peter M. Nardi and Beth E. Schneider, eds., *Social Perspectives in Lesbian and Gay Studies*. New York: Routledge, 1998, 100–133; Rust, Paula C. *Bisexuality and the Challenge to Lesbian Politics: Sex, Loyalty, and Revolution*. New York: New York University Press, 1995; Smith, Mark. "Ancient Bisexuality and the Interpretation of Romans 1:26–27." *Journal of the American Academy of Religion* 64:2 (1996), 223–56; Stekel, Wilhelm. (1934) *Bi-sexual Love*. Trans. James S. Van Teslaar. New York: Emerson, 1950; Stoller, Robert J. "The 'Bedrock' of Masculinity and Femininity: Bisexuality." In Jean Baker Miller, ed., *Psychoanalysis and Women*. Baltimore, Md.: Penguin, 1973, 273–84; Stoller, Robert J. (1973) "Facts and Fancies: An Examination of Freud's Concept of Bisexuality." In Jean Strouse, ed., *Women and Analysis: Dialogues on Psychoanalytic Views of Femininity*. New York: Grossman, 1974, 343–64; Storr, Merl. "Postmodern Bisexuality." *Sexualities* 2:3 (1999), 309–25; Storr, Merl, ed. *Bisexuality: A Critical Reader*. New York: Routledge, 1999; Trebilcot, Joyce. (1974) "Two Forms of Androgynism." *Journal of Social Philosophy* 8:1 (1977), 4–8. Reprinted in Mary Vetterling-Braggin, Frederick Elliston, and Jane English, eds., *Feminism and Philosophy*. Totowa, N.J.: Littlefield, Adams, 1977, 70–78; and Mary Vetterling-Braggin, ed., *"Femininity," "Masculinity," and "Androgyny": A Modern Philosophical Discussion*. Totowa, N.J.: Littlefield, Adams, 1982, 161–69; Tucker, Naomi, ed. *Bisexual Politics: Theories, Queries, and Visions*. New York: Harrington Park Press, 1995; Weise, Elizabeth Reba, ed. *Closer to Home: Bisexuality and Feminism*. Seattle, Wash.: Seal Press, 1992; Wilkinson, Sue. "Bisexuality 'A La Mode.'" *Women's Studies International Forum* 19:3 (1996), 293–301; Williams, Mark. *Sexual Pathways: Adapting to Dual Sexual Attraction*. Westport, Conn.: Praeger, 1999.

BOSWELL, JOHN (1947–1994). John Eastburn Boswell will always be associated with essentialism in the philosophy of sexuality, although he eschewed the term. An Ivy League–educated historian, a devout Catholic, and an openly gay man, Boswell dedicated much of his career to understanding **homosexuality**, especially in medieval Christian societies.

Boswell was born in Boston, Massachusetts. As a child, he traveled extensively, since his father was attached to the U.S. diplomatic corps, thereby beginning his acclaimed acquisition of languages. (He knew seventeen modern, medieval, and ancient languages.) Boswell attended the College of William and Mary and received his Ph.D. at Harvard (1975). He was hired by Yale, was eventually promoted to full professor, and was named A. Whitney Griswold Professor of History (1990). He published four books as well as numerous professional articles. He is best remembered for two books: *Christianity, Social Tolerance, and Homosexuality* (CSTH) and *Same-Sex Unions in Premodern Europe*.

When Boswell published CSTH (1980), little existed in print on homosexual history within either Christian or medieval studies. The available literature in English—by Derrick Bailey, **Vern L. Bullough**, and Michael Goodich—depicted the historical Christian response to same-sex eroticism as uniformly condemnatory. Boswell argued that since Christianity was born in an atmosphere of Greco-Roman tolerance of same-sex eroticism, early medieval Christians showed no real animosity toward it. Further, nothing in Christian Scripture or its early tradition required hostile assessments of homosexuality; such assessments derived from misreadings of Scripture. Only in the twelfth and thirteenth centuries did Christian writers formulate significant hostility toward homosexuality (for reasons Boswell could not explain). They read their hostility into Scripture, as some Christians have been doing ever since.

The response to CSTH was mixed. Some celebrated its reappraisal of religious and cultural traditions regarding homosexuality. On the cover of CSTH's first paperback edition, **Michel Foucault** (1926–1984) called the book "truly groundbreaking" and its analysis "unfailing erudition." Gay and lesbian Christians praised the book for providing them with a salvageable past and, especially, for "rescuing" the **Bible** by demonstrating the difficulties in translating culturally specific terms related to sexual behavior. Conservative Christians criticized CSTH as glossing over condemnations of same-sex behavior in both the earliest Christian era and in the Greek and Roman traditions. Boswell received negative reviews; to name but two, from James Brundage and Michael Sheehan, both medievalists who specialized in the history of Christian sexuality. Equally vehement in their condemnation of CSTH were some gay liberationists, who saw Boswell, in virtue of his Catholicism, as "whitewashing" the Catholic history of the persecution of homosexuals. Most scathing were writings by the Gay Academic Union, including *Homosexuality, Intolerance, and Christianity: A Critical Examination of John Boswell's Work* (1981). This was the first of several attempts to discredit Boswell. Wayne Dynes's 1990 *Encyclopedia of Homosexuality* was still antagonistic to Boswell's ideas.

Even though Foucault had praised CSTH, his writings were invoked to challenge another aspect of Boswell's work. In *History of Sexuality*, Foucault had written that "as defined by the . . . [medieval] canonical codes, sodomy was a category of forbidden acts" and "their perpetrator was nothing more than the juridical subject of them" and that it was only in the nineteenth century that the "homosexual became a personage" (43). Boswell, however, used "gay" to refer broadly and transhistorically to "persons who are conscious of erotic inclination toward their own gender as a distinguishing characteristic" (CSTH, 44). The bulk of scholarship was moving in the direction of Foucault's **social constructionism** and away from Boswell's essentialism.

A year before CSTH, Robert Padgug had argued that twentieth-century sexual categories were not the same as those in the past and are now shaped by modern capitalism. The point has been elaborated by, among others, David Halperin. It is no coincidence, he claims, that no ancient Greek or Latin terms are equivalent to our "homosexual" and "heterosexual" ("Sex before Sexuality"). Just as we have no word "pectoriphage" to identify someone who prefers eating chicken, because food preferences are not a meaningful distinction, the ancients did not categorize according to sexual object choice. Boswell's transcultural identification of all same-sex eroticism as "homosexuality" and all individuals so inclined as "gay" was judged anachronistic. Boswell was aware of the criticism that he had overemphasized the similarities between modern and past same-sex eroticism, but he seemed more concerned about the criticism that he had overemphasized the positive side of the early Christian tradition on same-sex eroticism. In his 1982 address to the Gay

Christian Movement in London ("Rediscovering Gay History"), Boswell defended himself against this criticism but not from the charge of anachronism, and he continued to refer to the people he discussed as "gay."

Perhaps Boswell thought he had sufficiently defended his view in CSTH. He admitted, in fact, that we "must be extremely cautious about projecting onto historical data ideas about gay people inferred from modern samples" (24), illustrating this with the relationship between male homosexuality and effeminacy, a phenomenon that varies culturally and historically. Boswell also urged that we "avoid transposing across temporal boundaries ideas about gay relationships which are highly culture-related" (25), providing the example of changing definitions of **marriage**. In a footnote, however, Boswell rejected the significance of the absence of sexual terminology in premodern societies: "English appears to have no real equivalent for the French term 'fiancé,' but this is certainly no indication that the idea of heterosexual engagement was unknown . . . prior to its adoption." He also denied that age-differentiated (pederastic) and gender-differentiated (crossdressing) same-sex eroticism were not "real homosexuality," offering the argument that "one must immediately wonder whether heterosexual relations between men and girls are any less heterosexual for the difference in age." He added, apparently alluding to his terminological usage as a *heuristic* device, that "the whole point of the homosexual/heterosexual distinction . . . is to subsume all varieties of erotic interest into categories of gender relations" (28). He concluded optimistically that "the difficulties of avoiding anachronistic projections . . . will be outweighed by the advantages" (30–31).

Perhaps those very advantages served as the greatest occasion for criticism of CSTH. For Boswell, the opportunity to talk about an assortment of sexual behaviors that we might today lump together as homosexuality was an advantage. His wide-ranging discussion included pederasty as practiced in ancient Athens and Rome (themselves two distinct forms), sexual practices related to gender violations (*viz.*, adult men who submitted to penetration, acting in what was deemed either an adolescent male or feminine role), and more egalitarian male bonds of "adoptive brothers" and comradeship. The men described in his sources were sometimes married or vowed to chastity at the same time that they conducted otherwise "gay" sexual lives. These behaviors are undoubtedly of interest to modern gay men seeking a history, and that was chief among the advantages for Boswell. But whether they should be considered ancient or medieval equivalents of current practices was, for his critics, precisely the point of contention.

The emphasis on men in CSTH yielded further criticism. Boswell assumed that the ancient and medieval take on male homosexuality applied also to lesbianism. But other scholars have insisted that premodern lesbianism has to be studied on its own terms. When ancients talked about female-female eroticism, they usually emphasized gender violations (Brooten, pt. 1). When medievals discussed it, they tended to see it within a context of egalitarian relationships (Matter; Murray). No female equivalent to classical pederasty existed, as far as we know, and if biblical justifications for condemning male homoeroticism are difficult to pin down in meaning, biblical justifications for condemning female homoeroticism are even sketchier (Miller).

The longest rebuttal Boswell gave to his constructionist detractors came in a 1983 essay, "Revolutions, Universals, and Sexual Categories." The debate, he ventured, was a form of the perennial philosophical dispute between nominalists, who believe categories are arbitrary, and realists, who believe they represent something real. Arguing that "there is no gay history" if the categories homosexual/heterosexual and gay/straight are merely inventions rather than genuine aspects of humanity, Boswell located himself firmly in the debate. But

Boswell also wanted to move beyond the debate, preferring to think that sexual categories can been viewed in three main ways: Type A, in which humans are seen as "capable of erotic and sexual interaction with either gender"; Type B, which postulates "two or more sexual categories, to which all human beings belong" through sexual object choice or sexual aim; and Type C, in which "one type of sexual response [is considered] normal (or 'natural' or 'moral' or all three) and all other variants abnormal ('unnatural,' 'immoral')" (23). For some societies, including ancient Greece, evidence exists for all three views.

The debate between essentialists and social constructionists was hottest among classicists. John Winkler (1943–1990) argued for a sharp discontinuity between ancient and modern sexual categories, since Athenians condemned only an adult man's willingness to be sexually penetrated. Craig Williams applied this notion to ancient Rome. Amy Richlin, however, asserted that the ancients still regarded sexually penetrated men as "real" persons. Further, since what was effectively condemned was a form of homosexuality, the condemnation could surely be called homophobic, even if it does not correspond to modern categories. Medieval historians seemed not to have been moved by the debate: Both Robert I. Moore and Jeffrey Richards described the persecution of "homosexuals" in their books on the hostility toward minorities in the Middle Ages. However, among medievalists in other disciplines, such as religious and literary studies (Frantzen; Jordan), Boswell's ideas were more roundly dismissed.

The debate was still raging when Boswell published *Same-Sex Unions* (SSU) in 1994. SSU's argument was as controversial as CSTH's and closely related to it: Not only had there been ritual unions of men in Greek and Roman antiquity similar to contemporary marriages, but Christians had adopted the ritual and utilized it to join men in same-sex unions performed in churches, until the end of the Middle Ages and, in some rural regions, beyond that.

The ceremony's survival in dozens of Christian liturgical books is clear enough, but the ceremony's significance is less clear. Boswell conceded that the language of these ceremonies did not authorize sex, but he did not expect it to: Ordinary marriage ceremonies do not mention sex, although everyone knows it will occur. Boswell showed that when the ceremony was eventually banned by the Church, authorities banned it precisely because they saw it legitimizing homosexual activity. Boswell's theoretical assumptions remained much the same in SSU. He reiterated his position that neither Greco-Roman culture nor early Christians had been hostile to homoeroticism. He assumed that the ceremony had been performed for women, too, although the evidence was slighter. About the constructionism/essentialism debate, he wrote: "[T]he apparently urgent, morally paramount distinction . . . between all heterosexual acts and relationships and all homosexual acts and relationships was largely unknown to the societies in which the unions first took place" (xxv). While he continued to use "homosexual" synonymously with "same sex" in SSU, he avoided "gay." The book fired fresh controversy. One notable review (Shaw) suggested that the ceremony was meant to cement political, not emotional or sexual, bonds. Another review saw the ceremonies as recognizing nonsexual **friendship**s or as a means of reconciling **military** rivals (Brown et al.).

Right about the time of Boswell's death, which followed SSU by only a few months, the debates dissipated. Perhaps it showed the reluctance of scholars to speak ill of the dead. Or maybe scholars tired of the endless repetition of the same points. More likely, a new generation of scholars came to the fore, ones nurtured on **queer theory** and who relished, rather than cringed at, the idea of assimilating past and modern identities. Defining "queer theory" in anything but broad terms is difficult, but as a historical method, it at least involves identifying with all individuals in the past who were conceived of as sexually different, especially those ridiculed, ostracized, or persecuted for their difference. So queer theorists can claim any number of ancient or medieval persons. Calling them "queer" does not necessarily assimilate them to modern gay or lesbian identities. But it does allow scholars to claim even celibate Christian saints as part of a "queer" past (Burrus). Boswell had little use for queer theory. Yet queer theorists, who have taken advantage of the heuristic value of his "essentialism," have been responsible for rescuing his work for the academic community.

The greatest tribute to Boswell's impact is that both CSTH and SSU spilled into popular culture (Dinshaw, 22–34). There was talk of filming a series for PBS on the topic, although it never came to fruition. When Colorado passed a law invalidating gay rights legislation (1992), Boswell presented a brief to Colorado's supreme court that aided in overturning the law. SSU had similar impact. Even before the book's release, Garry Trudeau's *Doonesbury* comic strip devoted several episodes to its argument. Christian gays and lesbians have availed themselves of the ceremonies, included in SSU, in gay-friendly churches. Both CSTH and SSU figured in judicial arguments against long-standing prohibitions of gay marriage and homosexual activity in "Western culture," which prompted Canada's supreme court to order (in 2003) the government to justify its refusal to marry same-sex couples. Future court decisions about same-sex marriage will almost certainly refer to Boswell, and he will deservedly continue to be discussed in scholarly works on homosexuality in ancient, early Christian, and medieval history.

See also Bible, Sex and the; Bullough, Vern L.; Foucault, Michel; Greek Sexuality and Philosophy, Ancient; Herdt, Gilbert; Heterosexism; Homosexuality, Ethics of; Marriage, Same-Sex; Orientation, Sexual; Queer Theory; Social Constructionism

REFERENCES

Bailey, Derrick S. *Homosexuality and the Western Christian Tradition*. London: Longman, 1955; Boswell, John. *Christianity, Social Tolerance, and Homosexuality: Gay People in Western Europe from the Beginning of the Christian Era to the Fourteenth Century*. Chicago, Ill.: University of Chicago Press, 1980; Boswell, John. "Rediscovering Gay History: Archetypes of Gay Love in Christian History." The Fifth Michael Harding Memorial Address (1982), Gay Christian Movement, London; Boswell, John. "Revolutions, Universals, and Sexual Categories." *Salmagundi*, nos. 58–59 (Fall 1982–Winter 1983), 89–113; Boswell, John. *Same-Sex Unions in Premodern Europe*. New York: Villard, 1994; Brooten, Bernadette. *Love between Women: Early Christian Responses to Female Homoeroticism*. Chicago, Ill.: University of Chicago Press, 1996; Brown, Elizabeth A. R., Claudia Rapp, and Brent Shaw. "Ritual Brotherhood in Ancient and Medieval Europe: A Symposium." *Traditio* 52 (1997), 261–381; Brundage, James. Review of *Christianity, Social Tolerance, and Homosexuality*, by John Boswell. *The Catholic Historical Review* 68:1 (1982), 62–64; Bullough, Vern L. *Homosexuality: A History*. New York: New American Library, 1979; Burrus, Virginia. *The Sex Lives of Saints: An Erotics of Ancient Hagiography*. Philadelphia: University of Pennsylvania Press, 2004; Dinshaw, Carolyn. *Getting Medieval: Sexualities and Communities, Pre- and Postmodern*. Durham, N.C.: Duke University Press, 1999; Dynes, Wayne R., ed. *The Encyclopedia of Homosexuality*, 2 vols. New York: Garland, 1990; Foucault, Michel. *The History of Sexuality*, vol. 1: *An Introduction*. Trans. Robert Hurley. New York: Vintage, 1978; Frantzen, Allen J. *Before the Closet: Same-Sex Love from "Beowulf" to "Angels in America."* Chicago, Ill.: University of Chicago Press, 1998; Gay Academic Union. *Homosexuality, Intolerance, and Christianity: A Critical Examination of John Boswell's Work*. <www.galha.org/ptt/lib/hic/bibliography.html> [accessed 15 November 2004]; Goodich, Michael. *The Unmentionable Vice: Homosexuality in the Later Medieval Period*. Santa Barbara, Calif.: ABC-Clio, 1979; Halperin, David. "Sex before Sexuality: Pederasty, Politics, and Power in

Classical Athens." In Martin Duberman, Martha Vicinus, and George Chauncey, Jr., eds., *Hidden from History: Reclaiming the Gay and Lesbian Past*. New York: New American Library, 1989, 37–53; Jordan, Mark. *The Invention of Sodomy in Christian Theology*. Chicago, Ill.: University of Chicago Press, 1997; Matter, E. Ann. "My Sister, My Spouse: Woman-Identified Women in Medieval Christianity." *Journal of Feminist Studies in Religion* 2:2 (1986), 81–93; Miller, James. "The Practice of Romans 1:26: Homosexual or Heterosexual?" *Novum Testamentum* 37:1 (1995), 1–11; Moore, Robert I. *The Formation of a Persecuting Society: Power and Deviance in Western Europe, 950–1250*. New York: Blackwell, 1987; Murray, Jacqueline. "Twice Marginal and Twice Invisible: Lesbians in the Middle Ages." In Vern L. Bullough and James Brundage, eds., *Handbook of Medieval Sexuality*. New York: Garland, 1996, 191–222; Padgug, Robert. "Sexual Matters: On Conceptualizing Sexuality in History." *Radical History Review* 20 (Spring–Summer 1979), 3–23; Richards, Jeffrey. *Sex, Dissidence and Damnation: Minority Groups in the Middle Ages*. London: Routledge, 1990; Richlin, Amy. "Not Before Homosexuality: The Materiality of the *Cinaedus* and the Roman Law against Love between Men." *Journal of the History of Sexuality* 3:4 (1993), 523–73; Shaw, Brent. "A Groom of One's Own? The Medieval Church and the Question of Gay Marriage." *The New Republic* (18–25 July 1994), 33–41; Sheehan, Michael. "Christianity and Homosexuality." [Review of *Christianity, Social Tolerance, and Homosexuality*, by John Boswell] *Journal of Ecclesiastical History* 33:4 (1982), 438–46; Williams, Craig. *Roman Homosexuality: Ideologies of Masculinity in Classical Antiquity*. New York: Oxford University Press, 1999; Winkler, John J. "Laying Down the Law: The Oversight of Men's Sexual Behavior in Classical Athens." In *The Constraints of Desire: The Anthropology of Sex and Gender in Ancient Greece*. New York: Routledge, 1990, 45–70.

Mathew Kuefler

ADDITIONAL READING

Boswell, John. "Categories, Experience, and Sexuality." In Edward Stein, ed., *Forms of Desire: Sexual Orientation and the Social Constructionist Controversy*. New York: Routledge, 1992, 133–73; Boswell, John. "Introduction" to Chris Galser, *Uncommon Calling: A Gay Man's Struggle to Serve the Church*. Louisville, Ky.: Westminster John Knox, 1988. Reprinted as "Logos and Biography" in Eugene F. Rogers, Jr., ed., *Theology and Sexuality: Classic and Contemporary Readings*. Oxford, U.K.: Blackwell, 2002, 356–61; Boswell, John. "Revolutions, Universals, and Sexual Categories." *Salmagundi*, nos. 58–59 (Fall 1982–Winter 1983), 89–113. Reprinted, with "Postscript" (1988), in Martin Duberman, Martha Vicinus, and George Chauncey, Jr., eds., *Hidden from History: Reclaiming the Gay and Lesbian Past*. New York: New American Library, 1989, 17–36; and John Corvino, ed., *Same Sex: Debating the Ethics, Science, and Culture of Homosexuality*. Lanham, Md.: Rowman and Littlefield, 1997, 185–202; Boswell, John. "Sexual and Ethical Categories in Premodern Europe." In David P. McWhirter, Stephanie A. Sanders, and June M. Reinisch, eds., *Homosexuality/Heterosexuality: Concepts of Sexual Orientation*. New York: Oxford University Press, 1990, 15–31; Bullough, Vern L. *Sexual Variance in Society and History*. New York: Wiley, 1976; Dinshaw, Carolyn. "Remembering and Forgetting Boswell." In *Getting Medieval: Sexualities and Communities, Pre- and Postmodern*. Durham, N.C.: Duke University Press, 1999, 22–34; Duberman, Martin, Martha Vicinus, and George Chauncey, Jr., eds. *Hidden from History: Reclaiming the Gay and Lesbian Past*. New York: New American Library, 1989; Gay Academic Union. "Bibliography of Reviews of *Christianity, Social Tolerance, and Homosexuality* (1985)." <www.galha.org/ptt/lib/hic/bibliography.html> [accessed 15 November 2004]; Hall, Richard. "Historian John Boswell on Gay Tolerance and the Christian Tradition." *The Advocate* (28 May 1981), 20–27; Halperin, David. *One Hundred Years of Homosexuality: And Other Essays on Greek Love*. New York: Routledge, 1990; Halsall, Paul. "John Boswell Page." In *People with a History: An Online Guide to Lesbian, Gay, Bisexual, and Trans History*. <www.fordham.edu/halsall/pwh/index-bos.html> [accessed 15 January 2004]; Hays, Richard B. "Relations Natural and Unnatural: A Response to John Boswell's Exegesis of Romans 1." *Journal of Religious Ethics* 14:1 (1986), 184–215; Hinkle, Christopher. "Boswell, John." In Timothy F. Murphy, ed., *Reader's Guide to Lesbian and Gay Studies*. Chicago, Ill.: Fitzroy Dearborn, 2000,

94–95; Hitt, Jack, Joan Blythe, John Boswell, Leon Botstein, and William Kerrigan. [Forum] "New Rules about Sex on Campus." *Harper's Magazine* (September 1993), 33–42. Reprinted as "Student-Professor Sexual Relations: A Forum Discussion." In Bruno Leone and Katie de Koster, eds., *Rape on Campus*. San Diego, Calif.: Greenhaven, 1995, 87–98; Kuefler, Mathew. "Male Friendship and the Suspicion of Sodomy in Twelfth-Century France." In Carol B. Pasternack and Sharon Farmer, eds., *Difference and Genders in the Middle Ages*. Minneapolis: University of Minnesota Press, 2003, 145–81; Kuefler, Mathew. *The Manly Eunuch: Masculinity, Gender Ambiguity, and Christian Ideology in Late Antiquity*. Chicago, Ill.: University of Chicago Press, 2001; Mass, Lawrence. "Sexual Categories, Sexual Universals: A Conversation with John Boswell." In *Homosexuality as Behavior and Identity: Dialogues of the Sexual Revolution*, vol. 2. New York: Haworth, 1990, 202–33; Padgug, Robert. "Sexual Matters: On Conceptualizing Sexuality in History." *Radical History Review* 20 (Spring–Summer 1979), 3–23. Reprinted in Edward Stein, ed., *Forms of Desire: Sexual Orientation and the Social Constructionist Controversy*. New York: Routledge, 1992, 43–67; and Martin Duberman, Martha Vicinus, and George Chauncey, Jr., eds., *Hidden from History: Reclaiming the Gay and Lesbian Past*. New York: New American Library, 1989, 54–64; Paglia, Camille. Review of *Same-Sex Unions in Premodern Europe*, by John Boswell. *Washington Post* (17 July 1994). <www.fordham .edu/halsall/pwh/bosrev-paglia.html> [accessed 16 February 2005]; Sedgwick, Eve Kosofsky. *Epistemology of the Closet*. Berkeley: University of California Press, 1990; Soble, Alan. "Correcting Some Misconceptions about St. Augustine's Sex Life." *Journal of the History of Sexuality* 11:4 (2002), 545–69. Rev. version, <www.uno.edu/~asoble/pages/augbos.htm> [accessed 17 November 2004]; Stein, Edward, ed. *Forms of Desire: Sexual Orientation and the Social Constructionist Controversy*. New York: Garland, 1990. Reprinted, New York: Routledge, 1992; Thomas, Keith. "Rescuing Homosexual History." *New York Review of Books* (4 December 1980), 26–29; Westermarck, Edward. "Christianity and Irregular Sex Relations." In *Christianity and Morals*. New York: Macmillan, 1939, 360–78.

BUDDHISM. While Buddhist philosophy is rich and wide-ranging, covering logic, metaphysics, semantics, psychology, ethics, and other traditional philosophical fields, it has been throughout its history ultimately soteriological in orientation. Buddhist philosophical enquiry may wander seemingly far from a concern for human suffering, indeed the suffering of all sentient beings. Nevertheless, the Buddha made clear his refusal to discuss various issues not pertinent to that concern.

Insofar as any stance on **sexual activity** can be properly thought of as Buddhist, it must be rooted in the basic tenets of Buddhist soteriology rather than merely reflect fleeting social conditions or individual views. On the other hand, the Buddha's (560–ca. 483 BCE) sermons, delivered in various locations in northern India, were not preoccupied with providing a coherent and comprehensive philosophical system, with well-defined terms and unambiguous principles, but with securing changes in the behavior and thought of his hearers that would conduce to easing their suffering. Hence, a good deal of reconstruction is an inevitable element of much exposition of Buddhist thought, especially in connection with the early writings. These writings, the *Tipitaka* ("Three Baskets"), were orally transmitted until inscribed on palm leaves around 33 BCE. They constitute the canon of the conservative Theravadan tradition, which holds them to be a record of Buddha's teaching. The vast literature of the various Mahayanan traditions originated in northern India, spreading to China (around the first century CE), Japan (around 600), and Tibet (around 700).

The *Dhammacakkappavattana* is traditionally regarded as the first sermon given by the Buddha after his Enlightenment, around the age of thirty-five. This sermon sketches the basic framework that unifies Buddhist soteriology, namely, the Four Noble Truths, and introduces its key concepts. The Second Noble Truth introduces the key concept of craving (*tanha* [Pali]; literally, "thirst"). It declares:

> This, bhikkhus, is the Noble Truth of the origin of suffering: it is this craving which leads to renewed existence, accompanied by delight and lust, seeking delight here and there; that is, craving for sensual pleasures, craving for existence, craving for extermination. (Bodhi, 1844)

In the Pali writings, craving for sensual pleasures is preeminent. Craving for sexual pleasures is, in turn, commonly used by the Buddha as an illustration of the craving for sensual pleasures. At least at a general philosophical level, any viable understanding of a Buddhist view on sexual activity must proceed through its connection with the Buddhist soteriological concept of craving (and the related concept of "clinging"—the craving to retain something). Even when craving is satisfied by obtaining what is craved, it merely generates a source of further suffering, the fear of losing that object. (One is reminded here of **Plato** [427–347 BCE], *Symposium*, 200b–e.)

Deep meditative techniques and metaphysical views developed as fundamental counters to all forms of craving and clinging. The Theravadan tradition's metaphysics is basically reductionist. The only genuine existents are the five impermanent, transient elements or aggregates (body, sensation, perception, volition, consciousness). The personal self is not a genuinely independent existent but a mere construction of these elements. Hence it is absurd to have those cravings and clingings (including those of a sexual nature) that are linked to something that does not "really" exist. On the other hand, the impermanent, transient nature of the elements, such as sensations, makes them inappropriate objects of craving and clinging. The Mahayanan traditions adopt a thoroughgoing antirealism, denying even that the Theravadan elements are real existents. Since nothing can be said "really" to exist, or to exist in its own right, but exists (especially in Tibetan traditions) only "by convention," there is nothing that we should crave or cling to. Meditative practice provides deep experiential confirmation and conviction, for the Theravadan, of the reduction of all things to the transient elements or, for the Mahayanan, of the merely conventional existence of all things. In either case, craving for the world is destroyed. Insofar as sexual activity involves craving for the transient or the unreal, it is destroyed by appropriate meditative realization.

As central as the concept or craving (and its cognates) are in Buddhist soteriology, they are rarely given any serious analysis. Thus, cravings are, at times, understood to be what one might regard as vicious or immoral desires or motivations, such as lust, anger, or greed. At other times, virtually any desire or motivation appears to count as a craving, as when Buddhist thinkers raise questions about desires for the plainly noble, such as for Enlightenment itself. At yet other times, such as when the teachings emphasize the role of the waywardness of the human mind as the source of suffering, cravings are seen as essentially uncontrollable or perhaps addictive desires. Given the Buddha's practical soteriological concerns, such variation in meaning is unproblematic, even helpful, but it is an obstacle to philosophical reconstruction. Hence, while a Buddhist stance on sexual activity must link it to "craving" and "clinging," this may, given the unsettled nature of just what they constitute, appear a more clear and demanding constraint than it really is.

In the Pali texts, the difference between the injunctions on sexual activity for the laity and injunctions for monks and nuns suggests two distinct ways that such activity bears on the path to Enlightenment. The ethical demands on the laity are captured in the Five Precepts, one of which proscribes sexual misconduct. This prohibition fits with karmic elements in Buddhism and to cravings such as lust that cause the suffering of others. The code of conduct for monks and nuns demands celibacy. While sexual activity may well disturb meditation and monastic peace, it is not in itself immoral. Pali texts suggest a more principled basis for the exclusion of sexual activity from the Path to Enlightenment, namely, an indissoluble bond between sexual activity and craving. The vehemence of the attack on sexual activity itself, as opposed to sexual misconduct, is seen in such passages as this one (from *Suttanipāta*; Hare, 124):

> On seeing craving, passion and disgust,
> Even desire for intercourse then failed:
> And pray! What bag of excrements is this?
> I had as lief not touch her with my foot!

The apparent misogyny of this passage is, theoretically at least, misleading, for a comparable description of the male form would be appropriate to dampen female ardor for the male. While there is no consistent stance in the Pali texts, various discourses suggest that sexual activity inescapably generates craving. In the *Alagaddūpama Sutta* the Buddha rejects as heretical Arittha's view that one can follow the Buddha's teachings while yet indulging in sensual pleasures (Nanamoli and Bodhi, 224 ff.).

One of the most significant and admired of the Pali discourses, the *Mahānidāna Sutta*, declares that in the meditative period that gave to rise his Enlightenment the Buddha came to understand the causal process by which suffering arises. While parts of this so-called Twelve Link process are controversial and obscure, one instructive section is largely uncontroversial. This describes the sequence in which contact, such as sexual contact, gives rise to sensation, which gives rise to a judgment of desirability, which in turn gives rise to craving, grasping, and ensuing suffering. A sound Buddhist stance on sexual activity must be reconciled with this basic aetiology of suffering. The *Alagaddūpama Sutta* implies that, at least with respect to sexual activity, the point of intervention to prevent the arising of suffering must be *prior* to contact. But this is at odds with central meditative practices that focus on the transition from sensation to craving. In the major Pali discourse, the *Satipatthāna Sutta*, the monk is encouraged to look on decaying bodies not with disgust and revulsion; rather "he abides independent, not clinging to anything in the world" (Walshe, 335). By analogy, sexual craving is to be avoided or eliminated not by eradicating exposure to sexual stimuli but by becoming able to experience these stimuli without generating craving for them.

Many passages in the Pali writings do dwell on the repulsiveness of the objects of **sexual desire**. Plainly this strategy operates at a more practical level than the metaphysical considerations mentioned above. By presenting the sexual stimulus in such a negative way, the power of the stimulus is diminished. The point, however, is not to promote asceticism, the fruitlessness of the practices of self-denial that the Buddha himself experienced during his search for Enlightenment. Rather, the Buddha taught a Middle Way between indulgence and asceticism.

In tandem, as it were, with the strategy of becoming able to experience the sexual stimulus yet not reacting with lust, in effect destroying the disposition of craving itself, there is the strategy of avoiding the stimulus. The Buddha encouraged monks to avoid even seeing women. This does not directly destroy the craving disposition but merely sidesteps the conditions of the display of the stimulus. It might be argued, however, that the lustful disposition is gradually weakened by a protracted absence of stimulation. Certainly, the Buddhist holds that indulging craving strengthens it.

Such practices as the observation of decaying corpses are clearly designed to destroy attachment to the body, to destroy "craving for existence." But if denial of attachment is to be reconciled with deeper, pervasive features of Buddhist teaching, attachment should not be replaced by repulsion or disgust. Attaining a balanced, calm, and undisturbed mind is a core element of all Buddhist traditions. Repulsion, disgust, and aversion disturb the mind just as surely as craving and clinging. Hence they, too, must be surmounted. While disgust may serve as a temporary antidote to craving, the goal is a Middle Way between these two, a state of mind that might be variously described as acceptance, wisdom, or the like.

The development of Mahayana Buddhism several centuries after the Buddha's death reemphasized and made more sophisticated elements left undeveloped in the Pali writings. Impermanence, given a role in establishing the inherent unquenchablility of desire, yields the more profound doctrine of emptiness. Compassion, one of the original Four Abodes, becomes far more significant. Powerful arguments against various forms of dualism are developed, and the soteriological consequences of this are extracted. The rejection of individuals as "independent selves" reflects earlier questioning of the reality of the personal self (see Siderits). These developments, combined with emphasizing the availability of Enlightenment for everyone, allowed for an elaboration of perspectives on sexuality that were largely subdued in the earlier teachings.

The extensively generalized and deepened understanding of craving and clinging is evident in various ways in the teachings of Zen Buddhism, arising in the twelfth century. Its iconoclasm prevents substituting more venerable subjects, such as the Dhamma, the Buddha, and rules of conduct, as objects of craving and clinging in the place of the more traditional sensual pleasures. This reflects an interpretation of the Second Noble Truth that emphasizes the attitude of craving itself as the source of suffering and the impediment to Enlightenment, rather than selected objects of the attitude, notably sensual pleasures. The point is nicely brought out in the Zen story (Reps, 28) about two monks, Tanzan and Ekido, who encounter a beautiful woman who is unable to cross a muddy section of road. Tanzan picks her up, carries her across, and sets her down at the appropriate point. Soon after, Ekido, unable to contain his annoyance, remonstrates with Tanzan for having physical contact. Tanzan replies, "I left the girl there. Are you still carrying her?" Ekido's uncompromising, immoderate adherence to rule displays an obsession with physical contact, while Tanzan is free from any trace of lingering effect despite the physical contact.

Zen's meditative techniques focus on "freeing the mind," and its attack on discursive thinking challenges the way fixity enters the functioning of the basic semantic concepts of meaning and truth. Its art and poetry spell out more positively than in the earlier literature a picture of a life free from craving and clinging. Spontaneity and naturalness replace reckless, uncompromising pursuit of goals, whether sensual or noble. Similarly, sexual activity that is engaged in free from conceptual overlay but simply allowed to occur as a natural, spontaneous phenomenon lacks the potential to generate suffering. Unlike the view suggested in the *Alagaddūpama*, the propensity for sexual activity to yield suffering is handled not by preventing sexual experiences but by preventing them from generating a craving for their repetition. This allows for a more consistent soteriology for craving, because the craving danger of the sensual pleasures of food and drink cannot be dealt with by precluding the experiences of eating and drinking. Rather, consistently with the instructions of the *Satipaṭṭhāna Sutta*, followers of the Buddha must learn how to experience these pleasures while "remaining independent, not clinging to anything in the world," that is, without developing cravings for them.

The Pali texts insist on expulsion from religious orders for certain homosexual activities, notably sexual penetration with emission. However, mutual **masturbation**, while serious, was not a ground for expulsion. In contrast, a strong tradition of "boy love" developed in esoteric Buddhism in Japan. Paul Shalow's study includes translations of texts describing a range of homosexual techniques, several of which use terminology also used for meditative postures. One particularly interesting passage, from Kitamura Kigin's (1624–1705) preface to his compilation *Rock Azaleas* (1667; translated in Shalow, 222), suggests that the acceptance of homosexual interactions may have been a way to reconcile Japanese Buddhism's more tolerant attitude to natural human functioning with the constraints of monastic life.

Sexuality is given far greater prominence in the writings of Buddhist Tantric adepts than in earlier traditions. As Roger Jackson brings out (90–94), adepts such as the eleventh-century Kānha speak explicitly of their sexual partners and their role in the adept's practices. Tantric pictorial representations at times display considerable erotic power, with figures in states of great bliss and abandon. It is tempting to equate this eroticism with a rejection of conventionality, construed as the clinging to fixed modes of behavior, including sexual conventions. But while this construal may do justice to that aspect of Buddhist teaching, it ignores the discipline and mental control fundamental to Buddhism. Indeed, without further explanation, such a treatment of sexuality is indistinguishable from unconstrained surrender to the forces of craving. On the other hand, given that Wisdom is seen in Mahayana Buddhism as the feminine aspect of Enlightenment, there is room, perhaps, for sexual partners to be seen as metaphorical representations of Wisdom and sexual congress as metaphor for the adept's engagement with Wisdom. But this hardly does justice to the many Tantric writings in which sexual activity is described in considerable and apt detail. Nor, of course, would it illuminate any legitimate role for sexual activity within Buddhist practice.

While the Pali texts may be wrong in denying the possibility of divorcing sexual activity from craving, doing so might reasonably be regarded as difficult in the extreme. Moreover, the temptation to claim such an achievement while still subject to mundane pleasures is a great and dangerous one. On the other hand, the Tantric adepts might reasonably be regarded as drawing out the implications of early teachings in their expectation that the inability to experience sexual stimuli without developing craving for them is a barrier to Enlightenment. The whole issue is overshadowed by the indeterminacy of the crucial concept "craving." Indeed, the Tantric tradition effectively recognizes this and commonly offers a rather specific determinant (for the male) of the presence of craving in sexual activity, namely, the occurrence of seminal emission. While this may be of great practical use, it does little to advance the philosophical explication of the concept.

See also Bataille, Georges; Catholicism, History of; Chinese Philosophy; Consequentialism; Desire, Sexual; Gnosticism; Greek Sexuality and Philosophy, Ancient; Hinduism; Indian Erotology; Jainism; Manichaeism; Tantrism

REFERENCES

Bodhi, Bhikkhu. *Connected Discourses*, vol. 2. Boston, Mass.: Wisdom Publications, 2000; Faure, Bernard. *The Power of Denial: Buddhism, Purity, and Denial*. Princeton, N.J.: Princeton University Press, 2003; Faure, Bernard. *The Red Thread: Buddhist Approaches to Sexuality*. Princeton, N.J.: Princeton University Press, 1998; Hare, Edward M., trans. *Woven Cadences of Early Buddhists: Sacred Books of the Buddhists*, vol. 15. London: Oxford University Press, 1945; Jackson, Roger R. "Ambiguous Sexuality: Imagery and Interpretation in Tantric Buddhism." *Religion* 22:1 (1992), 85–100; Nanamoli, Bhikkhu, and Bhikkhu Bodhi. *The Middle Length Discourses of the Buddha*. Boston, Mass.: Wisdom Publications, 1995; Plato. (ca. 380 BCE) *Symposium of Plato*. Trans. Tom Griffith. Berkeley: University of California Press, 1986, 1989; Reps, Paul. *Zen Flesh, Zen Bones*. London: Penguin, 1957; Shalow, Paul. "Kūkai and the Tradition of Male Love in Japanese Buddhism." In José I. Cabezón, ed., *Buddhism, Sexuality, and Gender*. Albany: State University of New

York Press, 1992, 215–30; Siderits, Mark. *Personal Identity and Buddhist Philosophy: Empty Persons*. Aldershot, U.K.: Ashgate, 2003; Walshe, Maurice. *Thus Have I Heard*. London: Wisdom Publications, 1987.

Len O'Neill

ADDITIONAL READING

Broido, Michael. "Killing, Lying, Stealing, and Adultery: A Problem of Interpretation in the Tantras." In Donald S. Lopez, Jr., ed., *Buddhist Hermeneutics*. Honolulu: University of Hawai'i Press, 1988, 71–118; Cabezón, José Ignacio. "Homosexuality and Buddhism." In Arlene Swidler, ed., *Homosexuality and World Religions*. Valley Forge, Pa.: Trinity Press, 1993, 81–101; Cabezón, José Ignacio, ed. *Buddhism, Sexuality, and Gender*. Albany: State University of New York Press, 1992; Clasquin, Michel. "Contemporary Theravada and Zen Attitudes to Human Sexuality: An Exercise in Comparative Ethics." *Religion* 22:1 (1992), 63–83; Dynes, Wayne R., and Stephen Donaldson, eds. *Asian Homosexuality*. New York: Taylor and Francis, 1992; Giles, James. "The No-Self Theory: Hume, Buddhism, and Personal Identity." *Philosophy East and West* 43:2 (1993), 175–200; Giles, James. *No Self to Be Found: The Search for Personal Identity*. Lanham, Md.: University Press of America, 1997; Goss, Robert E. "Buddhism." In Timothy F. Murphy, ed., *Reader's Guide to Lesbian and Gay Studies*. Chicago, Ill.: Fitzroy Dearborn, 2000, 100–101; Guenther, Herbert V. *The Tantric View of Life*. London: Shambhala, 1976; Gutschow, Kim. *Being a Buddhist Nun: The Struggle for Enlightenment in the Himalayas*. Cambridge, Mass.: Harvard University Press, 2004; Kajiyama, Yuichi. "Women in Buddhism." *Eastern Buddhist* [n.s.] 15:1 (1982), 53–70; Klein, Anne Carolyn. "Finding a Self: Buddhist and Feminist Perspectives." In Clarissa Atkinson, Constance Buchanan, and Margaret Miles, eds., *Shaping New Vision: Gender and Values in American Culture*. Ann Arbor, Mich.: UMI Research Press, 1987, 191–218. Reprinted in Charles Taliaferro and Paul J. Griffiths, eds., *Philosophy of Religion: An Anthology*. Malden, Mass.: Blackwell, 2003, 329–44; Marra, Michele. "The Buddhist Mythmaking of Defilement: Sacred Courtesans of Medieval Japan." *Journal of Asian Studies* 52:1 (1993), 49–65; Money, John. "Transcultural Sexology: Formicophilia, a Newly Named Paraphilia in a Young Buddhist Male." In *The Adam Principle. Genes, Genitals, Hormones, & Gender: Selected Readings in Sexology*. Buffalo, N.Y.: Prometheus, 1993, 334–40; Naylor, B. Christina. "Buddhas or Bitches: Nichiren's Attitude to Women." *Religious Traditions* 11 (1988), 63–76; Qvarnström, Olle, ed. *Jainism and Early Buddhism: Essays in Honor of Padmanabh S. Jaini*. Fremont, Calif.: Asian Humanities Press, 2003; Rahula, Walpola Sri. *What the Buddha Taught*. New York: Grove Press, 1986; Schuster, Nancy. "Women in Buddhism." In Arvind Sharma, ed., *Women in World Religions*. Albany: State University of New York Press, 1987, 105–33; Shaw, Miranda. *Passionate Enlightenment: Women in Tantric Buddhism*. Princeton, N.J.: Princeton University Press, 1994; Snelling, John. *The Buddhist Handbook*. London: Rider, 1987; Stevens, John. *Lust for Enlightenment: Buddhism and Sex*. Boston, Mass.: Shambhala, 1990; Stone, Jim. "Parfit and the Buddha: Why There Are No People." *Philosophy and Phenomenological Research* 48:3 (1988), 519–32; Stone, Jim. "Why There Still Are No People." *Philosophy and Phenomenological Research* 70:1 (2005), 174–92; Thomas, Paul. *Epics, Myths and Legends of India: A Comprehensive Survey of the Sacred Lore of the Hindus, Buddhists and Jains*, 11th ed. Bombay, India: D. B. Taraporevala, n.d.; Willis, Janice Dean. "Dakini: Some Comments on Its Nature and Meaning." In Janice Dean Willis, ed., *Feminine Ground: Essays on Women and Tibet*. Ithaca, N.Y.: Snow Lion Publications, 1987, 57–75; Wilson, Elisabeth. *Charming Cadavers: Horrific Figurations of the Feminine in Buddhist Hagiographic Literature*. Chicago, Ill.: University of Chicago Press, 1996; Wilson, Elisabeth. "The Female Body as a Source of Horror and Insight in Post-Ashokan Indian Buddhism." In Jane Marie Law, ed., *Religious Reflections on the Human Body*. Bloomington: Indiana University Press, 1995, 76–79.

BULLOUGH, VERN L. (1928–   ). Vern LeRoy Bullough was introduced at the 1965 meeting of the American Historical Association as "the historian who specialized in whores, queers, and perverts but who could also do some 'real' research occasionally" (see Bullough, "Problems of Research," 380). Thanks in large part to Bullough, historical research about **prostitution, homosexuality**, and other marginalized sexual behaviors is no longer considered less than "real" research.

Bullough was born in Salt Lake City and raised in Utah during the depression and World War II. He received his B.A. from the University of Utah (1951), M.A. from the University of Chicago (1951), Ph.D. from the University of Chicago (1954), and B.S. in nursing from California State University at Long Beach (1981). He held teaching positions at Youngstown University (1954–1959) and California State University (CSU) at Northridge (1959–1980), was dean of natural and social sciences (1980–1990) at the State University of New York College at Buffalo, and was Distinguished Professor (1987–1993) of the State University of New York. More recently, Bullough has served as an adjunct professor at CSU Northridge and the University of Southern California. (See Bullough and Bullough, "How We Got into Sex.")

Bullough opened up the study of sexuality for professional historians, who had been reluctant to touch on this traditionally taboo topic. In 1970, he helped organize and participated in the first session on sexual topics ever held at an American Historical Association conference. Bullough wrote or edited, often with his first wife (of forty-nine years) Bonnie Bullough (1927–1996), over twenty-five books on sexual topics and hundreds of journal articles. He has written about prostitution, gender, homosexuality, crossdressing, medieval sexuality, the history of sexual science and medicine, and **pornography**. Together, the Bulloughs in 1994 produced *Human Sexuality: An Encyclopedia*, the first encyclopedia about sexuality to appear in English in over thirty years, since **Albert Ellis** and Albert Abarbanel's 1961 *Encyclopedia of Sexual Behavior*. (Vern contributed thirty entries himself to this volume. It contains several philosophical essays, including an **overview of the philosophy of sex** by Russell Vannoy.) Vern and Bonnie Bullough also published extensively in nursing. He has collaborated as well with fellow historian James Brundage in editing two volumes devoted to medieval sexuality, *Sexual Practices and the Medieval Church* (1982) and *Handbook of Medieval Sexuality* (1996).

Although *History of Prostitution* appeared in 1964, Bullough considers his first important work on sex and gender to be *The Subordinate Sex: A History of Attitudes toward Women* (1973; revised in 1988, with Shelton and Slavin, as *The Subordinated Sex*). This book was the first overall historical survey about women; only later did feminist scholars publish heavily in this area. In both *Prostitution* and *Subordinate*, Bullough takes the approach common to all his writings, describing the historical forces that formed our customs and social beliefs and that still affect our attitudes. Some of Bullough's writings on women's issues have focused on fertility and **contraception**. He points out the influence of biological and medical factors on patterns of male-female inequality and how advances in science and medicine allow contemporary women to overcome prior limitations.

Bullough's *Sexual Variance in Society and History* (1976) broke new ground in presenting a comprehensive and sympathetic history of homosexuality and other stigmatized sexual practices, such as transvestism and **masturbation**. Bullough documented how, despite local official doctrine, sexual behavior throughout history and across cultures has varied widely. The early medieval church opposed homosexuality as a matter of theological principle yet tolerated it in practice (see also **John Boswell**'s [1947–1994] later work in this area). Bullough has always emphasized the complexity and "messiness" of real life and real people. Inevitably, there are contradictions between legal, religious, or political policies and writings and the thoughts and behaviors of ordinary people, tensions that are often oversimplified by historians.

Sexual Variance was soon followed by the 1977 book *Sin, Sickness, and Sanity*, one of the earliest contemporary pieces of scholarship to survey thought about sexuality over various historical periods. About sexual practices such as masturbation, homosexuality, **nudism**, and contraception, the Bulloughs demonstrated how a medical model developed in the nineteenth century characterized (on their view, erroneously) as sickness the sexualities that had been classified (again, on their view erroneously) for centuries by Christianity as sinfulness. Ongoing sexual research and theorizing in both the sciences and humanities has undermined many of these characterizations. By understanding the past, the Bulloughs maintain, we can discover the sources of our sexual attitudes and be in a position to separate the wheat from the chaff. The book was revised in 1995 and retitled *Sexual Attitudes: Myths and Realities*.

Cross Dressing, Sex, and Gender (1993) grew out of Bullough's long interest in gender and homosexuality (see also his anthology *Before Stonewall*). It was the first comprehensive historical work on the subject of crossdressing. In defending the view that crossgender tendencies should be more widely tolerated because within limits it is "normal" behavior, the book shows that dressing across gender boundaries has been widespread throughout history and that it comprises a complex set of psychological and social phenomena with no simple explanation. It is a candidate for therapeutic intervention only when it becomes a dysfunction, that is, involves intolerable interference with one's personal life or occupational responsibilities.

In much of Bullough's writing, he alludes to the impact of medicine and sex research on Western attitudes and culture. In *Science in the Bedroom* (1994), he focuses entirely on the history of sex research, starting with medicine in ancient Greece, continuing through the European predecessors of American work (for example, Jean Baptiste Parent-Duchâtelet [1790–1836], Magnus Hirschfeld [1868–1935], and **Havelock Ellis** [1859–1939]), and concluding with Alfred Kinsey (1894–1956) and his successors, Evelyn Hooker (1907–1996), William Masters (1915–2001), and Virginia Johnson, among others (see also Robinson). Developments in scientific knowledge have gradually eroded misconceptions about sexuality, but it has taken decades, even centuries, for attitudes to change. Again Bullough documents that sexual science has challenged traditional Western assumptions that sexual activity is a major cause of illness and crime. In this book, Bullough also interestingly depicts some sex researchers as complex human beings. For example, Havelock Ellis found sex fascinating and troublesome in his Victorian youth (including being attracted to urolagnia). He went into medicine because he thought it the only profession in which he could safely devote himself to the forbidden topic of sexuality (76–77). And the interest of family planning educator Marie Stopes (1880–1958) in studying sexuality resulted from the failure of her first marriage, annulled on the basis of nonconsummation (138).

Bullough has been active in numerous humanist organizations since the 1950s and is a Laureate of the International Academy of Humanism. In his writings, two central tenets of humanism come across strongly: a commitment to critical reason and factual evidence and toleration of diversity in ideas and behaviors. He has written repeatedly that by employing history to uncover and understand beliefs and behavior, we can trace the sources of mistaken ideas and bring more accurate findings to bear on our own dilemmas. Similarly, the scientific process of continual collection and critique of data also helps us avoid misconceptions and plan our future more rationally. Bullough's interweaving of the data and methods of science and the humanities has been valuable in breaking down boundaries between disciplines. Literature and creative writing (including pornography; see his "Research and Archival Value of Erotica/Pornography") can be rewarding sources of information about past sexual behavior and attitudes.

Bullough, no system builder, has not promoted through his writings any glamorous new theory about sexuality. "What is needed," he has written, "is not more theories but a more modest study of past attitudes" and, of course, of behavior (*Sin, Sickness, and Sanity*, 9). He has been willing to base his own studies on diverse sources, increasing the reach and wealth of both history and sexology. Bullough found religious writings, creative writing, and ethnological accounts to be illuminating sources of historical information about sexuality—the last two often overlooked by historians. He has sometimes characterized such historians as producing mere "historical poetry" (*Subordinate*, 12), that is, history derived from groundless assumptions and eager theories rather than real written records. In developing and promoting historical research about sexuality, Bullough has also stimulated other disciplines to realize the significance of history for their own studies.

See also Boswell, John; Dysfunction, Sexual; Ellis, Havelock; Feminism, French; Feminism, History of; Feminism, Lesbian; Feminism, Liberal; Feminism, Men's; Homosexuality, Ethics of; Homosexuality and Science; Paraphilia; Pornography; Prostitution; Sexology

REFERENCES

Boswell, John. *Christianity, Social Tolerance, and Homosexuality: Gay People in Western Europe from the Beginning of the Christian Era to the Fourteenth Century*. Chicago, Ill.: University of Chicago Press, 1980; Bullough, Bonnie, and Vern L. Bullough. "How We Got into Sex." In Bonnie Bullough, Vern L. Bullough, Marilyn A. Fithian, William E. Hartman, and Randy Sue Klein, eds., *Personal Stories of "How I Got into Sex": Leading Researchers, Sex Therapists, Educators, Prostitutes, Sex Toy Designers, Sex Surrogates, Transsexuals, Criminologists, Clergy, and More*... Amherst, N.Y.: Prometheus, 1997, 55–72; Bullough, Vern L. *The History of Prostitution*. New Hyde Park, N.Y.: University Books, 1964; Bullough, Vern L. "Problems of Research on a Delicate Topic: A Personal View." *Journal of Sex Research* 21:4 (1985), 375–86; Bullough, Vern L. "Research and Archival Value of Erotica/Pornography." In Martha Cornog, ed., *Libraries, Erotica, and Pornography*. Phoenix, Ariz.: Oryx, 1991, 99–105; Bullough, Vern L. *Science in the Bedroom: A History of Sex Research*. New York: Basic Books, 1994; Bullough, Vern L. *Sexual Variance in Society and History*. New York: Wiley, 1976; Bullough, Vern L. *The Subordinate Sex: A History of Attitudes toward Women*. Urbana, Ill.: University of Illinois Press, 1973; Bullough, Vern L., ed. *Before Stonewall: Activists for Gay and Lesbian Rights in Historical Context*. New York: Harrington Park/Haworth, 2002; Bullough, Vern L., and James Brundage, eds. *Handbook of Medieval Sexuality*. New York: Garland, 1996; Bullough, Vern L., and James Brundage, eds. *Sexual Practices and the Medieval Church*. Buffalo, N.Y.: Prometheus, 1982; Bullough, Vern L., and Bonnie Bullough. *Cross Dressing, Sex, and Gender*. Philadelphia: University of Pennsylvania Press, 1993; Bullough, Vern L., and Bonnie Bullough. *Sexual Attitudes: Myths and Realities*. Amherst, N.Y.: Prometheus, 1995; Bullough, Vern L., and Bonnie Bullough. *Sin, Sickness, and Sanity: A History of Sexual Attitudes*. New York: New American Library, 1977; Bullough, Vern L., and Bonnie Bullough, eds. *Human Sexuality: An Encyclopedia*. New York: Garland, 1994; Bullough, Vern L., Brenda Shelton, and Sarah Slavin. *The Subordinated Sex: A History of Attitudes toward Women*. Athens: University of Georgia Press, 1988; Ellis, Albert, and Albert Abarbanel, eds. *The Encyclopedia of Sexual Behavior*. New York: Hawthorne Books, 1961; Robinson, Paul. *The Modernization of Sex: Havelock Ellis, Alfred Kinsey, Williams Masters and Virginia Johnson*. New York: Harper and Row, 1976; Vannoy, Russell. "Philosophy and Sex." In Vern L. Bullough and Bonnie Bullough, eds., *Human Sexuality: An Encyclopedia*. New York: Garland, 1994, 442–49.

Martha Cornog

ADDITIONAL READING

Bullough, Bonnie. "Female Prostitution: Current Research and Changing Interpretations." *Annual Review of Sex Research* 7 (1996), 158–80; Bullough, Bonnie, and Vern L. Bullough. "Introduction: Female Prostitution: Current Research and Changing Interpretations." In James E. Elias, Vern L. Bullough, Veronica Elias, and Gwen Brewer, eds., *Prostitution: On Whores, Hustlers, and Johns*. Amherst, N.Y.: Prometheus, 1998, 23–44; Bullough, Bonnie, Vern L. Bullough, Marilyn A. Fithian, William E. Hartman, and Randy Sue Klein, eds. *Personal Stories of "How I Got into Sex": Leading Researchers, Sex Therapists, Educators, Prostitutes, Sex Toy Designers, Sex Surrogates, Transsexuals, Criminologists, Clergy, and More . . .* Amherst, N.Y.: Prometheus, 1997; Bullough, Vern L. "Art: Painting, Sculpture, and Other Visual Art." In Vern L. Bullough and Bonnie Bullough, eds., *Human Sexuality: An Encyclopedia*. New York: Garland, 1994, 43–50; Bullough, Vern L. "Christianity and Sexuality." In Ronald M. Green, ed., *Religion and Sexual Health: Ethical, Theological, and Clinical Perspectives*. Boston, Mass.: Kluwer, 1992, 3–16; Bullough, Vern L. "History, the Historian, and Sex." In Gary G. Brannigan, Elizabeth Rice Allgeier, and Albert Richard Allgeier, eds., *The Sex Scientists*. New York: Longman, 1998, 1–14; Bullough, Vern L. "History in Adult Human Sexual Behavior with Children and Adolescents in Western Societies." In Jay R. Feierman, ed., *Pedophilia: Biosocial Dimensions*. New York: Springer-Verlag, 1990, 69–90; Bullough, Vern L. "The History of Sex Research in the USA." Paper presented at the European Federation of Sexology meeting, Berlin (29 June 2000). Cited and discussed in Annette Fuglsang Owens, review of *Women's Sexualities: Generations of Women Share Intimate Secrets of Sexual Self-Acceptance*, by Carol Rinkleib Ellison. *Electronic Journal of Human Sexuality* 3 (25 July 2000). <www.ejhs.org/volume3/book7.htm> [accessed 17 August 2004]; Bullough, Vern L. *Homosexuality: A History*. New York: New American Library, 1979; Bullough, Vern L. "The Kinsey Scale in Historical Perspective." In David P. McWhirter, Stephanie A. Sanders, and June M. Reinisch, eds., *Homosexuality/Heterosexuality: Concepts of Sexual Orientation*. New York: Oxford University Press, 1990, 3–14; Bullough, Vern L. "Music and Sex." In Vern L. Bullough and Bonnie Bullough, eds., *Human Sexuality: An Encyclopedia*. New York: Garland, 1994, 413–15; Bullough, Vern L., and Bonnie Bullough. *Women and Prostitution: A Social History*. Buffalo, N.Y.: Prometheus, 1987; De Cecco, John P. "Vern L. Bullough (1928–   ): Making the Pen Mightier Than the Sword." In Vern L. Bullough, ed., *Before Stonewall: Activists for Gay and Lesbian Rights in Historical Context*. New York: Harrington Park/Haworth, 2002, 361–68; Elias, James E., Vern L. Bullough, Veronica Elias, and Gwen Brewer, eds. *Prostitution: On Whores, Hustlers, and Johns*. Amherst, N.Y.: Prometheus, 1998; Goodich, Michael. Review of *Sexual Variance in Society and History*, by Vern L. Bullough. *American Historical Review* 82:4 (1977), 921; Schoenwald, Richard L. Review of *The History of Prostitution*, by Vern L. Bullough. *American Historical Review* 70:3 (1965), 834–35.

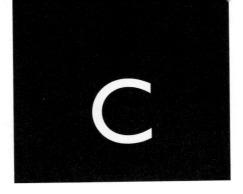

CASUAL SEX. Casual sex is often characterized as sex for the sake of sexual pleasure itself, rather than, say, for procreation, and is often contrasted with sex that expresses **love** or is done in a loving context. It involves **sexual desire** alone rather than sexual desire *and* love. Men, generally, engage in casual sex, or would like to, more than women—excluding female sex workers (for an evolutionary account of this difference, see Buss). When gay men engage in it, they often keep it impersonal, especially when otherwise involved in (non-monogamous) relationships (Blumstein and Schwartz, 295–97). Types of casual sex include one-night stands, orgiastic and "swinging" sex, anonymous encounters in bathhouses and the backrooms of bars (usually between gay men), encounters in Internet chat rooms (**cybersex**), and **prostitution**. Casual sex admits of both conceptual and normative questions. I start with the conceptual. It might seem easy to define "casual sex," but it is not. This, however, does not mean that "there is no such thing as a casual . . . sexual act" (Anscombe, 24).

No definition that relies only on behavioral criteria will work. Such a definition might capture some sexual acts that are casual, such as orgies, sex with animals (**bestiality**), and sex with human corpses (necrophilia), but it would not capture the difference between two couples, one that engages in oral sex casually and the other noncasually. There might be no behavioral differences between them. Beliefs or other mental states must figure in the definition.

One might define "casual sex" as "sexual activity for the sake of sexual pleasure only." It is not sex intended for procreation or the communication of love but solely for pleasure, as in recreational sex. This will not do. We can describe sex for pleasure as recreational if it occurs between two people in a loving relationship, but here it is not casual. Anthony Ellis defines "casual sex" as sex between partners who have no deep or substantial relationship (157). This definition does not specify the type of prior relationship that exists between the parties: that they are strangers, acquaintances, or friends. This is good because not only strangers engage in casual sex. Acquaintances sometimes do, and friends. But the definition fails. Suppose both parties believe that their sex will lead to a committed relationship. Even in the presence of these beliefs, the sexual act, on Ellis's definition, would still be casual. But it is plausible that the presence of these beliefs renders their sex not (fully) casual. It is likely a mark of casual sex that it be done without any beliefs that it be anything more than a sexual encounter.

Let us try this definition: "Casual sex is sexual activity engaged in with the understanding or belief that it will not lead to emotional commitments." One good thing about this definition is that it includes only "negative" mental states as necessary for sex to be casual. The inclusion of "positive" states leads to counterintuitive results. For example, suppose the positive intention "for the sake of sexual pleasure" is necessary. This yields the result that **sexual activity** between a prostitute and her client is not casual, because prostitutes typically are not motivated to engage in sex for their own pleasure. Thus, the motives and intentions of the parties must be left open: We should stipulate only that the parties understand that there is no future commitment.

"Understanding" is important. Suppose Monica has sex with Bill, hoping or desiring that it will lead to a love relationship. However, Monica understands that Bill has no such hope and that he does not desire to be in a relationship with her. Thus, Monica realizes that Bill is about to engage in casual sex, yet nevertheless hopes, against the odds, that it will lead somewhere. Despite her hopes, the sex between them is casual, for both realize that it is engaged in only for the sake of sex. Thus, while mental states are crucial for defining casual sex, we must carefully choose which ones to include. Certain hopes and desires should not factor into the definition.

This definition faces problems. First, must both parties involved have the above understanding? What if one person understands that the sexual encounter will not lead to a future commitment, while the other does not, or believes the opposite? Indeed, how would we describe a sexual encounter in which the parties, or at least one, have no beliefs one way or the other? Should we require that the parties *have* the belief that their sex will not lead to any commitment or that the parties have *no* belief that there will be a commitment? If the former, how strong must the belief be? Should the parties believe that their sex *will not*, or *probably* will not, lead to a commitment? Further, must these beliefs be genuine or veridical, or could they be self-deceptive or false? And how should we describe sex occurring between a person and an entity that cannot have beliefs: an animal, an inflated doll, a cadaver? Perhaps these sexual acts are not casual; at least the latter two are cases of **masturbation**, and masturbation might not be casual sex, due to the absence of a partner. But sex with an animal could not be dismissed so easily.

Second, the definition does not reflect the understanding of most people that casual sex involves one important positive motive, the desire for sexual pleasure. The definition does not mention this motive. However, there are many motives for casual sex, and thus most people's understanding might be mistaken. Third, the definition applies to a sexual act, **rape**, that might be, strictly speaking, casual, yet is not the first case that comes to mind when we think of casual sex. Marital and **date rape** (perhaps) aside, the rapist does not think of himself as forcing sex on a person while believing that this will lead to a committed relationship. Even if rape is casual sex because of this fact, this is not the way we usually think of rape or of casual sex. Fourth, it is worthwhile to reconsider whether it is necessary that a definition of "casual sex" refers to mental states. If the parties to a casual encounter do believe it will lead to an emotional commitment, but it does not, that failure would seem to be sufficient to describe their sex as casual.

Thus, the above definition does not capture *exactly* what we mean by "casual sex." Perhaps "casual sex" is too vague for precise analysis, and pinning down a definition might come at the cost of jettisoning some of our intuitions about it. There is, of course, the danger of confusing the concept of casual sex with promiscuity. Any definition of promiscuity must assert that it is sexual activity with different partners over time (Frederick Elliston [1944–1987], 225–26). Because casual sex does not entail multiple partners (a single one-night stand in a person's life might be casual), it is not the same as promiscuity. It might even be that promiscuity does not entail casual sex. Suppose one has sex with many partners while believing that this is the best way to secure a committed relationship. This person's sexual behavior is promiscuous, but because of the intention we would not necessarily describe it as casual. (Benatar [193–94] equates promiscuity and casual sex, but this is because he defines promiscuity as sex lacking romantic or emotional significance instead of in terms of sex with multiple partners.)

I turn, now, to normative issues. These can arise along three logically different axes: the moral versus the immoral, the sexually pleasurable versus the not pleasurable, and the normal versus the perverted.

Sometimes casual sex is morally wrong for reasons having nothing to do with its being casual. If two married people engage in casual sex (with persons other than their spouses), each also commits **adultery**. Insofar as adultery is wrong, their casual sex is wrong as adultery. Casual sex might also be wrong because it involves deception or coercion. If Tom falsely promises Nicole **marriage** if Nicole were to have sex with him, Nicole's **consent** is not genuine because it relies on false information. Tom has deceived her, and the ensuing sex would be morally wrong. If Sally tells the destitute Mark, who does not desire Sally, that she will not evict him and his children from their apartment if he were to have sex with her, the ensuing sex would be coerced and hence wrong (see Mappes, 180–83). Again, it is not wrong just because it is casual. Casual sex might also be wrong due to a lack of adequate communication. Suppose Edna and Skinner are about to have sex. Edna does not desire that it be more than casual but is unsure of Skinner's intentions. It might even be uncommon that the parties, excited by desire, know each other's intentions. If there is a moral obligation to disclose one's intentions, failure to do so would make casual sex wrong—although not because it is casual. Note that unclarity about intentions might be gendered; women, more than men, often use sexual encounters as preludes to relationships (Blumstein and Schwartz, 297).

Even if casual sex involves no deception or coercion, is not adulterous, and the parties clearly communicate their intentions, it still might be wrong in virtue of its consequences (an "external" reason for its wrongfulness), that is, harm to the parties involved and harm to other people. Two possible bad consequences of casual sex are contracting disease and unwanted pregnancy. These are consequences to the parties to the sexual act, but they might also affect other persons and society in general. Anthony Ellis claims that these effects are not morally relevant because they are "medical problems" (166). This is not exactly true. Some **sexually transmitted diseases** (e.g., HIV [human immunodeficiency virus]) present serious moral problems. Unwanted pregnancies also change one's life drastically, as pregnant teenage girls know. The parties to the sexual act should, morally and pragmatically, take precautions against disease and pregnancy. But that casual sex that leads to unwanted pregnancy or disease might be morally wrong does not show that casual sex itself is wrong.

It is not obvious what other bad consequences casual sex has. One possibility is that insofar as society applies a double standard to men and women, women who accept casual sex are seen as cheap ("sluts"), while men are not (Blumstein and Schwartz, 297). Such negative views about women might be a form of harm (for example, a blow to their "reputation"). However, the double standard is only a contingent and perhaps disappearing feature of our society. This may be why casual sex does not always cause negative judgments. Many female college students who engage in casual sex are not viewed negatively and so escape the double standard. Further, whether some people's judging a woman a "slut" harms her depends on how it affects her psychologically: Some woman can brush it off easily or even laugh at it. Moreover, the argument does not tell against casual sex between men.

Another possibility was suggested by **G.E.M. Anscombe** (1919–2001) in claiming that casual sex makes one "shallow" (24), perhaps by making practitioners incapable of forming meaningful, loving relationships (see Kristjansson). However, this argument applies primarily to promiscuous sex, not casual sex. It is difficult to see why a few casual sexual events in one's life would make one incapable of forming loving relationships. Further, the argument depends on the assumption that love relationships are crucial in a person's leading a good life. This might not be true. It seems that one can, logically and psychologically, lead a good life without such relationships (though perhaps not without **friendship**; Halwani, chaps. 2, 3). Indeed, **Albert Ellis** argues that "personality growth"—an increase in enlightened self-interest, self-acceptance, tolerance, flexibility, and acceptance of ambiguity and uncertainty—is "abetted and enhanced by sexual adventuring" (95). Casual sex, as a form of "sexual adventuring," might have these benefits. However, whether healthy or successful sexual adventuring *presupposes* these admirable personality traits, instead of enhancing them, is unclear. Further, the list of traits praised by Ellis is obviously value-laden and might not be fully accepted by other psychologists.

Casual sex might also be morally wrong for "internal" reasons. Some motives could make a casual sex act morally wrong. Having a one-night stand with a monk to humiliate him afterward about his lax virtue is wrong, since it is done out of the vicious intention to demean. Having sex with a teenage girl or a married woman to blackmail her is also wrong. But such motives are not part of casual sex itself. Some motives are, of course, good. A nurse or a friend might masturbate a willing quadruple amputee to orgasm out of kindness. Most casual sex is not done from such motives. Typically, it is done for sexual pleasure. What needs to be shown, to make the moral case against casual sex, is that the motive to achieve sexual pleasure is morally bad. Perhaps this motive leads one to neglect the needs of one's partner. If this refers to the partner's needs outside the context of the sexual act, then further argument must be provided to explain why this is morally objectionable; for in most of our dealings with people, we do not consider all their other needs. If, however, the needs are sexual and pertain to the casual sex event itself, the argument is likely unsound. It involves misunderstanding what a person typically feels in casual sex. He or she does not usually want another to be a passive body but wants full sexual interaction with that person. This usually takes the form of tending to the partner's sexual needs, even if partly for one's own sake (Goldman, 268–71; Soble, "Sexual Use," 229–32). Prostitution might be an exception, casual sex in which the client does not typically go out of his way to please the prostitute.

The crucial accusation on the grounds of base motives might be that sexual desire leads one to treat one's partner as less than fully human; desire focuses on one aspect of a person, his or her body, and on the sexual organs in particular. This is the accusation of **sexual objectification**. Note that to claim that casual sex is objectifyingly immoral need not turn on issues of motive. Casual sex might be objectifyingly immoral even if done out of non-lustful motives, as when a prostitute engages in sex with a client for the money. **Immanuel Kant** (1724–1804) claimed that whenever we sexually desire another, we do not desire the person as such but only his or her sexual parts (*Lectures*, 162–68). This leads to a problem: On this account of sexual desire, it is difficult for sexuality to satisfy Kant's Second Formulation of the Categorical Imperative: "Act in such a way that you treat humanity, whether in your own person or in the person of any other, always at the same time as an end and never simply as a means" (*Grounding*, Ak 4:429). Casual sex, from a Kantian perspective, involves one person's not only treating another as an object but also treating oneself the same way. Kant thought the only time that sexual activity was permissible, despite its objectification, was when it occurs within marriage.

In contemporary discussions of objectification (unlike Kant's), the focus is not on the agent's objectifying himself in the sexual act but on the agent's objectifying the other. Prostitution, **pornography**, and casual sex have been judged immoral because they involve objectification, that is, treating a person as an object. This is wrong because persons are not, or not *just*, objects. The main problem with objectification is that it reduces a person to the status of something less than human, like an animal or inanimate object. But we are not animals or objects, since we possess something special—rationality, inherent worth, dignity, autonomy, or an immaterial and eternal soul. But here we must be cautious. These attributions are not empirical in any straightforward way. For we find many humans to be irrational, lacking worth, or undignified. The claim that humans have a special ontological and hence moral status needs cogent defense. If it is false, casual sex would not be objectifying, because it could not reduce us to something we are not or fail to respect a status we do not have (see Soble, *Pornography*, chap. 2).

The second normative issue concerns the nonmoral goodness of casual sex. Is casual sex pleasurable? It might seem that a positive answer to this question is obvious, for people find a large, indefinite number of people desirable. Sexual activity is, under certain "normal" conditions, enjoyable. However, this does not mean that casual sex is always pleasurable. Just because the prospect of sex is exciting, it need not turn out satisfying and pleasurable. One might want to distinguish the pleasure that regular sexual partners experience and the pleasure that casual sex partners experience (see Moulton, 538–39; Soble, *Sexual Investigations*, 87–89). The sexuality of regular partners might be routine, but the parties know what to expect and can count on some satisfaction. Casual sex partners, however, do not know what to expect. While they might approach the encounter with anticipatory excitement (and indeed experience the pleasure of making contact with a new person), the ensuing sex might not be as satisfying as imagined: The partners do not know how to satisfy each other's particular needs or desires. Nevertheless, some types of casual sex might have higher probabilities of yielding satisfaction. Two examples are anonymous sex and sex within purely sexual relationships (say, between "fuck buddies")—the former because the expectations are minimal to begin with, the latter because the expectations are known. Note that **Sigmund Freud** (1856–1939) once speculated that both men (183) and women (186), for different psychological reasons, had some difficulty achieving full sexual satisfaction with their spouses, someone they loved. Men, in particular, often find casual sexual encounters more satisfying than sexual activity with their beloved and loving wives. This division between the sexual and the affectionate psychological currents implies a sexual problem with or disadvantage of marriage and long-term relationships (which, of course, may still offer other benefits). What Kant thought was terribly morally suspicious about sexuality Freud identifies as an important factor in satisfaction.

The third normative issue about casual sex concerns psychological normality and **sexual perversion**. There are some types of casual sex that might qualify as also being perverted, just like some casual sex is adulterous, harmful, and so forth. *If* shoe or panty fetishism is perverted, then any coupled casual sex involving gratification with shoes or panties will be perverted, but not because it is casual. A more interesting question is whether casual sex might be psychologically abnormal, even when it is morally permissible or pleasurable (or even *because* it is pleasurable). If the natural or normal way that sexual desire and activity progress is by aiming at or culminating in love (see **Roger Scruton**, chaps. 4, 10), then casual sex, perhaps by definition, would not be normal. However, given that we very often experience sexual desire directed at various people without love entering the scene at all (not even unconsciously), it seems that the very common event of casual sex is perfectly within the bounds of the psychologically normal. It is implausible to analyze the sexually normal so that many people turn out to be abnormal or perverted. Perhaps the philosopher who argues that casual sex is abnormal is not, after all, offering a psychological thesis but is telling us how he or she would *like* things to be (Primoratz, chap. 3).

Casual sex is difficult to define. We know that it has much to do with the lack of an emotional or loving commitment and much to do with seeking pleasure for its own sake. Other than that, a plausible definition immune to counterexamples is elusive. Casual sex does not seem to be morally wrong as such. The one plausible case to be made revolves around objectification. But there is room for dissent, and if casual sex is faulted for being objectifying, much else in the sexual domain must also be faulted. It might even be that some casual sex is "an act of charity which proclaims the glory of God" (Williams, 81–82).

See also Abstinence; Addiction, Sexual; Adultery; Anscombe, G.E.M.; Communication Model; Consequentialism; Cybersex; Ethics, Sexual; Ethics, Virtue; Evolution; Freud, Sigmund; Kant, Immanuel; Objectification, Sexual; Personification, Sexual; Perversion, Sexual; Prostitution; Psychology, Evolutionary; Rape, Acquaintance and Date; Rimmer, Robert; Russell, Bertrand; Sex Work; Utopianism

REFERENCES

Anscombe, G.E.M. "Contraception and Chastity." *The Human World*, no. 7 (1972), 9–30; Benatar, David. "Two Views of Sexual Ethics: Promiscuity, Pedophilia, and Rape." *Public Affairs Quarterly* 16:3 (2002), 191–201; Blumstein, Philip, and Pepper Schwartz. *American Couples: Money, Work, Sex*. New York: Morrow, 1983; Buss, David M. "Casual Sex." In *The Evolution of Desire: Strategies of Human Mating*. New York: Basic Books, 1994, 73–96; Ellis, Albert. "Sexual Adventuring and Personality Growth." In Herbert A. Otto, ed., *The New Sexuality*. Palo Alto, Calif.: Science and Behavior Books, 1971, 94–109; Ellis, Anthony. "Casual Sex." *International Journal of Moral and Social Studies* 1:2 (1986), 157–69; Elliston, Frederick. "In Defense of Promiscuity." In Robert Baker and Frederick Elliston, eds., *Philosophy and Sex*, 1st ed. Buffalo, N.Y.: Prometheus, 1975, 223–43; Freud, Sigmund. (1912) "On the Universal Tendency to Debasement in the Sphere of Love." In James Strachey, ed. and trans., *The Standard Edition of the Complete Psychological Works of Sigmund Freud*, vol. 11. London: Hogarth Press, 1953–1974, 177–90; Goldman, Alan. "Plain Sex." *Philosophy and Public Affairs* 6:3 (1977), 267–87; Halwani, Raja. *Virtuous Liaisons: Care, Love, Sex, and Virtue Ethics*. Chicago, Ill.: Open Court, 2003; Kant, Immanuel. (1785) *Grounding for the Metaphysics of Morals*. Trans. James Ellington. Indianapolis, Ind.: Hackett, 1993; Kant, Immanuel. (ca. 1780) *Lectures on Ethics*. Trans. Louis Infield. New York: Harper and Row, 1963; Kristjansson, Kristjan. "Casual Sex Revisited." *Journal of Social Philosophy* 29:2 (1998), 97–108; Mappes, Thomas A. "Sexual Morality and the Concept of Using Another Person." In Thomas A. Mappes and Jane S. Zembaty, eds., *Social Ethics: Morality and Social Policy*, 6th ed. Boston, Mass.: McGraw-Hill, 2002, 170–83; Moulton, Janice. "Sexual Behavior: Another Position." *Journal of Philosophy* 73:16 (1976), 537–46; Primoratz, Igor. *Ethics and Sex*. New York: Routledge, 1999; Scruton, Roger. *Sexual Desire: A Moral Philosophy of the Erotic*. New York: Free Press, 1986; Soble, Alan. *Pornography, Sex, and Feminism*. Amherst, N.Y.: Prometheus, 2002; Soble, Alan. *Sexual Investigations*. New York: New York University Press, 1996; Soble, Alan. "Sexual Use and What to Do about It: Internalist and Externalist Sexual Ethics." In Alan Soble, ed., *The Philosophy of Sex*, 4th ed. Lanham, Md.: Rowman and Littlefield, 2002, 225–58; Williams, Harry Abbott. "Theology and Self-Awareness." In A. R. Vidler, ed., *Soundings: Essays Concerning Christian Understanding*. Cambridge: Cambridge University Press, 1963, 67–101.

Raja Halwani

ADDITIONAL READING

Anscombe, G.E.M. "Contraception and Chastity." *The Human World*, no. 7 (1972), 9–30. Reprinted in HS (29–50). Reprinted, revised, in Michael Bayles, ed., *Ethics and Population*. Cambridge, Mass.: Schenkman, 1976, 134–53; Ben-Ze'ev, Aaron. *Love Online: Emotions on the Internet*. Cambridge:

Cambridge University Press, 2004; Birkhead, Tim. *Promiscuity: An Evolutionary History of Sperm Competition and Sexual Conflict*. London: Faber and Faber, 2000; Blackie, Michael. "Anonymous Sex." In Timothy F. Murphy, ed., *Reader's Guide to Lesbian and Gay Studies*. Chicago, Ill.: Fitzroy Dearborn, 2000, 47–49; Brecher, Edward M. "When Sexual Inhibitions Are Cast Off." In *The Sex Researchers*. Boston, Mass.: Little, Brown, 1969, 247–79; Cover, Rob. "Promiscuity." In Timothy F. Murphy, ed., *Reader's Guide to Lesbian and Gay Studies*. Chicago, Ill.: Fitzroy Dearborn, 2000, 472–73; Earle, W. J. "Depersonalized Sex and Moral Perfection." *International Journal of Moral and Social Studies* 2:3 (1987), 203–10. Reprinted in HS (67–74); Einon, Dorothy. "Are Men More Promiscuous Than Women?" *Ethology and Sociobiology* 15 (1994), 131–43; Ellis, Albert. "The Justification of Sex without Love." In *Sex without Guilt*. New York: Lyle Stuart, 1958, 66–86; Ellis, Anthony. "Casual Sex." *International Journal of Moral and Social Studies* 1:2 (1986), 157–69. Reprinted in HS (125–37); Elliston, Frederick. "In Defense of Promiscuity." In Robert Baker and Frederick Elliston, eds., *Philosophy and Sex*, 1st ed. Buffalo, N.Y.: Prometheus, 1975, 223–43. Reprinted in P&S3 (73–90); STW (146–58); Goldman, Alan. "Plain Sex." *Philosophy and Public Affairs* 6:3 (1977), 267–87. Reprinted in HS (103–23); POS1 (119–38); POS2 (73–92); POS3 (39–55); POS4 (39–55); Gould, Terry. *The Lifestyle: A Look at the Erotic Rites of Swingers*. New York: Firefly, 2000; Halwani, Raja. "Are One-Night Stands Morally Problematic?" *International Journal of Applied Philosophy* 10:1 (1995), 61–67; Lehrman, Sally. "The Virtues of Promiscuity." *AlterNet* (22 July 2002). <www.alternet.org/story.html?StoryID=13648> [accessed 16 February 2005]; LeMoncheck, Linda. *Loose Women, Lecherous Men: A Feminist Philosophy of Sex*. New York: Oxford University Press, 1997; Lesser, A. H. "Love and Lust." *Journal of Value Inquiry* 14:1 (1980), 51–54. Reprinted in HS (75–78); Mappes, Thomas A. (1985) "Sexual Morality and the Concept of Using Another Person." In Thomas A. Mappes and Jane S. Zembaty, eds., *Social Ethics: Morality and Social Policy*, 4th ed. New York: McGraw-Hill, 1992, 203–16. 5th ed., 1997, 163–76. 6th ed., 2002, 170–83. Reprinted in POS4 (207–23); Masters, William H., and Virginia E. Johnson. "Swinging Sex: Is There a Price to Pay?" In *The Pleasure Bond: A New Look at Sexuality and Commitment*. Boston, Mass.: Little, Brown, 1974, 140–75; Mayo, David. "An Obligation to Warn of HIV Infection?" In Alan Soble, ed., *Sex, Love, and Friendship: Studies of the Society for the Philosophy of Sex and Love 1977–1992*. Amsterdam, Holland: Rodopi, 1997, 447–53; Moulton, Janice. "Sexual Behavior: Another Position." *Journal of Philosophy* 73:16 (1976), 537–46. Reprinted in HS (91–100); POS1 (110–18); POS2 (63–71); POS3 (31–38); POS4 (31–38); Nussbaum, Martha C. "Objectification." *Philosophy and Public Affairs* 24:4 (1995), 249–91. Reprinted in POS3 (283–321); POS4 (381–419). Reprinted, revised, in *Sex and Social Justice*. New York: Oxford University Press, 1999, 213–39; O'Neill, Nena, and George O'Neill. *Open Marriage: A New Life Style for Couples*. New York: M. Evans, 1972; Reiss, Ira. "The Double Standard in Premarital Sexual Intercourse." *Social Forces* 34 (March 1956), 224–30; Rinehart, Paula. "Losing Our Promiscuity." In Patricia Beattie Jung and Shannon Jung, eds., *Moral Issues and Christian Responses*, 7th ed. Belmont, Calif.: Wadsworth, 2003, 74–82; Schofield, Michael. *Promiscuity*. London: Gollancz, 1976; Shalit, Wendy. *A Return to Modesty: Discovering the Lost Virtue*. New York: Free Press, 1999; Soble, Alan. "Sexual Use and What to Do about It: Internalist and Externalist Sexual Ethics." *Essays in Philosophy* 2:2 (2001). <www.humboldt.edu/~essays/soble.html> [accessed 17 November 2004]. Reprinted, rev., in POS4 (225–58); Stafford, J. Martin. "On Distinguishing between Love and Lust." *Journal of Value Inquiry* 11:4 (1977), 292–303. Reprinted in J. Martin Stafford, ed., *Essays on Sexuality and Ethics*. Solihull, U.K.: Ismeron, 1995, 53–64; Teichman, Jenny. "Intention and Sex." In Cora Diamond and Jenny Teichman, eds., *Intention and Intentionality: Essays in Honour of G.E.M. Anscombe*. Ithaca, N.Y.: Cornell University Press, 1979, 147–61; Vannoy, Russell. "Can Sex Express Love?" In Alan Soble, ed., *Sex, Love, and Friendship: Studies of the Society for the Philosophy of Sex and Love 1977–1992*. Amsterdam, Holland: Rodopi, 1997, 247–57; Vannoy, Russell. *Sex without Love: A Philosophical Exploration*. Buffalo, N.Y.: Prometheus, 1980; Winch, Peter, Bernard Williams, Michael Tanner, and G.E.M. Anscombe. "Discussion of 'Contraception and Chastity.'" In Michael D. Bayles, ed., *Ethics and Population*. Cambridge, Mass.: Schenkman, 1976, 154–63; Wolf, Naomi. *Promiscuities: A Secret History of Female Desire*. London: Vintage, 1998.

CATHOLICISM, HISTORY OF. Christian moral teachings on sexuality evolved somewhat haphazardly over the centuries, with successive generations appropriating earlier positions often based on very different premises. A series of fairly negative accretions, so to speak, were added one upon another until, in the eighteenth century, we arrive at an absolutely negative estimation of **sexual desire**. The teachings, for the most part, reflected the concerns of celibate men who, while pursuing a life of discipleship ("the state of spiritual perfection"), found sexual desires to be obstacles rather than aids in the pursuit of that perfection. The impact these teachings had on members of Christian cultures generally and Catholic cultures in particular remains to be learned. With reason, historian James Brundage has claimed: "The Christian horror of sex has for centuries placed enormous strain on individual consciences and self-esteem in the Western world" (9).

Sexual desires were not understood as belonging to, or needing to be included in, a broader understanding of human personality. Rather, they were as random and as precipitous as they were for anyone who does not have a consolidating concept like "sexuality." As arbitrary, powerful feelings, little about their nature lent their being conceptually incorporated into an overarching reality. The idea of venereal desires was as unstable as the experienced desires themselves. **Language**, too, hindered understanding sexual desires as belonging to a more holistic category. Pierre Payer's remarks on medieval ideas of sexuality apply also to the very beginning of the Christian era:

> A contemporary writer dealing with medieval ideas of sex faces a peculiar problem of language. Treatises entitled "On sex" are nowhere to be found, nor does one find talk about "sexuality," because medieval Latin had no terms for the English words "sex" and "sexuality." In the strictest sense, there are no discussions of sex in the Middle Ages. Whatever one might think of Michel Foucault's overall thesis about the development of the history of sexuality in the West, his claim about the relatively late date for the invention of sex and sexuality is, I believe, of paramount significance. The concept of sex or sexuality as an integral dimension of human persons, as an object of concern, discourse, truth, and knowledge, did not emerge until well after the Middle Ages. (14)

With that *caveat*, we turn now to the development of Christian teachings on sexual desires.

The Judaic tradition believed in the moral rightness of spousal sexual intimacy and procreation. It did not commend celibacy for its rabbinical leaders, except for communal movements like the Essenes, who practiced celibacy. Regarding sexual conduct, the Hebrew Scriptures regularly upheld fidelity and repeatedly prohibited sexual licentiousness. Like their neighboring communities, the Israelites were patriarchal, and women were, in effect, considered property.

In the Gospels, Jesus promoted the primacy of the **love** commandment and said very little about sexuality; an ethics of interiority that privileged the singleness of heart of the disciple was his major concern. Jesus acknowledged that celibacy was "only for those to whom it is given" (Matt. 19:10–12). Concerning gender, Luke asserted time and again the agency of women as supporters and companions of Jesus: on his mission (8:1–3), at his passion (23:27–31), at his death (23:49), and at his burial (23:54–56). Most notably, at a time when women's testimony had no legal force, women were the first to announce the Good News of Jesus's resurrection (24:1–11). Matthew (28:1–10) and John (20:11–18) privileged the testimony of Mary Magdalene as the first witness and preacher of the Good

News. For this reason many scholars (especially Cahill; Schüssler Fiorenza) find a nearly gender egalitarian approach to discipleship. Christians see in Acts of the Apostles, as the Church is born, that Mary the mother of Jesus (1:14) had a central role in receiving the Holy Spirit with the twelve apostles. Elsewhere, other women are accorded leadership positions (e.g., Rom. 16).

The Pauline letters express more interest in sexuality than the Gospels. Expecting that the "end times" were coming, **Saint Paul** (5–64?) commended celibacy for those who could wait (1 Cor. 7:39), **marriage** for those who could not. Marriage was a licit remedy for sexual desire, while celibacy was preferable for those wishing to be free of anxiety (1 Cor. 7:32). Paul's pragmatic view of marriage did not include procreation. Paul regarded homosexual activity as an attribute of the idolatrous, who failed to recognize the revelation of God in Jesus Christ (Rom. 1:26–27). Many ethicists (Hartwig; Jung and Smith) argue that Paul's position was not based on any necessary connection between **homosexuality** and idolatry but on a mere presumption that anyone who committed homosexual acts worshiped a false God. Marion Soards claims, however, "We cannot fault Paul's appraisal of homosexual behavior without denying the theological vision that informs his understanding of God and humanity" (26).

Paul's anticipation of the imminence of the "end time" proved mistaken, and Christians realized that they would have to develop a lifelong identity. This task was affected by the way Christianity esteemed the human body. While sharing with other traditions the belief in God as Creator and therein the goodness of the created world, Christianity distinguished itself by the Incarnation, the enfleshment of God. Its central liturgy revolved around eating the body and drinking the blood of its Savior; it defined the Church as the "Body of Christ"; and its hope was in the resurrection of the body. Not surprisingly, then, its most heated moral arguments were about gender, sexuality, and reproduction. Because Christianity took the human body seriously, the body became both sign and problem (Meeks, 130–49).

The Scripture scholar Rudolf Bultmann (1884–1976) wrote that, for Paul, *soma* ("body" in Greek) "belongs inseparably, constitutively, to human existence. . . . The only human existence there is—even in the sphere of the Spirit—is somatic existence" (192). Bultmann argues that the body is so integrated into human existence that the human does not have *soma* but is *soma*. For this reason, Paul never used *soma* about a corpse. *Soma* was used to combat the individualism of **Gnosticism** and provided the basis for the metaphysical unity of the person and for the possibility of relationships (Jewett, 458). Paul did distinguish *soma* from *sarx* ("flesh"), which referred to negative desires that keep us from God. **Michel Foucault** (1926–1984) ruminated on whether *sarx* captured in some sense the Christian understanding of sexuality (5). His suggestion helps us comprehend Christianity's esteeming the body while still having a "horror" of sexuality. Arguing, however, that Paul's distinction between *soma* and *sarx* was a cause of Christianity's negative view of sexuality would be difficult.

The appreciation of body (*soma*) is tied to the early Christian hope in the resurrection. Human fulfillment as embodied in the risen Christ is central for understanding the early Christians' hopes and moral responsibilities. From the second century, Christians "saw the integrated mortality of body and spirit as an anthropological necessity: only the immortality of the whole person can make our present struggle to integrate the body and spirit meaningful" (Daley, 32). Human destiny as defined in the Risen Christ provided the opportunity and the demand for all Christians to find in their own bodies the fullness of the Spirit of Christ. This task of personal integration was given greater impetus through the resolution of the controversy about the identity of Jesus. Integrating the divinity and humanity of Christ was the major theological project and accomplishment of the early Church: "The unity of Christ, possessor of two natures but remaining nonetheless one single persona, is . . . the main achievement of centuries of Christological and Trinitarian pugnacious investigations" (Stroumsa, 35). This had practical significance in the ascetical imitation of Christ, which called Christians to seek a unified self: Just as Christ brought divinity and humanity into one, Christians were to bring body and soul together. Integration became a key task for all early Christians, to "be an entity of body and soul, a Christ-bearing exemplar" (Stroumsa, 39–40).

This integration of body and soul was distinctive. In Greek thought, the self was separate from the body: To know oneself meant to attend to one's soul, often at the exclusion of the body. Thus when Christianity, believing humans are in God's image, made integrating the body and soul a theological expression of humanity's integrity and a normative task, it proposed to the Western world a new understanding of the person. "The discovery of the person as a unified composite of soul and body in late antiquity was . . . a Christian discovery" (Stroumsa, 44).

From this task of integration, Peter Brown found that "the Christian doctrine of sexuality as a privileged symptom of personal transformation was the most consequential rendering ever achieved of the ancient and Christian yearning for a single heart" ("Late Antiquity," 300). The singleness of heart is achieved by imitating Jesus Christ, who submitted to the will of God. In *Body and Society*, Brown relates how Christian doctrine freed citizens from Roman control of their bodies (428–47). Christian attitudes to sexuality delivered the deathblow to the ancient notion of the city as the arbiter of the body. Christian preachers endowed the body with intrinsic, inalienable qualities. The body was no longer a neutral, indeterminate outcrop of the natural world, whose usefulness and right to exist were subject predominantly to civic considerations of status and utility. Though Christianity did not give sexuality stability, it did give stability to the body.

Brown also claims that chastity played a decisive role in liberating women from the city. Women benefactresses in either a widowed or virginal state freed themselves from the claims of the city that they reproduce and became instead models of generosity in the life of the Church. For Christians, the paradox of the closed womb was that it was a sign of the benefactress's openness to Scripture, Christ, and the poor. Joyce Salisbury in *Church Fathers*, however, is less enthusiastic about the closed womb: Rather than a sign of freedom, it was another exercise of control. As the woman was to absent herself from **sexual activity**, likewise she was to remove herself from all worldly commerce. In particular, for the true virgin and good Christian woman, a silent mouth was the corollary to the chaste womb. The Christian community raised women to a privileged position for their chastity but also silenced them in return for that privilege.

Still, Paul's recommending sexual **abstinence** for those who could practice it left those who could not with needed resolution. How could venereal desires be incorporated into the person? Instead of seeing marriage, along with Paul, as resolving the fear of incontinence, the lifelong call to integration required a positive purpose for marital relations. For this reason, Christians turned to the Stoics, for whom sexual intercourse could be "brought under the rule of reason not by subduing it but by giving it a rational purpose, procreation. . . . With the adoption of the Stoic norm for sexual intercourse, the direction of **sexual ethics** was set for centuries to come" (Farley, 2367). The Stoic purpose came, however, with a price. Clement of Alexandria (ca. 150–215 CE), who maintained the moral legitimacy of marriage and argued that condemning marital sex was against the Gospels, held with the Stoics that sex for the sake of pleasure, even in marriage, was contrary to law and reason

(2.10.92). The "Alexandrian rule" about pursuing sex for pleasure would vex Christians for centuries.

The first time that sexual norms were developed was at the Council of Elvira in the early fourth century (300–303?), which dedicated nearly half of its eighty canons to sexual conduct. "The Elvira canons seem to represent an attempt to define a Christian self-identity. What made a Christian different from a pagan? Part of the answer, according to the Elvira canons, was that Christianity observed a strict code of sexual ethics" (Brundage, 70). Though it seems that nearly all clergy of the third century (whose marital status was known) were in fact married, Elvira was the first attempt to prohibit clerical marriage. In the fourth century, sexual ethics underwent further development as Church Fathers began writing specifically about venereal desires. Furthermore, Christianity, when it became the state religion in the fourth century, took on institutional control of the population in much the way pagan Rome had earlier controlled citizens' bodies. Finally, because integration or single-heartedness remained the moral imperative, many Fathers fashioned a normative framework from their personal experiences. In short, Christian sexual theology grew out of the struggles of major figures whose ascetical programs for integration encountered the impasse of their own sexual urges. This is most evident in the lasting impression **Saint Augustine** (354–430) made on Christianity.

Three broad strokes paint Augustine's vision of sexuality. First, against **Manichaeism** Augustine defended the moral rightness of marriage and of intercourse when engaged in for procreation. He believed that intercourse for any other reason was morally wrong, though not necessarily mortally sinful. Still, he believed that sexual desires were disordered but could be restored to a rational order by submitting them to the purpose of procreation. Second, in his later writings against Pelagianism, which rejected the necessity of redemption by Christ, Augustine developed a theology of original sin. He located the greatest effect of the sin in the basic disorder of sexual desire and placed the transmission of sin in the act of intercourse. Thus sex became inextricably and irreversibly contaminated with sin in Christian theology. Still, Augustine held that if a married couple had intercourse solely for procreation, they did not sin. If for mutual pleasure, they sinned, though only slightly. But if they intended to avoid procreation, they sinned mortally. Third, Augustine's troubling understanding of women and sexuality reflects the fact that theology was being shaped by men, for men, and based on men's self-understanding. Since many Fathers were hermits or monks, not only was their sexuality dispensable as they pursued integration, but their relationships with women as persons were also dispensable. Augustine "could not for the life of him think of any reason why woman should have been given to man than for the procreation of children" (Mahoney, 66).

A second look at Augustine, however, highlights other features. Augustine upheld the primacy of love in the moral tradition. He recognized the legitimacy of marital claims, particularly the conjugal debt, that is, that a spouse had a right to sexual relations. And as dark as his sexual views were, he was neither Manichaean nor Gnostic. Nor was he St. Jerome (340–420), for whom it was best for men to have as little relations with women as possible, whether as wife, concubine, or prostitute.

The Fathers' focus on procreation led to judgments about specific sex acts. If married persons must not intend contracepted sex, they also must not engage in anal or oral intercourse. In 342, the emperors Constantius and Constans outlawed such sexual activity as deviant. This same edict also prohibited homosexual activity and was incorporated into Theodosius's law in 390 and into the Theodosian Code in 438 (Crompton, 133–36). Social tolerance of homosexuality was thwarted by civil laws that specifically opposed it on the belief that effeminacy weakened the state. Hence the death penalty was imposed on any male who engaged in passive sexual activity. The Emperor Justinian (527–565), in implementing the edict of 342, expanded the death penalty to include all males involved in any homosexual activity.

At the same time, virginity became a significant Christian practice in a communal context. Sexual renunciation allowed women a freedom and a social role that marriage did not. Free of the real dangers of pregnancy, childbirth, and patriarchal dominance, these women could explore with other women a life with Christ in a setting largely ignored by the Fathers. Their communities, along with men's religious communities, were a case of Christianity's promoting a certain equality. The communities of the Benedictines are notable reminders of the development of the institutional environments in which Christian virginity flourished. Yet as monastic communities were developing, the sexual lives of monks came under scrutiny, especially with regard to the "vices" of the solitary life: **masturbation**, sexual **fantasy**, even nocturnal emission. Both John Cassian (365–433) and Caesarius of Arles (470–543) wrote extensively on the need to subdue all influence of sexuality in the growth toward spiritual perfection. There were no writings against masturbation prior to Cassian. It was simply not considered a sexual offense (Brundage, 83, 103, 109–10; Cappelli, 77–132).

The positions of the Fathers and early Councils and the later laws of the Roman Empire were constitutive elements in the formation of Christian moral teaching on sexual activity. At the end of the sixth century, another format for moral teaching appeared, handbooks for confession. At first, these were an attempt to establish fair penances for the monastic practice of confessing sins and receiving absolution. These "penitentials" were developed from the sixth to the twelfth century by abbots throughout Britain and continental Europe. By considering the seriousness of the sin, the attending circumstances, and the spiritual maturity of the sinner, they sought to offer standard penances for the same type of action by the same type of agent. Since most of those who assumed the practice of confessing were monks, sexual sins were predominantly about solitary and same-sex activity. In the penitentials, these topics received great attention and, through them, monks were taught to be preoccupied with fears of same-sex desire, masturbation, other "impure thoughts," and nocturnal emission. When one compares the penance of one abbot's penitential with another, a certain appreciation of context arises. Most were concerned with the "dignity" of the male and were considerably harsher on passive anal or oral intercourse, more grievous activities than taking another man's wife. In the pursuit of spiritual perfection, the issue of single-heartedness or purity was paramount. Penitentials also considered the activities of nuns, though they considered lesbian relations less seriously sinful. In rural communities the sins of **bestiality** were considered in detail.

In the early thirteenth century, Pope Innocent III imposed on the entire Church the Easter duty. For the first time, every Christian was required to confess her or his sinfulness at least once annually. Henry Charles Lea, the great Protestant historian, called this the most significant legislation in the history of the Church (I:230). Prior to Innocent III's edict, most Christians did not confess particular acts as sinful. That practice was reserved for those pursuing a life of spiritual perfection. But by the thirteenth century, being absolved of one's sinfulness was the key to salvation, and specific acts finally became the focus of ordinary Christians trying to understand whether they were among the saved. So the penitentials were replaced by more comprehensive and sophisticated "confessional" manuals.

The penitentials were designed mostly for abbots and others hearing the confessions of monks and nuns, but the confessional manuals of the thirteenth century were, for the

Church, universal. The injunctions that once fell against monks and nuns pursuing spiritual perfection were now applied to the laity, and although confessional penances considered not only the sin but also the rank of the sinner (clergy, nobility, serf, etc.), certain sins were still distinguished solely by their matter as grave. Masturbation, for instance, which was never a serious matter in the first four centuries, was now considered gravely sinful. The original genesis of that judgment depended precisely on the vocational choice of the monk who abandoned his sexuality for the sake of the ascetical life, yet what was a sin for an ascetic of forty years in the eighth century became a sin of the same gravity for a boy of twelve in the thirteenth. Similarly, whatever concern the empire may have had about homosexual behavior and whatever policing it might have done about it, now, through the annual confession, the Church could police and socially control the behavior of those with same-sex attractions—not only in the monastery but anywhere. The Church was now able to put "the fear of God" in everyone. In short, whatever sexual teachings prompted anxiety in monks and nuns as they pursued spiritual perfection became sources of anxiety in the laity. The difference, of course, was that there was no context of the pursuit of spiritual perfection for most of the laity. Whereas the monk might fear damnation because he did not strive adequately to realize his vocational choice, the layman of fifty now feared damnation because he masturbated or had impure thoughts.

Just as penitentials before Innocent III were little concerned with women's solitary vices or same-sex attractions, the confessional manuals after Innocent III were just as disinterested, if the women were not affecting the well-being of men. Nonetheless, caution is required about the self-understanding of persons regarding their sexual desires. Joyce Salisbury argues that we are only beginning to learn the testimonies of women, particularly religious, and are finding that their read on sexuality and women is quite positive and hardly like that of the Fathers, abbots, and canonists ("Gendered Sexuality"). Similarly, Jacqueline Murray admonishes against presuming that the available writings give us any accurate idea of even the "average" male's self-understanding. Historical research, having been dominated by these sin manuals, has not yet yielded adequate access to the common person's ideas.

The penitential and confessional manuals eventually made their way into the canonical manuals. The eleventh century marks the beginning of early canonical collections that would serve as the foundation for later canon law, and the twelfth century marks their significant development. These texts considered, for the most part, the penalties to be applied against clergy who were not sexually continent. But they also condemned any sexual activity that was not procreative or did not take place in marriage. Gratian's *Decretum* (ca. 1140) bears witness to this (Brundage, 235–42; Noonan, 196–97, citing *Decretum* 2.32.2.1–3).

At this time there spawned a prominent conceptual category, "sins against nature." Ivo (1040–1116) defined in his *Decretum* unnatural intercourse as "the use of a member not granted for this" (9.110). Fusing Augustine's *On Marriage and Concupiscence* (2.20) with *Against the Second Answer of Julian* (5.17), Ivo declared: "To act against nature is always unlawful and beyond doubt more flagrant and shameful than to sin by a natural use in fornication or adultery" (9.106). John Noonan comments that Ivo's work is a milestone in the development of Church teaching in part because Ivo brings Augustine's texts into focus to establish the gravity of sins against nature (172–73). About sins against nature, Noonan writes:

> In the theological development of the thirteenth century, anal intercourse, oral intercourse, coitus interruptus, and departure from the assumed position in

intercourse were all analyzed as instances of the marital sin against nature. I do not believe it anachronistic to assume that the twelfth-century writers had such acts as referents for their catch-all phrase. In many of the later writers, too, the variety of sins comprehended by the "sin against nature" can only be inferred from a study of common theological usage. There is never any attempt to provide a biological description of the acts condemned. Medical terms are eschewed. The vagina is usually described as "the vessel" or "the fit vessel." Ejaculation is often described as "pollution." The term "coitus interruptus" is never employed, but the usual description is "outside the fit vessel." (224)

Noonan also notes that "sodomy and coitus interruptus are often treated as two varieties of the sin against nature" (226). As examples of those who wrote about both, he cites William Peraldus (d. ca. 1274), Jean Gerson (1363–1429), and Antoninus (1389–1459).

Teachings on same-sex relationships were treated particularly under the sin against nature. Though Augustine earlier had mentioned (ca. 397) that those citizens of Sodom who violated the "male" angels acted against nature (*Confessions* 3.8.15), the notion of sinning against nature received its first extended discussion in *The Book of Gomorrah* by Peter Damian (1007–1072). Damian devoted a section to the topic of the different types of person who sin against nature.

Four types of this form of criminal wickedness can be distinguished in an effort to show you the totality of the whole matter in an orderly way: some sin with themselves alone [masturbation]; some by the hands of others [mutual masturbation]; others between the thighs [interfemoral intercourse]; and finally, others commit the complete act against nature [anal intercourse]. The ascending gradation among these is such that the last mentioned are judged to be more serious that the preceding. (29)

Damian's concern is specifically with fellow monks committing these sins (Jordan, *Sodomy*, 57–66).

What was defined as nature, and why one sin was understood as graver than another, varied. Robert of Sorbonne (1201–1274), for instance, wrote that the closer one is related to a person, the more seriously one sinned; because masturbation is the worst form of **incest**, the sin of masturbation is the gravest (Glorieux, 54–57; Jordan, *Ethics*, 101). Later, Peter of Poitiers (1130–1205) agreed and dedicated a lengthy passage to the "monster of masturbation" (Jordan, *Sodomy*, 105). Albert the Great (1206–1280) bestowed on same-sex intercourse a triple condemnation: It was a sin against grace, as condemned in the Old and New Testaments; it was a sin against reason; and it was a sin against nature, because it "contradicts the natural impulse to species continuity" (Jordan, *Sodomy*, 126).

What links these sins together as unnatural was that the semen went elsewhere than into its fit vessel; that is what constituted their unnaturalness. Further, semen did not pertain to the male *per se* but more appropriately to the future of the species. Thus **Saint Thomas Aquinas** (1224/25–1274) wrote in *Summa contra gentiles*:

The seed, although superfluous as to the conservation of the individual, is yet necessary to the propagation of the species, while other superfluities, such as excrement, sweat, urine, and the like, are necessary for nothing. Hence the emission of the latter concerns only the good of the individual. But not only this is required in the emission of the seed; it is also required that it be emitted to be of use in generation, to which coitus is ordained. . . . The disordered emission of seed is contrary to the good of nature, which is the conservation of the species. (bk. III, chap. 122)

Thomas elaborated this view in his later work, the *Summa theologiae*, in which he stated that venereal use "is highly necessary to the common good, which is the conservation of the human race" (II.II.153.3). Here Thomas developed the natural teleology of (the male) reproductive organ as belonging to the common good and laid the groundwork for supposing that our reproductive organs existed not for ourselves but for the propagation of the species (see Noonan, 244 ff.; and on semen, Lutterbach).

The sin against nature became a clear marker in the "moral" manuals of the sixteenth to the twentieth centuries that follow the confessional manuals of the twelfth to the sixteenth (Kosnick et al., 43–44). From Albert and Thomas until the twentieth century, the moral treatises distinguished between sexual sins "in accordance with nature" and those "contrary to nature." The former sins included heterosexual fornication, **adultery**, incest, **rape**, and abduction; the latter sins (bestiality, masturbation, contracepted coitus, anal and oral intercourse) were, in general, more grievous, in virtue of the "common good" value the tradition placed on semen.

Sins against nature received further treatment by being coupled with two other concepts: intrinsic evil and "parvity of matter." Intrinsic evil was a fourteenth-century concept that characterized particular actions as absolutely, always wrong, regardless of circumstances, an *a priori* evaluation that removed from consideration any question of their moral legitimacy. Actions were put into this category either because they were against nature and/or because the agent had no right to the exercise of the activity (see Ugorji). Classic examples of the latter included lying or the direct killing of the innocent. Instances of unnatural acts satisfied both criteria, since in performing an unnatural act one exercised a forbidden activity. The category of intrinsic evil, then, closed debate about the licitness of any sexual act in which a man's semen was emitted elsewhere than in his wife's vagina.

Nonetheless, the issue of the degree of the sinfulness was still open. The question arose whether any sin of lust could be considered a light matter or had what the manualists called "parvity of matter." Since Aquinas, sins of lust were considered always mortally sinful. Subsequent to the scholastics, fifteenth- and sixteenth-century casuists, influenced by nominalism and therefore not inclined to the concept of intrinsically evil actions, entertained specific cases and varying circumstances. On their account, if actions were not to involve the illicit emission of semen and if the pleasure felt in the action was constitutive of the intention to engage licitly in conjugal relations, then such actions could be considered light or venially sinful or, in some cases, not sinful at all. Likewise, kisses, or passing fantasies that did not linger or become a *delectatio morosa*, were also, in some instances, not considered mortal sins. Martin the Master (1432–1482), Jean Mair (1467–1550), Martin of Azplicueta (1495–1586), and Thomas Sanchez (1550–1610) were among the major casuists who could imagine that these fairly marginal sexual actions were morally light or permitted (see Vereecke).

Though the *Catechism of the Council of Trent* (1566) did not enter the discussion of these more specific issues, it presented marriage among the seven sacraments and defined its three goods as "mutual assistance," "procreation," and "an antidote to avoid the sins of lust." For the most part, the *Catechism* attended to the indissolubility of marriage (338–55). It addressed venereal desires specifically in its treatment of the Sixth Commandment, where it began with the observation: "The bond between man and wife is one of the closest, and nothing can be more gratifying to both than to know that they are objects of mutual and special affection." However, it immediately warned the pastor not to go into too much detail when explaining the sins of the commandment, lest he "inflame corrupt passion." The *Catechism* also recommended purity for all and dedicated almost all its comment (without detail) to the filthy sin of impurity (431–39).

Among theologians writing in the moral manuals, the question of "parvity of matter" continued unabated. In 1612 the Superior General of the Society of Jesus (the Jesuits) condemned the position that excused from mortal sin some slight pleasure in deliberately sought venereal desires. Not only did he bind Jesuits to obey the teaching under pain of excommunication, but he imposed on them the obligation to expose the Jesuits who violated even the spirit of the decree (Boyle, 14–16). These and other sanctions dissuaded moralists from entertaining the lightness or licitness of circumstantial exceptions, as earlier casuists had done. By 1750 the moral manualists locked into place the teaching that all sexual desires and subsequent activity were always mortally sinful unless they were the conjugal action of spouses that was in itself left open to procreation. Therein they assimilated into the tradition the claims that sins against the Sixth and Ninth Commandments had no parvity of matter. It is striking that this position did not apply to the other commandments.

"Parvity of matter," "intrinsic evil," and the absolute wrongness of "sins against nature" combined to isolate venereal desires. Moreover, the teleology of the reproductive organs as belonging to the common good, the right of the spouse to claim the marital debt, and the denial of the right of the agent to use his or her sexual organs for anything other than marital procreation isolated even the sexual organs—especially from the human person. Just as the monk in the first millennium sought through ascetical practices to integrate himself body and soul, but at the cost of dispensing with his sexual desires, so, too, in the second millennium after the imposition of the Easter duty, celibate Church theologians deprived the laity of the idea that sexual pleasure could be legitimate and any sense that their sexual desires could ever lead to anything good. The theologians replaced the natural inclination to satisfy those desires with a mortal fear of them and a moral pathology of sexuality itself. The Gospel summons to love and the early Church's call to be one in mind and body developed well throughout the centuries, but they never touched in any way on human sexual desire. To the contrary, as Christianity advanced, it achieved a virtual moral quarantining of sex.

See also Abortion; Abstinence; Augustine (Saint); Bestiality; Bible, Sex and the; Boswell, John; Buddhism; Catholicism, Twentieth- and Twenty-First Century; Desire, Sexual; Foucault, Michel; Gnosticism; Homosexuality, Ethics of; Judaism, History of; Marriage; Masturbation; Natural Law (New); Paul (Saint); Perversion, Sexual; Protestantism, History of; Roman Sexuality and Philosophy, Ancient; Social Constructionism; Thomas Aquinas (Saint)

REFERENCES

Augustine. *Opera Omnia.* Ed. Cornelius Mayer. Charlottesville, N.C.: InteLex, 1997; Boyle, Patrick. *Parvitas Materiae in Sexto in Contemporary Catholic Thought.* Lanham, Md.: University Press of America, 1987; Brown, Peter. *The Body and Society: Men, Women, and Sexual Renunciation in Early Christianity.* New York: Columbia University Press, 1988; Brown, Peter. "Late Antiquity." In Paul Veyne, ed., *A History of Private Life,* vol. 1: *From Pagan Rome to Byzantium.* Cambridge, Mass.: Harvard University Press, 1987, 235–311; Brundage, James A. *Law, Sex, and Christian Society in Medieval Europe.* Chicago, Ill.: University of Chicago Press, 1987; Bultmann, Rudolf. "Soma." In Rudolf Bultmann, ed., *Theology of the New Testament,* vol. 1. London: SCM, 1952, 192–203; Cahill, Lisa Sowle. *Sex, Gender, and Christian Ethics.* Cambridge: Cambridge University Press, 1996; Cappelli, Giovanni. *Autoerotismo: Un problema morale nei primi secoli cristiani?* Bologna, Italy: Edizioni Dehoniano, 1986; *Catechism of the Council of Trent for Parish Priests Issued by Order of Pope*

Pius V. Trans. John A. McHugh and Charles J. Callan. New York: Joseph F. Wagner, 1934; Clement of Alexandria. (ca. 190) *Christ the Educator* [*Paidagogus*]. Trans. Simon P. Wood. New York: Fathers of the Church, 1954; Crompton, Louis. *Homosexuality and Civilization*. Cambridge, Mass.: Harvard University Press, 2003; Daley, Brian. "The Ripening of Salvation." *Communio* 17 (Spring 1990), 27–49; Damian, Peter. *The Book of Gomorrah*. Ed. Pierre Payer. Waterloo, Can.: Wilfrid Laurier University Press, 1982; Farley, Margaret. "Sexual Ethics." In Warren Reich, ed., *Encyclopedia of Bioethics*, rev. ed., vol. 5. New York: Simon Schuster Macmillan, 1995, 2363–75; Foucault, Michel. *The History of Sexuality*, vol. 2: *The Use of Pleasure*. Trans. Robert Hurley. New York: Pantheon, 1985; Glorieux, Palémon. *Aux origins de la Sorbonne*, vol. 1: *Robert de Sorbon*. [Études de philosophie médiévale, LIII.] Paris: J. Vrin, 1965; Hartwig, Michael. *The Poetics of Intimacy and the Problem of Sexual Abstinence*. New York: Peter Lang, 2000; Ivo. *Opera Omnia*. Paris: Laurentium Cottereau, 1647; Jewett, Robert. *Paul's Anthropological Terms*. Leiden: Brill, 1971; Jordan, Mark D. *The Ethics of Sex*. Oxford, U.K.: Blackwell, 2002; Jordan, Mark D. *The Invention of Sodomy in Christian Theology*. Chicago, Ill.: University of Chicago Press, 1997; Jung, Patricia Beattie, and Ralph F. Smith. *Heterosexism: An Ethical Challenge*. Albany: State University of New York Press, 1993; Kosnick, Anthony, William Carroll, Agnes Cunningham, Ronald Modras, and James Schulte. *Human Sexuality: New Directions in American Catholic Thought*. New York: Paulist Press, 1977; Lea, Henry Charles. *The History of Auricular Confession and Indulgences in the Latin Church*, 3 vols. Philadelphia, Pa.: Lea Brothers, 1896. Reprint, Westport, Conn.: Greenwood Press, 1968; Lutterbach, Hubertus. "Die Sexualtabus in den Bussbüchern." *Saeculum* 46:2 (1995), 216–48; Mahoney, John. *The Making of Moral Theology: A Study of the Roman Catholic Tradition*. New York: Oxford University Press, 1987; Meeks, Wayne A. *The Origins of Christian Morality: The First Two Centuries*. New Haven, Conn.: Yale University Press, 1993; Murray, Jacqueline. "Hiding Behind the Universal Man: Male Sexuality in the Middle Ages." In Vern L. Bullough and James A. Brundage, eds., *Handbook of Medieval Sexuality*. New York: Garland, 1996, 123–52; Noonan, John T., Jr. *Contraception: A History of Its Treatment by the Catholic Theologians and Canonists*. Cambridge, Mass.: Harvard University Press, 1965; Payer, Pierre J. *The Bridling of Desire: Views of Sex in the Later Middle Ages*. Toronto, Can.: University of Toronto Press, 1993; Peter of Poitiers. *Summa de Confessione: Compilatio praesens*. Ed. Jean Longère. Turnhout, Belgium: Brepols, 1980; Salisbury, Joyce. *Church Fathers, Independent Virgins*. London: Verso, 1991; Salisbury, Joyce. "Gendered Sexuality." In Vern L. Bullough and James A. Brundage, eds., *Handbook of Medieval Sexuality*. New York: Garland, 1996, 81–102; Schüssler Fiorenza, Elisabeth. *In Memory of Her: A Feminist Theological Reconstruction of Christian Origins*. New York: Continuum, 1983; Soards, Marion. *Scripture and Homosexuality: Biblical Authority and the Church Today*. Louisville, Ky.: Westminster John Knox, 1995; Stroumsa, Gedaliahu. "*Caro salutis cardo*: Shaping the Person in Early Christian Thought." *History of Religions* 30 (August 1990), 25–50; Thomas Aquinas. *Opera Omnia*. Paris: Librairie Philosophique J. Vrin, 1989; Ugorji, Lucius Iwejuru. *The Principle of Double Effect: A Critical Appraisal of Its Traditional Understanding and Its Modern Reinterpretation*. Frankfurt am Main, Ger.: Peter Lang, 1985; Vereecke, Louis. *De Guillaume d'Ockham à Saint Alphonse de Liguori: Études d'histoire de la théologie morale moderne, 1300–1787*. Rome, Italy: Alfonsianum University, 1986.

James F. Keenan

ADDITIONAL READING

Ariès, Philippe. "St. Paul and the Flesh." In Philippe Ariès and André Béjin, eds., *Western Sexuality: Practice and Precept in Past and Present Times*. Trans. Anthony Forster. New York: Blackwell, 1985, 36–39; Baldwin, John W. "Consent and the Marital Debt: Five Discourses in Northern France around 1200." In Angeliki E. Laiou, ed., *Consent and Coercion to Sex and Marriage in Ancient and Medieval Societies*. Washington, D.C.: Dumbarton Oaks, 1993, 257–70; Benko, Stephen. *Pagan Rome and the Early Christians*. Bloomington: Indiana University Press, 1984; Brown, Peter. (1967) *Augustine of Hippo: A Biography*, rev. ed. London: Faber and Faber, 2000; Brundage, James A. "Sex and Canon Law." In Vern L. Bullough and James A. Brundage, eds., *Handbook of Medieval Sexuality*. New York: Garland, 1996, 33–50; Bullough, Vern L. "Christianity and Sexuality." In Ronald M. Green, ed.,

Religion and Sexual Health: Ethical, Theological, and Clinical Perspectives. Boston, Mass.: Kluwer, 1992, 3–16; Bullough, Vern L., and James A. Brundage, eds. *Handbook of Medieval Sexuality.* New York: Garland, 1996; Burrus, Virginia. (1979) *Jerome, Chrysostom, and Friends: Essays and Translations,* 2nd ed. New York: Mellen Press, 1982; Burrus, Virginia. *The Sex Lives of Saints: An Erotics of Ancient Hagiography.* Philadelphia: University of Pennsylvania Press, 2004; Clark, Elizabeth A., and Herbert Richardson, eds. *Women and Religion: A Feminist Sourcebook of Christian Thought,* 1st ed. New York: Harper and Row, 1977. Revised and expanded ed., *Women and Religion: The Original Sourcebook of Women in Christian Thought.* San Francisco, Calif.: HarperCollins, 1996; Daley, Brian. *The Hope of the Early Church.* New York: Cambridge University Press, 1991; Edwards, Robert R., and Stephen Spector, eds. *The Olde Daunce: Love, Friendship, Sex, and Marriage in the Medieval World.* Albany: State University of New York Press, 1991; Farley, Margaret A. "Sexual Ethics." In Warren Reich, ed., *Encyclopedia of Bioethics,* vol. 4. New York: Free Press, 1978, 1575–89; Farley, Margaret A. "Sexual Ethics." In Warren Reich, ed., *Encyclopedia of Bioethics,* rev. ed., vol. 5. New York: Simon Schuster Macmillan, 1995, 2363–75; Fuchs, Eric. (1979) *Sexual Desire and Love: Origins and History of the Christian Ethic of Sexuality and Marriage.* Trans. Marsha Daigle. New York: Seabury Press, 1983; Grisez, Germain, Joseph Boyle, John Finnis, William E. May, and John C. Ford. *The Teaching of "Humanae Vitae": A Defense.* San Francisco, Calif.: Ignatius Press, 1988; Harrington, Daniel, and James F. Keenan. *Jesus and Virtue Ethics: Building Bridges between New Testament Studies and Moral Theology.* Lanham, Md.: Sheed and Ward, 2002; Hawkes, Gail. *Sex and Pleasure in Western Culture.* Malden, Mass.: Polity, 2004; Keenan, James F. "The Casuistry of John Mair." In James F. Keenan and Thomas A. Shannon, eds., *The Context of Casuistry.* Washington, D.C.: Georgetown University Press, 1995, 85–102; Keenan, James F. "Christian Perspectives on the Human Body." *Theological Studies* 55:2 (1994), 330–46; Keenan, James F. "The Open Debate: Moral Theology and the Lives of Gay and Lesbian Persons." *Theological Studies* 64:1 (2003), 127–50; Keenan, James F., ed. *Catholic Ethicists on HIV/AIDS Prevention: Thirty-seven Theologians from around the World Show How Roman Catholic Moral Traditions Can Mediate the Clash of Values in HIV Prevention.* New York: Continuum, 2000; Lutterbach, Hubertus. *Sexualität im Mittelalter: Eine Kulturstudie anhand von Bussbüchern des 6. bis 12. Jahrhunderts.* Cologne, Ger.: Böhlau Verlag, 1999; McNeill, John T., and Helena M. Gamer. *Medieval Handbooks of Penance: A Translation of the Principal Libri Poenitentiales and Selections from Related Documents.* New York: Columbia University Press, 1938; Murray, Jacqueline. "Twice Marginal and Twice Invisible: Lesbians in the Middle Ages." In Vern L. Bullough and James A. Brundage, eds., *Handbook of Medieval Sexuality.* New York: Garland, 1996, 191–222; Nolan, John Gavin. *Jerome and Jovinian.* Washington, D.C.: Catholic University of America, 1956; Noonan, John T., Jr. (1965) *Contraception: A History of Its Treatment by the Catholic Theologians and Canonists,* enlarged ed. Cambridge, Mass.: Harvard University Press, 1986; Pagels, Elaine. *Adam, Eve, and the Serpent.* New York: Vintage, 1988; Payer, Pierre J. "Confession and the Study of Sex in the Middle Ages." In Vern L. Bullough and James A. Brundage, eds., *Handbook of Medieval Sexuality.* New York: Garland, 1996, 3–32; Payer, Pierre J. *Sex and the Penitentials: The Development of a Sexual Code, 550–1150.* Toronto, Can.: University of Toronto Press, 1984; Porter, Jean. *Divine and Natural Law: Reclaiming the Tradition for Christian Ethics.* Grand Rapids, Mich.: Eerdmans, 1999; Portmann, John. *Sex and Heaven: Catholics in Bed and Prayer.* New York: Palgrave Macmillan, 2003; Ranke-Heinemann, Uta. (1988) *Eunuchs for the Kingdom of Heaven: Women, Sexuality, and the Catholic Church.* Trans. Peter Heinegg. New York: Penguin, 1990; Stone, Lawrence. "Sex in the West." *The New Republic* (8 July 1985), 25–37; Tentler, Thomas. *Sin and Confession on the Eve of the Reformation.* Princeton, N.J.: Princeton University Press, 1977; Westermarck, Edward. *Christianity and Morals.* London: Kegan Paul, Trench, Trubner; New York: Macmillan, 1939.

CATHOLICISM, TWENTIETH- AND TWENTY-FIRST-CENTURY. Twentieth-century Roman Catholic treatment of sexuality involved both major changes in attitude and few, but significant, developments in official teaching. The principal issues

spotlighted were **contraception**, clerical celibacy, divorce, gender roles, **homosexuality**, reproductive technologies, **abortion**, and sex outside marriage.

During the twentieth century the social, economic, and technological contexts of human sexuality underwent tremendous changes. Populations exploded and moved from rural to urban settings and from multigenerational to nuclear families. New technologies drastically reduced infant and child mortality; they also yielded reliable contraception, safer abortion, and medical remedies for infertility. Education became increasingly gender-neutral, while the global economy forced millions of married women into wage labor. By the 1980s, AIDS (acquired immunodeficiency syndrome) had reached pandemic levels. The collective impact of these events was to pressure the Catholic Church (and other religions) to develop new approaches to sexuality, **marriage**, and family.

Catholic teaching on sexuality was also affected by changes in Catholic moral theology. Sexuality had traditionally been treated with suspicion and almost exclusively as a moral problem. One change in moral theology that emerged in the second half of the twentieth century was that sex *per se* came to be treated less negatively; specifically, theological mention of sexuality began to occur not only within discussions of sin but also in connection with the goodness of creation and even as a manifestation of Christian **love**. This shift to a more nuanced treatment of sex resulted from a broader shift in Catholic moral theology that began in the late nineteenth century and continued into the twentieth, particularly in the work of Bernard Haring (1912–1998) and Josef Fuchs (1912–   ). These German theologians, building on new interpretations of the New Testament, stressed the law of love—for example, the Sermon on the Mount—as the center of Catholic moral theology, rather than the legalism of the traditional moral manuals used in the education of clergy. At the same time, the neo-Thomist movement, especially strong in France, stressed the good, rather than that which is commanded, as the primary ethical category (McBrien, 908–9). These new emphases led to reevaluations of sexuality.

But while new theological work reflected larger shifts in moral theology, the revolution in Catholic attitudes and practice was not generated only by theologians. Laity played a major role, especially in Europe and the United States, due largely to the vast increase in education that occurred during the twentieth century. On this foundation, middle-class laypersons built careers involving complex, responsible decision making affecting whole societies. The education and careers of increasing numbers of laity gave them confidence in interpreting marital sexuality and sustained the willingness to support their interpretations against what they perceived as clerical interpretations not based in experience.

The 1917 *Code of Canon Law* contained three definitions regarding marriage that reflected past Church teachings; these would become hotly contested later in the century:

> 1013.1 The primary end of marriage is the procreation and education of children; its secondary end is mutual help and the allaying of concupiscence.

> 1013.2 The essential properties of marriage are unity and indissolubility, which acquire a peculiar firmness in Christian marriage by reason of its sacramental character.

> 1081.2 Matrimonial consent is an act of the will by which each party gives and accepts a perpetual and exclusive right over the body, for acts which are themselves suitable for the generation of children.

In subsequent disputes, many theologians and bishops would reshuffle the primary and secondary ends, so that both procreation and mutual help were primary ends and allaying concupiscence a secondary end. "Mutual help" was redefined as developing a loving and intimate relationship of trust, in contrast to its earlier, more pragmatic form, as cooperation developing out of the shared work of rearing children. The indissolubility of marriage would also be challenged in the following decades as people not only lived longer but became more individuated through the multiplication of decisions they were forced to make about themselves in late modern conditions.

The first major teaching about sexuality of the twentieth century was Pope Pius XI's (1857–1939; pope, 1922–1939) 1930 encyclical *Casti connubii* defending marriage against modernity. This encyclical insisted that matrimony is both a divine institution and an act of human will requiring **consent**. In matrimony, "the souls of the contracting parties are joined and knit together more directly and more intimately than are their bodies, and that not by any passing affection of sense or spirit, but by a deliberate and firm act of the will" (*Casti*, #7). This two-becomes-one understanding of marriage, as primarily a contract instead of a relationship, lay beneath many later disputes about sex. If marriage were a contract oriented to procreation and the education of children, then lack of love, trust, or intimacy would not be relevant to the continuation of the marriage; the contract was not about feelings or human relationships. In the encyclical, Pius disapproved of conceiving marital unity as grounded in affectionate feeling, which for him was temporary and unreliable. During the following decades his understanding of marriage came to be judged inadequate, both for failing to acknowledge the need for intimacy at the core of contemporary marriage and for positing that marital unity was based on male headship.

Casti connubii itself began a movement away from canon law on marriage by blurring the line between marriage's primary and secondary ends:

> The mutual inward moulding of husband and wife, this determined effort to perfect each other, can in a very real sense . . . be said to be the chief reason and purpose of matrimony, provided matrimony be looked at not in the restricted sense as instituted for the proper conception and education of the child, but more widely as the blending of life as a whole and mutual exchange and sharing thereof. (#24)

This was a shift away from the traditional impersonal, contractual understanding of marriage. No longer did "perfecting the spouse" mean only showing respect and consideration for the other and praying for the spouse's virtue. *Casti connubii* began a transformation of "perfecting the spouse" toward an intimate, mutually dependent relationship in which spousal love supported virtue and the expansion of virtue and love into other relationships.

Though Church law and teaching insisted that marriage was a contract oriented to procreation, the Church had never taught that married couples had an obligation to engage in intercourse to generate children. Spouses were to provide sex on demand (the marriage debt) to allay temptation to sexual sin by the other spouse (marital sexual activity was *remedium ad concupiscentiae*), but if neither spouse demanded sex, couples were praised for completely avoiding it. Some bishops, influenced by lives of some saints and the writings of theologians such as **Saint Augustine** ([354–430]; *Epistles*, 262:4; *On the Good of Marriage*, chaps. 3, 6; see Clark) and Hugh of St. Victor ([1096–1141]; 7, 9, 11; see Ranke-Heinemann, 97, 164–67), continued openly to advocate "Josephite marriages" in which the couple disavowed all sexual intercourse (supposedly like Mary and Joseph). Standard homiletic fare for much of the twentieth century was the encouragement given to couples by priests to abstain from sex before receiving communion, during Lent, on certain holy days, and periodically as penance and moral discipline (Ranke-Heinemann,

98–100, 143–46, 195). Many referred to **Saint Paul** ([5–64?]; 1 Cor. 7:1–5) on the subject of sexual **abstinence** but emphasized not Paul's conclusion—that couples should resume sex after prayer—but his assumption that sexual abstinence enabled prayer.

Another sign of the beginning of a shift in the treatment of primary and secondary ends of marriage was *Casti connubii*'s discussion of secondary ends. While the *Code of Canon Law* named as secondary ends of marriage "mutual help" and "allaying of concupiscence," Pius XI wrote:

> For in matrimony as well as in the use of matrimonial rights there are also secondary ends, such as mutual aid, the cultivating of mutual love, and the quieting of concupiscence. (#59c)

The repetition of "mutual" indicates the shift, as does the addition of "the cultivating of mutual love." As the training and roles of men and women became more alike between the mid-nineteenth century and mid-twentieth century, mutuality in marriage became more possible and more common.

While Pius XI began the slide toward a more interpersonal understanding of marriage, *Casti connubii* also held to various past teachings. He insisted on marriage's indissolubility (#21, #34, #35), on limiting the use of the sexual faculties to matrimony and only with procreative intent (#54, #55, #59), and on sexual complementarity: Wives owed obedience to husbands and belonged in the home (#74). This last theme was repeated in his 1937 *Divini redemptoris* (#71). The sexes were so different, for Pius XI, that he condemned co-education as promiscuous for ignoring the fact that "nature . . . fashions the two [sexes] quite different in organism, in temperament, in abilities" (*Divini illius magistri*, #72).

On each of these topics Pius XI's immediate successors saw changes in terms of practice, if not in law or theological teaching. While the official ban on divorce endured throughout the entire century, in many parts of the world a great many unhappy marriages were annulled by recognizing a significant original defect in the union (see Foster). On the issue of contraception, Pius XII (1876–1958; pope, 1939–1958) initiated a major step away from procreative possibility as necessary for licit sex in marriage. His "Allocution to Midwives" (1951) permitted, for couples with compelling moral reasons to limit births, the use of the "rhythm method" (or "natural family planning"), a technique based on abstinence during the woman's fertile period. Pius XII thereby redirected moral censure from "contraceptive intent" to "illicit means of contraception." He continued to insist on the restriction of **sexual activity** to marriage and to differentiate contraception from abortion. But the newly allowed practice had effects: Large Catholic families, which in the 1940s and 1950s were a sign of virtuous parental self-sacrifice and obedience to Catholic teaching, began disappearing after 1960 and by the 1970s no longer distinguished Catholics from Protestants and Jews in much of the United States and Europe. Allowing natural family planning also gave "cover" to Catholic families who used forbidden contraceptive means as well.

Pius XII also softened somewhat the **language** of his predecessors by speaking not so much about the "false" equality of women (cf. *Casti*, #74) as about women's spiritual equality, coupled with a highly romanticized pedestalization of women as mothers. Women were equal in the eyes of God—what really counted—but their most significant role was as the center of family, not as workers in the world. His successors John XXIII (1881–1963; pope, 1958–1963) and Paul VI (1897–1978; pope, 1963–1978) supported a rise in the status of women. However, both understood women within the restrictive framework of sexual complementarity, which at least for John meant functional inequality. In his first encyclical (1959), John XXIII wrote, "Within the family, the father stands in God's place. He must lead and guide the rest by his authority and the example of his good life" (*Ad petri cathedram*, 509; for translation problems, see Gudorf, *Catholic Social Teaching*, 337). And in *Convenuti a Roma* (1961), he wrote, "It is true that living conditions tend to bring about almost equality of the sexes. Nevertheless, while their justly proclaimed equality of rights must extend to all the claims of personal and human dignity, it does not in any way imply equality of function" (611). Thus John XXIII only haltingly and inconsistently inserted language about practical lived equality into discussions of women in family, society, and church.

Because it occurred during the development of oral contraceptives, Pius XII's shift from contraceptive intent to means raised expectations of further liberalization and more questioning of Natural Law arguments concerning sexuality. Thus the very pope who most romanticized fertility and large families (see Gudorf, *Catholic Social Teaching*, 272–308) inaugurated a thirty-year period in which the Church gradually recognized that overpopulation (see Hanigan; Vatican Council II, #50), poverty, and medical threats to life and health (and not merely depravity, as taught by Pius XI) pressed couples to limit family size. Eventually, Vatican references to responsible parenthood pointed not to a noncontraceptive norm with limited personal, medical—not social—exceptions but rather to a family planning norm that countenanced officially licit contraceptive means.

Vatican II's *Pastoral Constitution* insisted that the decision to have children belonged to parents and should reflect the welfare of the whole family, the material and spiritual conditions of the times, and the interests of society and the Church (#50). A Pontifical Commission appointed by John XXIII in 1962 to study the matter issued its conclusions in 1966, as well as a minority report. The Commission recommended that the morality of marital sexual acts "does not depend upon the direct fecundity of each and every particular act" but instead on the character of the marital relationship, which should be chaste and loving (II, 2). However, Paul VI's *Humanae vitae* (1968) expressed the traditional view, in the minority report, that the unitive and procreative aspects of marital sexual intercourse were morally inseparable; every coital act must therefore be open to procreation. This "inseparability" principle was exhaustively debated over the next two decades. It was defended by the Vatican both in terms of scholastic teaching and in terms of Church authority, and Pius XI was invoked: "No difficulty can arise that justifies the putting aside of the law of God which forbids all acts intrinsically evil. There is no possible circumstance in which husband and wife cannot, strengthened by the grace of God, fulfill faithfully their duties and preserve in wedlock their chastity unspotted" (*Casti*, #61).

Among many theological responses to *Humanae vitae* was *Human Sexuality* (Kosnick et al.), commissioned by the Catholic Theological Society of America. As did other contemporary theology, this report stressed personhood, integrity, and intimacy in human relationships and rejected the conclusion of *Humanae vitae*. (For one sustained Catholic defense of the encyclical, see Grisez et al.) Many Catholic theologians argued that **Saint Thomas Aquinas**'s (1224/25–1274) own treatment of sexuality was not guided by his general theological method but was the principal area of his thought that constituted an exception to this method. Usually led by reason as the guide to moral behavior, Thomas in this one area, sexuality, abandoned the guide of reason. He feared that while reason was strong enough to throw light in other areas of life, it was not strong enough to overcome the distortions powerfully introduced by **sexual desire** (Fuchs, 671). Consequently, in sexuality, instead of defining humans in terms of their ability to use reason, Thomas turned to physicalism, particularly the work of Ulpian (d. 228), who understood human sexuality as essentially **animal sexuality** (Curran, *Themes*, 165–80). In this approach to understanding human sexuality, biology and biological urges alone indicated God's will—that sex be procreative (see Beis).

For modern revisionists, Thomas had simply been wrong about sex. As created by God, human sexuality is more than brute biology: It involves psychology, relationships, responsibility, conscience. They asked, Why should biology—the fact that sometimes, but not nearly always, sexual intercourse results in pregnancy—take precedence over human psychology, the interior knowledge, for example, of young newlyweds that they would be better parents if they postponed procreation until they had formed a stable partnership and were better able to support and educate a family? Physicalism did not deal with the wholeness or complexity of the human person. Thomas, who spent virtually his entire life monastically confined, might be excused for ignorance about marital sex; still, late-twentieth-century married couples' experience of sexual desire was not (as he imagined) of a drive undeniable and uncontrollable by reason. Married couples experience, instead, desire domesticated and thwarted: desire aimed only at each other and thwarted by the practical needs of everyday life—to get children off to school, to get themselves to work, to get enough sleep to be able to repeat the routine the next morning. The satisfaction of the sexual desire of married couples is often postponed as a result of lacking time or **privacy** or fearing pregnancy (Kaiser, 229).

The firestorm of controversy following *Humanae vitae* was new in modern Catholicism, as sexuality was debated in public forums and newspapers and magazines, both Catholic and non-Catholic (see Cohen; Watt). Most Catholics in the developed world might have turned a deaf ear to official teaching and employed artificial contraception even without the supportive, dissenting views of bishops and theologians; indeed, by 1980 most Catholic women of reproductive age in the developed world did so. But the existence of widespread theological dissent became public knowledge in the United States when Reverend Charles Curran was dismissed from the Theology Faculty at the Catholic University of America (see Haring), and articles in Catholic newspapers appeared, written by dissenters such as theologian Rosemary Ruether and Patricia Crowley, a laywoman who had served on the Pontifical Commission (Kaiser, 137, 187–91). The publicity of theological dissent gave laypersons the comfort of knowing they were not alone, that other people of faith, including theologians, priests, and bishops, were alongside them.

In Europe national hierarchies issued statements outlining the possibility of and conditions for legitimate dissent from *Humanae vitae* (Curran, *Catholic Moral Tradition*, 211). But many bishops in the United States attempted to enforce the new teaching, especially against priests. The issue was exceptionally difficult for priests, who dealt with the laity in the confessional. Many priests heard heartbreaking stories from young couples who had more children than they could afford to raise comfortably, who felt forced to pick fights and avoid each other, even during crisis times in which they needed mutual support, to avoid another pregnancy. Some priests refused to enforce the teaching and advised couples to ignore it and use contraception. Initially provoked by contraception, dissent expanded to other areas of Church teaching. But during the papacy (1978–2005) of John Paul II (**Karol Wojtyła** [1920–2005]) the legitimacy of any dissent from papal teaching, not only on contraception or even gender/sexuality, was regularly called into question by the Vatican (e.g., *Veritatis splendor*, 1993).

The disruption of traditional sources of intimacy in modern society, especially shifts from extended to nuclear families and toward increasing geographical mobility, left marriage as the virtually exclusive location of interpersonal intimacy. This had effects on clerical celibacy. In earlier social patterns, which had different gender roles, most people found intimacy in nonsexual relationships with others of the same sex and with whom they shared interests, training, and work. In the modern pattern, in which intimacy came to be more closely associated with marriage and sexual relationships, clerical celibacy became problematic: It meant sacrifice and interpersonal isolation, which in turn could produce psychological dysfunction, including alcoholism. Together with Vatican II's elevation of the role of the laity and the simultaneous decrease in sex negativity, the identification of interpersonal intimacy with sexual relationships triggered a large, sustained exodus of priests from the priesthood. Religious orders were affected less than secular clergy, but priests, sisters, and brothers in religious life also left at high rates, most of them to marry. Those who left were disproportionately young or middle-aged. Despite calls to reverse the trend through optional celibacy and allowing married priests to continue in pastoral ministry, the Church hierarchy insisted on celibacy, while acknowledging that it was a matter of discipline, not theology. The exodus of clergy and the religious continued throughout the 1960s and 1970s. By the 1990s most developed nations not only had a severe priest shortage, but their largest priest cohorts were at retirement age.

Nevertheless, the Church was not willing to extend ordination to women (see Paul VI, *Ministeria quaedam*, 1972; *Chers fils*, 1976; John Paul II, *Ordinatio sacerdotalis*, 1994). Indeed, much of Paul VI's language about the role of women was reminiscent of that used by Pius XII and John XXIII. Further, in 1976 the Congregation for the Doctrine of the Faith responded to the growing call for women priests by issuing *Inter Insigniores*, signed by Paul VI. It gave three principal arguments against the ordination of women: Jesus had chosen only men as apostles; the Church had chosen only men to be priests; and since Jesus was male and priests are a sign of Jesus, priests must be male. All three reasons were immediately challenged, and dissent became rife. In both North America and Europe support for women priests rose significantly instead of declining. "In 1974, 29% of [U.S.] Catholics favored women's ordination. By 1985 . . . 47% did. In 1992 and in polls since, about two-thirds of Catholics—and in at least one poll, 80% of those under 35—agreed that women should be ordained" (Bannan).

The 1976 letter, *Chers fils*, also addressed love in marriage. Paul VI insisted that while love plays a lofty and necessary role in marriage, it does not affect the law. People sometimes lay undue emphasis on conjugal love and the perfection of the spouses, neglecting children as a basic value of marriage and making love so important that they open the door to divorce. In opposition to this trend, Paul VI declared that consent makes marriage. Once consent produces a juridical effect, the wills of the consenting partners have no power to affect that juridical reality. In 1975, the Congregation for the Doctrine of the Faith issued its "Declaration on Certain Questions in Sexual Ethics," which largely reiterated Paul VI's traditional teaching: Licit sexual acts occurred only in marriage, and the unitive and procreative aspects of sex are inseparable (#5).

The *Declaration* defended the teaching on intrinsically evil acts—that some physical acts are always mortally sinful—and rejected fundamental "option theology," which pictured the human person as developing over time, taking on new layers of personhood through cultivating good, mature habits and becoming generally oriented toward the good and not normally at constant risk of mortal sin. The *Declaration*, to the contrary, presented virtue as much more precarious in everyday moral life, contending that even well-intentioned persons could suddenly commit an intrinsically evil act. **Masturbation**, for example, and other such misuses of the sexual faculty were traditionally understood to be intrinsically evil. The *Declaration* reiterated this stance (#10). Many theologians retorted that, according to scientific studies, masturbation begins in infancy and is prerational. It is therefore better understood not as sexual sin but as an immature form of sexuality gradually transformed into fully mature adult sexual giving (Curran, *Themes*, 180–81). In this view masturbation would be sinful only when preferred over shared sexual giving. (The two theses about masturbation received abundant confirmation by most of **sexology** and psychology.) The *Declaration* resisted, reaffirming that "masturbation is an intrinsically and seriously disordered act" because (harking back to Thomas) it violates the intended purpose of sexuality, that is, procreation (#8). The question to what extent sterile marital intercourse abides by or violates this same purpose of the sexual faculty has continued to plague moral theology (consider Finnis, 1066–68; Jung and Smith, 38, 146, 200–201n.4, 218n.10; Koppelman, 46–50).

The discussion of the fault of masturbation, its being nonprocreative, naturally brings to mind homosexuality. Social science research indicated that many homosexual persons were aware of homosexual attraction prior to the age of reason, which undermined the traditional Catholic moral understanding of homosexuality as the perverse choice of an act not natural to human persons. The *Declaration* for the first time recognized some distinctions among persons who commit homosexual acts and specifically recognized the existence of homosexual **orientation** (Curran, *History*, 140–46). In particular, the *Declaration* recognized a distinction between those persons having innate homosexual instincts and those whose same-sex tendencies are transitory or situational, a distinction that was interpreted by some as an acknowledgment by the Church that homosexual desire/orientation and perhaps homosexual acts were not immoral if the orientation were innate and not chosen. A document later issued by the Congregation for the Doctrine of the Faith (1987) under John Paul II denied that interpretation: "Although the particular inclination of the homosexual person is not a sin, it is a more or less strong tendency ordered toward an intrinsic moral evil, and thus the inclination itself must be seen as an objective disorder" ("Care of Homosexual Persons," #3). No explanation *how* this orientation was an objective disorder was forthcoming. The Congregation seemed to be applying the traditional formula "objectively wrong but not subjectively culpable." But this formula is properly applied to acts, and an orientation is not an act.

In the last decades of the twentieth century, the civil rights of homosexual persons were the center of controversy, especially in the United States and Europe. Catholic authorities were opposed to recognizing homosexuality as a status to be protected from discrimination, though periodically the Church condemned violence against gays and lesbians. The Congregation's 1992 document, "Discrimination against Homosexuals," asserted:

> "Sexual orientation" does not constitute a quality comparable to race, ethnic background, etc., in respect to non-discrimination. Unlike these, homosexual orientation is an objective disorder. There are areas in which it is not unjust discrimination to take orientation into account, for example, in the placement of children for adoption or foster care, in employment of teachers or athletic coaches, and in military recruitment.

While "Care of Homosexual Persons" found it "deplorable that homosexual persons have been and are the object of violent malice in speech or in action," it implied that these "irrational and violent reactions" are provoked by those who condone homosexuality and claim it is not disordered.

Defense of Church teaching on sexuality was a cornerstone of John Paul II's papacy, beginning with *Familaris consortio* (1981), which defended marital indissolubility, the superiority of virginity over marriage (#11, #13), the unacceptability of trial marriages (#81), and the need to exclude from sacramental reception remarried divorced persons (#84). But *Familiaris* also defended the equality of women (#22–#23). Conservative on sex, John Paul II made extraordinary changes in Church teaching about gender. The headship of husbands over wives in the family is rooted in the **Bible**, both in Genesis 3:16, where God tells Eve, "[Y]our desire shall be for your husband, and he shall rule over you," and in Paul: "Wives, be subject to your husbands as to the Lord" (Eph. 5:22). While John XXIII had reaffirmed men's headship of women, and Paul VI had avoided the subject, in 1988 John Paul II decisively rejected male headship (*Mulieris dignitatem*). Paul interpreted God's words to Eve in Genesis not as God's stating the punishment for sin but as a prediction of the evil that human sin had introduced. But for John Paul II, as Christ is the new Adam who saves humanity from the consequences of sin, Christ restored the original equality of male and female (*Mulieris*, #10). John Paul II even reinterpreted Paul's commanding wives to be subject to husbands as a singular way of speaking that "is to be understood and carried out in a new way: as a mutual subjection out of reverence for Christ" (#24). Thus the attempt of the Church to accommodate modernity has had mixed success. Church teaching shifted from women's inequality and subjection to women's equality with men in society and family but not in the Church itself. For many inside and outside the Church, it remains unconvincing that women are fully equal to men yet unable to resemble Christ sufficiently for ordination.

The Vatican has held fast to understanding sexuality as centrally important in human personality, an idea new in the nineteenth century, and has retained sexual complementarity. This is doubly ironic: For most of Christian history, sexuality was not understood as central to personality at all (see Augustine, *De Trinitate*, 12.7.12), and late modern culture has pushed sex/gender to the periphery of human identity by minimizing sex differences, even to the point of opening sex to individual choice (Gudorf, "Erosion of Sexual Dimorphism"). The shift in Church teaching that occurred in the last half of the twentieth century from legal, contractual language to more personalist language regarding marriage and sexuality ended the demonization of sexual pleasure (see Gudorf, *Body, Sex, and Pleasure*; Jung) that had been endemic in Christian theology. But the shift has not been able to disguise the discordance between Church teaching on sexual morality and popular, experientially based, sexual morality.

See also Abstinence; Anscombe, G.E.M.; Catholicism, History of; Completeness, Sexual; Contraception; Heterosexism; Kant, Immanuel; Love; Marriage; Marriage, Same-Sex; Masturbation; Natural Law (New); Reproductive Technology; Sexuality, Dimensions of; Thomas Aquinas (Saint); Wojtyła, Karol (Pope John Paul II)

REFERENCES

Augustine. (401–402) *De bono coniugali (On the Good of Marriage)*. Trans. Patrick G. Walsh. Oxford, U.K.: Clarendon Press, 2001; Augustine. (420) *De Trinitate (On the Trinity)*. Trans. by Stephen McKenna. Cambridge: Cambridge University Press, 2002; Augustine. *Epistles*. Trans. Sister Wilfrid Parsons. *The Fathers of the Church*, vol. 6. Washington, D.C.: Catholic University of America, 1964; Bannan, Regina. "Impact of Catholic Feminist Dissent." Women's Ordination Conference Homepage. <www.womensordination.org/pages/art_impact.html> [accessed 10 January 2005]; Beis, Richard H. "Contraception and the Logical Structure of the Thomist Natural Law Theory." *Ethics* 75:4 (1965), 277–84; Clark, Elizabeth A. "'Adam's Only Companion': Augustine and the Early Christian Debate on Marriage." *Recherches Augustiniennes* 21 (1986), 139–62; Cohen, Carl. "Sex, Birth Control, and Human Life." *Ethics* 79:4 (1969), 251–63; Congregation for the Doctrine of the

Faith (The Sacred). "Care of Homosexual Persons." *Acta Apostolicae Sedis* 79 (1987), 543–54; Congregation for the Doctrine of the Faith (The Sacred). *"Inter Insigniores"* [Declaration on the Question of the Ordination of Women to the Ministerial Priesthood]. *Acta Apostolicae Sedis* 69 (1977), 98–116; Congregation for the Doctrine of the Faith (The Sacred). *"Persona Humana*: Declaration on Certain Questions in Sexual Ethics." (1975). <www.vatican.va/roman_curia/congregations/cfaith/documents/rc_con_cfaith_doc_19751229_persona-humana_en.html> [accessed 10 January 2005]; Congregation for the Doctrine of the Faith (The Sacred). "Responding to Legislative Proposals on Discrimination against Homosexuals." *Origins* 22:10 (1992), 94–96; Curran, Charles E. *The Catholic Moral Tradition Today: A Synthesis*. Washington, D.C.: Georgetown University Press, 1999; Curran, Charles E. *History and Contemporary Issues: Studies in Moral Theology*. New York: Continuum, 1996; Curran, Charles E. *Themes in Fundamental Moral Theology*. Notre Dame, Ind.: University of Notre Dame Press, 1977; Finnis, John. "Law, Morality, and 'Sexual Orientation.' " *Notre Dame Law Review* 69:5 (1994), 1049–76; Foster, Michael Smith. *Annulment: The Wedding That Was. How the Church Can Declare a Marriage Null*. New York: Paulist Press, 1998; Fuchs, Josef. "Natural Law." In Judith Dwyer, ed., *The New Dictionary of Catholic Social Thought*. Collegeville, Minn.: Liturgical Press, 1994, 669–75; Grisez, Germain, Joseph Boyle, John Finnis, William E. May, and John C. Ford. *The Teaching of "Humanae Vitae": A Defense*. San Francisco, Calif.: Ignatius Press, 1988; Gudorf, Christine E. *Body, Sex, and Pleasure: Reconstructing Christian Sexual Ethics*. Cleveland, Ohio: Pilgrim Press, 1994; Gudorf, Christine E. *Catholic Social Teaching on Liberation Themes*. Washington, D.C.: University Press of America, 1980; Gudorf, Christine E. "The Erosion of Sexual Dimorphism: Challenges to Religion and Religious Ethics." *Journal of the American Academy of Religion* 69:4 (2001), 863–91; Hanigan, James. "Population." In Judith Dwyer, ed., *The New Dictionary of Catholic Social Thought*. Collegeville, Minn.: Liturgical Press, 1994, 760–62; Haring, Bernard. "The Curran Case: Conflict between Rome and a Moral Theologian." Trans. Benedict Neeman. In Charles E. Curran and Richard A. McCormick, eds., *Readings in Moral Theology No. 6: Dissent in the Church*. Mahwah, N.J.: Paulist Press, 1988; Hugh of St. Victor. (ca. 1135) *De sacramentis*. Trans. Roy J. Deferrari. Cambridge, Mass.: Mediaeval Academy of America, 1951; John XXIII (Pope). *"Ad petri cathedram."* *Acta Apostolicae Sedis* 51 (1959), 509–10; translation: *The Pope Speaks* 5:4 (1959), 368; John XXIII (Pope). *"Convenuti a Roma."* *Acta Apostolicae Sedis* 53 (1961), 610–12; translation: *The Pope Speaks* 7:4 (1962), 344–46; John Paul II (Pope). *"Familiaris consortio."* *Acta Apostolicae Sedis* 74 (1982), 81–191; John Paul II (Pope). *"Mulieris dignitatem."* *Acta Apostolicae Sedis* 80:13 (1988), 1653–1729; translation: Publication No. 244-6, Office of Publishing and Promotion Services, United States Catholic Conference, Washington, D.C., 1988; John Paul II (Pope). *"Ordinatio sacerdotalis"* ("On Women's Ordination"). Apostolic Letter (22 May 1994). *Acta Apostolicae Sedis* 86 (1994); *Origins* 24:4 (1995), 49–53; John Paul II (Pope). *"Veritatis splendor."* *Acta Apostolicae Sedis* 85 (1993), 1134–1228; Jung, Patricia Beattie. "Sanctifying Women's Pleasure." In Patricia Beattie Jung, Mary E. Hunt, and Radhika Balakrishnan, eds., *Good Sex: Feminist Perspectives from the World's Religions*. New Brunswick, N.J.: Rutgers University Press, 2001, 77–95; Jung, Patricia Beattie, and Ralph F. Smith. *Heterosexism: An Ethical Challenge*. Albany: State University of New York Press, 1993; Kaiser, Robert Blair. *The Politics of Sex and Religion*. Kansas City, Mo.: Leaven Press, 1985; Koppelman, Andrew. "Homosexual Conduct: A Reply to the New Natural Lawyers." In John Corvino, ed., *Same Sex: Debating the Ethics, Science, and Culture of Homosexuality*. Lanham, Md.: Rowman and Littlefield, 1997, 44–57; Kosnick, Anthony, William Carroll, Agnes Cunningham, Ronald Modras, and James Schulte. *Human Sexuality: New Directions in American Catholic Thought*. New York: Paulist Press, 1977; McBrien, Richard. *Catholicism*. San Francisco, Calif.: HarperCollins, 1994; *The 1917 Pio-Benedictine Code of Canon Law*. Trans. and ed. Edward N. Peters. San Francisco, Calif.: Ignatius Press, 2001; Paul VI (Pope). *"Chers fils."* *Acta Apostolicae Sedis* 68 (1976), 197–201; translation: *The Pope Speaks* 21:2 (1976), 162–66; Paul VI (Pope). *"Humanae vitae."* *Acta Apostolicae Sedis* 60:9 (1968), 481–503; translation: *Catholic Mind* 66 (September 1968), 35–48; Paul VI (Pope). *"Ministeria quaedam."* *Acta Apostolicae Sedis* 64 (1972), 529–55; translation: *The Pope Speaks* 17:3 (1972), 257–61; Pius XI (Pope). *"Casti connubii"* ("On Christian Marriage"). *Acta Apostolicae Sedis* 22 (1930), 539–92; translation: *Catholic*

Mind 29:2 (1931), 21–64; Pius XI (Pope). *"Divini illius magistri."* *Acta Apostolicae Sedis* 22 (1930), 49–86; Pius XI (Pope). *"Divini redemptoris."* *Acta Apostolicae Sedis* 29 (1937), 65–106; Pius XII (Pope). "Allocution to Midwives." *Acta Apostolicae Sedis* 43 (1951), 835–54; Pontifical Commission for Population, Family, and Birth. *Commission Final Report* (June 1966). In Robert Blair Kaiser, *The Politics of Sex and Religion.* Kansas City, Mo.: Leaven Press, 1985, appendix B, 248–58; Ranke-Heinemann, Uta. (1988) *Eunuchs for the Kingdom of Heaven: Women, Sexuality, and the Catholic Church.* Trans. Peter Heinegg. New York: Doubleday, 1990; Vatican Council II. *"Gaudium et Spes*: The Pastoral Constitution on the Church in the Modern World." *Acta Apostolicae Sedis* 58 (1966), 1025–1120. Vatican translation in David J. O'Brien and Thomas A. Shannon, eds., *Catholic Social Thought: The Documentary Heritage.* Maryknoll, N.Y.: Orbis Books, 1992, 164–237; Watt, E. D. "Professor Cohen's Encyclical." *Ethics* 80:3 (1970), 218–21.

Christine E. Gudorf

ADDITIONAL READING

Berry, Jason. (1992) *Lead Us Not into Temptation.* Urbana: University of Illinois Press, 2000; Böckle, Franz, and Jacques-Marie Pohier, eds. *Sexuality in Contemporary Catholicism.* New York: Seabury, 1976; Cahill, Lisa Sowle. *Sex, Gender, and Christian Ethics.* Cambridge: Cambridge University Press, 1996; Canadian Conference of Bishops. "Pastoral Letter Regarding Same-Sex Marriage." *Origins* 32:27 (2002), 445–46; Carmody, Denise, and John Carmody. "Homosexuality and Roman Catholicism." In Arlene Swidler, ed., *Homosexuality and World Religions.* Valley Forge, Pa.: Trinity Press, 1993, 135–48; Cohen, Carl. "Sex, Birth Control, and Human Life." *Ethics* 79:4 (1969), 251–63. Reprinted in P&S1 (150–65); P&S2 (185–99); Congregation for the Doctrine of the Faith (The Sacred). "Considerations Regarding Proposals to Give Legal Recognition to Unions between Homosexual Persons." *Origins* 33:14 (2003), 445–46; Congregation for the Doctrine of the Faith (The Sacred). *"Donum vitae."* *Acta Apostolicae Sedis* 80 (1988), 70–162; Cozzens, Donald. *Sacred Silence: Denial and Crisis in the Church.* Collegeville, Minn.: Liturgical Press, 2002; Curran, Charles E. "Fertility Control: Ethical Issues." In Warren T. Reich, ed., *Encyclopedia of Bioethics,* 2nd ed. New York: Macmillan, 1995, 832–39; Curran, Charles E. *Moral Theology at the End of the Century.* Milwaukee, Wis.: Marquette University Press, 1999; Daly, Mary. *The Church and the Second Sex.* New York: Harper Colophon, 1968; Finnis, John. "Law, Morality, and 'Sexual Orientation.'" *Notre Dame Law Review* 69:5 (1994), 1049–76. Reprinted, revised, in *Notre Dame Journal of Law, Ethics, and Public Policy* 9:1 (1995), 11–39. Reprinted, revised, in John Corvino, ed., *Same Sex: Debating the Ethics, Science, and Culture of Homosexuality.* Lanham, Md.: Rowman and Littlefield, 1997, 31–43; France, David. *Our Fathers: The Secret Life of the Catholic Church in an Age of Scandal.* New York: Broadway, 2004; Furey, Pat, and Jeannine Gramick, eds. *The Vatican and Homosexuality.* New York: Crossroad, 1988; Gudorf, Christine E. "Encountering the Other: The Modern Papacy on Women." In Charles E. Curran, Margaret A. Farley, and Richard McCormick, eds., *Feminist Ethics and the Catholic Moral Tradition.* New York: Paulist Press, 1996, 66–89; Jenkins, Philip. *Pedophiles and Priests: Anatomy of a Contemporary Crisis.* New York: Oxford University Press, 1996; John Paul II (Pope). "Authentic Concept of Conjugal Love." *Origins* 28:37 (1999), 654–56; John Paul II (Pope). *"Evangelium vitae."* *Origins* 24:42 (1995), 689–727; John Paul II (Pope). "The Ratified and Consummated Sacramental Marriage." *Origins* 29:34 (2000), 553–55; Jung, Patricia B., and Thomas A. Shannon, eds. *Abortion and Catholicism: The American Debate.* New York: Crossroad, 1988; Keenan, James F., ed. *Catholic Ethicists on HIV/AIDS Prevention: Thirty-seven Theologians from around the World Show How Roman Catholic Moral Traditions Can Mediate the Clash of Values in HIV Prevention.* New York: Continuum, 2000; McCormick, Richard A. "Human Sexuality: Toward a Consistent Ethical Method." In John A. Coleman, ed., *One Hundred Years of Catholic Social Thought.* Maryknoll, N.Y.: Orbis, 1991, 189–97; Olyan, Saul M., and Martha C. Nussbaum, eds. *Sexual Orientation and Human Rights in American Religious Discourse.* New York: Oxford University Press, 1998; Paul VI (Pope). *"Humanae vitae."* *Acta Apostolicae Sedis* 60:9 (1968), 481–503; *Catholic Mind* 66 (September 1968), 35–48. Reprinted in Claudia Carlen, ed.,

The Papal Encyclicals 1958–1981. Raleigh, N.C.: Pierian Press, 1990, 223–36; and P&S1 (131–49); P&S2 (167–84); P&S3 (96–105); Pontifical Council for the Family. "Family, Marriage, and 'De Facto' Unions." *Origins* 30:30 (2001), 473–88; Ratzinger, Joseph (Cardinal). "Letter to the Bishops of the Catholic Church on the Collaboration of Men and Women in the Church and in the World." (31 May 2004) <www.usccb.org/collaboration.pdf> and <www.freerepublic.com/focus/f-religion/1182483/posts> [accessed 20 April 2005]; Regan, A. "Lust." In *New Catholic Encyclopedia*, vol. 8. New York: McGraw-Hill, 1967, 1081–85; Steinfels, Margaret O'Brien. "This Crisis through the Laity's Lens." *Origins* 32:7 (2002), 110–13; Swidler, Leonard, and Arlene Swidler, eds. *Women Priests: A Catholic Commentary on the Vatican Declaration.* New York: Paulist Press, 1977; Thielicke, Helmut. *The Ethics of Sex.* Trans. John W. Doberstein. New York: Harper and Row, 1964; Von Hildebrand, D. "Sex." In *New Catholic Encyclopedia*, vol. 13. New York: McGraw-Hill, 1967, 147–50; Werth, Barry. "Father's Helper: How the Church Used Psychiatry to Care for—and Protect—Abusive Priests." *The New Yorker* (9 June 2003), 61–67.

CELIBACY. *See* Abstinence

CHASTITY. *See* Abstinence

CHINESE PHILOSOPHY. The most explicit discussions of sex in Chinese philosophy occur in texts that present theories and instructions regarding the use of sexual technique for the purpose of self-cultivation. Though self-cultivation is almost exclusively associated in Western ethics with cultivation of the mind in its various facets, no such boundary exists in the Chinese tradition. Moral self-cultivation is as much physiological as psychological. This is largely due to the metaphysics of the Dao (also Romanized "Tao") or "the Way," which is the conceptual center for any indigenous Chinese ethical theory, regardless of school identification. Hence, it is central for both Confucian as well as Daoist theorizing.

The chief conception of the Way that emerges in philosophical texts is that of an ineffable, transcendent, and primary principle that refracts mysteriously into expressible and knowable forms in the world (Roth, 101–68). The Way is primary in several ways: as cosmological origin, as metaphysical underpinning, and as normative foundation. Though details vary, it is commonly held that the Way expresses itself in the knowable world through at least three important subprinciples: the Yin and the Yang (a binary set of principles describable as "the feminine" and "the masculine") and Qi ("Ch'i"), the energizing or vitalizing influence. Yin and Yang are not quite tangible, but they are associated with a diversity of detectable characteristics. Yin characteristics include the moist, dark, cold, low, supple, and weak aspects of things, while Yang includes the dry, bright, hot, high, hard, and strong. Qi is more clearly a sort of substance that varies in quality from a thick or nearly solid fluidity to a vaporous or ephemeral spirit. Yin and Yang are, in the order of things, somewhat prior to Qi in the sense that they can inform Qi: One may speak of a heavier "Yin-Qi" and a lighter "Yang-Qi," conforming to the characteristics that a particular locus of Qi exhibits (Needham, 34–67).

These three principles infuse and articulate all sublunary processes: physical, social, and psychological. The mind or "heart-mind" (*xin/hsin*) is regarded as operating within the same purview of Yin, Yang, and Qi as the rest of the body. Activities deemed in the contemporary West as "mental"—perception, belief, emotion, aesthetic judgment, and desire—are distributed via attribution throughout the body in Chinese discussions. The heart-mind's special power, from occupying the seat of moral judgment to the more prosaic task of Qi storage, varies from one moral-physiological account to the next. So moral self-cultivation may involve whatever aspects of bodily attunement are necessary, in a particular account, for attaining the proper arrangement or activity of Qi as the embodied form of the Way. The range of practices for attunement to the Way runs from Confucian rituals of daily life to Daoist dietary practices. Self-cultivation may also involve regimented application of rare, naturally occurring substances and elixirs or substances produced by alchemical processes (Needham, 20–129; Schipper, 160–82).

The texts that include sexual technique as a means to self-cultivation cannot be classified as indisputably Daoist, but they resonate better with certain texts that can. In particular, seminal Daoist texts such as the *Daodejing* (*Tao Te Ching*) and the *Zhuangzi* (*Chuang Tzu*) seem either partially or obliquely concerned with the heights that may be attained through forms of breathing and other techniques of body control. Most consonant with Daoism is the fact that sexual technique serves the goal of preserving one's original Dao-given vitality, the results of which include notable longevity or even immortality. Daoist texts tend to include other extraordinary results of preserving the vitality of the Way, from levitation to effortless political influence. And, finally, there are visible, radiant effects on the skin and countenance, phenomena also found in Confucian texts (Harper, 548–57). All these effects represent unfettered possession and expression of the Way. Because of Qi's central role in embodying the Way, sexual technique, along with breath control, calisthenics, or meditation, aims at the dual task of preserving the Qi with which one is endowed and manipulating or exercising one's body to be a maximally effective organism for the activity of Qi in its Yin and Yang aspects.

The traditions of sexual technique extant from at least the second century BCE to the present involve instructions for men that emphasize, during sex with women, sperm retention and recirculation. Sperm is an important form of Qi's refined essence, which is called "Jing" ("Ching"). Jing is Qi in one of its purest, most potent forms. Hence the generation and controlled circulation of sperm is, for a man, especially effective for accumulating the vitality of the Way. Sexual technique in such service involves two foci. First, a man requires a female partner from which to draw in Yin, or feminine, Qi essence. To be successful in this, the man must arouse and stir up the woman's essence through foreplay that is regimented by knowledge of the vessels and channels in which the essence rests and flows. The woman must be brought to climax, or near climax, to release her essence through vaginal secretion, which the man's penis is then thought to absorb. The man's second focus is controlling his own climax. He must not ejaculate or otherwise allow seminal seepage. During his climax he should redirect the accumulated sexual essence—both his own sperm that is generated during sex and the absorbed feminine essence—"inward," so that it travels up his spine to the brain where Jing is stored (Harper, 566–93; Needham, 192–201; Shapiro, 553–74).

There are relatively few discussions of the way in which sexual technique may be useful for women. Indeed, there are some texts that warn explicitly against allowing women to have knowledge of such regimens. But in the discussions that are instructive to women, the principles are largely the same. A woman may benefit from controlled sexual arousal (though some of the success of this seems to depend on the manipulations of a male partner) and by controlling her own climax. She may, as a result, redirect the essences generated in her breasts up the spine and into her brain (Needham, 205–7).

Sexual techniques involving sperm retention were in obvious tension with the concern to provide progeny in Confucianism, the primary philosophical support for the traditional cult of ancestry in China. Though recorded theories of human nature, ethical motivation, ideal political organization, and self-cultivation are varied and complex, one of the main social concerns for two millennia of Confucians has been the maintenance of fairly rigid and hierarchical social roles and rank distinctions. This was particularly true regarding the unit of patriarchal lineage, the extended family. The key function of sex within a broadly Confucian framework was the production of heirs to the line of male descendants, who were responsible for honoring ancestors with ceremonial rituals as well as with moral and social success. Because of Confucianism's status as state ideology through much of imperial Chinese history, it had widespread influence on attitudes regarding sex and associated practices. Two major elements of Chinese sexual history, broadly construed, may be understood through Confucianism's concern with primogeniture: same-sex relationships and footbinding.

Male same-sex sexual relations are recorded from as early as the Shang period (ca. sixteenth to eleventh century BCE) and continue until the Middle Ages—with little or no documented censure (Hinsch, 15–54). Some of the early lack of censure may have to do with the fact that "documentation" largely involved records of rulers and their underlings. However, rulers tend to be the main object of criticism in early Confucian texts, so that explanation only goes so far. To the extent that same-sex relationships among males are regarded disfavorably, the reasons tend to invoke concerns that apply to both same-sex and other-sex relationships that threaten to compromise the ethical or political virtue of one or both parties. In fact, some same-sex relationships were praised and eulogized in earlier historical references because from them positive moral and political lessons could be learned about loyalty and the depth of emotional attachment between a ruler and favored subject (Hinsch). Such references seem to take for granted that such same-sex relationships could occur alongside the relationships with wives and concubines that were sufficient for producing heirs.

References to same-sex relationships between women are much less common until the Ming (1368–1644) and Qing (1644–1911; "Ch'ing") dynasties, when attitudes began to be more antagonistic toward both male and female same-sex partnering. In fictional accounts, even in the novels of female writers, women's same-sex sexual activities are trivialized as youthful play, or they seem modeled on other-sex relationships through the motif of crossdressing (Wu, 4 ff.). In any case, a woman's duty to provide heirs for a man seems beyond question.

Legal documents as well, during the Ming and Qing dynasties, began to reflect a gradual coalescence of antagonism toward same-sex male relationships. Examination of laws during these late dynasties concerning anal penetration of men by men indicates that by then negative attitudes toward **homosexuality** were forming, based on the loss of status (through humiliation or social debasement) that a penetrated man suffers. Ming laws concerning heterosexual sexual misconduct exclusively targeted **adultery** and the sexual assault of girls and women by men, while laws about sex among males exclusively targeted anal penetration, consensual or nonconsensual. Initially, in the Ming, these laws are a subcategory of laws linked (by legal analogy) to dishonorable forms of assault during an altercation—more specifically, pouring foul substances into the mouth of one's antagonist. These laws evolve later, in the Qing, into laws under the broader category of sexual assault. However, they carried lighter sentences if the victim was a male who had already lost honorable male status, either through previous anal penetration (consensual or nonconsensual) or from having impersonated a woman in, for example, drama or **prostitution** (Sommer, 143–68). This suggests that attitudes against homosexuality had less to do with norms about "natural" and "unnatural" sex and more to do with male-centered social hierarchy norms. It also suggests that legally acceptable sexual penetration of women reflected their presumptive lower status.

The practice of footbinding, however, reflected even more directly the status and role of women in a broadly Confucian social order (Blake, 694–700). Footbinding involved methodical binding of each foot of a young girl starting around three years of age and continuing into womanhood, for the rest of her life. It involved binding the toes under toward the heel of the foot with silk bands, so that the foot—through the breakage of bones, the sloughing off of injured flesh, and healing—would form a smaller foot of roughly three inches in length. The practice seems to have occurred with varying fashionability from the Tang dynasty (618–906; "T'ang") to the late Qing, when it was almost completely abolished. Footbinding seems to have reached its height of prestige and popularity in the Ming dynasty, during which it became a highly eroticized feminine affect.

Footbinding incorporated multifarious philosophical and political attitudes that contributed to its eroticization, an important set of which related to securing the myth of ethnic Han Chinese cultural superiority (Blake, 689–90; Ko, 12–16). Ethnically Han Chinese held power in most of the dynasties of Chinese history (the Mongols [Yuan dynasty, 1271–1368] and Manchus [Qing] were the exceptions) and believed in their moral superiority as originators of Chinese culture, including the moral, social, and political aspects of Confucianism. Footbinding, an elaborate and painstaking "adornment" of women's feet, represented a highly cultivated specialization of women's role and rank within the complex of Confucian culture. A woman of virtuous refinement did not require large or strong feet for her most important social and ethical contribution: producing male heirs to the ancestral line. But footbinding seems to have been a particularly ethnic Han expression of Confucianism's relegation of women's function and virtue to exclusively domestic matters. Non-Han dynasties such as the Qing embraced Confucian social norms but ultimately rejected footbinding along with other Ming dynasty appearance-code customs, regarding them as merely definitive of Han Chinese ethnic identity. Hence they could be discarded without harm to the Confucian manner of rule.

Though undocumented, legend has it that the famed neo-Confucian Zhu Xi ("Chu Hsi," 1130–1200) of the Song (Sung) dynasty (960–1279) actively introduced and promoted footbinding as an important facet of Confucian social ordering (Ko, 14). By the time of the late Qing dynasty, the prominent Confucian poet and writer Gong Zizhen ("Kung Tzuchen," 1792–1841) severely criticized the practice, along with opium trafficking and sycophantic ministers, as damaging the state's adherence to the Way (De Bary and Lufrano, 180–84).

Footbinding resisted explicit codification even during favorable dynasties, largely due to its status, in practice, as a woman's concern, one that was conceived alternately on the model of sartorial adornment or as preparation for menstruation, dutiful sex, and childbirth (Blake, 683–90). The practice was passed from grown women to girls in the spatial and moral interior of the household. Overt, public enforcement of the practice was, it seems, neither necessary nor desirable. The high social status that Han culture succeeded in placing on footbinding created resistance to early Qing attempts to eradicate it. Manchu women during the Qing may even have taken to the fashion of platform shoes to imitate the appearance of bounded gait. The cultural refinement and "interior" virtue that the binding of feet was meant to indicate must have partially influenced its erotic appeal (Levy). A woman's gendered attractiveness depended on her possessing, or at least appearing to possess, feminine virtues.

Looking at the practice from the perspective of the women and girls who endured it, we can discern that an important moral motivation for it was probably present in the perceived duty that women had to control their bodies. In light of their role in the all-important Confucian task of providing future celebrators of the ancestral lineage, women's achieving mastery over their bodily desires through the practiced discipline of pain would have been valuable to them. This aspect of footbinding may contribute to explaining why the tradition survived for as long as it did and was as widely practiced as it was—in the absence of any sign of overt, coercive male control over the practice and despite the excruciating pain involved.

See also Beauty; Catholicism, History of; Consequentialism; Dworkin, Andrea; Genital Mutilation; Greek Sexuality and Philosophy, Ancient; Hinduism; Indian Erotology; Jainism; Manichaeism; Plato; Sadomasochism; Tantrism

REFERENCES

Blake, C. Fred. "Footbinding in Neo-Confucian China and the Appropriation of Female Labor." *Signs* 19 (Spring 1994), 676–712; De Bary, William Theodore, and Richard Lufrano. *Sources of Chinese Tradition*, 2nd ed., vol. 2. New York: Columbia University Press, 2000; Harper, Donald. "The Sexual Arts of China as Described in a Manuscript of the Second Century B.C." *Harvard Journal of Asiatic Studies* 47:2 (1987), 539–93; Hinsch, Bret. *Passions of the Cut Sleeve: The Male Homosexual Tradition in China*. Berkeley: University of California Press, 1990; Ko, Dorothy. "The Body as Attire: The Shifting Meanings of Footbinding in Seventeenth-Century China." *Journal of Women's History* 8:4 (1997), 8–27; Levy, Howard S. *The Lotus Lovers: The Complete History of the Curious Erotic Custom of Footbinding in China*. Buffalo, N.Y.: Prometheus, 1992; Needham, Joseph. *Science and Civilisation in China*, vol. 5: *Chemistry and Chemical Technology*, part 5: *Spagyrical Discovery and Invention: Physiological Alchemy*. Cambridge: Cambridge University Press, 1983; Roth, Harold. *Original Tao: Inward Training (Nei-yeh) and the Foundations of Taoist Mysticism*. New York: Columbia University Press, 1999; Schipper, Kristofer. *The Taoist Body*. Trans. Karen C. Duval. Berkeley: University of California Press, 1993; Shapiro, Hugh. "The Puzzle of Spermatorrhea in Republican China." *Positions* 6:3 (1998), 551–96; Sommer, Matthew H. "The Penetrated Male in Late Imperial China: Judicial Construction and Social Stigma." *Modern China* 23:2 (1997), 140–80; Wu, H. Laura. "Through the Prism of Male Writing: Representation of Lesbian Love in Ming-Qing Literature." *Nan Nü* 4:1 (2002), 1–34.

Manyul Im

ADDITIONAL READING

Beurdeley, Michel, ed. *The Clouds and the Rain: The Art of Love in Ancient China*. London: Hammond and Hammond, 1969; Chan, Connie S. "Don't Ask, Don't Tell, Don't Know: Sexual Identity and Expression among East Asian-American Lesbians." In Bonnie Zimmerman and Toni A. H. McNaron, eds., *The New Lesbian Studies: Into the Twenty-first Century*. New York: Feminist Press at CUNY, 1996, 91–97; Cheng, Chung-Ying, and Nicholas Bunnin, eds. *Contemporary Chinese Philosophy*. Oxford, U.K.: Blackwell, 2002; Dynes, Wayne R., and Stephen Donaldson, eds. *Asian Homosexuality*. New York: Taylor and Francis, 1992; Gonzalez-Crussi, Frank. "The Conditions for Seduction, According to an Old Chinese Text." In *On the Nature of Things Erotic*. San Diego, Calif.: Harcourt Brace Jovanovich, 1988, 119–39; Hinsch, Bret. *Women in Early Imperial China*. Lanham, Md.: Rowman and Littlefield, 2002; Holmgren, Jennifer. "Myth, Fantasy, or Scholarship: Images of the Status of Women in Traditional China." *The Australian Journal of Chinese Affairs*, no. 6 (July 1981), 147–70; Ishihara, Akira, and Howard S. Levy. *The Tao of Sex*. New York: Harper and Row, 1970; Lee, Grant S. "Taoism." In Ruth Chadwick, ed., *Encyclopedia of Applied Ethics*, vol. 4. San Diego, Calif.: Academic Press, 1998, 305–10; Leibniz, Gottfried. (1716) *Discourse on the Natural*

Theology of the Chinese. Trans. and ed. Henry Rosemont, Jr., and Daniel J. Cook. Honolulu: University of Hawai'i Press, 1977; Lieu, Samuel N. C. (1985) *Manichaeism in the Later Roman Empire and Medieval China: A Historical Survey,* 2nd ed. Tübingen, Ger.: J.C.B. Mohr, 1992; Lopez, Donald S., Jr. *Religions of China in Practice.* Princeton, N.J.: Princeton University Press, 1996; McMahon, Keith. *Misers, Shrews, and Polygamists: Sexuality and Male-Female Relations in Eighteenth-Century Fiction.* Durham, N.C.: Duke University Press, 1995; Ng, Vivien W. "Ideology and Sexuality: Rape Laws in Qing China." *Journal of Asian Studies* 46:1 (1987), 57–70; Ng, Vivien W. "Looking for Lesbians in Chinese History." In Bonnie Zimmerman and Toni A. H. McNaron, eds., *The New Lesbian Studies: Into the Twenty-first Century.* New York: Feminist Press at CUNY, 1996, 160–64; Roth, Harold. "Evidence for Stages of Meditation in Early Taoism." *Bulletin of the School of Oriental and African Studies, University of London* 60:2 (1997), 295–314; Su Tzu. *Su Tzu's Chinese Philosophy Page.* <mars.superlink.net/~fsu/philo.html> [accessed 19 May 2005]; Tao, Julia Po-Wah Lai. "Confucianism." In Ruth Chadwick, ed., *Encyclopedia of Applied Ethics,* vol. 1. San Diego, Calif.: Academic Press, 1998, 597–608; Van Gulik, Robert Hans. *Sexual Life in Ancient China: A Preliminary Survey of Chinese Sex and Society from ca. 1500 B.C. till 1644 A.D.* Leiden, Holland: Brill, 2003; Wawrytko, Sandra A. "Homosexuality and Chinese and Japanese Religions." In Arlene Swidler, ed., *Homosexuality and World Religions.* Valley Forge, Pa.: Trinity Press, 1993, 199–230.

CLITORIDECTOMY. *See* Genital Mutilation

CODES OF ETHICS. *See* Ethics, Professional Codes of

COERCION (BY SEXUALLY AGGRESSIVE WOMEN). Female sexual aggression is a controversial topic. It is difficult to define, challenging to measure, and even, according to some, dangerous to study. Nevertheless, a modest body of literature about sexually aggressive women exists.

Sexual aggression can be defined as behavior that attempts to make another person engage in **sexual activity** despite their unwillingness to do so (Krahe et al.). Sexual aggression typically involves verbal, psychological, or economic pressure; manipulation made possible by intoxication; or physical force or its threat. Sexual aggression thus covers a broad range of acts from deception to physical compulsion. "Sexual aggression" and "sexual coercion" are often used interchangeably (Struckman-Johnson and Struckman-Johnson, "Dynamics and Impact"). Female sexual aggression, which may constitute **rape**, is the performance of any of these behaviors by a woman.

Knowledge about sexually aggressive women would be deeper were this topic studied rigorously. But inquiry has been and continues to be questioned. The study of the coercion or rape of men by women might "delegitimize women's experiences of rape" and thereby constitute backlash against **feminism** (Stock, 178–79). In particular, investigating sexually aggressive women might trivialize men's rape of women by, for example, encouraging the assumption that both sexes have similar experiences of sexual victimization (see Muehlenhard). But the most significant challenge to research on sexually aggressive women is likely the belief that only men are capable of sexual aggression.

One historically fundamental criterion of rape has been the perpetrator's being male and the victim's being female. Common law defined rape as a felony committed by men on women. (The first gender-neutral rape statute in the United States was Michigan's [1974]; see Posner and Silbaugh, 5–7.) Women have traditionally been perceived as too gentle, small, weak, and disinterested in sex to engage in sexual aggression. Sex-role norms that mandate that men should initiate sexual activity and women should control or resist these initiatives contribute to the belief that women are not sexually aggressive (Anderson and Struckman-Johnson, 11). Accepting stereotypes of men as aggressive and women as passive might justify or excuse male lack of self-control and attendant aggressive behavior. Further, if women see their coercing men as "normal," men may also see their coercing women as "normal," and more women will be victimized. Studying sexually aggressive women undermines these stereotypes.

The belief that women are not sexually aggressive occasioned a defect in early studies: Questionnaires asked only women to report victimization and only men to report perpetration (Allgeier and Lamping). Research results thus reinforced the notion that women are not sexually aggressive. More recent instruments ask men and women to report both victimization and perpetration (e.g., O'Sullivan et al.). This methodology permits female sexual aggression to be discovered and studied.

Research on female sexual aggression has focused on college-age women committing acts against men in their peer group. In six studies involving over 1,300 women, between 1.6 and 7.1 percent reported using physical force to have sexual contact with a man. From 0.5 to 52.4 percent reported taking advantage of an intoxicated man or using coercive tactics (persistent verbal arguments, fondling, removing his or her clothing, blackmail). Between 3.7 and 15.6 percent of 607 men in five studies reported being physically forced or threatened with force by a woman wanting sex; from 12.5 to 66 percent reported having unwanted sex due to a woman's coercion or an alcohol- or drug-induced inability to resist (Anderson and Melson).

The most common behavior in female sexual aggression is persisting in advances by sexually arousing their partners (Struckman-Johnson et al.). The second most common tactic involves deception and emotional manipulation (lies about **love**, calling their partners gay, threats to break up). These personal violations may very well be traumatic for the male (Struckman-Johnson and Struckman-Johnson, "Men's Reactions"). Women also take advantage of men too intoxicated to resist. But women are unlikely to use physical force (grabbing, slapping, sitting on their partner). In the continuum from persistent sexual arousal, through deception and emotional maneuvers, to exploiting someone's drunkenness, and on to employing physical force or its threat, the behaviors of sexual aggression are plausibly increasingly unethical (and illegal). Although men's rates of sexual aggression overall are higher, both men and women employ all the tactics on the continuum and similarly so, except physical force or its threat (O'Sullivan et al.). Female sexual aggression might, therefore, be seen as less unethical. It might also be less unethical if men are not harmed by it.

Whether the acts of sexually aggressive women harm men is controversial. Men might not be offended by sexually demanding women. Men might even benefit from the sexual excitement, the opportunity to experience a **fantasy**, or feeling sexually desired (Struckman-Johnson and Struckman-Johnson, "Dynamics and Impact"). One study found that men's reactions to female sexual aggression are not as adverse as women's reactions to male sexual aggression: 42 percent of the men (verses 6 percent of the women) reported not being upset (O'Sullivan et al.). If men are happy to succumb, studying female sexual aggression might be much ado about nothing.

However, men who encounter sexually aggressive women might not acknowledge their adverse reactions; doing so would violate an internalized sex-role stereotype of male physical and psychological invulnerability (Krahe et al.). Several studies document men's trauma and subsequent **sexual dysfunction**, depression, anxiety, and damage to self-esteem due to female sexual aggression (see calderwood; Larimer et al.; Sarrel and Masters). One estimate is that 20 percent who encounter female sexual aggression experience significant negative emotional effects (Struckman-Johnson and Struckman-Johnson, "Men's Reactions"). If men are harmed by sexually aggressive women but are in denial, should we convince them that they have been victimized? (Some women would never have thought that they had been sexually harassed or raped until convinced by others.) Alternatively, if men are not harmed by female sexual aggression, should we not unearth the mechanism of their resilience and teach it to women?

Research on sexually aggressive women has spurred debate about a double standard: Female sexual aggression tends to be judged more leniently than the same acts committed by a man. Legal codes place many female sexually aggressive behaviors below the threshold for rape even when they involve physical force or a weapon (Anderson and Savage). If a woman locks a man in her room and tries to undress him, her action is likely to be seen in common thinking as **seduction**. The same actions performed by a man are likely to be labeled "attempted rape."

This double standard has significant implications. Thirty-six percent of men report that when they were minors they had sexual contact with adult women (Anderson and Sorensen). If this happened between a twelve-year-old girl and a nineteen-year-old man, it would be statutory rape. Should it be statutory rape if the older partner is female? Perhaps not, according to the double standard. Similarly, consider incidents in which one person takes sexual advantage of another too intoxicated to resist. As a result of early research on sexual aggression on college campuses (e.g., Koss et al.), men who reportedly took sexual advantage of intoxicated women were labeled "date rapists." Recent surveys show that from about 30 to 50 percent of women said that they had initiated sex with a man when his judgment was impaired by alcohol or drugs (Anderson, "Variations"; Anderson and Sorensen). This behavior on the part of a man is ubiquitously stigmatized as **date rape** and carries punishments ranging from dismissal from school to incarceration. Are we ready to define 30 to 50 percent of college women as date rapists and institute the same punishments for them?

In the twenty-first century, areas for exploration of female sexual aggression include the characteristics of the men chosen as targets; men's reactions, including token resistance; and women's social and biologically based motives for sexual aggression (see Anderson and Struckman-Johnson, 79–93). Female sexual aggression against women is also worth investigating (see Girshick; Struckman-Johnson and Struckman-Johnson, "Sexual Coercion"). Another question to be resolved is whether sexually aggressive women have personality traits that can be relied on to identify them (say, by parents wishing to assess the girls their teenaged sons date; by men wanting to avoid—or possibly find—a predatory partner). No definitive profile has yet emerged. Some evidence indicates that sexually aggressive women are more likely than others to have been sexually abused, to have hostile personalities, and to believe that relationships between men and women are adversarial (Anderson, "Correlates"; Craig-Shea). Paradoxically, perhaps, sexually aggressive women are also more likely to have progressive beliefs about women's roles, to have a greater desire for power, and to be more highly motivated to seek intimacy (Clements-Schreiber et al.; Zurbriggen).

See also Addiction, Sexual; Consent; Feminism, Men's; Flirting; Harassment, Sexual; Incest; Law, Sex and the; Objectification, Sexual; Pedophilia; Rape; Rape, Acquaintance and Date; Seduction; Violence, Sexual

REFERENCES

Allgeier, Elizabeth R., and Jennifer Lamping. "Theories, Politics, and Sexual Coercion." In Peter B. Anderson and Cindy Struckman-Johnson, eds., *Sexually Aggressive Women: Current Perspectives and Controversies.* New York: Guilford, 1998, 49–75; Anderson, Peter B. "Correlates of College Women's Self-Reports of Heterosexual Aggression." *Sexual Abuse: A Journal of Research and Treatment* 8:2 (1996), 121–32; Anderson, Peter B. "Variations in College Women's Heterosexual Initiation Strategies." *Sexual Abuse: A Journal of Research and Treatment* 10:4 (1998), 283–92; Anderson, Peter B., and Dyan Melson. "From Deviance to Normalcy: Women as Sexual Aggressors." *Electronic Journal of Human Sexuality* 5 (23 October 2002). <www.ejhs.org/volume5/deviance011.htm> [accessed 3 January 2004]; Anderson, Peter B., and Jane Savage. "Social, Legal, and Institutional Responses to Heterosexual Aggression by College Women." Paper presented at the National Women's Studies Association Conference (21 June 2003), New Orleans, La.; Anderson, Peter B., and William Sorensen. "Male and Female Differences in Reports of Women's Heterosexual Initiation and Aggression." *Archives of Sexual Behavior* 28:3 (1999), 285–95; Anderson, Peter B., and Cindy Struckman-Johnson, eds. *Sexually Aggressive Women: Current Perspectives and Controversies.* New York: Guilford, 1998; calderwood, deryck. "The Male Rape Victim." *Medical Aspects of Human Sexuality* 21 (May 1987), 53–55; Clements-Schreiber, Michele, John K. Rempel, and Serge Desmarais. "Women's Sexual Pressure Tactics and Adherence to Related Attitudes: A Step toward Prediction." *Journal of Sex Research* 35:2 (1998), 197–205; Craig-Shea, Mary. "When the Tables Are Turned: Verbal Sexual Coercion among College Women." In Peter B. Anderson and Cindy Struckman-Johnson, eds., *Sexually Aggressive Women: Current Perspectives and Controversies.* New York: Guilford, 1998, 94–104; Girshick, Lori B. *Woman-to-Woman Sexual Violence: Does She Call It Rape?* Boston, Mass.: Northeastern University Press, 2002; Koss, Mary, Christine Gidycz, and N. Wisnieski. "The Scope of Rape: Incidence and Prevalence of Sexual Aggression and Victimization in a Sample of Higher Education Students." *Journal of Consulting and Clinical Psychology* 55:2 (1987), 162–70; Krahe, Barbara, Renate Scheinberger-Olwig, and Steffen Bieneck. "Men's Reports of Nonconsensual Sexual Interactions with Women: Prevalence and Impact." *Archives of Sexual Behavior* 32:2 (2003), 165–76; Larimer, Mary, Amy Lydum, Britt Anderson, and Aaron Truner. "Male and Female Recipients of Unwanted Sexual Contact in a College Sample: Prevalence Rates, Alcohol Use, and Depression Symptoms." *Sex Roles* 40:3–4 (1999), 295–308; Muehlenhard, Charlene L. "The Importance and Danger of Studying Sexually Aggressive Women." In Peter B. Anderson and Cindy Struckman-Johnson, eds., *Sexually Aggressive Women: Current Perspectives and Controversies.* New York: Guilford, 1998, 19–48; O'Sullivan, Lucia, E. Sandra Byers, and Larry Finkleman. "A Comparison of Male and Female College Student's Experiences of Sexual Coercion." *Psychology of Women Quarterly* 22:2 (1998), 177–95; Posner, Richard A., and Katharine B. Silbaugh. *A Guide to America's Sex Laws.* Chicago, Ill.: University of Chicago Press, 1996; Sarrel, Philip M., and William H. Masters. "Sexual Molestation of Men by Women." *Archives of Sexual Behavior* 11:2 (1982), 117–31; Stock, Wendy. "Women's Sexual Coercion of Men: A Feminist Analysis." In Peter B. Anderson and Cindy Struckman-Johnson, eds., *Sexually Aggressive Women: Current Perspectives and Controversies.* New York: Guilford, 1998, 169–84; Struckman-Johnson, Cindy, and David Struckman-Johnson. "The Dynamics and Impact of Sexual Coercion of Men by Women." In Peter B. Anderson and Cindy Struckman-Johnson, eds., *Sexually Aggressive Women: Current Perspectives and Controversies.* New York: Guilford, 1998, 121–43; Struckman-Johnson, Cindy, and David Struckman-Johnson. "Men's Reactions to Female Sexual Coercion." *Psychiatric Times* 17:3 (2001). <www.mhsource.com/pt/mensreact.html> [accessed 23 January 2004]; Struckman-Johnson, Cindy, and David Struckman-Johnson. "Sexual Coercion Reported by Women in Three Midwestern Prisons." *Journal of Sex Research* 39:3 (2002), 217–28; Struckman-Johnson, Cindy, David Struckman-Johnson, and Peter B. Anderson. "Tactics of Sexual Coercion: When Men and Women Won't Take

No for an Answer." *Journal of Sex Research* 40:1 (2003), 76–86; Zurbriggen, Eileen. "Social Motives and Cognitive Power-Sex Associations: Predictors of Aggressive Sexual Behavior." *Journal of Personality and Social Psychology* 78:3 (2000), 1–23.

Peter B. Anderson and Cindy Struckman-Johnson

ADDITIONAL READING

Anderson, Peter B. "Women's Motives for Heterosexual Initiation and Aggression." In Peter B. Anderson and Cindy Struckman-Johnson, eds., *Sexually Aggressive Women: Current Perspectives and Controversies.* New York: Guilford, 1998, 79–93; Anderson, Peter B., and Ronelle Aymami. "Reports of Female Initiation of Sexual Contact: Male and Female Differences." *Archives of Sexual Behavior* 22:4 (1993), 335–43; Bennett, Ruth. "Men Also Feel Coerced into Having Sex, New University Study Finds." *The Times-Picayune* [New Orleans] (19 August 1999), E11 [Newhouse News Service]; Burton, David. "Male Adolescents: Sexual Victimization and Subsequent Sexual Abuse." *Child and Adolescent Social Work Journal* 20:4 (2003), 277–96; Denov, Myriam. "The Myth of Innocence: Sexual Scripts and the Recognition of Child Sexual Abuse by Female Perpetrators." *Journal of Sex Research* 40:3 (2003), 303–14; Feibert, Martin, and L. M. Tucci. "Sexual Coercion: Men Victimized by Women." *Journal of Men's Studies* 6:2 (1998), 127–33; Gilbert, Neil. "Realities and Mythologies of Rape." *Society* 29 (May–June 1992), 4–10; Kahn, Arnold, Jennifer Jackson, Christine Kully, Kelly Badger, and Jessica Halvorsen. "Calling It Rape: Differences in Experiences of Women Who Do or Do Not Label Their Sexual Assault as Rape." *Psychology of Women Quarterly* 27:3 (2003), 233–43; Koss, Mary P., and Kenneth E. Leonard. "Sexually Aggressive Men: Empirical Findings and Theoretical Implications." In Neil M. Malamuth and Edward Donnerstein, eds., *Pornography and Sexual Aggression.* Orlando, Fla.: Academic Press, 1984, 213–32; Masters, William H. "Sexual Dysfunction as an Aftermath of Sexual Assault of Men by Women." *Journal of Sex and Marital Therapy* 12:1 (1986), 35–45; Menard, Kim, Gordon Nagayama Hall, Amber Phung, Marian Gherbial, and Lynette Martin. "Gender Differences in Sexual Harassment and Coercion in College Students." *Journal of Interpersonal Violence* 18:10 (2003), 1222–39; Mezey, Gillian, and Michael King, eds. *Male Victims of Sexual Assault.* Oxford, U.K.: Oxford University Press, 1992; Muehlenhard, Charlene L., and Stephen Cook. "Men's Self-Reports of Unwanted Sexual Activity." *Journal of Sex Research* 24:1–4 (1988), 58–72; Muehlenhard, Charlene L., Debra E. Friedman, and Celeste M. Thomas. "Is Date Rape Justifiable? The Effects of Dating Activity, Who Initiated, Who Paid, and Men's Attitudes toward Women." *Psychology of Women Quarterly* 9:3 (1985), 297–310; Muehlenhard, Charlene L., Irene G. Powich, Joi L. Phelps, and Laura M. Givsi. "Definitions of Rape: Scientific and Political Implications." *Journal of Social Issues* 48:1 (1992), 23–44; Muehlenhard, Charlene L., and Jennifer L. Schrag. "Nonviolent Sexual Coercion." In Andrea Parrot and Laurie Bechhofer, eds., *Acquaintance Rape: The Hidden Crime.* New York: John Wiley, 1991, 115–28; O'Sullivan, Lucia, and E. Sandra Byers. "Eroding Stereotypes: College Women's Attempts to Influence Reluctant Male Sexual Partners." *Journal of Sex Research* 30:3 (1993), 270–82; Patai, Daphne, and Noretta Koertge. *Professing Feminism: Cautionary Tales from the Strange World of Women's Studies.* New York: Basic Books, 1994. *Professing Feminism: Education and Indoctrination in Women's Studies*, new and expanded ed. Lanham, Md.: Lexington, 2003; Roiphe, Katie. *The Morning After: Sex, Fear, and Feminism on Campus.* New York: Little, Brown, 1993; Sommers, Christina Hoff. *Who Stole Feminism? How Women Have Betrayed Women.* New York: Simon and Schuster, 1994. Expanded paperback ed., 1995; Struckman-Johnson, Cindy. "Forced Sex on Dates: It Happens to Men, Too." *Journal of Sex Research* 24:1–4 (1988), 234–41; Struckman-Johnson, Cindy. "Male Victims of Acquaintance Rape." In Andrea Parrot and Laurie Bechhofer, eds., *Acquaintance Rape: The Hidden Crime.* New York: John Wiley, 1991, 192–214; Struckman-Johnson, Cindy, and David Struckman-Johnson. "Men Pressured and Forced into Sexual Experience." *Archives of Sexual Behavior* 23:1 (1994), 93–114; Struckman-Johnson, Cindy, and David Struckman-Johnson. "Men's Reactions to Hypothetical Forceful Advances from Women: The Role of Sexual Standards, Relationship Availability, and the Beauty Bias." *Sex Roles* 37:5–6 (1997), 319–33.

COMMUNICATION MODEL. With varying degrees of intensity, frequency, and subtlety, human **sexual activity** expresses and communicates a wide range of emotions, attitudes, and desires. This will surprise no one. What might be surprising is the claim, made by some philosophers, that interpersonal communication is essential to human sexuality. The search for essences has been common in philosophy since **Plato** (427–347 BCE), and one fundamental issue in the philosophy of sex is the question of the essence or nature of sexuality. The issues are at once taxonomic, conceptual, and metaphysical. Does sex have a distinct *telos* (purpose) in terms of which we can explicate its nature?

Many philosophers have offered answers to these questions. Consider these four models or theories. First, the reproductive model asserts that the natural purpose of sex is procreation, a view historically associated with Roman Catholicism, as in **Saint Thomas Aquinas** (1224/25–1274). Second, the romantic (or metaphysical) model, advanced by nearly everyone from the author of Genesis 2:23–24 and Plato's Aristophanes (*Symposium*, 192c–e) to your Aunt Martha, connects sex with **love** or **marriage** or a "union of souls." Third, the pleasure model emphasizes the physical pleasure, satisfaction, or release of tension of sexuality. This model derives from **Sigmund Freud** (1856–1939) and has been recently elaborated in different ways (see Goldman; Gray; Primoratz). Fourth, the communication model understands sexuality in terms of **language** and communication. Although this model has been suggested by many philosophers (for example, by **Irving Singer** in 1973; *Goals*, 20), it has been most fully articulated by Robert C. Solomon.

Each model of human sexuality characterizes the nature and purpose of sex and hence can be used to develop a list of necessary and sufficient conditions for classifying activity as sexual or, more flexibly, to identify some acts as paradigmatically sexual, others as borderline sexual, and others as nonsexual. The models also typically furnish moral standards and criteria of deviant or perverted sex. By privileging heterosexual coitus, the reproductive model judges homosexual acts both deviant and immoral. The romantic model privileges sex with love or sex within marriage, thereby marginalizing **casual sex**. The pleasure (or, to use Goldman's terminology, "plain sex") model rejects these two models on the grounds that they add to sexuality something analytically extraneous to it; the model focuses, instead, only on the pleasure that sexuality affords. The communication model sees sexual activity as essentially intersubjective and takes as paradigmatic acts in which people use body language to express feelings and attitudes, including love, trust, tenderness, affection, anger, hatred, indifference, fear, shyness, shame, embarrassment, passivity, dependence, submissiveness, domination, and possessiveness.

Solomon finds precedent for the communication model in Jean-Paul Sartre (1905–1980) and **Thomas Nagel**, though neither philosopher explicitly states it. For Sartre, whose own views derive from **G.W.F. Hegel** (1770–1831), sexuality is intersubjective, expressive, and antagonistic. It is intersubjective because **sexual desire** is inherently directed toward another person (rather than, for example, one's own pleasure). It is expressive of one's freedom and subjectivity through the desire to possess, objectify, and dominate the other. And it is antagonistic because sexual relations are conflicts between two people, each of whom attempts to express his or her freedom at the expense of the other (*Sartre*, 499–500, 508, 516–19; see Oaklander). Solomon rejects the dispiriting Sartrean inevitability of antagonism but accepts the Sartrean structure of sexuality: its intersubjectivity and expressivity (*Love*, 268–77; "Sex, Contraception," 106–7; "Sex and Perversion," 94–95). Nagel also draws on Sartrean intersubjectivity, fashioning an account of sexual desire as involving reflexive, mutual perception. My sexual desire is for you, for some particular you, but my desire is also that you desire me. In part, your desire for me results from your recognizing my desire for you. Similarly, my desire for you, and my sexual arousal, in part results from my recognizing your desire for me. This system of mutual perception includes the communication of one's desire and intention to arouse the other. Solomon argues ("Sex and Perversion," "Sexual Paradigms") that while Nagel is right about the role of reciprocal communication in sexuality, Nagel limits communication too severely: Much more is expressed by sexuality than sexual desire and an intention to arouse.

In arguing for the superiority of the communication model, Solomon provides criticisms of the others. The reproductive model is too narrow, because much of what people do when they have sexual relations is peripheral to or even contrary to reproduction ("Sex and Perversion," 270). Similarly, the romantic model is too narrow. Only sometimes do sexual experiences rise to the heights of a "union," and besides, the notion of a union is too vague or poetic (*Love*, 74; "Sex, Contraception," 106; "Sex and Perversion," 276). Solomon is most vociferous about the deficiencies of the pleasure model. First, it is too broad, finding sexuality wherever pleasure is found—a kind of hedonistic pansexualism ("Sex and Perversion," 275). Second, the pleasure model violates a principle articulated by **Aristotle** (384–322 BCE) and endorsed by Solomon: Pleasure is not the goal or purpose of human activity but an accompaniment of natural, good, or rational activity (*Nicomachean Ethics*, I.8, 1099a; X.5, 1176a; X.7, 1177a). Third, insofar as the pleasure model focuses on orgasm, it makes **masturbation** the paradigmatic and eminently preferable sexual activity ("Sex, Contraception," 105; "Sex and Perversion," 275–76; "Sexual Paradigms," 96 [on this argument, see Hamilton, 132–33; Moulton; Soble, 84–87]). Fourth, the pleasure model fails to account for the significance of sex in our lives. In privileging pleasure, the model portrays sexual activity as if it were "scratching an itch." For Solomon, "our sexual behavior is never 'without meaning' . . . and every sexual act has its significance" ("Sex, Contraception," 105; *Love*, 84, 248; see Morgan's essays).

These criticisms of the pleasure model point toward what Solomon believes is the best account of human sexuality, the communication model. According to Solomon,

> Sexuality is primarily a means of communicating with other people, a way of talking to them, of expressing our feelings about ourselves and them. It is essentially a language, a body language, in which one can express gentleness and affection, anger and resentment, superiority and dependence far more succinctly than would be possible verbally. . . . If sexuality is a means of communication, it is not surprising that it is *essentially* an activity performed with other people. ("Sex and Perversion," 279)

The communication model offers a teleological account of human sexuality: The essential nature of sex is to serve the purpose of interpersonal communication. Sex is **language**, the primary purpose of which is communication. It is, specifically, a nonverbal body language in which the basic unit of expression is the gesture ("Sex and Perversion," 280; "Sexual Paradigms," 90). In stressing the expression of attitudes and emotions by sexuality, this model explains why sexuality can be supremely significant for us. It is important because communicating attitudes and emotions is important.

Christopher Hamilton finds this suggestion especially pertinent nowadays and gives it a quasi-theological twist. Because sexual activity can express mutual acceptance and forgiveness, "in an age of decay of religious belief, there may lie secretly in the modern obsession with sex a kind of longing for a redemption no longer available in traditional terms" (140). While endorsing a version of the communication model, Rush Rhees makes a similar point, with a psychological rather than theological emphasis: "[S]ex is something between people; a form of communication (if the word has any shape left). Awakening and bewilderment are both connected with this. . . . I doubt if we talk or think of sex as communication now. And if we look round—if we look elsewhere—this is not surprising. We need not wonder if it stays superficial" (154). Simon Blackburn, too, finds Solomon's model "illuminating" (138n.58) but prefers communal music-making as the paradigm of communication rather than verbal conversation: "In conversations we can branch out in all directions, and we devote conscious thought to what we say. Such a model misses out the domination by the body. So in general, a better comparison is to music-making, where the reciprocal sensitivities can be more or less unconscious, and also for that matter where difficulties such as timing are perhaps more salient" (89).

On the communication model, two-party sex, specifically mutual touch and intercourse, is the paradigm case, since sex is essentially interpersonal communication (Solomon, "Sex and Perversion," 282). But the partners might be of either sex; what matters is that the partner's sexuality is communicative, not their gender or **sexual orientation**. Thus there is nothing deviant about **homosexuality**. In **sexual perversion** there is a communication breakdown; it is sexuality that misfires in its communicative aim ("Sex and Perversion," 282–83) and not a matter of anatomy or physiology (as in Aquinas and other Catholic philosophers). Thus heterosexual oral and anal sex, items in the "vocabulary" of the language of sex, are also not perverted. Even if not deviant, sex between people who have known each other for a long time might be unsatisfying, because they are now only repeating the same old messages to each other (Solomon, "Sexual Paradigms," 344; but see Johnson, 308–9; Moulton, 538–39, 544–45).

For Solomon, however, solitary masturbation is deviant, since it renounces interpersonal communication. Masturbation is like talking to oneself or writing a letter to someone but not mailing it; it is "empty and without content" ("Sex and Perversion," 283). Group sex can, of course, be communicative, but it is complicated—"like trying to hold several conversations at once or working on several books at the same time"—and so risks muddying the messages conveyed and missing the special communicative intimacy offered by two-party sex. Fetishism might be either an enrichment of one's erotic vocabulary or, if obsessively exclusive, an impoverishment. Voyeurs might "have nothing to say" on their own, though they might be "good listeners." Acts of **pedophilia** are like "carrying on an adult conversation with a child who does not have the vocabulary to understand," while **bestiality** is like talking to "a dog who nods dumb agreement to every proposal." To the extent that these acts deviate from the paradigm case of interpersonal communication, they do not fulfill sexuality's essential purpose ("Sex and Perversion," 283–86).

The communication model has received considerable critical attention (from Goldman; Moulton; Primoratz; Soble; Wilder; but see Leibowitz's defense). One objection is that this model is itself too narrow. The view that the primary purpose of sex *qua* language is communication ignores many normal and customary purposes besides communication that language serves. We may use language to clarify our thoughts (for ourselves, even if sometimes for others); to "think out loud"; to record our experiences and thoughts, as in a diary; to take part in a ritual or artistic performance; to tell stories, in which the author's sincerity is often beside the point; and perhaps most important, to express ourselves without communicating or intending to communicate with others. (Language, then, can provide enjoyment in itself; it is not only instrumentally valuable.) If sex is compared with language, a richer conception of language leads to a richer conception of sex (see Steiner, 39–41; on writing and masturbation, see Derrida, 144–57). The implications are striking: If we eliminate the model's exclusive focus on interpersonal communication, the grounds for privileging two-party sex and marginalizing masturbation disappear (Primoratz, *Ethics and Sex*, 38; Soble, 78–79; Wilder, 100–102).

Nevertheless, perhaps the inherent purpose of language *is* communication. This claim, that the purpose of language should be understood instrumentally, as interpersonal communication, is an unsupported assumption of the model. One might speculate, from the perspective of **evolution**, about the communicative adaptiveness of language (see Hauser), but inferences from this to philosophical claims about language's inherent purpose are tenuous. Indeed, it may be doubted, given the various purposes we have when using language in all its forms, that language has any inherent purpose, beyond its adaptive functions. This point could be made about sex, too: The search for the inherent purpose of sex, apart from its biological role in procreation, given the multitude of purposes we have when engaging in sex, may be doomed. This does not (yet) mean that language and sex have no nature. But the instrumental ("means-ends") conception of language and sex presupposed by the communication model is misleading. Conceptions of sex that focus not on its instrumental efficacy but on its intrinsic qualities (as in Goldman and Primoratz) might be more plausible. Solomon's instrumentalism shows itself well regarding masturbation, which for him is only "essential as an ultimate retreat" ("Sex and Perversion," 283). *Homo ludens* gets short shrift.

The treatment of pleasure in the communication model is also problematic. On Solomon's view, sexual pleasure is an accompaniment or by-product of sexual activity, not its purpose. The communication model attempts to explain the meaningfulness and importance of sex in terms of sexuality's expressive powers, but all it can say, apparently, about *why* sex is pleasurable is that we derive pleasure from interpersonal communication. It is probably more accurate to talk about the many different pleasures of both communication and sexuality, even if there is some overlap. Indeed, the pleasures of sex might be mostly physical, not communicative (see Vannoy). Both sexual activity and conversation, of course, create and nurture intimacy, but the pleasures of sexual intimacy are more deeply rooted in the body than the pleasures of intimate talk. While the pleasures of artful verbal intercourse are undeniable, they rarely include the intensity and ecstasy of sexual pleasures. Although it understands sexuality as body language, the communication model leads, oddly, to a disembodied, even unsexy, view of sexual pleasure.

Another problem with versions of the communication model, which it shares with other models, is their essentialism; in claiming that sex is essentially a language used to express interpersonal feelings, the model assumes that sex indeed has an essence. But this essentialism, the idea that sex has a single, distinctive, definitive *telos*, is contestable (as suggested by Solomon himself in another articulation of the model; "Sex, Contraception," 99–102). Perhaps human sexuality, as claimed by **social constructionism**, has no essence. The communication model does provide a powerful metaphor for sex. It throws light on the expressive capacities of sexuality that are neglected or poorly construed by other models. Were it shorn of its essentialism, it would still illuminate much of what is interesting and delightful about sex.

See also Completeness, Sexual; Cybersex; Descartes, René; Existentialism; Flirting; Hegel, G.W.F., Lacan, Jacques; Language; Masturbation; Nagel, Thomas; Perversion, Sexual; Scruton, Roger; Sexuality, Dimensions of; Social Constructionism

REFERENCES

Aristotle. (ca. 325 BCE?) *Nicomachean Ethics*. Trans. Terence Irwin. 2nd ed. Indianapolis, Ind.: Hackett, 1999; Blackburn, Simon. *Lust: The Seven Deadly Sins*. New York: Oxford University

Press/New York Public Library, 2004; Derrida, Jacques. (1967) *Of Grammatology*. Trans. Gayatri Chakravorty Spivak. Baltimore, Md.: Johns Hopkins University Press, 1974; Goldman, Alan. "Plain Sex." *Philosophy and Public Affairs* 6:3 (1977), 267–87; Gray, Robert. "Sex and Sexual Perversion." *Journal of Philosophy* 75:4 (1978), 189–99; Hamilton, Christopher. *Living Philosophy: Reflections on Life, Meaning and Morality*. Edinburgh, Scot.: Edinburgh University Press, 2001; Hauser, Marc. *The Evolution of Communication*. Cambridge, Mass.: MIT Press, 1996; Johnson, Charles W. "Body Language." In Alan Soble, ed., *Sex, Love, and Friendship*. Amsterdam, Holland: Rodopi, 1997, 299–311; Leibowitz, Flo. " 'Sexual Paradigms' Twenty Years Later." In Alan Soble, ed., *Sex, Love, and Friendship*. Amsterdam, Holland: Rodopi, 1997, 33–36; Morgan, Seiriol. "Dark Desires." *Ethical Theory and Moral Practice* 6:4 (2003), 377–410; Morgan, Seiriol. "Sex in the Head." *Journal of Applied Philosophy* 20:1 (2003), 1–16; Moulton, Janice. "Sexual Behavior: Another Position." *Journal of Philosophy* 73:16 (1976), 537–46; Nagel, Thomas. "Sexual Perversion." *Journal of Philosophy* 66:1 (1969), 5–17; Oaklander, L. Nathan. "Sartre on Sex." In Alan Soble, ed., *The Philosophy of Sex: Contemporary Readings*, 1st ed. Totowa, N.J.: Littlefield, Adams, 1980, 190–206; Plato. (ca. 380 BCE) *The Symposium*. Trans. Walter Hamilton. New York: Penguin, 1951; Primoratz, Igor. *Ethics and Sex*. London: Routledge, 1999; Primoratz, Igor. "Sexual Morality: Is Consent Enough?" *Ethical Theory and Moral Practice* 4:3 (2001), 201–18; Rhees, Rush. (1971–1972) "The Tree of Nebuchadnezzar." In D. Z. Phillips, ed., *Moral Questions*. New York: St. Martin's Press, 1999, 151–58; Sartre, Jean-Paul. (1943) *Being and Nothingness: An Essay on Phenomenological Ontology*. Trans. Hazel E. Barnes. New York: Philosophical Library, 1956; Singer, Irving. (1973) *The Goals of Human Sexuality*. New York: Schocken, 1974; Soble, Alan. *Sexual Investigations*. New York: New York University Press, 1996; Solomon, Robert C. *Love: Emotion, Myth and Metaphor*. Garden City, N.J.: Anchor Press, 1981; Solomon, Robert C. "Sex and Perversion." In Robert B. Baker and Frederick A. Elliston, eds., *Philosophy and Sex*, 1st ed. Buffalo, N.Y.: Prometheus, 1975, 268–87; Solomon, Robert C. (1987) "Sex, Contraception, and Conceptions of Sex." In G. Lee Bowie, Meredith W. Michaels, and Kathleen Higgins, eds., *Thirteen Questions in Ethics*, 2nd ed. Fort Worth, Tex.: Harcourt Brace, 1992, 95–107; Solomon, Robert C. "Sexual Paradigms." *Journal of Philosophy* 71:11 (1974), 336–45; Steiner, George. (1975) *After Babel*, 3rd ed. Oxford, U.K.: Oxford University Press, 1998; Vannoy, Russell. *Sex without Love: A Philosophical Exploration*. Buffalo, N.Y.: Prometheus, 1980; Wilder, Hugh. "The Language of Sex and the Sex of Language." In Alan Soble, ed., *The Philosophy of Sex: Contemporary Readings*, 1st ed. Totowa, N.J.: Littlefield, Adams, 1980, 99–109.

Hugh Wilder

ADDITIONAL READING

Berkowitz, Leonard J. "Sex: Plain and Symbol." In Alan Soble, ed., *Sex, Love, and Friendship*. Amsterdam, Holland: Rodopi, 1997, 279–87; Card, Claudia. "The Symbolic Significance of Sex." In Alan Soble, ed., *Sex, Love, and Friendship*. Amsterdam, Holland: Rodopi, 1997, 289–96; Goldman, Alan. "Plain Sex." *Philosophy and Public Affairs* 6:3 (1977), 267–87. Reprinted in HS (103–23); POS1 (119–38); POS2 (73–92); POS3 (39–55); POS4 (39–55); Gray, Robert. "Sex and Sexual Perversion." *Journal of Philosophy* 75:4 (1978), 189–99. Reprinted in POS1 (158–68); POS3 (57–66); POS4 (57–66); Hamilton, Christopher. "Sex." In *Living Philosophy: Reflections on Life, Meaning and Morality*. Edinburgh, Scot.: Edinburgh University Press, 2001, 125–41; Johnson, Edward. "Lovesexpressed." In Alan Soble, ed., *Sex, Love, and Friendship*. Amsterdam, Holland: Rodopi, 1997, 259–63; Ketchum, Sara Ann. "The Good, the Bad, and the Perverted: Sexual Paradigms Revisited." In Alan Soble, ed., *The Philosophy of Sex: Contemporary Readings*, 1st ed. Totowa, N.J.: Littlefield, Adams, 1980, 139–57; Lawrence, D. H. (1927) "Making Love to Music." In Harry T. Moore, ed., *Sex, Literature, and Censorship*. New York: Twayne, 1953, 40–46; Moore, Gareth. "Sexual Needs and Sexual Pleasures." *International Philosophical Quarterly* 35:2 (1995), 193–204; Moulton, Janice. "Sexual Behavior: Another Position." *Journal of Philosophy* 73:16 (1976), 537–46. Reprinted in HS (91–100); POS1 (110–18); POS2 (63–71); POS3 (31–38); POS4 (31–38); Nagel, Thomas.

"Sexual Perversion." *Journal of Philosophy* 66:1 (1969), 5–17. Reprinted in P&S1 (247–60); POS1 (76–88). Reprinted, revised, in Thomas Nagel, *Mortal Questions*. Cambridge: Cambridge University Press, 1979, 39–52; and POS2 (39–51); POS3 (9–20); POS4 (9–20); STW (105–12); Oaklander, L. Nathan. "Sartre on Sex." In Alan Soble, ed., *The Philosophy of Sex: Contemporary Readings*, 1st ed. Totowa, N.J.: Littlefield, Adams, 1980, 190–206; Pierce, Christine. "Review Essay: Philosophy." *Signs* 1:2 (1975), 487–503; Pineau, Lois. "Date Rape: A Feminist Analysis." *Law and Philosophy* 8:2 (1989), 217–43. Reprinted in Hugh LaFollette, ed., *Ethics in Practice: An Anthology*, 1st ed. Cambridge, Mass.: Blackwell, 1997, 418–28; 2nd ed., 2002, 410–17; Leslie P. Francis, ed., *Date Rape: Feminism, Philosophy, and the Law*. State College: Pennsylvania State University Press, 1996, 1–26; HS (483–509); Primoratz, Igor. "Sex as Language." In *Ethics and Sex*. London: Routledge, 1999, 34–40; Purdy, Laura M. Review of *The Philosophy of Sex* [1st ed.], edited by Alan Soble. *Philosophical Investigations* 4:4 (1981), 68–70; Rhees, Rush. "Sexuality" (1962–1963), "The Tree of Nebuchadnezzar" (1971–1972), and "Chastity" (1963). In D. Z. Phillips, ed., *Moral Questions*. New York: St. Martin's Press, 1999, 139–50, 151–58, 159–63; Solomon, Robert C. "Heterosex." In Earl E. Shelp, ed., *Sexuality and Medicine*, vol. 1: *Conceptual Roots*. Dordrecht, Holland: Reidel, 1987, 205–24; Solomon, Robert C. (1981) *Love: Emotion, Myth, and Metaphor*. Buffalo, N.Y.: Prometheus, 1990; Solomon, Robert C. *The Passions*. Garden City, N.Y.: Anchor/Doubleday, 1976; Solomon, Robert C. "Sex, Contraception, and Conceptions of Sex." In S. F. Spicker, W. B. Bondeson, and H. T. Engelhardt, eds., *The Contraceptive Ethos*. Dordrecht, Holland: Reidel, 1987, 223–40. Reprinted in G. Lee Bowie, Meredith W. Michaels, and Kathleen Higgins, eds., *Thirteen Questions in Ethics*, 2nd ed. Fort Worth, Tex.: Harcourt, Brace, Jovanovich, 1992, 95–107; Solomon, Robert C. "Sexual Paradigms." *Journal of Philosophy* 71:11 (1974), 336–45. Reprinted in HS (81–90); POS1 (89–98); POS2 (53–62); POS3 (21–29); POS4 (21–29); Solomon, Robert C., and Kathleen M. Higgins, eds. *The Philosophy of (Erotic) Love*. Lawrence: University Press of Kansas, 1991; Steindorff, Carrie M. "Communication and Sexuality." In Vern L. Bullough and Bonnie Bullough, eds., *Human Sexuality: An Encyclopedia*. New York: Garland, 1994, 131–35; Vannoy, Russell. "Can Sex Express Love?" In Alan Soble, ed., *Sex, Love, and Friendship*. Amsterdam, Holland: Rodopi, 1997, 247–57; Vogler, Candace. "Sex and Talk." *Critical Inquiry* 24 (Winter 1998), 328–65; Wilder, Hugh. "The Language of Sex and the Sex of Language." In Alan Soble, ed., *The Philosophy of Sex: Contemporary Readings*, 1st ed. Totowa, N.J.: Littlefield, Adams, 1980, 99–109. Reprinted in SLF (23–31).

COMPLETENESS, SEXUAL. In the Catholic sexual theology of **Saint Thomas Aquinas** (1224/25–1274), one type of "sin of lechery," indeed the worst kind, includes all those human sexual activities that are "incompatible with the purpose of the sex-act." By this he means that some sexual acts cannot, due to their anatomical form or physiological nature, result in conception and procreation (e.g., **bestiality**, **masturbation**, heterosexual and homosexual oral sex and anal intercourse). "In so far as generation is blocked," Aquinas writes, "we have unnatural vice, which is any complete sex-act from which of its nature generation cannot follow" ("Specific Kinds of Lust," *Summa theologiae* 2a2ae, ques. 154, art. 1; 207; the Latin may not be as specific as this translation: "[C]ontra naturam, quod est in omni actu venereo ex quo generatio sequi non potest"). A "complete" sexual act, for Aquinas, seems to be one in which a penis ejaculates, most usually, but not necessarily, into a vagina. Even today this is an ordinary, not uncommon sense of "complete," even if phallocentric. (A *complete* act "indicat[es] a venereal movement brought to its term usually accompanied by pleasure amounting to a climax"; Regan, 1083.) Heterosexual fellatio, which might in some cases be merely preparatory to the procreative sex act of a penis ejaculating into a vagina, would be sinful as an "unnatural vice" (yet complete), were the act, occurring separately from the coital act, to induce ejaculation outside the proper vessel, so that "generation cannot follow."

Note three things about Aquinas's concept of completeness and his view of the purpose of sex: The ejaculation of the penis into a vagina is the mark of *natural* human sexuality (ejaculation elsewhere, where the "complete" act cannot result in conception, is unnatural); the ejaculation of the penis into a vagina is, therefore, also a requirement of the *moral* (in Natural Law ethics, unnatural sexual acts are immoral); and what Aquinas judges to be natural and hence moral in human sexuality depends on anatomical and physiological considerations, the sorts of biological features that humans share with other animals.

After the medievals, of course, much has been written about the natural, as well as the moral, in human sexuality (for some of this history, see Soble, *The Philosophy of Sex and Love* and *Sexual Investigations*). In 1969, **Thomas Nagel**, in his frequently cited essay "Sexual Perversion," made a contribution to our trying to understand the sexually natural and perverted, a contribution that mostly implicitly draws on the **phenomenology** and **existentialism** of **G.W.F Hegel** (1770–1831), Jean-Paul Sartre (1905–1980), and Maurice Merleau-Ponty (1908–1961), as well as the late-nineteenth-century or early-twentieth-century "psychological turn" in the approach to **sexual perversion** associated with **Sigmund Freud** (1856–1939).

On Nagel's view, a notion of "completeness" applies to human sexuality, but completeness is a *psychological* instead of, as in Aquinas, a physiological notion and has nothing to do with ejaculation. Nagel's appropriation of the concept "completeness" from the Catholic canon law tradition is ironic, since he mostly turns Aquinas on his head. (Yet **Irving Singer** complains about Nagel's notion of completeness that it "neglect[s]" termination, resolution, and satisfaction [80]. That, however, was Nagel's "neologistic" point. Singer prefers a broadly Thomistic notion of completeness, which includes but goes beyond orgasm [78–84].) Even so, completeness *is*, for Nagel—in his sense—the mark of natural human sexuality. However, incompleteness has no moral implications. Along with many others in a non-Catholic, liberal tradition, Nagel denies that an act's being unnatural makes it for that reason alone immoral. Nagel, then, employs "complete" and "incomplete" in a different sense and hence offers a different view of what is natural/perverted in human sexuality. For Aquinas, for example, a man's masturbating to completion on a female shoe is unnatural and perverted *because* the act cannot result in procreation. For Nagel, the act is not in a psychological sense complete, and it is this failure to abide by a psychological standard that makes the act perverted, not the fact that the act is not procreative in form or intent.

Nagel acknowledges that his notion of complete, or psychologically natural, sexuality was suggested to him by Sartre's *Being and Nothingness* (1943; see "Concrete Relations with Others," 361–430). The core of Nagel's theory is that a person *X* becomes aroused sexually not merely by sensing (touching, smelling) the body of another person *Y* (that much is true of less sophisticated **animal sexuality**). More important, the person *X* becomes sexually aroused by noticing that the other person *Y* is sexually aroused by sensing *X*. In a Sartrean way of putting it, *X* feels himself or herself becoming flesh, or embodied, or incarnated in response to the sexual gaze of the other. (Or in a somewhat Hegelian way of putting it, my consciousness of myself as a sexual being results from my realizing that your consciousness acknowledges my sexuality.) The sexual phenomenon to which Nagel draws our attention—a spiral of arousal in which each participant is aroused by noticing the arousal of the other person—is absent from the sexuality of other animals. As opposed to Aquinas, who attempts to determine what is natural in human sexuality by looking at what animals and humans have in common (*viz.*, that coitus leads to procreation), Nagel, in elucidating specifically human natural sexuality, focuses on how animals and humans differ.

Nagel's provocative thesis is that each person's mutually recognizing and then responding to, with increased desire and arousal, the other's desire and arousal is "completeness," the central feature of any psychologically natural sexual interaction. Sex is incomplete or "truncated" (and hence constitutes sexual perversion) to the extent that these reciprocally reinforcing sexual perceptions are absent. In voyeurism, for example, the male voyeur is aroused only by his detached sexual perceptions of the other and not by perceiving that she is aroused by noticing his desire for her. (Indeed, that is exactly what the voyeur wants to avoid. See Soble, *Philosophy of Sex and Love*, 39.) As partial confirmation of Nagel's thesis (he wants his notion of sexual perversion to match ordinary intuitions to some significant degree), the *Diagnostic and Statistical Manual of Mental Disorders* of the American Psychological Association classifies voyeurism as a **paraphilia**, a mental sexual disorder (DSM-IV, 532; sec. 302.82). For Nagel, perversion is sexuality that lacks psychological completeness, although he adds, again in agreement with DSM, that incomplete sexuality is strictly perversion only when it is a person's preferred manner of sexual expression. Nagel's idea is that a person who engages in incomplete sex because nothing else is available (or for the money) is not necessarily a "pervert" even though he or she might perform perverted sexual acts.

Sara Ruddick, in an essay published in 1971 as "On Sexual Morality" and revised in 1975 as "Better Sex," provides an account of psychological sexual completeness that is fundamentally the same as Nagel's, although she more explicitly describes it using the terminology of Merleau-Ponty. Note that neither Nagel nor Ruddick employs psychological completeness to *define* sex, so that for both philosophers incomplete sex still counts as sex, although sex that is abnormal, deficient, or flawed in some way. It is here, regarding the sort of flaw involved in incompleteness, that Ruddick diverges from Nagel. First, Ruddick denies that psychological completeness has anything to do with sexual perversion, which she explains in the biological terms of Aquinas. (For a critique and a defense of the type of sexual teleology found in Ruddick, see Priest and Baltzly, respectively.) Thus, for Ruddick, physiological completeness (ejaculation into a vagina), not psychological completeness, is the clue to the sexually natural and the perverted. As in Aquinas, voyeuristic **sexual desire**s are perverted on her view when they are divorced from the "natural object" or "standard aim" of sexual desire—heterosexual intercourse. Homosexual sexual interactions, as long as they are psychologically complete—which Nagel has no doubt they are—are not perverted in his account. But Ruddick's biological criterion entails that **homosexuality** is perverted. The "saving grace" for her view may be that she rejects, with Nagel against Aquinas, the claim that unnatural or perverted sex has by itself moral significance.

Second, Ruddick claims (again parting ways with Nagel) that psychological completeness is beneficial to the persons involved in such a sexual interaction. She suggests that psychologically complete sexual acts promote our psychological well-being. Further, by joining people together in a reciprocal psychological experience, complete sex helps people overcome the contrast between self and other that often underlies moral conflict; complete sex produces emotional responses in the partners that can eventually generate **love** and the values that flow from it; and complete sex has the Kantian virtue of involving respect for persons. Nagel, by contrast, argues (almost as an afterthought, at the very end of his essay) that *incomplete* sex may be "good" sex in both the nonmoral and moral senses of "good": Incomplete sex can be very exciting, and there is nothing morally wrong with it just because it is incomplete. (See Soble, *Sexual Investigations*, 74–75, for difficulties in claiming that completeness has moral significance in the ways claimed by Ruddick. Ruddick slides illicitly from Nagel's merely descriptive or *ontological* meaning of "sensing a person" to a very different *moral* meaning of "sensing a person.")

Many scholars have discussed the notion of psychological completeness. **Roger Scruton** seems to be one of Nagel's few fans, acknowledging and relying on his account of completeness in *Sexual Desire* (24, 126). Simon Blackburn, too, is a fan, although the philosophical link he draws between **Thomas Hobbes**'s (1588–1679) account of sex and Nagel's completeness is tenuous (88–89). Sara Ann Ketchum was an early critic of Nagel, arguing that another ingredient, "mutuality," must be added to reciprocity in the description of psychologically complete sex. Arnold Davidson worries about Nagel's suggestion that sexual perversion arises in a person through distorting influences that occur during psychosexual development and about whether that approach is consistent with Nagel's phenomenology of sexual arousal (91–94). Joseph Margolis argues that Nagel must have failed in his attempt to provide an account of sexual perversion that owed nothing to social attitudes or customs (297–300)—since no account of sexual perversion could do so. Robert Gray argues that Nagel wrongly analytically linked sexual desire to **sexual activity**; on Gray's alternative view, an activity is sexual if and only if it produces sexual pleasure. Alan Soble raises problems about the judgments of solitary masturbation that seem to follow from how Nagel and Ruddick employ completeness. He rejects the implication in Nagel that masturbation is perverted, in part by showing how even solitary masturbation could be psychologically complete ("Masturbation," 78–80). He also argues against Ruddick's view that masturbation is morally inferior sex (*Sexual Investigations*, 75). Janice Moulton proposes that psychological completeness, being aroused by the arousal of the other, may be primarily a feature of sexual encounters between (relative) strangers and may not play much of a role in sexual acts between long-standing partners. (We should be reluctant to infer that only novel sexual encounters are natural and that sex engaged in by stable couples has the aura of perversion.) Alan Goldman opines that thinking of sexual relations as involving Sartrean reciprocal interpersonal awareness overintellectualizes sex (277). Robert Solomon criticizes Nagel for missing the whole point of sexuality: the communication of attitudes, feelings, and emotions. Nagel, for Solomon, gets the partners to the stage of mutual arousal, then fails to ask what the point of this arousal is.

Despite all this criticism, Nagel's and Ruddick's notions of sexual completeness still might reveal something about human sexual experience. What that is, however, is not obvious. As Soble has argued,

> Completeness is not definitive of the sexual; plenty of genuine but incomplete sexual activity occurs. Completeness is not a mark of the natural . . . since on that criterion we would have to judge perverted too many ordinary sexual behaviors. . . . There is no equivalence between a sexual act's being pleasurable and its being complete. And completeness is not [convincingly] a measure of morality. Then how does completeness figure in sexuality? [Perhaps] not at all. (*Sexual Investigations*, 76)

Further philosophical work on psychological completeness may show us in what sense complete sex is an "ideal" noncontingently significant in human sexuality.

See also Catholicism, History of; Communication Model; Cybersex; Desire, Sexual; Existentialism; Freud, Sigmund; Leibniz, Gottfried; Nagel, Thomas; Objectification, Sexual; Paraphilia; Perversion, Sexual; Phenomenology; Psychology, Twentieth- and Twenty-First-Century; Scruton, Roger; Sexology

REFERENCES

American Psychiatric Association. *Diagnostic and Statistical Manual of Mental Disorders*, 4th ed. [DSM-IV] Washington, D.C.: Author, 1994; Baltzly, Dirk. "Peripatetic Perversions: A Neo-Aristotelian

Account of the Nature of Sexual Perversion." *The Monist* 85:1 (2003), 3–29; Blackburn, Simon. *Lust: The Seven Deadly Sins*. New York: Oxford University Press/New York Public Library, 2004; Davidson, Arnold I. "Styles of Reasoning, Conceptual History, and the Emergence of Psychiatry." In Peter Galison and David J. Strump, eds., *The Disunity of Science: Boundaries, Contexts, and Power*. Stanford, Calif.: Stanford University Press, 1996, 75–100; Goldman, Alan. "Plain Sex." *Philosophy and Public Affairs* 6:3 (1977), 267–87; Gray, Robert. "Sex and Sexual Perversion." *Journal of Philosophy* 75:4 (1978), 189–99; Ketchum, Sara Ann. "The Good, the Bad, and the Perverted: Sexual Paradigms Revisited." In Alan Soble, ed., *The Philosophy of Sex: Contemporary Readings*, 1st ed. Totowa, N.J.: Littlefield, Adams, 1980, 139–57; Margolis, Joseph. "The Question of Homosexuality." In Robert B. Baker and Frederick A. Elliston, eds., *Philosophy and Sex*, 1st ed. Buffalo, N.Y.: Prometheus, 1975, 288–302; Moulton, Janice. "Sexual Behavior: Another Position." *Journal of Philosophy* 73:16 (1976), 537–46; Nagel, Thomas. (1969) "Sexual Perversion." In *Mortal Questions*. Cambridge: Cambridge University Press, 1979, 39–52; Priest, Graham. "Sexual Perversion." *Australasian Journal of Philosophy* 75:3 (1997), 360–72; Regan, A. "Lust." In *New Catholic Encyclopedia*, vol. 8. New York: McGraw-Hill, 1967, 1081–85; Ruddick, Sara. (1971) "Better Sex." In Robert B. Baker and Frederick A. Elliston, eds., *Philosophy and Sex*, 2nd ed. Buffalo, N.Y.: Prometheus, 1984, 280–99; Sartre, Jean-Paul. (1943) *Being and Nothingness: A Phenomenological Essay on Ontology*. Trans. Hazel Barnes. New York: Washington Square Press, 1956; Scruton, Roger. *Sexual Desire: A Moral Philosophy of the Erotic*. New York: Free Press, 1986; Singer, Irving. *Sex: A Philosophical Primer*. Lanham, Md.: Rowman and Littlefield, 2001; Soble, Alan. "Masturbation: Conceptual and Ethical Matters." In Alan Soble, ed., *The Philosophy of Sex: Contemporary Readings*, 4th ed. Lanham, Md.: Rowman and Littlefield, 2002, 67–94; Soble, Alan. *The Philosophy of Sex and Love: An Introduction*. St. Paul, Minn.: Paragon House, 1998; Soble, Alan. *Sexual Investigations*. New York: New York University Press, 1996; Solomon, Robert C. "Sexual Paradigms." *Journal of Philosophy* 71:11 (1974), 336–45; Thomas Aquinas. (1265–1273) *Summa theologiae*, vol. 43. Cambridge, U.K.: Blackfriars, 1964–1976.

Alan Soble

ADDITIONAL READING

American Psychiatric Association. *Diagnostic and Statistical Manual of Mental Disorders*, text revision of the 4th ed. [DSM-IV-TR] Washington, D.C.: Author, 2000; Blackburn, Simon. "Hobbesian Unity." In *Lust: The Seven Deadly Sins*. New York: New York Public Library/Oxford University Press, 2004, 87–92; Davidson, Arnold I. "Styles of Reasoning, Conceptual History, and the Emergence of Psychiatry." In Peter Galison and David J. Strump, eds., *The Disunity of Science: Boundaries, Contexts, and Power*. Stanford, Calif.: Stanford University Press, 1996, 75–100. Reprinted, abridged, as "Conceptual History and Conceptions of Perversions," in P&S2 (476–86); Goldman, Alan. "Plain Sex." *Philosophy and Public Affairs* 6:3 (1977), 267–87. Reprinted in HS (103–23); POS1 (119–38); POS2 (73–92); POS3 (39–55); POS4 (39–55); Gray, Robert. "Sex and Sexual Perversion." *Journal of Philosophy* 75:4 (1978), 189–99. Reprinted in POS1 (158–68); POS3 (57–66); POS4 (57–66); Levy, Donald. "Perversion and the Unnatural as Moral Categories." *Ethics* 90:2 (1980), 191–202. Reprinted, revised, in POS1 (169–89); Margolis, Joseph. *Negativities: The Limits of Life*. Columbus, Ohio: Merrill, 1975; Merleau-Ponty, Maurice. (1945) *Phenomenology of Perception*. Trans. Colin Smith. New York: Routledge and Kegan Paul, 1962; Moulton, Janice. "Sexual Behavior: Another Position." *Journal of Philosophy* 73:16 (1976), 537–46. Reprinted in HS (91–100); POS1 (110–18); POS2 (63–71); POS3 (31–38); POS4 (31–38); Nagel, Thomas. "Sexual Perversion." *Journal of Philosophy* 66:1 (1969), 5–17. Reprinted in P&S1 (247–60); P&S2 (268–79); POS1 (76–88). Reprinted, revised, in Thomas Nagel, *Mortal Questions*. Cambridge: Cambridge University Press, 1979, 39–52; in Eugene F. Rogers, Jr., ed., *Theology and Sexuality: Classic and Contemporary Readings*. Oxford, U.K.: Blackwell, 2002, 125–36; and P&S3 (326–36); POS2 (39–51); POS3 (9–20); POS4 (9–20); STW (105–12); Primoratz, Igor. "Sexual Perversion." *American Philosophical Quarterly* 34:2 (1997): 245–58; Rogers, Eugene F., Jr., ed. Introduction to "Sexual Perversion," by Thomas Nagel. In *Theology and Sexuality: Classic and Contemporary Readings*. Oxford,

U.K.: Blackwell, 2002, 125; Ruddick, Sara. "On Sexual Morality." In James Rachels, ed., *Moral Problems: A Collection of Philosophical Essays*, 2nd ed. New York: Harper and Row, 1971, 16–34. Reprinted, revised, as "Better Sex," in Robert B. Baker and Frederick A. Elliston, eds., *Philosophy and Sex*, 1st ed. Buffalo, N.Y.: Prometheus, 1975, 83–104; P&S2 (280–99); and, abridged, in Judith A. Boss, ed., *Analyzing Moral Issues*, 3rd ed. New York: McGraw-Hill, 2005, 368–77; Singer, Irving. "Completeness and Reciprocity." In *Sex: A Philosophical Primer*. Lanham, Md.: Rowman and Littlefield, 2001, 78–84; Soble, Alan. "Philosophies of Masturbation." In Martha Cornog, author and ed., *The Big Book of Masturbation: From Angst to Zeal*. San Francisco, Calif.: Down There Press, 2003, 149–66; Soble, Alan. "Psychological Perversion." In *The Philosophy of Sex and Love: An Introduction*. St. Paul, Minn.: Paragon House, 1998, 38–41; Solomon, Robert C. "Sexual Paradigms." *Journal of Philosophy* 71:11 (1974), 336–45. Reprinted in HS (81–90); POS1 (89–98); POS2 (53–62); POS3 (21–29); POS4 (21–29).

CONFUCIANISM. *See* Chinese Philosophy

CONSENT. We are not interested in "consent" as a freestanding concept. We are interested in it because the presence of consent can be *morally transformative*, and we want to know when and to what extent that is so. To say that consent is morally transformative is to say that consent "alters the normative relations in which others stand with respect to what they may do" (Kleinig, 300). It alters a person's duties, rights, and privileges. Just as a person *B*'s consent transforms a physician's cutting into flesh from battery to permissible surgery, *B*'s consent may provide moral or legal legitimation for a sexual act with *B* by *A* that would not be legitimate without consent. Taking off a woman's clothes without her consent, which might be **rape** or assault, differs from taking them off with consent, during a romantic encounter (Schulhofer, 278; Toobin, 42). *B*'s consent to *A*'s doing *X* might also transform the obligations and rights of third parties: If *B* consents to *A*'s doing *X* with *B*, it might be wrong for *C* to interfere, and if *B* refuses to consent, *C* might acquire an obligation to interfere.

Problems about consent to sex arise because people sometimes desire to have sex with others who do not (ever or at that time) desire to have sex with them. But what is the moral and legal significance of consent? Should it always be criminal, or is it always immoral, to engage in sexual relations in the absence of another's consent? When is consent morally transformative or valid? What sorts of pressure put on *B* by *A* vitiate the voluntary nature of, and so *invalidate*, *B*'s consent? Is *B*'s consent invalidated by *A*'s deception or *B*'s immaturity, mental **disability**, or intoxication?

In considering the significance of consent, we should distinguish three questions: (1) When are sexual relations morally unworthy? (2) When are sexual relations morally impermissible? And (3) when should sexual relations be illegal? The contrast between the first two is between sexual acts that are undesirable or not ideal and those that are morally wrong. Although sex between a prostitute and a customer might not be morally laudable, it might be morally permissible. The answers to (2) and (3) are not identical. There are good *moral* reasons why an act's being morally wrong should not be sufficient for it to be illegal. The law is a blunt and expensive instrument to be invoked with great reluctance (Wertheimer, *Consent to Sexual Relations*, chap. 1). It might be morally wrong (not simply not ideal) for *A* to gain *B*'s consent to sex by lying about his affections, but there are moral reasons for not regarding *A*'s behavior as so objectionable as to warrant the law's involvement.

"Consensual minimalism" is the view that engaging in **sexual activity** is morally and legally permissible if and only if both parties consent (see Primoratz). That is, the mutual consent of the parties is required for any sex between them to be permissible, and the permissibility of their sexual activity is assured simply by the presence of mutual consent (in the absence of negative externalities, as when A or B is married to C).

It is widely claimed (Schulhofer, chap. 1) that consent to sex has not always been a necessary condition of legal permissibility, because most rape statutes, for many years, required the presence of *force*. Moreover, it was for many years not criminal to engage in sex with one's wife without her concurrent consent. Yet despite appearances to the contrary, the law might have regarded consent as necessary. After all, having sex with an unconscious or under-age person, neither of whom can consent, was a crime. The law might have required force because it presumed (dubiously) consent in the absence of force. Even the marital exclusion was based on the (dubious) notion that getting married provided *ex ante* consent for one's spouse to engage in sexual relations at will.

Setting the law aside, there are good reasons for regarding mutual consent as necessary and sufficient for the moral permissibility of sexual relations. Requiring consent is consistent with protecting a person's *negative autonomy*, so that a person can control the conditions under which others may engage in sexual relations with him or her. Respecting persons' autonomy demands that we never treat them only as a means but always as an end. On some readings of this "formula of humanity" (from **Immanuel Kant** [1724–1804], Ak 4:429), A does not treat B only as a means if A regards B's rational, voluntary consent as a precondition of their sexual activity. Further, regarding consent as sufficient for the moral permissibility of sexual activity enhances a person's *positive autonomy*. When consent is sufficient, the parties interact with each other on terms they themselves regard as satisfactory, thereby again exercising control over their lives. In this case, A shows respect for B, and for B's decision to engage in sex with A, by taking B's consent seriously, as decisive (Soble, "Sexual Use," 237–38). Consensual minimalism may also be supportable on utilitarian grounds if, as seems likely, nonconsensual transactions do not increase overall utility and consensual transactions enhance the utility of the parties.

Is consensual minimalism correct? First, consent is not *always* necessary for morally permissible sexual contact. If two people are involved in a relationship in which sexual contact is a normal feature, it is arguably permissible for one person to initiate low-level sexual contact without the other's consent and then move to a marginally higher level of intimacy without prior consent, as long as he or she does not persist if asked to stop. There might also be cases in which even coitus is permissible without concurrent and competent consent:

> *Sleep.* A and B have been dating for several months. On this occasion, they had "wonderful" sex the night before. B, who has been sound asleep, awakens to find A on top of and inside her. A says, "Good morning." B smiles back and says, "Good morning."

If A's action is morally permissible, then consent is not always necessary, unless we adopt the fiction that B has hypothetically consented or claim that retrospective consent (B's smiling "good morning") can legitimize a prior nonconsensual action. In other cases, B might give *ex ante* consent to sexual intercourse without giving concurrent and competent consent:

> *Rohypnol conception.* A and B are good friends. B wishes to become pregnant and wants A to father her child but does not want to experience intercourse

with *A*. She tells *A* that he should penetrate her while she is unconscious from rohypnol.

These cases are exceptions. Even if consent is not strictly necessary for morally permissible sex, it is generally necessary.

Second, consent would not be sufficient to render sexual relations permissible if other necessary conditions must be satisfied (see Seiriol Morgan). According to some (sexually conservative) people, sex is permissible only if the partners are of different sexes, are married, engage only in penis-vagina intercourse, or perform coitus without **contraception**. From a different (more sexually liberal) perspective, sexual relations are permissible only if the sexuality is not commercial, is rooted in intimacy or equality, is communicative or reciprocal, or is not exploitative or objectifying (see Chamallas; Pineau). Conservatives often argue that some such conditions should be required by law. Liberals sometimes argue that their preferred conditions are necessary to render sexual relations morally permissible but rarely argue that they should be incorporated into the law. By contrast to both, consensual minimalism appeals to "motivational pluralism," claiming that it is permissible for people to engage in sex for a variety of reasons (pleasure, conception, **love**, money, curiosity) and in a variety of ways (tender, rough, one-sided, same-sex, in groups), as long as the parties give sufficiently voluntary, informed, competent consent.

What sort of phenomenon is morally transformative consent? There are two accounts of the ontology of consent. On the *subjective* view, consent is a psychological phenomenon: A person consents if and only if he or she has the relevant mental state (Alexander). On the *performative* view, consent is behavioral: A person consents if and only if he or she gives a token of or expresses consent in an appropriate way (Kleinig). It is plausible that a suitably qualified performative view is closer to the truth (Wertheimer, *Consent*, chap. 7). If *B*'s consent is morally transformative because it changes *A*'s reasons for action, it is difficult to see how *B*'s mental state, by itself, could do that job. Consider:

> *Guilt.* Unbeknownst to *A*, *B* wants *A* to have intercourse with her without her consent because she feels guilty about saying yes. While *B* says, "No, please don't," *A* holds *B* down and penetrates *B*.

On the subjective view, because *B* wants to be raped, she consented ("internally"), and *A* merely did what *B* wanted *A* to do, even if *A* did not realize that. On the performative view, *A* proceeded wrongly. To be sure, tokens of consent are morally significant because they are reliable indicators of ("internal") desires, intentions, and choices. But since consent alters one's normative relations with other people, public indication of one's will is required, which is absent in this case and required by the performative view.

How can a person communicate or token consent? There are three ways: by a verbal act, by a nonverbal act, and through silence or inaction. Some argue that verbal permission to sexual activity should be required (Remick). Others argue that we should require one person to obtain affirmative indication of another's consent but think that a verbal permission rule imposes too much formality and artificiality (Schulhofer, 272). But nothing problematic follows from construing any form of behavior or omission as a consent token so long as its meaning is clear and the person can indicate to the contrary if it is not.

> *Smile.* *A* and *B* have been dating. They have not had intercourse. *A* proposes that they go to his apartment. *B* agrees. Once inside, *A* points to his bedroom and says, "How about we go there?" *B* smiles and follows *A* into the bedroom but says nothing.

If *B* did not intend to consent to sexual relations and says, "I'm sorry, I didn't know you meant *that*," there should be little confusion whether she has consented to sex, even if it was reasonable for *A* to believe temporarily that she had (see Archard, 32).

Some have suggested that we can resolve the question of when sexual relations are permissible through the principle "no means no." But the difficult issues are not about whether *B* has said yes or no. The difficult questions concern whether "yes" means "yes." For even if *B* unambiguously says yes, her consent might not be valid or morally transformative. The most important task of a theory of consent to sexual relations is to develop a general account of the *principles of valid consent* (PVC), the principles by which we determine whether *B*'s yes renders *A*'s proceeding permissible. PVC takes two forms: the principles of valid consent for morality and the principles of valid consent for the law (Wertheimer, *Consent*). Both forms are moral principles, but the moral principles that indicate when consent should be regarded as legally valid are not identical to the principles that indicate when a person's consent renders another's action morally permissible.

The choice among competing versions of PVC must be sensitive to considerations that pull in opposite directions. To the extent that we seek to protect an agent's negative autonomy, we should set high standards for what qualifies as valid consent. (We might say that a mentally retarded woman cannot give valid consent.) But setting high standards for what counts as valid consent might encroach on an agent's positive autonomy, on her ability to realize her goals and purposes. (Setting high standards for PVC might prevent a mentally retarded woman from experiencing sexual pleasure and intimacy.) The main point is that PVC is the output of our moral reasoning. We must decide when to regard consent as valid, and we cannot do that simply by looking "inside" the concept of consent.

When do the PVC regard a person's consent as invalid? Here we provide only a rough sketch of the issues. A person's consent is invalid if it is coerced or not voluntary. What does that mean? We can set aside cases in which *B* does not token consent *at all*, as when *B* is unconscious or is physically overpowered. The present issue concerns cases in which *B* makes some sort of rational decision to acquiesce in the face of *A*'s actions. Sometimes *A* threatens physical force if *B* does not acquiesce:

> *Force*. *A* at first overpowers *B* physically and holds her down despite *B*'s attempts to resist; but then *A* threatens her with additional force if she continues to resist.

> *Charade*. *A* approaches *B* on the street, puts a gun to her back, and says, "We're walking up to my apartment." When they arrive, he says, "You and I are going to play a game. You are going to ask me to screw you. Act well, and I won't hurt you. Resist, and I'll kill you." *B* takes off her clothes and says, "I want you."

These cases present no theoretical problems. When *A* coerces *B* by the use or threat of physical force, *B*'s consent, no matter how explicit, is not valid. Here "yes" does not mean "yes."

Not all cases of *A*'s application of pressure to obtain consent from *B* are as easy to resolve. Consider:

> *Abandonment*. *A* and *B* drive to a secluded spot in *A*'s car. *B* resists *A*'s advances. *A* says, "Have sex with me or I will leave you here."

> *Indecent Proposal*. *A* says to *B*, "I'll give you $1,000,000 if you spend the night having sex with me."

Dating. A and B have been dating for some time but have not yet had sexual relations. A says, "I'm not willing to continue dating you if we don't have sex, so either we have sex or I'm terminating the relationship."

Lecherous Millionaire. B's child needs expensive medical treatment. A proposes to pay for the treatment if B will have sex with him twice a week for a year.

Lower Grade. A professor, A, says to B, "Have sex with me, or I will give you a grade lower than your work deserves."

Higher Grade. A professor, A, says to B, "Have sex with me, and I will give you a grade higher than your work deserves."

In which cases is B's consent valid? Some argue that A coerces B into sex when B has "no reasonable alternative" but to accept A's proposal, in which case B's consent might be invalid in all these cases. But the most important factor in determining when coercive proposals nullify consent's transformative power is whether what A proposes to do if B does not accept A's proposal would violate B's rights or whether A proposes not to do for B what A has an obligation to do for B (Wertheimer, *Coercion*, chap. 12). Thus A's proposal is arguably coercive in *Abandonment, Lower Grade, Force,* and *Charade.* It is not coercive in *Indecent Proposal, Dating, Lecherous Millionaire,* and *Higher Grade*; in none of these cases does A propose to violate B's rights or deny something to B to which B is entitled.

Some have argued that A coerces B when A makes an offer to B that is "too good to refuse" (*Indecent Proposal, Lecherous Millionaire*). There *is* a sense in which one is forced to do that to which there is no reasonable alternative. Moreover, this feeling is intense when the less attractive alternative is highly unsatisfactory. But it does not follow that such choices are coerced in a morally relevant way. To see this, consider:

Gangrene. A patient's leg is gangrenous, and she must choose between amputation and death. She understands the alternative. Because she does not want to die, she signs the consent form.

Although B might reasonably believe that she has no choice but opting for amputation, we do not say that B's consent to amputation is invalid; that is because no one has proposed to violate her rights if she refuses to consent to the amputation.

The previous example is important. In choosing among possible versions of PVC, we must consider what principles should be applied to the difficult and nonideal circumstances in which people find themselves. Women agree, sometimes reluctantly, to sexual relations they would reject under more favorable conditions. But we do not enhance their welfare or autonomy by denying the transformative power of their consent by denying that in these cases "yes" means "yes." If we say that B's consent should not be regarded as valid in *Lecherous Millionaire,* then A will not make any proposal, the result B is most concerned to avoid. Defending a version of PVC that prevents people from consenting to transactions that move them from an unfortunate to a better (or less unfortunate) situation is difficult.

That a proposal is coercive does not in itself establish how it should be evaluated legally. Although B's consent token does not make sexual intercourse morally permissible in *Lower Grade* or *Abandonment,* it is another question whether the law should regard A as having committed a sexual crime, **sexual harassmen**t, or some other offense. If the law should regard these cases as sexual offenses (even if it does not now do so), we might want to regard them as sexual extortion rather than rape (Wertheimer, *Consent,* chap. 8).

How would PVC handle deception? Consider:

Gynecologist. A physician, *A*, tells *B* that he will insert an instrument into her vagina. Instead, *A* inserts his penis.

Twins. One twin, *A*, whose identical twin is married to *B*, slips into *B*'s bed while she is half asleep. *B*, believing *A* is her husband, has sex with him.

Affection. *A* and *B* are dating. *A* makes advances. *B* says, "I don't want to go farther unless you really care about me." *A* falsely says that he does.

Single. *A* and *B* meet in a night class and go out on several dates. *B* makes it clear that she never has sex with married men. *A* falsely tells *B* that he is single.

Vasectomy. *A* makes advances to *B*, who tells *A* she will accept only if *A* wears a condom. *A* falsely tells *B* that he has had a vasectomy.

Cure. *A*, a hospital employee, tells *B* her blood tests indicate that she has a serious disease curable either by expensive and painful surgery or by intercourse with a donor (*A* himself) who has been injected with a serum. *A* and *B* meet in a hotel and have intercourse (*Boro v. Superior Court*).

The standard view is that *A* commits *fraud in the factum* when *B* is deceived about what is done (*Gynecologist*); *A* commits *fraud in the inducement* when *B* consents to what she believes to be intercourse but does so because she is deceived about certain facts, such as the purpose of intercourse, *A*'s nominal identity, *A*'s characteristics, or *A*'s mental states (Joel Feinberg [1926–2004], 300).

Although deception typically renders agreements voidable in commercial contexts, and while consent must be *informed* in many medical contexts, *caveat amator* has long been the legal principle for sex. Several states criminalize deception with respect to a **sexually transmitted disease** or impersonation of a husband, but those exceptions aside, the law has been permissive with respect to sexual deception. Moreover, prevailing moral norms might be only somewhat less permissive. We might think it sleazy, a case of nonideal sex, if a male lies about his marital status or affections to get a woman into bed, but many do not think this a particularly serious matter. Still, it is arguable that sex obtained by deception should be regarded as morally impermissible, whatever the best legal approach. Again, "yes" does not necessarily mean "yes."

Note a crucial difference between coercion and deception. Whereas coercion typically gives rise to an aversive experience, deception typically gives rise to no aversive experience at the time of sexual relations and might not cause an aversive experience *ex post* if it is not discovered. On an experiential view of the harm of nonconsensual sex, it is harmful just in case it causes an aversive experience, which it often does, but it would not be harmful in those cases in which the victim does not experience anything aversive. On an objective view, *A* has harmed *B*'s interest in sexual autonomy or violated *B*'s rights even if *B* did not experience that harm. To the extent that we adopt an experiential account of harm, sexual deception is properly regarded as less serious than coerced sex. On an objective view, deception may be a very serious matter (Wertheimer, *Consent*, chaps. 5, 9).

Even if *B*'s consent is given willingly and there is no deception, *B*'s token of consent is morally transformative, and "yes" means "yes," only if *B* is suitably competent, that is, has the requisite emotional and cognitive capacities. There are several ways in which *B*'s competence might be suspect, including age, retardation, false preferences, and intoxication.

When and why should we regard a minor's consent as invalid? In principle, we could evaluate a person's competence by reference to the capacities relevant to the decision. We allow youngsters to make decisions if their decisions are not likely to be seriously harmful. Is it harmful for young girls to engage in what would otherwise be described and experienced as consensual sex? This is an empirical question, and the answer will be a function of the age of the parties, the age span between them, social attitudes toward sex by minors, and so on.

Whereas some feminists are concerned to protect young girls from consenting to "devastatingly harmful [sexual] interactions" (Oberman, 72), they also advocate allowing young girls to choose to have abortions. It is not easy to see why a fourteen-year-old should be regarded as sufficiently mature to make an **abortion** decision but not sufficiently mature to make a sexual decision. Not easy, but not impossible. The capacities needed to make reasonable decisions about engaging in sex are not identical to those needed to make reasonable decisions about abortion. Further, the positive autonomy costs are different. Refusing to treat a minor's consent to sex as valid requires her to abstain from sexual relations (as well as requiring that others abstain from having sex with her). These positive autonomy costs are not trivial but are arguably not excessive. By contrast, refusing to treat a minor's consent to abortion as valid requires her to carry a fetus to term, to seek her parents' permission, or to appeal to a court. Thus we might have more reason to err on the side of positive autonomy regarding abortion than regarding sex.

Mental retardation presents similar issues (Wertheimer, *Consent*, chap. 10). We want to protect the mentally retarded against predators. If the retarded are likely to suffer as a result of consenting to sex, that is reason to regard their consent as invalid. But we also have reason to advance their positive autonomy. To say that the mentally retarded cannot consent, or that their "yes" does not mean "yes," is to deny them intimacy and sexual pleasure permanently.

It might also be argued that a woman's consent to sex should not be regarded as valid if rooted in false or distorted preferences or beliefs, because women are socialized to consent to sex that they do not enjoy or to enjoy what they should not enjoy (Wertheimer, *Consent*, chap. 10). It is possible that women consent to sexual relations that do not serve their deepest interests (West). If so, is this consent transformative? Maybe, maybe not. Some women inappropriately sacrifice their interests for the sake of others or excessively identify their interests with those of others. But consider religious beliefs. Taking freedom of religion seriously means allowing people to act on religious beliefs even when they are false and their actions do not serve their interests. A similar claim could be made about false sexual beliefs or preferences.

There is at least one important exception to this rule: sex between psychotherapists and patients (Wertheimer, *Exploitation*, chap. 6). Even though a woman's consent to sexual relations with her psychotherapist is not always distorted by transference or always harmful, the risks are high. Moreover, even benevolently motivated psychotherapists experience countertransference and might not be well positioned to determine when a sexual relationship will be benign. It is therefore probably best to adopt a *per se* rule that treats all patient consent to sexual relations as invalid.

Intoxication can also compromise a person's competence to consent (Wertheimer, *Consent*, chap. 11). Because an intoxicated agent lacks the capacities normally required by ascriptions of responsibility, we would not treat intoxicated consent as valid, at least if the intoxication is not self-induced:

> *Spiked*. A woman, *B*, attends a fraternity party. There is a bowl of punch that has been spiked with vodka but is labeled nonalcoholic. *B* has several glasses of punch and becomes drunk. When *A* proposes that they go to his room, she agrees.

But is it permissible for a male to have sexual relations with a woman who tokens consent while *voluntarily* intoxicated? It could be argued that if *B*'s intoxication is self-induced, we should treat *B* as responsible for her intoxicated behavior, and that includes treating her as responsible for her consent. And if people should be held responsible for wrongful acts committed while intoxicated (driving while drunk through a crowd on the sidewalk), perhaps we should also treat *B*'s consent as valid.

> *Fraternity Party*. A college freshman, *B*, has never had much to drink. She attends a fraternity party and is offered punch. She asks, "Does this have alcohol?" *A* responds, "Absolutely." *B* has several glasses and becomes drunk for the first time in her life. When *A* proposes that they go to his room, *B* agrees.

But even if we should hold *B* responsible for her behavior when intoxication is self-induced, it is another question whether we should treat *B*'s consent as valid. Ascriptions of responsibility are open-ended: To be held morally responsible for one's choices is not to be required to internalize *all* the consequences of that behavior. If one chooses to smoke, one voluntarily assumes an extra risk of cancer, but it does not follow that one should bear all the medical costs of disease.

Consider other contexts:

> *Biopsy*. Before meeting with her physician to get the results of a biopsy, *B* gets intoxicated. Her physician proposes surgery. *B* signs the consent form.

Many would argue that we should not regard *B*'s consent as valid, that a physician cannot say, "She was drunk when she came in; she's responsible for her intoxication, not I." Current legal doctrine holds that a contract made by an intoxicated person is voidable "if the other party has reason to know that the intoxicated person is unable to act in a reasonable manner in relation to the transaction" (Calamari and Perillo, 329). Many states prohibit tattooing an intoxicated person even when the intoxication is voluntary. These contexts do not show that PVC would treat intoxicated consent to sexual relations as *in*valid. They do suggest that we should not assume that PVC would treat such consent as valid. Moreover, they show that we cannot insist that we treat *B*'s consent as valid just because we hold people responsible for wrongdoing committed while intoxicated. The mental capacities required for responsibility for criminal wrongdoing might be different from and less robust than the capacities required for responsibility for consent.

Once again, we must balance protecting negative and positive autonomy. The pleasures of alcohol and sex are so closely intertwined for some people that requiring contemporaneous sober consent to sexual relations would be unduly restrictive of positive autonomy. Such an approach would not be endorsed by many women. It is an open question how PVC should treat intoxicated consent to sex.

One more interesting moral question is, When *should* a person consent to sex? Given asymmetry of desire for sexual intercourse, should the less desirous party consent more often than he or she would prefer? One possible answer is that partners could view the frequency, and perhaps the type, of sexual relations as a matter to be governed by principles of distributive justice (Wertheimer, "Consent and Sexual Relations," 109–12; Soble, *Sexual*

Investigations, 53–55). Partners do decide how a wide variety of benefits and burdens should be distributed between them, such as household chores, child care, and where to dine. If regarding these matters as subject to principles of distributive justice is reasonable, principles of distributive justice might also apply to sex. These principles would probably require that partners compromise on a frequency that is less than one person prefers and more than the other prefers. Hence, one partner might decide to have sexual relations he or she does not otherwise desire.

Objections can be raised against applying principles of distributive justice to sexual frequency. It has been claimed that women should never consent to sexual relations they do not want (see Robin Morgan). This objection begs the question whether a woman should *want* sexual relations for moral reasons. It might be said that many activities that are not desired are candidates for moral deliberation, but sex is different. As a practical matter, it might be self-defeating for partners to engage in sex for morally conscientious reasons of fairness: *A* will not enjoy sex when he believes *B* consents because she wants to be fair. This is an empirical question, and the notion might very well be false. It might also be argued that even if one *would* enjoy sex motivated by fairness, one *should not* enjoy such relations. But if *A* may properly enjoy sex motivated by *B*'s desire to conceive, why should it be wrong when *B* is motivated by moral reasons? Motivational pluralism seems relevant here. Of course, appeals to justice, however meritorious, might generate a decline in a relationship's quality. When a couple frames sexual issues in terms of justice, this might weaken intimacy, benevolence, and mutual identification. This, too, is an empirical question.

See also Bestiality; Coercion (by Sexually Aggressive Women); Communication Model; Consequentialism; Contraception; Disability; Harassment, Sexual; Hegel, G.W.F.; Incest; Law, Sex and the; Liberalism; MacKinnon, Catharine; Pedophilia; Rape; Rape, Acquaintance and Date; Seduction

REFERENCES

Alexander, Larry. "The Moral Magic of Consent (II)." *Legal Theory* 2:3 (1996), 165–74; Archard, David. *Sexual Consent*. Boulder, Colo.: Westview, 1998; *Boro v. Superior Court*. 163 Cal. App. 1224; 210 Cal. Rptr. 122 (1985); Calamari, Joseph, and Joseph Perillo. *Contracts*, 3rd ed. St. Louis. Mo.: West, 1987; Chamallas, Martha. "Consent, Equality, and the Legal Control of Sexual Conduct." *Southern California Law Review* 61:4 (1988), 777–862; Feinberg, Joel. *The Moral Limits of the Criminal Law*, vol. 3: *Harm to Self*. New York: Oxford University Press, 1986; Kant, Immanuel. (1785) *Grounding for the Metaphysics of Morals*. Trans. James Ellington. Indianapolis, Ind.: Hackett, 1993; Kleinig, John. "Consent." In Lawrence C. Becker and Charlotte B. Becker, eds., *Encyclopedia of Ethics*, 2nd ed., vol. 1. New York: Routledge, 2001, 299–304; Morgan, Robin. "Theory and Practice: Pornography and Rape." In *Going Too Far: The Personal Chronicle of a Feminist*. New York: Random House, 1977, 163–69; Morgan, Seiriol. "Dark Desires." *Ethical Theory and Moral Practice* 6:4 (2003), 377–410; Oberman, Michelle. "Turning Girls into Women: Re-evaluating Modern Statutory Rape Law." *Journal of Criminal Law and Criminology* 85:1 (1994), 15–79; Pineau, Lois. "Date Rape: A Feminist Analysis." *Law and Philosophy* 8:2 (1989), 217–43; Primoratz, Igor. "Sexual Morality: Is Consent Enough?" *Ethical Theory and Moral Practice* 4:3 (2001), 201–18; Remick, Lani Anne. "Read Her Lips: An Argument for a Verbal Consent Standard in Rape." *University of Pennsylvania Law Review* 141:3 (1993), 1103–51; Schulhofer, Stephen. *Unwanted Sex: The Culture of Intimidation and the Failure of Law*. Cambridge, Mass.: Harvard University Press, 1998; Soble, Alan. *Sexual Investigations*. New York: New York University Press, 1996; Soble, Alan. "Sexual Use and What to Do about It: Internalist and Externalist Sexual Ethics." In Alan Soble, ed., *Philosophy of Sex*, 4th ed. Lanham, Md.: Rowman and Littlefield, 2002, 225–58; Toobin, Jeffrey. "The Consent Defense." *The New Yorker* (1 September 2003), 40–44, 87; Wertheimer, Alan. *Coercion*. Princeton, N.J.: Princeton University Press, 1987; Wertheimer, Alan. "Consent and Sexual

Relations." *Legal Theory* 2:2 (1996), 89–112; Wertheimer, Alan. *Consent to Sexual Relations*. Cambridge: Cambridge University Press, 2003; Wertheimer, Alan. *Exploitation*. Princeton, N.J.: Princeton University Press, 1996; West, Robin. "The Harms of Consensual Sex." *American Philosophical Association Newsletters* 94:2 (1995), 52–55.

Alan Wertheimer

ADDITIONAL READING

Alexander, Larry, ed. *Special Issue: Sex and Consent*, parts I and II. *Legal Theory* 2:2–3 (1996), 87–264; Appelbaum, Paul S., Charles W. Lidz, and Alan Miesel. *Informed Consent: Legal Theory and Clinical Practice*. New York: Oxford University Press, 1987; Archard, David. "Exploited Consent." *Journal of Social Philosophy* 25 (1994), 92–101. Reprinted in Leslie P. Francis, *Sexual Harassment as an Ethical Issue in Academic Life*. Lanham, Md.: Rowman and Littlefield, 2001, 212–18; Archard, David. "The Limits of Consensuality I: Incest, Prostitution, and Sado-masochism." In *Sexual Consent*. Boulder, Colo.: Westview, 1998, 98–115; Archard, David. "The Limits of Consensuality II: The Age of Sexual Consent." In *Sexual Consent*. Boulder, Colo.: Westview, 1998, 116–29; Archard, David. " 'A Nod's as Good as a Wink': Consent, Convention, and Reasonable Belief." *Legal Theory* 3:3 (1997), 273–90; Baker, Brenda M. "Understanding Consent in Sexual Assault." In Keith Burgess-Jackson, ed., *A Most Detestable Crime: New Philosophical Essays on Rape*. New York: Oxford University Press, 1999, 49–70; Belliotti, Raymond. *Good Sex: Perspectives on Sexual Ethics*. Lawrence: University Press of Kansas, 1993; Belliotti, Raymond. "A Philosophical Analysis of Sexual Ethics." *Journal of Social Philosophy* 10:3 (1979), 8–11; Belliotti, Raymond. "Sexual Intercourse between Consenting Adults Is Always Permissible." In Louis P. Pojman, ed., *The Moral Life: An Introductory Reader in Ethics and Literature*. New York: Oxford University Press, 2000, 681–89; Brett, Nathan. "Sexual Offences and Consent." *Canadian Journal of Law and Jurisprudence* 11:1 (1998), 69–88; Brundage, James A. "Implied Consent to Intercourse." In Angeliki E. Laiou, ed., *Consent and Coercion to Sex and Marriage in Ancient and Medieval Societies*. Washington, D.C.: Dumbarton Oaks, 1993, 245–56; Burgess-Jackson, Keith. "Statutory Rape: A Philosophical Analysis." *Canadian Journal of Law and Jurisprudence* 8:1 (1995), 139–58. Reprinted in HS (463–82); Crowley, Ray. " 'Consent Condoms'? No Thanks." *Spiked* (4 July 2001). <www.spiked-online.com/Articles/00000002D16E.htm> [accessed 31 August 2004]; Culver, Charles M., and Bernard Gert. "Competence." In Jennifer Radden, ed., *The Philosophy of Psychiatry: A Companion*. New York: Oxford University Press, 2004, 258–70; Davis, Michael. "Setting Penalties: What Does Rape Deserve?" *Law and Philosophy* 3:1 (1984), 61–110; Doniger, Wendy. "Sex, Lies, and Tall Tales." *Social Research* 63:3 (1996), 663–99; Doniger, Wendy. *Splitting the Difference: Gender and Myth in Ancient Greece and India*. Chicago, Ill.: University of Chicago Press, 1999; Faden, Ruth R., and Tom L. Beauchamp. *A History and Theory of Informed Consent*. New York: Oxford University Press, 1986; Feinberg, Joel. *The Moral Limits of the Criminal Law*, 4 vols. New York: Oxford University Press, 1984–1988; Gauthier, Jeffrey A. "Consent, Coercion, and Sexual Autonomy." In Keith Burgess-Jackson, ed., *A Most Detestable Crime: New Philosophical Essays on Rape*. New York: Oxford University Press, 1999, 71–91; Hickman, Susan, and Charlene L. Muehlenhard. "By the Semi-Mystical Appearance of a Condom: How Young Women and Men Communicate Sexual Consent in Heterosexual Situations." *Journal of Sex Research* 36:3 (1999), 258–72; Husak, Douglas N., and George C. Thomas III. "Date Rape, Social Convention, and Reasonable Mistakes." *Law and Philosophy* 11:1 (1992), 95–126; Kramer, Karen M. "Rule by Myth: The Social and Legal Dynamics Governing Alcohol-Related Acquaintance Rapes." *Stanford Law Review* 47 (1994), 115–60; Laiou, Angeliki E., ed. *Consent and Coercion to Sex and Marriage in Ancient and Medieval Societies*. Washington, D.C.: Dumbarton Oaks, 1993; Lim, Grace, and Michael Roloff. "Attributing Sexual Consent." *Journal of Applied Communication Research* 27:1 (1999), 1–24; MacKinnon, Catharine A. "Rape: On Coercion and Consent." In *Toward a Feminist Theory of the State*. Cambridge, Mass.: Harvard University Press, 1989, 171–83; Malm, H. M. "The Ontological Status of Consent and Its Implications for the Law on Rape." *Legal Theory* 2:2 (1996), 147–64; Mappes,

Thomas A. (1985) "Sexual Morality and the Concept of Using Another Person." In Thomas A. Mappes and Jane S. Zembaty, eds., *Social Ethics: Morality and Social Policy*, 4th ed. New York: McGraw-Hill, 1992, 203–16. 5th ed., 1997, 163–76. 6th ed., 2002, 170–83. Reprinted in POS4 (207–23); McGregor, Joan. *Is It Rape? On Acquaintance Rape and Taking Women's Consent Seriously*. Aldershot, U.K.: Ashgate, 2005; Mill, John Stuart. (1859) *On Liberty*. Ed. Elizabeth Rapaport. Indianapolis, Ind.: Hackett, 1978; Muehlenhard, Charlene L., and Jennifer L. Schrag. "Nonviolent Sexual Coercion." In Andrea Parrot and Laurie Bechhofer, eds., *Acquaintance Rape: The Hidden Crime*. New York: John Wiley, 1991, 115–28; O'Neill, Onora. "Between Consenting Adults." *Philosophy and Public Affairs* 14:3 (1985), 252–77. Reprinted in *Constructions of Reason: Explorations of Kant's Practical Philosophy*. Cambridge: Cambridge University Press, 1989, 105–25; Pateman, Carole. "Women and Consent." *Political Theory* 8:2 (1980), 149–68. Reprinted in *The Disorder of Women: Democracy, Feminism, and Political Theory*. Cambridge: Cambridge University Press, 1989, 71–89; Pineau, Lois. "Date Rape: A Feminist Analysis." *Law and Philosophy* 8:2 (1989), 217–43. Reprinted in Leslie P. Francis, ed., *Date Rape: Feminism, Philosophy, and the Law*. State College, Pa.: Pennsylvania State University Press, 1996, 1–26; HS (483–509); Posner, Richard A. "Coercive Sex." In *Sex and Reason*. Cambridge, Mass.: Harvard University Press, 1992, 383–404; Posner, Richard A., and Katharine B. Silbaugh. "Age of Consent." In *A Guide to America's Sex Laws*. Chicago, Ill.: University of Chicago Press, 1996, 44–64; Primoratz, Igor. *Ethics and Sex*. London: Routledge, 1999; Sample, Ruth. *Exploitation: What It Is and Why It's Wrong*. Lanham, Md.: Rowman and Littlefield, 2003; Soble, Alan. "Antioch's 'Sexual Offense Policy': A Philosophical Exploration." *Journal of Social Philosophy* 28:1 (1997): 22–36. Reprinted in David Boonin and Graham Oddie, eds., *What's Wrong? Applied Ethicists and Their Critics*. New York: Oxford University Press, 2005, 241–49; POS4 (323–40); Soble, Alan. "Sexual Use and What to Do about It: Internalist and Externalist Sexual Ethics." *Essays in Philosophy* 2:2 (2001). <www.humboldt.edu/~essays/soble.html> [accessed 17 November 2004]. Reprinted, revised, in POS4 (225–58); Stavis, Paul F., and Leslie W. Walker-Hirsch. "Consent to Sexual Activity." In Robert D. Dinerstein, Stanley S. Herr, and Joan L. O'Sullivan, eds., *A Guide to Consent*. Washington, D.C.: American Association on Mental Retardation, 1999, 57–67; Steutel, Jan, and Ben Spiecker. "Sex Education, State Policy and the Principle of Mutual Consent." *Sex Education* 4:1 (2004), 49–62; Wertheimer, Alan. "Consent and Sexual Relations." *Legal Theory* 2:2 (1996), 89–112. Reprinted in POS4 (341–66); Wertheimer, Alan. "What Is Consent? And Is It Important?" *Buffalo Criminal Law Review* 3:2 (2001), 557–83; West, Robin. "Authority, Autonomy, and Choice: The Role of Consent in the Moral and Political Visions of Franz Kafka and Richard Posner." *Harvard Law Review* 99:2 (1985), 384–428; West, Robin. "A Comment on Consent, Sex, and Rape." *Legal Theory* 2:3 (1996), 233–51; West, Robin. "The Harms of Consensual Sex." *American Philosophical Association Newsletters* 94:2 (1995), 52–55. Reprinted in Thomas A. Mappes and Jane S. Zembaty, eds., *Social Ethics: Morality and Social Policy*, 6th ed. Boston, Mass.: McGraw-Hill, 2002, 184–88; and POS3 (263–68); POS4 (317–22); West, Robin. "Sex, Harm, and Impeachment." In Leonard V. Kaplan and Beverly I. Moran, eds., *Aftermath: The Clinton Impeachment and the Presidency in the Age of Political Spectacle*. New York: New York University Press, 2001, 129–49; West, Robin. "Unwelcome Sex: Toward a Harm-Based Analysis." In Catharine A. MacKinnon and Reva B. Siegel, eds., *Directions in Sexual Harassment Law*. New Haven, Conn.: Yale University Press, 2004, 138–52.

CONSEQUENTIALISM. Consequentialism asserts that an act's consequences are of paramount importance in determining whether the act is morally right or wrong. It maintains that a morally acceptable act must have good or beneficial consequences or, at least, must on balance produce better consequences than the other options available to the agent. If all options produce both desirable and undesirable consequences, the morally preferred act is the one that produces more good than bad. (The term "consequentialism" was coined by one of the theory's critics, **G.E.M. Anscombe** [1919–2001]; see her "Modern Moral Philosophy," 12; Diamond, 75.)

Consequentialism has two basic varieties: *agent-centered* and *other-person-centered* consequentialism. The former is *egoism*, the latter *altruism*. An ethical egoist will argue that any sexual behavior that benefits (on balance and in the long run) the agent is morally permissible. However, concern for the welfare of others, exclusively or inclusively, is, we ordinarily believe, inherent in the concept of ethics. If we expect agents to include others' welfare in their ethical deliberations, egoism cannot be considered an ethical theory (see Odell, *On Consequentialist Ethics*, 70–72; see also Sidgwick, 508). Several consequentialist theories fall within altruism. Each one morally judges various sexual acts according to its own unique perspective.

The most influential form of consequentialism is *utilitarianism*, primarily associated with Jeremy Bentham (1748–1832), John Stuart Mill (1806–1873), and Henry Sidgwick (1838–1900), although many other philosophers have defended it. Utilitarians in the twentieth century include **Bertrand Russell** (1872–1970; *Human Society*, 92–98; see Odell, *On Russell*, 69–81), who often discussed sexuality (see *Marriage and Morals*), and G. E. Moore (1873–1958), whose theory of practical ethics obliged us to act in accordance with the amount of good our actions produce (25, 147–48; see Odell, *On Moore*, 70–78). Bentham's utilitarianism, a *hedonism*, understood "good" as pleasure. Although Mill was also a hedonist, he differed from Bentham over the extension of pleasure. Bentham did not distinguish between the *quantity* and the *quality* of pleasure (*Principles of Morals*, 30–32). Mill did. On his view, the pleasure derived from reading Socrates was a *higher*-quality pleasure than that derived from sensuous activities, such as having sex (*Utilitarianism*, 21–13). Utilitarianism had its counterpart in antiquity in the work of Epicurus (341–270 BCE; see his "Letter to Menoeceus," 31–32). He was an egoistic hedonist (unlike Bentham and Mill, who were altruists), who promoted the goal of maximizing personal pleasure. Utilitarianism appeared earlier in Eastern philosophy than in the West (see Boss, 281–83). It is incorporated into the doctrines of the founder of **Buddhism**, Siddhattha Gotama (ca. 560–483 BCE), and Chinese philosopher Mo Tzu (b. ca. 500 BCE).

Utilitarianism has various formulations (William Frankena [1908–1994], 35–43). *Act* and *rule* utilitarianism are the most influential, but *general* utilitarianism is also worthy of consideration. Act utilitarianism (AU) claims that each act is to conform to the principle of utility; that is, every act should produce the greatest possible balance of good over evil. Act utilitarians apply the utilitarian principle (UP) "Maximize the good in the world" directly to every situation to determine moral obligation. Let us here distinguish also between *objective* and *subjective* act utilitarianism. The former morally judges an act in terms of its actual consequences. But no one can always accurately foresee the future; we are ordinarily satisfied with well-grounded predictable consequences. For this reason the AU principle becomes "Always act to maximize the *expectable* good," which is *subjective* AU.

Rule utilitarianism (RU) claims that actions are to be judged by reference to a set of rules that are themselves justified by UP. Agents who are concerned with whether they should perform an act are obliged to determine what the rule is regarding that act. For example, if the rule "never harm a dog" is justified by UP, then harming dogs is always wrong, even if AU would judge some individual harms to dogs acceptable. (By the way, AU does not always preclude following rules, and RU may not be distinguishable from some types of AU; see Brandt; Hooker; Johnson.) *General* utilitarianism (GU) claims that all acts are to be judged by the generalized utilitarian principle "Always act in a fashion that would, if everybody did likewise, produce the greatest possible balance of good over evil." The general utilitarian asks, in counterfactual Kantian fashion, what would happen were everyone to do the act in question. But the general utilitarian differs from **Immanuel Kant** (1724–1804) in the sequel. Kant would have us ask whether it would still be logically or naturally possible to act in that way (*Groundwork*, Ak 401–404; in Paton, 69–71); the general utilitarian asks how favorable the consequences would be.

Practice consequentialism, although rooted in utilitarianism, differs from all three forms (see Attfield; Odell "Practice Consequentialism."). One version, *folk-based practice* consequentialism (FBPC), maintains that (1) most if not all acceptable moral rules are formulations of intricate and interrelated practices that promote harmonious coexistence among human beings; (2) these moral rules are abbreviations of the lengthy formulations that would be required to describe fully the complicated set of prescriptions and prohibitions that comprise our ethical practices; (3) we are culturally, perhaps naturally, disposed to justify our actions in consequentialist fashion; (4) these underlying moral practices or "folk" ethics provide the foundation for all forms of consequentialism; and (5) the folk ethical practices incorporated by practice consequentialism are empirically verifiable (Odell, *On Consequentialist Ethics*, 117–50). FBPC is an account of the way things are or have come to be, and so (metaethically) it is naturalistic and in that sense objective. "The behavior it prescribes is behavior which—even if it does not maximize the good—is revealed by mankind's history to at least have had *much better* consequences for humanity than have accrued when our behavior infringes its precepts" (Odell, *On Consequentialist Ethics*, 90). Thus folk ethics is envisioned as an empirical technique for producing more human happiness and contentment than otherwise. (Mill comes the closest of any historical figure to advocating practice consequentialism; *Utilitarianism*, 25.)

Considering an example will illuminate the differences between these consequentialisms. Suppose that a close friend has engaged in a sexual act of which she is ashamed, you know about it, and a third party asks you if she did it. AU would have you try to determine if your telling this particular lie about your friend's conduct would increase or decrease the good; if your estimate is that it would increase the good (or prevent a decrease), the lie is right. RU implies that you should tell the truth to the third party, because (or if) there is a rule against lying that has been justified by UP (and no *exceptions* have evolved in the rule). GU would have you ask what would happen if everyone lied in such cases (described in a reasonable similar way). If you answer that lying in such cases, if done generally, would lead to bad consequences (say, an increase in distrust in the world), you should tell the truth. FBPC would remind you that our actual or folk practice about lying permits one to lie under various circumstances, and this may very well be one of them, for our practice surrounding lying recognizes the importance of shielding friends. For FBPC, cases that are taken to be exceptions to a rule (say, by RU) are already covered by the practices or moral rules that our abbreviations designate and so do not count as exceptions at all.

Now consider how these consequentialisms handle sexual acts: premarital sex, **adultery, masturbation**, orgies, **prostitution, homosexuality**, even voyeurism, exhibitionism, **incest, rape, pedophilia, bestiality**, and necrophilia. It is one thing for an activity to be repulsive and disgusting; it is another thing for it to be ethically wrong. Only the latter concerns us.

Act utilitarians would treat sexual events on a case-by-case basis. If they were Benthamite hedonists, they would define "good" as pleasure and "bad" as pain. The person following AU has to predict the pleasure an act is expected to produce (when finally attained) and subtract from this any pain it is expected to produce or that arises in the pursuit of the pleasure. This calculation determines how one should act (see Bentham, *Principles of Morals*, 30–32). Since for the victim the pain and misery of rape, pedophilia, and incest seem to outweigh the temporary pleasure the agent experiences, especially when we take into account the persisting psychological damage done to the victim, such acts would be judged immoral. Presumably, RU, GU, and FBPC would agree that behaviors grossly harmful to unwilling participants are morally wrong, although each would give its own characteristic justification for that judgment.

As long as homosexuality is safely practiced, and both participants are willing, it is hard to imagine that the pain would outweigh the pleasure. (In consensual homosexual **sado-masochism**, the pleasure one gets from enduring the pain would have to offset the pain.) Still, it might be argued that a prohibition of homosexuality (legal, social, or religious) is valid on GU grounds: If everyone were to behave purely homosexually, the human species (in the absence of artificial **reproductive technology**) would die out—which we assume is a bad consequence. Bentham argued against this prohibition (see Corvino, 315). He pointed out that if this reasoning were accepted by religiously inspired opponents of homosexuality, it would also entail that the holy religious practice of **abstinence**, or celibacy, should also be prohibited. According to Bentham, "If then merely out of regard to population it were right that pederasts should be burnt alive, monks ought to be roasted alive by a slow fire" ("Paederasty," 357). Judgments about incest will depend crucially on the particulars of the case. A situation in which a father of forty engages in **sexual activity** with a daughter of ten to sixteen is very much different from a situation in which the father (or brother) is fifty-five and the daughter (or sister) is well into middle age. If precautions are taken against pregnancy and venereal disease, their **consent** manifests sophisticated understanding of the events, and they are secure in thinking they would feel no guilt or express no recriminations afterward, hedonistic act utilitarian theory would not condemn their sexual activity.

Mutual consent and the absence of harm can be utilized to justify even some bestiality and necrophilia. Suppose a female ape in heat persistently backs up to a human male. Assuming that in this case the ape's behavior signals consent, and that she thoroughly enjoys the event, hedonistic AU would not complain. Or suppose—admittedly a fanciful example—that two heterosexual or homosexual lovers are inclined toward necrophilia and agree to allow the surviving partner to utilize the other's cadaver for sex. Many find such an act repulsive. It is also illegal. But it would appear to be permissible for hedonistic AU. The participation of consenting adults and producing more pleasure than pain (which is closely linked to the presence of consent) seem to be all that are required for the moral permissibility of a wide variety of sexual acts. Masturbation does not involve the consent of others (unless it is mutual masturbation), and it certainly gives much more pleasure than pain—unless one overdoes it.

This *caveat* should remind us that the pursuit of pleasure can be counterproductive and harmful in the long run. Seeking sexual experiences *ad libitum*, with no limits at all, can lead us to ignore other, sometimes more important, aspects of life. The possibility of a productive, contented life turns on our willingness to restrain passion. The relentless pursuit of pleasure can diminish or destroy one's ability to pursue a satisfying life—even in a Benthamite hedonistic sense, let alone a Millian sense, of pleasure as the good. Societies founded on the altruistic principle that we are obliged to maximize the good, where the good is hedonistic pleasure (Sodom and Gomorrah), are likely to collapse from self-indulgence.

Mill maintains that everyone should be free to strive to satisfy their individual tastes and to accomplish their personal goals, "so long as what we do does not harm" our "fellow creatures" and even if "they should think our conduct foolish, perverse, or wrong" (*On Liberty*, 12). Mill's sentiment has become very popular and has often been applied to sexual "experiments in living." (But see the lengthy reply by one of his contemporaries, James Fitzjames Stephen [1829–1894].) Mill himself, however, says very little about sexuality, and when he does, his coverage, as would be true of most Victorian gentlemen, is clothed in carefully chosen nonoffensive vocabulary. In one passage in *On Liberty* (chap. iv), he remarks that even though he personally does not find polygamy agreeable, the consent of the women who participate in group marriage to one man, with all that that implies about their sexual lives, is the significant consideration. About "fornication" he contends that it "must be tolerated"—only tolerated, neither recommended nor encouraged. Given that fornication must be tolerated (as being consensual and harming no one), Mill constructs (chap. v, "Applications") an argument defending gambling houses and pimping:

> On the side of toleration it may be said that the fact of following anything as an occupation, and living or profiting by the practice of it, cannot make that criminal which would otherwise be admissible; that the act should either be consistently permitted or consistently prohibited; that if the principles which we have hitherto defended are true, society has no business, *as* society, to decide anything to be wrong which concerns only the individual; that it cannot go beyond dissuasion, and that one person should be as free to persuade, as another to dissuade. (100)

Mill does not let the matter rest on this argument, however; he also constructs an argument for the opposing view:

> In opposition to this it may be contended, that although the public, or the State, are not warranted in authoritatively deciding, for purposes of repression or punishment, that such or such conduct affecting only the interests of the individual is good or bad, they are fully justified in assuming, if they regard it as bad, that its being so or not is at least a disputable question: that, this being supposed, they cannot be acting wrongly in endeavoring to exclude the influence of solicitations which are not disinterested, of instigators who cannot possibly be impartial—who have a direct personal interest on one side, and that side the one which the State believes to be wrong, and who confessedly promote it for personal objects only. There can surely, it may be urged, be nothing lost, no sacrifice of good, by so ordering matters that persons shall make their election, either wisely or foolishly, on their own prompting, as free as possible from the arts of persons who stimulate their inclinations for interested purposes of their own. . . . It is true that the prohibition is never effectual, and that, whatever amount of tyrannical power may be given to the police, gambling-houses [or brothels!] can always be maintained under other pretenses; but they may be compelled to conduct their operations with a certain degree of secrecy and mystery, so that nobody knows anything about them but those who seek them; and more than this society ought not to aim at. (101)

At the end, Mill may be espousing a zoning policy that would segregate those interested in gambling or prostitution from those not similarly inclined, a policy designed both to prevent harm and to permit chosen activities to occur. Although Mill finds the arguments in favor of prohibition forceful, he refuses to decide if they are "sufficient to justify the moral anomaly of punishing the accessory when the principal is (and must be) allowed to go free;

of fining or imprisoning the procurer, but not the fornicator—the gambling-house keeper, but not the gambler" (101).

Another issue that Mill tackled was the threat to person freedom raised by the fact that some people are repulsed or disgusted, morally or physically, by the behaviors of others (*On Liberty*, chap. iv). For example, some people experience nausea when witnessing the public display of sexual behavior, heterosexual or homosexual. Some even experience discomfort of a spiritual sort from knowing that heterosexual or homosexual anal and oral sex is occurring—right down the street in someone's home. Should these considerations matter in the morality and legality of offensive behavior? Mill thought not. Too much person freedom is at stake in allowing the tender sensibilities of some to trump the freedoms, sexual and otherwise, of others. This issue reemerged and was hotly debated in the 1960s, especially between H.L.A. Hart (1907–1992) and Patrick Devlin—both parties claiming to be representing the utilitarian position in some form or another (as did Fitzjames Stephen). "Morality and the law" and the credentials of "the offense principle" occupied center stage in this flurry of philosophical activity (see Joel Feinberg [1926–2004]; Wasserstrom).

There is no end to the objects to which humans have aversions. Some cannot stand to think about eating, for example, okra, blue cheese, opossum, asparagus, or sushi. Such facts hardly warrant prohibition of these edibles. Anal and oral sex, orgies, bondage, and so forth, like edibles, are subject to individual taste. But not only can one acquire tolerance for such activities and edibles; one might also come to crave them. Further, often in human history what is regarded as wrong or repulsive at one period is at another time not only condoned but applauded. Hence prohibition is counterproductive, and the variability and changeability of human likes and dislikes seem to call for a principle of freedom that tolerates the offensive. Note that this problem is generated within hedonistic consequentialisms. Nonhedonistic consequentialisms, such as FBPC, may be able to minimize its importance by defining the goal of moral rules as making it possible for humans to live together in harmony (Odell, *On Consequentialist Ethics*, 118, 122–24, 126–29, 143–46).

Rule utilitarianism may not be nearly as permissive as act utilitarianism, but much depends on social circumstances and empirical facts. (These sorts of questions are discussed by Atkinson.) It might have been possible to argue successfully in the early to middle part of the twentieth century that a rule prohibiting premarital sex was justified by utilitarian considerations. Following such a rule might well have had, in general, better consequences than its violation, namely, helping to prevent unwanted pregnancy, illegitimate births, illegal and dangerous **abortion**s, and the spread of (prepenicillin) **sexually transmitted diseases**. The costs of the frustrations of abstinence were, arguably, too slight to offset the disadvantages. But biomedical advances in **contraception** and antibiotics have made it possible to avoid pregnancy and disease without abstaining from sexual activity. Hence, it seems that a utilitarian argument can be made that the rule "no premarital sex at all" should be replaced by "premarital sex only with proper precautions against pregnancy and disease." Of course, now that antibiotic-resistant strains of venereal disease bacteria are increasing, and some diseases (herpes, AIDS [acquired immunodeficiency syndrome]) are caused by viruses against which we have little medical protection, the argument for a rule prohibiting premarital (and other) sex may still have some strength.

The general utilitarian employs the principle "Always act in a fashion that would, if everybody did likewise, produce the greatest possible balance of good over evil" to determine the morality of sexual acts. We are to inquire what the consequences would be if everyone engaged in incest or prostitution or public sex or homosexuality. "Unsophisticated" GU might argue that homosexuality is wrong because if each and every person were homosexual, humanity would die out. This is an unsophisticated GU because, as Bentham pointed out, it would imply that all those committed to abstinence would be immoral. "Sophisticated" GU argues that what is in question, instead, is what would happen *if everyone had the right to choose* for themselves. The GU argument might then proceed to claim that allowing individuals the right to choose among actions that are not harmful to others is the only way to ensure the greatest possible balance of good over evil. For this reason, sophisticated GU is likely to argue that masturbation, premarital sex, homosexuality, and group sex, since they involve freedom of choice, are permissible (if practiced safely). Sophisticated GU is also likely to argue that rape, incest, and adultery have harmful consequences for others and are therefore immoral. It is, however, possible, even if not very likely, for sophisticated GU to oppose masturbation, premarital sex, and so forth, on the grounds of wanting to avoid disharmony, the evil that would be generated by a clash with religious segments of society that oppose such behaviors.

FBPC, which holds that our ethical principles are generalizations of practices that have been empirically confirmed to promote harmonious coexistence among humans, and that are subject to modification when circumstances warrant, treats sexual acts as any other acts are. FBPC takes cognizance of the fact that humans are an evolving species. Our understanding and concepts of what best promotes harmonious coexistence are dynamic and flexible. Our ethical practices tend to evolve along with our increasing knowledge, and the conceptual adaptations that result from that knowledge are largely responsible for this **evolution**. But our ethical practices lag behind our increased knowledge and conceptual modifications, largely the result of religious and political forces that resist change and promote the *status quo* out of both fear and a desire for control. For FBPC, our practice concerning lying is well founded; unless we oppose lying in most circumstances, we cannot live together harmoniously. FBPC considers adultery unethical because it involves lying and deception. As is true for other consequentialisms, FBPC acknowledges that the consequences of promiscuity without proper safeguards, rape, and child molestation can be disastrous. But, for FBPC, for humans to live together in harmony, each individual's self-directed desires and actions, when those desires and actions do not jeopardize the well-being of others, must be granted high priority (Odell, *On Consequentialist Ethics*, 152–82). For this reason, FBPC finds justification for a variety of sexual practices that have often been prohibited or judged immoral. For example, FBPC implies that time is on the side of homosexuals. Many people who were opposed to homosexuality no longer object to it. Religious conservatives will likely never accept homosexuality, but what is important is that the majority of secular conservatives will eventually accept it. In general, FBPC claims that most arguments invoked in the past for calling a sexual activity perverse or abnormal are weak. For example, group sex does not inevitably lead to divorce for married couples who engage in it, and it can enhance both the quality of their lives and their intimacy. Engaging in group sex requires honesty and, as a result, can bring two people closer together.

See also Addiction, Sexual; Bestiality; Casual Sex; Consent; Diseases, Sexually Transmitted; Ellis, Albert; Ethics, Sexual; Fantasy; Firestone, Shulamith; Incest; Kant, Immanuel; Law, Sex and the; Liberalism; Nudism; Pedophilia; Rape, Acquaintance and Date; Reproductive Technology; Russell, Bertrand; Westermarck, Edward

REFERENCES

Anscombe, G.E.M. "Modern Moral Philosophy." *Philosophy* 33 (January 1958), 1–19; Atkinson, Ronald. *Sexual Morality*. London: Hutchinson, 1965; Attfield, Robin. *Value, Obligation, and*

Meta-Ethics. Amsterdam, Holland: Rodopi, 1995; Bentham, Jeremy (1784–1816?) "An Essay on Paederasty." In Robert B. Baker, Kathleen Wininger, and Frederick A. Elliston, eds., *Philosophy and Sex*, 3rd ed. Buffalo, N.Y.: Prometheus, 1984, 350–64; Bentham, Jeremy. (1789) *The Principles of Morals and Legislation*. Darien, Conn.: Hafner, 1970; Boss, Judith. *Ethics for Life*. Mountain View, Calif.: Mayfield, 2001; Brandt, Richard B. *A Theory of the Good and the Right*. Oxford, U.K.: Clarendon Press, 1979; Corvino, John. "Why Shouldn't Tommy and Jim Have Sex? A Defense of Homosexuality." In James E. White, ed., *Contemporary Moral Problems*, 7th ed. Belmont, Calif.: Wadsworth, 2002, 308–18; Devlin, Patrick. *The Enforcement of Morals*. Oxford, U.K.: Oxford University Press, 1965; Diamond, Cora. "Anscombe, G[ertrude] E[lizabeth] M[argaret]." In Lawrence C. Becker and Charlotte B. Becker, eds., *Encyclopedia of Ethics*, 2nd ed., vol. 1. New York: Routledge, 2001, 74–77; Epicurus. (ca. 300 BCE) "The Letter to Menoeceus." In Whitney J. Oates, ed., *The Stoic and Epicurean Philosophers: The Complete Extant Writings of Epicurus, Epictetus, Lucretius, and Marcus Aurelius*. New York: Random House, 1940, 3–66; Feinberg, Joel. *The Moral Limits of the Criminal Law*, vol. 2: *Offense to Others*. New York: Oxford University Press, 1985; Frankena, William. *Ethics*. Englewood Cliffs, N.J.: Prentice-Hall, 1973; Hart, H.L.A. (1962). *Law, Liberty and Morality*. Stanford, Calif.: Stanford University Press, 1963; Hooker, Brad. "Rule Consequentialism, Incoherence, Fairness." *Proceedings of the Aristotelian Society* 95 (1995), 19–35; Johnson, Conrad. *Moral Legislation: A Legal-Political Model for Indirect Consequentialist Reasoning*. Cambridge: Cambridge University Press, 1990; Kant, Immanuel. (1785) *Groundwork of the Metaphysic of Morals*. Trans. H. J. Paton. New York: Harper Torchbooks, 1964; Mill, John Stuart. (1859) *On Liberty*. New York: Appleton-Century-Crofts, 1947; Mill, John Stuart. (1863) *Utilitarianism*. Indianapolis, Ind.: Bobbs-Merrill, 1957; Moore, G. E. (1903) *Principia Ethica*. Cambridge: Cambridge University Press, 1959; Odell, S. Jack. *On Consequentialist Ethics*. Belmont, Calif.: Wadsworth, 2003; Odell, S. Jack. *On Moore*. Belmont, Calif.: Wadsworth, 2001; Odell, S. Jack. *On Russell*. Belmont, Calif.: Wadsworth, 2000; Odell, S. Jack. "Practice Consequentialism: A New Twist on an Old Theory." *Utilitas* 13:1 (2001), 86–105; Russell, Bertrand. *Human Society in Ethics and Politics*. New York: Simon and Schuster, 1955; Russell, Bertrand. (1929) *Marriage and Morals*. New York: Liveright, 1970; Sidgwick, Henry. (1874) *The Methods of Ethics*, 7th ed. London: Macmillan, 1907; Stephen, James Fitzjames. (1873) *Liberty, Equality, Fraternity*. London: Cambridge University Press, 1967; Wasserstrom, Richard A., ed. *Morality and the Law*. Belmont, Calif.: Wadsworth, 1971.

S. Jack Odell

ADDITIONAL READING

Abbey, Ruth. "Odd Bedfellows: Nietzsche and Mill on Marriage." *History of European Ideas* 23:2–4 (1997), 81–104; Anscombe, G.E.M. "Modern Moral Philosophy." *Philosophy* 33 (January 1958), 1–19. Reprinted in *The Collected Philosophical Papers of G.E.M. Anscombe*, vol. 3: *Ethics, Religion and Politics*. Oxford, U.K.: Blackwell, 1981, 26–42; Arrow, Kenneth J. (1951) *Social Choice and Individual Values*, 2nd ed. New Haven, Conn.: Yale University Press, 1963; Bentham, Jeremy. "An Essay on Paederasty." In Robert B. Baker and Frederick A. Elliston, eds., *Philosophy and Sex*, 2nd ed. Buffalo, N.Y.: Prometheus, 1984, 353–69; P&S3 (350–64); Bentham, Jeremy. "Offences against One's Self: Paederasty." *Journal of Homosexuality* 3 (1978), 383–405; continued in *Journal of Homosexuality* 4 (1978), 91–107; Brandt, Richard B. "Moral Obligation and General Welfare." *Ethical Theory: The Problems of Normative and Critical Ethics*. Englewood Cliffs, N.J.: Prentice-Hall, 1959, 380–406; Corvino, John. "Justice for Glenn and Stacy: On Gender, Morality, and Gay Rights." In James P. Sterba, ed., *Social and Political Philosophy: Contemporary Perspectives*. New York: Routledge, 2001, 300–318; Corvino, John. "Why Shouldn't Tommy and Jim Have Sex?" In John Corvino, ed., *Same Sex: Debating the Ethics, Science, and Culture of Homosexuality*. Lanham, Md.: Rowman and Littlefield, 1997, 3–16. Reprinted in James E. White, ed., *Contemporary Moral Problems*, 7th ed. Belmont, Calif.: Wadsworth, 2002, 308–18. Revised and reprinted as "Homosexuality: The Nature and Harm Arguments" in POS3 (137–48); POS4 (135–46); Crisp, Roger. "Teachers in an Age of Transition: Peter Singer and J. S Mill." In Dale Jamieson, ed., *Singer and His Critics*.

Oxford, U.K.: Blackwell, 1999, 85–102; Feinberg, Joel. "Harm and Offense." In Lawrence C. Becker and Charlotte B. Becker, eds., *Encyclopedia of Ethics*, 2nd ed., vol 2. New York: Routledge, 2001, 652–55; Feinberg, Joel. " 'Harmless Immoralities' and Offensive Nuisances." In Norman S. Care and Thomas K. Trelogan, eds., *Issues in Law and Morality*. Cleveland, Ohio: Press of Case Western Reserve University, 1973, 83–109. Reprinted in Joel Feinberg, *Rights, Justice, and the Bounds of Liberty: Essays in Social Philosophy*. Princeton, N.J.: Princeton University Press, 1980, 69–109; Feinberg, Joel. *The Moral Limits of the Criminal Law*, 4 vols. New York: Oxford University Press, 1984–1988; Ferguson, Frances. *Pornography, the Theory: What Utilitarianism Did to Action*. Chicago, Ill.: University of Chicago Press, 2004; Haber, Joram Graf, ed. *Absolutism and Its Consequentialist Critics*. Lanham, Md.: Rowman and Littlefield, 1994; Hooker, Brad. "The Collapse of Virtue Ethics." *Utilitas* 14:1 (2002), 22–40; Hursthouse, Rosalind. "Virtue Ethics vs. Rule-Consequentialism: A Reply to Brad Hooker." *Utilitas* 14:1 (2002), 41–53; Kristjansson, Kristjan. "Casual Sex Revisited." *Journal of Social Philosophy* 29:2 (1998), 97–108; Lyons, David. "Utilitarianism." In Lawrence C. Becker and Charlotte B. Becker, eds., *Encyclopedia of Ethics*, 2nd ed., vol. 3. New York: Routledge, 2001, 1737–44; Mill, John Stuart. (1869) *The Subjection of Women*. In Alice Rossi, ed., *Essays on Sex Equality: John Stuart Mill and Harriet Taylor Mill*. Chicago, Ill.: University of Chicago Press, 1970, 123–242; Mill, John Stuart. (1863) *Utilitarianism with Critical Essays*. Ed. Samuel Gorovitz. Indianapolis, Ind.: Bobbs-Merrill, 1971; Mohr, Richard D. "Four Millian Arguments for Gay Rights." In *Gays/Justice: A Study of Ethics, Society, and Law*. New York: Columbia University Press, 1988, 137–61; Railton, Peter. "Alienation, Consequentialism, and the Demands of Morality." *Philosophy and Public Affairs* 13:2 (1984), 134–71; Scarre, Geoffrey. "Utilitarianism." In Ruth Chadwick, ed., *Encyclopedia of Applied Ethics*, vol. 4. San Diego, Calif.: Academic Press, 1998, 439–49; Scheffler, Samuel. *The Rejection of Consequentialism*. Oxford, U.K.: Oxford University Press, 1982; Scheffler, Samuel, ed. *Consequentialism and Its Critics*. Oxford, U.K.: Oxford University Press, 1988; Sen, Amartya, and Bernard Williams, eds. *Utilitarianism and Beyond*. Cambridge: Cambridge University Press, 1982; Shanley, Mary Lyndon. "Marital Slavery and Friendship: John Stuart Mill's *The Subjection of Women*." *Political Theory* 9:2 (1981), 229–47. Reprinted in Mary Lyndon Shanley and Carole Pateman, eds., *Feminist Interpretations and Political Theory*. University Park: Pennsylvania State University Press, 1991, 164–80; Skipper, Robert. "Mill and Pornography." *Ethics* 103:4 (1993), 726–30; Slote, Michael. "Consequentialism." In Lawrence C. Becker and Charlotte B. Becker, eds., *Encyclopedia of Ethics*, 2nd ed., vol. 1. New York: Routledge, 2001, 304–7; Smart, J.J.C., and Bernard Williams. *Utilitarianism: For and Against*. Cambridge: Cambridge University Press, 1973; West, Henry R. *An Introduction to Mill's Utilitarian Ethics*. New York: Cambridge University Press, 2004.

CONSTRUCTIONISM. *See* Social Constructionism

CONTRACEPTION. Contraception can be achieved by timing and alteration of sexual intercourse and by barriers, devices, and medications. Some types of contraception function by preventing sperm from fertilizing ova. Other types disrupt the life cycle of early human gestation life forms, destroying them. The word "contraception" thus encompasses both the prevention of fertilization and the destruction of early human gestational life forms. Some of this destruction is accomplished by abortifacients, agents that disrupt a pregnancy by interfering with gestation after implantation of the preembryo in the uterine wall.

Ethical issues surrounding contraception came to prominence in the late 1960s and early 1970s (see Curran; Noonan, "Contraception"). Indeed, the ethical controversy over contraception played a role in the creation of the field of bioethics (see Jonsen), which developed into a large segment of the field of applied philosophical ethics. Contraception became ethically controversial, and has remained so, because there are competing, well-made arguments about the moral status of early human gestational life forms. These arguments come from secular philosophical ethics and from theological ethics or moral theology, which appeals to transcendent, sacred sources of moral standards and judgments.

Ethical issues in contraception concern mainly two topics. The first is the morality of sexual intercourse and whether contraception during intercourse (in the sense of preventing sperm from fertilizing ova) is permissible. The second is the moral status of fertilized ova, preembryos (developing fertilized ova not yet implanted in the uterine wall), embryos, and fetuses that are sometimes destroyed by contraceptive methods.

Ethical issues about preventing the fertilization of ova *in vivo* arise mainly in moral theology, that of Roman Catholicism in particular (for this history, see Noonan, *Contraception*). Roman Catholic moral theology draws on revelation in sacred texts, on the authoritative teachings of the Church, and on human reason. Like other Christian faiths, Roman Catholicism holds that God, in creating the world, made laws to which nature conforms. Since the laws originate in God, the font of all goodness, the laws are morally good. Natural laws thus not only establish how and why things happen in the world; they establish as well norms for moral judgments about what ought to happen in the world. Human behavior that violates the laws of nature is thus morally unacceptable.

Roman Catholicism is distinctive in teaching that natural law can be discovered on the basis of reason alone, unaided by faith, a claim that rests on appeals to scientific accounts of nature. Natural law creates objective moral standards of behavior and therefore grounds and directs moral judgment for everyone. The proposition that contraception—in the sense of taking deliberate steps designed, and therefore intended, to prevent sexual intercourse between a man and a woman from resulting in the fertilization of an ovum—violates natural law is one such moral judgment that binds all people capable of using reason, regardless of whether they share the theological commitments and convictions of the Roman Catholic faith, community, and tradition.

The Roman Catholic understanding of natural law developed long before Charles Darwin's (1809–1882) theory of "blind" **evolution** and differential reproductive success, the introduction of the concept of biological variability, and the resulting rejection of teleology (purpose in nature) in biological science. The older biology, with deep roots in the metaphysics of **Aristotle** (384–322 BCE), accepted teleology. Indeed, the older Roman Catholic Natural Law ethics (as found in, for example, **Saint Thomas Aquinas** [1224/25–1274]) cannot be understood apart from teleology.

The word "teleology" comes from a Greek root, *telos*, which means "end" or "purpose." In Aristotelian metaphysics, the end or purpose of a thing involves the perfection of its nature, the perfection of the kind of thing it is. Natural kinds—dogs, horses, human beings— have an ultimate purpose, their perfection, that they are designed by their Creator to achieve. (That this designer God exists can be established by reason, criticism of such arguments notwithstanding.) Activities also have natural ends they are designed to achieve; the achievement of these ends is essential to the goodness of those activities. These well-defined purposes of activities can be discovered by empirical investigation and reasoned reflection. Each activity has well-defined ends or purposes that are its naturally designed fulfillment or perfection. While the realization of these ends makes that activity good, the activity loses its moral worth when the ends are not realized.

According to Natural Law moral theory, if an activity is undertaken by human beings with the intent to disrupt or prevent the occurrence of the natural end for which God designed it, that activity violates natural law and is morally illicit. In the discourse of reason, the activity is judged ethically impermissible and prohibited. In theological discourse, the activity is labeled sinful and prohibited as well.

Roman Catholicism brings this way of thinking about the natural purposes of human activities to bear on sexual intercourse. Coitus between a man and woman has as its natural ends the uniting of a man and woman in marriage and procreating children. These ends are built into the reproductive organs of human beings. An activity during or following sexual intercourse that is designed and intended to prevent these natural ends from occurring is ethically impermissible; such activity would violate, as reason shows, the Natural Law standard that rightly governs and regulates sexual intercourse between a man and woman and *makes it morally good*. Interrupting sexual intercourse before male ejaculation (*coitus interruptus* or *coitus reservatus*) and use of douches, barrier techniques, and devices or medications that prevent sperm from fertilizing ova are ethically impermissible. They violate the unitive and procreative purposes of sexual intercourse between a man and woman. (Indeed, for a contemporary thinker in this tradition, Pope Paul VI [1897–1978], what is precisely wrong with contraception is that it deliberately *separates* the unitive end *from* the procreative end, whereas in God's design the two were meant to accompany each other inseparably. See "*Humanae vitae*.")

Natural Law reasoning invokes a teleological understanding of human biology: Biological activities have well-defined natural purposes. Biology after Darwin has been based on biological variability, a concept that rejects natural teleology in favor of the view that life forms and their organs and organ systems have *multiple* functions, none of which can be pinpointed as their one central purpose or end. (Think of the multiple purposes of the fingers—eating, writing, playing the piano, signaling, using a digit to clear a nostril or ear canal, some of which ends humans invented, taking advantage of biological structure.) None of these functions is definitive of the activity and therefore cannot serve to underwrite the thesis, central to teleology, that organs or organ systems have built-in ends. After Darwin, biology became a science of "functions," of variably patterned, purposeless, multiple processes of organ systems and organisms. A biological science that eschews teleology and ultimate ends has been successful in developing powerful explanations of phenomena. The intellectual and moral authority of reason unaided by faith requires appeal to the best science available. Modern biological science thoroughly rejects teleological conceptions of nature in general and of human physiology in particular. It therefore appears that the Roman Catholic objections to activities that are designed and intended to prevent fertilization of ova cannot be translated into the secular discourse of reason and therefore into philosophical ethics. This means that such objections lack intellectual and moral authority outside the Roman Catholic faith community.

There have been ongoing disputes within Roman Catholicism about the Church's teaching on contraception as announced in the 1968 papal encyclical "*Humanae vitae*" (Paul VI). This encyclical was issued after an interdisciplinary, international group had been convened to consider ethical challenges regarding contraception after the introduction of oral contraceptives or "birth-control pills." Paul VI rejected the advice of this commission, appointed by his predecessor, Pope John XXIII (1881–1963), to liberalize the Church's teaching on contraception. This led to a deep split within the Church between Paul VI and, on the other side, both theologians and laypersons who challenged the reasoning and conclusions of "*Humanae vitae*" (see Noonan, *Contraception*). Some of these theologians, such as Warren T. Reich (the editor-in-chief of the first two editions of the *Encyclopedia of Bioethics*), and laypersons such as André Hellegers (1926–1979), who founded the Kennedy Institute of Ethics at Georgetown University, and Daniel Callahan, who founded the Institute for Society, Ethics, and the Life Sciences (The Hastings Center) in New York, played major roles in the development of the new field of bioethics.

Secular, philosophical ethics proffers no particular objection to activities, devices, barriers, or medications that prevent the fertilization of ova. No line of reasoning establishes with final intellectual and moral authority—as pre-Darwinian Natural Law reasoning could—that clear and unalterable standards of moral judgment and behavior can be discovered in this matter. In contemporary philosophical bioethics, therefore, there is essentially no ongoing discussion of the ethics of contraception in the first of its two senses. However, ethical controversy continues about the second sense of contraception—preventing the fertilized ova from continuing cell division, migrating through the fallopian tubes to the uterus, implanting in the uterine wall, or the gestation of the embryo into a fetus. This ethical controversy is fueled by competing claims about the moral status of these early human life forms, a controversy that arises in the ethics of **abortion** as well.

To say that an entity has "moral status" means that others have obligations to it not to destroy it, to protect it from injury or destruction, and/or to nurture its continuing existence. Moral status can be self-generated, in which case an entity has independent moral status. Claiming that an entity has independent moral status requires an argument to show that some feature or features of the entity, which it has independently of other entities, generate the entity's moral status. For example, Kantian philosophers (disciples of **Immanuel Kant** [1724–1804]) argue that, in virtue of being rational and self-conscious, persons generate independent moral status. Moral status can also be conferred on one entity by another entity, in which case the first entity has dependent moral status. For example, some religious traditions hold that a creator God made human beings. As God's creatures or His property, all human beings have dependent moral status. In philosophical ethics, independent moral status is generally stronger than dependent moral status. In moral theology, by contrast, dependent moral status that originates in God's act of creation is stronger than any independent moral status.

The distinction between these two types of moral status is crucial for understanding the competing lines of argument that shape the controversy over early life forms. In philosophical ethics, claims that an entity has independent moral status require at the very least that the entity in question is sentient—it displays conscious awareness and can experience pain. Both awareness and pain require the existence of a functioning nervous system. Human gestational life forms of up to about three weeks (around the time of implantation in the uterine wall and development into an embryo) do not have nervous systems, so they cannot be considered sentient. They therefore cannot be considered to have independent moral status. This has obvious implications for the morality of contraceptive devices that destroy gestational life forms prior to three weeks.

Some philosophers have argued that, during human gestation, human life forms gradually acquire moral status, an ethical concept expressed in the discourse of "graded moral status" (see Strong). However, advocates of this line of philosophical argument do not think that graded moral status begins until later in pregnancy. Graded moral status therefore appears to have no application to the ethics of contraception that involves the destruction of early gestational human life forms.

Appeals to dependent moral status are not limited by whether the entity in question is capable of sentience. In particular, theological lines of reasoning that hold that God's creative act and power are under no such constraint can successfully claim that these early human life forms have dependent moral status. Advocates of this line of reasoning are therefore justified in claiming that these early human life forms have a God-given right to life. In public debates about the morality of abortion, often left unexpressed are the necessarily theological origins of a discourse of a "right to life" and its limitation to lines of reasoning appealing to dependent, not independent, moral status. The result has been to confuse public debate, not advance it.

Faith communities and traditions are, of course, free to instruct their members about the immorality of contraceptive methods that violate dependent moral status and the right to life that it generates. But in a pluralistic society such theological lines of reasoning have limited intellectual and therefore moral authority. Further, they cannot be translated into secular, philosophical discourse, because philosophical discourse is not obligated to accept accounts of a creator God as the origin of dependent moral status and because it cannot support, for reasons mentioned above, claims that very early gestational human life forms have independent moral status. As a result, contraceptive methods, including abortifacients that involve destruction of early human life forms, are not ethically controversial in philosophical ethics. But they can be controversial for some—but by no means all—faith communities and traditions.

Emergency contraception involves the use of medication administered immediately after unprotected sexual intercourse (whether voluntary or coerced) and can involve the destruction of early gestational human life forms (Cook and Dickens; Faundes et al.). Consideration of this issue requires the introduction of the concepts of individual and organizational conscience (McCullough and Chervenak, 111–12).

Matters of conscience concern our basic values and moral convictions, by which we live our lives and give meaning to them. Some of our values and convictions are rightly regarded as inviolable, either in all circumstances or only with very rare exceptions. To require an individual to act against his or her individual conscience is ordinarily regarded as ethically unacceptable, since such action would damage that individual's moral integrity. One exception is an individual in a well-defined social role that creates a duty to act in a certain way and no one else is available who can act. Every physician has an inescapable professional obligation in the informed **consent** process to inform women who have had unprotected sexual intercourse that there are medically reasonable alternatives to pregnancy (McCullough and Chervenak, 198–200). At the same time, physicians with conscience-based objections to abortion and therefore to abortifacients should not be obligated to violate their individual consciences; there are other physicians who do not have such objections and who can provide a prescription for emergency contraception and supervise its administration.

Not only individuals have consciences that others are obligated to respect; organizations can, too. In particular, health-care organizations supported by faith communities rightly base their mission and services on the values and convictions that define their supporting faith community. Many faith community–supported health-care organizations exist in the United States, and some, notably those sponsored by Roman Catholic and some Southern Baptist faith communities, do not permit termination of pregnancy or prescription of abortifacients for emergency contraception. In U.S. law and public policy this avoidance of abortion and abortifacients is allowed out of respect for organizational conscience, *when* the exercise of that conscience does not deny patients necessary medical care.

Emergency contraception presents ethical issues for such faith community–supported organizations and physicians who work in and for them. Physicians have an inescapable obligation in the disclosure component of the informed consent process to present to every patient all the medically reasonable alternatives to the patient for the management of her condition or problem. Emergency contraception is safe and effective and therefore is a medically reasonable alternative for managing the sequellae of unprotected sexual intercourse. If so, organizational policy that prohibits such disclosure on the basis of organizational conscience is ethically impermissible. The health-care organization cannot escape its share in the physician's fiduciary responsibilities to patients.

Both individuals and organizations can, however, justifiably place limits on the services provided to patients if two well-recognized conditions are met: Patients are informed about those limits and are free to seek medical care elsewhere. For voluntary emergency contraception these two conditions can be met. Women can elect to seek their medical care from physicians outside of faith-supported clinics and hospitals. If they seek care from such an organization, they can be rapidly informed about limits on services and immediately referred to physicians or clinics that provide this service. For emergency contraception following sexual assault, the condition of a voluntary choice by the woman cannot reasonably be met. Women who use emergency medical services or call the police after sexual assault are taken to the nearest emergency center—for the very good reason that their psychic and physical injuries, which may be life-threatening, require immediate medical or surgical attention. **Rape** involves more than sexual intercourse. Its sequellae are psychically and physically critical, not allowing luxurious "shopping" around for medical care facilities that are not restricted by organizational conscience.

The only way for an emergency center, situated in a faith-supported hospital that asserts organizational conscience–based objections to providing emergency contraception, to maintain its organizational integrity would be to work with local emergency medical services and police departments to ensure that sexual assault victims are transported to emergency centers that do not have organizational conscience objections. In large metropolitan areas this may be a practical solution, provided that the diversion does not result in a medically unacceptable delay in access to emergency center medical services; faith-supported hospitals are obligated, due to their fiduciary responsibility to patients who do not seek their services voluntarily, to provide immediate and effective referral. However, some sexual assault victims are not stable enough to be transferred to another facility. In such cases the federal Emergency Medical Treatment and Active Labor Act (1986) prohibits their transfer, and current standards of care would require administration of emergency contraception to women who consent to it. Damage to organizational integrity may therefore be an unavoidable risk for faith-supported hospitals that operate emergency centers. This issue becomes prominent when public hospitals are purchased by faith-supported hospitals or when the latter are given contracts to manage and staff the former. Whether faith-supported hospitals adhere to their fiduciary responsibilities to sexual assault victims who cannot be transferred is at least an open question and a serious health policy issue that has not been resolved in the United States.

See also Abortion; Anscombe, G.E.M.; Bible, Sex and the; Catholicism, Twentieth- and Twenty-First-Century; Consent; Evolution; Natural Law (New); Perversion, Sexual; Privacy; Psychology, Evolutionary; Rape; Reproductive Technology; Sex Education; Wojtyła, Karol (Pope John Paul II)

REFERENCES

Cook, R. J., and B. M. Dickens. "Access to Emergency Contraception." *Journal of Obstetrics and Gynaecology of Canada* 25:11 (2003), 914–16; Curran, Charles E. "Fertility Control: Ethical Issues." In Warren T. Reich, ed., *Encyclopedia of Bioethics*, 2nd ed. New York: Macmillan, 1995, 832–39; Faundes A., V. Brache, and F. Alverez. "Emergency Contraception—Clinical and Ethical Aspects." *International Journal of Gynaecology and Obstetrics* 82:3 (2003), 297–305; Jonsen, Albert. *The Birth of Bioethics.* New York: Oxford University Press, 2000; McCullough, Laurence B., and Frank A. Chervenak. *Ethics in Obstetrics and Gynecology.* New York: Oxford University Press, 1994; Noonan, John. "Contraception." In Warren T. Reich, ed., *Encyclopedia of Bioethics.* New York: Macmillan, 1978, 204–16; Noonan, John. (1965) *Contraception: A History of Its Treatment by the Catholic Theologians and Canonists,* enlarged ed. Cambridge, Mass.: Harvard University Press, 1986; Paul VI (Pope). "*Humanae vitae.*" *Catholic Mind* 66 (September 1968), 35–48; Reich, Warren T., ed. (1978) *Encyclopedia of Bioethics,* 2nd ed. New York: Macmillan, 1995; Strong, Carson. *Ethics in Reproductive and Perinatal Medicine: A New Framework.* New Haven, Conn.: Yale University Press, 1997.

Laurence B. McCullough

ADDITIONAL READING

Anscombe, G.E.M. [Elizabeth]. "Contraception and Chastity." *The Human World,* no. 7 (1972), 9–30. Reprinted in Michael D. Bayles, ed., *Ethics and Population.* Cambridge, Mass.: Schenkman, 1976, 134–53; Anscombe, G.E.M. "You Can Have Sex without Children: Christianity and the New Offer." In *Ethics, Religion, and Politics.* Minneapolis: University of Minnesota Press, 1981, 82–96; Beis, Richard H. "Contraception and the Logical Structure of the Thomist Natural Law Theory." *Ethics* 75:4 (1965), 277–84; Cahill, Lisa Sowle. "Grisez on Sex and Gender: A Feminist Theological Perspective." In Nigel Biggar and Rufus Black, eds., *The Revival of Natural Law: Philosophical, Theological and Ethical Responses to the Finnis-Grisez School.* Aldershot, U.K.: Ashgate, 2000, 242–61; Callahan, Joan C. "Birth-Control Ethics." In Ruth Chadwick, ed., *Encyclopedia of Applied Ethics,* vol. 1. San Diego, Calif.: Academic Press, 1998, 335–51; Cohen, Carl. "Sex, Birth Control, and Human Life." *Ethics* 79:4 (1969), 251–63. Reprinted in P&S1 (150–65); P&S2 (185–99); Cook, R. J., B. M. Dickens, C. Ngwena, and M. I. Plata. "Ethical and Legal Issues in Reproductive Health: The Legal Status of Emergency Contraception." *International Journal of Gynecology and Obstetrics* 75 (2001), 185–91; Dickens, B. M. "Reproductive Health Services and the Law and Ethics of Conscientious Objection." *Medical Law* 20:2 (2001), 283–93; Feldman, David. M. (1968) *Marital Relations, Birth Control, and Abortion in Jewish Law.* New York: Schocken, 1974; FIGO [International Federation of Obstetrics and Gynecology] Committee for the Ethical Aspects of Human Reproduction and Women's Health. "Ethical Guidelines Regarding Privacy and Confidentiality in Reproductive Medicine; Testing for Genetic Predisposition to Adult Onset Disease; Guidelines in Emergency Contraception." *International Journal of Gynecology and Obstetrics* 77 (2002), 171–75; Geach, Mary. "Marriage: Arguing to a First Principle in Sexual Ethics." In Luke Gormally, ed., *Moral Truth and Moral Tradition: Essays in Honour of Peter Geach and Elizabeth Anscombe.* Dublin, Ire.: Four Courts Press, 1994, 177–93; Glenmullen, Joseph. *The Pornographer's Grief and Other Tales of Human Sexuality.* New York: HarperCollins, 1993; Grisez, Germain. *Contraception and the Natural Law.* Milwaukee, Wis.: Bruce, 1964; Grisez, Germain, Joseph Boyle, John Finnis, William E. May, and John C. Ford. *The Teaching of "Humanae Vitae": A Defense.* San Francisco, Calif.: Ignatius Press, 1988; John Paul II (Pope). "*Evangelium Vitae.*" *Origins* 24:42 (1995), 689–727; Kosnick, Anthony, William Carroll, Agnes Cunningham, Ronald Modras, and James Schulte. *Human Sexuality: New Directions in American Catholic Thought.* New York: Paulist Press, 1977; Lowe, Pam. "Contraception and Heterosex: An Intimate Relationship." *Sexualities* 8:1 (2005), 75–92; Nicholson, Susan T. *Abortion and the Roman Catholic Church.* Knoxville, Tenn.: Religious Ethics, 1978; Paul VI (Pope). "*Humanae vitae.*" *Acta Apostolicae Sedis* 60:9 (1968), 481–503; *Catholic Mind* 66 (September 1968), 35–48. Reprinted in Claudia Carlen, ed., *The Papal Encyclicals 1958–1981.* Raleigh, N.C.: Pierian Press, 1990, 223–36; and P&S1 (131–49); P&S2 (167–84); P&S3 (96–105); Pius XI (Pope). "*Casti connubii*" ("On Christian Marriage"). *Catholic Mind* 29:2 (1931), 21–64; Singer, Irving, and Josephine Singer. "Periodicity of Sexual Desire in Relation to Time of Ovulation in Women." *Journal of Biosocial Science* 4 (November 1972), 471–81; Stubblefield, Anna. "Contraceptive Risk-taking and Norms of Chastity." *Journal of Social Philosophy* 27:3 (1996), 81–100; Watt, E. D. "Professor Cohen's Encyclical." *Ethics* 80:3 (1970), 218–21; Wilson, George B. "Christian Conjugal Morality and Contraception." In Francis X. Quinn, ed., *Population Ethics.* Washington,

D.C.: Corpus Books, 1968, 98–108; Winch, Peter, Bernard Williams, Michael Tanner, and G.E.M. Anscombe. "Discussion of 'Contraception and Chastity.' " In Michael D. Bayles, ed., *Ethics and Population*. Cambridge, Mass.: Schenkman, 1976, 154–63.

CYBERSEX. "Cybersex" is sometimes construed broadly to refer to a burgeoning array of erotically charged activities mediated by communications and information technology. These activities include, among other things, viewing sexually explicit videos online, sending by e-mail or instant messages flirtatious comments to a classmate, posting a personal profile on a Web site in search of an offline date, and bartering with an international sex trafficker (for these and others, see Döring; Hughes).

Analyses of cybersex in the broad sense feature in examinations of how new information technologies affect the meaning, experience, and politics of human sexuality and embodiment. Michael Heim regards Western culture's enthusiasm for computer technology as itself a Neo-Platonic expression of *eros*. Hubert Dreyfus invokes Maurice Merleau-Ponty (1908–1961) to lament the flight into cyberspace, away from the face-to-face encounters that ground trust and commitment. Others have variously developed neutral or more positive accounts of information technology, sexual embodiment, and the "postmodern" self (Haraway; Plant; Stone; Turkle). Zillah Eisenstein analyzes online sex within a broader discussion of new information technologies and global power relations.

More often, "cybersex" refers more narrowly to a "social interaction between at least two people who are exchanging real-time digital [video, audio, text-based] messages to become sexually aroused. People send provocative and erotic messages to each other, with the purpose of bringing each other to orgasm as they masturbate in real time" (Ben-Ze'ev, 5). Less restrictively, cybersex can be defined as a "computer mediated interpersonal interaction in which the participants are sexually motivated, meaning they are seeking sexual arousal and satisfaction" (Döring, 4). This definition encompasses both virtual reality–based cybersex and text-based cybersex.

Virtual reality–based cybersex involves "entering into a three-dimensional, audiovisual and tactile virtual reality via a full-body data suit and data helmet" (Döring, 5). As imagined by Howard Rheingold,

> [After] you put on your 3D glasses, you slip into a lightweight . . . bodysuit. . . . Embedded in the inner surface of the suit . . . is an array of intelligent sensor-effectors—a mesh of tiny tactile detectors coupled to vibrators of varying degrees of hardness, hundreds of them per square inch, that can receive and transmit a realistic sense of tactile presence, the way the audio and visual displays transmit a realistic sense of visual and auditory presence. . . . Now, imagine plugging your whole sound-sight-touch telepresence system into the telephone network. You see a lifelike but totally artificial visual representation of your own body and your partner's. . . . Your partner(s) can move independently in the cyberspace, and your representations are able to touch each other, even though your physical bodies might be continents apart. (346)

Though bodysuits were not available very early in the twenty-first century, prototype remote-controlled, computer-mediated sex toys were (Stein).

In "video-based cybersex," participants in online video conferences "take off their clothing, expose their bodies (especially their sexual organs) and watch each other during masturbation" (Döring, 5–6). In commercial video-based cybersex, clients pay to view a model via livecam; the clients e-mail or telephone directions for what the model should do (Hughes, 143–44; Rossney). "Text-based cybersex" involves the real-time exchange of short, explicit text messages in which "participants describe body characteristics to one another, verbalize sexual actions and reactions, and make believe that virtual happenings are real" (Döring, 6). Text-based cybersex requires a networked computer with suitable software and "an affinity for erotic verbalization, quick reading and typing skills, good writing ability, and a strong power of imagination" (Döring, 10). Text-based cybersex can be sorted into "TinySex" and "Hot Chat."

TinySex takes place in a MUD (Multi-user Domain), a computer-generated environment, having a particular theme, in which many persons can interact simultaneously. Once logged on, a person is represented in the MUD by a virtual character, established in a fictional self-description.

> MUDs put you in virtual spaces in which you are able to navigate, converse, and build. . . . For example, if I am playing the character named ST . . . any words I type after the command "say" will appear on all players' screens as "ST says." Any actions I type after the command "emote" will appear after my name just as I type them, as in "ST waves hi" or "ST laughs uncontrollably." I can "whisper" to a designated character and only that character will be able to see my words. (Turkle, 11)

The MUD program thus converts a character's first-person comments and actions into third-person reports on others' monitors.

Hot Chat is text-based cybersex that uses a chat program. Chat forums can be found on online services such as America OnLine and Compuserve as well as on the Internet, using Internet Relay Chat (IRC) channels that allow multiple users to connect to a live discussion. A person posts real-time messages to a virtual meeting place, where others are present and conversing. One then often withdraws to a private venue with a direct person-to-person connection to exchange more explicit sexual messages.

Some features of cybersex raise the conceptual question: Is cybersex really sex? Text-based cybersex *seems* at most carnal knowledge by description, not acquaintance (see **Bertrand Russell** [1872–1970]), as there is no "direct" bodily contact between participants. Though some text-based cybersex employs real-time messaging, some employs e-mail with significant time delays between sending and receiving erotic messages. (See Allan's *Lisa_33* for a twenty-first-century epistolary novel on this.) TinySex in MUDs sharpens the question whether writing first-person descriptions of the sexual activities of a virtual character or persona is tantamount to engaging in **sexual activity**. The possibility of virtual reality (VR) bodysuits, which would allow people to "feel" and see each other's body via an atypical electronic pathway, raises questions about the boundaries of the body and the locus of sexual union. Cybersex thus raises questions like: What is "sexual activity"? What is good sex? What is the relationship between imagined and real sexual acts? What is the relationship between one's personae in various venues and one's self?

Recent empirical studies suggest that many university students have tried cybersex (over 40 percent, according to Boies). Interpreting current data on whether students count cybersex as "sex" is tricky. According to one study, almost all students count vagina-penis coitus as "having sex," but very few (3.7 percent) describe **masturbation** in these terms, even when the masturbators are in the same room, and almost none (2.4 percent) so describe masturbation during computer contact or phone conversation (Randall and Byers, 91–92). Again, just over a third (34.1 percent) of the students agree that same-room masturbation involves a "sexual partner," but only half that (15.2 percent) say this about cybersex. Perhaps students take intercourse as the paradigm case of "real sex" and treat phone sex and cybersex as "less real" or "less sex," to the extent that they differ from direct flesh-to-flesh contact. Thus, masturbation with someone other than the beloved is slightly less likely to be described as being "unfaithful" if it is mediated by computer (78.7 percent) than if the masturbators are in the same room (94.5 percent). This leaves a puzzle: Despite strongly denying that masturbation during computer contact is "having sex" (97.6 percent) or involves a "sexual partner" (84.8 percent), the students (78.7 percent) did regard such cybersex with a third party as being "unfaithful." Perhaps most students put cybersex in the same class of sexual activity as solitary masturbation and believe that faithfulness requires abstention from any type of sexual activity that does not involve the beloved.

Conventionally, paradigmatic sexual activity requires direct physical contact, at least two people touching each other or two patches of epidermis rubbing against each other ("skin-to-skin contact"; Portmann, 231). Since there is no physical contact in Hot Chat, perhaps it belongs in the same category as the exchange of erotic letters, telephone sex, or coauthored **pornography** about the sex lives of virtual personae and not as sex between the writers/authors. Participants in Hot Chat, however, report that it can be as physically and emotionally compelling as paradigmatic sex, despite the absence of normal multisensory cues (Ben-Ze'ev, chap. 1). Sandy Stone suggests that phone sex might be arousing just because of the *dearth* of cues: "In phone sex, once the signifiers begin to 'float' loose from their moorings in a particularized physical experience, the most powerful attractor becomes the client's idealized fantasy. In this circumstance narrow bandwidth becomes a powerful asset, because extremely complex fantasies can be generated from a small set of cues" (94–95). The same may apply to Hot Chat. Further, Hot Chat sometimes leads to later offline trysts, so it might be classed as foreplay—sexual activity anticipatory of direct physical contact. But, and perhaps more to the point, Hot Chat might be categorized as sex proper, for even if the participants do not touch each other, what matters is that each is sexually aroused by the other's response to their text messages. If arousal rather than physical contact is central to the "sexual," phone sex and Hot Chat can be genuine sex. **Thomas Nagel**'s account of "natural" sex in terms of mutual arousal—which, in one of his examples, occurs by the people looking at each other through mirrors—seems pertinent here.

Anyway, it is not clear that direct physical contact is necessary for sexual activity: Sex using a dental dam or condom is not less sex for being safer (by preventing direct contact). As Nigel Warburton points out, sex between two people swathed in Saran wrap is still sex. The analytic problems here lie in both "direct" and "contact." Alan Goldman, for example, claims that "sexual desire is desire for contact with another person's body and for the pleasure which such contact brings; sexual activity is activity which tends to fulfill such desire of the agent. . . . [I]t is not a desire for a particular sensation detachable from its causal context, a sensation which can be derived in other ways" (268). On this view, cybersex—like experiences involving pornography—would be only "an imaginative substitute for the real thing" (270). Goldman's account, however, relies on an unexplicated notion of physical contact. Does half as much sex occur if participants are half-naked (or half-clothed)? An interesting feature of cyberspace is that it calls into question ordinary notions of "physical contact."

TinySex raises complex questions about the attribution of acts and agency. In a MUD, one assumes a named, fictional persona ("Pooh") by posting a self-description that need not match one's actual appearance, character, or species ("a stout and reliable bear"). The creator of Pooh types speech, actions, and reactions to be attributed to the persona "Pooh," not to the creator, the "author" of the Pooh character. For the sake of erotic arousal, Pooh's creator may initiate an encounter between Pooh and another persona, Piglet, scripted by another pseudonymous author. So "who it is that is communicating becomes unclear, and whether passion is being simulated or transmitted through the MUD becomes truly problematic" (Reid, 341). That MUD players find such encounters sexually arousing confirms, according to some, the postmodern claims that the self is multiple and fragmentary and that sex is an exchange of signifiers (Dibbell, 382; Turkle, 14–15).

One might argue that the question, "Has the author of Pooh had sex with Piglet?" is as wrongheaded as, "Did Shakespeare kill Macduff?" We can assert "Pooh had sex with Piglet" if the transcript of the MUD supports this reading, just as we can assert that "Macbeth killed Macduff " if the text of *Macbeth* supports that reading. No real sex took place in the MUD, any more than real killing occurs onstage at Stratford. Pooh's actions in the MUD do not reflect on the author's character, any more than Macbeth's actions in the play reflect on the actor playing Macbeth. But this line of thought does not sufficiently acknowledge the fact that the author of Pooh derived erotic pleasure, and perhaps masturbated, in response to what Pooh and Piglet did together in the MUD. Thus, "when this cyberspace self becomes the vehicle for real-life sexual arousal, what you think of as your 'real-life self' becomes implicated in whatever sexuality you experience on-line. Even if this cyberspace self is entirely fantastical . . . there is always some kind of 'real self' that is implicated insofar as you believe you had a role in deciding which fantasy persona to take on" (herrup, 245).

Perhaps TinySex, too, should be categorized as a kind of collaborative pornography, not sex proper. Still, even if TinySex may be closer to games or artistic improvisation than it is to sex, how we play games and improvise reflects our values, tastes, and moral personality. For example, consider a "virtual rape" in which a MUD player hijacks other players' characters and forcibly makes them perform unwanted sexual acts, distressing the characters' authors and onlookers (see Dibbell, 393; Turkle, 15). The decision to hijack a character and the subsequent indifference to the distress caused count against the virtue of the hijacking player. Here questions about the ethics of **fantasy** arise (see Neu).

Other questions are raised by VR bodysuits. Suppose that while wearing a VR bodysuit, your senses are being stimulated by the actions of someone in a bodysuit elsewhere. You respond not to a verbal description of the other's arousal but to sensory stimuli originating from the other's body, through a long and nonstandard causal chain. Might we see the VR suit as a prosthesis (glasses? stilts?) that extends the body's reach? It has been argued, to the contrary, that "digital machines of the late twentieth century are not [merely] add-on parts that serve to augment an existing human form. Quite beyond their own perceptions and control, bodies are continually engineered by the processes in which they engage" (Plant, 182). VR sex, then, should not be assimilated to sex with discrete tools (say, a dildo); rather, the immersive multimedia technology of VR changes the very boundaries of our bodies. On the other hand, a standard disproof of sexual infidelity has been to show that one (or one's body) was nowhere near the alleged sexual partner at the time sex was said to have occurred. So perhaps VR sex is not sex but only simulates it. This question is not idle: For those who believe that sex should occur only within monogamous relationships, determining whether cybersex is sex is important.

VR bodysuits, like Hot Chat, also create a gap between the **phenomenology** of sexual arousal and the other's body as the direct causal origin of arousing stimuli. Indeed, VR sex with another person might be qualitatively indistinguishable from "asymmetrical" VR sex, where there is no other person involved (and even indistinguishable from another type of asymmetrical sex: masturbation with fantasies of the other person). Warburton counts VR sex as sex where it involves awareness of the other's arousal through a fairly direct causal path. (Awareness of the other's arousal is the central ingredient of Nagel's account of psychologically normal sex.) Douglas Adeney allows that asymmetrical VR sex might only be fake sex but still preferable to no sex at all or even to real sex: to avoid transmitting diseases or because real sex is sometimes unsatisfying.

Similar questions arise from the possibility of being erotically aroused by a computer program—another form of asymmetry. Turkle (88 ff.) records the case of a student who flirts with the intelligent agent, Julia, which is programmed to generate appropriate e-mail responses to syntactic and semantic cues in incoming e-mails. For example, when asked, "Do you like doing X?" Julia generates a response through transformation rules replacing "you" with "I" and question formats with answer formats: "Yes, I *love* doing X." The student believes he is seducing a real woman. Robert Solomon argues that sex is paradigmatically communication between two people employing body **language** (60); if your partner cannot understand your communication, the sexual interaction is defective. Someone who advances Solomon's **communication model** of sexuality might want to distinguish between genuine and fake (say, Chinese box) communications to argue that the computer Julia cannot really understand the meaning of your typed symbols and hence that sex with "her" is either impossible or horribly semantically deviant (perhaps perverted, in a Solomonesque way). However, sex with a human sex worker who does not speak her client's language is still sex, even if the prostitute has merely memorized rote phrases from the john's language. So perhaps genuine understanding is necessary only for good sex. Instead, Solomon might in this case emphasize expressive body language, which in many cases is more important than verbal communication. The nonlinguistic body from any country *shows* that it is aroused; one need not say "I am aroused" in French or Arabic to express that message.

Cybersex, broadly defined, covers a wide range of phenomena in need of careful moral analysis. Data on the extent and nature of Internet usage for sexual purposes are available (Boies), as are studies of the impact of the Internet on sociability, courtship, and sexuality more generally (Kraut and Lundmark). Popular moralists and scholars have focused on pornography, particularly child pornography (and its putative link with online pedophile rings), virtual child pornography (Levy), cybersex **addiction**, cybersexual infidelity (Adamse and Motta; Fein and Schneider), online **sexual harassment**, including virtual stalking (Adam), and sexual trafficking of persons and images (Adam; Hughes). Discussion of ethical issues regarding the design of virtual environments (Brey; Ford) might be usefully applied to the design of interactive sex games (for example, Playboy CD-ROMs) and VR bodysuits.

Cybersex in its narrow sense also raises moral concerns. Because procreation cannot result from cybersex (or from masturbation or contracepted coitus), cybersex is, in the tradition of Roman Catholicism, among other religions, unnatural and hence immoral. But by the same token it carries no risk of unwanted pregnancy. Nor does it transmit venereal disease while providing pleasure. Yet cybersex cannot yield the benefit of wanted children and other advantages of "contact" sexuality. For **consequentialism**, these costs and benefits should influence the moral evaluation of cybersex. Other features of cybersex may matter. In entirely text-based cybersex, access to the other's body is always mediated by a textual representation under the other's control. For such cybersex to continue, at least one participant must continue typing, and that person's experience of immersion in sexual embodiment is constrained (temporarily or intermittently, at least). This feature of cybersex raises normative questions about authenticity, spontaneity, or alienation from one's body. On the other hand, text-based cybersex provides an opportunity to establish both **consent** and preferences as well as to announce and document promises and intentions, all concepts that play key roles not only in libertarian and liberal **sexual ethics** but also in some forms of deontology.

Cyberspace offers anonymous, discreet access to many potential cybersexual partners with a wide array of proclivities. That cybersex may be anonymous or pseudonymous raises questions about accountability and personal integrity, although these concerns arise in offline contexts, too. Sexual liberals welcome the broadening of opportunities for safe sexual experiences, especially for stigmatized sexual minorities, and favor expanding popular access to and reduced censorship or regulation of cyberspace. Exactly these opportunities are regarded with moral suspicion by sexual conservatives. Feminist theorists articulate a wide range of views about cyberspace and women's empowerment (see Döring).

Conceptual and metaphysical questions recur in moral debates about cybersex and interpersonal relationships. If one holds that the only proper occasion for sexual activity is within a committed relationship and that cybersex really is sex, then one must resolve the question whether a relationship conducted wholly online can count as a committed relationship (Collins; Dreyfus, 82–89). Similarly, if one thinks that sex is permissible only if it is an expression of **love**, one must then determine whether the virtual meeting of two minds can satisfy this condition or, instead, requires actually living together. Again, how should we judge virtual sex, which limits mutual physical vulnerability, if sex is morally valuable as expressing or deepening trust?

Cybersex underlines difficult questions about the relation between sex and gender, and their importance, particularly for those who believe only heterosex is permissible. If your partner in cybersex, who, unbeknownst to you, is anatomically male, consistently and convincingly described himself as female, while you, also anatomically male, described yourself as male to him, have you engaged in immoral gay cybersex or morally permissible heterosexual cybersex? What if your partner, when challenged, sincerely claims to be a woman trapped inside a man's body? Is her online self-presentation as female an expression of authenticity or culpably deceptive?

The epistemic features of cybersex allow profound deception, which go beyond familiar offline artifice to one's enhance sex appeal, such as cosmetics, elevator shoes, fibs about one's wealth, and so on (Bruckman; Reid). Cybersex allows more dramatic deceptions about one's anatomical sex, physical ability and age, and status. In one, much-discussed case from the early 1980s, when Internet bulletin boards were still novel, a shy male psychiatrist passed online as a feisty disabled woman who gave out lots of advice and seduced several of her online friends (Stone, 65–81; Van Gelder). Some of his/her friends were devastated by this betrayal, but others were less upset. Sorting out what honesty requires in cyberspace is complicated by the variety of online contexts and expectations. In a realm where people know that deception is commonplace and easy, deception may lose some of its immoral zing. Indeed, part of the appeal of TinySex is that it allows deceptive but consensual role-playing.

One might dismiss cybersex as the pursuit of simulated pleasures and as the repudiation of the risks and responsibilities of real relationships with actual embodied others. (This is a common objection to masturbation and pornography; see Nussbaum, 309.) However, occasional cybersex may benefit one's real-life partnerships by providing a safe venue "like a flight simulator" to practice transferable skills (Warburton). Further, cybersex may be an attempt to resist or escape the unfair and unchosen limits the real world imposes. If, for example, as a matter of bad luck one happens to be ugly by conventional standards of **beauty**, in a society that treats the ugly as sexual pariahs, one might find in cyberspace a community where beauty is defined differently or where one can fictionally present oneself as attractive. (For a similar defense of **prostitution**, see Califia.) If sex has an important place in a flourishing life, we should not dismiss cybersex as trivial.

See also Activity, Sexual; Addiction, Sexual; Adultery; Casual Sex; Communication Model; Completeness, Sexual; Existentialism; Fantasy; Friendship; Lacan, Jacques; Language; Liberalism; Love; Masturbation; Orientation, Sexual; Prostitution; Sex Work

REFERENCES

Adam, Alison. "Cyberstalking and Internet Pornography: Gender and the Gaze." *Ethics and Information Technology* 4:2 (2002), 133–42; Adamse, Michael, and Sheree Motta. *On-Line Friendships, Chatroom Romance, and Cybersex: Your Guide to Affairs of the Net.* Deerfield Beach, Fla.: Health Communication, 1996; Adeney, Douglas. "Evaluating the Pleasures of Cybersex." *Australasian Journal of Professional and Applied Ethics* 1:1 (1999), 69–79; Allan, Dan. *Lisa_33: A Novel.* New York: Viking, 2003; Ben-Ze'ev, Aaron. *Love Online: Emotions on the Internet.* Cambridge: Cambridge University Press, 2004; Boies, Sylvain C. "University Students' Uses of and Reactions to On-line Sexual Information and Entertainment: Links to Online and Offline Sexual Behaviour." *Canadian Journal of Human Sexuality* 11:2 (2002), 77–89; Brey, Philip. "The Ethics of Representation and Action in Virtual Reality." *Ethics and Information Technology* 1:1 (1999), 5–14; Bruckman, Amy S. "Gender Swapping on the Internet." In Peter Ludlow, ed., *High Noon on the Electronic Frontier: Conceptual Issues in Cyberspace.* Cambridge, Mass.: MIT Press, 1996, 317–25; Califia, Pat. "Whoring in Utopia." In *Public Sex: The Culture of Radical Sex.* Pittsburgh, Pa.: Cleis Press, 1994, 242–48; Collins, Louise. "Emotional Adultery: Cybersex and Commitment." *Social Theory and Practice* 25:2 (1999), 243–70; Dibbell, Julian. "A Rape in Cyberspace; or How an Evil Clown, a Haitian Trickster Spirit, Two Wizards, and a Cast of Dozens Turned a Database into a Society." In Peter Ludlow, ed., *High Noon on the Electronic Frontier: Conceptual Issues in Cyberspace.* Cambridge, Mass.: MIT Press, 1996, 375–95; Döring, Nicola. "Feminist Views of Cybersex: Victimization, Liberation, and Empowerment." *CyberPsychology and Behavior* 3:5 (2000), 863–84. <www.liebertpub.com/CPB/> [accessed 8 September 2004]; Dreyfus, Hubert L. *On the Internet.* New York: Routledge, 2001; Eisenstein, Zillah. *Global Obscenities: Patriarchy, Capitalism, and the Lure of Cyberfantasy.* New York: New York University Press, 1998; Fein, Ellen, and Sherrie Schneider. *The Rules for Online Dating: Capturing the Heart of Mr. Right in Cyberspace.* New York: Simon and Schuster, 2002; Ford, Paul J. "A Further Analysis of the Ethics of Representation in Virtual Reality: Multi-User Environments." *Ethics and Information Technology* 3:2 (2001), 113–21; Goldman, Alan. "Plain Sex." *Philosophy and Public Affairs* 6:3 (1977), 267–87; Haraway, Donna. (1985) "A Manifesto for Cyborgs." In Linda J. Nicholson, ed., *Feminism/Postmodernism.* New York: Routledge, 1990, 190–233; Heim, Michael. *The Metaphysics of Virtual Reality.* New York: Oxford University Press, 1993; herrup, mocha jean. "Virtual Identity." In Rebecca Walker, ed., *To Be Real: Telling the Truth and Changing the Face of Feminism.* New York: Doubleday, 1995, 239–51; Hughes, Donna M. "The Use of New Communications and Information Technologies for Sexual Exploitation of Women and Children." *Hastings Women's Law Journal* 13:1 (2002), 129–48; Kraut, Robert, and Vicki Lundmark (HomeNet Group). "Internet Paradox: A Social Technology That Reduces Social Involvement and Psychological Well-Being?" *American Psychologist* 53:9 (1998), 1017–31; Levy, Neil. "Virtual Child Pornography: The Eroticization of Inequality." *Ethics and Information Technology* 4:4 (2002), 319–23; Nagel, Thomas. "Sexual Perversion." In Alan Soble, ed., *The Philosophy of Sex: Contemporary Readings*, 2nd ed. Savage, Md.: Rowman and Littlefield, 1991, 39–51; Neu, Jerome. "An Ethics of Fantasy?" *Journal of Theoretical and Philosophical Psychology* 22:2 (2002), 133–57; Nussbaum, Martha C. "Objectification." In Alan Soble, ed., *The Philosophy of Sex: Contemporary Readings*, 3rd ed. Lanham, Md.: Rowman and Littlefield, 1997, 283–321; Plant, Sadie. *Zeros + Ones:*

Digital Women + the New Technoculture. London: Fourth Estate, 1997; Portmann, John. "Chatting Is Not Cheating." In John Portmann, ed., *In Defense of Sin.* New York: Palgrave, 2002, 223–41; Randall, Hilary E., and E. Sandra Byers. "What Is Sex? Students' Definitions of Having Sex, Sexual Partner, and Unfaithful Sexual Behaviour." *Canadian Journal of Human Sexuality* 12:2 (2003), 87–96; Reid, Elizabeth M. "Text-Based Virtual Realities: Identity and the Cyborg Body." In Peter Ludlow, ed., *High Noon on the Electronic Frontier: Conceptual Issues in Cyberspace.* Cambridge, Mass.: MIT Press, 1996, 327–45; Rheingold, Howard. *Virtual Reality: The Revolutionary Technology of Computer-Generated Artificial Worlds—and How It Promises to Transform Society.* New York: Simon and Schuster, 1992; Rossney, Robert. "The Next Best Thing to Being There." *Wired* 3:5 (1995). <www.wired.com/wired/archive/3.05/best.html> [accessed 27 September 2004]; Russell, Bertrand. (1912) "Knowledge by Acquaintance and Knowledge by Description." In *The Problems of Philosophy.* Oxford, U.K.: Oxford University Press, 1959, 46–59; Solomon, Robert. "Sexual Paradigms." In Alan Soble, ed., *The Philosophy of Sex: Contemporary Readings,* 2nd ed. Savage, Md.: Rowman and Littlefield, 1991, 53–62; Stein, Joel. "Will Cybersex Be Better Than Real Sex?" *Time* 155:25 (19 June 2000), 62, 64; Stone, Sandy [Stone, Allucquère Rosanne] *The War of Desire and Technology at the Close of the Mechanical Age.* Cambridge, Mass.: MIT Press, 1995; Turkle, Sherry. *Life on the Screen: Identity in the Age of the Internet.* New York: Simon and Schuster, 1995; Van Gelder, Lindsy. (1985) "The Strange Case of the Electronic Lover." In Rob Kling, ed., *Computerization and Controversy: Value Conflicts and Social Choices,* 2nd ed. San Diego, Calif.: Academic Press, 1996, 533–46; Warburton, Nigel. "Virtual Fidelity." *Cogito* (November 1996), 193–99.

Louise Collins

ADDITIONAL READING

Adeney, Douglas, and John Weckert. "Virtual Sex." *Res Publica* 4:2 (1995), 7–16; Braidotti, Rosi. "Cyberfeminism with a Difference." Universiteit Utrecht. <www.let.uu.nl/womens_studies/rosi/cyberfem.htm> [accessed 8 September 2004]; Branscomb, Anne Wells. "Internet Babylon? Does the Carnegie Mellon Study of Pornography on the Information Superhighway Reveal a Threat to the Stability of Society?" *Georgetown Law Journal* 83 (1995), 1935–57; Burnett, Robert, and P. David Marshall. *Web Theory: An Introduction.* New York: Routledge, 2003; Butterworth, Dianne. (1993) "Wanking in Cyberspace: The Development of Computer Porn." In Stevi Jackson and Sue Scott, eds., *Feminism and Sexuality: A Reader.* New York: Columbia University Press, 1996, 314–20; Califia, Pat. "Whoring in Utopia." In *Public Sex: The Culture of Radical Sex.* Pittsburgh, Pa.: Cleis Press, 1994, 242–48. Reprinted in POS4 (475–81); Cavalier, Robert J., ed. *The Impact of the Internet on Our Moral Lives.* Albany: State University of New York Press, 2005; Cooper, Al, ed. *Cybersex: The Dark Side of the Force.* New York: Brunner-Routledge, 2000; Cooper, Al, ed. *Sex and the Internet: A Guide Book for Clinicians.* New York: Brunner-Routledge, 2002; Cooper, Joel, and Kimberlee D. Weaver. *Gender and Computers: Understanding the Digital Divide.* Mahwah, N.J.: Erlbaum, 2003; Delmonico, David L. "Sex on the Superhighway: Understanding and Treating Cybersex Addiction." In Patrick J. Carnes and Kenneth M. Adams, eds., *Clinical Management of Sex Addiction.* New York: Brunner-Routledge, 2002, 239–54; Denizet-Lewis, Benoit. "Friends, Friends with Benefits, and the Benefits of the Local Mall." *New York Times Magazine* (30 May 2004), 30, 35, 54–59; Dyson, Esther. *Release 2.0: A Design for Living in the Digital Age.* New York: Broadway Books, 1997; Estlund, David M. "The Visit and the Video: Publication and the Line between Sex and Speech." In David M. Estlund and Martha C. Nussbaum, eds., *Sex, Preference, and Family: Essays on Law and Nature.* New York: Oxford University Press, 1997, 126–47; Goldman, Alan. "Plain Sex." *Philosophy and Public Affairs* 6:3 (1977), 267–87. Reprinted in HS (103–23); POS1 (119–38); POS2 (73–92); POS3 (39–55); POS4 (39–55); Green, Eileen, and Alison Adam, eds. *Virtual Gender: Technology, Consumption, and Identity.* New York: Routledge, 2001; Hayles, Katherine N. *How We Became Posthuman: Virtual Bodies in Cybernetics, Literature, and Informatics.* Chicago, Ill.: University of Chicago Press, 1999; Horn, Stacy. *Cyberville: Clicks, Culture, and the Creation of an Online Town.* New York: Warner Books, 1998; Hughes, Donna M. "The Internet and Sex Industries: Partners in

Global Sexual Exploitation." *IEEE Technology and Society Magazine* (Spring 2000), 35–42. <www.uri.edu/artsci/wms/hughes> [accessed 14 October 2004]; Hughes, Donna M. "Prostitution Online." *Journal of Trauma Practice* 2:3–4 (2003), 115–32. <www.uri.edu/artsci/wms/hughes/prostitution_online.pdf> [accessed 21 September 2004]; Hughes, Donna M. "Sex Tours via the Internet." *Agenda: A Journal about Women and Gender*, no. 28 (1996), 71–76; Johnson, Peter. "Pornography Drives Technology: Why Not to Censor the Internet." *Federal Communications Law Journal* 49:3 (1996–1997). <www.law.indiana.edu/fclj/pubs/v49/no1/johnson.html> [accessed 8 September 2004]; Kantrowitz, Barbara. "Men, Women, and Computers." *Newsweek* (16 May 1994), 48–55; King, C. Richard. "Siren Scream of Telesex: Speech, Seduction, and Simulation." *Journal of Popular Culture* 30:3 (1996), 91–101; Kipnis, Laura. "Fantasy in America: *The United States v. Daniel Thomas DePew*." In *Bound and Gagged: Pornography and the Politics of Fantasy in America*. New York: Grove Press, 1996, 3–63; Kraut, Robert, and Vicki Lundmark (HomeNet Group). "Social Impact of the Internet: What Does it Mean?" *Communications of the ACM* 41:12 (1998), 21–22; Leiblum, Sandra, and Nicola Döring. "Internet Sexuality: Known Risks and Fresh Chances for Women." In Al Cooper, ed., *Sex and the Internet: A Guide Book for Clinicians*. New York: Brunner-Routledge, 2002, 19–45; Ludlow, Peter, ed. *High Noon on the Electronic Frontier: Conceptual Issues in Cyberspace*. Cambridge, Mass.: MIT Press, 1996; MacKinnon, Catherine A. "Vindication and Resistance: A Response to the Carnegie Mellon Study of Pornography in Cyberspace." *Georgetown Law Journal* 83:4 (1995), 1959–67; Maheu, Marlene M., and Rona B. Subotnik. *Infidelity on the Internet: Virtual Relationships and Real Betrayal*. Naperville, Ill.: Sourcebooks, 2001; Meyer, Carlin. "Reclaiming Sex from the Pornographers: Cybersexual Possibilities." *Georgetown Law Journal* 83 (1995), 1969–2008; Miller, Laura. "Women and Children First: Gender and the Settling of the Electronic Frontier." In James Brook and Iain A. Boal, eds., *Resisting the Virtual Life: The Culture and Politics of Information*. San Francisco, Calif.: City Lights Books, 1995, 49–57; Nagel, Thomas. "Sexual Perversion." *Journal of Philosophy* 66:1 (1969), 5–17. Reprinted in P&S1 (247–60); P&S2 (268–79); POS1 (76–88). Reprinted, revised, in Thomas Nagel, *Mortal Questions*. Cambridge: Cambridge University Press, 1979, 39–52; and P&S3 (326–36); POS2 (39–51); POS3 (9–20); POS4 (9–20); STW (105–12); Newitz, Annalee. "Cracking the Code to Romance." *Wired* 12:6 (2004). <www.wired.com/wired/archive/12.06/dating.html> [accessed 8 September 2004]; Nussbaum, Martha C. "Objectification." *Philosophy and Public Affairs* 24:4 (1995), 249–91. Reprinted in POS3 (283–321); POS4 (381–419). Reprinted, revised, in *Sex and Social Justice*. New York: Oxford University Press, 1999, 213–39; Patterson, Zabet. "Going On-line: Consuming Pornography in the Digital Eta." In Linda Williams, ed., *Porn Studies*. Durham, N.C.: Duke University Press, 2004, 104–23; Perry, Ruth, and Lisa Greber. (1990) "Women and Computers: An Introduction." In Barbara Laslett, Sally Gregory Kohlstedt, Helen Longino, and Evelynn Hammonds, eds., *Gender and Scientific Authority*. Chicago, Ill.: University of Chicago Press, 1996, 155–82; Pollitt, Katha. "Webstalker: When It's Time to Stop Checking on Your Ex." *The New Yorker* (19 January 2004), 38–42; Posner, Richard A., and Katharine B. Silbaugh. "Obscene Communication." In *A Guide to America's Sex Laws*. Chicago, Ill.: University of Chicago Press, 1996, 217–32; Rimm, Marty. "Marketing Pornography on the Information Superhighway: A Survey of 917,410 Images, Descriptions, Short Stories, and Animations Downloaded 8.5 Million Times by Consumers in Over 2000 Cities in Forty Countries, Provinces, and Territories." *Georgetown Law Journal* 83 (1995), 1849–1934; Sampaio, Anna, and Janni Aragon. "Filtered Feminisms: Cybersex, E-Commerce, and the Construction of Women's Bodies in Cyberspace." *Women's Studies Quarterly* 3–4 (2001), 126–47; Schiesel, Seth. "The Internet's Wilder Side." *New York Times* (6 May 2004), G1, G6; Schiesel, Seth. "Voyager to a Strange Planet." *New York Times* (12 June 2003), G1, G9; Schneider, Jennifer. "Effects of Cybersex Addiction on the Family: Results of a Survey." In Al Cooper, ed., *Cybersex: The Dark Side of the Force*. New York: Brunner-Routledge, 2000, 31–58; Schneider, Jennifer, and Robert Weiss. *Cybersex Exposed: Simple Fantasy or Obsession?* Center City, Minn.: Hazelden, 2001; Small, Meredith F. "The Naked Ape in Cyberspace." In *What's Love Got to Do with It?* New York: Anchor Books, 1995, 203–8; Solomon, Robert C. "Sexual Paradigms." *Journal of Philosophy* 71:11 (1974), 336–45. Reprinted in HS (81–90); POS1 (89–98); POS2 (53–62); POS3 (21–29); POS4 (21–29); Spender, Dale. *Nattering on the Net: Women, Power and Cyberspace*. Melbourne, Australia: Spinifex Press, 1996; Van Gelder, Lindsy. "The Strange Case of the Electronic Lover." In Charles Dunlop and Rob Kling, eds., *Computerization and Controversy: Value Conflicts and Social Choices*, 1st ed. San Diego, Calif.: Academic Press, 1991, 364–75; Wajcman, Judy. *Technofeminism*. Malden, Mass.: Polity, 2004; Wysocki, Diane Kholos. "Let Your Fingers Do the Talking: Sex on the Adult Chat-line." *Sexualities* 1:4 (1998), 425–52.

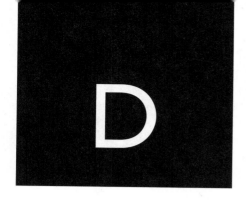

DARWIN, CHARLES. *See* Evolution

DATE RAPE. *See* Rape, Acquaintance and Date

DESCARTES, RENÉ (1596–1650). French philosopher René Descartes, who also did groundbreaking work in mathematics and science, was born in La Haye, Touraine. He lost his mother in infancy, suffered from frail health, was educated by the Jesuits at La Flèche, never married, lived in several countries without settling down, led a private and quiet life, maintained voluminous correspondence with virtually all the major minds of Europe, and died in Stockholm shortly after going to Sweden to be philosopher-in-residence at the court of Queen Christina (1626–1689). Descartes had a brief affair with a Dutch servant, Helène Jans, about which he remarked, "Only a little while ago I was young; I am a man and did not take a vow of chastity, and have never claimed to pass as better behaved than other men" (Rodis-Lewis, 138). Descartes acknowledged their daughter, Francine (1635–1640), arranged for them to live near him (despite frequently moving), and was deeply grieved by Francine's early death.

Descartes is best known in philosophy for his contributions to epistemology and metaphysics, particularly for his radical mind-body dualism (see *Meditations*), according to which the mind is a thinking, conscious, substance (*res cogitans*), and the body is only matter extended in space (*res extensa*). This view constituted a profound break with philosophy in the tradition of **Aristotle** (384–322 BCE) and **Thomas Aquinas** (1224/25–1274); it entailed rejecting teleology (purposiveness) in nature and committed Descartes to explaining bodily processes mechanistically. Descartes viewed life as a kind of heat produced in the organs of the body by a process similar to fermentation. In his account of reproduction, each of the sexes produces a sort of seminal fluid that acts as a kind of yeast for the other, thereby generating the heat that is the essence of life. Male and female thus have equal parts to play (*Description of the Human Body*, 322). Although Descartes's philosophical innovations threatened to undercut the metaphysical foundations of the tradition's understanding of sexuality, his views about **love**, desire, and sexuality remained conventional. He discussed these in letters and his last book, *Passions of the Soul*. This book grew out of his correspondence with Princess Elizabeth of Bohemia (1618–1680), who had been pressing Descartes to explain how mind, a *res cogitans*, could interact or join with body, a *res extensa*.

The passions are important for understanding the way mind and body are joined, for they are "so close and so internal to our soul that it cannot possibly feel them unless they are truly as it feels them to be" (*Passions*, art. 26). Yet passions are "caused, maintained and strengthened by some movement of the spirits" (art. 27; "spirits" refers to animal spirits, i.e., tiny, fast-moving particles involved in perception and movement). They "dispose our soul to want the things which nature deems useful for us, and to persist in this volition; and the same agitation of the spirits which normally causes the passions also disposes the body to make movements which help us to attain these things" (art. 52). Far from judging the passions evil, Descartes says, "I have found almost all of them to be good and to be so useful to this life that our soul would have no reason to wish to remain joined to its body for even one minute if it could not feel them" (letter to Pierre Chanut [1601–1662], 1 November 1646; *Oeuvres*, vol. IV, 538). "[P]ersons whom the passions can move most deeply are capable of enjoying the sweetest pleasures of this life" (art. 212).

There are, for Descartes, six primitive passions: wonder, love, hate, desire, joy, and sadness. Love is "an emotion of the soul caused by a movement of the spirits that prompts (*inciter*) the soul to join itself in volition (*de volunté*) to objects that appear agreeable" (*Passions*, art. 79; translation by author [see *Oeuvres*, vol. XI, 387]). More precisely, love is "the assent by which we consider ourselves henceforth as joined with what we love in such a manner that we imagine a whole, of which we take ourselves to be only one part, and the thing loved to be the other" (art. 80). Love covers a wide variety of phenomena, ranging from the prenatal infant's love for food to our love for God (letter to Chanut, 1 February 1647; Kenny, 211–15). It is commonly associated with a mysterious heat around the heart and a tendency to open our arms as if to embrace something (Kenny, 209). (Descartes provides much fanciful physiology but oddly never mentions the genitals, even though **sexual desire** must obviously involve them.) Sometimes in the "whole" or "union" of love we regard ourselves as the larger, more important part. However, we might also regard ourselves as the less important part, as happens with a father's love for his child and a soldier's love for his country. In these cases, we are ready to sacrifice even our lives for the other. We perceive other people as capable of becoming a "second self" (*un autre soi-même*; art. 90). Love thus enables the soul to break out of its isolation and egoism. (For Descartes on love, see Beavers; Frierson. Other philosophers who propose a "union" account of love or desire include **Plato** [427–347 BCE], Michel Montaigne [1533–1592], **G.W.F. Hegel** [1770–1831], and Robert Nozick [1938–2002]; see Soble.)

Desire is forward-looking and moves us to attain a good or avoid an evil. Sexual desire is a result of normal maturation. "Nature has established a difference of sex in human beings, as in animals lacking reason, and with this she has also implanted certain impressions in the brain which bring it about that at a certain age and time, we regard ourselves as deficient—as forming only one half of a whole, whose other half must be a person of the opposite sex." When we observe something attractive in another person, our soul "feel[s] towards that one alone all the inclination which nature gives it to pursue the good which it represents as the greatest we could possibly possess" (*Passions*, art. 90). The physical causes that move us to love one person more than another, even before we know their merit, are dispositions or arrangements of the parts of our brain sometimes, but not always, caused by previous experiences (letter to Chanut, 6 June 1647; *Oeuvres*, vol. V, 56–57).

Passions based on attraction, being perceived through the senses, strongly affect the soul, but they are also "the most deceptive of the passions, against which we must guard ourselves most carefully" (*Passions*, art. 85). Love is more powerful than hatred, and disordered love is more harmful than hatred because there is "more danger in being united with, and almost transformed into, a thing which is bad than in being separated in volition from one that is good" (letter to Chanut, 1 February 1647; Kenny, 216). Citing a poem about Paris setting Troy ablaze to cool his passion for Helen, Descartes remarks that the greatest evils of love are those done only for the pleasure of the beloved or oneself.

Mastery of the passions is the key to happiness. Knowledge of what is truly good is essential, and we should not desire with passion what does not depend on us (a decidedly Stoic element in Descartes). We cannot control our passions directly, since we continue to feel them until the agitation of spirits subsides, so we need to manage them indirectly. Descartes offers a variety of practical suggestions for doing so. Sometimes we must wait them out, refraining from action, directing our attention to something else. Over time we can retrain ourselves and acquire new habits. Sometimes merely realizing the cause of some inclination may free us from it, as Descartes's realization that he was drawn to cross-eyed people because of his childhood love for a cross-eyed girl freed him from feeling this inclination any more (letter to Chanut, 6 June 1647; *Oeuvres*, vol. V, 56–58).

Human sexuality is rooted in the body, and longing for a member of the opposite sex arises naturally in our development. We were made this way by a benevolent God, so we know it is for our good. We have, however, no detailed knowledge about the almighty's purposes, so specific norms governing sexual behavior must come from revelation or social convention.

See also Aristotle; Desire, Sexual; Fichte, Johann Gottlieb; Hegel, G.W.F.; Hume, David; Leibniz, Gottfried; Love; Plato; Roman Sexuality and Philosophy, Ancient; Schopenhauer, Arthur; Spinoza, Baruch; Thomas Aquinas (Saint)

REFERENCES

Beavers, Anthony. "Desire and Love in Descartes' Late Philosophy." *History of Philosophy Quarterly* 6:3 (1989), 279–94; Descartes, René. (1664) *Description of the Human Body*. In John Cottingham, Robert Stoothoff, and Dugald Murdoch, eds., *The Philosophical Writings of Descartes*, vol. 1. Cambridge: Cambridge University Press, 1985, 314–24; Descartes, René. (1641) *Meditations on First Philosophy, with Selections from the Objections and Replies*, revised ed. Trans. and ed. John Cottingham. Cambridge: Cambridge University Press, 1996; Descartes, René. *Oeuvres de Descartes*, revised ed., 12 vols. Ed. Charles Adam and Paul Tannery. Paris: Vrin, 1964–1976; Descartes, René. *The Passions of the Soul*. In Charles Adam and Paul Tannery, eds., *Oeuvres de Descartes*, vol. XI. Paris: Vrin, 1967, 327–488; Descartes, René. *The Passions of the Soul*. (1649) In John Cottingham, Robert Stoothoff, and Dugald Murdoch, eds., *The Philosophical Writings of Descartes*, vol. 1. Cambridge: Cambridge University Press, 1985, 328–404; Frierson, Patrick. "Learning to Love: From Egoism to Generosity in Descartes." *Journal of the History of Philosophy* 40:3 (2002), 313–38; Kenny, Anthony, ed. *Descartes: Philosophical Letters*. Trans. Anthony Kenny. Minneapolis: University of Minnesota Press, 1981; Rodis-Lewis, Geneviève. *Descartes: His Life and Thought*. Trans. Jane Todd. Ithaca, N.Y.: Cornell University Press, 1998; Soble, Alan. "Union, Autonomy, and Concern." In Roger Lamb, ed., *Love Analyzed*. Boulder, Colo.: Westview, 1997, 65–92.

Celia Wolf-Devine

ADDITIONAL READING

Beavers, Anthony F. "Passion and Sexual Desire in Descartes." *Philosophy and Theology* 12:2 (2000), 223–43; revision of "Passion and Sexual Desire in Descartes." *Philosophy and Theology* 2:5 (disk suppl. no. 1), 1988; Bordo, Susan. "The Cartesian Masculinization of Thought." In Sandra Harding and Jean O'Barr, eds., *Sex and Scientific Inquiry*. Chicago, Ill.: University of Chicago Press, 1987, 247–64; Bordo, Susan. *The Flight to Objectivity: Essays on Cartesianism and Culture*. Albany: State University of New York Press, 1987; Bordo, Susan, ed. *Feminist Interpretations of*

Descartes. University Park: Pennsylvania State University Press, 1999; Cottingham, John G., ed. *The Cambridge Companion to Descartes*. Cambridge: Cambridge University Press, 1992; Cottingham, John, Robert Stoothoff, and Dugald Murdoch, eds. *The Philosophical Writings of Descartes*. Vols. 1 and 2: Trans. John Cottingham, Robert Stoothoff, and Dugald Murdoch. Cambridge: Cambridge University Press, 1985. Vol. 3: *The Correspondence*: Trans. John Cottingham, Robert Stoothoff, Dugald Murdoch, and Anthony Kenny. Cambridge: Cambridge University Press, 1991; Damasio, Antonio. *Descartes' Error: Emotion, Reason, and the Human Brain*. New York: Avon, 1994; Descartes, René. *Les Passions de 'Âme*. Introduction and notes by Geneviève Rodis-Lewis. Paris: Librairie Philosophique J. Vrin, 1955; Freud, Sigmund. (1929) "Some Dreams of Descartes': A Letter to Maxime Leroy." In *The Standard Edition of the Complete Psychological Works of Sigmund Freud*, vol. 21. Trans. James Strachey. London: Hogarth Press, 1953–1974, 203–4; Gombay, Andre, and Byron Williston, eds. *Passion and Virtue in Descartes*. Amherst, N.Y.: Humanity Books, 2003; Matheron, Alexander. "Amour, digestion, et puissance selon Descartes." *Revue philosophique de la France et de l'etranger*, no. 4 (1988), 433–45; Montaigne, Michel. (1572/1595) "On Affectionate Relationships." In M. A. Screech, ed. and trans., *The Essays of Michel de Montaigne*. London: Penguin, 1991, 205–19; Morgan, Vance. *Foundations of Cartesian Ethics*. Atlantic Highlands, N.J.: Humanities Press, 1994; Nozick, Robert. "Love's Bond." In *The Examined Life*. New York: Simon and Schuster, 1989, 68–86. Reprinted in STW (231–40); Nye, Andrea. *The Princess and the Philosopher: Letters of Elizabeth of the Palatine to René Descartes*. Lanham, Md.: Rowman and Littlefield, 1999; Seidel, George. *Knowledge as Sexual Metaphor*. Selinsgrove, Pa.: Susquehanna University Press, 2000; Stern, Karl. *The Flight from Woman*. New York: Farrar, Straus and Giroux, 1965. Reprint, New York: Noonday Press, 1970; Voss, Stephen. "Cartesian Love." Forthcoming. Information available at <voss@boun.edu.tr>.

DESIRE, SEXUAL. The combination of a powerful phenomenology and multiple layers of social meaning makes sexual desire an inevitable but challenging subject for philosophical analysis. In sexual desire the forces of biology and culture rise simultaneously to the level of consciousness, focusing our thoughts, invading our imaginations, and flooding our bodies with anticipation and excitement. But our thoughts, imaginations, and bodies have been instructed by family, church, and state, all of which demand a stake in how sexual desire is expressed and satisfied. Philosophical reflections on sexual desire have three foci. First, philosophers seek a proper place for sexual desire within prior theories of human nature and human society. Second, they are concerned to understand the complex relationships between sexual desire and other sexual concepts; sexual pleasure, **sexual activity**, **sexual perversion**, and sexual arousal all have intimate ties to sexual desire. Finally, philosophers provide analyses of the concept, hoping to get a glimpse of what sexual desire is, itself, in the fog of special interests that seek to regulate sexual attitudes and practices.

Early discussions of sexual desire were concerned to situate it within a wider normative setting, invariably with an eye to regulation and reform. Nonetheless, it is possible to discern in outline the characteristic features of sexual desire. **Plato** (427–347 BCE) located sexual desire among the bodily appetites, capable of regulation by reason, and so with a proper (if subordinate) place in a just person's soul. In his *Symposium*, the priestess Diotima instructs Socrates that, with increased wisdom, a felt desire (*eros*) for "one beautiful body only" (210b) develops into a desire for "converse with the true beauty simple and divine" (211e) of which that one body is only a tarnished reflection. To aid our better selves in the control of sexual desire, the Stoic Emperor Marcus Aurelius (121–180 CE) recommended that we see the goal of sexual desire for what it truly is: the mere "attrition of an entrail and a convulsive expulsion of mere mucus" (bk. VI, 13).

With the transition from Hellenistic to Christian philosophy, sexual desire was transformed from a part of the soul in need of restraint to a demon in need of exorcism. **Saint Augustine** (354–430) portrayed the insubordination of sexual desire (and the sexual organs) as proof of our fallen state (bk. XIV, chap. 17), and he speculates that, in their original sinless state, Adam and Eve would have engaged in sexual intercourse without the involuntary responses that make it passionately pleasurable for fallen, postlapsarian humans. If there was pleasure in sex, it was comparable to the pleasure in gardening (bk. XIV, chap. 23), and only the wish to fulfill their duty, to obey God's command to "be fruitful and multiply," provided Adam and Eve with a reason to engage in intercourse (not, as commonly with us, the anticipation of body-convulsing orgasms). **Thomas Aquinas** (1224/25–1274) surmised that Adam and Eve would have found sex even more pleasurable than we do, but the prospect of such pleasure would not have excited them to "lust" (*Summa theologiae* Ia, ques. 98, art. 2, reply 3). Sexual desire, as lust, disappears from Eden because only reproduction, not pleasure, is the goal of prelapsarian sexual activity.

Immanuel Kant (1724–1804) held that because sexual desire is not desire for the whole person, it led to treating the other as an object and hence to the "debasement of humanity" (156)—unless it was first sheltered by the covenant of **marriage**. But under that shelter, Kant generously allowed that the pleasures of sex were so considerable that it would be "altogether too scrupulous to forbid married couples those intimacies which are not immediately connected with propagation" (22). **Arthur Schopenhauer** (1788–1860) contended that "the sexual impulse" is always subservient to a biological imperative, but that "nature can only attain its ends by implanting a certain illusion in the individual . . . so that when he serves the species he imagines he is serving himself" (vol. 2, 345–46). The identification of the true aim of sexual desire (propagation of the species) exposes as illusory the experience of the individual, who only imagines that he "seeks the heightening of his own pleasure" (347). Here, as with Plato, it is tempting to conjecture that the elevation of the aims of sexual desire to a higher metaphysical purpose is meant to lend it a respectability that it otherwise lacks. To that extent, Schopenhauer's analysis may still be rooted in a concern for the reformation of sexual attitudes.

In the twentieth century, philosophical accounts of sexual desire reached a new level of sophistication in Jean-Paul Sartre's (1905–1980) phenomenological analysis of sexual desire and experience in *Being and Nothingness*. Much subsequent work (e.g., Roger Taylor, **Thomas Nagel**, James Giles) shows his direct influence. On Sartre's view, sexual desire is desire for a "double reciprocal incarnation" (508) of two persons. We desire another person, whose consciousness will respond involuntarily to our caresses by flooding into and enlivening her body. As her consciousness fills her flesh under our touch, she transforms into an object for us. In the process, our own consciousness responds to her, and we are incarnated and objectified in return. The goal of sexual desire is a fully reciprocal absorption of two consciousnesses into the flesh of two bodies. In Sartre's development of this idea, our desires aim at an ideal they never fully achieve, and by falling short of the ideal, our sexual practices inevitably collapse into one or another form of sexual perversion (515–16; see Oaklander). In his seminal essay "Sexual Perversion," Nagel proposed a less pessimistic, but deeply Sartrean, account of perversion, which stimulated serious reflection on the nature of sexual desire for the next generation of philosophers. (It was critiqued immediately by Robert Solomon.) On Nagel's view, as on Sartre's, sexual desire has an ideal aim essentially involving another person; so long as we desire part of the ideal, our desire for it will be sexual, but to the extent that we desire anything less than the whole, our desire will be perverse.

Recent philosophical discussions of sexual desire address two closely related problems. First, there is the conceptual or analytic problem of determining what constitutes a desire *as* sexual. An illuminating conceptual analysis will help clarify the related concepts of sexual activity, sexual pleasure, and sexual perversion. Second, given the multiple layers of historical and cultural investment in the control of sexual desire, it seems a properly philosophical task to identify and unmask any mythologies or illusions that obscure our view of it. These two concerns are inseparable if "analysis" is understood as the sifting of what is universal or essential in sexual desire from its historically and culturally local guises (Goldman, 267). But the idea has also been defended that sexuality is "socially constructed," in which case there is nothing universal to be discovered behind the many masks worn by sexual desire (see **Michel Foucault** [1926–1984], *History*, 150–57; "Sex, Power"). **Social constructionism** need not deny biological realities; more plausibly, it often contends that what qualifies as sexual desire emerges only after our biological urges are subjected to socialization.

Two assumptions frame conceptual analyses of sexual desire. First, all desires that are "sexual" are assumed to share features in virtue of which they are included in the category. Second, it is assumed that desires are best categorized by identifying their "objects," that is, the aims or objectives of subjects who experience the desires. Jointly, these assumptions imply that saying what constitutes a desire as "sexual" requires locating a common object (or type of object) for all instances of sexual desire. As Solomon expresses the idea, "Sexual desire is distinguished, like all desires, by its aims and objects" (337).

It is of only limited help in identifying the objects of sexual desire to ask people what they desire, since our sincere avowals of desire will reveal a wildly heterogeneous assortment of acts and partners. The *avowed objects* of sexual desire will include pleasure, the infliction of pain, the exercise of power, feelings of vulnerability, or simply peeking through keyholes. In seeking a common factor in the midst of this variety, philosophical analysis is motivated by the idea that our prephilosophical avowals of sexual desire fail to provide a sufficiently unifying description of its many objects. Further, and more dramatically, there is Plato's idea that we are typically mistaken about *which* objects or activities we sexually desire. Philosophers thus seek to describe a *constitutive object* of desire, that is, an object-type such that desiring any object of this type is necessary and sufficient for constituting the desire as sexual.

There are two natural candidates for the constitutive object of desire: sexual pleasure and sexual activity. One proposal counts the concept of sexual pleasure as the more basic concept, then characterizes sexual desire as a desire for a *sui generis* sexual pleasure. On such a view, the constitutive sexual pleasures are a species of culturally universal bodily sensations, prior to any accretion of social meanings (Goldman, 267; Primoratz, 43, 46; Soble, *Sexual Investigations*, 123–24). But the concept of pleasure is itself a scene of disagreement. If sexual pleasure consists in bodily sensations, and sexual desire is desire for sexual pleasure, then our sexual activities and our sexual partners are means to other ends. We may care about our lovers in other, nonsexual, ways, but such concern will not be essential for sexual desire. If these sensations could be produced by electrical stimulation of the brain, sexual acts and partners would be sexually dispensable.

Following **Aristotle** (384–322 BCE), both Solomon (341) and Gareth Moore (203) recommend a more robust model of sexual pleasure. We can distinguish the bodily sensations that *result from* an activity and the pleasure (enjoyment) *taken in* it. In this model, the enjoyment to be had in a particular activity is intrinsically tied to the activity. The pleasures associated with reading a novel or making **love** are distinct kinds of pleasure, but only because the activities are of distinct kinds. If so, producing in other ways the bodily sensations that accompany these activities will not constitute enjoying the activities. Now, if sexual pleasure is enjoying an activity, then our concept of sexual pleasure is parasitic on the prior concept of sexual activity. Thus sexual desire would be better analyzed by reference to the distinctive sorts of activities desired and not to the sensations the activities produce.

Characterizing the constitutive objects of sexual desire as "sexual activity" requires first sorting sexual from nonsexual activities. Any effort at sorting will be problematic, because the activities we ordinarily count as sexual are themselves heterogeneous, ranging from a sensuous kiss to sodomy, wearing furs, or inflicting pain. The existence of sexual perversions threatens to explode any coherent category of distinctively sexual activities (see Gray). In principle, any activity might be the object of a sexual desire. Furthermore, the object of one person's sexual desire might be the object of another person's nonsexual desire. When Sambian boys perform fellatio on adult males as part of a ritual for attaining masculinity by insemination, informants insist that the practice is not sexual but akin to breast-feeding (**Gilbert Herdt**, 62, 69–70). If we can accept this, we should also accept that the adult male's desire is paternal, not sexual.

Such examples encourage social constructionists (Shrage, 350–51; contrast Soble, *Sexual Investigations*, 124–26, 154–55) but can also suggest that the desires that motivate our activities should be given a more prominent place in our understanding of other sexual concepts. A desire to touch another person's genitals in administering a medical examination need not be sexual, but a desire to fondle them is, even if the two activities are behaviorally indistinguishable. We might, however, distinguish touching and fondling in terms of their psychological origins (say, their motivations; Neu, 207–8). If fondling is physically indistinguishable from nonsexual touching, it is plausible that sexual fondling must be identified as the sexual activity it is in terms of the sexual desire it expresses or reveals. If so, the concept of sexual desire is conceptually prior to the concept of sexual activity.

These considerations are far from conclusive, but it is easy to see how sexual desire could be pivotal in the effort to understand other sexual concepts. If distinctively sexual pleasure is identifiable only in terms of the distinctively sexual activities we enjoy, and if sexual activities are identifiable only in terms of the sexual desires that enervate them, we first need to know what constitutes a desire as sexual.

One issue dividing philosophers is whether a description of the constitutive object of sexual desire should make essential reference to the experiences of other persons. Central to Sartre's account was the idea that the goals of sexual desire are essentially interpersonal: To have sexual desire is to desire to incarnate the consciousness of another person. Sartre was not the first to insist on the interpersonal nature of sexual desire. **Thomas Hobbes** (1588–1679) had earlier characterized it as "two appetites together, to please and to be pleased," in which he discerned the "delight men take in delighting" ("Human Nature," chap. 9, sec. 15). Such delight cannot be had without others and cannot be desired without incorporating the experiences of others into the contents of our desires.

This idea has provoked a fruitful debate: Those who assign importance to the interpersonal character of sexual desire (Simon Blackburn; Giles; Nagel; **Roger Scruton**; Solomon) have lined up against those who emphasize the more solipsistic pleasures of sex (Primoratz, 42–46; Soble, *Sexual Investigations*, 80–90) or those wishing to restore respectability to anonymous sexual encounters or **masturbation**. Resolving this debate may require, among other things, a fuller exploration of sexual **fantasy** (Soble, "Introduction," 16–17). Masturbation is typically accompanied by fantasy, the content of which may better reflect the true objects of our desires than does our actual sexual practice. If the content of sexual fantasy includes other persons and their experiences, solitary masturbation may not express a solipsistic desire (see Solomon, 343). Conversely, persons with truly solipsistic desires might be thought to employ fantasies about solitary masturbation to aid in their sexual interactions with others.

This issue divides philosophers who already agree that sexual desire is desire for sexual pleasure; the relevant pleasure may itself be either solipsistic or, as Hobbes thought, interpersonal ("delight in delighting"). Seiriol Morgan, for whom sexual pleasure is the constitutive aim of sexual desire, defends pluralism about sexual pleasure, arguing that it comes in different forms in different scenarios, ranging from solipsistic pleasures to pleasures laden with interpersonal meaning (7). Moore also counts both sorts of pleasures as sexual but argues that only "relational pleasures . . . occurring within a relationship between specific persons" can qualify as the objects of a sexual *desire*. The more solipsistic pleasures are better viewed as the relief of a bodily urge, in which other persons serve as "scratching posts for [a] sexual itch" (202).

Accounts of the constitutive object also disagree about whether sexual desire has as its object a *particular* individual or is, instead, unfocused, with generic objects. A desire for a glass of water is not usually for a particular glass of water but for something generic, and many different glasses of water would satisfy it. But a sexual desire for Reneé is not a desire for just any Reneé. Nagel (8) and Scruton (76, 78–82, 90) argue that sexual desire is "nontransferable," that the object of sexual desire is not replaceable by another as object of that desire. A desire to have sex with a tall person is not a sexual desire unless it focuses on a particular tall person. If the direction of our interest shifts to other persons, we have not transferred our original desire to a new object but have gained a new desire.

This might appear to be only a concern with individuating and counting sexual desires, but also at stake is our understanding of what the *satisfaction* of sexual desire consists. If (1) the satisfaction of a sexual desire consists in sexual pleasure (or the release of sexual tension) and (2) the object of a sexual desire is *whatever* satisfies it, then sexual desire has a generic object. Blackburn employs both (1) and (2) to argue that a randy sailor, returning to shore after long **abstinence**, desires only "relief from womanlessness. But that can be a genuine [sexual] desire or lust" (106). By contrast, Moore rejects (1), arguing that we should count the satisfaction that any generic person could bring as the *relief of a felt bodily urge* (or "need") and not the *satisfaction of desire* (203). In effect, Moore distinguishes lust (randiness), which can be assuaged by generic partners, from desire, which can be satisfied only by the particular person who is its object.

In a closely related maneuver, the fundamental assumption that sexual desire is to be analyzed by identifying a constitutive object has also been challenged. Some philosophers locate the defining feature of sexual desire not in its objects but in its accompanying phenomenological or physiological states. On such a view, we can say that sexual desires have as their objects just the variety of persons or activities that we prephilosophically avow. But what constitutes desires for those persons or activities as sexual are the distinctive bodily states employed to identify the desires, not the distinctive objects of those desires.

According to Jerome Shaffer, the defining feature of sexual desire is that the occurrence of certain bodily states will "constitute the satisfaction or fulfilment of the desire" (186), even though "the desire is not for the particular state that will constitute satisfaction of it" (184). Shaffer thus accepts (1) but rejects (2). His idea is subtle and best clarified with the help of an analogy. Hunger is an objectless bodily state, associated with (but not identical to) a desire to eat. Nonetheless, the satisfaction of our hunger can sometimes be the satisfaction of a desire to eat. This allows us to define a subset of desires to eat (those satisfied by satiating our hunger) without reference to the particular dishes desired. Similarly, Shaffer maintains that in sexual desire we do not envision a particular object of desire in advance (its object is thus generic), but we find that particular bodily arousals or occurrences will satisfy our desire. In these cases, our desire is sexual.

In a related strategy, what constitutes a desire as sexual is not the object at which it aims, or the bodily events that satisfy it, but the distinctive property in virtue of which the object is found to be desirable. An analogy will again be helpful. A desire to exercise is a desire to engage in any of countless activities bearing little resemblance to one another, but all of which are desired for their effect on our physical health. Many of these activities can be immensely enjoyable, and if chosen for pleasure, they will still be good exercise. But if chosen for pleasure, our desire for them will not be a desire for exercise. Similarly, a sexual desire will be a desire for any activity whatsoever, provided that the activity is found desirable in virtue of its anticipated effects on our bodily states of sexual arousal (see Jacobsen). If two persons desire the same activity, but one desires it for the effect it has on bodily arousal, while the other desires it for the money it pays, only the first has a sexual desire. Both these proposals (Shaffer's and Jacobsen's) give an essential role to sexual arousal, which is itself conceived as an objectless state distinct from, and conceptually prior to, sexual desire. The challenge to both views is to distinguish between sexual and nonsexual bodily arousal without employing the concept of sexual desire.

Ongoing debates concern the kind of object needed to constitute a desire for it as sexual but also whether sexual desire can best be defined by its objects. In the effort to address such questions, philosophers find themselves inextricably entangled with a knot of sexual concepts, including sexual pleasure, activity, fantasy, arousal, and perversion. Understanding sexual desire will involve unraveling the entire knot. Such concerns seem increasingly remote from the more overt interest of earlier philosophers in sexual reform, but that appearance may be deceptive. We have seen that analyses of sexual desire typically discount or redescribe our avowed objects of desire and presume that a desire is constituted as sexual by some fact about its object that falls outside the purview of the person who experiences the desire. But if Oedipus had known the truth about the object of his sexual desire (that she was his mother), that knowledge would have ended his desire. Any genuinely informative new description of the objects of our desires can transform our desires—they can be heightened, diminished, or extinguished by our changing perspective on their objects. This seemed evident to Marcus Aurelius, whose less-than-enticing description of sexual intercourse was intended to dampen our desire for it. If changing our beliefs about what we desire can change our desires, then philosophical analyses of sexual desire may still be implicated in the ancient project of sexual reform that was initiated by Plato, Aurelius, and Augustine.

See also Activity, Sexual; Aristotle; Augustine (Saint); Buddhism; Catholicism, History of; Communication Model; Completeness, Sexual; Existentialism; Fantasy; Foucault, Michel; Herdt, Gilbert; Hobbes, Thomas; Hume, David; Indian Erotology; Kant, Immanuel; Masturbation; Nagel, Thomas; Perversion, Sexual; Plato; Protestantism, History of; Schopenhauer, Arthur; Scruton, Roger; Social Constructionism; Thomas Aquinas (Saint)

REFERENCES

Aristotle. (ca. 325 BCE?) *Nicomachean Ethics*. Trans. David Ross. Oxford, U.K.: Oxford University Press, 1980; Augustine. (413–427) *The City of God*. Trans. Henry Bettenson. London: Penguin, 1984; Aurelius, Marcus. (167 CE) *Meditations*. Trans. and ed. A.S.L. Farquharson. New York: Knopf,

1946; Blackburn, Simon. *Lust: The Seven Deadly Sins*. New York: Oxford University Press/New York Public Library, 2004; Foucault, Michel. *The History of Sexuality*, vol. 1: *An Introduction*. Trans. Robert Hurley. New York: Vintage, 1978; Foucault, Michel. "Sex, Power, and the Politics of Identity." In Paul Rabinow, ed., *Ethics: Subjectivity and Truth*. [*Essential Works of Foucault 1954–1984*, vol. 1] New York: New Press, 1994, 163–73; Giles, James. "A Theory of Love and Sexual Desire." *Journal for the Theory of Social Behaviour* 24:4 (1994), 339–57; Goldman, Alan. "Plain Sex." *Philosophy and Public Affairs* 6:3 (1977), 267–87; Gray, Robert. "Sex and Sexual Perversion." *Journal of Philosophy* 75:4 (1978), 189–99; Herdt, Gilbert. "Fetish and Fantasy in Sambia Initiation." In Gilbert Herdt, ed., *Rituals of Manhood: Male Initiation in Papua New Guinea*. Berkeley: University of California Press, 1982, 44–97; Hobbes, Thomas. (1640) *The Elements of Law Natural and Politic*. Ed. J.C.A. Gaskin. Oxford, U.K.: Oxford University Press, 1994; Jacobsen, Rockney. "Arousal and the Ends of Desire." *Philosophy and Phenomenological Research* 53:3 (1993), 617–32; Kant, Immanuel. (ca. 1762–1794) *Lectures on Ethics*. Trans. Peter Heath. Ed. Peter Heath and J. B. Schneewind. Cambridge: Cambridge University Press, 1997; Moore, Gareth. "Sexual Needs and Sexual Pleasures." *International Philosophical Quarterly* 35:2 (1995), 193–204; Morgan, Seiriol. "Sex in the Head." *Journal of Applied Philosophy* 20:1 (2003), 1–16; Nagel, Thomas. "Sexual Perversion." *Journal of Philosophy* 66:1 (1969), 5–17; Neu, Jerome. "Freud and Perversion." In Jerome Neu, ed., *The Cambridge Companion to Freud*. Cambridge: Cambridge University Press, 1991, 175–208; Oaklander, L. Nathan. "Sartre on Sex." In Alan Soble, ed., *The Philosophy of Sex: Contemporary Readings*, 1st ed. Totowa, N.J.: Rowman and Littlefield, 1980, 190–206; Plato. (ca. 380 BCE) *Symposium of Plato*. Trans. Tom Griffith. (1986) Berkeley: University of California Press, 1989; Primoratz, Igor. *Ethics and Sex*. London: Routledge, 1999; Sartre, Jean-Paul. (1943) *Being and Nothingness: A Phenomenological Essay on Ontology*. Trans. Hazel Barnes. New York: Washington Square Press, 1956; Schopenhauer, Arthur. (1818/1844/1859) *The World as Will and Idea*, 2 vols. Trans. Richard B. Haldane and John Kemp. London: Routledge and Kegan Paul, 1883; Scruton, Roger. *Sexual Desire: A Moral Philosophy of the Erotic*. New York: Free Press, 1986; Shaffer, Jerome A. "Sexual Desire." *Journal of Philosophy* 75:4 (1978), 175–89; Shrage, Laurie. "Should Feminists Oppose Prostitution?" *Ethics* 99:2 (1989), 347–61; Soble, Alan. "An Introduction to the Philosophy of Sex." In *The Philosophy of Sex: Contemporary Readings*, 1st ed. Totowa, N.J.: Rowman and Littlefield, 1980, 1–56; Soble, Alan. *Sexual Investigations*. New York: New York University Press, 1996; Solomon, Robert. "Sexual Paradigms." *Journal of Philosophy* 71:11 (1974), 336–45; Taylor, Roger. "Sexual Experiences." *Proceedings of the Aristotlean Society* 68 (1967–1968), 87–104; Thomas Aquinas. (1265–1273) *Summa theologiae*, 60 vols. Trans. Blackfriars. Cambridge, U.K.: Blackfriars, 1964–1976.

Rockney Jacobsen

ADDITIONAL READING

Baier, Glen. "A Proper Arbiter of Pleasure: Rousseau on the Control of Sexual Desire." *Philosophical Forum* 30:1 (1999), 249–68; Benn, Piers. "Is Sex Morally Special?" *Journal of Applied Philosophy* 16:3 (1999), 235–45; Dillon, Martin C. "Erotic Desire." *Research in Phenomenology* 15 (1985), 145–63; Frye, Marilyn. "Lesbian 'Sex.'" In Jeffner Allen, ed., *Lesbian Philosophies and Cultures*. Albany: State University of New York Press, 1990, 305–15. Reprinted in *Willful Virgin: Essays in Feminism 1976–1992*. Freedom, Calif.: Crossing Press, 1992, 109–19; and Anne Minas, ed., *Gender Basics: Feminist Perspectives on Women and Men*, 1st ed. Belmont, Calif.: Wadsworth, 1993, 328–33; Fuchs, Eric. (1979) *Sexual Desire and Love: Origins and History of the Christian Ethic of Sexuality and Marriage*. Trans. Marsha Daigle. New York: Seabury Press, 1983; Giles, James. *The Nature of Sexual Desire*. Westport, Conn.: Praeger, 2004; Giles, James. "Sartre, Sexual Desire, and Relations with Others." In James Giles, ed., *French Existentialism: Consciousness, Ethics, and Relations with Others*. Amsterdam, Holland: Rodopi, 1999, 155–73; Goldman, Alan. "Plain Sex." *Philosophy and Public Affairs* 6:3 (1977), 267–87. Reprinted in HS (103–23); POS1 (119–38); POS2 (73–92); POS3 (39–55); POS4 (39–55); Gray, Robert. "Sex and Sexual Perversion." *Journal of*

Philosophy 75:4 (1978), 189–99. Reprinted in POS1 (158–68); POS3 (57–66); POS4 (57–66); Hamilton, Christopher. "Sex." In *Living Philosophy: Reflections on Life, Meaning and Morality.* Edinburgh, Scot.: Edinburgh University Press, 2001, 125–41; Herdt, Gilbert. *Rituals of Manhood: Male Initiation in Papua New Guinea.* Berkeley: University of California Press, 1982; Hocquenghem, Guy. *Homosexual Desire.* Trans. Daniella Dangoor. London: Allison and Busby, 1978. Durham, N.C.: Duke University Press, 1993; Ketchum, Sara Ann. "The Good, the Bad and the Perverted: Sexual Paradigms Revisited." In Alan Soble, ed., *The Philosophy of Sex: Contemporary Readings,* 1st ed. Totowa, N.J.: Rowman and Littlefield, 1980, 139–57; Koertge, Noretta. "Constructing Concepts of Sexuality: A Philosophical Commentary." In David McWhirter, Stephanie Sanders, and June Reinisch, eds., *Homosexuality/Heterosexuality: Concepts of Sexual Orientation.* New York: Oxford University Press, 1990, 387–97; Levine, Steven. "Re-exploring the Concept of Sexual Desire." *Journal of Sex and Marital Therapy* 28:1 (2002), 39–51; MacKinnon, Catharine A. "Desire and Power: A Feminist Perspective." In Cary Nelson and Lawrence Grossberg, eds., *Marxism and the Interpretation of Culture.* Urbana: University of Illinois Press, 1988, 105–21; Martin, Christopher F. J. "Are There Virtues and Vices That Belong Specifically to the Sexual Life?" *Acta Philosophica* 4:2 (1995), 205–21; Morgan, Seiriol. "Dark Desires." *Ethical Theory and Moral Practice* 6:4 (2003), 377–410; Moulton, Janice. "Sexual Behavior: Another Position." *Journal of Philosophy* 73:16 (1976), 537–46. Reprinted in HS (91–100); POS1 (110–18); POS2 (63–71); POS3 (31–38); POS4 (31–38); Nagel, Thomas. "Sexual Perversion." *Journal of Philosophy* 66:1 (1969), 5–17. Reprinted in P&S1 (247–60); POS1 (76–88). Reprinted, revised, in Thomas Nagel, *Mortal Questions.* Cambridge: Cambridge University Press, 1979, 39–52; and POS2 (39–51); POS3 (9–20); POS4 (9–20); STW (105–12); Neu, Jerome. "Freud and Perversion." In Jerome Neu, ed., *The Cambridge Companion to Freud.* Cambridge: Cambridge University Press, 1991, 175–208. Reprinted in *A Tear Is an Intellectual Thing: The Meanings of Emotion.* New York: Oxford University Press, 2000, 144–65; STW (87–104). Original publication in Earl E. Shelp, ed., *Sexuality and Medicine,* vol. 1: *Conceptual Roots.* Dordrecht, Holland: Reidel, 1987, 153–84; Nussbaum, Martha C. "Constructing Love, Desire, and Care." In David M. Estlund and Martha C. Nussbaum, eds., *Sex, Preference, and Family: Essays on Law and Nature.* New York: Oxford University Press, 1997, 17–43; Oaklander, L. Nathan. "Sartre on Sex." In Alan Soble, ed., *The Philosophy of Sex: Contemporary Readings,* 1st ed. Totowa, N.J.: Rowman and Littlefield, 1980, 190–206; Ruddick, Sara. "On Sexual Morality." In James Rachels, ed., *Moral Problems: A Collection of Philosophical Essays,* 2nd ed. New York: Harper and Row, 1971, 16–34. Reprinted, revised, as "Better Sex," in Robert B. Baker and Frederick A. Elliston, eds., *Philosophy and Sex,* 1st ed. Buffalo, N.Y.: Prometheus, 1975, 83–104; P&S2 (280–99); Shaffer, Jerome A. "Sexual Desire." *Journal of Philosophy* 75:4 (1978), 175–89. Reprinted in SLF (1–12); Shrage, Laurie. "Is Sexual Desire Raced? The Social Meaning of Interracial Prostitution." *Journal of Social Philosophy* 23:1 (1992), 42–51; Shrage, Laurie. "Should Feminists Oppose Prostitution?" *Ethics* 99:2 (1989), 347–61. Reprinted in HS (275–89); POS3 (323–38); POS4 (435–50); STW (71–80); Singer, Irving, and Josephine Singer. "Periodicity of Sexual Desire in Relation to Time of Ovulation in Women." *Journal of Biosocial Science* 4 (November 1972), 471–81; Soble, Alan. "Analysis." In *Sexual Investigations.* New York: New York University Press, 1996, 111–42; Soble, Alan. "Sexual Concepts." In *The Philosophy of Sex and Love.* St. Paul, Minn.: Paragon House, 1998, 3–25; Solomon, Robert. "Sexual Paradigms." *Journal of Philosophy* 71:11 (1974), 336–45. Reprinted in HS (81–90); POS1 (89–98); POS2 (53–62); POS3 (21–29); POS4 (21–29); Sullivan, John P. "Philosophizing about Sexuality." *Philosophy of the Social Sciences* 14:1 (1984), 83–96; Taylor, Roger. "Sexual Experiences." *Proceedings of the Aristotlean Society* 68 (1967–1968), 87–104. Reprinted in POS1 (59–75).

DISABILITY. The *Diagnostic and Statistical Manual of Mental Disorders* of the American Psychiatric Association uses "mental retardation" for a disorder that begins before age eighteen and is characterized by significant limitations in both intellectual functioning (IQ of 70 or below) and adaptive behavior in at least two different skill areas (e.g., self-care, work, interpersonal functioning; 39–46). The American Association on Mental Retardation (AAMR) uses the same label and roughly the same definition. However, the AAMR manual (*Mental Retardation*, xii, 5) notes that individuals with mental retardation and their advocates are searching for a less stigmatizing term. In other English-speaking countries, particularly the United Kingdom (Leicester and Cooke, 182–83) and Australia (Foreman, 310), "mental retardation" is seen as deeply offensive and as misdescribing the disability. Other terms have been used: "intellectual disability" and "learning disability." The former might be preferable, because significantly subaverage intellectual functioning is a major criterion of the disability, while the latter might lead to confusing this disability with specific learning disorders (e.g., in reading, mathematics).

What are the central ethical issues regarding the sexuality of individuals with intellectual disabilities? And how are these issues different from ethical issues pertaining to the sexuality of the physically disabled? In the late twentieth century, at least in much of the West, the religiously inspired position, that only sexual acts that in normal circumstances can result in reproduction are morally proper, was challenged, if not replaced, by more liberal **sexual ethics**. Consistently with this development, the majority of social service and health professionals began to recognize that individuals with disabilities, whether intellectual or physical, are, like other people, sexual beings who should be able to express their sexuality independently of the possibility of procreation (Dixon and Dixon, 450; Fairbairn et al., 35–37). Although "sexual rights" are widely taken for granted, how they should be understood is unclear. Are they freedom rights, welfare rights, or some combination? Further, different meanings of "sexual rights" may be morally appropriate depending on the group we have in mind: the intellectually disabled, the physically disabled, the nondisabled.

A central characteristic of a liberal democracy is that its citizens have the right to arrange their lives according to their own beliefs and values. This basic civil liberty can be specified in terms of freedom rights that pertain to different spheres of life: the right to spend one's money as one sees fit (the sphere of financial affairs), the right to chose or refuse medical therapy on the basis of one's conception of the good (the sphere of health care), and among many others, the right to decide whether to engage in **sexual activity** (the sphere of sexuality). Freedom rights or self-determination rights should be distinguished from welfare rights, which are rights to various kinds of benefits: the right of citizens to a minimum income and to decent and accessible health care, and the right of specific groups to sexual services. Both freedom and welfare rights generate duties in others to behave in certain ways, but they differ in important respects. Freedom rights are "negative" rights; they entail duties in others *not* to interfere with or render impossible the action that the right-holder is entitled to perform. Welfare rights are "positive" rights; they entail duties in others to *do* certain things, namely, provide benefits or assist the right-holder in getting that to which he or she is entitled. The requirements for being holders of freedom and welfare rights are different. A precondition for welfare rights is the capacity to suffer (or having interests that can be preserved, protected, or promoted), whereas a precondition for freedom rights is having the mental equipment for exercising these rights, that is, the capacity for making competent choices.

Regarding the intellectually disabled, the status of freedom rights is central in ethical discussions. Should they have the same self-governance rights as everyone else? If not, do they lack freedom rights in all life spheres, or are they holders of at least some self-determination rights, for example, the right to arrange their sexual lives? Philosophers have infrequently addressed these ethical questions; when they do, they reluctantly ascribe freedom rights to the intellectually disabled (Downie; Murphy; Wikler). Usually they argue that these persons, in virtue of their intellectual limitations, lack the capacities required for being freedom rights holders. By contrast, many psychologists, especially those who support "normalization and deinstitutionalization," oppose denying people with intellectual disabilities self-determination rights, as long as their disability is only moderate (IQ 35–40 to 50–55) or mild (50–55 to 70) (Boddington and Podpadec, 178). They are inclined to interpret the right of these persons to express their sexuality as a self-governance right. Regarding the physically disabled, however, welfare rights are the central issue. Should they have the same package of welfare rights as everyone else? Or should they have additional benefits, including assistance in expressing their sexuality? Assuming that they are not intellectually disabled, they should not be denied self-determination rights. Rather, the question is whether their right to express their sexuality entails not only a freedom right to pursue their sexual interests but also welfare rights, say, the right to be transported to one's sex partner, the right to special equipment, and the right to financial assistance for employing prostitutes or sex therapists.

The central role of freedom rights in ethical discussions about the intellectually disabled does not exclude consideration of their welfare rights. That these people lack some capacity for competent decision making and therefore are not full bearers of self-determination rights may justify special welfare rights. Perhaps intellectually disabled people who are not competent to decide how to lead their sexual lives should be offered **sex education** and social skills training to enhance their competence (Khemka and Hickson, 24; Stavis and Walker-Hirsch, 62). Or perhaps they have sexual welfare rights to be guided and protected by surrogate decision makers, who make decisions on their behalf, preferably according to what the disabled would have chosen were he or she competent (Des Noyers Hurley and O'Sullivan, 48–52; O'Sullivan). That welfare rights are central to issues about the physically disabled similarly does not mean that freedom rights are insignificant. Indeed, freedom rights might partially justify welfare rights: Freedom rights to express one's sexuality may be worthless if physical disabilities impede its exercise.

Modern moral philosophy can justify ascribing sexual welfare rights to the physically disabled, to eliminate obstacles to sexual fulfillment, in different ways. Utilitarianism, for example, might appeal to the doctrine of "diminishing marginal utility," arguing that total utility will be increased if money or other resources are taken from the rich, for whom the loss of a little in effect amounts to losing nothing, and given to the poor, for whom gaining that same amount is an enormous increase in utility (see Broome, 434; Hare, 164–65). Given, for almost anyone, the significance of sexuality, and given diminishing marginal utility, utilitarianism seems to justify governmental redistribution of resources for the satisfaction of the sexual welfare rights of the disabled (see Brandt, 316–19). Alternatively, special welfare rights for the disabled might be justified, at least indirectly, by Rawlsian social contract theory (see Murphy). The parties in the original position, reasoning behind a veil of ignorance, do not know whether they will be handicapped; hence, to protect their potential interests, they might select principles of social justice that secure these welfare rights. However, according to John Rawls (1921–2002), the parties in the original position represent citizens who have the moral, intellectual, and physical capacities that enable them to be fully cooperating members of society. Contracting parties so described would at that stage ignore the interests of those who suffer from serious illness or are severely handicapped. Determining what is owed to them is not done in the original position but during the later legislative stage that draws out more specific content from the two principles of justice (*Political Liberalism*, 20–21, 74, 184). Rawls did write earlier that the mentally disabled were entitled to "equality" (*Theory of Justice*, 510), but he left that sentiment vague.

Competent persons have freedom rights because they are presumed to be the best judges of their own good (John Stuart Mill [1806–1873], chap. 4, 74), and so individual well-being is a fundamental value served by competent individuals' having freedom rights in various spheres (Buchanan and Brock, 29–36). Consenting to sexual activity that enhances one's well-being and refusing to engage in acts that are detrimental are, typically, competent decisions. This prudential criterion of competency is usually presupposed in empirical research on the capacities of the intellectually disabled to give informed **consent**. If, in an experimental setting, they are asked to indicate which choice the protagonist in a hypothetical story should make, their opting for choices favoring the best interest of the protagonist is taken as showing decision-making skills (Hickson et al.; Khemka and Hickson). This makes sense, as far as it goes, for without being able to understand the nature and consequences of sexual activity, and without having a capacity to determine and weigh the advantages and disadvantages of different options, a person is not a competent decision maker.

However, some courts in the United States understand competence in sexual decision making also in terms of appreciating the moral dimensions of sexual behavior (Sundram and Stavis, 259), and a survey of randomly selected psychologists found that many tend to accept moral factors as indicators of competency (Hill Kennedy and Niederbuhl). Thus whether a decision is competent depends on both its prudential and moral aspects. Although research on competent decision making focuses on prudential dimensions, moral dimensions are also important. Parents refrain from giving a child freedom to make sexual decisions if the child's ability to make moral judgments is still flawed. In particular, the reasoning powers required for being a competent decision maker include, from a secular or liberal perspective, being able to evaluate whether one's decisions are consistent with respecting the freedom rights of others. Being able to apply this principle is tantamount to being able to assess sexual behavior in terms of the principle of mutual consent. The interesting thing is that the abilities to reason morally and prudentially are similar to the capacities that Rawls (*Political Liberalism*, 19, 103–4) considers constitutive of being a fully cooperating member of society: the capacity for a sense of justice and the capacity for a conception of the good, respectively.

In liberal democratic societies every adult citizen has the freedom rights covered by Rawls's first principle of justice. From this it may be deduced that in liberal democracies a presumption of *global* competence for all adult persons is widely accepted (Buchanan and Brock, 21). Can this global status of competence be accorded to those who are intellectually disabled? The severely (IQ 20–25 to 35–40) and profoundly (below 20–25) intellectually disabled do not qualify. Although some people with severe intellectual disabilities do engage in mutual sexual behavior, including intercourse, their capacity for making prudentially or morally competent decisions is seriously impaired, to such an extent that a presumption of global incompetence is justified (Kaeser). The moderately or mildly disabled are different. What is repeatedly emphasized in publications on the sexuality of these individuals is that their professional care providers often experience tension between respecting the personal choices of their clients and protecting them from harm (Hill Kennedy and Niederbuhl; Morris et al.; Stavis and Walker-Hirsch; Sundram and Stavis). Practitioners struggle to balance their duty to protect the well-being and safety of their clients and their duty to advocate for the right of their clients to make choices. This balancing suggests that many care providers accept neither the presumption of global competence nor the presumption of global incompetence. They might be right. What seems the best strategy for people with mild or moderate intellectual impairment is examining in each instance whether they have the capacity to choose the option that both serves their own well-being and does not contravene morality, including, importantly, the principle that others have the right to give or withhold consent.

If particular disabled persons lack the capacity for competent sexual decision making, and hence cannot be regarded as holders of sexual self-governance rights, is that sufficient reason for disallowing all sexual activity among them? In U.S. **law**, sex between intellectually disabled people who lack the ability to consent might be criminal (Kaeser, 35, 41), although they are unlikely to be prosecuted (Sundram and Stavis, 260). Care providers who permit them to engage in sex are liable to criminal prosecution (Sundram and Stavis, 261). But if individuals with impaired decision-making capacities engage in sexual activity that clearly promotes their well-being, why prevent it (as long as we take measures on their behalf to ensure that pregnancy or the transmission of disease does not occur)? Prohibition merely on the basis of religious convictions is arguably inconsistent with the fundamental moral principle of beneficence. Thus there is reason to take seriously that surrogate decision makers be empowered to employ their authority and responsibility to choose the options that best serve the well-being of disabled people, not only in medical, educational, and residential matters but also regarding sexuality (Kaeser; Spiecker and Steutel).

See also Consent; Consequentialism; Dysfunction, Sexual; Ethics, Sexual; Incest; Pedophilia; Prostitution; Psychology, Twentieth- and Twenty-First-Century; Queer Theory; Rape; Sex Work; Sexology

REFERENCES

American Association on Mental Retardation. *Mental Retardation: Definition, Classification, and Systems of Supports*, 10th ed. Washington, D.C.: Author, 2002; American Psychiatric Association. *Diagnostic and Statistical Manual of Mental Disorders*, 4th ed. Washington, D.C.: Author, 1994; Boddington, Paula, and Tessa Podpadec. "Who Are the Mentally Handicapped?" *Journal of Applied Philosophy* 8:2 (1991), 177–90; Brandt, Richard B. *A Theory of the Good and the Right*. Oxford, U.K.: Clarendon Press, 1979; Broome, John. "Economic Analysis." In Lawrence C. Becker and Charlotte B. Becker, eds., *Encyclopedia of Ethics*, 2nd ed., vol. 1. New York: Routledge, 2001, 432–39; Buchanan, Allen B., and Dan W. Brock. *Deciding for Others: The Ethics of Surrogate Decision Making*. Cambridge: Cambridge University Press, 1989; Des Noyers Hurley, Anne, and Joan L. O'Sullivan. "Informed Consent for Health Care." In Robert D. Dinerstein, Stanley S. Herr, and Joan L. O'Sullivan, eds., *A Guide to Consent*. Washington, D.C.: American Association on Mental Retardation, 1999, 39–55; Dixon, Dwight, and Joan K. Dixon. "Physical Disabilities and Sex." In Vern L. Bullough and Bonnie Bullough, eds., *Human Sexuality: An Encyclopedia*. New York: Garland, 1994, 450–57; Downie, Robin S. "Ambivalence of Attitude to the Mentally Retarded." In Ronald S. Laura and Adrian F. Ashman, eds., *Moral Issues in Mental Retardation*. London: Croom Helm, 1985, 29–42; Fairbairn, Gavin, Denis Rowley, and Maggie Bowen. *Sexuality, Learning Difficulties and Doing What's Right*. London: David Fulton, 1995; Foreman, Phil. Review of *Mental Retardation* [American Association on Mental Retardation]. *Journal of Intellectual and Developmental Disability* 28:3 (2003), 310–11; Hare, Richard M. *Moral Thinking: Its Levels, Method and Point*. Oxford, U.K.: Clarendon Press, 1981; Hickson, Linda, Harriet Golden, Ishita Khemka, Tiina Urv, and Salifu Yamusah. "A Closer Look at Interpersonal Decision-Making Adults with and without Mental Retardation." *American Journal on Mental Retardation* 103:3 (1998), 209–24; Hill Kennedy, Carrie, and John Niederbuhl. "Establishing Criteria for Sexual Consent Capacity." *American Journal on Mental Retardation* 106:6 (2001), 503–10; Kaeser, Fred. "Can People with Severe Mental Retardation Consent to Mutual Sex?" *Sexuality and Disability* 10:1 (1992), 33–42; Khemka, Ishita, and Linda Hickson. "Decision-Making by Adults with Mental Retardation in Simulated Situations of Abuse."

Mental Retardation 38:1 (2000), 15–26; Leicester, Mal, and Pam Cooke. "Rights Not Restrictions for Learning Disabled Adults: A Response to Spiecker and Steutel." *Journal of Moral Education* 31:2 (2002), 181–87; Mill, John Stuart. (1859) *On Liberty*. Ed. Elizabeth Rapaport. Indianapolis, Ind.: Hackett, 1978; Morris, C. Donald, John M. Niederbuhl, and Jeffrey M. Mahr. "Determining the Capability of Individuals with Mental Retardation to Give Informed Consent." *American Journal on Mental Retardation* 98:2 (1993), 263–72; Murphy, Jeffrie G. "Rights and Borderline Cases." In Loretta Kopelman and John C. Moskop, eds., *Ethics and Mental Retardation*. Dordrecht, Holland: Reidel, 1984, 3–17; O'Sullivan, Joan L. "Adult Guardianship and Alternatives." In Robert D. Dinerstein, Stanley S. Herr, and Joan L. O'Sullivan, eds., *A Guide to Consent*. Washington, D.C.: American Association on Mental Retardation, 1999, 7–37; Rawls, John. *Political Liberalism*. New York: Columbia University Press, 1993; Rawls, John. *A Theory of Justice*. Cambridge, Mass.: Harvard University Press, 1971; Spiecker, Ben, and Jan Steutel. "Sex between People with 'Mental Retardation': An Ethical Evaluation." *Journal of Moral Education* 31:2 (2002), 155–69; Stavis, Paul F., and Leslie W. Walker-Hirsch. "Consent to Sexual Activity." In Robert D. Dinerstein, Stanley S. Herr, and Joan L. O'Sullivan, eds., *A Guide to Consent*. Washington, D.C.: American Association on Mental Retardation, 1999, 57–67; Sundram, Clarence J., and Paul F. Stavis. "Sexuality and Mental Retardation: Unmet Challenges." *Mental Retardation* 32:4 (1994), 255–64; Wikler, Daniel. "Paternalism and the Mildly Retarded." In Rolf Sartorius, ed., *Paternalism*. Minneapolis: University of Minnesota Press, 1983, 83–94.

Jan Steutel and Ben Spiecker

ADDITIONAL READING

Barry, Brian M. *The Liberal Theory of Justice: A Critical Examination of the Principle Doctrines in* A Theory of Justice *by John Rawls*. Oxford, U.K.: Clarendon Press, 1973; Bayles, Michael D. "Equal Human Rights and Employment for Mentally Retarded Persons." In Ronald S. Laura and Adrian F. Ashman, eds., *Moral Issues in Mental Retardation*. London: Croom Helm, 1985, 11–27; Cea, Christine D., and Celia B. Fisher. "Health Care Decision-Making by Adults with Mental Retardation." *Mental Retardation* 41:2 (2003), 78–87; Crux, Felix de la, and Gerard D. LaVeck, eds. *Human Sexuality and the Mentally Retarded*. New York: Brunner/Mazel, 1973; Culver, Charles M., and Bernard Gert. "Competence." In Jennifer Radden, ed., *The Philosophy of Psychiatry: A Companion*. New York: Oxford University Press, 2004, 258–70; Daniels, Norman, ed. *Reading Rawls: Critical Studies of* A Theory of Justice. New York: Basic Books, 1974; Freeman, Samuel R., ed. *The Cambridge Companion to Rawls*. New York: Cambridge University Press, 2003; Hayes, Susan C. "The Ethics of De-Institutionalisation—and Afterwards." In Ronald S. Laura and Adrian F. Ashman, eds., *Moral Issues in Mental Retardation*. London: Croom Helm, 1985, 43–55; Hickson, Linda, and Ishita Khemka. "Decision Making and Mental Retardation." In Laraine Masters Glidden, ed., *International Review of Research in Mental Retardation*, vol. 22. San Diego, Calif.: Academic Press, 1999, 227–65; Hill Kennedy, Carrie. "Assessing Competency to Consent to Sexual Activity in the Cognitively Impaired Population." *Journal of Forensic Neuropsychology* 1:3 (1999), 17–33; Kahn, Russi F. "Mental Retardation and Paternalistic Control." In Ronald S. Laura and Adrian F. Ashman, eds., *Moral Issues in Mental Retardation*. London: Croom Helm, 1985, 57–68; Khemka, Ishita, and Linda Hickson. "Decision-Making by Adults with Mental Retardation in Simulated Situations of Abuse." *Mental Retardation* 38:1 (2000), 15–26; Margolis, Joseph. "Applying Moral Theory to the Retarded." In Loretta Kopelman and John C. Moskop, eds., *Ethics and Mental Retardation*. Dordrecht, Holland: Reidel, 1984, 19–35; Murphy, Jeffrie G. "Do the Retarded Have a Right Not to Be Eaten?" In Loretta Kopelman and John C. Moskop, eds., *Ethics and Mental Retardation*. Dordrecht, Holland: Reidel, 1984, 43–46; Spicker, Paul. "Mental Handicap and Citizenship." *Journal of Applied Philosophy* 7:2 (1990), 139–51; Steutel, Jan, and Ben Spiecker. "Reasonable Paternalism and the Limits of Sexual Freedom: A Response to Greenspan and Leicester and Cooke." *Journal of Moral Education* 31:2 (2002), 189–94; Wertheimer, Alan. "Retardation." In *Consent to Sexual Relations*. Cambridge: Cambridge University Press, 2003, 223–26; Wolff, Robert Paul. *Understanding Rawls: A Reconstruction and Critique of* A Theory of Justice. Princeton, N.J.: Princeton University Press, 1977.

DISEASES, SEXUALLY TRANSMITTED. Philosophical and moral issues arise concerning sexually transmitted diseases (STDs) including, from the early 1980s, acquired immunodeficiency syndrome (AIDS). Some of these questions have to do with testing people for STDs, **privacy** and confidentiality surrounding a person's disease status, discrimination against those with STDs, and the conducting of research about STDs.

STDs have long had a curious social interpretation: They have been considered signs of depravity, sinfulness, and God's punishment. They have been throughout history the diseases contracted by the immoral as their just deserts. Allan Brandt has remarked that "social values continue to define the sexually transmitted diseases as uniquely sinful" (202). STDs, in particular syphilis until the 1940s and AIDS late in the twentieth century and beyond, stigmatize infected individuals (see Gilman).

In the nineteenth century, during a period of U.S. colonialism and black slavery, syphilis was believed to come from Africa. Africans had "exotic" bodies and were "hypersexual," in virtue of which, in America, they were believed to be at high risk for syphilis. An especially egregious case of racial discrimination occurred in the Tuskegee Syphilis Study in the early 1930s, in which syphilitic African Americans were observed without medical intervention, even after the discovery of penicillin, until they died (*Final Report*; Gilman, 100; Levine, 78). During the 1970s, the morally repugnant disease of choice was genital herpes. This was, however, short-lived because "the symptomology of this viral disease was too trivial to warrant such an association over the long run" (Gilman, 98) and because AIDS soon entered the scene.

When AIDS was recognized as a clinical entity, it became the perfect morally repugnant disease: It was associated with two already stigmatized groups, promiscuous homosexual males and intravenous drug users (Gunderson et al., 9–10; see Krauthammer, 19). AIDS carried stigma with it because, in the popular understanding of the disease, it was transmitted by sinful and perverted **sexual activity** (e.g., gay male anal intercourse) and equally disreputable African American male drug abuse. AIDS, we know, is not a typical STD, and perhaps not precisely an STD at all, although AIDS raises issues that apply to all STDs and, indeed, to disease in general (see Sontag). Contracting AIDS does not require engaging in bodily fluid–mixing sexual contact (blood transfusions are another source), yet AIDS was categorized as an STD because a frequent and visible cause of it was gay homosexual activity (Gilman, 90). As a result, to the popular or religious mind, the cure for AIDS was not to be found in medical science but in moral rectitude. A "conservative movement attacked what it perceived as a Sodom-like collapse of morals," and a sexual panic set in "[u]nder the rallying cry of reestablishing 'family values'" (Groneman, 151, 176). AIDS was not seen as presenting only prudential concerns resolvable by engaging in "safer" sex and eventually by medical science. Instead, sex was turned into something both bad and dangerous, "to be tolerated and redeemed, if at all, only within an abiding relation for which it serves as a token or symbol—a relation not merely of monogamy . . . but a relation of exclusive marriage" (Mohr, 253).

AIDS, like syphilis, was a plague of cities, which traditionally (and biblically, e.g., Sodom and Gomorrah) have been regarded as harborers of disease, degeneracy, and moral pollution. Regarding AIDS, only particular city dwellers were sinful: homosexuals, heroin addicts, and Haitians—to be Haitian in New York was to *be* an AIDS carrier. Indeed, in the popular perception of the disease, "the major risk factor in acquiring AIDS [was] *being a particular type of person*, rather than *doing particular things*" (Treichler, 44). Public perception blamed the victim for the disease, and many from the radical Religious Right believed God was punishing evildoers. Even scientists exhibited "homophobia, stereotyping, confusion, doublethink, them-versus-us, blame-the-victim, wishful thinking"—all the "popular forms of semantic legerdemain about AIDS" (Treichler, 37). But the AIDS problem became far more poignant when the "morally innocent," in the sense of the Religious Right itself (fetuses and infants; hemophiliacs and other recipients of blood transfusions) became infected with HIV (human immunodeficiency virus). In response, some voiced the sane warning that AIDS was also a heterosexual disease. Others focused on (or scapegoated) the male bisexual, "a homosexual *posing* as a heterosexual—acting as the secret conveyor of the diseases of the former to the healthy bodies of the latter" (Grover, 21). Sexually insatiable and possessing uncontrollable, predatory impulses, the male bisexual "corrupted" the heterosexual population. But, of course, so did the heterosexual intravenous drug user.

Many of the ethical and policy issues concerning AIDS did not become significant until AIDS was perceived as a threat to the general, that is, heterosexual, population. Funding for AIDS research and education began to rise substantially only when this population was threatened. "If AIDS funding were aimed simply at preventing the deaths of intravenous drug users, it would not be nearly as well motivated as it indeed is" (Mohr, 229). What seems to keep it motivated is not only gay male cases of AIDS but the spread of AIDS to women and to heterosexuals in general and the fact that the "morally innocent" (fetuses, neonates, recipients of blood transfusions, those injured in hospital accidents; see Murphy; Sim) have come down with the disease.

One question is whether the government should act paternalistically, through legislation or other policies, to prevent people from engaging in risky behavior, thereby protecting them from becoming infected with the AIDS-inducing virus, HIV, and harming themselves. It is widely accepted that the state may use the law to attempt to protect people from being harmed by the behavior of other persons who might maliciously or through deception expose them unwillingly to HIV (see Posner and Silbaugh; contrast Mayo). But a strong justification is required for the state to interfere with liberty of action to protect persons from themselves. (For the classic statement of this position, see John Stuart Mill [1806–1873], *On Liberty*.) Since, for example, "[t]he case for general contagion cannot be made" and it is unlikely that people contract the disease "mysteriously or through casual contact" (Mohr, 219)—if it were, the state could intervene—the question is whether the government should shut down bathhouses (or take other steps) as a way to protect people from exposing themselves to the disease.

At least sometimes the state *might* be justified in enacting paternalistic legislation (for discussion, see Joel Feinberg [1926–2004]). One example is making the purchase of certain drugs depend on having a physician's prescription. Moreover, the state might be able to enact legislation that is in effect paternalistic but do so by pointing out the indirect harms to other people that the state wants to prevent. For example, the law in many jurisdictions requires individuals to use seatbelts or wear motorcycle helmets, on the grounds that accidents without seatbelts or helmets indirectly cause harm to other people by prompting an increase in insurance costs or taxes. Whether the state is justified in, say, regulating bathhouses to prevent this type of indirect harm is unclear. Paternalistic legislation might be justified in protecting the general good health of a society, something important if people are going to lead autonomous, flourishing lives. Drug regulation, therefore, might be permissible, although probably not banning fast food. It can be argued that *if* putting oneself at risk for AIDS (or some other disease) during sexual activity were similar to driving a race car, exploring uncharted caves, or climbing a mountain (see Mohr, 229), then this sexual activity should not be prohibited on paternalistic grounds. In this case, the assessment of the value of the activity should be left to the individual—and society is off the hook to provide funding for research or for medical care required by the damage suffered by either unfortunate spelunkers or unlucky sexual actors.

Considerations of public health, even if not powerful enough to justify paternalism, might justify testing individuals to determine whether they are HIV-positive. Testing for AIDS became available in 1983, when researchers were able to isolate and culture HIV-infected T-cells. Once HIV could be grown in cell lines, protein could be extracted from inactivated virus to use in an HIV-antibody test (Grover, 20). Various procedures for AIDS testing exist, each having moral and social implications: mandatory, universal testing; mandatory testing of select populations; AIDS testing as part of "routine" testing; anonymous testing; and what is called "completely unlinked" testing.

Should there be mandatory, universal testing as a matter of policy for the sake of public health? There are powerful objections to this procedure, including the invasion of privacy that would be involved and the extreme financial cost. (Add to that the expense of counseling those individuals who test positive.) Further, as in other testing scenarios, the danger cannot be avoided that those recently infected people who get false negatives will be less concerned about practicing "safer" sex with partners who also test negative (Gunderson et al., 53).

What about mandatory testing of select populations? Even though the problem of false negatives remains, there might there be good reasons (some paternalistic) to test, say, **marriage** applicants or pregnant women. Knowledge of test results can be a precautionary warning, giving prospective brides and grooms a basis for making more rational decisions about proceeding with marriage. Note that the selective testing of potential marriage partners would reveal, until **same-sex marriage** is widespread, the incidence of AIDS only among those who participate in the "privileged" heterosexual institution of marriage (Mohr, 254). Mandatory prenatal HIV testing is another possibility. Some argue that there may be medical benefits to the pregnant woman and her fetus; but since the pregnant woman faces possible social and psychological harms, should she test positive, this testing should be handled the same way that prenatal diagnosis for fetal abnormalities has been handled, namely, as a decision made by the pregnant woman (see Walters).

What about selective mandatory testing of members of "high-risk" groups? The notion, however, of a "high-risk" group may merely stereotype and discriminate. A gay man who never engages in unprotected sex (and there may be many) or an intravenous (IV) drug user who never uses dirty needles (and there may be many) is not at high risk, despite public prejudice. Hence "high-risk group member" is not equivalent to "gay man" or "IV drug user," and if so, it is difficult to make sense of "high-risk group." Some heterosexuals who engage in **casual sex** might fall into that classification, but not necessarily (if they routinely engage in protected or safe sex). Some groups are already subject to mandatory AIDS testing, for example, U.S. **military** recruits and active duty personnel. The reason that such testing is required for the health of the armed forces community may be plausible. But it has been claimed, to the contrary, that military AIDS testing "simply badgers the antibody positive soldier until he admits he's queer and then discharges him" for *that* reason (Mohr, 258).

What about testing for AIDS during routine testing for other conditions? Hospital patients due for surgery, for example, are often tested for HIV without their knowledge and hence in the absence of informed **consent** (Gunderson et al., 42). Some argue that such routine HIV testing of hospital patients should not require informed consent but should be treated like other simple and routine blood tests. It has many benefits, including revealing potentially dangerous situations for hospital workers. Further, it is impractical to expect explicit consent for every test administered to a hospital patient. Others argue that because the psychological and other costs of testing positive for HIV are so high, patients should have a right to refuse to undergo the test (see Reamer's anthology).

Another reason against testing without consent is that doing so threatens privacy and confidentiality, which are widely regarded as important values, especially with respect to a person's medical status. (Consider the federal Health Insurance Privacy and Portability Act, enacted in 1996.) The traditional argument in favor of confidentiality is that protected communication between patient and physician is necessary for optimal medical care; without it, patients might be reluctant to make themselves vulnerable by sharing personal information with physicians.

Anonymous testing is a procedure for HIV testing that is sensitive to concerns about privacy and confidentiality. The results of anonymous tests are known only by the persons tested. Since public health officials believe it is important for people to know their HIV status, funding has been provided for anonymous testing and subsequent counseling (Gunderson et al., 46). Of course, mere testing and knowledge of one's HIV status does not prevent the spread of AIDS. The HIV-infected person must exercise self-control and abstain from unsafe sexual activities. Finally, there is "completely unlinked" testing, in which no one at all knows the identity of those whose test results are positive or negative. This procedure is used to screen donated blood.

When people receive bad news about their health, they typically turn to family and friends for support. Most people expect that their loved ones will respond in a caring and concerned way. However, when the news is that the person is HIV-positive, even loved ones sometimes respond with fear and hostility. Compounding the problem is that disclosing that one is infected is often followed by loved ones asking *how* one got infected. The infected person may be reluctant to answer personal questions about a delicate matter, especially if it means revealing ("coming out") his or her **sexual orientation**. This makes the infected person, already psychologically vulnerable, a possible object of discriminatory behavior even within the family.

Further, information about one's HIV status is often shared by health-care workers with insurance companies and employers, who might use that information to make decisions negatively affecting the infected person. Insurance companies argue that if cigarette smokers, for example, pay higher premiums, since they are more likely to require medical care, then HIV-positive status should also be taken into account, for the same reason. On this view, it is not unfair discrimination to determine who is medically compromised (e.g., HIV-positive; high cholesterol levels) by asking questions, checking medical records, or requiring medical tests. In reply, some argue that climbing mountains and other high-risk behaviors (even just crossing the street!) are not taken into account when setting insurance premiums, so HIV status should not be taken into account, either. Further, the dissemination of such information could result in the loss of one's job, another form of what some would claim is unfair discrimination (Gunderson et al., 166).

Employers do worry about the HIV status of their employees, in light of its possible effect on insurance costs, lost time from work due to illness and medical treatments, the expense of training new employees, and discrimination emanating from other employees and customers. For example, consider a restaurant owner who loses customers because patrons find out that a server or cook is HIV-positive. The infected person poses no health risk to co-workers or customers by virtue of this illness, yet it is incredibly difficult to change public perceptions, fears, and prejudices (Gunderson et al., 183).

There are also controversial issues regarding AIDS research. Many AIDS vaccine trials are conducted in the developing world, especially Africa. As Carol Levine points out, such research often violates a principle of justice in medical research that requires distributing the benefits of research to those who bear the risks. Many countries where trials are conducted have grossly inadequate and underfunded health-care systems and so do not have the resources to distribute vaccines, monitor, and treat the population (100). In response, some argue that subjects in these trials would not receive any benefits at all if vaccine trials were not conducted in their countries, and so they are receiving in some ways better care as research subjects than they would have otherwise received. Others question whether AIDS experiments should include placebo or control groups, because azidothymidine (AZT) is a drug that provides some known benefit. Trials comparing groups of HIV-positive persons receiving AZT and groups receiving a placebo began in 1986 but were discontinued—in response to protest and for much the same reason that testing penicillin on syphilis was abandoned.

See also Abstinence; Adultery; Bisexuality; Casual Sex; Consent; Cybersex; Heterosexism; Homosexuality, Ethics of; Homosexuality and Science; Law, Sex and the; Liberalism; Military, Sex and the; Privacy; Prostitution; Queer Theory; Sex Education

REFERENCES

Brandt, Allan. *No Magic Bullet: A Social History of Venereal Disease in the United States since 1880*. New York: Oxford University Press, 1987; Feinberg, Joel. *The Moral Limits of the Criminal Law*, vol. 3: *Harm to Self*. New York: Oxford University Press, 1986; *Final Report of the Tuskegee Syphilis Study Ad Hoc Advisory Panel*. Washington, D.C.: U.S. Public Health Service, 1973; Gilman, Sander. "AIDS and Syphilis: The Iconography of Disease." In Douglas Crimp, ed., *AIDS: Cultural Analysis, Cultural Activism*. Cambridge, Mass.: MIT Press, 1988, 87–108; Groneman, Carol. *Nymphomania: A History*. New York: Norton, 2000; Grover, Jan Zita. "AIDS: Keywords." In Douglas Crimp, ed., *AIDS: Cultural Analysis, Cultural Activism*. Cambridge, Mass.: MIT Press, 1988, 17–30; Gunderson, Martin, David Mayo, and Frank Rhame. *AIDS: Testing and Privacy*. Salt Lake City: University of Utah Press, 1989; Krauthammer, Charles. "The Politics of a Plague." *The New Republic* (1 August 1983), 18–21; Levine, Carol. "AIDS and the Ethics of Human Subjects Research." In Frederic G. Reamer, ed., *AIDS and Ethics*. New York: Columbia University Press, 1991, 77–104; Mayo, David. "An Obligation to Warn of HIV Infection?" In Alan Soble, ed., *Sex, Love, and Friendship*. Amsterdam, Holland: Rodopi, 1997, 447–53; Mill, John Stuart. (1859) *On Liberty*. Ed. Elizabeth Rapaport. Indianapolis, Ind.: Hackett, 1978; Mohr, Richard D. *Gays/Justice: A Study of Ethics, Society, and Law*. New York: Columbia University Press, 1988; Murphy, Timothy F. "Health Care Workers with HIV." In *Ethics in an Epidemic: AIDS, Morality, and Culture*. Berkeley: University of California Press, 1994, 93–107; Posner, Richard A., and Katharine B. Silbaugh. "Transmission of Disease." In *A Guide to America's Sex Laws*. Chicago, Ill.: University of Chicago Press, 1996, 72–82; Reamer, Frederic G., ed. *AIDS and Ethics*. New York: Columbia University Press, 1991; Sim, J. "AIDS, Nursing, and Occupational Risk: An Ethical Analysis." *Journal of Advanced Nursing* 17:5 (1992), 569–75; Sontag, Susan. *AIDS and Its Metaphors*. New York: Farrar, Straus and Giroux, 1989; Treichler, Paula A. (1987) "AIDS, Homophobia, and Biomedical Discourse: An Epidemic of Signification." In Douglas Crimp, ed., *AIDS: Cultural Analysis, Cultural Activism*. Cambridge, Mass.: MIT Press, 1988, 31–70; Walters, LeRoy. "Ethical Issues in the Prevention and Treatment of HIV Infection and AIDS." *Science* 239 (5 February 1988), 597–603.

Carol V. Quinn

ADDITIONAL READING

"AIDS: The Emerging Ethical Dilemmas." *Hastings Center Report* [Special Supp.] 15:4 (1985); Bayer, Ronald. "Gays and the Stigma of Bad Blood." *Hastings Center Report* 13:2 (1983), 5–7; Bazell, Robert. "The History of an Epidemic." *The New Republic* (1 August 1983), 14–18; Carter, Julian B. "Birds, Bees, and Venereal Disease: Toward an Intellectual History of Sex Education." *Journal of the History of Sexuality* 10:2 (2001), 213–49; Cohen, Elliot D., and Michael Davis, eds. *AIDS: Crisis in Professional Ethics.* Philadelphia, Pa.: Temple University Press, 1994; Colter, Ephen Glenn, Wayne Hoffman, Eva Pendleton, Alison Redick, and David Serlin, eds. *Policing Public Sex: Queer Politics and the Future of AIDS Activism.* Boston, Mass.: South End Press, 1996; Crimp, Douglas, ed. *AIDS: Cultural Analysis, Cultural Activism.* Cambridge, Mass.: MIT Press, 1988; Elbaz, Sohair W., and William Pardue. "A Bibliography on AIDS and Professional Ethics." In Elliot D. Cohen and Michael Davis, eds., *AIDS: Crisis in Professional Ethics.* Philadelphia, Pa.: Temple University Press, 1994, 253–69; Elwood, William N. *Power in the Blood: A Handbook on AIDS, Politics, and Communication.* Mahwah, N.J.: Erlbaum, 1999; Fee, Elizabeth. (1988) "Venereal Disease: The Wages of Sin?" In Kathy Peiss and Christina Simmons, eds., *Passion and Power: Sexuality in History.* Philadelphia, Pa.: Temple University Press, 1989, 178–98; Feinberg, Joel. *The Moral Limits of the Criminal Law,* 4 vols. New York: Oxford University Press, 1984–1988; Feldman, Douglas, and Thomas Johnson, eds. *The Social Dimensions of AIDS: Method and Theory.* New York: Praeger, 1986; *Final Report of the Tuskegee Syphilis Study Ad Hoc Advisory Panel.* Washington, D.C.: U.S. Public Health Service, 1973. Reprinted in Stanley Joel Reiser, Arthur J. Dyck, and William J. Curran, eds., *Ethics in Medicine: Historical Perspectives and Contemporary Concerns.* Cambridge, Mass.: MIT Press, 1977, 316–21; Gillet, Grant. "AIDS and Confidentiality." *Journal of Applied Philosophy* 4 (1987), 15–20; Herdt, Gilbert H., ed. *Sexual Cultures and Migration in the Era of AIDS.* Oxford, U.K.: Oxford University Press, 1997; Humber, James M., and Robert F. Almeder, eds. *Biomedical Ethics Reviews, 1988: AIDS and Ethics.* Clifton, N.J.: Humana Press, 1989; Johnson, Diane, and John F. Murray. "AIDS without End." *New York Review of Books* (18 August 1988), 57–63; Keenan, James F., ed. *Catholic Ethicists on HIV/AIDS Prevention: Thirty-seven Theologians from around the World Show How Roman Catholic Moral Traditions Can Mediate the Clash of Values in HIV Prevention.* New York: Continuum, 2000; Landesman, Sheldon. "AIDS and the Duty to Protect." *Hastings Center Report* 17 (February 1987), 22–23; Lebacqz, Karen, and Deborah Blake. "Safe Sex and Lost Love." In Elizabeth Stuart and Adrian Thatcher, eds., *Christian Perspectives on Sexuality and Gender.* Grand Rapids, Mich.: Eerdmans, 1996, 263–70; Lee, Robert E. *AIDS in America: Our Chances, Our Choices.* New York: Whitston, 1987; Leishman, Katie. "AIDS and Syphilis." *The Atlantic* (January 1988), 17–26; Lieberson, Jonathan. "Anatomy of an Epidemic." *New York Review of Books* (18 August 1983), 17–22; McIlvenna, Ted, ed. *The Complete Guide to Safer Sex.* Fort Lee, N.J.: Barricade Books, 1992; Mello, Jeffrey. *AIDS and the Law of Workplace Discrimination.* Boulder, Colo.: Westview, 1995; Mohr, Richard D. "The AIDS Crisis: Ethics in Dark Times." In *Gays/Justice: A Study of Ethics, Society, and Law.* New York: Columbia University Press, 1988, 215–73; Mohr, Richard D. "AIDS, Gays, and State Coercion." *Bioethics* 1:1 (1987), 35–50. Reprinted in HS (257–72); Mohr, Richard D. "What to Do and Not to Do about AIDS." In *A More Perfect Union: Why Straight America Must Stand Up for Gay Rights.* Boston, Mass.: Beacon, 1994, 97–111; Murphy, Timothy F. "AIDS." In Ruth Chadwick, ed., *Encyclopedia of Applied Ethics,* vol. 1. San Diego, Calif.: Academic Press, 1998, 111–22; Murphy, Timothy F. "AIDS: Literature." In Timothy F. Murphy, ed., *Reader's Guide to Lesbian and Gay Studies.* Chicago, Ill.: Fitzroy Dearborn, 2000, 33–37; Murphy, Timothy F. *Ethics in an Epidemic: AIDS, Morality, and Culture.* Berkeley: University of California Press, 1994; Murphy, Timothy F. *Gay Science: The Ethics of Sexual Orientation Research.* New York: Columbia University Press, 1997; Murphy, Timothy F. "Is AIDS a Just Punishment?" *Journal of Medical Ethics* 14:3 (1988), 154–60; Overall, Christine, ed. *Perspectives on AIDS: Ethical and Social Issues.* New York: Oxford University Press, 1991; Padgug, Robert A. "Gay Villain, Gay Hero: Homosexuality and the Social Construction of AIDS." In Kathy Peiss and Christina Simmons, eds., *Passion and Power: Sexuality in History.* Philadelphia, Pa.: Temple

University Press, 1989, 293–313; Philipson, Tomas J., and Richard A. Posner. *Private Choices and Public Health: The AIDS Epidemic in an Economic Perspective*. Cambridge, Mass.: Harvard University Press, 1993; Pierce, Christine. "AIDS and *Bowers v. Hardwick*." In Alan Soble, ed., *Sex, Love, and Friendship*. Amsterdam, Holland: Rodopi, 1997, 435–45; Pierce, Christine, and Donald VanDeVeer, eds. *AIDS: Ethics and Public Policy*. Belmont, Calif.: Wadsworth, 1988; Rechy, John, and Jonathan Lieberson. "An Exchange on AIDS." *New York Review of Books* (13 October 1983), 43–45; Ryan, Michael, and Avery Gordon. *Body Politics: Disease, Desire, and the Family*. Boulder, Colo.: Westview, 1994; Sartorius, Rolf, ed. *Paternalism*. Minneapolis: University of Minnesota Press, 1983, 83–94; Shilts, Randy. *And the Band Played On: Politics, People, and the AIDS Epidemic*. New York: St. Martin's Press, 1988; Singer, Linda. (posthumous) *Erotic Welfare: Sexual Theory and Politics in the Age of Epidemic*. Ed. Judith Butler and Maureen MacGrogan. New York: Routledge, 1993; Smith, Richard L. *AIDS, Gays, and the American Catholic Church*. Cleveland, Ohio: Pilgrim Press, 1994; Stanton, Domna C., ed. *Discourses of Sexuality: From Aristotle to AIDS*. Ann Arbor: University of Michigan Press, 1992; Steinbock, Bonnie. "Harming, Wronging, and AIDS." In James M. Humber and Robert F. Almeder, eds., *Biomedical Ethics Reviews, 1988: AIDS and Ethics*. Clifton, N.J.: Humana Press, 1989, 27–43; Treichler, Paula A. "AIDS, Homophobia, and Biomedical Discourse: An Epidemic of Signification." *Cultural Studies* 1:3 (1987), 263–305; Treichler, Paula A. *How to Have a Theory in an Epidemic: Cultural Chronicles of AIDS*. Durham, N.C.: Duke University Press, 1999; Watney, Simon. "Missionary Position: AIDS, Africa, and Race." In Russell Ferguson, Martha Gever, Trinh T. Minh-Ha, and Cornel West, eds., *Out There: Marginalization and Contemporary Culture*. Cambridge, Mass.: MIT Press, 1990, 89–103; Watney, Simon. "The Spectacle of AIDS." In Douglas Crimp, ed., *AIDS: Cultural Analysis, Cultural Activism*. Cambridge, Mass.: MIT Press, 1988, 71–86; Weeks, Jeffrey. "AIDS and the Regulation of Sexuality." In *Making Sexual History*. Oxford, U.K.: Blackwell, 1999, 142–62; Weeks, Jeffrey. "Living with AIDS." In *Invented Moralities: Sexual Values in an Age of Uncertainty*. New York: Columbia University Press, 1995, 15–20; Ziporyn, Terra. *Disease in the Popular American Press: The Case of Diphtheria, Typhoid Fever, and Syphilis, 1870–1920*. Westport, Conn.: Greenwood Press, 1988.

DWORKIN, ANDREA (1946–2005). Born to secular Jewish parents and raised in Camden, New Jersey, Andrea Dworkin became a radical "second-wave" feminist. By Dworkin's own account (*Life and Death*, 3–38), her work was informed by a series of negative personal experiences, including sexual assault at age nine, again by doctors at the Women's House of Detention in New York in 1965 (after an arrest for protesting the Vietnam War), work as a prostitute, and **marriage** to a battering husband whom she left in 1971. While Dworkin self-identified as a lesbian, since 1974 she lived with a gay male partner, writer John Stoltenberg, whom she married in 1998. Understandably, the main theme of Dworkin's work is male violence against women. This violence is a defining feature of our male-supremacist culture, in which **rape**, **prostitution**, and **pornography** are inevitable expressions of gender norms.

Dworkin's writings are primarily aimed at social change rather than intellectualizing. She describes her first book as "a political action where revolution is the goal" (*Woman Hating*, 17). What one finds in her writings is not so much philosophical theorizing as calls to action. Thus it is difficult to summarize the abstract theory to which she is committed and from which she draws arguments against the sexism she finds in our culture. What is clear is her desire to eliminate binary concepts of gender and their oppressive effects. (This perhaps dissolves the apparent tension in identifying as lesbian yet having a man as life partner.) In particular, Dworkin urges the destruction of a female gender role that involves masochism, self-hatred, and passivity. She sees male supremacy constructed and reinforced in our culture through the sexist structuring of public institutions and private interactions, locating three crucial foci of male supremacy in action: pornography, sexual intercourse, and rape. These are her central concerns. Her work includes seven monographs of feminist analyses, three collections of essays and speeches, a memoir (*Heartbreak*), two novels (*Ice and Fire*; *Mercy*), and a book of short stories (*New Woman's Broken Heart*), all of which explore these themes.

Pornography. Dworkin is well known for her antipornography writing and activism. This began with her analysis of pornography in *Woman Hating* and continued with a series of essays in *Our Blood* and *Letters from a War Zone* and her first full-length treatment, *Pornography: Men Possessing Women*. In *Woman Hating* she actually had positive things to say about the pornography of the 1960s and early 1970s, pointing out that its graphic depictions and celebrations of oral sex and female genitals helped "break down barriers to the realization of a full sexuality" (79). But in *Right-wing Women* she asserted that all feminists, to be feminists, had to be antipornography. Dworkin's campaign against pornography with lawyer **Catharine MacKinnon** has drawn much attention. In 1983, they drafted an ordinance for the Minneapolis City Council that treated pornography as a form of sex discrimination, making its production and distribution a ground for civil rights action. The ordinance defines pornography as the graphic, sexually explicit subordination of women (Dworkin and MacKinnon, *Pornography and Civil Rights*, 36). This contrasts with the standard legal framework, which Dworkin and MacKinnon view as mistaken in its focus on *obscenity* as pornography's problematic feature. Dworkin identifies the wrong of pornography in the harm it does to women. Women who participate in its production are coerced, entrapped, and exploited. In her view, these women are working as prostitutes and are, like prostitutes, being objectified and dehumanized merely for the pleasure of men. Consumption of pornography also causes harm through its involvement in rape, battery, **sexual harassment**, abuse, and reinforcement of women's second-class status. Dworkin views pornography as one of, perhaps the, central means by which male supremacy in our society is constructed and perpetuated (*Right-wing Women*, 226–27).

The Minneapolis ordinance was twice passed by the City Council but vetoed by the mayor. Civil libertarians, including many feminists, vigorously opposed the ordinance. The basis of their objection was the claim that freedom of speech is fundamental in free, democratic societies. Curtailment of this freedom is justifiable only when some variety of speech can be shown to be sufficiently harmful and when the limits imposed on it are not vague or overbroad. The ordinance, they argued, failed on both grounds. Indeed, the unconstitutionality of the ordinance was upheld by the Seventh Circuit Court of Appeals in *American Booksellers Association v. Hudnut* and affirmed by the U.S. Supreme Court (see MacKinnon and Dworkin, *In Harm's Way*, 462–82).

Dworkin (as well as MacKinnon) finds these arguments unpersuasive, believing that the free speech rights of men must not be treated as more important than the rights of women to be free from sexual abuse. She is equally unmoved by the claim that insufficient evidence exists establishing the harms of pornography, asserting that the hearings conducted about the ordinance provided compelling evidence (*In Harm's Way*). Certainly the hearings revealed that some women who participated in the production of pornography were harmed by intimidation and violence. The hearings also established that some women have been abused and sexually assaulted by men who consume pornography and that pornography is sometimes incorporated into this abuse (Russell, "Pornography and Violence").

What this establishes about a pornography-harm causal connection is not clear. Correlation alone does not demonstrate causation (see Soble, 144–50).

Dworkin replies that pornography is not like many other factors frequently present in abuse and rape, saying of men who perpetrate these crimes that "the directions [they] followed are found in pornography. . . . [T]hey are not found anywhere else" (*Pornography*, xxvi). Dworkin does not, however, merely assume that pornography causes men to assault women sexually through a simple process of mimicking pornography's content. Dworkin's model is more sophisticated: Pornography purportedly affects men's attitudes, through its coupling of sexual pleasure with objectifying, degrading, or violent images of women, such that men become more likely to abuse women. Pornography "plays a big part in normalizing the ways in which [women] are demeaned and attacked" (*Life and Death*, 133). The mechanisms through which this alleged normalization occurs are those proposed by, among others, sociologist Diana Russell, who argues that exposure to pornography predisposes some men to desire rape and undermines inhibitions against acting on rape fantasies (*Dangerous Relationships*, 121). The status of the empirical evidence here is contentious, though Dworkin clearly accepts Russell's interpretation.

In addition to being accused of naiveté about the sexual assault–pornography connection, Dworkin has also been accused of reinforcing sexist norms by portraying women, in and out of pornography, as passive victims. However, Dworkin is not antisexual, nor does she assume male sexuality is intrinsically harmful. She condemns pornography because it expresses objectionable views of women and sexuality, but she believes that merely intellectually rejecting those views is not enough. We cannot reject these views yet continue to produce and consume the pornography that expresses them; we must eliminate pornography, not just read or view it in light of nonsexist beliefs. But Dworkin does not advocate the abolition of all sexually explicit material. Her own fiction contains graphic, sometimes violent, descriptions of sex. This, of course, raises the question of the distinction between pornography and unobjectionable sexual material. The ordinance defines pornography as the sexually explicit *subordination* of women, so what must be distinguished are depictions that subordinate and those that do not. Dworkin understands subordination to be the "active placing of someone in an unequal position or in a position of loss of power" (*Pornography and Civil Rights*, 39). This might be uncontroversial, but the guidance it provides seems weak. Dworkin does not think that drawing the distinction is difficult in practice: No "pornographer has any trouble knowing what to make" (*Pornography and Civil Rights*, 36). Her optimism in the face of the complexity of the issue seems unwarranted.

Dworkin's perception of pornography stems from the analysis of cultural gender norms she presents in *Woman Hating*. There she approaches pornography as cultural material from which we can discern the principles that structure our gendered concepts of sexuality. But her analysis also starts with another form of material: fairy tales. These contain the gender roles that children learn and adults never overcome. Fairy tales, as she reads them, tell us that only two kinds of women exist. Good women (Sleeping Beauty, Cinderella) are passive, sleeping, innocent, helpless victims, while bad women (the Queen, the Wicked Stepmother) are active, devouring, awake, powerful. Men in fairy tales, on the other hand, are all heroes, all good, even when they do bad. Fairy tales, then, tell us that men and women are "different, absolute opposites" (47). In women, **beauty**, passivity, and victimization are desirable. In women, action and power are evil and must be destroyed. Whatever men do is good, because men do it. The moral of fairy tales is that "happiness for a woman is to be passive, victimized, destroyed, or asleep" (49).

The link for Dworkin is that "[p]ornography, like fairy tales, tells us who we are" (*Woman Hating*, 53; see Stoltenberg, 120–21). But its ideas are not confined to books and magazines; they structure the real world of human relations. To establish this, Dworkin discusses cultural practices that play out the sexist messages she has perceived, such as European witch-burning and Chinese footbinding. Witch-burning manifests the principles that ugliness, knowledge, action, and independence are dangerous in women, in need of punishment, worthy of death. Footbinding shows the value and beauty of women identified with **disability**, dependency, and passivity. These are clear examples of misogynist cultural practices. According to Dworkin, however, they are continuous with contemporary female beauty practices, the result of the glorification of culturally mandatory and continual body modification that requires tolerating, even romanticizing, self-inflicted pain. This is one source of the masochism Dworkin finds in the constructed feminine personality. More generally, women become masochistic as the result of conforming to social rules of femininity that degrade them as persons. This is especially noteworthy because women's masochism is "the mechanism which assures that the system of male supremacy will continue to operate as a whole even if parts of the system itself break down or are reformed. . . . [It] must be rooted out from the inside before women will ever know what it is to be free" (*Our Blood*, 61).

Another theme appears in Dworkin's analysis of *Suck*, a countercultural pornographic magazine of the 1960s. The depiction of sexuality she finds there contains the same gender principles encoded in fairy tales. Dworkin argues that the sexual revolution was not revolutionary but reactionary in its reinforcement of masculinist culture and binary gender roles. This analysis is extended in her essay "Why So-Called Radical Men Love and Need Pornography" (*Letters*, 214–21). Dworkin argues that men rightly fear the **sexual violence** they recognize in each other; to ensure their own safety, they arrange things so that sexual violence is directed against women as a class. Traditional sexual prohibitions against **homosexuality** and female promiscuity reinforce this class system. Weakening them therefore weakens the gender class system. The male radicals of the 1960s thus endangered their own social superiority by promoting sexual freedom. Faced with the choice between continuing the fight for freedom and shifting allegiance back to male supremacy, they chose the latter. This accounts for the subsequent proliferation of pornography and its increasing misogyny. Pornography only looks like it promotes women's sexual freedom; in fact, it contains the same sexist messages as fairy tales. It functions as propaganda to keep women in their place and is thereby backlash against **feminism**. This thesis is, of course, debatable. The proliferation of pornography is unlikely an effect of a small group of men reacting to feminism. Pornography is also unlikely to be effective against women's liberation, since the messages it expresses are ambiguous; to what extent woman-hating messages are in pornography, and whether they are understood to be there by consumers, is difficult to decide. Further, much pornography does not depict fairy-tale women but celebrates women who are independent, active, and powerful.

Sexual Intercourse. Dworkin generally doubts the contribution of the sexual revolution to the liberation of women. She claims that neither oral **contraception** nor promiscuity help liberate women but, instead, perpetuate women's oppression. They make women "more accessible, more open to exploitation" (*Woman Hating*, 81; see also MacKinnon, *Feminism Unmodified*, 144–45, and *Toward a Feminist Theory*, 190). The possibility of pregnancy and prohibitions against promiscuity gave women some power to refuse men's sexual demands. Removing them without making more fundamental changes only further disempowers women. Their accurately perceiving this, according to Dworkin, explains why right-wing women embrace traditional gender roles. They recognize that the liberation offered by the Left is no liberation at all. These women "see that within the system in which they live they cannot make their bodies their own, but they can agree to privatized male ownership: keep it one-on-one, as it were" (*Right-wing Women*, 69). Even though this response will not promote the liberation of women either, the sexual revolution does not go far enough in its recommendation that women adopt a male pattern of sexuality free of commitment and in its valorization, for both men and women, of a promiscuous, objectifying sexual style (see Callahan). Furthermore, for Dworkin, behaving like men makes women oppressors. Liberation requires more fundamental changes.

A change in our model of sexuality is necessary. Dworkin therefore suggests that sexual intercourse itself is a politically suspicious practice in our current cultural context. Her analysis of intercourse categorizes it as a central experience of **objectification** and oppression endured by women and through which male supremacy is taught and learned. Our culture's concepts of gender and sexuality make penetration an act of conquering, possession, and violation that turns women into objects for men's ownership and control. This objectification is at the same time "the normal use of a woman, her human potentiality affirmed by it, and a violative abuse" (*Intercourse*, 122). So long as men have power over women and male sexuality is constructed as dominating and controlling, heterosexual coitus will have this negative character.

The meaning of intercourse is, for Dworkin, independent of the meaning individual acts of intercourse might have for the participants. Even feminist men dominate and control women when they have intercourse with them; even women who experience coital pleasure and not violation or domination are violated and dominated. Social power relations determine the negative meaning of intercourse, not the individual's intentions or feelings. "Intercourse occurs in a context of a power relation that is pervasive and incontrovertible" and, moreover, "most men have controlling power over what they call *their* women—the women they fuck" (*Intercourse*, 125–26). The social power of men is enacted in and reinforced through coitus and is a central aspect of its meaning, despite what we experience. Whatever one makes of the claim that social context solely determines the meanings of actions (surely there is much to worry about here), a weaker reading of Dworkin has her saying only that individuals do not have complete freedom to fix the meanings of their actions. In sex, as in **language**, we must fashion meaning out of the materials at hand. Still, the cultural materials related to coitus might not be as univocal as Dworkin believes, and her pessimism about intercourse might not be fully justified.

Dworkin entertains the idea that intercourse must be abandoned to break the hold that the model of dominance, invasion, and possession has over us, arguing men may have to "give up their precious erections and begin to make love as women do together" (*Our Blood*, 13). As early as *Woman Hating*, she extols androgynous sexuality: "[A]ndrogynous fucking requires the destruction of all conventional role-playing . . . and of the personality structures dominant-active ('male') and submissive-passive ('female')" (185). The philosophy of sexuality Dworkin advances, then, makes genuine human sexuality depend on genuine human freedom—freedom from arbitrary and oppressive gender roles. Until these are eradicated, coitus will retain its negative meaning and function as a classroom of male supremacy. Ethical and humane intercourse might be possible in the future, but only after we achieve real freedom.

Rape. Calls for freedom occur repeatedly in Dworkin's writings: not only freedom from gender roles and pornography but also from rape. For Dworkin, rape is, along with pornography and intercourse, one of three focal elements of male supremacy. The prominence of rape in the history of Western culture (see Brownmiller) is important in Dworkin's thoughts about intercourse: The violation and possession of intercourse is only a short step from rape. Dworkin's blurring the line between consensual intercourse and rape is intentional (*Intercourse*, 136–38; see MacKinnon, *Toward*, 146, 174–75). It derives from her belief that women have been socially and legally unable to give or withhold **consent** to sex through much of human history. This inability does not derive from some deficit in women but from the social and legal negation of their autonomy and personhood. If women are not afforded the same rights as men, if they are legally chattel, if economic and social circumstances curtail their choices, and if they are socialized to be passive and masochistic, then women will hardly be in a position to grant or withhold genuine consent.

Unified by men's right of access to women's bodies, consensual intercourse and violent rape are thereby points on the same continuum. All "consensual" heterosexual sex is for women some form of sexual-economic bargain. This is clear in prostitution, which vividly expresses the economic exploitation of women. Dworkin asserts that prostitutes are coerced by the system of male supremacy even when they are not intimidated or forced into particular acts of prostitution. Women cannot voluntarily prostitute themselves any more than they can genuinely consent to "normal" intercourse. Indeed, Dworkin connects prostitution and rape: Prostitution "in and of itself is an abuse of a woman's body" and "is more like gang rape than it is like anything else" (*Life and Death*, 141).

Dworkin's writings on rape concentrate on the meanings and implications of historical and contemporary laws about rape, sexual assault, and marriage. She also argues that rape is the inevitable expression of masculine sexuality as constructed in Western culture. Rape and sexual assault are not merely acts done by "psychopaths or deviants from our social norms" but are "committed by exemplars of our social norms" (*Our Blood*, 45). Rape and assault are caused by our normative definitions of men as aggressive, dominant, and powerful and women as passive, submissive, and powerless. Thus, we must eliminate these cultural definitions. Again, Dworkin unearths the problems our gender norms generate.

Dworkin points out that women have been treated in law and by custom as the property of their fathers or husbands. This remained in the law of rape until only quite recently. Marital rape became criminal in all fifty states only in 1993, and thirty-three states still retained some exceptions to their marital rape laws in 2003 (Bennice and Resick). Previously, men had a legal right of sexual access to their wives. Wives did not have the power to refuse. On Dworkin's view, this situation was just part of a pattern of regulation of sexual conduct that normalized coercive relations between the sexes, a pattern that included treating compliance as consent, admitting victims' sexual history in defense of a rape charge, and requiring physical injury as proof of rape. A cultural belief that women want to be raped, which is often expressed in pornographic and mainstream portrayals of women as deserving, inviting, and enjoying rape, also normalizes sexual violence. Perhaps novelistic and cinematic depictions of a woman's enjoying rape should not be read uncritically as endorsements. Even so, Dworkin insists that in our culture "rape becomes the signet of romantic love" and so "remains our primary model for heterosexual relating" (*Our Blood*, 29). In her early work, she argued that the solution to the problem of rape lay in part in the revision of rape laws. Progress has been made on this front, and Dworkin should get some credit. Her writing as a revolutionary act has had an effect.

Critics of Dworkin do recognize that accusing her of "man-hating" in her opposition to pornography and intercourse misunderstands her, however natural the accusation is, given her strong convictions and the force of her expression (compare the careful Nussbaum with the less careful Mullarkey). The real targets of Dworkin's contempt are the norms of masculinity and femininity we have constructed in our commitment to binary concepts of gender and the violent, misogynist sexuality both men and women inherit as a result. This perspective fuels her campaigns against rape and pornography and her pessimistic analysis of the sexual revolution of the 1960s.

See also Beauty; Chinese Philosophy; Consent; Ethics, Sexual; Feminism, Lesbian; Feminism, Liberal; Fichte, Johann Gottlieb; Firestone, Shulamith; Genital Mutilation; Hobbes, Thomas; MacKinnon, Catharine; Objectification, Sexual; Pornography; Prostitution; Rape; Rape, Acquaintance and Date; Sadomasochism; Sex Work

REFERENCES

American Booksellers Association v. Hudnut. 771 F. 2d 323 (1985); Bennice, Jennifer A., and Patricia A. Resick. "Marital Rape: History, Research, and Practice." *Trauma, Violence, and Abuse* 4:3 (2003), 228–46; Brownmiller, Susan. *Against Our Will: Men, Women, and Rape.* New York: Simon and Schuster, 1975; Callahan, Sidney. "Abortion and the Sexual Agenda." *Commonweal* (25 April 1986), 232–38; Dworkin, Andrea. *Heartbreak: The Political Memoir of a Feminist Militant.* New York: Basic Books, 2002; Dworkin, Andrea. *Ice and Fire: A Novel.* New York: Weidenfeld and Nicolson, 1987; Dworkin, Andrea. *Intercourse.* New York: Free Press, 1987; Dworkin, Andrea. *Letters from a War Zone: Writings, 1976–1987.* London: Secker and Warburg, 1988; Dworkin, Andrea. *Life and Death: Unapologetic Writings on the Continuing War against Women.* New York: Free Press, 1997; Dworkin, Andrea. *Mercy.* London: Secker and Warburg, 1990; Dworkin, Andrea. *The New Woman's Broken Heart.* San Francisco, Calif.: Frog in the Well, 1980; Dworkin, Andrea. *Our Blood: Prophecies and Discourses on Sexual Politics.* New York: Harper and Row, 1976; Dworkin, Andrea. *Pornography: Men Possessing Women.* New York: Penguin Books, 1989; Dworkin, Andrea. *Right-wing Women.* New York: Perigee Books, 1983; Dworkin, Andrea. *Woman Hating.* New York: Dutton, 1974; Dworkin, Andrea, and Catharine A. MacKinnon. *Pornography and Civil Rights: A New Day for Women's Equality.* Minneapolis, Minn.: Organizing Against Pornography, 1988; MacKinnon, Catharine A. *Feminism Unmodified: Discourses on Life and Law.* Cambridge, Mass.: Harvard University Press, 1987; MacKinnon, Catharine A. *Toward a Feminist Theory of the State.* Cambridge, Mass.: Harvard University Press, 1989; MacKinnon, Catharine A., and Andrea Dworkin, eds. *In Harm's Way: The Pornography Civil Rights Hearings.* Cambridge, Mass.: Harvard University Press, 1997; Mullarkey, Maureen. "Hard Cop, Soft Cop." *The Nation* 244:21 (30 May 1987), 720–26; Nussbaum, Martha. "Rage and Reason." *The New Republic* 217:6–7 (11 August 1997), 36–42; Russell, Diana E. H. *Dangerous Relationships: Pornography, Misogyny, and Rape.* Thousand Oaks, Calif.: Sage, 1998; Russell, Diana E. H. "Pornography and Violence: What Does the New Research Say?" In Laura Lederer, ed., *Take Back the Night: Women on Pornography.* New York: William Morrow, 1980, 218–38; Soble, Alan. *Pornography, Sex, and Feminism.* Amherst, N.Y.: Prometheus, 2002; Stoltenberg, John. *Refusing to Be a Man: Essays on Sex and Justice.* Portland, Ore.: Breitenbush Books, 1989.

Sarah Hoffman

ADDITIONAL READING

Always Causing Legal Unrest. "The Andrea Dworkin Web Site." <www.nostatusquo.com/ACLU/dworkin/> [accessed 24 November 2004]; Allen, Amy. "Rethinking Power." *Hypatia* 13:1 (Winter 1998), 19–40; Baldwin, Margaret. "The Sexuality of Inequality: The Minneapolis Pornography Ordinance." *Law and Inequality: A Journal of Theory and Practice* 2:2 (1984), 629–53; Callahan, Sidney. "Abortion and the Sexual Agenda." *Commonweal* (25 April 1986), 232–38. Reprinted in POS3 (151–64); POS4 (177–90); Carse, Alisa L. "Pornography: An Uncivil Liberty?" *Hypatia* 10:1 (1995), 155–82; Douglass, Carol Ann. "What We're Trying to Save: Thoughts after Reading

Catharine A. MacKinnon's *Feminism Unmodified* and Andrea Dworkin's *Intercourse." Off Our Backs* 17 (June 1987), 14–15; Dworkin, Andrea. "Against the Male Flood: Censorship, Pornography, and Equality." In Patricia Smith, ed., *Feminist Jurisprudence*. New York: Oxford University Press, 1993, 449–66; Dworkin, Andrea. *Scapegoat: The Jews, Israel, and Women's Liberation*. New York: Free Press, 2000; Dworkin, Andrea. "Why So-Called Radical Men Love and Need Pornography." In Laura Lederer, ed., *Take Back the Night: Women on Pornography*. New York: William Morrow, 1980, 148–54; Ferguson, Frances. "Pornography: The Theory." *Critical Inquiry* 21:3 (1995), 670–95; Ferguson, Frances. "Sade and the Pornographic Legacy." *Representations* 36 (Autumn 1991), 1–21; Gilbert, Harriet. "So Long as It's Not Sex and Violence: Andrea Dworkin's *Mercy*." In Lynne Segal and Mary McIntosh, eds., *Sex Exposed: Sexuality and the Pornography Debate*. New Brunswick, N.J.: Rutgers University Press, 1993, 216–29; Harrold, Deborah. "Review of *Intercourse*, by Andrea Dworkin." *Ethics* 99:3 (1989), 670–71; Jakobsen, Janet. "Agency and Alliance in Public Discourse about Sexualities." *Hypatia* 10:1 (1995), 133–54; Jenefsky, Cindy, and Ann Russo. *Without Apology: Andrea Dworkin's Art and Politics*. Boulder, Colo.: Westview, 1998; Jones, Ann. "Review of *Right-wing Women*, by Andrea Dworkin." *Political Science Quarterly* 98:3 (1983), 547–48; Kaveney, Roz. "Review Article: Dworkin's *Mercy*." *Feminist Review* 38 (Summer 1991), 77–85; MacKinnon, Catharine A. (1982) "Linda's Life and Andrea's Work." In *Feminism Unmodified: Discourses on Life and Law*. Cambridge, Mass.: Harvard University Press, 1987, 127–33; Manning, Rita C. "Redefining Obscenity." *Journal of Value Inquiry* 22 (1988), 193–205; Merck, Mandy. "Bedroom Horror: The Fatal Attraction of *Intercourse*." *Feminist Review* 30 (Autumn 1988), 89–103. Reprinted as "The Fatal Attraction of *Intercourse*" in *Perversions: Deviant Readings*. New York, Routledge, 1993, 195–216; Moorcock, Michael. "Fighting Talk" [interview with Andrea Dworkin]. *New Statesman and Society* (April 1995), 16–17; Nussbaum, Martha. "Equity and Mercy." *Philosophy and Public Affairs* 22:2 (1993), 83–126; Pagnattaro, Marisa Anne. "The Importance of Andrea Dworkin's *Mercy*: Mitigating Circumstances and Narrative Jurisprudence." *Frontiers* 19:1 (1998), 147–66; Pannick, David. "Puffing Up the Porn." [Review of *Pornography: Men Possessing Women*, by Andrea Dworkin] *The Listener* (3 December 1981), 690; Picart, Caroline J. "Rhetorically Reconfiguring Victimhood and Agency: The Violence against Women Act's Civil Rights Clause." *Rhetoric and Public Affairs* 6:1 (2003), 97–125; Porter, Roy. "Signor Cock." [Review of *Intercourse*, by Andrea Dworkin] *London Review of Books* 9:12 (25 June 1987), 7; Rosen, Jeffrey. "Review of *In Harm's Way: The Pornography Civil Rights Hearings*, by Andrea Dworkin and Catherine A. MacKinnon." *The New Republic* 218:26 (29 June 1998), 25–35; Russell, Diana E. H. "Pornography and Rape: A Causal Model." *Political Psychology* 9:1 (1988), 41–73. Revised version in Diana E. H. Russell, ed., *Making Violence Sexy: Feminist Views on Pornography*. New York: Teachers College Press, 1993, 120–50; Shellrude, Kathleen. "Coming between the Lines: A Fresh Look at the Writings of Anti-Porn and Whore Feminists." *Canadian Woman Studies* 20:4 (2001), 41–47; Steiner, Wendy. "Declaring War on Men." [Review of *Mercy*, by Andrea Dworkin] *New York Times Book Review* (15 September 1991), 11; Sternhell, Carol. Review of *Ice and Fire* and *Intercourse*, by Andrea Dworkin. *New York Times Book Review* (3 May 1987), 3, 50; Superson, Anita M. "Right-wing Women: Causes, Choices, and Blaming the Victim." *Journal of Social Philosophy* 24:3 (1993), 40–61; Vadas, Melinda. "The Pornography/Civil Rights Ordinance v. The BOG: And the Winner Is . . .?" *Hypatia* 7:3 (1992), 94–109; Winship, Janice. "Review of *Pornography: Men Possessing Women*, by Andrea Dworkin, and *Pornography and Silence*, by Susan Griffin." *Feminist Review* 11 (Summer 1982), 97–100; Wolfe, Alan. Review of *Pornography: Men Possessing Women*, by Andrea Dworkin. *The New Republic* 202:8 (19 February 1990), 27–32.

DYSFUNCTION, SEXUAL. Sexual dysfunctions are impairments to a person's desire for or ability to perform sexual acts. During the twentieth century, psychotherapeutic, behavioral, medical, and pharmacological treatments for sexual dysfunctions were developed. The American Psychiatric Association's *Diagnostic and Statistical Manual of Mental Disorders* (DSM) identifies sexual dysfunctions as disruptions to the normal pattern of **sexual desire** and to the psychological and physiological changes that characterize sexual arousal and response. These disruptions may be lifelong or acquired and may affect all or only specific sexual situations. They may result from psychological factors, medical conditions, and substance use or abuse, including therapeutic drug-taking (DSM-IV, 493–95).

Sexual dysfunctions are conceptualized as deviations from biologically based patterns of desire and activity (Slowinski, 540). Sex therapist Helen Singer Kaplan (1929–1995) claimed that people needed healthy and responsive genital organs because they were driven naturally toward genital arousal and orgasm (*New Sex Therapy*, 63, 145). Individuals would be sexually dysfunctional if their genitals did not respond to erotic stimulation (Bancroft, 372), or if they did not enjoy or desire genital gratification. Since the 1960s, **sexual activity** has been seen as a birthright of every person, one that promotes quality of life and facilitates meaningful relationships (Irvine, 191, 223; Mayers et al., 269). Sexual dysfunctions thus threaten psychological security, since "if sex does not happen in the expected ways we accuse ourselves, or are accused by our lovers, of being impotent . . . frigid . . . uncaring, or even hostile. This makes what happens in bed a test of our adequacy as men and women" (Apfelbaum, 5). Most people experience intermittent failure of the ability to perform sexually, and 41 percent of women and 34 percent of men reportedly suffer ongoing difficulties with sexual functioning (Dunn et al., 519–24).

Scientific interest in sexual dysfunctions began in the nineteenth century with the emergence of systematic studies of sexuality and sexual pathology. Sex researchers such as Richard von Krafft-Ebing (1840–1902), **Havelock Ellis** (1859–1939), and **Sigmund Freud** (1856–1939) established a platform for the mid-twentieth-century surveys of sexual behavior conducted by Alfred Kinsey (1894–1956) and his colleagues (LoPiccolo and Heiman; Weeks, 61–95). William Masters (1915–2001) and Virginia Johnson contributed to our understanding of sexual dysfunction by describing a four-stage human sexual response cycle: excitement, plateau, orgasm, and resolution (*Human Sexual Response*, chap. 1). Masters and Johnson studied the bodily changes undergone during sexual activity. They believed that successful treatment of sexual difficulties required accurate physiological knowledge about human sexual responses, and they have been credited with ending the "dark ages"of the scientific study of sexuality (Kaplan, *New Sex Therapy*, 3). Masters and Johnson acknowledged that their standardized physiological stages of sexual response ignored individual gradations and psychogenic aspects. They claimed nonetheless to have provided a natural framework for understanding sexual functioning.

Masters and Johnson's approach to the treatment of sexual inadequacies emphasized short-term behavioral and educative techniques designed to overcome psychological blockages and conditioned physiological responses impeding sexual release. They taught couples to give pleasure to each other in nonthreatening contexts. This contrasted with psychoanalytic treatments derived from Freud, which required lengthy therapy to unravel deep-seated psychic disorders presumed to underlie sexual dysfunctions (Kleinplatz, "What's New," 97). Masters and Johnson recognized anxiety as impeding sexual performance, but they emphasized genital malfunctions and ignored disorders of desire (Kaplan, "Sexual Aversion," 65). Kaplan expanded Masters and Johnson's typology to include dysfunctions of desire. She combined their excitement and plateau stages into a single arousal phase, kept Masters and Johnson's third stage as the orgasm phase, dropped the resolution stage, and added a desire phase at the beginning of the cycle. The response cycle described in DSM-IV includes desire, excitement or arousal, orgasm, and resolution, which is a hybrid of the schemas of Masters and Johnson and Kaplan. Disorders may affect any one of these phases or several at once (Basson, 378; DSM-IV, 493–95).

Some sexual dysfunctions are manifested differently in men and women. Arousal phase disorders in women involve insufficient vaginal lubrication and swelling to enable completion of sexual activity, whereas in men arousal phase disorders involve inability to attain or maintain an adequate erection (DSM-IV, 500, 502). Orgasmic disorders in women involve delayed or absent orgasm following sexual excitement; in men they include loss of erection prior to ejaculation, premature ejaculation, and inability to ejaculate or experience orgasm. Dyspareunia, which affects both men and women, is genital pain associated with intercourse. Vaginismus is an involuntary muscular contraction of the outer vagina that makes penetration impossible (DSM-IV, 511–15).

Dysfunctions of the desire phase of the response cycle, known as hypoactive sexual desire disorder, are thought to be more prevalent among women and involve lack of interest in or aversion to sexual activity. Kaplan believed that healthy individuals have a physiologically based desire for genital stimulation and orgasm, normally achieved through heterosexual coitus, regardless of their cultural context (*Disorders of Sexual Desire*, xviii, 60). Sexual desire is not seen here as an optional personal taste or a culturally conditioned preference but as a biologically mandated requirement for normalcy.

DSM-IV emphasizes that sexual dysfunctions should not be diagnosed unless they cause psychic distress or interpersonal difficulties. This requirement protects individuals from being labeled dysfunctional independently of their subjective dissatisfaction with their sexual experiences or performance. At the same time, however, the necessity of distress or difficulty for a diagnosis of sexual dysfunction must be understood in light of the influence of sociocultural factors in constructing personal conceptions of adequate sexuality. People arguably do not measure their own sexual desires and activities against natural drives felt within their bodies or against desires they know intuitively they should have. Rather, they learn socially generated expectations about supposedly natural sexuality from their culture, and they may use these expectations to assess themselves and others. Complaints of personal distress about sexual performance thus may not reflect natural feelings or objective judgments but may express expectations learned from society. People may believe they are supposed to feel sexual desire and be distressed by its absence, or they may experience difficulties in relationships with others who have learned to expect them to feel desire and to seek genital gratification. As a result, if medical doctors and sex therapists accept persons' reports of distress about their desires or performance as evidence of fundamental disorders, they risk reinforcing merely socially established expectations about sexuality (Irvine, 222; Kleinplatz, "Critique," 117–18).

The sexual response cycle conceptualizes normal sex as embodying a natural sequence that is, arguably, masculinist, heterosexist, and dominated by reproductive coitus. The cycle presumes that inherently erotic situations naturally provoke genital responses that, once generated, can and should lead to completion in orgasm, usually through penile-vaginal intercourse. Any sexual acts that fulfill only part of this cycle presumably are incomplete and inadequate.

Feminist writers have criticized the response cycle for not reflecting women's sexual experience and for reducing sexuality to orgasmic coitus. The idea that the sexual cycle, once initiated, should lead to orgasm is questionable (Tiefer, 6). The response cycle does not always progress from desire to orgasm, since desire often results from (rather than leads to) sexual encounters with others (Basson, 379). The centrality of coital orgasm also has been challenged: Sexual intercourse without orgasm is enjoyed by many women, for whom orgasm is neither an expectation of nor an incentive to sexual activity and for whom its lack is not necessarily distressing (Anderson, 106–7). The complete response cycle may reflect only the preferences of persons devoted to a particular style of sexual gratification.

Nonheterosexuals also enjoy noncoital sexual experiences and argue that the genital, orgasmic focus of the response cycle assumes that the form of sexual satisfaction must be constant regardless of **sexual orientation** (Boyle, 74). People with physical disabilities or medical disorders that make coitus difficult or impossible also challenge the imperative for coital orgasm and the focus on genitality. Coital orgasm is not always essential for subjectively gratifying experiences, and a lack of interest in or ability to engage in coitus or to exhibit genital responses similar to the coital does not necessarily make a person sexually dysfunctional.

Another criticism of the response cycle is that it defines sexual adequacy in terms of the kinds of genital responses needed for reproduction. Literature dealing with erectile dysfunction, for example, assumes that men naturally need and want penile erections to penetrate and ejaculate within vaginas. Men are expected to maintain erections long enough not only to ejaculate through vaginal thrusting but also in that way to provoke orgasms in women. Since women also are expected to lubricate sufficiently to facilitate penile penetration, successful completion of the sexual cycle is tied to reproductive genital intercourse. Kaplan claimed that sexual desire serves reproduction by provoking people to "to impregnate, [and] to be impregnated" (*Disorders*, 78). On her view, male engorgement "transforms the small, flaccid urinary penis into the large, rigid reproductive phallus," and lubrication "transforms the tight, dry vaginal potential space into a well-lubricated open receptacle for the phallus" (*New Sex Therapy*, 15, 19). The sexual response cycle thus begins with sexual desire and leads sequentially to coital orgasm that is reproductive in form, even if reproduction is blocked by the use of **contraception**.

Many treatments of sexual arousal disorders aim to facilitate coital orgasm (Nicholson, 38). Definitions of disorders often do not mention coitus directly; for example, "erectile disorder" is defined as the incapacity of a man to maintain "an erection sufficient for satisfactory sexual performance" (Gajewski, 288; DSM-IV, 502). Nevertheless, while the form that a satisfactory performance should take is left open, it is commonly assumed by therapists to be coital orgasm (Daker-White and Donovan, 100). People with difficulties reaching orgasm during coitus often are counseled to masturbate, first by themselves and then with their partner, to progress to coitus. Orgasm achieved through **masturbation** in itself is not taken to resolve the dysfunction; this is only a step on the way to coitus (Anderson, 121–22).

Homosexuality is no longer considered a sexual dysfunction (or **paraphilia**), since the 1970s (Conrad and Schneider, 208–9). But same-sex sexual activity is assumed to involve the same body parts, sensations, and physical reactions as heterosexual coitus and to occur with the same frequency as among heterosexuals. This perspective could indirectly desexualize gays and lesbians: They could be judged dysfunctional not by virtue of their sexual orientation but because the style and frequency of their sexual acts deviate from a heterosexual model. Hypoactive sexual desire disorder, for example, supposedly is more prevalent among lesbians than heterosexuals (Nichols, 162). Referred to as "lesbian bed death," this is often explained by the lack of a male to generate sexual desire, resulting in infrequent sexual interaction. However, the idea that lesbians are prone to sexual desire disorders arguably depends on a socially determined definition of sexuality (see Frye). Lesbian sexuality need not be genitally focused, and lesbian couples often pursue nongenital contact as sexually valuable goals in themselves rather than as steps on the way to orgasm (see Iasenza). Nongenital and nonorgasmic bodily contact is often not recognized as sexual activity, but this contact can be as fulfilling sexually to the people involved as coitus is to some heterosexuals (Nichols, 164). Many heterosexual women also enjoy sexuality without coitus or even without genital arousal (Basson et al., 222; McConaghy, 185; Nicholson and Burr, 1737).

Physical disabilities and medical conditions can play a role in and influence the course of sexual dysfunctions. DSM-IV notes that various sexual dysfunctions can result from a general medical condition (515–18): diabetes mellitus, heart disease, or hypertension may cause male erectile disorders. Medically caused dysfunctions pose special problems, since they are not directly susceptible to behavioral or psychotherapeutic treatments. Unless the underlying condition is alleviated, the sufferers may be forced to live with a significant sexual deficit. The popularity of sildenafil citrate (Viagra) arises in part from its claimed ability to improve performance in men with medically caused erectile impairments. There is an ongoing search for drugs that will have similar effects in alleviating sexual disorders in women (Fourcroy; Hartley and Tiefer).

Some therapists believe that persons suffering from medically caused genital dysfunctions can obtain relief without necessarily having to rectify their deficient genital responses. If genuine sexual pleasure is obtainable by noncoital, nonorgasmic, or nongenital activities, then enjoyable, adequate sexual functioning need not exhibit standard genital responses (LoPiccolo, 43). People with spinal injuries, for example, have described orgasms centered in nongenital parts of the body (Wilkerson, 48). Were these kinds of experiences accepted as sexual, the experiential scope of functional sexuality would be widened.

Sexual dysfunctions are understood largely in the context of sexuality as a naturally given and universally constant domain of human experience. The pharmacological and short-term treatment methods that are currently popular deal predominantly with physical symptoms and surface psychological blockages instead of underlying issues. Little attention is paid to theoretical challenges to the etiology of sexuality and its disorders, to the contribution of social context, and to varying conceptions (of course, value-laden and philosophical) of "ideal" sexual experience and performance. The study and treatment of sexual dysfunctions as a field arguably fails to confront the narrow socially established understanding of normal sexuality.

See also Addiction, Sexual; Bullough, Vern L.; Disability; Feminism, Men's; Money, John; Paraphilia; Perversion, Sexual; Philosophy of Sex, Overview of; Queer Theory; Sexology; Sherfey, Mary Jane; Singer, Irving; Social Constructionism

REFERENCES

American Psychiatric Association. *Diagnostic and Statistical Manual of Mental Disorders*, 4th edition. [DSM-IV] Washington, D.C.: Author, 1994; Anderson, Barbara L. "Primary Orgasmic Dysfunction: Diagnostic Considerations and Review of Treatment." *Psychological Bulletin* 93:1 (1983), 105–36; Apfelbaum, Bernard. "What the Sex Therapies Tell Us about Sex." In Peggy J. Kleinplatz, ed., *New Directions in Sex Therapy: Innovations and Alternatives*. Philadelphia, Pa.: Brunner-Routledge, 2001, 5–28; Bancroft, John. (1983) *Human Sexuality and Its Problems*, 2nd ed. Edinburgh, Scot.: Churchill Livingstone, 1989; Basson, Ruth. "The Female Sexual Response Revisited." *Journal of Obstetrics and Gynaecology Canada* 22 (May 2000), 378–82; Basson, R., S. Leiblum, L. Brotto, L. Derogatis, J. Fourcroy, K. Fugl-Meyer, A. Graziottin, J. R. Heiman, E. Laan, C. Meston, L. Schover, J. van Lankveld, and W. Weijmar Schultz. "Definitions of Women's Sexual Dysfunction Reconsidered: Advocating Expansion and Revision." *Journal of Psychosomatic Obstetrics and Gynecology* 24:4 (2003), 221–29; Boyle, Mary. "Sexual Dysfunction or Heterosexual Dysfunction?" *Feminism and Psychology* 3:1 (1993), 73–88; Conrad, Peter, and Joseph W. Schneider. *Deviance and Medicalization: From Badness to Sickness*. St. Louis, Mo.: Mosby, 1980; Daker-White, Gavin, and Jenny Donovan. "Sexual Satisfaction, Quality of Life, and the Transaction of Intimacy in Hospital Patients' Accounts of Their (Hetero)sexual Relationships." *Sociology of Health and Illness* 24:1 (2002), 89–113; Dunn, Kate M., Peter R. Croft, and Geoffrey I. Hackett. "Sexual Problems: A Study of the Prevalence and Need for Health Care in the General Population." *Family Practice* 15:6 (1998),

519–24; Fourcroy, Jean L. "Female Sexual Dysfunction Potential for Pharmacotherapy." *Drugs* 63:14 (2003), 1445–57; Frye, Marilyn. "Lesbian 'Sex.'" In Jeffner Allen, ed., *Lesbian Philosophies and Cultures*. Albany: State University of New York Press, 1990, 305–15; Gajewski, Jerzy B. "Sexual Effects of Medications and Their Interaction: Implication for Men with Physical Disabilities or Chronic Illness." *Canadian Journal of Human Sexuality* 7:3 (1998), 287–94; Hartley, Heather, and Leonore Tiefer. "Taking a Biological Turn: The Push for a 'Female Viagra' and the Medicalization of Women's Sexual Problems." *Women's Studies Quarterly* 31:1–2 (2003), 42–54; Iasenza, Suzanne. "Lesbian Sexuality Post-Stonewall to Post Modernism: Putting the 'Lesbian Bed Death' Concept to Bed." *Journal of Sex Education and Therapy* 25:1 (2000), 59–70; Irvine, Janice M. *Disorders of Desire: Sex and Gender in Modern American Sexology*. Philadelphia, Pa.: Temple University Press, 1990; Kaplan, Helen Singer. *Disorders of Sexual Desire and Other New Concepts and Techniques in Sex Therapy*. New York: Brunner/Mazel, 1979; Kaplan, Helen Singer. *The New Sex Therapy: Active Treatment of Sexual Dysfunction*. New York: Times Books/Random House, 1974; Kaplan, Helen Singer. "Sexual Aversion Disorder: The Case of the Phobic Virgin, or an Abused Child Grows Up." In Raymond C. Rosen and Sandra R. Leiblum, eds., *Case Studies in Sex Therapy*. New York: Guilford Press, 1995, 65–80; Kleinplatz, Peggy J. "A Critique of the Goals of Sex Therapy, or the Hazards of Safer Sex." In Peggy J. Kleinplatz, ed., *New Directions in Sex Therapy: Innovations and Alternatives*. Philadelphia, Pa.: Brunner-Routledge, 2001, 109–31; Kleinplatz, Peggy J. "What's New in Sex Therapy? From Stagnation to Fragmentation." *Sexual and Relationship Therapy* 18:1 (2003), 95–106; LoPiccolo, Joseph. "The Prevention of Sexual Problems in Men." In George W. Albee, Sol Gordon, and Harold Leitenberg, eds., *Promoting Sexual Responsibility and Preventing Sexual Problems*. Hanover, N.H.: University Press of New England, 1983, 39–65; LoPiccolo, Joseph, and Julia Heiman. "Cultural Values and the Therapeutic Definition of Sexual Function and Dysfunction." *Journal of Social Issues* 33:2 (1977), 166–83; Masters, William H., and Virginia E. Johnson. *Human Sexual Response*. Boston, Mass.: Little, Brown, 1966; Mayers, Kathleen S., Daniel H. Heller, and Jessica A. Heller. "Damaged Sexual Self-Esteem: A Kind of Disability." *Sexuality and Disability* 21:4 (2003), 269–82; McConaghy, Nathaniel. *Sexual Behavior Problems and Management*. New York: Plenum, 1993; Nichols, Margaret. "Sexual Desire Disorder in a Lesbian-Feminist Couple: The Interaction of Therapy and Politics." In Raymond C. Rosen and Sandra R. Leiblum, eds., *Case Studies in Sex Therapy*. New York: Guilford, 1995, 161–75; Nicholson, Paula. "Feminism and the Debate about Female Sexual Dysfunction: Do Women Really Know What They Want?" *Sexualities, Evolution, and Gender* 5:1 (2003), 37–39; Nicholson, Paula, and Jennifer Burr. "What Is 'Normal' about Women's (Hetero)sexual Desire and Orgasm? A Report of an In-depth Interview Study." *Social Science and Medicine* 57:9 (2003), 1735–45; Slowinski, Julian W. "Sexual Dysfunction." In Vern L. Bullough and Bonnie Bullough, eds., *Human Sexuality: An Encyclopedia*. New York: Garland, 1994, 540–42; Tiefer, Leonore. "Historical, Scientific, Clinical, and Feminist Criticisms of 'The Human Response Cycle' Model." *Annual Review of Sex Research* 2 (1991), 1–23; Trimmer, Eric. *Basic Sexual Medicine: A Textbook of Sexual Medicine and an Introduction to Sex Counselling Techniques*. London: Heinemann Medical, 1978; Weeks, Jeffrey. *Sexuality and Its Discontents: Meanings, Myths, and Modern Sexualities*. London: Routledge and Kegan Paul, 1985; Wilkerson, Abby. "Disability, Sex Radicalism, and Political Agency." *NWSA Journal* 14:3 (2002), 33–57.

Joseph A. Diorio

ADDITIONAL READING

American Psychiatric Association. *Diagnostic and Statistical Manual of Mental Disorders*, 4th ed., text rev. [DSM-IV-TR] Washington, D.C.: Author, 2000; Berman, Helene, Dorothy Harris, Rick Enright, Michelle Gilpin, Tamzin Cathers, and Gloria Bukovy. "Sexuality and the Adolescent with a Physical Disability: Understandings and Misunderstandings." *Issues in Comprehensive Pediatric Nursing* 22:4 (1999), 183–96; Breggin, Peter Robert. "Sex and Love: Sexual Dysfunction as a Spiritual Disorder." In Earl E. Shelp, ed., *Sexuality and Medicine*, vol. 1: *Conceptual Roots*. Dordrecht, Holland: Reidel, 1987, 243–66; Brownworth, Victoria A., and Susan Raffo, eds. *Restricted Access:*

Lesbians on Disability. Seattle, Wash.: Seal Press, 1999; Candib, Lucy, and Richard Schmitt. "About Losing It: The Fear of Impotence." In Larry May, Robert Strikwerda, and Patrick D. Hopkins, eds., *Rethinking Masculinity: Philosophical Explorations in Light of Feminism*, 2nd ed. Lanham, Md.: Rowman and Littlefield, 1996, 211–34; De Vito, Scott. "On the Value-Neutrality of the Concepts of Health and Disease: Unto the Breach Again." *Journal of Medicine and Philosophy* 25:5 (2000), 539–67; DeLamater, John D., and Janet Sibley Hyde. "Essentialism vs. Social Constructionism in the Study of Human Sexuality." *Journal of Sex Research* 35:1 (1998), 10–18; Earle, Sarah. "Disability, Facilitated Sex, and the Role of the Nurse." *Journal of Advanced Nursing* 36:3 (2001), 433–40; Frye, Marilyn. "Lesbian 'Sex.'" In Jeffner Allen, ed., *Lesbian Philosophies and Cultures*. Albany: State University of New York Press, 1990, 305–15. Reprinted in *Willful Virgin: Essays in Feminism 1976–1992*. Freedom, Calif.: Crossing Press, 1992, 109–19; and Anne Minas, ed., *Gender Basics: Feminist Perspectives on Women and Men*, 1st ed. Belmont, Calif.: Wadsworth, 1993, 328–33; Giami, Alain. "Sexual Health: The Emergence, Development, and Diversity of a Concept." *Annual Review of Sex Research* 13 (2002), 1–35; Hartman, William E., and Marilyn A. Fithian. *Treatment of Sexual Dysfunction: A Bio-Psycho-Social Approach*. Long Beach, Calif.: Center for Marital and Sexual Studies, 1972; Jannini, E. A., C. Simonelli, and A. Lenzi. "Sexological Approach to Ejaculatory Dysfunction." *International Journal of Andrology* 25:6 (2002), 317–32; Jehu, Derek. *Sexual Dysfunction: A Behavioural Approach to Causation, Assessment, and Treatment*. Chichester, U.K.: Wiley, 1979; King, Michael. "The Duke of Dysfunction." *New Zealand Listener* (4 April 1998), 18–21; Kinsey, Alfred, Wardell Pomeroy, and Clyde Martin. *Sexual Behavior in the Human Male*. Philadelphia, Pa.: W. B. Saunders, 1948; Kinsey, Alfred, Wardell Pomeroy, Clyde Martin, and Paul Gebhard. *Sexual Behavior in the Human Female*. Philadelphia, Pa.: W. B. Saunders, 1953; Kleinplatz, Peggy J., ed. *New Directions in Sex Therapy: Innovations and Alternatives*. Philadelphia, Pa.: Brunner-Routledge, 2001, 109–31; Korenman, Stanley G. "Sexual Function and Dysfunction." In Jean D. Wilson, Daniel W. Foster, Henry M. Kronenberg, and P. Reed Larson, eds., *Williams Textbook of Endocrinology*, 9th ed. Philadelphia, Pa.: W. B. Saunders, 1998, 927–38; Lipsith, Josie, Damian McCann, and David Goldmeier. "Male Psychogenic Sexual Dysfunction: The Role of Masturbation." *Sexual and Relationship Therapy* 18:4 (2003), 447–71; LoPiccolo, Joseph. "Direct Treatment of Sexual Dysfunction in the Couple." In John Money and Herman Musaph, eds., *Handbook of Sexology*. Amsterdam, Holland: Excerpta Medica, 1977, 1227–44; Masters, William H., and Virginia E. Johnson. *Human Sexual Inadequacy*. Boston, Mass.: Little, Brown, 1970; Meston, Cindy M., and Andrea Bradford. "A Brief Review of the Factors Influencing Sexuality after Hysterectomy." *Sexual and Relationship Therapy* 19:1 (2004), 5–14; Minton, Henry L. "American Psychology and the Study of Human Sexuality." *Journal of Psychology and Human Sexuality* 1:1 (1988), 17–34; Mona, Linda R. "Sexual Options for People with Disabilities: Using Personal Assistance Services for Sexual Expression." *Women and Therapy* 26:3–4 (2003), 211–22; Moynihan, Ray. "The Making of a Disease: Female Sexual Dysfunction." *British Medical Journal* 326:7379 (2003), 45–47; Nadelson, Carol C., and David B. Marcotte. *Treatment Interventions in Human Sexuality*. New York: Plenum, 1983; Payne, Barbara P. "Sex and the Elderly: No Laughing Matter." In Elizabeth Stuart and Adrian Thatcher, eds., *Christian Perspectives on Sexuality and Gender*. Grand Rapids, Mich.: Eerdmans, 1996, 367–76; Rosen, Raymond C. "Looking Beyond Erectile Dysfunction: The Need for Multi-Dimensional Assessment of Sexual Dysfunction." *European Urology Supplements* 2:10 (2003), 9–12; Rosen, Raymond C., and Sandra R. Leiblum, eds. *Case Studies in Sex Therapy*. New York: Guilford, 1995; Simons, Jeffrey S., and Michael P. Carey. "Prevalence of Sexual Dysfunctions: Results from a Decade of Research." *Archives of Sexual Behavior* 30:2 (2001), 177–219; Soble, Alan. "Health." In *Sexual Investigations*. New York: New York University Press, 1996, 143–74; Tepper, Mitchell S. "Sexuality and Disability: The Missing Discourse of Pleasure." *Sexuality and Disability* 18:4 (2000), 283–90; Tevlin, Helen E., and Sandra R. Leiblum. "Sex-Role Stereotypes and Female Sexual Dysfunction." In Violet Franks and Esther Rothblum, eds., *The Stereotyping of Women: Its Effects on Mental Health*. New York: Springer, 1983, 129–50; Tiefer, Leonore. "Historical, Scientific, Clinical, and Feminist Criticisms of 'The Human Response Cycle' Model." *Annual Review of Sex Research* 2 (1991), 1–23. Reprinted in *Sex Is Not a Natural Act and Other*

Essays, 2nd ed. Boulder, Colo.: Westview, 2004, 41–61; Wakefield, Jerome. "Female Primary Orgasmic Dysfunction: Masters and Johnson versus DSM-III-R on Diagnosis and Incidence." *Journal of Sex Research* 24:1–4 (1988), 363–77; Winton, Mark Alan. "Paradigm Change and Female Sexual Dysfunctions: An Analysis of Sexology Journals." *Canadian Journal of Human Sexuality* 10:1–2 (2001), 19–24.

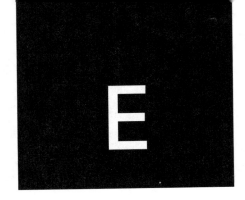

ECONOMIC ANALYSIS OF SEXUALITY. *See* Posner, Richard

EDUCATION, SEX. *See* Sex Education

ELLIS, ALBERT (1913–   ). In the 1940s, psychologist Albert Isaac Ellis galloped way ahead of the sexual revolution. Even now, it has not caught up with him.

Born in Pittsburgh, Pennsylvania, Ellis as a youngster developed strong intellectual interests. Yearning to be the Great American Novelist, he majored in business at the City College of New York to make a quick fortune and then devote himself to writing ("Psychotherapy without Tears," 109). Graduating in 1934 during the Great Depression with no fortune in sight, he took a brief job as a political propagandist and conquered his public speaking phobia by drawing on philosophy and psychology and forcing himself to give speeches. Encouraged, he tackled his shyness with girls by starting conversations with a hundred young women in the Bronx Botanical Gardens. Only one agreed to a date, then reneged, but Ellis lost his fear completely (Dryden, 134–36).

During subsequent unemployment, odd jobs, and a ten-year position with a novelty firm, Ellis wrote twenty unpublished novels, plays, and poems and heavily researched works about **love** and sex. Deeply absorbed in the "sex-family revolution" while developing expertise in helping friends answer their sex questions, he decided to get formal credentials in counseling. He received a master's in clinical psychology (Columbia, 1943) and began private practice in New York while working on his Ph.D. (Columbia, 1947). In 1948–1949, he maintained private practice while also holding faculty positions (New York University, Rutgers) and a clinical appointment (Northern New Jersey Mental Hygiene Clinic). Ellis was chief psychologist for the New Jersey State Diagnostic Center (1949–1950) and the New Jersey Department of Institutions and Agencies (1950–1952).

By 1952, Ellis's psychoanalytic practice had become full-time, with specialization in sex and **marriage** counseling. By 1955 he was disillusioned with psychoanalysis and developed Rational Therapy (now "Rational Emotive Behavioral Therapy," REBT), a cognitive-behavioral approach applicable to problems beyond sex and marriage. Psychoanalysis, he came to believe, spent too much time analyzing free association, dreams, and the client's past and too little time examining the client's irrational beliefs (*Reason and Emotion*, rev. ed., 234–36). Ellis's work as a therapist convinced him that while disturbance may have roots in the past, current thinking and behavior maintain disturbance. Reading (as a teenager) **Sigmund Freud** (1856–1939) on sex helped Ellis "loosen up and . . . consider practically all forms of noncoercive sex permissible" (Reiss and Ellis, 176), yet he disagreed with Freud that sexual problems were a major cause of emotional problems. Indeed, the reverse is more likely (Reiss and Ellis, 181). Ellis has admitted that Freud made genuine contributions in describing human psychological defenses (Dryden, 108), and he emulated the high value Freud placed on rationality (Wiener, 145–47). Ellis also admired the philosophy of scientific rationality espoused by Alfred Jules Ayer (1910–1989) and Karl Popper (1902–1994) (*Reason*, 123; *Reason*, rev. ed., 175).

According to REBT theory, emotional disturbance derives largely from "musturbation," the client's self-propagated perfectionistic demands that the world *must* be different than it is. These "musts" can be unlearned and the demands downgraded to desires. Ellis's first book based on REBT principles was *How to Live with a Neurotic* (1957). A few years later, Ellis and fellow therapist Robert Harper wrote a comprehensive self-help book, *A Guide to Rational Living* (1961), which became the REBT lay classic. They claimed that fighting the battle against perfectionistic demands requires perseverance but yields happiness and peace of mind. REBT was probably not the earliest form of cognitive-behavioral therapy, though it was the first to become widely known. It inspired other psychotherapists to develop cognitive-based therapies, and today most psychotherapists use cognitive-behavior techniques, including challenging clients' irrational or mistaken ideas. Ellis's theory can be illustrated by his approach to **masturbation**. On his view, masturbation is abnormal if it is someone's sole satisfying sexual outlet, despite the availability of coupled sexual activity, or if someone masturbates in the absence of desire, or if it is done in a "self-sabotaging and/or socially-destructive manner" (*Sex without Guilt in the 21st Century*, 6–10, 171). One goal of therapy is to help clients avoid self-sabotaging masturbation, such as doing it in public. Another is to help clients distraught about their masturbation correct their irrational beliefs about this "harmless and quite beneficial sex act" (10).

In 1959, Ellis founded the Institute for Rational Living (later the Institute for Rational-Emotive Therapy, now the Albert Ellis Institute). Since then, he has maintained a marathon professional schedule: treating patients, writing books (he has authored or edited over seventy-five) and papers, overseeing REBT trainees, running workshops, and lecturing around the world. Ellis was briefly married, twice. From 1965 to 2002 he maintained a partnership with psychotherapist Janet Wolfe. In 1988, Ellis praised her: "Although I was a pioneering psychotherapist-feminist before I met her, she has helped me deepen my pro-feminist attitudes and has contributed greatly . . . to the application of [REBT] to women's and men's sex role issues" (Wiener, 124). Ellis raised doubts about the vaginal orgasm ("Is the Vaginal Orgasm a Myth?"; *If This Be Sexual Heresy*, 134) well before the research of William Masters (1915–2001) and Virginia Johnson (*Human Sexual Response*, 66–67). He always crusaded for women's sexual freedom as well as men's.

Ellis's first book, *Folklore of Sex* (1951), analyzed sexual attitudes in the American mass media for one day, January 1, 1950, and complemented Alfred Kinsey's (1894–1956) study of behavior. Ellis alleged that Americans were deeply conflicted about sexuality, which they viewed simultaneously as appalling and appealing. This ambivalence has unfortunate effects: chaotic national policies about sexual matters, reduction of even "legitimate" sexual enjoyment, ignorance of sexual biology, personality disturbances, **sexual dysfunction**, and lack of support for **contraception** and **sex education**. Ellis advocated remedies in some twenty books about sexuality over the next thirty years. His famous *Sex without Guilt* (1958) championed a liberal approach (reminiscent of the utilitarianism of John Stuart Mill [1806–1873]) to **adultery**, masturbation, and censorship: "Every human being . . . should have the right to as much (or as little) . . . sex enjoyments as he prefers—as long as . . . he does not needlessly, forcefully, or unfairly interfere with the sexual (or non-sexual) rights and satisfactions of others" (170–71). But a person needs to curb sexual activities "so that they do not too seriously offend the sensibility of his relatives, friends, lovers, neighbors, employers, etc. [or] . . . he will often find himself in socio-economic difficulties" (172). In the third edition of *Sex without Guilt* ("In the 21st Century"; 2003), Ellis contends that Americans might now be less sexually conservative in their attitudes, but recalcitrant fears block adequate sex education and the prevention and treatment of sexual problems. Government funds promote **abstinence** education, not sex education, and little is earmarked for research on enhancing erotic experience (67–69).

Ellis's sexual advocacy books were popular but shocking. They attracted criticism from professional colleagues, were censored by publishers and advertisers, received few reviews, and were even banned (Reiss and Ellis, 164, 178–80; Wiener, 105–7). The scholarly *Encyclopedia of Sexual Behavior* (1961) garnered him considerably more respect (see Lessa's review). The first genuine sex encyclopedia since Victor Robinson's (1886–1947) *Encyclopaedia Sexualis* (1936), it stood alone for over thirty years, until **Vern L. Bullough** and Bonnie Bullough's (1927–1996) *Human Sexuality*. Composed by over ninety contributors in the arts, sciences, and humanities, the encyclopedia was widely cited for several decades. Ellis, who wrote 4 of the 111 entries, considers it "one of my best publications" (Reiss and Ellis, 165).

Of the great twentieth-century sexologists whose work liberalized sexual attitudes, including **Havelock Ellis** (1859–1939), Alfred Kinsey (1894–1956), William Masters and Virginia Johnson, only Ellis wrote highly readable, entertaining books for the public, including manuals on love and sex. Two focused on men (*Sex and the Single Man*, 1963; revised, *Sex and the Liberated Man*, 1976) and two on women (*Intelligent Woman's Guide to Man-hunting*, 1963; revised, *Intelligent Woman's Guide to Dating and Mating*, 1979). In a friendly, frank, and authoritative style, Ellis wrote about how men and women can overcome inhibitions about sex, learn how to meet partners, and enjoy masturbation, petting, and other activities while being responsible about contraception, **sexually transmitted diseases**, and ethical concerns like **consent** and deception. Other books were directed to couples: *Art and Science of Love* (1960; revised, 1966) was a manual of sex techniques, while *Creative Marriage*, coauthored with Harper (1961; reprinted as *Guide to Successful Marriage*, 1977), adapted his sexual prescriptions to relationships. *The Civilized Couple's Guide to Extramarital Adventure* (1972) elaborated Ellis's carefully qualified liberal views about adultery that had been pronounced earlier (*Sex without Guilt*, 43–55; "Healthy and Disturbed Reasons for Having Extramarital Relations"). The term "civilized adultery," wrote Ellis, is one "I coined some years ago to describe extramarital arrangements where both participants [in the marriage] are entirely open and aboveboard" (*Civilized Couple's Guide*, 25–26). Ellis maintains that sexually open marriages beneficially expanded opportunities for sex, love, and personality growth (see "Sexual Adventuring"; *Sex without Guilt in the 21st Century*, 199–209). He also points out disadvantages, including disapproval, the expense of money and time, and dishonesty.

Ellis's first book about REBT for therapeutic professionals, *Reason and Emotion in Psychotherapy* (1962), included four chapters on the application of REBT to marital problems, premarital counseling, frigidity, impotence, and "fixed homosexuality." Thirty years later, Ellis prepared a revised edition in the Talmudic spirit, adding commentaries, updates, and several new chapters; this came at the expense of the sex chapters, which were eliminated. Gradually, Ellis shifted from writing about sexuality except within REBT contexts. "I have said just about all I have to say about the subject," he declared in 1985 (Wiener, 88–89). His books after the 1980s focused on educating professionals about REBT and helping the public apply REBT to aging, alcoholism, anger, anxiety, child rearing, death and dying, fear of flying, overeating, stress, and procrastination. (His extensive roster of self-help books began before, and probably helped ignite, the later explosion of the genre.) Ellis's most recent major work on the application of REBT to sex is *Dating, Mating, and Relating* (2003, coauthored with Harper). *Sex without Guilt in the 21st Century*, which incorporates an REBT framework, is his first book exclusively on sex in twenty-five years.

Ellis credits philosophy for inspiring his sexual views and the development of REBT. He has often quoted Epictetus's (ca. 55–135) dictum from the *Enchiridion*, that we are disturbed not by things but by the view we take of them (13). He appreciated several Stoic ideas: the distinction between the changeable and unchangeable and the wisdom of accepting the latter with equanimity; the influence of thought on emotion; and the responsibility for contributing to the common welfare. From the Epicureans, he drew the concept of responsible enjoyment as a rational goal of human life (*Reason*, rev. ed., 64–65). REBT's technique of forcefully questioning irrational beliefs is based on the Socratic elenchus. Other philosophers Ellis has credited (*Reason*, rev. ed., 48, 53, 60, 64; *Guide to Rational Living*, 3rd ed., 5; Dryden, 132) include Lao-Tzu (ca. 600 BCE), Buddha (560–ca. 483 BCE), Confucius (ca. 551–479 BCE), Heraclitus (ca. 540–480 BCE), Democritus (ca. 460–370 BCE), Zeno of Citium (ca. 335–263 BCE), Cicero (106–43 BCE), Seneca (ca. 3 BCE–65 CE), Marcus Aurelius (121–180), **Baruch Spinoza** (1632–1677), **Immanuel Kant** (1724–1804), Ralph Waldo Emerson (1803–1882), **Søren Kierkegaard** (1813–1855), Henry David Thoreau (1817–1862), John Dewey (1859–1952), George Santayana (1863–1952), **Bertrand Russell** (1872–1970), Martin Buber (1878–1965), Paul Tillich (1886–1965), **Martin Heidegger** (1889–1976), and Jean-Paul Sartre (1905–1980).

In *Psychology Today*, Ellis was described as "a force to be reckoned with, both as a person and as a professional . . . renowned as much for his colorful language and strong opinions as for his innovations in therapy" (Epstein, 67). Always willing to use Anglo-Saxon words, as when calling humans "fallible, fucked-up, and full of frailty" ("Psychotherapy without Tears," 116), Ellis once polled an audience after a complaint was made about his obscenities. When only 3 out of 200 wanted him to stop saying "fuck," he invited the three objectors to leave (Trimpey, 85–86). Although some mental health practitioners and laypersons assess Ellis's profanity and strong therapeutic style as inappropriate or counterproductive (Yankura and Dryden, 104–5), Ellis contends that earthy **language** allows him to cut through clients' pretenses (Warga, 57).

In Darrell Smith's survey of psychologists, Ellis was ranked as the second most influential psychotherapist (after Carl Rogers [1902–1987]; Freud was third). A more recent paper that lists the 100 "most eminent psychologists of the 20th century" fails to mention him (Haggbloom et al.). Perhaps this means that Ellis's ideas are now taken for granted, like those of behaviorist John B. Watson (1878–1958), also not one of the elect. As the prime exemplar of his philosophy, Ellis has apparently enjoyed his ninety years as a single-minded, eccentric, controversial, and responsible hedonist. "I'm very happy. I like my work . . . going around the world, teaching the gospel according to St. Albert . . . [a]nd seeing clients, doing group therapy, writing books" (Epstein, 75).

See also Adultery; Bullough, Vern L.; Casual Sex; Consequentialism; Freud, Sigmund; Liberalism; Masturbation; Psychology, Twentieth- and Twenty-First-Century; Rimmer, Robert; Russell, Bertrand; Sexology; Sherfey, Mary Jane

REFERENCES

Bullough, Vern L., and Bonnie Bullough, eds. *Human Sexuality: An Encyclopedia.* New York: Garland, 1994; Dryden, Windy. *A Dialogue with Albert Ellis: Against Dogma.* Bristol, Pa.: Open University

Press, 1991; Ellis, Albert. (1960) *The Art and Science of Love*, revised ed. New York: Lyle Stuart, 1966; Ellis, Albert. *The Civilized Couple's Guide to Extramarital Adventure*. New York: Wyden, 1972; Ellis, Albert. *The Folklore of Sex*. New York: Charles Boni, 1951; Ellis, Albert. "Healthy and Disturbed Reasons for Having Extramarital Relations." In Gerhard Neubeck, ed., *Extramarital Relations*. Englewood Cliffs, N.J.: Prentice-Hall, 1969, 153–61; Ellis, Albert. "How I Manage to Be a *Rational* Rational Emotive Behavior Therapist." In Albert Ellis and Shawn Blau, eds., *The Albert Ellis Reader: A Guide to Well-Being Using Rational Emotive Behavior Therapy*. New York: Citadel Press/Kensington, 1998; Ellis, Albert. *How to Live with a Neurotic*. New York: Crown, 1957; Ellis, Albert. *If This Be Sexual Heresy*. New York: Tower Publications, 1966; Ellis, Albert. *The Intelligent Woman's Guide to Dating and Mating*. Secaucus, N.J.: Lyle Stuart, 1979; Ellis, Albert. *The Intelligent Woman's Guide to Man-hunting*. New York: Lyle Stuart, 1963; Ellis, Albert. "Is the Vaginal Orgasm a Myth?" In A. P. Pillay and Albert Ellis, eds., *Sex, Society, and the Individual*. Bombay, India: International Journal of Sexology Press, 1953, 155–62; Ellis, Albert. "Psychotherapy without Tears." In Arthur Burton, ed., *Twelve Therapists*. San Francisco, Calif.: Jossey-Bass, 1972, 103–26; Ellis, Albert. *Reason and Emotion in Psychotherapy*. New York: Lyle Stuart, 1962. Revised ed., New York: Birch Lane Press, 1994; Ellis, Albert. *Sex and the Liberated Man*. Secaucus, N.J.: Lyle Stuart, 1976; Ellis, Albert. *Sex and the Single Man*. New York: Lyle Stuart, 1963; Ellis, Albert. *Sex without Guilt*. New York: Lyle Stuart, 1958; Ellis, Albert. *Sex without Guilt in the 21st Century*. Fort Lee, N.J.: Barricade Books, 2003; Ellis, Albert. "Sexual Adventuring and Personality Growth." In Herbert A. Otto, ed., *The New Sexuality*. Palo Alto, Calif.: Science and Behavior Books, 1971, 94–109; Ellis, Albert, and Albert Abarbanel, eds. *The Encyclopedia of Sexual Behavior*, 2 vols. New York: Hawthorn Books, 1961; Ellis, Albert, and Robert A. Harper. *Creative Marriage*. Secaucus, N.J.: Lyle Stuart, 1961. Reprinted, *A Guide to Successful Marriage*. North Hollywood, Calif.: Wilshire Books, 1977; Ellis, Albert, and Robert A. Harper. *Dating, Mating, and Relating: How to Build a Healthy Relationship*. New York: Kensington/Citadel, 2003; Ellis, Albert, and Robert A. Harper. (1961) *A Guide to Rational Living: Third Edition, Thoroughly Revised and Updated for the Twenty-First Century*. Hollywood, Calif.: Wilshire, 1997; Epictetus. *Handbook of Epictetus*. Trans. Nicholas P. White. Indianapolis, Ind.: Hackett, 1983; Epstein, Robert. "The Prince of Reason." *Psychology Today* 34:1 (January 2001), 66–76; Haggbloom, Steven J., Renee Warnick, Jason E. Warnick, Vinessa K. Jones, Gary L. Yarbrough, Tenea M. Russell, Chris M. Borecky, Reagan McGahhey, John L. Powell, Jamie Beavers, and Emmanuelle Monte. "The 100 Most Eminent Psychologists of the 20th Century." *Review of General Psychology* 6:2 (2002), 139–52; Lessa, William A. Review of *The Encyclopedia of Sexual Behavior*, edited by Albert Ellis and Albert Abarbanel. *American Anthropologist* 63:6 (1961), 1395–96; Masters, William H., and Virginia E. Johnson. *Human Sexual Response*. Boston, Mass.: Little, Brown, 1966; Reiss, Ira L., and Albert Ellis. *At the Dawn of the Sexual Revolution: Reflections on a Dialogue*. New York: AltaMira/Rowman and Littlefield, 2002; Robinson, Victor, ed. *Encyclopaedia Sexualis: A Comprehensive Encyclopaedia-Dictionary of the Sexual Sciences*. New York: Dingwall-Rock, 1936; Smith, Darrell. "Trends in Counseling and Psychotherapy." *American Psychologist* 37:7 (1982), 802–9; Trimpey, John. "Plain Speaking." In Dominic DiMattia and Leonor Lega, eds., *Will the Real Albert Ellis Please Stand Up? Anecdotes by His Colleagues, Students, and Friends Celebrating His 75th Birthday*. New York: Institute for Rational-Emotive Therapy, 1990, 85–86; Warga, Claire. "You Are What You Think." *Psychology Today* 22:9 (September 1988), 55–58; Wiener, Daniel N. *Albert Ellis: Passionate Skeptic*. New York: Praeger, 1988; Yankura, Joseph, and Windy Dryden. *Albert Ellis*. London: Sage, 1994.

Martha Cornog

ADDITIONAL READING

Altman, Meryl. "Everything They Always Wanted You to Know: The Ideology of Popular Sex Literature." In Carole S. Vance, ed., *Pleasure and Danger: Exploring Female Sexuality*. London: Routledge and Kegan Paul, 1984, 115–30; Ayer, Alfred Jules. (1946) *Language, Truth, and Logic*. New York: Dover, 1952; Bernard, Michael E., and Raymond DiGiuseppe, eds. *Inside Rational-Emotive*

Therapy: A Critical Appraisal of the Theory and Therapy of Albert Ellis. New York: Academic Press, 1989; Blau, Shawn F. "Conspiracy of the 'Musts.' " [Review of *Reason and Emotion in Psychotherapy: A Comprehensive Method of Treating Human Disturbances*, by Albert Ellis, 2nd ed.] *Contemporary Psychology* 43:2 (1998), 103–4; DiMattia, Dominic, and Leonor Lega, eds. *Will the Real Albert Ellis Please Stand Up? Anecdotes by His Colleagues, Students, and Friends Celebrating His 75th Birthday*. New York: Institute for Rational-Emotive Therapy, 1990; Ellis, Albert. "Art and Sex." In Albert Ellis and Albert Abarbanel, eds., *The Encyclopedia of Sexual Behavior*, vol. 1. New York: Hawthorn, 1961, 161–79. 2nd ed., New York: Jason Aronson, 1973, 161–79; Ellis, Albert. "How I Became Interested in Sexology and Sex Therapy." In Bonnie Bullough, Vern L. Bullough, Marilyn A. Fithian, William E. Hartman, and Randy Sue Klein, eds., *Personal Stories of "How I Got into Sex": Leading Researchers, Sex Therapists, Educators, Prostitutes, Sex Toy Designers, Sex Surrogates, Transsexuals, Criminologists, Clergy, and More . . .* Amherst, N.Y.: Prometheus, 1997, 131–40; Ellis, Albert. "Is the Vaginal Orgasm a Myth?" In A. P. Pillay and Albert Ellis, eds., *Sex, Society, and the Individual*. Bombay, India: International Journal of Sexology Press, 1953, 155–62. Reprinted in Manfred F. DeMartino, ed., *Sexual Behavior and Personality Characteristics*. New York: Grove Press, 1963, 348–60; Ellis, Albert. "Masturbation." *Journal of Social Therapy* 1:3 (1955), 141–43. Reprinted, abridged, in Manfred F. DeMartino, ed., *Sexual Behavior and Personality Characteristics*. New York: Grove Press, 1963, 255–57; Ellis, Albert, and Albert Abarbanel, eds. *The Encyclopedia of Sexual Behavior*, 2 vols. New York: Hawthorn, 1961. New and revised 2nd ed., New York: Hawthorn, 1967. 2nd ed. (1 vol.), New York: Jason Aronson, 1973; Ellis, Albert, and Shawn Blau, eds. *The Albert Ellis Reader: A Guide to Well-Being Using Rational Emotive Behavior Therapy*. New York: Citadel Press/Kensington, 1998; Ellis, Albert, and Robert O. Conway. *The Art of Erotic Seduction*. New York: Lyle Stuart, 1969; Ellis, Albert, and Robert A. Harper. *A Guide to Rational Living in an Irrational World*. Englewood Cliffs, N.J.: Prentice-Hall, 1961. *A Guide to Rational Living: Third Edition, Thoroughly Revised and Updated for the Twenty-First Century*. Hollywood, Calif.: Wilshire, 1997; Farrell, Warren. "A Tapestry of Alternatives." [Review of *Sex and the Liberated Man*, by Albert Ellis] *Contemporary Psychology* 23:4 (1978), 269; Green, Adam. "The Human Condition: Ageless, Guiltless." *The New Yorker* (13 October 2003), 42–43; Korman, Sheila. "The Intelligent Woman's Guide to Dating and Mating." [Review] *Journal of Marriage and the Family* 43:2 (1981), 479; Nielsen, Stevan L., W. Brad Johnson, and Albert Ellis. *Counseling and Psychotherapy with Religious Persons: A Rational Emotive Behavior Therapy Approach*. Mahwah, N.J.: Erlbaum, 2001; O'Neill, Nena, and George O'Neill. *Open Marriage: A New Life Style for Couples*. New York: M. Evans, 1972; Orleans, Myron. "Sex and the Liberated Man, by Albert Ellis." [Review] *Contemporary Psychology* 7:2 (1978), 204; Oxhorn, Richard. "Albert Ellis and Robert A. Harper[,] A New Guide to Rational Living." *Contemporary Psychology* 21:3 (1976), 220; Popper, Karl R. (1934) *The Logic of Scientific Discovery*. Trans. Karl Popper, Julius Freed, and Lan Freed. New York: Harper and Row, 1968; Rorer, Leonard G. "Attacking Arrant Nonsense Forthrightly." [Retrospective review of *Reason and Emotion in Psychotherapy*, by Albert Ellis, 1st ed.] *Contemporary Psychology* 43:9 (1998), 597–600.

ELLIS, HAVELOCK (1859–1939).

Henry Havelock Ellis was born in Croydon (London), England in 1859. He died at the age of eighty, two months before **Sigmund Freud** (1856–1939), then also residing in England. Both were cremated at Golders Green.

At seven, Ellis accompanied his father, a sea captain, on a voyage around the world. On the coast of Peru, "I first gained full self-consciousness" (*My Life*, 61). He says this in the context of recounting some sexual experiences but insists on their (or his) innocence. Also on this trip, he pushed the ship's cat overboard, but such impulses "are always liable to arise in childhood; they clearly have little significance and should not be treated too seriously" (62). Ellis's analysis of his own motivations often exhibits this mixture of candor and superficiality. At sixteen he took a second voyage with his father, but after four months it was decided that he should remain in Australia. He spent his Australian years as a school-teacher and tutor. He found religious doubts pulling him away from his mother's conventional piety. He also experienced his first waking orgasm, in response (argues Grosskurth, 39) to a passage about female urination. In Australia, he later claimed, he recognized the study of sex as his life's work.

Returning to England at twenty to study medicine as preparation for his rather undefined career as scholar of sex, Ellis was drawn into London cultural life and began writing about literary and scientific subjects as well as frequenting groups concerned with advanced social thinking. In 1890 his first two books were published: a literary study, *The New Spirit*, "the programme of all my life's work," and a scientific treatise, *The Criminal*, "the first application of *The New Spirit*" (quoted in Grosskurth, 123). In 1894, Ellis published *Man and Woman*, examining familiar prejudices and stereotypes, discarding many, and seeking explanations for others. He criticized fashionable ideas about women's inferiority, but many critics feel, like Fraser Harrison, that "it is impossible to read his *Man and Woman* today without seeing it as part of that Victorian tradition which sought to assign to women a social role secondary to that of men" (106).

In 1896, Ellis's study of **homosexuality**, produced with Renaissance historian (and *sub rosa* homosexual rights activist) John Addington Symonds (1840–1893), was published in German. Before the English version could appear, objection from the estate of Symonds required that his name and much of his material be removed, so Ellis's *Sexual Inversion* did not appear until 1897. Disgraced homosexual writer Oscar Wilde (1856–1900) had just been released from prison. Grosskurth notes,

> *Sexual Inversion* was an unprecedented book. Never before had homosexuality been treated so soberly, so comprehensively, so sympathetically. To read it today is to read the voice of common sense . . . ; to read it then was . . . to be affronted by a deliberate incitement to vice of the most degrading kind. . . . Ellis was . . . the first person to write a book in English which treated homosexuality as neither a disease nor a crime. (185)

The volume was suppressed and the bookseller put on trial. Henceforth Ellis published most of his studies in the psychology of sex in America instead of England. Though Ellis judged his autobiography "the only book of mine I expect to be remembered" (quoted in Grosskurth, 430), the massive and erudite *Studies* is unquestionably his *magnum opus*. In its final order, it consists of seven volumes: (1) *The Evolution of Modesty/The Phenomena of Sexual Periodicity/Auto-Erotism* (1899, 1900, 1910); (2) *Sexual Inversion* (1897, 1901, 1915); (3) *Analysis of the Sexual Impulse/Love and Pain/The Sexual Impulse in Women* (1903); (4) *Sexual Selection in Man* (1905); (5) *Erotic Symbolism/The Mechanism of Detumescence/The Psychic State in Pregnancy* (1906); (6) *Sex in Relation to Society* (1910, 1937); and (7) *Eonism and Other Supplementary Studies* (1928). Despite its methodological defects, it exerted a major impact on the science of sex, changing attitudes and influencing the approach of subsequent writers. Canadian novelist Robertson Davies (1913–1995) submits that in the *Studies* "Ellis wrote the greatest work of literature which is also a work of science in the English tongue, after Robert Burton's *Anatomy of Melancholy*" (95).

Ellis was from his youth in self-conscious reaction against the constraints and hypocrisies of Victorian life. In his first book, Ellis celebrates what he sees as the

> growing willingness to search out the facts of things, and to found life upon them, broadly and simply, rather than to shape it to the form of unreasoned and traditional ideals. . . . [For] it must be among our chief ethical rules to see that

we build the lofty structure of human society on the sure and simple foundations of man's organism. (*New Spirit*, 8)

Ellis devoted his career to defending and elaborating this nonreductive biological realism. His studies focus on identifying basic facts of sexual life, in their variety and complexity, as a prelude to aligning social life to those realities. In his "General Preface" (1897) to the *Studies*, Ellis views his work as a secular analogue to the theological treatment of sex, one that will replace the "non-natural and unwholesome basis of asceticism" with the "open-air light of science" (vol. I, xxix). He says:

We want to get into possession of the actual facts, and from the investigation of the facts we want to ascertain what is normal and what is abnormal from the point of view of physiology and of psychology. We want to know what is naturally lawful under the various sexual chances that may befall man, not as the born child of sin, but as a naturally social animal. What is a venial sin against nature, what is a mortal sin against nature? The answers are less easy to reach than the theologians' answers. (vol. I, xxix–xxx)

Ellis also challenges Victorian ideas when he insists on the importance of the "play function" of sex ("the most alarming of all Ellis's ideas"; Davies, 93), which entails a separation of sex from reproduction. Through his personal relationship with American reproductive-rights pioneer Margaret Sanger (1883–1966), Ellis exerted an influence on the birth-control movement. But because sex cannot always be separated from reproduction, Ellis steadfastly supported eugenics.

In contrast to Freud, Ellis insisted that his concern was normal sexuality, but he believed that anomalous individuals, whether genius or pervert, help us understand what is, or what can become, normal. Great artists and thinkers help us to discover reality and adapt to it, and "it is the intimate thought and secret emotions of such men that become the common property of after generations" (*New Spirit*, viii). Ellis also rejects, at least for his own case, central Freudian ideas, such as repression:

There was no occasion for such repression.... There was no need for it ... because the veil of impassive reserve with which I concealed the whole of my intimate personal life rendered repression ... superfluous.... This fact now seems to me of immense significance for the whole of my life; it is, from one point of view, the key to all my work and my whole attitude towards the world. I have never repressed anything. What others have driven out of consciousness ... as being improper or obscene, I have maintained and even held in honour. (*My Life*, 83)

Sometimes, what Ellis rejects in Freud is the transformation of a concept originally introduced by Ellis himself. For example, in 1898 and later, Ellis discusses "auto-erotism," which he describes as "spontaneous sexual emotion generated in the absence of an external stimulus" (*Auto-Erotism*, 161; see *Eonism*, 363). The auto-erotic thus does not include sexual phenomena involving heterosexual or homosexual partners or various fetish objects (*Auto-Erotism*, 161), which Ellis deals with separately in the *Studies*. It does include, but is not limited to, **masturbation** in the absence of such external stimuli; erotic dreams, for example, Ellis calls "the type of auto-erotic activity" (*Eonism*, 362).

In *Three Essays on the Theory of Sexuality*, Freud explicitly adopts the term "auto-erotic" from Ellis but complains that from the psychoanalytic perspective "the essential point is not the genesis of the excitation, but the question of its relation to an object" (181; note added in 1920). A similar process of terminological adaptation occurs with "narcissism." Freud first attributes the term to Paul Näcke (1851–1913) but later credits Ellis (*Three Essays*, 218; note added in 1920; see "Narcissism," 73). Ellis sees himself as responsible "for the first generalized description of this psychological attitude, and for the invocation of Narcissus" but concedes that "the 'ism' was appended by Näcke" (*Eonism*, 356).

With both terms, however, deeper differences of meaning are at issue. Reviewing the development of "the conception of narcissism," Ellis writes:

> For me Narcissism was the extreme form of auto-erotism . . . a term devised to cover all the spontaneous manifestations of the sexual impulse in the absence of a definite outer object to evoke them. . . . For the psycho-analyst "auto-erotism" generally means sexual activity directed towards the self as its object. . . . [But] if we divert the term "auto-erotism" to this use we have no term left to cover the objectless spontaneous sexual manifestations for which the term was devised. (*Eonism*, 362–63)

And he complains that "while I had regarded all these manifestations [of auto-erotism and narcissism] as . . . not of invariable occurrence in the life of every individual, Freud sought to establish them as almost inevitable stages in the development towards adult sexual maturity" (*Eonism*, 363).

Through his broad reading and extensive acquaintance with leaders in the arts, sciences, and politics, Ellis was exposed to many influences. Scientific ones include George Drysdale (1826–1904), an early defender of **contraception**; eugenics pioneer Francis Galton (1822–1911); and James Hinton (1822–1875), whose work nurtured Ellis's mystical tendencies and made him more aware of women's needs. Literary influences include Benedetto Croce (1866–1952), John Henry Newman (1801–1890), Walter Pater (1839–1894), François Rabelais (1494–1553), **Jean-Jacques Rousseau** (1712–1778), and Hippolyte Taine (1828–1893). Some of the most important influences, however, are highly personal.

> I have said that probably in childhood I was sexually normal. But I think I can trace a slight fibre of what, if possibly normal in childhood, is commonly held—though this I doubt since I have found it so common—not to be so when it persists or even develops after puberty. I mean . . . urolagnia, which never developed into a real perversity nor ever became a dominant interest and formed no distinguishable part of the chief love-interests of my life. . . . Later my vision of this function became in some degree attached to my feeling of tenderness towards women—I was surprised how often women responded to it sympathetically—and to my conception of beauty, for it was . . . a part of the yet unrecognised loveliness of the world, which we already recognise in fountains. (*My Life*, 85)

He describes an experience with a nurse when he was a baby, and later experiences with his mother as an adolescent, as well as his favorite sister Louie's blunt characterization of his mother's behavior: "She was flirting with you!" (*My Life*, 55, 85–86). Ellis both minimizes and emphasizes the importance of these experiences:

> It was not until the age of sixteen that this trait became a conscious and active, though always subordinate, element in my mind. . . . It proved of immense intellectual benefit to me, for it was the germ of a perversion and enabled me to understand the nature of perversions. (*My Life*, 86–87)

From his relationships with his mother, sister, and wife, Ellis learned how closely **perversion**s stood to ordinary experience.

For historian Paul Robinson, Ellis's *Studies* "established the basic moral categories for nearly all subsequent sexual theorizing." Ellis is the key figure in the emergence of "sexual modernism" at the turn of the twentieth century, standing "in the same relation to modern sexual theory as . . . Albert Einstein to modern physics" (Robinson, 3). Even Ellis's ambivalent biographer Grosskurth allows that he "undoubtedly stands as the major transitional figure in establishing the preoccupations and methodology of later sexual investigation" (219).

Ellis undermined the Victorian conception of sex, defending homosexuality and masturbation. Though he persisted in venerating motherhood, Ellis defended the "love rights" of women in an era that took female sexual unresponsiveness for granted.

> Freud confessed that he was still bewildered as to what women really wanted. Ellis would have been ready with an answer: a more fulfilled sensual life. This, above all, he had learned from Hinton—an awareness of women's needs; and this awareness has been the greatest factor in the sexual revolution of the twentieth century. (Grosskurth, 225)

Ellis made specific discoveries, such as the association of female **sexual desire** with menstruation and the idea of erogenic (erogenous) zones later popularized by psychoanalysis. He opened up many paths for investigation, even if his methods had their limitations. Davies puts those limitations in perspective: "Later writers on sexual subjects have complained that taken as a whole, they [the *Studies*' autobiographical sketches] do not cover a very wide range of society or a very large number of people. But they were the first things of their kind, and they are excellent reading still. . . . It was a great part of Ellis's genius that he was able to call forth such documents" (94).

Most important, perhaps, was the liberating effect of Ellis's attitudes. Edward Brecher recalls that "reading 'The Evolution of Modesty' has been an unforgettable experience for countless men and women (myself included), enabling them to transcend the limitations of the sexual perspective prevailing in their own time and place" (4). And after quoting Ellis's reflection in old age—"I cannot see now a girl walking along the street, with her free air, unswathed limbs, her gay and scanty raiment, without being conscious of a thrill of joy that in my youth was unknown. I can today feel in London as in earlier days I scarcely could even in Paris, that I am among people who are growing to be gracious and human"—Brecher comments, "No man alive or dead contributed more to that change than Havelock Ellis himself " (48–49).

Ellis's credentials as literary critic and social scientist seem secure, but though celebrated as the "sage of sex" and "philosopher of love," his qualifications as philosopher are debatable. "Ellis's erudition was breathtaking," says Brecher, "but much of his wisdom can with little loss be summed up in one brief sentence: everybody is not like you, your loved ones, and your friends and neighbors" (4). Social scientists during the first half of the twentieth century often tried (incoherently) to base tolerance on relativism. Ellis, too, tends to assume that "a broader view of the phenomena teaches us to suspend judgment" (*Studies*, vol. I, xxxiii).

Does it? In the concluding section of "The Evolution of Modesty," Ellis summarizes five "factors" in modesty: the female animal's gesture of sexual refusal, the fear of arousing disgust, the concern about ceremonial incorrectness (based on fear of magic influence), the development of ornament and clothing, and the conception of women as property (*Studies*, vol. I, 80). He then turns to the question whether modesty increases with social progress and suggests it does not. "Among savages, modesty is far more radical and invincible than among *the civilized.*" Modesty is emphasized most "in *a new and crude civilization.*" He suggests that "the disappearance of misplaced signs of modesty" is a "mark of *increasing civilization.*" He suggests that in "older and more *mature civilizations,*" such as Greece and Rome, Japan, or France, modesty "becomes subservient to human use." He notes that "modesty is a much more invincible motive among the lower social classes than among the *more cultivated classes.*" And he suggests that "in the *fully-developed* human being self-respect itself holds in check any excessive modesty" (vol. I, 81; italics added). On a single page, Ellis invokes half a dozen times an undefined normative notion of superior development that ranges loosely across individuals, social classes, and civilizations. He thus enlists the prejudices of his reader, a nineteenth-century believer in social hierarchy, to promote his own ideas that too much modesty is not necessarily a good thing, that forms of modesty may become outdated, and that true modesty must be subordinate to appropriate purposes ("human use").

The factors of modesty, Ellis says, "are based on emotions which make little urgent appeal save to races in a savage or barbarous condition." In the reader's "advanced civilization," he suggests, disgust has been mitigated by knowledge, ceremonial correctness has been reduced to etiquette, the conception of women as property has been surpassed, and sexual refusal is not really relevant. "Thus civilization tends to subordinate, if not to minimize, modesty," is his conclusion—almost. For modesty is also "the necessary foundation for all love's most exquisite audacities," he adds. "Without modesty, we could not have, nor rightly value at its true worth, that bold and pure candor which is at once the final revelation of love and the seal of its sincerity" (*Studies*, vol. I, 82).

We may question both thesis and argument, but what ultimately astonishes in Ellis is his erudition. At the top of one page, he says, "Of the Araucanian women of Chile, Treutler has remarked . . . ," and at the bottom, "Thus I have been told of a ballet-girl who thinks . . . while Fanny Kemble, in her *Reminiscences,* tells of an actress" (*Studies*, vol. I, 81). It is the scope and variety and salience of reference that astound. Ellis's views do not commend themselves because they have been established by analytical argument. On that level, at most of the crucial points his arguments beg the question. Nonetheless, Ellis's work deserves serious attention in difficult matters that require subtle judgment. His mastery and synthesis impress, more than his analysis.

The comment of Ellis's last companion, Françoise Lafitte-Cyon (a.k.a. Françoise Delisle; 1886–1974), on his urolagnia is telling: "It was part of our normality" (quoted in Brecher, 33; Grosskurth, 284). She summed up, in a letter to Sanger, the essential lesson she had learned from Ellis, "that there is not one sexual anomaly which cannot be transformed into beauty when there is love and art in both lovers" (Grosskurth, 285). Ellis helped many view sexual anomalies as "a part of the yet unrecognised loveliness of the world." Not everyone would consider what he saw loveliness, but Ellis, who believed "it is logically contradictory ideas that are the most valuable" (*Dance of Life*, 97), would hardly have cared whether we call what he did "philosophy."

See also Abstinence; Bestiality; Bullough, Vern L.; Freud, Sigmund; Homosexuality and Science; Hume, David; Masturbation; Perversion, Sexual; Psychology, Twentieth- and Twenty-First-Century; Sexology; Westermarck, Edward

REFERENCES

Brecher, Edward M. "The First of the Yea-Sayers." In *The Sex Researchers.* Boston, Mass.: Little, Brown, 1969, 3–49; Davies, Robertson. "Havelock Ellis as a Man of Letters." In *A Voice from the*

Attic: Essays on the Art of Reading. New York: Viking, 1972, 90–95; Ellis, Havelock. *The Criminal*. London: Walter Scott, 1890. 4th ed., 1910; Ellis, Havelock. *The Dance of Life*. Boston, Mass.: Houghton Mifflin, 1923; Ellis, Havelock. *Man and Woman: A Study of Human Secondary Sexual Characters*. London: Walter Scott, 1894. 8th ed., London: Heinemann, 1934; Ellis, Havelock. *My Life: Autobiography of Havelock Ellis*. Boston, Mass.: Houghton Mifflin, 1939; Ellis, Havelock. *The New Spirit*. London: Bell, 1890. New York: Boni and Liveright, n.d.; Ellis, Havelock. (1897–1928) *Studies in the Psychology of Sex*. New York: Random House, 1936. (Four, later two, volumes; paginated according to the original seven volumes); Freud, Sigmund. (1914) "On Narcissism: An Introduction." In *The Standard Edition of the Complete Psychological Works of Sigmund Freud*, vol. 14. Trans. James Strachey. London: Hogarth Press, 1953–1974, 73–102; Freud, Sigmund. (1905) *Three Essays on the Theory of Sexuality*. In *The Standard Edition of the Complete Psychological Works of Sigmund Freud*, vol. 7. Ed. and trans. James Strachey. London: Hogarth Press, 1953–1974, 125–245; Grosskurth, Phyllis. *Havelock Ellis: A Biography*. New York: Knopf, 1980; Harrison, Fraser. *The Dark Angel: Aspects of Victorian Sexuality*. New York: Universe Books, 1977; Robinson, Paul. "Havelock Ellis." In *The Modernization of Sex: Havelock Ellis, Alfred Kinsey, William Masters and Virginia Johnson*. New York: Harper and Row, 1976, 1–41.

Edward Johnson

ADDITIONAL READING

Ashby, Hope E. "Ellis, Havelock." In Vern L. Bullough and Bonnie Bullough, eds., *Human Sexuality: An Encyclopedia*. New York: Garland, 1994, 183; Bland, Lucy, and Laura Doan, eds. *Sexology in Culture: Labelling Bodies and Desires*. Chicago, Ill.: University of Chicago Press, 1998; Bland, Lucy, and Laura Doan, eds. *Sexology Uncensored: The Documents of Sexual Science*. Chicago, Ill.: University of Chicago Press, 1998; Brome, Vincent. *Havelock Ellis, Philosopher of Sex: A Biography*. London: Routledge and Kegan Paul, 1979; Calder-Marshall, Arthur. *The Sage of Sex: A Life of Havelock Ellis*. New York: G. P. Putnam's Sons, 1959; Cameron, J. M. "Sex in the Head." *New York Review of Books* (13 May 1976), 19–28; Collis, John Stewart. *Havelock Ellis, Artist of Life: A Study of His Life and Work*. New York: W. Sloane, 1959; Ellis, Havelock. *Affirmations*. London: Walter Scott, 1898. 3rd ed., 1926; Ellis, Havelock. *Fountain of Life*. Boston, Mass.: Houghton Mifflin, 1930; Ellis, Havelock. *Little Essays of Love and Virtue*. London: Black, 1922; Ellis, Havelock. *More Essays of Love and Virtue*. London: Constable, 1931; Ellis, Havelock. (1939) "My Credo." In *The Genius of Europe*. New York: Rinehart, 1951, 3–13. Reprint, Westport, Conn.: Greenwood Press, 1974; Ellis, Havelock. *The Nationalization of Health*. London: Fisher Unwin, 1892; Ellis, Havelock. *Sex and Marriage: Eros in Contemporary Life*. Ed. John Gaworth. New York: Random House, 1951; Ellis, Havelock. *The Task of Social Hygiene*. London: Constable, 1912; Garton, Stephen. *Histories of Sexuality*. London: Taylor and Francis, 2004; Goldberg, Isaac. *Havelock Ellis: A Biographical and Critical Survey*. New York: Simon and Schuster, 1926; Jackson, Margaret. "Eroticizing Women's Oppression: Havelock Ellis and the Construction of the 'Natural.'" In *The Real Facts of Life: Feminism and the Politics of Sexuality c. 1850–1940*. London: Taylor and Francis, 1994, 106–28; Nottingham, Chris. *The Pursuit of Serenity: Havelock Ellis and the New Politics*. Amsterdam, Holland: University Press, 1999; Peterson, Houston. *Havelock Ellis: Philosopher of Love*. Boston, Mass.: Houghton Mifflin, 1928; Robinson, Paul. *The Freudian Left: Wilhelm Reich, Geza Roheim, Herbert Marcuse*. New York: Harper and Row, 1969; Rowbotham, Sheila, and Jeffrey Weeks. (1977) *Socialism and the New Life: The Personal and Sexual Politics of Edward Carpenter and Havelock Ellis*. London: Longwood, 1980; Shalit, Wendy. *A Return to Modesty: Discovering the Lost Virtue*. New York: Free Press, 1999; Tougaw, Jason. "Havelock Ellis." In Timothy F. Murphy, ed., *Reader's Guide to Lesbian and Gay Studies*. Chicago, Ill.: Fitzroy Dearborn, 2000, 199–200; Weeks, Jeffrey. "Havelock Ellis and the Politics of Sex Reform." In *Making Sexual History*. Oxford, U.K.: Blackwell, 1999, 17–52; Wortis, Joseph. *Fragments of an Analysis with Freud*. New York: Simon and Schuster, 1954.

ENGELS, FRIEDRICH. *See* Marxism

EROTICA. *See* Pornography

ESSENTIALISM. *See* Social Constructionism

ETHICS OF HOMOSEXUALITY. *See* Homosexuality, Ethics of

ETHICS, PROFESSIONAL CODES OF. Any occupation seeking professional status—accountants, advertisers, architects, bankers, brokers, engineers, financial planners, insurance agents, public officials, personal trainers, realtors, even zookeepers—subscribes to some sort of professional code. These self-regulatory canons, guidelines, principles, and rules are a relatively recent phenomenon. Medicine, the first occupation to style itself a "profession" in the modern sense of the term—that is, a self-regulating occupation of highly educated members who are publicly committed to the service of others—was also the first to formulate formal codes of professional ethics. The American Medical Association (AMA) adopted the first national code of medical ethics at its founding convention in 1847. Over a half-century later, in 1908, the American Bar Association (ABA) adopted the first formal code of professional legal ethics, the "Canons of Professional Ethics." Medicine thus provided a model upon which law and other professions built.

In drafting their first codes of ethics, medical practitioners did not start from scratch. Instead, they drew from a moral tradition resting on precepts that came from the "Hippocratic oath." This oath, written sometime in the fourth century BCE, has been preserved in the form of unpunctuated texts, like the following fragment:

> [A]nd I will use regimens for the benefit of the ill in accordance with my ability and my judgment but from [what is] to their harm or injustice I will keep [them] and I will not give a drug that is deadly to anyone if asked [for it] nor will I suggest the way to such a counsel and likewise I will not give a woman a destructive pessary and in a pure and holy way I will guard my life and my *techne*. (Von Staden)

The text's lack of punctuation permitted later readers to interpret it in a variety of ways. Roman Stoics, medieval and modern Christians, and contemporary pro-life advocates, for example, read this passage as categorically prohibiting **abortion**. Following this tradition, nineteenth- and early-twentieth-century medical societies typically incorporated prohibitions against abortion into their codes of professional ethics. Yet, situated in its historical context, this reading is questionable. The Greeks of the period were not protective of the fetus: They practiced infanticide by exposure of unwanted newborns, and other Hippocratic texts discuss abortion techniques. It is likely that the prohibition on using a "destructive pessary" was intended as an admonition against using abortifacients that endanger maternal health or life, "even if asked" to do so. The prohibition can thus be read as an extension of the admonition against giving deadly drugs. The point to appreciate is that the unpunctuated original Greek text is superlatively malleable and sustains multiple readings.

Four features of the text of the Hippocratic oath dealing with sex and gender were preserved by professional codes: (1) the oath's male chauvinist presumptions, (2) its prohibitions on sexual relations, (3) its explicit gender egalitarianism, and (4) its requirement of confidentiality.

(1) The male chauvinism of ancient Greek society is naturally reflected in the text of the oath. Its **language** is unambiguously male chauvinist, presuming that the practice of medicine was the exclusive prerogative of fathers and sons. The professional codes of ethics of the nineteenth century preserved these chauvinist presumptions. In mid-century (1849), Elizabeth Blackwell (1821–1910) challenged the idea of medicine as an exclusively male prerogative, becoming the first woman in the United States (perhaps anywhere) to receive a medical degree from a regular medical college. Other women followed and soon began to seek admission to the AMA—only to hit a barrier erected by the presumptive male chauvinism of the language of professional ethics. The AMA's 1847 code is studded with such statements as, "All practitioners of medicine, their wives and children . . . are entitled to gratuitous services" (AMA 1847, chap. II, art. II, sec. 1), which presume that practitioners are male. In 1868 the AMA's Committee on Ethics was asked to determine whether the AMA's code of ethics excluded women from medicine. Dispatching with tradition and literalism, the all-male committee determined that gender was *not* grounds for exclusion from membership. In 1871, on a vote of 83 to 26, the AMA's House of Delegates admitted women members. In 1873 the British Medical Association (which lacked a formal code of ethics) also admitted its first woman member, Elizabeth Garrett Anderson (1836–1917), who was also the first British woman physician.

Law was less welcoming to women than medicine. The first woman to become a practicing lawyer in the United States (perhaps anywhere) was Myra Colby Bradwell (1831–1894), editor of the *Chicago Legal News*. Bradwell passed the Illinois bar exam with honors in 1869 but was nonetheless denied admission to the bar. In 1873 the U.S. Supreme Court upheld this decision. Eventually, however, the Illinois bar relented, admitting Bradwell in 1890; two years later she received a license to practice before the U.S. Supreme Court. Yet despite the progress made by Anderson, Blackwell, Bradwell, and other women pioneers, law, medicine, and other professions were largely inhospitable to women until the U.S. civil rights legislation of the 1960s, which catalyzed a worldwide movement of egalitarian reform. Today, the AMA encourages "medical schools and other medical institutions . . . to increase the number of women in leadership positions" (*Code of Medical Ethics*, §9.035).

(2) Perhaps the most famous line dealing with sex in the Hippocratic oath states, "[I]nto as many houses as I may enter I will go for the benefit of the ill while being far from all voluntary and destructive injustice especially from sexual acts both upon women's bodies and upon men's both of the free and of the slaves" (Von Staden). It is likely that this unequivocal prohibition of sexual relations was necessitated by the observational and empirical nature of Hippocratic medicine, which required physicians to physically observe, probe, and touch the human body. The oath recognizes that these acts can have sexual overtones and makes it clear to physicians, to patients, and to the public that the goal of physical examination is to benefit the sick person, not to serve the interests of the physician or to gratify his sexual appetites. These explicit prohibitions, however, also serve to implicitly define as permissible a nonsexual interpretation of acts that would otherwise be understood as sexual. Taboos against touching or examining the naked body stultified the development of empirical, observationally based medicine in many cultures (for example, Imperial China). By formally and publicly emphasizing beneficial intent, while articulating a strong

prohibition against sexual relations with patients, the oath appears to have served an essential role in legitimating the sort of physical examinations essential to scientific medicine.

Virtually every modern code of medical ethics has preserved this feature of Hippocratic ethics (see, for example, AMA *Code*, §8.14). Section 2.1 of the American Psychiatric Association's (APA) code of ethics is exceptionally explicit:

> The necessary intensity of the treatment relationship may tend to activate sexual and other needs and fantasies on the part of both patient and psychiatrist, while weakening the objectivity necessary for control. Additionally, the inherent inequality in the doctor-patient relationship may lead to exploitation of the patient. Sexual activity with a current or former patient is unethical.

The AMA extends the prohibition to apply to any behavior that might be considered sexual or **sexual harassment**, and the prohibition encompasses a patient's relatives and significant others (§8.145). It also prohibits physicians in a supervisory role from having sexual relations with those people that they supervise (§3.08). The ABA, too, recognizes the conflict of interest implicit in sexual relations between lawyers and clients. Rule 1.8 proscribes such relations: "A lawyer shall not have sexual relations with a client unless a consensual sexual relationship existed between them when the client-lawyer relationship commenced."

These explicit prohibitions on sexual relations between medical practitioners and patients, and between lawyers and clients, stand in marked contrast to codes of ethics of other professional bodies. The American Association of University Professors' (AAUP) Statement on Professional Ethics, for example, merely requires professors "to avoid any exploitation, harassment, or discriminatory treatment of students," and it repeats this admonition with respect to fellow faculty members. The statement leaves open, to the potentially self-serving interpretive imaginations of readers, the question of whether sexual advances, or a sexual relationship between faculty members and students or supervisors and subordinates, should be considered "exploitation, harassment, or discriminatory." The contrast between the AAUP code and the AMA, APA, and ABA codes on this point is noteworthy.

(3) Another remarkable feature of the fragment of the oath quoted above is that the scope of the commitment to "benefit the ill" and to abstain from "all voluntary and destructive injustice" extends to women as well as men, the enslaved as well as the free. Ancient Greece was a culture of gender inequality. Women had little role in public life and tended to be segregated in specially designated areas of the household. Slaves had no rights, and in elite households slave boys and girls could be passed around as party favors for visiting male guests. By extending the prohibition on sexual relationships to slaves, the oath implies that the physician's duty to benefit the ill crosses caste, class, and status lines, applying equally to all patients, female or male, slave or free. Stoic and Christian interpreters were to emphasize this reading. A strong egalitarian commitment to benefit patients, irrespective of gender, class, status, race, religion, or ethnicity, thus became part of the Hippocratic tradition.

Later codes of professional medical ethics preserved this feature of the Hippocratic tradition. These issues were resurrected during the early years of the AIDS (acquired immunodeficiency syndrome) epidemic (the 1980s), when some physicians refused to treat HIV (human immunodeficiency virus)-positive patients, who were often gay or intravenous drug users. The AMA responded by inserting the following statement in its code of ethics: "A physician may not ethically refuse to treat a patient whose condition is within the physician's current realm of competence solely because the patient is seropositive for HIV. Persons who are seropositive should not be subjected to discrimination based on fear or prejudice" (*Code*, §9.131). Similarly, a strong commitment to client representation in legal ethics requires lawyers to represent and to act as a diligent and zealous advocate for clients, irrespective of "the client's political, economic, social, or moral views or activities" (ABA, *Model Rules of Professional Conduct*, 1.2).

(4) The text of the oath also asserts a commitment to confidentiality: "[A]nd about whatever I may see or hear in treatment or even without treatment, in the life of human beings—things that should not ever be blurted out outside—I will remain silent holding such things to be unutterable [sacred, not to be divulged]." Christian commentators, mindful of the sanctity of confession (instituted by the Lateran Council in 1215), have tended to interpret the Hippocratic tradition as requiring a near-absolute commitment to confidentiality. The AMA's 1847 *Code of Ethics* expressly links confidentiality to sex and gender, noting that because "a medical man is under the strongest obligations of secrecy," even "the female sex should never allow feelings of shame and delicacy to prevent them from disclosing . . . symptoms and causes of complaint peculiar to them" (chap. I, art. II, sec. 4). However, the 1847 *Code* also notes that confidential secrets may be disclosed when it is "imperatively required to do so" (chap. I, art. I, sec. 2). The current AMA *Code* also offers a strong but qualified commitment to confidentiality. "The information disclosed to a physician during the course of the relationship between physician and patient is confidential to the greatest extent possible. . . . The physician should not reveal confidential communications or information without the express consent of the patient, unless required to do so by law" (§5.05). Rule 1.6 of the ABA's *Model Rules* offers a similar commitment to limited confidentiality, permitting lawyers to breach confidentiality when it is likely to save lives, to prevent crimes, or when required by court orders.

The professions have always provoked suspicion. They have often been condemned as monopolizing conspiracies that sustain orthodoxy, suppress competition, and feign self-regulation to arrogate privileges for themselves, even as they stave off external regulation. While there is a measure of truth in all these charges, professional codes formally commit professional societies and their membership to ethical ideals and standards, stating what is permissible and prohibited in a format that can be adjudicated, analyzed, decried, debated, enforced, interpreted, invoked, protested, reinterpreted, repealed, and revoked. Professional morality is thus neither a matter of individual conscience nor a question of what is traditionally "the done thing." It is a matter of what the profession expressly states before its own membership and the public.

Compare, for example, the AAUP's advice on sexual relationships with that of the AMA. Whereas the AMA states unequivocally that supervisory personnel may not have sexual relations with or date subordinates or patients, the AAUP is vague on supervisor-supervisee and faculty-student relationships. May a thesis supervisor date, or have sexual relations with, the person being supervised? May a faculty member date, or have sexual relations with, a graduate or undergraduate student? The professor-student and supervisor-subordinate relationships involve an asymmetry of power and significant potential for exploitation, similar to the physician-patient and the lawyer-client relationships. Yet the AAUP code does not provide guidance. Similarly, occupations not having any formal code of ethics at all offer no formal guidance for their members or the public.

It is sometimes suggested that the statements in professional codes are merely window dressing: They neither reflect nor effectively regulate the actual practices of a profession, and they tend, moreover, to be antiquated and self-serving. While these claims have some validity, the public nature of professional codes of ethics, which are typically available via the Internet, opens them to assessment, critique, and correction by the public, as well as by the profession itself. The AMA's original statement about physician's obligations to treat HIV-infected individuals, for example, allowed squeamish doctors to opt out. As soon as these guidelines were published, however, critiques from the gay community and from within the profession itself prompted the AMA's House of Delegates to enact the new, tougher guidelines of §9.131.

Professional standards, moreover, are enforceable, not only by the professions themselves but also by external accrediting and regulatory bodies and, in common-law jurisdictions like Britain and the United States, by courts of law. Anyone who incurs damages caused by a breach of the self-imposed duties that professions formalize in their codes of ethics may sue for redress in civil court. The commitments that a profession makes for its membership in its published codes of ethics are made before the world, and the world at large has the opportunity to hold professionals accountable to them.

See also Activity, Sexual; Coercion (by Sexually Aggressive Women); Ethics, Sexual; Ethics, Virtue; Greek Sexuality and Philosophy, Ancient; Harassment, Sexual; Rape, Acquaintance and Date

REFERENCES

American Association of University Professors. *Statement on Professional Ethics* (1987). <www.aaup.org/statements/Redbook/Rbethics.htm> [accessed 20 September 2004]; American Bar Association. *Model Rules of Professional Conduct*. Chicago, Ill.: Author, 2003; American Bar Association. *2004 Compendium of Professional Responsibility, Rules, and Standards*. Chicago, Ill.: Author, 2004; American Medical Association. (1847) *Code of Ethics*. In Robert B. Baker, Stephen R. Latham, Arthur L. Caplan, and Linda L. Emanuel, eds., *The American Medical Ethics Revolution: How the AMA's Code of Ethics Has Transformed Physicians' Relationships to Patients, Professionals, and Society*. Baltimore, Md.: Johns Hopkins University Press, 1999, 324–34; American Medical Association, Council on Ethics and Judicial Affairs. *Code of Medical Ethics: Current Opinions with Annotations, 2004–2005*. Chicago, Ill.: American Medical Association, 2004; American Psychiatric Association. *Opinions of the Ethics Committee on the Principles of Medical Ethics with Annotations Especially Applicable to Psychiatry*. Arlington, Va.: Author, 2001; American Psychiatric Association. *The Principles of Medical Ethics with Annotations Especially Applicable to Psychiatry*. Arlington, Va.: Author, 2001; Von Staden, Heinrich. " 'In a Pure and Holy Way': Personal and Professional Conduct in the Hippocratic Oath." *Journal of the History of Medicine and Allied Sciences* 51 (1996), 406–8.

Robert Baker

ADDITIONAL READING

Carroll, Mary Ann, Henry G. Schneider, and George R. Wesley. *Ethics in the Practice of Psychology*. Englewood Cliffs, N.J.: Prentice-Hall, 1985; "Code of Ethics for Prostitutes." *Coyote Howls* 5:1 (1978), 9; Garrett, Tanya. "Inappropriate Therapist-Patient 'Relationships.' " In Robin Goodwin and Duncan Cramer, eds., *Inappropriate Relationships: The Unconventional, the Disapproved, and the Forbidden*. Mahwah, N.J.: Erlbaum, 2002, 147–70; Goldman, Alan H. *The Moral Foundations of Professional Ethics*. Totowa, N.J.: Rowman and Littlefield, 1980; Lebacqz, Karen. *Professional Ethics: Power and Paradox*. Nashville, Tenn.: Abingdon Press, 1985; Masters, William H., Virginia E. Johnson, and Robert C. Kolodny, eds. *Ethical Issues in Sex Therapy and Research*. Boston, Mass.: Little, Brown, 1977; Porter, Roy. "A Touch of Danger: The Man-Midwife as Sexual Predator." In G. S. Rousseau and Roy Porter, eds., *Sexual Underworlds of the Enlightenment*. Chapel Hill: University of North Carolina Press, 1988, 206–32; Posner, Richard A., and Katharine B. Silbaugh. "Abuse of Position of Trust or Authority." In *A Guide to America's Sex Laws*. Chicago, Ill.: University of

Chicago Press, 1996, 111–28; Pritchard, Jane. "Codes of Ethics." In Ruth Chadwick, ed., *Encyclopedia of Applied Ethics*, vol. 1. San Diego, Calif.: Academic Press, 1998, 527–33; Risen, Candace B., and Stanley E. Althof. "Professionals Who Sexually Offend: A Betrayal of Trust." In Raymond C. Rosen and Sandra R. Leiblum, eds., *Case Studies in Sex Therapy*. New York: Guilford, 1995, 368–79; "Sexual Misconduct, Guidelines and Codes of Ethics for the American Medical Association, American Swimming Coaches Association, and Antioch College." In Robert Trevas, Arthur Zucker, and Donald Borchert, eds., *Philosophy of Sex and Love: A Reader*. Upper Saddle River, N.J.: Prentice-Hall, 1997, 373–93.

ETHICS, SEXUAL. In the first quarter of the twentieth century, British philosopher **Bertrand Russell** (1872–1970) expressed an idea that is *prima facie* agreeable enough: "[S]exual relations should be a mutual delight, entered into solely from the spontaneous impulse of both parties" (*Marriage and Morals*, 121). Who would object to "mutual delight"? The "spontaneous impulse," however, even if "of both," may cause us to pause. What contrasts with spontaneous impulse? That is, if this is what sexual relations should be, what should they not be? In effect, Russell has already told us, in general terms. His "solely," if taken literally (let us not patronize Russell by discounting this word), means that a necessary condition of proper or permissible **sexual activity** is that it is "entered into" with or through only one reason or motive: spontaneous impulse. Entering into sexual relations for *any* other sole reason is something that should never happen. Let us assume that Russell means that if spontaneous impulse is missing, something has gone wrong, and that as long as spontaneous impulse is present, and is one of the reasons or motives of the sexual event, then the presence of another, contemporaneously operating reason or motive does not by itself make the event objectionable. When a sexual act is motivated by spontaneous impulse, *con* or *sans* additional accompanying reasons or motives, it still must be evaluated, for Russell does not claim that a sexual act's arising from spontaneous impulse is sufficient for it to be acceptable. But note that a standard counterexample, and one of the strongest, to the claim of sufficiency, the immorality of **adultery**—X and Y's acting on their spontaneous impulses for each other when either is married to Z—is not clearly a situation that Russell would countenance as a counterexample.

So, what are the reasons or motives that, if present while spontaneous impulse is absent, would make sexual relations objectionable? It would be difficult to compose a comprehensive and definitive list of *all* the other reasons or motives people might have to engage in sex, but there are some obvious candidates. (1) "Because you have a gun at my head." This case exhibits neither "mutual delight" nor "spontaneous impulse of both," through coercion and/or the absence of **consent**. (2) "Because I need the money." This case also violates the two clauses, but whether through coercion and/or the absence of consent is not clear. (See Mappes on the "exploitation" in such cases.) Indeed, Russell does have mercenary sex, or **prostitution**, in mind—but also situations in which a woman agrees to **marriage**, and hence sex, because she will be economically better off married or will avoid being worse off. "The intrusion of the economic motive into sex is . . . disastrous" (121), Russell writes. (3) "Because if I, a wife and mother of a young child, do not have sex with you, my husband, even though I am exhausted from a day's labor or prefer to watch television or read a book tonight before bed, you will have yet another gripe against me and will, if I refuse too often, leave me, abandon me, as you have reminded me time and again, and I fear for myself and my child, whom I might not be able to support adequately without your income." It is a fair bet that Russell was talking about this scenario when he wrote that "the total amount of undesired sex endured by women is probably greater in marriage than in prostitution" (122). If he was, he was already inspired by a radical vision popularized half a century later in Second Wave **feminism**. Friedrich Engels (1820–1895), however, had taken this logic one step further fifty years before Russell, when he claimed that in capitalism a married woman *is* a prostitute, one who has been compelled to sell her body once and for all into "slavery" instead of selling it on a "piece-work" basis (*Origin*, 82; see Emma Goldman [1869–1940], 179; Jaggar). Whereas Russell keeps marriage and prostitution distinct, and sees both the prostitute and the wife in sexual dire straights, Engels conflates the two, thereby making the point more dramatically.

Robin Morgan is the Second Wave feminist writer most closely associated with this theme. (During First Wave feminism, it was Victoria Woodhull [1838–1927]; see "Tried as by Fire," 40; **Andrea Dworkin** [1946–2005], 135–36.) In her essay "Theory and Practice: Pornography and Rape," Morgan defines "**rape**" and then illustrates it:

> [R]ape exists any time sexual intercourse occurs when it has not been initiated by the woman, out of her own genuine affection and desire.... How many millions of times have women had sex "willingly" with men they didn't want to have sex with?... How many times have women wished just to sleep instead or read or watch the Late Show?... Most of the decently married bedrooms across America are settings for nightly rape. (165–66)

Although Russell sensed something very wrong in the marriage bedroom, he was not ready to call it "rape" (probably the thought never occurred to him). Why does Morgan call these daily events "rape"? The fundamental idea is that genuinely consensual, uncoerced participation in sexual activity, without a hint of pressure, requires the ability of each party freely to say no or to refuse without any recrimination, retaliation, or yelling; that, in turn, requires substantial equality between the parties. Given that in patriarchy, or a social/economic/political regime of male dominance, an enormous differential in privilege and power exists between men and women, women's consent to heterosexual activity is largely chimerical. Morgan would like heterosexual intercourse to occur only out of the woman's own "genuine affection and desire" (something akin to Russell's spontaneous impulse) because she is apprehensive that otherwise the woman will be pressured—since in patriarchy she is the social, economic, and sexual subordinate of the man—in both subtle and not-so-subtle ways to engage in sexual activity in which she really prefers not to engage. If sex occurs only when the woman herself desires it, only when she wants it precisely out of her own **sexual desire** (as evidenced by her initiating the act), and not for any other reason, then we can speak about unsullied, rape-free heterosexuality. Russell likely would agree, even if he would not speak of "rape."

We can explore and assess Russell's and Morgan's provocative views in a number of ways. (See **Irving Singer** for another list of evaluative criteria.) First, we can inquire whether, or to what extent, they have uncovered something morally reprehensible about sexual relations. Sexual acts have long been the subject of moral assessment, not only by religious thinkers but also by secular ethicists. In theory, a sexual act (a token or a type) might be morally obligatory, permissible, supererogatory, or wrong. In evaluating a sexual act along this dimension, we can take into account many complex factors, including the nature of the act in question, its structure, its effects, the state of mind of the actors, the antecedents of the act, and the context in which it occurs. Russell and Morgan are making claims within this "moral dimension," the domain of sexual ethics. We will return to the issue of the plausibility of their moral pronouncements.

Second, we can examine an act's nonmoral quality, which can be given a narrow technical meaning: Does the act provide pleasure (nonmoral goodness) or is it tedious, boring, unenjoyable, uncomfortable (nonmoral badness)? Although moral rightness and nonmoral goodness are distinct things, some connection exists between them: For many ethicists, that an act produces nonmoral value is a plus in its moral favor (although not always decisive). We can presume that Russell and Morgan are distressed that women endure, and have to endure, much "undesired" nonmorally bad sex. That is, not only are women under pressure to engage in sex, but also the sex they do engage in unwillingly does not please them. This is not to say that the situation of women, in the Russell-Morgan view, would be improved were their undesired and coerced sexual acts to bring them sexual pleasure. It is to say that women should be able to participate in sex that is both morally right and nonmorally good. Indeed, much of the reason why sex is nonmorally bad for women is that it is not sex that they would choose to do, were they to have a real choice.

The third thing we can examine about an act is its legality: Is it in the **law** permissible or prohibited? This, of course, varies by jurisdiction and is distinct from judgments of both moral and nonmoral goodness: Some sexual acts that are nonmorally good (e.g., adultery, occasionally) are often legally or morally proscribed; some acts that are morally wrong (again, adultery) might not be illegal. Still, the legal status of an act may have an impact on its morality, for example, if there is a *prima facie* moral duty to obey the law. Suppose that Morgan is right that "most . . . decently married bedrooms . . . are settings for nightly rape." Should not the police and the courts become involved? They do not, because the law uses a different definition of "rape," in which a woman's having no desire for the act and her not initiating it are irrelevant. The central question for the law is whether she did not consent, was physically forced into the act, or was severely threatened. The law does not recognize the sorts of pressures that Morgan has in mind as being intense enough or a type of force that makes subsequent sexual activity rape. Maybe the law employs incorrect notions of rape, consent, force, and threat. These definitions are not written in stone, and in part because they are "essentially contested concepts" (Reitan) they can be changed by, for example, political and legislative activity. Note that the way Morgan defines "rape" supports her thesis that **pornography** contributes causally to the rape of women by men (which is what she means by "pornography is the theory, rape is the practice"). The wider or more inclusive the definition of rape we utilize—or the wider the definition of pornography—it will be that much easier to find a causal connection between them.

Fourth, we can investigate sex acts pragmatically by appraising their nonmoral goodness and badness in a broad sense that goes beyond pleasure or its absence. To mention only a few pragmatic considerations: Some sexual acts are medically innocuous (no chance of contracting a **sexually transmitted disease** or of damaging tissue exists), psychologically safe (the parties will not experience guilt feelings, anxiety, or regret afterward), or have desirable and sometimes intended consequences (the act cements their **love** or leads to a child). Other sexual acts are not safe, or even hazardous, medically or psychologically, or have unwanted consequences (again, pregnancy). Pragmatic considerations, clearly, have an impact on our moral judgments. To the extent that Morgan is right that there is a large disparity between the powers and privileges of men and women, women will be especially vulnerable to losing out or suffering in terms of these pragmatic costs and benefits, being exposed to medically unsafe sex, psychologically traumatic sex, and disruptive pregnancies. Conception as one possible, even hoped for, result of sexual activity raises a question for the Russell-Morgan approach: What if a woman, or both the man and the woman, engage in intercourse motivated only or predominantly by a wish for a child? Russell would have to say that as long as they are motivated by both a wish for a child and spontaneous impulse, their coitus could be acceptable. Morgan would have to say something similar: As long as the woman initiates coitus out of her own "genuine affection and desire," the additional reason of wanting to become pregnant would not make the act objectionable. Still, one must wonder about a perspective on sexual morality that judges deficient an act of intercourse in which both the man and the woman do it *only* for the sake of the child-to-be. One need not be a Roman Catholic to express that wonder; one might be a Secular Pluralist about motives.

Finally, sexual acts can be evaluated as biologically or psychologically natural or unnatural ("perverted," "kinky"). For some ethicists, the naturalness of sexual activity is very important to its morality (Roman Catholics), while for others it is altogether irrelevant (Secular Humanists). Is it possible that both the man and the woman are spontaneously motivated by sexual impulses to engage in what psychiatry calls a **paraphilia**? There is no doubt that they could be spontaneously moved to engage in what Roman Catholicism considers unnatural sexual acts, for that religion, with qualifications, counts almost anything other than penis-vagina intercourse as unnatural, for example, oral sex to orgasm. (See **Saint Thomas Aquinas** [1224/25–1274], *Summa theologiae*, vol. 43, 2a2ae, ques. 154, art. 1–12.) It would seem to be a happy yet unlikely coincidence that a male foot fetishist would stumble upon a woman who yearned to have her feet pampered. There is nothing in principle, however, in Russell's view that rules out a **Havelock Ellis** (1859–1939) meeting a Françoise Lafitte-Cyon (1886–1974), after which they sexually enjoy urolagnia together, where spontaneous impulse is their motive. By contrast, it might seem bizarre for a woman, abiding by Morgan's principle, to initiate sexually perverted acts with a man out of her own genuine desire, for the psychiatric **perversion**s are associated nearly exclusively with male sexuality. Further, three scenarios in which a woman might be expected to participate in paraphiliac activity do not satisfy Morgan's principle. (1) She caves into the pressure that the man applies in his attempt to satisfy his perverse desires with her. This case is no different from her caving into his pressure to engage in "normal" intercourse when she prefers to watch TV or go to sleep. (2) She willingly engages in his perversion(s) because she knows that doing so will bind him to her, offering her the domestic stability she favors (see Greer, 152). Even though this procedure might benefit her in the long run and bring her contentment, it violates Morgan's principle, for the woman's motive—to attain security—is one of many wrong motives for engaging in sex. (3) A woman might (often does) participate in men's sexual perversions because doing so—as a professional dominatrix, for example—brings in a tidy sum (see Theroux). Again, this is one of many reasons for engaging in sexual activity that is rejected by Morgan's principle, even if the woman's income is sky high, even if her profession thereby permits her the luxury of maintaining independence from men (and other women), even if as an autonomous and successful businesswoman she can diversify, invest, write books, travel at whim, and lead an otherwise full and satisfying life.

There is yet another motive a woman might have for engaging in rocky road, or even vanilla, sexual activity with her husband: out of her "genuine affection" for him, even if it is not especially accompanied by sexual desire. The wording of Morgan's principle— "and," not "or"—implies that a woman's attending to her husband's sexual yearnings just because she loves him is unacceptable. Russell's principle has that implication as well. (Morgan might add that her "loving" him is only an aspect of her patriarchal indoctrination, as is her interest in anything heterosexual to begin with, and hence could not be "genuine." [See Adrienne Rich.] Under conditions of patriarchy, Morgan's principle might very well be vacuous. Only after the dismantling of patriarchy could women finally say that their desires, whatever they turn out to be, are genuinely their own. Perhaps **Catharine MacKinnon** takes this position.) Further, such catering or attending to a man's sexual desires is not usually done at the initiative of the woman but at the request of the man. Morgan's principle rules out, then, a woman's making a pure gift of sexual activity to her husband on his birthday or their anniversary. The battle of the sexes, rooted mildly in biology and fostered, exaggerated by culture, here becomes nuclear.

No sane ethicist (the **Marquis de Sade** does not count as an ethicist) denies that X's forcing Y to perform a sexual act by brandishing a loaded gun or by physically overpowering the smaller, weaker Y does something morally reprehensible. But to derive from that truth that only one motive for engaging in sexual activity is permissible—either Russell's spontaneous impulse or Morgan's initiating sex out of one's genuine affection and desire—would seem to be a great leap of logic. Perhaps these two principles can be construed as stating an ideal, but if so, that concedes that other motives, even if not the best, may be unobjectionable. Instead of stating such stringent principles, a relaxed ethicist would offer something like: Every person should engage in sexual activity only when he or she *wants* to, where "wants" neither reduces to nor is equivalent to what Russell and Morgan proposed. The point is that "wants" by itself does not establish that some motives or reasons for engaging in sexual activity are better or worse than any others. More argument is required to work out the details, but at least restrictions on motives or reasons are not built right into the very principle governing sexual behavior. It is not ruled out immediately, even though some of these reasons might be ruled out eventually, that we may engage in sexual activity merely to make the other person happy, or just to make ourselves happy, or to make the baby-to-be happy later, or to relieve boredom, or to get some exercise, or to keep in practice (use it or lose it), or to make some money, or to win a bet, or to pay off a debt, or as a way to congratulate the Bar Mitzvah boy, or his father. (See Annie Sprinkle's list of 101 benefits of sexual activity.)

One other thing: Russell and Morgan, in their determination to protect the well-being and freedom of women, may have overlooked the way in which it is counterproductive to restrict sex to times when women are motivated by their own genuine or spontaneous desire. We, both men and women, can be dominated, overpowered, reduced to slavery, in a very real sense as much by the other's bodily and mental **beauty**, those features of persons that elicit our own genuine desire for them or provokes spontaneous impulse, as by the other's brute strength or malicious threats. Except the gun at one's head and extreme economic need, nothing undermines one's autonomy as much as being compelled or propelled by the combination of sexual desire and genuine affection for the object of one's attention. What we need is a little detachment, some lightness, a spot of relief from Morgan's and Russell's too-heavy sexual motives, and this is something provided by our having and acting on a wide variety of reasons when we decide to engage in sexual activity.

See also Adultery; Casual Sex; Consent; Consequentialism; Ethics, Virtue; Fantasy; Feminism, History of; Feminism, Lesbian; Feminism, Men's; Flirting; Hobbes, Thomas; Homosexuality, Ethics of; Kant, Immanuel; MacKinnon, Catharine; Marxism; Objectification, Sexual; Pedophilia; Philosophy of Sex, Overview of; Philosophy of Sex, Teaching the; Pornography; Prostitution; Rape; Seduction; Sex Work; Sexuality, Dimensions of; Wojtyła, Karol (Pope John Paul II)

REFERENCES

Dworkin, Andrea. *Intercourse*. New York: Free Press, 1987; Engels, Frederick. (1884) *The Origin of the Family, Private Property, and the State*. New York: International Publishers, 1942. Peking,

China: Foreign Languages Press, 1978; Goldman, Emma. "The Traffic in Women." In *Anarchism and Other Essays*. (1910) New York: Dover, 1969, 177–94; Greer, Germaine. *The Female Eunuch*. New York: Bantam, 1971; Jaggar, Alison M. "Prostitution." In Alan Soble, ed., *The Philosophy of Sex: Contemporary Readings*, 1st ed. Totowa, N.J.: Rowman and Littlefield, 1980, 348–68; Mappes, Thomas. (1985) "Sexual Morality and the Concept of Using Another Person." In Thomas A. Mappes and Jane S. Zembaty, eds., *Social Ethics*, 4th ed. New York: McGraw-Hill, 1992, 203–26; Morgan, Robin. (1974) "Theory and Practice: Pornography and Rape." In *Going Too Far: The Personal Chronicle of a Feminist*. New York: Random House, 1977, 163–69; Reitan, Eric. "Rape as an Essentially Contested Concept." *Hypatia* 16:2 (2001), 43–66; Rich, Adrienne. "Compulsory Heterosexuality and Lesbian Existence." *Signs* 5:4 (1980), 631–60; Russell, Bertrand. *Marriage and Morals*. London: George Allen and Unwin, 1929; Singer, Irving. "Criteria of Sexual Goodness." In *Sex: A Philosophical Primer*. Lanham, Md.: Rowman and Littlefield, 2001, 65–101; Sprinkle, Annie. "The Benefits of Sex." <www.anniesprinkle.org/html/writings/101_uses.html> [accessed 15 February 2005]; Theroux, Paul. "Nurse Wolf." *The New Yorker* (15 June 1998), 50–63; Thomas Aquinas. (1265–1273) *Summa theologiae*, 60 vols. Cambridge, U.K.: Blackfriars, 1964–1976; Woodhull, Victoria C. (1874) "Tried as by Fire." In *The Victoria Woodhull Reader*. Ed. Madeleine B. Stern. Weston, Mass.: M & S Press, 1974 [pages not consecutively numbered].

Alan Soble

ADDITIONAL READING

Alpert, Rebecca T. "Guilty Pleasures: When Sex Is Good Because It's Bad." In Patricia Beattie Jung, Mary E. Hunt, and Radhika Balakrishnan, eds., *Good Sex: Feminist Perspectives from the World's Religions*. New Brunswick, N.J.: Rutgers University Press, 2001, 31–43; Goldman, Emma. "The Traffic in Women." Anarchy Archives (Web site). <dwardmac.pitzer.edu/Anarchist_Archives/goldman/aando/traffic.html> [accessed 2 June 2005]; Halwani, Raja. "Sexual Morality." In Timothy F. Murphy, ed., *Reader's Guide to Lesbian and Gay Studies*. Chicago, Ill.: Fitzroy Dearborn, 2000, 534–37; Halwani, Raja. *Virtuous Liaisons: Care, Love, Sex, and Virtue Ethics*. Chicago, Ill.: Open Court, 2003; Jacoby, Susan. (1983) "Sexual Revenge." In Christina Sommers and Fred Sommers, eds., *Vice and Virtue in Everyday Life: Introductory Readings in Ethics*, 3rd ed. Fort Worth, Tex.: Harcourt Brace Jovanovich, 1993, 420–29; Jaggar, Alison M. "Prostitution." In Alan Soble, ed., *The Philosophy of Sex: Contemporary Readings*, 1st ed. Totowa, N.J.: Rowman and Littlefield, 1980, 348–68. Reprinted in POS2 (259–80); Jordan, Mark D. *The Ethics of Sex*. Oxford, U.K.: Blackwell, 2002; Jung, Patricia Beattie, and Shannon Jung, eds. "Sexual Ethics." In *Moral Issues and Christian Responses*, 7th ed. Belmont, Calif.: Wadsworth, 2003, 51–101; Kant, Immanuel. "Duties towards the Body in Respect of Sexual Impulse." In *Lectures on Ethics*. Trans. Louis Infield. New York: Methuen, 1930. Indianapolis, Ind.: Hackett, 1980, 162–71. Reprinted in POS4 (199–205); STW (140–45); Mappes, Thomas A. (1985) "Sexual Morality and the Concept of Using Another Person." In Thomas A. Mappes and Jane S. Zembaty, eds., *Social Ethics: Morality and Social Policy*, 4th ed. New York: McGraw-Hill, 1992, 203–16. 5th ed., 1997, 163–76. 6th ed., 2002, 170–83. Reprinted in POS4 (207–23); Murphy, Jeffrie G. "Some Ruminations on Women, Violence, and the Criminal Law." In Jules Coleman and Allen Buchanan, eds., *In Harm's Way: Essays in Honor of Joel Feinberg*. Cambridge: Cambridge University Press, 1994, 209–30; Nussbaum, Martha C. "Sex in the Head." [Review of *Sexual Desire: A Moral Philosophy of the Erotic*, by Roger Scruton] *New York Review of Books* (18 December 1986), 49–52; Regan, A. "Lust." In *New Catholic Encyclopedia*, vol. 8. New York: McGraw-Hill, 1967, 1081–85; Rich, Adrienne. "Compulsory Heterosexuality and Lesbian Existence." *Signs* 5:4 (1980), 631–60. Reprinted in *Blood, Bread, and Poetry: Selected Prose 1979–1985*. New York: Norton, 1986, 23–75; and Henry Abelove, Michèle Aina Barale, and David M. Halperin, eds., *The Lesbian and Gay Studies Reader*. New York: Routledge, 1993, 227–54; Ruddick, Sara. "On Sexual Morality." In James Rachels, ed., *Moral Problems: A Collection of Philosophical Essays*, 2nd ed. New York: Harper and Row, 1971, 16–34. Reprinted, revised, as "Better Sex," in Robert B. Baker and Frederick A. Elliston, eds., *Philosophy and Sex*, 1st ed. Buffalo, N.Y.: Prometheus, 1975,

83–104; P&S2 (280–99); and, abridged, in Judith A. Boss, ed., *Analyzing Moral Issues*, 3rd ed. New York: McGraw-Hill, 2005, 368–77; Scruton, Roger. "Sexual Morality." In *Sexual Desire: A Moral Philosophy of the Erotic*. New York: Free Press, 1986, 322–47; Singer, Peter, ed. "Sexual Morality." In *Ethics*. Oxford, U.K.: Oxford University Press, 1994, part I.B.iii, 93–112; Soble, Alan. "Ethics." In *Sexual Investigations*. New York: New York University Press, 1996, 1–59; Soble, Alan. "The Love Gambit." In *Pornography, Sex, and Feminism*. Amherst, N.Y.: Prometheus, 2002, 173–83; Soble, Alan. "Pornography and the Social Sciences." *Social Epistemology* 2:2 (1988), 135–44. Reprinted in POS2 (317–31); POS4 (421–34); Spencer, Daniel T. *Gay and Gaia: Ethics, Ecology, and the Erotic*. Cleveland, Ohio: Pilgrim Press, 1996; Thielicke, Helmut. *The Ethics of Sex*. Trans. John W. Doberstein. New York: Harper and Row, 1964; Tuana, Nancy, and Laurie Shrage. "Sexuality." In Hugh LaFollette, ed., *The Oxford Handbook of Practical Ethics*. Oxford, U.K.: Oxford University Press, 2003, 15–41; Wertheimer, Alan. "Consent and Sexual Relations." *Legal Theory* 2:2 (1996), 89–112. Reprinted in POS4 (341–66); West, Robin. "A Comment on Consent, Sex, and Rape." *Legal Theory* 2:3 (1996), 233–51; Wojtyła, Karol. (Pope John Paul II) *Love and Responsibility*. New York: Farrar, Straus and Giroux, 1981.

ETHICS, VIRTUE. Starting in the 1950s, some philosophers, such as **G.E.M. Anscombe** (1919–2001), Philippa Foot, and Bernard Williams (1929–2003), became dissatisfied with moral philosophy. They thought too much emphasis was being put on the evaluation of action and not enough on other dimensions of morality, such as character and living a good life. This spawned a movement among many philosophers to reinvestigate Greek ethics, and contemporary virtue ethics was born (see Statman, 3–7). "Virtue ethics" refers to moral philosophy that relies centrally on the notion of "virtue" (or the virtues). Virtue ethics is independent of, and perhaps rivals, traditional moral theories such as utilitarianism and Kantianism. Note, however, that "[t]he recent use of 'virtue ethics' to distinguish one standpoint within ethics from others would have been unintelligible in Greek philosophy, for which, since a virtue was an excellence . . . and ethics concerned excellences of character, all ethics was virtue ethics" (MacIntyre, 1757).

One way virtue ethics is distinctive is that it begins with natural facts about human beings and derives from these a view about what a moral life for humans is (see Foot; Hursthouse, *On Virtue Ethics* [*OVE*], pt. 3). The virtues are important because they link up with the good life and human flourishing. Most ancient Greek philosophers, including **Aristotle** (384–322 BCE), agreed that virtue was necessary for human happiness. Aristotle did not think virtue was sufficient or being virtuous ensured flourishing. Many contemporary virtue ethicists defend Aristotle, though some shy away from both the necessity and sufficiency claims. They argue only that the virtues are one's best bet for flourishing (Hursthouse, *OVE*, pt. 3). One *can* flourish without the virtues, but the odds are against it. If so, a virtue is a character trait that one generally needs to flourish.

Classic examples of virtues include courage, temperance, wisdom, justice, and generosity. Contemporary philosophers include care, compassion, pity, self-respect, and respect. There is no agreed on definition of "virtue," but the consensus is that a virtue is a character trait that disposes its possessor to feel and act rightly. Consider courage, a disposition to defend important goods in the face of risks. If a courageous person comes across a drowning child, she knows that something important, a human life, is in jeopardy. If she is a mediocre swimmer, saving the child is risky. In jumping into the water to rescue the child, she acts well. She would also experience the appropriate emotions. She would feel fear, given the risks, yet she would also feel confident in her ability to save the child.

The virtues are infused with practical wisdom, an intellectual virtue that helps the agent recognize what is good, important, and worthy about life, and helps the agent see what to do in a given situation. Practical wisdom thereby "triggers" particular virtues. The virtuous (and, so, wise) agent "sees" that the drowning situation requires courage and, *ceteris paribus*, acts courageously.

There are vices that correspond to the virtues. When Aristotle claims that virtue is a state that lies in a mean (1107a), he is usually understood to assert that for every virtue there are two vices, one of excess, one of deficiency. The virtue of courage lies in the mean between exhibiting too much fear and too little (or none). However, Aristotle also claims that when one acts virtuously, one acts for the right reason, at the right time, toward the right people, and in the right way (*Nicomachean Ethics*, 1106b20–23, 1109a28, 1115b17). This implies that not every virtue corresponds to exactly two vices. Some virtues might admit of more than two vices by allowing more than one way a person could act wrongly, more than one wrong reason for acting, and more than one wrong person toward whom one acts (Hursthouse, "A False Doctrine of the Mean").

Does virtue ethics have anything interesting to say about sexuality? (This was something about which Aristotle said virtually nothing.) We must first see how virtue ethics treats the evaluation of acts. One view is that an act is right if and only if it is one that a virtuous agent would characteristically do (Hursthouse, *OVE*, 28). "Characteristically" is meant to rule out cases in which the agent acts out of character: when he or she is sick, sad, or depressed. Given the virtue of temperance, the virtue concerned with the right use and experience of bodily pleasures, virtue ethics does not reject **sexual activity** as such. The question is whether virtue ethics forbids certain sexual acts, whether these are acts that a virtuous person would not characteristically do.

Some sexual acts are clearly forbidden: **Rape** is wrong because, among other things, it is unjust. A virtue ethicist agrees that some criteria for the permissibility of sexual acts, such as free **consent** and the absence of deception, are necessary. But if this were all that virtue ethics had to say about sexual morality, it would not add anything to the enterprise. A more interesting question is whether there are vices that lead an agent to commit sexual acts that are wrong precisely because they stem from vice. Suppose Don is greedy. He has millions, yet wants more. Having exhausted other avenues for making money, he sells his sexual services. When Don has sex with clients, the transactions are mutually consensual and involve no deception. But a virtue ethicist might claim that these acts are wrong because they stem from greed. Thus sexual acts might be wrong if they emanate from vices, such as selfishness, cowardice, and cruelty (see Morgan).

Since temperance is *the* virtue concerned with the proper use and experience of bodily pleasure, it holds pride of place in discussions of sexuality. Temperance is often an agent-oriented virtue, one that concerns its possessor's welfare, unlike justice, which concerns what others are owed. Because pleasure is natural to human beings, virtue ethics does not shun it but requires that it be experienced moderately. What does "moderately" mean? One view is that the temperate person consumes food and drink, and engages in sex, in moderate *amounts*—neither too much nor too little. Doing so is arguably important for mental and physical health. Yet this view makes it difficult (even humorous) to evaluate sexual acts. Is the third sexual act in a week wrong because it crosses the line? If one goes a month without sex, has one crossed the line in the other direction?

Temperance is also often other-oriented. Suppose Caligula discovers his sister naked and writhing in wanton sexual heat. She attempts to seduce him, arguing that if Egyptian siblings engage in sex, why can't they? Caligula, however, is temperate. Even though he finds his sister attractive, his temperance, which allows him to recognize and abide by the wrongness of **incest**, prevents him from enjoying her. By contrast, Nero very much desires sexual intercourse with *his* sister. He has no scruples about engaging in incest because he is intemperate. Acts that stem from intemperance are wrong because the intemperate agent's desires lead him to desire wrong things. However, even if an agent does not act on these desires, he might still be intemperate for having them.

The Nero example shows, perhaps, that some sexual acts are always wrong; a temperate person would never do them. Aristotle held that an intemperate person desires the wrong things (1118b25, 1119a15). **Thomas Aquinas** (1224/25–1274) agreed but thought that any sexual activity other than procreative sex within **marriage** was sinful (in part because "inordinate"; *Summa theologiae* 2a2ae, ques. 154), a view promulgated by other traditionalists. For Peter Geach, temperance implies engaging in sex only with one's spouse in a faithful marriage. Through sex we transmit original sin, and only marital sex neutralizes "the corruption of sex in fallen man." Hence sex outside marriage is "poison" (Geach, 146–47). We need to investigate whether other sexual acts square with virtue ethics: rape, **adultery**, incest, promiscuity, **casual sex**, **prostitution**, **sadomasochism**, **bestiality**, and necrophilia. I cowardly leave incest, bestiality, sadomasochism, and necrophilia to the reader. Rape is the easiest. Within virtue ethics, rape is always wrong, no matter what character trait it stems from, whether intemperance, lust for revenge, assertion of power, or other vices. Rape is wrong, in part, for *sexual* reasons: The intemperate person violates another's sexual autonomy.

Adultery might be wrong because an intemperate person is willing, out of **sexual desire**, to break promises made to a spouse. But even if an adulterous act violated no promise, it might still be wrong through intemperance. A temperate person would have no desire to engage in such acts *because* the acts are adulterous; at the very least, he or she would not give such desires any value or weight (Carr, "Chastity and Adultery," 368–70). The question, then, is whether desiring to engage in adultery *is* intemperate. Some argue that this need not be so, because adulterous desires are in themselves normal and natural. Insofar as we do not break promises (and so forth), adultery is not necessarily intemperate (Halwani, chap. 3).

Now consider promiscuity, that is, having a large number of casual sexual encounters. This is wrong from a traditional or religious viewpoint, and liberals would condemn it when it involved coercion or deception. If virtue ethics were to judge promiscuity wrong, it would argue on different grounds, such as that promiscuity is intemperate. Promiscuity, however, need not stem from other-oriented intemperance or other vices; one need not bribe or connive others into sex, for example. If so, the only option is to argue that promiscuity, or the desire for it, fosters vice (or, as I examine later, is incompatible with agent-oriented temperance).

The argument requires evidence that promiscuous people tend to become vicious. But even if we gathered a large sample of vicious promiscuous people, we would still need to show that their promiscuity played a causal role in their viciousness. If one became promiscuous because one was depressed, then promiscuity would not be the cause of any later viciousness but another sign of one's mental or moral downfall. Ideal would be tracing a large sample of people who start off in life as decent people, who become promiscuous, then become vicious. Substantiating a connection from promiscuity to vice is empirically difficult. We should also keep in mind that people become promiscuous at an age *after* their characters have been formed. Hence, by the time one is promiscuous, one is already largely on one's way to being virtuous or vicious. Since virtues and vices are stable character traits, how promiscuous sex could endanger the virtues is unclear.

Is prostitution, selling and buying sexual activity, wrong according to virtue ethics? Not necessarily (Halwani, chap. 3). Clients might seek prostitutes because they have a healthy sex drive and do not have the time for or interest in one-night stands or relationships. Or they might be sexually undesirable: facially repulsive, old, or deformed. There is no reason to think that clients of prostitutes are typically motivated by vice. Most prostitutes engage in sex for money. However, unless the desire for money is itself vicious, prostitution is not wrong if selling sexual services does not in itself indicate vice. Some cases of prostitution might be vicious, but not necessarily because they are prostitution.

What about **sexual perversion**? **Pedophilia** betokens a lack of sensitivity to children's needs and their inability to consent to sex. Exhibitionism and voyeurism show lack of respect for others' autonomy. If a person has sexual desires for any of these practices, he is not fully virtuous: He has at least one vice, or his desires are incompatible with at least one virtue (see Baltzly, 17–25). Sadomasochistic sexual acts might also manifest a vice, cruelty, in those who practice them. However, most sadomasochists (unlike the heroes of the **Marquis de Sade** [1740–1814]) do not practice wanton brutality. Instead, they play out scripted acts, involving actions agreed on in advance, and so sadomasochism involves respect for the consent and autonomy of the parties. One complicating factor is that some sadomasochists have desires for playing morally dubious roles, such as being a Nazi or a slave. These desires might indicate the lack of some virtue or the presence of some vice.

Sexual orientation is another issue. Homosexual acts, like heterosexual acts, might be done virtuously or viciously. And it seems that a homosexual orientation poses no moral difficulty. Why should sexual orientation indicate the presence of vice or absence of virtue? However, arguing that a homosexual orientation is problematic is possible. On one version of virtue ethics, a character trait is a virtue only if it is likely to promote its possessor's survival, enjoyment, and freedom from pain; the functioning of the social group; and the species' survival (Hursthouse, *OVE*, 198–201). Given the last condition, homosexual orientation might be a vice (Hooker, 36–37). But having a homosexual orientation tells us little about the sexual behavior of its possessor. Whether someone with a homosexual orientation procreates, and how he or she procreates, depends on many factors and is never ruled out. **Homosexuality** does not by itself signify that a person is a defective human being (Hursthouse, "Virtue Ethics vs. Rule-Consequentialism," 43–46).

Are there sex acts that contravene agent-oriented temperance? Maybe promiscuity is incompatible with temperance: It is "too much" sex. Because agent-oriented temperance protects a person's own physical and mental health, we must ask how "too much" sex endangers these goods. Aside from **sexually transmitted disease** (which is avoidable), it is hard to see how "too much" is dangerous. However, the mental dangers are real: not that a promiscuous person might become crazy but that he or she might become a slave to sexual desire. Reason would not rule and would play merely the role of fulfilling sexual desire by procuring yet another encounter. Must this happen? It is possible to imagine someone who enjoys sex but does not want to be involved in a relationship. This person might rationally plan his life so that, along with other activities that are commonly regarded as fulfilling, he engages in promiscuity. If so, not all promiscuity would indicate psychological or moral defect and not all would be intemperate (Halwani, chap. 3). However, promiscuity might be incompatible with healthy maturation if some psychological theories, such as **Sigmund Freud**'s (1856–1939), are true (see Carr, "Freud and Sexual Ethics").

This analysis applies equally to prostitution and morally permissible forms of sexual perversion. However, it will not work for immoral acts, such as rape, voyeurism, and exhibitionism. It is implausible that a person is agent-oriented temperate as long as he rationally plans his life such that appropriate room is made for these activities. Is a man temperate if raping others does not undermine his rational abilities to pursue a worthwhile life? No. For virtue ethics, rationality is not a means-end concept. It has a built-in moral dimension to it, whereby a virtuous person has wisdom that allows him or her to seek what is worthy in life, which rules out immoral actions. Agent-oriented temperance, like other virtues, is parasitic on a normative concept of rationality (see Foot, chap. 4; Quinn, chaps. 11, 12; Sherman, chap. 3).

One complication should be mentioned: With respect to sexual desires that need not indicate lack of virtue or the presence of vice, it might still be the case that they endanger some external goods necessary for flourishing. According to Aristotle (1099b–1102a) and most contemporary versions of virtue ethics, having the virtues is not enough for flourishing. One also needs goods without which one either cannot flourish or cannot easily (or at all) practice virtue. Having money is essential for the practice of some virtues, such as generosity and charity, and is essential for a person's life to go smoothly. Some sexuality might imply a lack of important external goods. The desire for casual sex, bestiality, or fetishistic acts might undermine the ability to sustain romantic relationships (see Kristjansson). The argument depends on whether the desire in question *is* incompatible with the external good in question (why cannot two people have a healthy relationship and include shoe fetishism as part of their sex?) and on whether the endangered external good is necessary for flourishing (is romantic **love** always a good thing?). (See Halwani, chaps. 2, 3.)

Contemporary virtue ethicists and philosophers whose views are closely allied with virtue ethics fall roughly into two groups. The conservatives include Anscombe, John Finnis (a Thomist), Peter Geach, and **Roger Scruton** (a sort of Aristotelian). All condemn sex outside of marriage. The nonconservative group might include Martha Nussbaum, an Aristotelian who has not declared herself a virtue ethicist. Nussbaum swings between liberal and illiberal views; compare her defense of prostitution (288–97) with her critique of anonymous casual sex (236–37). Other virtue ethicists—Philippa Foot, Rosalind Hursthouse, Michael Slote, Christine Swanton—have not systematically discussed sexuality.

See also Abstinence; Adultery; Aristotle; Casual Sex; Ethics, Sexual; Greek Sexuality and Philosophy, Ancient; Judaism, History of; Natural Law (New); Sexuality, Dimensions of; Thomas Aquinas (Saint)

REFERENCES

Anscombe, G.E.M. "Contraception and Chastity." *The Human World*, no. 7 (1972), 9–30; Aristotle. (ca. 325 BCE?) *Nicomachean Ethics*. Trans. Terence Irwin. Indianapolis, Ind.: Hackett, 1985; Baltzly, Dirk. "Peripatetic Perversions: A Neo-Aristotelian Account of the Nature of Sexual Perversion." *Monist* 85:1 (2003), 3–29; Carr, David. "Chastity and Adultery." *American Philosophical Quarterly* 23:4 (1986), 363–71; Carr, David. "Freud and Sexual Ethics." *Philosophy* 62, no. 241 (July 1987), 361–73; Finnis, John. "Law, Morality, and 'Sexual Orientation.'" *Notre Dame Law Review* 69:5 (1994), 1049–76; Foot, Philippa. *Natural Goodness*. Oxford, U.K.: Oxford University Press, 2001; Geach, Peter T. "Temperance." In *The Virtues: The Stanton Lectures 1973–74*. Cambridge: Cambridge University Press, 1977, 131–49; Halwani, Raja. *Virtuous Liaisons: Care, Love, Sex, and Virtue Ethics*. Chicago, Ill.: Open Court, 2003; Hooker, Brad. "The Collapse of Virtue Ethics." *Utilitas* 14:1 (2002), 22–40; Hursthouse, Rosalind. "A False Doctrine of the Mean." *Proceedings of the Aristotelian Society* 81 (1980–1981), 57–72; Hursthouse, Rosalind. *On Virtue Ethics*. New York: Oxford University Press, 1999; Hursthouse, Rosalind. "Virtue Ethics vs. Rule-Consequentialism: A Reply to Brad Hooker." *Utilitas* 14:1 (2002), 41–53; Kristjansson, Kristjan. "Casual Sex Revisited." *Journal of Social Philosophy* 29:2 (1988), 97–108; MacIntyre, Alasdair. "Virtue Ethics." In Lawrence C. Becker and Charlotte B. Becker, eds., *Encyclopedia of Ethics*, 2nd ed., vol. 3. New York: Routledge,

2001, 1757–63; Morgan, Seiriol. "Dark Desires." *Ethical Theory and Moral Practice* 6:4 (2003), 377–410; Nussbaum, Martha. *Sex and Social Justice*. New York: Oxford University Press, 1999; Quinn, Warren. *Morality and Action*. Cambridge: Cambridge University Press, 1993; Scruton, Roger. *Sexual Desire: A Moral Philosophy of the Erotic*. New York: Free Press, 1986; Sherman, Nancy. *The Fabric of Character: Aristotle's Theory of Virtue*. Oxford, U.K.: Clarendon Press, 1989; Slote, Michael. *Morals from Motives*. New York: Oxford University Press, 2001; Statman, Daniel, ed. *Virtue Ethics: A Critical Reader*. Washington, D.C.: Georgetown University Press, 1997; Swanton, Christine. *Virtue Ethics: A Pluralistic View*. Oxford, U.K.: Oxford University Press, 2003; Thomas Aquinas. (1266–1273) *Summa theologiae* [1a–1ae, ques. 55–89; 2a2ae, ques. 1–170]. Cambridge, U.K.: Blackfriars, 1964–1976.

Raja Halwani

ADDITIONAL READING

Annas, Julia. *The Morality of Happiness*. New York: Oxford University Press, 1993; Anscombe, G.E.M. [Elizabeth]. "Contraception and Chastity." *The Human World*, no. 7 (1972), 9–30. Reprinted in Michael D. Bayles, ed., *Ethics and Population*. Cambridge, Mass.: Schenkman, 1976, 134–53; and HS (29–50); Carr, David. *Educating the Virtues: An Essay on the Philosophical Psychology of Moral Development and Education*. London: Routledge, 1991; Carr, David, and Jan Steutel, eds. *Virtue Ethics and Moral Education*. London: Routledge, 1999; Carroll, Mary Ann. "Sexual and Other Activities and the Ideal Life." In Alan Soble, ed., *Sex, Love, and Friendship*. Amsterdam, Holland: Rodopi, 1997, 215–21; Charland, Louis C. "Character: Moral Treatment and the Personality Disorders." In Jennifer Radden, ed., *The Philosophy of Psychiatry: A Companion*. New York: Oxford University Press, 2004, 64–77; Crisp, Roger, and Michael Slote, eds. *Virtue Ethics*. Cambridge: Cambridge University Press, 1998; Darwall, Stephen, ed. *Virtue Ethics*. Oxford, U.K.: Blackwell, 2002; Dent, Nicholas J. H. *The Moral Psychology of the Virtues*. New York: Cambridge University Press, 1984; Finnis, John. "Law, Morality, and 'Sexual Orientation.'" *Notre Dame Law Review* 69:5 (1994), 1049–76. Reprinted, revised, in *Notre Dame Journal of Law, Ethics, and Public Policy* 9:1 (1995), 11–39. Reprinted, revised, in John Corvino, ed., *Same Sex: Debating the Ethics, Science, and Culture of Homosexuality*. Lanham, Md.: Rowman and Littlefield, 1997, 31–43; Foot, Philippa. (1978) *Virtues and Vices and Other Essays in Moral Philosophy*. Oxford, U.K.: Oxford University Press, 2003; Halwani, Raja. "Care Ethics and Virtue Ethics." *Hypatia* 18:3 (2003), 161–92; Halwani, Raja. "Outing and Virtue Ethics." *Journal of Applied Philosophy* 19:2 (2002), 141–54; Halwani, Raja. "Virtue Ethics and Adultery." *Journal of Social Philosophy* 29:3 (1998), 5–18. Reprinted in David Benatar, ed., *Ethics for Everyday*. Boston, Mass.: McGraw-Hill, 2002, 226–40; Halwani, Raja, ed. *Sex and Ethics: Essays on Sexuality, Virtue, and the Good Life*. London: Palgrave/Macmillan, 2006; Harman, Gilbert. "Virtue Ethics without Character Traits." In Alex Byrne, Robert Stalnaker, and Ralph Wedgwood, eds., *Fact and Value: Essays on Ethics and Metaphysics for Judith Jarvis Thomson*. Cambridge, Mass.: MIT Press, 2001, 117–27; Harrington, Daniel, and James F. Keenan. *Jesus and Virtue Ethics: Building Bridges between New Testament Studies and Moral Theology*. Lanham, Md.: Sheed and Ward, 2002; Hauerwas, Stanley. "Gay Friendship." In Eugene Rogers, ed., *Theology and Sexuality*. Oxford, U.K.: Blackwell, 2002, 289–305; Hauerwas, Stanley, and Allen Verhey. "From Conduct to Character: A Guide to Sexual Adventure." In Elizabeth Stuart and Adrian Thatcher, eds., *Christian Perspectives on Sexuality and Gender*. Grand Rapids, Mich.: Eerdmans, 1996, 175–81; Hursthouse, Rosalind. "A False Doctrine of the Mean." *Proceedings of the Aristotelian Society* 81 (1980–1981), 57–72. Reprinted in Nancy Sherman, ed., *Aristotle's Ethics: Critical Essays*. Lanham, Md.: Rowman and Littlefield, 1999, 105–19; Kruschwitz, Robert B., and Robert C. Roberts, eds. *The Virtues: Contemporary Essays in Moral Character*. Belmont, Calif.: Wadsworth, 1987; MacIntyre, Alasdair. *After Virtue*, 2nd ed. Notre Dame, Ind.: University of Notre Dame Press, 1984; Martin, Christopher F. J. "Are There Virtues and Vices That Belong Specifically to the Sexual Life?" *Acta Philosophica* 4:2 (1995), 205–21; Martin, Mike. *Love's Virtues*. Lawrence: University Press of Kansas, 1996; Meilaender, Gilbert. *The Theory and Practice of Virtue*. Notre

Dame, Ind.: University of Notre Dame Press, 1984; Pincoffs, Edmund. *Quandaries and Virtues.* Lawrence: University Press of Kansas, 1986; Putman, Daniel. "Sex and Virtue." *International Journal of Moral and Social Studies* 6:1 (1991), 47–56; Shalit, Wendy. *A Return to Modesty: Discovering the Lost Virtue.* New York: Free Press, 1999; Sherman, Nancy. *Making a Necessity of Virtue: Aristotle and Kant on Virtue.* Cambridge: Cambridge University Press, 1997; Sihvola, Juha. "Aristotle on Sex and Love." In Martha Nussbaum and Juha Sihvola, eds., *The Sleep of Reason: Erotic Experience and Sexual Ethics in Ancient Greece and Rome.* Chicago, Ill.: University of Chicago Press, 2002, 200–221; Slote, Michael. *Goods and Virtues.* Oxford, U.K.: Oxford University Press, 1990; Solomon, Robert C. "The Virtue of Love." In Peter A. French, Theodore E. Uehling, Jr., and Howard K. Wettstein, eds., *Ethical Theory: Character and Virtue. Midwest Studies in Philosophy* 13 (1988), 12–31. Reprinted as "The Virtue of (Erotic) Love," in Robert C. Solomon and Kathleen Higgins, eds., *The Philosophy of (Erotic) Love.* Lawrence: University Press of Kansas, 1991, 492–518; STW (241–55); Solomon, Robert C. "The Virtues of a Passionate Life: Erotic Love and 'the Will to Power.' " *Social Philosophy and Policy* 15:1 (1998), 90–118; Sommers, Christina. "Teaching the Virtues." *American Philosophical Association Newsletter on Teaching Philosophy* 90:2 (1991), 42–44; Sommers, Christina Hoff, and Fred Sommers, eds. (1985, 1989) *Vice and Virtue in Everyday Life: Introductory Readings in Ethics*, 3rd ed. Fort Worth, Tex.: Harcourt Brace Jovanovich, 1993. 6th ed., Belmont, Calif.: Wadsworth, 2004; Steutel, Jan. "Virtues and Human Flourishing: A Teleological Justification." In David Carr, ed., *Education, Knowledge and Truth: Beyond the Postmodern Impasse.* London: Routledge, 1998, 129–42; Trianosky, Gregory. "What Is Virtue Ethics All About? Recent Work on the Virtues." *American Philosophical Quarterly* 27:4 (1990), 335–44; Wallace, James. *Virtues and Vices.* Ithaca, N.Y.: Cornell University Press, 1978; Watson, Gary. "On the Primacy of Character." In Owen Flanagan and Amelie Oksenberg Rorty, eds., *Identity, Character, and Morality: Essays in Moral Psychology.* Cambridge, Mass.: MIT Press, 1993, 449–69. Reprinted in Daniel Statman ed., *Virtue Ethics: A Critical Reader.* Washington, D.C.: Georgetown University Press, 1997, 56–81; Winch, Peter, Bernard Williams, Michael Tanner, and G.E.M. Anscombe. "Discussion of 'Contraception and Chastity.' " In Michael D. Bayles, ed., *Ethics and Population.* Cambridge, Mass.: Schenkman, 1976, 154–63; Young, Charles. "Aristotle on Temperance." *Philosophical Review* 97:4 (1988), 521–42.

EVOLUTION. In the theory of evolution, organisms result from a long, slow, natural (lawful) process of development from other, probably simpler, organisms and, ultimately, perhaps from inorganic matter. This idea arose in the 1700s but caught fire in 1859 when Charles Darwin (1809–1882) published *On the Origin of Species*, in which he proposed that natural selection brought on by the struggle for existence was the mechanism of change. Evolution received a boost early in the twentieth century, when the newly discovered principles of heredity, Mendelian genetics, were fused with Darwinian selection. Thus was born the modern-day theory.

"Sex," a matter of intense interest and importance to evolutionists, refers to a species' having two types, male and female, both necessary for reproduction. The earth is 4.5 billion years old; life dates from just under 4 billion years. The arrival of sex and the flowering of complex life forms about 500 million years ago (the Cambrian Explosion) may have been linked. Although most organisms are not sexual, most "higher" organisms (plants and animals) are.

In *Origin*, Darwin was concerned with the evolutionary reasons for sex. From his grandfather Erasmus Darwin (1731–1802), a late-eighteenth-century evolutionist, he got the insight that sex was linked to variation in organisms and changing environmental conditions. Response to change requires a supply of new variation, and sexual reproduction shakes up the factors of heredity so that new variations appear. This idea was incorporated into natural selection. More organisms are born than can survive and, more important, than can reproduce. Struggle for space, food, and mates ensues. Some organisms, the "fit," succeed in this competition; others lose, so differential reproduction takes place between them. Evolutionary consequences occur if the fit have heritable traits that the unfit lack, traits that are key in determining their success. Evolution will be in the direction of traits that help in the struggle, leading to adaptations such as the hand and eye.

Although Darwin thought variations were random, he also thought that the variation-producing process, an important component of which is sex, was adaptive (he did not know how). He never asked why only two sexes exist, instead of three or more (perhaps he realized that getting two together is trouble enough), but he did explain sex ratios—why there is roughly a 50:50 distribution. Thinking in terms of what we call an "evolutionarily stable strategy," Darwin argued that if one sex became rare, an adaptive advantage would accrue to parents having offspring of this sex, until a balance was regained. This theory is now accepted, although Darwin, having introduced it in *Descent of Man* (1871), later decided he was wrong. The idea finally took root in 1930 when Ronald A. Fisher (1890–1962) reintroduced it in his *Genetical Theory of Natural Selection* (142–43).

A related phenomenon that concerned Darwin was organisms that have foregone or been deprived of sex. As opposed to the co-discoverer of natural selection, Alfred Russel Wallace (1823–1913), Darwin insisted that selection works not for the group but for the individual. Whereas Wallace saw the mule's sterility as an adaptation preserving the integrity of the parent species (horse, donkey), Darwin thought, as we do, that this sterility was a by-product of the mating of animals with incompatible reproductive systems. What, though, about the sterility of female castes in social insects? Given natural selection, a mechanism that stresses reproduction, why are they sterile? (Note that such species are not sexually balanced.) Darwin proposed that nests were "superorganisms" and that selection works on the whole as if it were an individual. Particular insects are parts of an organism rather than organisms in their own right.

Drawing on animal and plant breeding, Darwin proposed another evolutionary mechanism, sexual selection (*Descent*, vol. 1, 253–423; vol. 2, 1–384; *Origin*, 87–90). He noticed that breeding primarily for economic features (coat, flesh) corresponded to natural selection, and breeding secondarily for fanciful features (fighting ability, **beauty**) corresponded to another kind of selection in which economics yields to within-species reproductive ends. Breeders or fanciers aim for brute force (fighting cocks) or beauty (pigeons), and Darwin saw that this secondary selection likewise has two forms. Although he knew that the forms could operate with either sex, he labeled them "male combat" and "female choice" sexual selection. Deer antlers result from the first form, peacock tail feathers from the second.

In *Origin*, Darwin did not make much of sexual selection, but it later played a significant role in his thinking. In the 1860s, Wallace became a convinced spiritualist, contending that many human features, such as intelligence and hairlessness, could not have been produced by natural selection. Darwin agreed. But instead of opting for extrascientific causes, Darwin argued that sexual selection yielded these features and many others, including racial and sexual differences. Darwin, notoriously, had a Victorian view of male-female differences and expressed in *Descent of Man* conventional sentiments about the sexes: "Man is more courageous, pugnacious, and energetic than woman, and has a more inventive genius" (vol. 2, 316). Women have "greater tenderness and less selfishness" (326). You could be reading a novel by Charles Dickens.

Darwinian evolutionary theory is not inherently sexist (see Ruse, "Is Darwinism Sexist?").

Wallace never much cared for sexual selection. It was too anthropomorphic for his tastes, insofar as it supposed that peacocks have the same standard of beauty as we. Further, it conflicted with his notion that selection is not for the individual but the group. In the case of female choice sexual selection, Wallace argued that rather than the male being bright, the female is drab. This allows her to escape detection when raising her family, while bright nesting birds would attract predators. For Wallace, this accounts for much sexual dimorphism (*Contributions*, 45–129). About humans, however, Wallace reversed himself, influenced by Edward Bellamy's (1850–1898) futuristic novel *Looking Backward*. Bellamy thought that young women will eventually control reproduction, so that war will vanish because they will choose to mate only with nonviolent males. Perhaps Wallace's endorsement of the view that human progress depends ultimately on female sexual selection (*Studies*, vol. 2, 507) was as touchingly naive as his enthusiasm for spiritualism. But Wallace was a prominent Victorian evolutionist who did not share Darwin's sexism. He would have been comfortably at home in any contemporary women's studies program. (As would Sarah Blaffer Hrdy, a student of the sociobiologist E. O. Wilson, who has presented a feminist picture of human evolution; see her *Mother Nature*; *The Woman That Never Evolved*.)

Evolutionists did not again approach fundamental questions about sex until the 1960s. One spur was realizing Darwin's correctness about the level at which natural selection operates. Although group selection is not impossible (a view defended by Stephen Jay Gould [1941–2002]), the presumption must be that selection works for the individual's benefit. (But see Dawkins, who presses the view that the unit of selection is the gene.) One reason is that of two competing organisms, one selfish, one altruistic, the selfish one will succeed. This does not mean that organisms will not help others out of enlightened self-interest, conscious or otherwise. But that is another matter.

If individual selection is the norm, a colossal question about sex arises: Why does sex exist at all? In the vast majority of cases, the female does all or most of the child rearing. How does she benefit? Why should she not asexually propagate 100 percent of her own genes in preference to 50 percent of hers and 50 percent of those of a biological stranger? Only if she does so for the group would sexual reproduction make sense. Since the 1960s, much evolutionary thought addressed this problem: how sex is adaptive to sexed individuals or, rather, how it is beneficial to individual females. No fully satisfactory or generally accepted answer exists.

John Maynard Smith (1920–2004) suggested that we ask two questions, one about the origin of sex and another about its maintenance (70). Due to sex, organisms tend to be diploid; they carry two sets of chromosomes, matched against each other. In sexual reproduction, after some shuffling, one set of chromosomes is passed on. Having two sets of chromosomes might benefit the individual: Defective chromosomes can be remedied or concealed by the other. This might answer Smith's first question. But why does sex persist? Why, if given the choice, do sexed organisms not revert to asexuality? Some species reproduce both asexually and sexually (some amphibians). Why do they not become altogether asexual? Why do aphids, which reproduce asexually all summer, reproduce sexually in the winter?

Various solutions have been proposed. Perhaps genes (or DNA [deoxyribonucleic acid] molecules) are vulnerable, and sex enables them to be repaired. Or perhaps the sexual shuffling of genes is valuable for the individual. On the negative side, if there is no sex, individual lines accumulate bad mutations until further existence is impossible ("Muller's ratchet"). On the positive side, if the environment is highly variable, it pays a female to have many different offspring, some of which will survive and reproduce. William Hamilton (1936–2000) argued, however, that even if the external environment is not variable, individuals are still under attack from parasites, which reproduce and evolve more rapidly than their hosts. The shuffling of genes in sexual reproduction makes the hosts "moving targets" (Hamilton et al.). After a parasite adapts to a host, the host reproduces; because its offspring are slightly different, the parasite must start over. Hamilton supports his view by pointing out that sexual organisms often have bright displays to show off their physical fitness, convincing potential mates that they prevail in combating parasites (see also Thornhill and Gangestad). Further, if sex is difficult to eliminate, it might persist simply as an unfortunate legacy of the past. George Williams argues that this might explain continued mammalian sexuality (102–3). It might also explain why females, making the best of a bad lot, try to involve males in parenting. Sometimes this is effective, as with birds whose nests are open to attack and who migrate seasonally, which together yield a premium on raising offspring quickly. That requires a parenting father.

There has been some success regarding sex ratios. Although a 50:50 distribution is expected, it does not always occur. Fisher indicated that ratios will be distorted if producing one sex requires more work than producing the other (141–43). And Hamilton's hypotheses about hymenoptera (ants, bees, wasps) are influential. Whereas females are produced by fertilized eggs (and, so, are diploid), males are produced by unfertilized eggs (and are haploid). This causes unbalanced ratios and, moreover, solves Darwin's puzzle about hymenopteran sterility, without dubiously saying that the nest is the individual organism. Due to the diploid-haploid system, females are 50 percent related to their female offspring but 75 percent related to their sisters. (Sisters receive an identical set of genes from their shared haploid fathers.) Hence, according to individual selection, females are better off raising fertile sisters than fertile daughters. Sterility is an individual adaptation, saving the workers from expending energy on producing daughters rather than fertile females.

Hamilton also explained, by "local mate competition," why distorted ratios occur in other situations ("Extraordinary Sex Ratios"). If brothers compete for the same mates, mothers do not benefit from having many sons. Any son will do. For insurance reasons, mothers cannot have only one son, but a bias in favor of females is expected. Empirical studies have confirmed this; and experiments have vindicated Hamilton's fingering individual selection. Indeed, sex ratios reveal individual/group selection differences clearly. Generally, a group does not need every male. The job could be and is in fact done by fewer than 50 percent (even 10 percent). So group selection would favor females. But if this occurred in the group, individual mothers would gain, were all their offspring male, and individual selection would force the 10 percent figure higher. The distribution's usually being 50:50 shows that individual selection is operating.

For a century after *Origin* and *Descent*, most biologists agreed with Wallace about sexual selection. No one denied it absolutely, due to sexual selection through male combat. But female choice sexual selection was thought unduly anthropomorphic. With the reemphasis in the 1960s on individual selection and the recognition that interesting problems involve not only physical characteristics but also behavior, renewed interest in sexual selection emerged, as something significant in the "battle of the sexes." (For contemporary treatments of sexual selection, see Miller; Perper.) Explaining and understanding sexual dimorphism has been successful. The basic, Darwinian, premise was that the sexes have different strategies for ensuring that mating furnishes offspring. To use stock market language, males hold penny stocks, while females favor blue chips. Less metaphorically, males produce many sperm and can fertilize many females, whereas females produce (often far) fewer eggs and hence fewer offspring. Further, they often must care for them alone.

Obviously, not all females care for their young. But the general rule is that males are promiscuous and females choosy (or "coy"; Wilson, 125). So the male strategy is to push toward polygyny (one male, multiple females), whereas females resist. Males can copulate, pass on sperm, and move on. Females are stuck with the fertilized egg and child rearing. Males did not always get their way; otherwise they would have won the battle of the sexes, and mothers would have had only sons. Overall, there must be a balance or a draw. Still, tension arises between the sexes as both seek supremacy.

There are subtle ways of winning. For instance, females may sometimes benefit, and so be winners, by sharing a winning male. They will receive more direct care—an alpha male can offer more to each of his mates than a beta male can to just one mate—and their sons will inherit his advantageous traits. This situation (polygyny) may also skew sex ratios. When males compete, they may win big or lose completely. But even the lowest female will have some offspring if males are promiscuous, not choosy. Hence, healthy mothers skew their offspring toward males, unhealthy mothers toward females. Although empirical evidence confirms that in many mammals their physiology works to this end, not all species will be polygamous. Birds often tend toward monogamy, through the pressure to raise offspring quickly. Sometimes polyandry (multiple males, single females) prevails, if males can reproduce only this way. The dunnocks, hedge sparrows, often exhibit this relationship, for the female can manipulate males to achieve help at the nest.

One controversial area of evolutionary theory has been its application to humans. With Darwin, evolutionists claim that selection is key in producing in humans adaptations directed to the individual. Since human and mammalian biology are similar, this application has led to loose talk about male dominance and the like (e.g., Goldberg), which elicited hostile reactions by those who felt threatened or belittled. Many countered that culture permitted humans to escape biology: Everything we do is socially constructed with little connection to the purported dictates of genes (e.g., Lewontin et al.).

The truth is, reasonably, somewhere in the middle. Sexual selection has undoubtedly operated on humans, as it operated on our closest relatives, the great apes. A good sign of a polygynous tendency is that males tend to be larger than females; witness red deer, elephant seals, gorillas. Humans manifest this dimorphism, which suggests that we are at least mildly polygynous. (Many societies have this arrangement.) However, polygyny is not inevitable. Tibetan and Inuit societies tend toward polyandry as a result of the difficulty of scraping a living and raising offspring. The evidence seems to show that in more prosperous societies women have higher status and the tendency is toward monogamy. But caution is needed. The United States practices (serial) monogamy, in which older, successful men have second wives and more children, and so the United States mimics openly polygynous societies. And, as DNA testing establishes, being in a socially defined monogamous marriage does not imply biological (sexual) fidelity. More research is needed before the conclusion can be reached that modern Americans have shucked off their biology—or want to. (This is not to deny that human males are involved in child care and hence that there is selective pressure to stay in some kind of relationship with one's children.)

Humans follow other biological patterns. Various factors, including infanticide, skew sex ratios according to socioeconomic status. In some upper-level Indian castes, girls growing to maturity are practically unknown, whereas in lower castes the converse is the tendency (at least, resources are poured into girls). A much discussed question concerns the human equivalent of hymenopteran sterility: the 10 percent of the population that is primarily homosexual (see Ruse, *Homosexuality*). Although homosexuals are not sterile, their lifestyles favor fewer offspring. This is anomalous, evolutionarily speaking. **Sexual orientation** is surely a multifactored end product, yet increasing evidence indicates a role for biology. On one hypothesis, the hymenopteran model is very appropriate: Homosexuals reproduce by proxy, through aiding close relatives. Another possibility is that, as with diseases such as sickle-cell anemia, **homosexuality** figures into a genetic trade-off, so that some family members can be "superheterosexuals." Homosexuality is not necessarily a disease, but we should not naively pretend there is no cost for more natural functioning. This is probably the implication of any theory like Darwin's that makes reproduction central; reproduction is biologically ideal, even if it is not necessarily morally ideal. (No Darwinian must assert that smallpox virus reproduction is morally good.)

Criticism, even if less vehement than previously, still haunts the application of evolution to humans. But evolutionary theory has always been controversial, so this state of affairs is not unusual. Evolutionary theory has contributed mightily to our understanding of sex, although issues remain to engage future generations.

See also Animal Sexuality; Beauty; Bestiality; Fichte, Johann Gottlieb; Firestone, Shulamith; Hegel, G.W.F.; Homosexuality, Ethics of; Homosexuality and Science; Perversion, Sexual; Psychology, Evolutionary; Schopenhauer, Arthur; Sherfey, Mary Jane; Social Constructionism; Spencer, Herbert; Westermarck, Edward

REFERENCES

Bellamy, Edward. (1888) *Looking Backward: 2000–1887.* Foreword by Erich Fromm. New York: New American Library, 1960; Darwin, Charles. *The Descent of Man,* 2 vols. London: John Murray, 1871; Darwin, Charles. *On the Origin of Species.* London: John Murray, 1859; Dawkins, Richard. (1976) *The Selfish Gene,* 2nd ed. New York: Oxford University Press, 1989; Fisher, Ronald A. *The Genetical Theory of Natural Selection.* Oxford, U.K.: Oxford University Press, 1930; Goldberg, Steven. *The Inevitability of Patriarchy.* New York: Morrow, 1974; Gould, Stephen Jay. *The Structure of Evolutionary Theory.* Cambridge, Mass.: Harvard University Press, 2002; Hamilton, William D. "Extraordinary Sex Ratios." *Science* 156:3774 (28 April 1967), 477–88; Hamilton, William D., Robert Axelrod, and Robert Tanese. "Sexual Reproduction as an Adaptation to Resist Parasites." *Proceedings of the National Academy of Sciences, USA* 87:9 (1990), 3566–73; Hrdy, Sarah Blaffer. *Mother Nature: A History of Mothers, Infants, and Natural Selection.* New York: Pantheon Books, 1999; Hrdy, Sarah Blaffer. *The Woman That Never Evolved.* Cambridge, Mass.: Harvard University Press, 1981; Lewontin, Richard C., Steven Rose, and Leon J. Kamin. *Not in Our Genes: Biology, Ideology, and Human Nature.* New York: Pantheon, 1984; Miller, Geoffrey. *The Mating Mind: How Sexual Choice Shaped the Evolution of Human Nature.* New York: Doubleday, 2000; Perper, Timothy. "Theories and Observations on Sexual Selection and Female Choice in Human Beings." *Medical Anthropology* 11:4 (1989), 409–54; Ruse, Michael. *Homosexuality: A Philosophical Inquiry.* New York: Blackwell, 1988; Ruse, Michael. "Is Darwinism Sexist? (And If It Is, So What?)." In Noretta Koertge, ed., *A House Built on Sand: Exposing Postmodernist Myths about Science.* New York: Oxford University Press, 1998, 119–29; Smith, John Maynard. *The Evolution of Sex.* Cambridge: Cambridge University Press, 1978; Thornhill, Randy, and Gangestad, S. W. "Human Facial Beauty: Averageness, Symmetry, and Parasite Resistance." *Human Nature* 4:3 (1993), 237–69; Wallace, Alfred Russel. *Contributions to the Theory of Natural Selection: A Series of Essays.* London: Macmillan, 1870; Wallace, Alfred Russel. *Studies: Scientific and Social,* 2 vols. London: Macmillan, 1900; Williams, George C. *Sex and Evolution.* Princeton, N.J.: Princeton University Press, 1975; Wilson, Edward O. *On Human Nature.* Cambridge, Mass.: Harvard University Press, 1978.

Michael Ruse

ADDITIONAL READING

Barash, David P. "Evolution as a Paradigm for Behavior." In Michael S. Gregory, Anita Silvers, and Diane Sutch, eds., *Sociobiology and Human Nature.* San Francisco, Calif.: Jossey-Bass, 1978,

13–32; Birkhead, Tim. *Promiscuity: An Evolutionary History of Sperm Competition*. Cambridge, Mass.: Harvard University Press, 2000; Blackwell, Antoinette Brown. (1875) "Sex and Evolution." In Alice S. Rossi, ed., *The Feminist Papers: From Adams to de Beauvoir*. New York: Columbia University Press, 1973, 356–77; Blackwell, Antoinette Brown. *The Sexes throughout Nature*. New York: G. P. Putnam's Sons, 1875; Bowler, Peter J. (1984, 1989) *Evolution: The History of an Idea*, 3rd ed. Berkeley: University of California Press, 2003; Caulfield, Mina Davis. "Sexuality in Human Evolution: What Is 'Natural' in Sex?" *Feminist Studies* 11:2 (1985), 343–63; Darwin, Charles. *The Descent of Man, and Selection in Relation to Sex*. London: John Murray, 1871. Photoreproduction: Princeton, N.J.: Princeton University Press, 1981; Darwin, Charles. (1872) *The Expression of the Emotions in Man and Animal*. Chicago, Ill.: University of Chicago Press, 1965; Darwin, Erasmus. (1794–1796) *Zoonomia; or, The Laws of Organic Life*, 3rd ed. London: J. Johnson, 1801; Degler, Carl N. *In Search of Human Nature: The Decline and Revival of Darwinism in American Social Thought*. New York: Oxford University Press, 1991; Ellis, Havelock. (1897–1928) *Studies in the Psychology of Sex*, vol. 4: *Sexual Selection in Man*. Philadelphia, Pa.: F. A. Davis, 1905; Etcoff, Nancy. *Survival of the Prettiest: The Science of Beauty*. New York: Doubleday, 1999; Fisher, Elizabeth. *Woman's Creation: Sexual Evolution and the Shaping of Society*. Garden City, N.Y.: Anchor Books, 1979; Fisher, Helen E. *The Sex Contract: The Evolution of Human Behavior*. New York: Morrow, 1982; Gould, Stephen Jay. "Cardboard Darwinism." *New York Review of Books* (25 September 1986), 47–54; Gould, Stephen Jay. "Freudian Slip." *Natural History* 96:2 (1987), 14–21; Gould, Stephen Jay. "Male Nipples and Clitoral Ripples." In *Bully for Brontosaurus: Reflections in Natural History*. New York: Norton, 1991, 124–38; Hamer, Dean, and Peter Copeland. *The Science of Desire: The Search for the Gay Gene and the Biology of Behavior*. New York: Simon and Schuster, 1994; Hamilton, William D. *The Narrow Roads of Gene Land: The Collected Papers of W. D. Hamilton*. New York: W. H. Freeman/Spektrum, 1996; Hersey, George L. *The Evolution of Allure: Sexual Selection from the Medici Venus to the Incredible Hulk*. Cambridge, Mass.: MIT Press, 1996; Himmelfarb, Gertrude. "Social Darwinism, Sociobiology, and the Two Cultures." In *Marriage and Morals among the Victorians*. New York: Knopf, 1986, 76–93; Hrdy, Sarah Blaffer, C. Davison Ankney, and Richard C. Lewontin. "Women versus the Biologists: An Exchange." *New York Review of Books* (14 July 1994), 54–55; Hubbard, Ruth. "Have Only Men Evolved?" In Ruth Hubbard, Mary Sue Henifin, and Barbara Fried, eds., *Women Look at Biology Looking at Women: A Collection of Feminist Critiques*. Boston, Mass.: G. K. Hall, 1979, 7–36. Reprinted in Ruth Hubbard, Mary Sue Henifin, and Barbara Fried, eds., *Biological Woman—The Convenient Myth*. Cambridge, Mass.: Schenkman, 1982, 17–45; in Sandra Harding and Merrill Hintikka, eds., *Discovering Reality: Feminist Perspectives on Epistemology, Metaphysics, Methodology, and Philosophy of Science*. Dordrecht, Holland: Reidel, 1983, 45–69; and Janet A. Kourany, ed., *Scientific Knowledge: Basic Issues in the Philosophy of Science*, 2nd ed. Belmont, Calif.: Wadsworth, 1998, 225–42; Johnson, Phillip E. (1991) *Darwin on Trial*. Downers Grove, Ill.: InterVarsity, 1993; Jones, Owen D. "Sex, Culture, and the Biology of Rape: Toward Explanation and Prevention." *California Law Review* 87:4 (1999), 827–941; Kitcher, Philip. "Two Cheers for Homosexuality." In *Vaulting Ambition: Sociobiology and the Quest for Human Nature*. Cambridge, Mass.: MIT Press, 1985, 243–52; Lewontin, Richard C. "Women versus the Biologists." *New York Review of Books* (7 April 1994), 31–35; McIver, Tom. *Anti-Evolution*. Baltimore, Md.: Johns Hopkins University Press, 1992; Michod, Richard E. *Eros and Evolution: A Natural Philosophy of Sex*. Reading, Mass.: Addison-Wesley, 1995; Michod, Richard E., and Bruce R. Levin, eds. *The Evolution of Sex: An Examination of Current Ideas*. Sunderland, Mass.: Sinauer, 1988; Miller, Geoffrey. "Sexual Selection and the Mind: A Talk with Geoffrey Miller." John Brockman, ed. and publ. *Edge* 41 (26 May 1998). <www.edge.org/3rd_culture/miller/index.html> [accessed 8 October 2004]; Orr, H. Allen. "The Descent of Gould." *The New Yorker* (30 September 2002), 132–38; Radcliffe Richards, Janet. "Natural Premises and Political Conclusions." In *Human Nature after Darwin: A Philosophical Introduction*. London: Routledge, 2000, 223–42; Regan, Pamela C. "Functional Features: An Evolutionary Perspective on Inappropriate Relationships." In Robin Goodwin and Duncan Cramer, eds., *Inappropriate Relationships: The Unconventional, the Disapproved, and the Forbidden*. Mahwah, N.J.: Erlbaum, 2002, 25–42; Rice, Lee, and Steven Barbone. "Hatching Your

Genes Before They're Counted." In Alan Soble, ed., *Sex, Love, and Friendship*. Amsterdam, Holland: Rodopi, 1997, 89–98; Ritvo, Lucille. *Darwin's Influence on Freud: A Tale of Two Sciences*. New Haven, Conn.: Yale University Press, 1990; Roughgarden, Joan. *Evolution's Rainbow: Diversity, Gender, and Sexuality in Nature and People*. Berkeley: University of California Press, 2004; Ruse, Michael. "Are There Gay Genes? Sociobiology Looks at Homosexuality." *Journal of Homosexuality* 4:1 (1981), 5–34. Reprinted as "Are There Gay Genes? Sociobiology and Homosexuality" in SLF (61–86); Ruse, Michael. *Darwin and Design: Does Evolution Have a Purpose?* Cambridge, Mass.: Harvard University Press, 2003; Ruse, Michael. *The Darwinian Revolution: Science Red in Tooth and Claw*. Chicago, Ill.: University of Chicago Press, 1979; Ruse, Michael. (2000) *The Evolution Wars: A Guide to the Debates*. New Brunswick, N.J.: Rutgers University Press, 2001; Ruse, Michael. *Homosexuality: A Philosophical Inquiry*. New York: Blackwell, 1988; Ruse, Michael. "Is Homosexuality Bad Sexuality?" In Robert M. Stewart, ed., *Philosophical Perspectives on Sex and Love*. New York: Oxford University Press, 1995, 113–24; Ruse, Michael. *Is Science Sexist? And Other Problems in the Biomedical Sciences*. Dordrecht, Holland: Reidel, 1981; Ruse, Michael. (1979) *Sociobiology: Sense or Nonsense?* 2nd ed. Dordrecht, Holland: Reidel, 1985; Ruse, Michael. *Taking Darwin Seriously: A Naturalistic Approach to Philosophy*. New York: Blackwell, 1986. Reprinted, Amherst, N.Y.: Prometheus, 1998; Salmon, Catherine, and Donald Symons. *Warrior Lovers: Erotic Fiction, Evolution, and Female Sexuality*. New Haven, Conn.: Yale University Press, 2001; Slotten, Ross A. *The Heretic in Darwin's Court: The Life of Alfred Russel Wallace*. New York: Columbia University Press, 2004; Stanford, Craig B. "Darwinians Look at Rape, Sex, and War." *American Scientist* 88:4 (2000), 360–68; Sterelny, Kim, and Paul E. Griffiths. *Sex and Death: An Introduction to Philosophy of Biology*. Chicago, Ill.: University of Chicago Press, 1999; Sussman, Robert W., and Audrey R. Chapman, eds. *The Origins and Nature of Sociality*. New York: Aldine de Gruyter, 2004; Symons, Donald. *The Evolution of Human Sexuality*. New York: Oxford University Press, 1979; Symons, Donald. "On the Use and Misuse of Darwinism in the Study of Human Behavior." In Jerome Barkow, Leda Cosmides, and John Tooby, eds., *The Adapted Mind: Evolutionary Psychology and the Generation of Culture*. New York: Oxford University Press, 1992, 137–59; Waal, Frans B. M. de. *Chimpanzee Politics: Power and Sex among Apes*. London: Cape, 1982; Walsh, Anthony. "Love and Sex." In Vern L. Bullough and Bonnie Bullough, eds., *Human Sexuality: An Encyclopedia*. New York: Garland, 1994, 369–73; Wilson, Holly. "Kant's Evolutionary Theory of Marriage." In Jane Kneller, ed., *Autonomy and Community*. Albany: State University of New York Press, 1998, 283–306.

EVOLUTIONARY PSYCHOLOGY. *See* Psychology, Evolutionary

EXISTENTIALISM. "Existentialist" is most often used as a covering term for a number of European thinkers who came after **G.W.F. Hegel** (1770–1831) and whose writings investigate human existence, choice, and individual responsibility. They take as their point of departure the concrete individual striving to realize a meaningful life. They emphasize that we find ourselves thrown into a world we did not make, born at a time and place we did not choose, and compelled to face numerous challenges, including the anguish of choice, the inevitability of death, and the complexity of relations (even sexual) with others. They urge authenticity, responsibility, and self-realization, and scorn self-deception, hypocrisy, and unreflective conformity to the norms of one's society. In the area of sex and **love**, they deliberate, in particular, about the problem of reconciling self-realization and personal fulfillment with authenticity toward others.

The central figures of existentialism include the philosophers **Søren Kierkegaard** (1813–1855), **Friedrich Nietzsche** (1844–1900), Karl Jaspers (1883–1969), Gabriel Marcel (1889–1973), **Martin Heidegger** (1889–1976), Jean-Paul Sartre (1905–1980), Simone de Beauvoir (1908–1986), Maurice Merleau-Ponty (1908–1961), and novelist Albert Camus (1913–1960). Other figures (among them philosophers, theologians, poets, and novelists) associated with existentialism include Fyodor Dostoyevsky (1821–1881), Lev Shestov (1836–1938), Rainer Maria Rilke (1875–1926), Martin Buber (1878–1965), Franz Kafka (1883–1924), José Ortega y Gasset (1883–1955), and Paul Tillich (1886–1965). Even if we consider only the central figures, generalizing about existentialism beyond the common threads mentioned above is difficult. The "existentialists" are a diverse assortment of thinkers. Some, like Kierkegaard and Marcel, were deeply religious. Others, like Nietzsche, Sartre, Beauvoir, and Camus, were atheists. Some were Marxists, others harsh critics of **Marxism**. Kierkegaard was a royalist. Heidegger was a member of the Nazi party. Even the name "existentialist" is problematic. Marcel coined the term "*existentialiste*" in 1943, but Heidegger and Camus consistently refused that label.

In the final analysis, it is Sartre and Beauvoir to whom the classification "existentialist" remains most firmly attached. Former lovers, intimate friends, and close collaborators, Beauvoir and Sartre continued to identify themselves as existentialists well into the 1960s and sometimes used the word "existentialism" as a label for their own philosophy. In 1963, Jaspers, who had played a major role in the formation of twentieth-century existentialism, remarked, "There is no existentialism. There is Sartre" (Suhl, 272).

Søren Kierkegaard. Kierkegaard, the first existentialist, maintained a polite silence about the physical aspects of sex but wrote at length about heterosexual love. His first major work, *Either/Or* (*E/O*; 1843), was inspired in part by reflections on a momentous event in his own love life. He had just broken off his engagement with eighteen-year-old Regine Olsen (1822–1904), despite their mutual love and the entreaties of Regine and her father not to abandon her. Part I of *Either/Or* looks at life and love through the eyes of various personae whose stage of existence is "aesthetic." Among the constitutive characteristics of aesthetic existence are passion to live one's life poetically; need for variety, novelty, and change; endless striving for self-fulfillment; antipathy toward duty as a restriction on freedom; and the perpetual threat of boredom.

Although erotic love is a preoccupation of aesthetic existence, its forms are limited. One is the art of **seduction**, which Kierkegaard explores through the legendary Don Juan, especially as portrayed by Wolfgang Amadeus Mozart (1756–1791) in *Don Giovanni*, as well as through his own fictional persona, Johannes, in "Diary of a Seducer" (*E/O*, vol. 1). Kierkegaard's John is more a seducer of souls than bodies. He disdains **rape** as momentary, imagined enjoyment and aims instead at the seduction of freedom. "No, if one can bring it to a point where a girl has but one task for her freedom, to give herself, so that she feels her whole happiness in this, so that she practically begs for this devotedness and yet is free—only then is there enjoyment" (*E/O*, vol. 1, 342). This view anticipates Sartre's interpretation of love and reflects Kierkegaard's success at persuading Regine to give up another suitor, Fritz Schlegel (1817–1896), and become devoted to him.

Another erotic option for aesthetic existence is lifelong love of a person one has lost or never possessed. Even when **marriage** is possible, separation is preferable to marriage, for it preserves the ideality and inspiration of first love untarnished by time and the dullness of domestic duty. Victor Eremita, the imaginary persona credited (by Kierkegaard) with editing *Either/Or*, explains it as follows:

> Many a man became a genius because of a girl, . . . many a man became a poet because of a girl, many a man became a saint because of a girl—but he did not become a genius because of the girl he got, for with her he became only a

cabinet official; . . . he did not become a poet because of the girl he got, for because of her he became only a father; he did not become a saint because of the girl he got, for he got none at all. . . . If a woman's ideality were in itself inspiring, then the one who inspires would have to be the one to whom he is bound for life. Life expresses it another way. It says: In a negative relationship woman makes man productive in ideality. (*Stages on Life's Way*, 59)

In Part II of *Either/Or*, another persona, Judge William, offers a contrary view. He argues that marriage is the "the transfiguration of the first love and not its annihilation, is its friend, not its enemy" (*E/O*, vol. 2, 31). Christian marriage, he claims, far from excluding the passion and ideality of erotic love, preserves these "pagan" joys and elevates them to a higher level of fulfillment. The married man has not killed time but has saved it and preserved it in eternity. The married man who truly does this lives poetically. However, marriage of this kind is possible only in the "ethical" stage of existence. To reach that stage, the aesthetic individual must make the leap from amorality, where no either/or has permanent significance, to an ethical point where each is judged against standards of good and evil (see also Kierkegaard's *Works of Love* [1847]).

Repetition and *Fear and Trembling*, published later in 1843, suggest Kierkegaard's hope that he might yet find a way to be reunited with Regine. *Fear* delineates a "religious" stage of existence distinct from both aesthetic and ethical existence. The book's hero is Abraham, who obeys God's command to sacrifice his son Isaac, thereby destroying his own happiness and violating his ethical duty to family and tribe. Kierkegaard breathes new life into this biblical tale by imagining Abraham as a knight of faith determined to carry out God's command in fear and trembling, yet hopeful that Isaac will be restored to him, since for God all things are possible. Although Kierkegaard had yet to develop his analysis of Christendom as an obstacle to becoming a Christian, he was drawn to a religious vocation that seemed incompatible with marriage. Thus, to comprehend the faith of Abraham was to comprehend the possibility of being reunited with the woman whose love he needed to sacrifice. But Kierkegaard's own story had a different ending. Regine married her former suitor and rejected Kierkegaard's effort to establish a brotherly relationship with her new family. Kierkegaard never married. When he died, he left what remained of his possessions to Regine, with a brief testament stating that his engagement to her was as binding as marriage.

Friedrich Nietzsche. Nietzsche's observations on sex, love, and marriage are terse, scattered, and difficult to unify. Near the beginning of his first book, *The Birth of Tragedy* (1872), he celebrates the genius of classical Greek drama in reconciling the Apollonian spirit of measure and order with the drunken passion and raw sexuality of Dionysian revelry. He contrasts the Greeks' dramatic festivals in honor of Dionysus with festivals from Rome to Babylon, "to say nothing here of the modern," where sexual licentiousness overwhelmed all family life and revelers indulged in "that horrible mixture of sensuality and cruelty," "the real 'witches brew' " (*Birth of Tragedy*, 39). He also speaks of the sublimation (*sublimieren*) of sexual energy and declares, "[T]he degree and kind of man's sexuality reach up into the ultimate pinnacle of his spirit" (*Beyond Good and Evil*, 81). Yet he does not develop a theory of human nature that treats sexual energy as a principal source of motivation in human affairs. Walter Kaufmann (1921–1980) argues that Nietzsche came to see sexuality as "merely a foreground of something else that is more basic and hence preserved in sublimation: the will to power" (222).

Nietzsche's disparaging remarks about women, love, and marriage in his later works have generally been taken as reliable evidence of his mature convictions, but this blanket interpretation can be challenged. Ruth Abbey argues that the works of Nietzsche's middle period (1878–1882) suggest that "marriage can be based on reason rather than sexual passion, that it can and should resemble friendship, and that it can and should have a pedagogical function. And, in adducing this ideal of marriage, he comes very close to early feminist-liberal thinking about marriage" (90). Yet attempts to tame Nietzsche's stormy thoughts on the sexes may be too optimistic.

Consider Nietzsche's unusually long discussion in "Woman and Child." In the opening pages he says that "[t]he perfect woman is a higher type of human than the perfect man"; "good marriage is based on a talent for friendship"; "[m]en who are too intellectual need marriage every bit as much as they resist it like a bitter medicine"; the critical test of a successful marriage is "being able to have good conversations with this woman into old age" (*Human, All Too Human*, 195–99). But as the section progresses, his observations become gloomier: The idolization of love was originally devised by women to heighten their power, but having become trapped in their own net, they are now more deceived and disappointed than men. He finds women more devious, mercurial, contradictory, and vengeful than men. This could all be changed, since "one can in a few centuries educate women to be anything, even men," but those centuries would be racked with intellectual and social chaos that would make men furious (205). He worries about the differences between the sexual appetites of men and women and surmises that it would be asking too much of a good wife (friend, help-mate, mother, manager, businesswoman) to be a concubine as well. He doubts that living with a woman can be good for a free spirit. He compares the happiness of marriage to the fibrous trap of a spider's web. He asserts that becoming too close to a person (be it a lover or a friend) is like "touching a good etching with our bare fingers; one day we have poor, dirty paper in our hands and nothing more" (206).

The last year of Nietzsche's middle period, 1882, coincides with his ragged relationship with Louise von Salomé (1861–1937), the vivacious, young daughter of a Russian general. It is questionable whether Nietzsche proposed marriage to Lou, as she later claimed (Hayman, *Nietzsche*, 246), but there is ample evidence that he fell in love with her. Their situation soon became hopelessly complicated. Paul Rée (1849–1901), who had introduced Nietzsche to Lou and proposed a Platonic *ménage à trois*, also fell in love with her. In Lucerne, the three had their photograph taken. It shows Lou kneeling in a farmer's cart, holding a whip in one hand, ropes tied to Nietzsche and Rée in the other. Nietzsche was upset when he learned that Lou had shown the photograph to other people and angered by his sister's report of what Lou had told her about his ungentlemanly behavior. In the ensuing months, Nietzsche became sicker and more miserable. He wrote to Lou, renouncing all intimacy, "if only I can feel certain that where we feel *united* is where ordinary souls cannot reach" (Hayman, *Nietzsche*, 253). Like Kierkegaard, Nietzsche came to regard the end of his one real love affair as a heroic sacrifice. After living with Rée for several years, Salomé married the Orientalist Friedrich Carl Andreas (1846–1930) and later became Rilke's mistress and a friend and disciple of **Sigmund Freud** (1856–1939).

In 1883, Nietzsche completed Parts I and II of *Thus Spoke Zarathustra*. Here Nietzsche endorses chastity for those to whom it comes naturally and marriage as the means by which a couple may produce something higher than themselves. But his comments on women and love are contemptuous and misogynistic. "Everything about woman, is a riddle, and everything about woman has one solution: that is pregnancy." "A real man wants two things: danger and play. Therefore, he wants woman as the most dangerous plaything." "The happiness of man is: I will. The happiness of woman is: he wills." "You are going to women? Do not forget the whip!" "Bitterness lies in the cup of even the best love." "And your marriage concludes many brief follies as a long stupidity" (177–79, 181–83). Nietzsche's later writings do little to temper this misogyny.

Jean-Paul Sartre. In the twentieth century, the French existentialists dominate the debate on sexuality. Sartre includes erotic relations in his stories, plays, novels, and biographies, but his principal contribution is the chapter "Concrete Relations with Others" in *Being and Nothingness* (*L'être et le néant*, 361–430). Here he argues that **sexual desire** is central to the ontology of human existence, not just as a "fact of life" but as one basic way (along with love, hate, masochism, and sadism) that each human being attempts to deal with the freedom of others. This argument is closely connected to his ontology and theory of bad faith (Kamber, *On Sartre*).

Sartre's ontology is founded on his analysis of consciousness as a nonsubstantial awareness (being-for-itself) of a substantial being other than itself (being-in-itself). But being-for-itself is doubly dependent on being-in-itself, for to be awareness of the latter it must exist as a body (consciousness incarnate) in the midst of the world. He also claims that human beings have a preontological comprehension of the existence of the other. This comprehension has nothing to do with calculations of probability; it is a matter of "factual necessity" (*Being*, 250–51) and is made concrete by our embodiment. Because I exist as a body, I am subject to the permanent possibility of being seen by the other. Sartre insists, "We *encounter* the Other; we do not constitute him" (250). In particular, the look (*le regard*) of the other can make me take the other's point of view on myself: It can objectify my subjectivity, transcend my freedom, and steal my world. For Sartre, the essence of shame is not the recognition of "doing something wrong" but the apprehension of being-for-others. "My original fall," says Sartre, "is the existence of the Other. Shame—like pride—is the apprehension of myself as a nature . . . a given attribute of this being which I am for the Other" (263).

Although Sartre denies that humans have a nature or essence, he argues that we are commonly disposed to act in the following ways: (1) to flee the anguish of freedom and responsibility through bad faith (self-deception); (2) to seek to overcome the contingency of our existence by becoming the foundation of our own being; and (3) to strive to assimilate, transcend, or possess the freedom of others through concrete relations such as love and sexual desire. Indeed, every desire (or motive) that a person has is an expression of that person's fundamental choice of being (*what* that person desires to be), and every fundamental choice is an expression of our common human desire to be God! By "God" Sartre means an "in-itself-for-itself," a consciousness that is its own cause or foundation. Such a being is a contradiction, it cannot exist anywhere, yet we strive in vain to become the impossible. According to Sartre, most people spend their lives in bad faith passionately seeking to complete their projects of being and thereby escape freedom and contingency. "Man," declares Sartre, "is a useless passion" (*Being*, 615).

"Concrete Relations with Others" is one part of this grand argument. It examines the possibility of winning the struggle between my subjectivity and that of the other either by assimilating (through love or masochism), ignoring (through indifference), or objectifying (through desire or sadism) the other's freedom. It treats these attitudes as modes of bad faith and concludes that all must fail. The ideal of love is to recover myself in the look of the other by making myself so fascinating that I become "the whole world" for my beloved. I try to captivate the freedom of my beloved without curbing that freedom, and my beloved's love fills with me joy, for I feel that it justifies my contingent existence: The beloved wills that I be what I am. But love, says Sartre, is "an ideal out of reach" (377); it is a game of mirrors, an infinite regress of wishing to be loved. The real benefit is not mutual justification as the object-limit of each other's freedom but a fragile détente of mutual subjectivity, a détente that can be broken at any time or spoiled by a third party. Masochism, for Sartre, is a desperate attempt to grasp what love cannot by "causing myself to be absorbed by the Other and losing myself in his subjectivity in order to get rid of my own" (377). But this fails as well. The masochist adopts an instrumental (hence subjective) attitude toward the other; he manipulates the other to treat him as an object but remains mired in his own subjective humiliation.

The failure of assimilation brings Sartre to **objectification**. The first candidate is ignoring the freedom of others by treating people as though they were objects in the world. This is possible in a mechanical fashion, but it requires living against the grain of experience, for the look is always there. It also fails as a project of bad faith since the other's "disappearance" increases my awareness of being an unjustifiable subjectivity wholly responsible for myself.

A more plausible candidate is sexual desire. Sartre notes that "existential philosophies have not believed it necessary to concern themselves with sexuality. Heidegger, in particular, does not make the slightest allusion to it in his existential analytic with the result that his 'Dasein' appears to us as asexual" (*Being*, 383). This prompts him to state, "The fundamental problem of sexuality can therefore be formulated thus: is sexuality a contingent accident bound to our physiological nature, or is it a necessary structure of being-for-itself-for-others?" (384). Sartre observes that infants, eunuchs, and the elderly can have sexual desires even though they lack the physiology for ejaculation and orgasm. Indeed, sexuality lasts from birth to death. It is more basic than gender or any particular practice. What, then, is the object of sexual desire? The desired body, of course, but not just as a material object; it is the body of the other "as an organic totality in situation with consciousness at the horizon" (386). However, to realize my desire for the other's body I must rely on my own body in an unusual way: I must let my body clog my consciousness so that I can experience the carnality of another person through my own carnality. "I make myself flesh *in the presence of the Other in order to appropriate* the Other's flesh" (389). This is particularly evident in the caress. The caress is not a simple stroking: It is a ritual of reciprocal incarnation. "[T]he caress reveals the flesh by stripping the body of its action, by cutting it off from the possibilities which surround it" (390). It is no accident that desire, while aiming at the body as a whole, focuses on masses of flesh (breasts, buttocks, thighs) that are barely capable of spontaneous movement. The "true goal of desire" is "the full pressing together of the flesh of two people" (396). The failure of sexual desire arises from the contingency of particular sexes, sex organs, coitus, and orgasm. Coitus brings about "the rupture of that reciprocity of incarnation which was precisely the unique goal of desire" (398). It moves sex to the instrumental plane and ends in disappointment. The pleasure of orgasm is the death of desire.

Sadism is the attempt to incarnate the other's freedom and subjectivity through violence rather than reciprocal carnality. Sexual desire aims to make the other flesh through pleasure, sadism through pain. The type of incarnation sought by the sadist is the obscene; he aims at compelling the victim to assume postures that betray impotence. More than that, "what he wants to knead with his hands and bend under his wrists is the Other's freedom" (*Being*, 403). Sartre denies that the motivation of the sadist is a thirst for power. His purpose is not to suppress the freedom of his tortured victim but to force that freedom to identify with tortured flesh. Ironically, the success of the sadist defeats his purpose. Once the incarnation is achieved and the victim reduced to a panting body, the sadist is confronted with flesh without purpose. If he wishes now to possess that flesh, he must become flesh himself through sexual desire. But sadism fails for another reason as well: Freedom is in principle out of reach. "The sadist discovers his error when his victim *looks* at him" (405). The freedom he has abased through pain and cries for mercy has not disappeared. Another attitude, hate, aims at the death of the other, and thus the termination of the other's freedom. But even death does not eliminate what the other has been or the hater's responsibility.

Any evaluation must give due credit to the breadth and originality of Sartre's argument, yet many points invite criticism (see, for example, Giles). Although Sartre begins by saying there are two fundamental attitudes (assimilation and objectification), he adds hate as a third and has trouble justifying the pairing of subcategories such as love and masochism. He develops a plausible case for the ontological character of sexual desire but suggests without proof that all attitudes toward the other are fundamentally sexual (*Being*, 406–7). With respect to sexual desire itself, his insistence that its true goal is "the full pressing together of the flesh of two people" (396), rather than acts involving particular organs, seems counterintuitive. James Giles tries to rescue and amend Sartre's insight by pointing to the intimacy between mother and infant (165). But Sartre's account of sexuality may be compromised by his effort to relate ontology to physiology without considering social and evolutionary history. It is also possible that Sartre's analysis reflects the limitations of his own sexual experience. He remarks elsewhere, "I was more a masturbator of women than a copulator. . . . For me what mattered most in a sexual relationship was embracing, caressing, moving my lips over a body. . . . I came erect quickly, easily: I made love often, but without very much pleasure" (Hayman, *Sartre*, 144).

A disturbing feature of Sartre's argument is his eagerness to demonstrate the failure and futility of all concrete relations between human beings. Since most people, Sartre included, succeed in establishing intimate and deeply satisfying long-term relationships with other people, all this talk of failure and futility seems melodramatic. For Marcel, concrete relations with others begin with an infant's smile in response to a mother's care. It is the child's first contact with the outside world and the foundation of its personal identity. Fidelity in the mature individual can triumph over tragedy and absence, even the absence we call death (152). In Sartre's defense, it could be argued that he is speaking solely about bad-faith attitudes. Sartre says in a footnote, "These considerations do not exclude the possibility of an ethics of deliverance and salvation. But this can be achieved only after a radical conversion which we cannot discuss here" (*Being*, 412). Perhaps the root problem is not the struggle between consciousnesses striving for primacy in a shared world but the vain attempt to extract from being-for-others the impossible ideal of bad faith. Sartre never wrote an essay on authentic love or sexuality, but Thomas Flynn tries to block out the essential features by drawing on Sartre's later works. Merleau-Ponty challenges Sartre's confinement of sexuality to inauthentic relations with others, by endeavoring to show that sexuality and its ambiguities are "co-extensive with life" (169). Tillich finds the key to sexual authenticity in the joining of libido with both *eros*, the desire for union with a bearer of values, and with *philia*, the love of an I for a Thou (28–32).

Simone de Beauvoir. Simone de Beauvoir's *The Second Sex* (1949) argues that the chief obstacle to authentic interpersonal relations between men and women is not alterity (otherness) *per se* but socially constructed alterity. Woman is defined with reference to man, not he to her: "[S]he is the incidental, the inessential as opposed to the essential. He is the Subject, he is the Absolute—she is the Other" (xxii). In contrast to Sartre's theory that bad faith (as the desire to be God) is fundamental to being human, Beauvoir contends, "It is not a mysterious essence that compels men and women to act in good or bad faith, it is their situation that inclines them more or less toward the search for truth" (xxxiii). She attempts to show that the principal reasons (and remedies) for the failure of love between men and women are neither biological nor ontological but social and economic.

"[I]n human society nothing is natural" (*Second*, 725), but since the history of women is the history of people who have no memory of independence, no religion or culture of its own, no sense of common identity, and who are tied biologically to their oppressors, the condition of women has come to seem like nature itself. "[W]oman has always been man's dependent, if not his slave; the two sexes have never shared the world equally" (xxvi). In matters of love and sex, the male is expected to be active, the aggressor, the female passive, the prey. We speak of a man's potency but describe women as frigid or hot. While this distinction has a basis in physiological differences, it has been transformed through culture into a pervasive conception of men as "transcendent" (free agents) and women as "immanent" (objects to be acted on). Beauvoir finds an attractive alternative in female **homosexuality**. "Woman's homosexuality is one attempt among others to reconcile her autonomy with the passivity of her flesh. . . . [A]ll women are naturally homosexual" (407). But she also sees the possibility of sexual harmony between men and women "not in refinement of technique" but in "mutual generosity of body and soul" (402). For this to happen, a woman must "regain her dignity as a transcendent and free subject while assuming her carnal condition" (402).

The publication of *The Second Sex* provoked ridicule and anger from the French bourgeoisie. Beauvoir's lover, American novelist Nelson Algren (1909–1981), told her: "You've won. You've made all the right enemies" (Bair, 408). But the book had difficulty attracting dependable friends. Despite early praise by feminists, *The Second Sex* was widely regarded as a work of secondary importance until after Beauvoir's death. Feminists of the mid-1970s and 1980s tended to see the work as phallocentric, overly indebted to Sartre, and privileging traditionally male activities. Some were troubled by the apparent inconsistency between Beauvoir's advocacy of independence and her devotion to Sartre. Her habit of putting him first undermined her relationship with Algren and may have led her to underestimate her own potential as a philosopher. Although she had come to accept Sartre's casual womanizing, she was pained by his deeper attachments and fought to maintain her place as his most trusted companion. Perhaps *The Second Sex* was her vision of an authenticity that eluded her grasp. Margaret Simons has helped a new wave of scholars focus on the text and appreciate the originality of Beauvoir's philosophy.

Albert Camus. Camus also touches on authenticity in love and sex. The protagonist of *The Stranger* (1942) is an authentic sensualist, but free of the poetic imperative and endless striving that characterized Kierkegaard's aesthetes. Meursault delights in the cheerful company, good looks, smells, and sexual caresses of a young woman (Marie) he has met at the beach on the day of his mother's funeral. He lives in the present without pretense, guile, or normative principles. He tells Marie "love" has no meaning for him, but he agrees to marry since it does not make any difference to him. Later, in prison awaiting execution, he stops thinking about Marie, "since apart from our bodies, now separated, there wasn't anything to keep us together or even to remind us of each other" (115). Yet Meursault's love of the physical world remains undiminished. In pouring out his anger at the prison chaplain, he declares that "none of his [religious] certainties was worth one hair of a woman's head" (120).

The Plague (1946) suggests that acting out of love for one's beloved is as morally authentic as acting out of sympathy for human suffering (Kamber, *On Camus*). The protagonist,

Dr. Rieux, has chosen to stay in Oran to fight the plague, though his wife is dying in a far-off sanatorium. A young journalist, Rambert, is determined to escape the quarantined city to be reunited with his lover. Rambert tells Rieux, "What interests me is living and dying for what one loves," but then wonders, "Maybe I'm all wrong in putting love first." "No," Rieux says vehemently, "you are *not* wrong" (149–50).

The Fall (1956) draws a savage picture of inauthentic love. The protagonist, Jean-Baptiste Clamence, who paraded as a paragon of magnanimity before his fall into self-knowledge, was an avid seducer of bodies and souls. Always successful with women, he sometimes amused himself by persuading his lovers, before leaving them, to swear eternal fidelity. When he tries to fall in love, he cannot. "For more than thirty years I had been in love exclusively with myself. What hope was there of losing such a habit? I didn't lose it" (100).

The Fall brings us back to the challenge faced by all existentialists in dealing with love and sex: reconciling self-realization and personal fulfillment with authenticity toward others. Camus's portrait of the faithless Clamence, the hypocritical would-be moralist who ignores the cries of a woman who has thrown herself into the Seine, is also a self-portrait. Camus knew that his wife Francine Faure Camus (1914–1979) was tormented by his infidelities and that they were part of the reason for her suicide attempts. When he showed Francine his unfinished manuscript, she remarked, "You're always pleading the causes of all sorts of people, but do you ever hear the screams of people who are trying to reach you?" (Todd, 342).

See also Bataille, Georges; Completeness, Sexual; Desire, Sexual; Feminism, French; Fichte, Johann Gottlieb; Hegel, G.W.F.; Heidegger, Martin; Hobbes, Thomas; Kant, Immanuel; Kierkegaard, Søren; Lacan, Jacques; Leibniz, Gottfried; Nagel, Thomas; Nietzsche, Friedrich; Paglia, Camille; Phenomenology; Poststructuralism; Sadomasochism

REFERENCES

Abbey, Ruth. "Odd Bedfellows: Nietzsche and Mill on Marriage." *History of European Ideas* 23:2–4 (1997), 81–104; Bair, Deirdre. *Simone de Beauvoir: A Biography*. New York: Summit Books, 1990; Beauvoir, Simone de. (1949) *The Second Sex*. Trans. and ed. Howard M. Parshley. New York: Vintage, 1989; Camus, Albert. (1956) *The Fall*. Trans. Justin O'Brien. New York: Vintage, 1962; Camus, Albert. (1946) *The Plague*. Trans. Stuart Gilbert. New York: Random House, 1948; Camus, Albert. (1942) *The Stranger*. Trans. Matthew Ward. New York: Vintage, 1989; Flynn, Thomas. "Inauthentic and Authentic Love in Sartrean Existentialism." In David Goicoechea, ed., *The Nature and Pursuit of Love: The Philosophy of Irving Singer*. Buffalo, N.Y.: Prometheus, 1995, 209–20; Giles, James. "Sartre, Sexual Desire, and Relations with Others." In James Giles, ed., *French Existentialism: Consciousness, Ethics, and Relations with Others*. Amsterdam, Holland: Rodopi, 1999, 155–73; Hayman, Ronald. *Nietzsche: A Critical Life*. New York: Oxford University Press, 1980; Hayman, Ronald. (1987) *Sartre: A Biography*. New York: Carroll and Graf, 1992; Kamber, Richard. *On Camus*. Belmont, Calif.: Wadsworth, 2002; Kamber, Richard. *On Sartre*. Belmont, Calif.: Wadsworth, 2001; Kaufmann, Walter. *Nietzsche: Philosopher, Psychologist, Antichrist*. Princeton, N.J.: Princeton University Press, 1974; Kierkegaard, Søren. (1843) *Either/Or*, 2 vols. Ed. and trans. Howard V. Hong and Edna H. Hong. Princeton, N.J.: Princeton University Press, 1987; Kierkegaard, Søren. (1843) *Fear and Trembling* and *Repetition*. Ed. and trans. Howard V. Hong and Edna H. Hong. Princeton, N.J.: Princeton University Press, 1983; Kierkegaard, Søren. (1845) *Stages on Life's Way*. Ed. and trans. Howard V. Hong and Edna H. Hong. Princeton, N.J.: Princeton University Press, 1988; Kierkegaard, Søren. (1847) *Works of Love: Some Christian Reflections in the Form of Discourses*. Ed. and trans. Howard V. Hong and Edna H. Hong. Princeton, N.J.: Princeton University Press, 1995; Marcel, Gabriel. (1940) *Creative Fidelity* [*Du refus à l'invocation*]. Trans. Robert Rosthal. New

York: Farrar, Straus and Giroux, 1964; Merleau-Ponty, Maurice. (1945) *The Phenomenology of Perception.* Trans. Colin Smith. London: Routledge and Kegan Paul, 1962; Nietzsche, Friedrich. (1886) *Beyond Good and Evil.* Trans. with commentary, Walter Kaufmann. New York: Vintage, 1966; Nietzsche, Friedrich. (1872) *The Birth of Tragedy* and *The Case of Wagner.* Trans. Walter Kaufmann. New York: Vintage, 1967; Nietzsche, Friedrich. (1878) *Human, All Too Human: A Book for Free Spirits.* Trans. Marion Faber with Stephen Lehmann. Lincoln: University of Nebraska Press, 1984; Nietzsche, Friedrich. (1883/1892) *Thus Spoke Zarathustra.* In *The Portable Nietzsche.* Ed. and trans. Walter Kaufmann. New York: Viking, 1954, 121–439; Sartre, Jean-Paul. (1943) *Being and Nothingness: An Essay on Phenomenological Ontology.* Trans. Hazel E. Barnes. New York: Philosophical Library, 1956; Simons, Margaret. *Beauvoir and "The Second Sex": Feminism, Race, and the Origins of Existentialism.* Lanham, Md.: Rowman and Littlefield, 1999; Simons, Margaret, ed. *Feminist Interpretations of Simone de Beauvoir.* University Park: Pennsylvania State University Press, 1995; Suhl, Benjamin. *Jean-Paul Sartre: The Philosopher as Literary Critic.* New York: Columbia University Press, 1970; Tillich, Paul. *Love, Power, and Justice: Ontological Analyses and Ethical Applications.* Oxford, U.K.: Oxford University Press, 1960; Todd, Olivier. (1997) *Albert Camus: A Life.* Trans. Benjamin Ivry. New York: Carroll and Graf, 2000.

Richard Kamber

ADDITIONAL READING

Acocella, Joan. "The Frog and the Crocodile: Love Letters from the Woman behind 'The Second Sex.'" *The New Yorker* (23 and 31 August 1998), 144–52; Bair, Deirdre. *Simone de Beauvoir: A Biography.* New York: Summit, 1990; Beauvoir, Simone de. (1981) *Adieux: A Farewell to Sartre.* Trans. Patrick O'Brian. New York: Pantheon, 1984; Beauvoir, Simone de. (1959) *Brigitte Bardot and the Lolita Syndrome.* Trans. Bernard Frechtman. New York: Reynal, 1960; Beauvoir, Simone de. (1947) *The Ethics of Ambiguity.* Trans. Bernard Frechtman. Secaucus, N.J.: Citadel Press/Philosophical Library, 1948; Beauvoir, Simone de. (1990) *Letters to Sartre.* Trans. Quintin Hoare. New York: Arcade, 1992; Beauvoir, Simone de. (1951–1952) "Must We Burn Sade?" Trans. Annette Michelson. In Austryn Wainhouse and Richard Seaver, comps., *The Marquis de Sade: The 120 Days of Sodom and Other Writings.* New York: Grove Press, 1966, 3–64; Buber, Martin. (1922) *I and Thou* [*Ich und du*]. Trans. Walter Kaufmann. New York: Scribner's, 1970; Camus, Albert. (1942) *The Myth of Sisyphus and Other Essays* [*Le mythe de Sisyphe: Essai sur l'absurde*]. Trans. Justin O'Brien. New York: Knopf, 1955; Collins, Marjorie L., and Christine Pierce. "Holes and Slime: Sexism in Sartre's Psychoanalysis." *Philosophical Forum* 5:1–2 (1973–1974), 112–27; Contat, Michel, and Michel Rybalka. *The Writings of Jean-Paul Sartre,* vol. 1: *A Biographical Life.* Trans. Richard C. McCleary. Evanston, Ill.: Northwestern University Press, 1974; Diamond, Malcolm Luria. *Martin Buber, Jewish Existentialist.* New York: Oxford University Press, 1960; Dostoyevsky, Fyodor. (1864) *Notes from Underground.* Trans. Richard Pevear. New York: Knopf, 2004; Dillon, M. C. *Beyond Romance.* Albany: State University of New York Press, 2001; Dillon, M. C. "Merleau-Ponty on Existential Sexuality: A Critique." *Journal of Phenomenological Psychology* 11:1 (1980), 67–81; Dillon, M. C. "Sex, Time, and Love: Erotic Temporality." *Journal of Phenomenological Psychology* 18:1 (1987), 33–48. Reprinted in SLF (313–25); Giles, James, ed. *French Existentialism: Consciousness, Ethics, and Relations with Others.* Amsterdam, Holland: Rodopi, 1999; Hayman, Ronald. *Sartre: A Biography.* New York: Simon and Schuster, 1987. Reprinted, New York: Carroll and Graf, 1992; Heath, Peter L. "Nothing." In Paul Edwards, ed., *The Encyclopedia of Philosophy,* vol. 5. New York: Macmillan, 1967, 524–25; Heinämaa, Sara. "Simone de Beauvoir's Phenomenology of Sexual Difference." *Hypatia* 14:4 (1999), 114–32; Heinämaa, Sara. *Toward a Phenomenology of Sexual Difference: Husserl, Merleau-Ponty, Beauvoir.* Lanham, Md.: Rowman and Littlefield, 2003; Jaspers, Karl. (1913) *General Psychopathology.* Trans. J. Hoenig and Marian W. Hamilton. Chicago, Ill.: University of Chicago Press, 1963; Kafka, Franz. *Parables and Paradoxes.* Trans. Clement Greenberg, Ernst Kaiser and Eithne Wilkins, Willa and Edwin Muir, and Tania and James Stern. Ed. Nahum N. Glatzer. New York: Schocken, 1946; paperback ed., 1961; Kierkegaard, Søren. (1843) *Repetition: An*

Essay in Experimental Psychology. Trans. Walter Lowrie. Princeton, N.J.: Princeton University Press, 1941; Lingis, Alphonso. *Libido: The French Existential Theories.* Bloomington: Indiana University Press, 1985; Manser, Anthony. *Sartre: A Philosophic Study.* London: Althone, 1966; Mathis, Glen A. "Touch and Vision: Rethinking with Merleau-Ponty Sartre on the Caress." *Philosophy Today* 23 (Winter 1979), 321–28; McBride, William L. "Sartre's Debt to Kierkegaard." In Martin J. Matuštík and Merold Westphal, eds., *Kierkegaard in Post/Modernity.* Bloomington: Indiana University Press, 1995, 18–42; Merck, Mandy. "Marilyn Monroe by Gloria Steinem, Brigitte Bardot by Simone de Beauvoir." In *Perversions: Deviant Readings.* New York: Routledge, 1993, 61–85; Merleau-Ponty, Maurice. (1964) *The Visible and the Invisible.* Trans. Alphonso Lingis. Ed. Claude Lefort. Evanston, Ill.: Northwestern University Press, 1964; Mitchell, Juliet. (1974) "Simone de Beauvoir: Freud and the Second Sex." In *Psychoanalysis and Feminism: Freud, Reich, Laing, and Women.* New York: Vintage, 1975, 305–18; Murdoch, Iris. *Sartre: Romantic Rationalist.* New Haven, Conn.: Yale University Press, 1953; Nagel, Thomas. "Sexual Perversion." *Journal of Philosophy* 66:1 (1969), 5–17. Reprinted in P&S1 (247–60); POS1 (76–88). Reprinted, revised, in Thomas Nagel, *Mortal Questions.* Cambridge: Cambridge University Press, 1979, 39–52; and POS2 (39–51); POS3 (9–20); POS4 (9–20); STW (105–12); Nietzsche, Friedrich. (1901) *The Will to Power.* Trans. Walter Kaufmann and R. J. Hollingdale. New York: Random House, 1967; Oaklander, L. Nathan. (1977) "Sartre on Sex." In Alan Soble, ed., *The Philosophy of Sex: Contemporary Readings,* 1st ed. Totowa, N.J.: Rowman and Littlefield, 1980, 190–206; Ortega y Gasset, José. (1941) *History as a System and Other Essays toward a Philosophy of History.* Trans. Helene Weyl. New York: Norton, 1961; Ortega y Gasset, José. (1940) *On Love: Aspects of a Single Theme.* Trans. Toby Talbot. New York: Meridian Books, 1957; Park, See-Young. "D. H. Lawrence Unbuttoned: *Aaron's Rod, Kangaroo,* and the Influence of Lev Shestov." In Paul Poplawski, ed., *Writing the Body in D. H. Lawrence: Essays on Language, Representation, and Sexuality.* Westport, Conn.: Greenwood Press, 2001, 79–91; Prose, Francine. "Lou Andreas-Salomé." In *The Lives of the Muses: Nine Women and the Artists They Inspired.* New York: HarperCollins, 2002, 139–85; Rice, Lee C. "Freud, Sartre, Spinoza: The Problematic of the Unconscious." *Giornale di Metafisica* 17:1 (1995), 87–106; Rilke, Rainer Maria. (1910) *The Notebooks of Malte Laurids Brigge.* Trans. Stephen Mitchell. New York: Vintage, 1990; [Andreas-]Salomé, Lou. (1894) *Friedrich Nietzsche in seinen Werken.* Translated as *Nietzsche* by Siegfried Mandel (1988). Urbana: University of Illinois Press, 2001; Sartre, Jean-Paul. (1939) *The Emotions: Outline of a Theory.* Trans. Bernard Frechtman. New York: Philosophical Library, 1948; Sartre, Jean-Paul. (1939) *Intimacy and Other Stories (Le mur).* Trans. Lloyd Alexander. New York: New Directions, 1948; Sartre, Jean-Paul. (1952) *Saint Genet: Actor and Martyr.* Trans. Bernard Frechtman. New York: George Braziller, 1963; Sartre, Jean-Paul. (1960) *Search for a Method.* Trans. Hazel E. Barnes. New York: Knopf, 1963; Sartre, Jean-Paul. *Witness to My Life: The Letters of Jean-Paul Sartre to Simone de Beauvoir, 1926–1939.* Ed. Simone de Beauvoir. Trans. Lee Fahnestock and Norman Macafee. New York: Scribner's, 1992; Schwarzer, Alice. *After* The Second Sex: *Conversations with Simone de Beauvoir.* Trans. Marianne Howarth. New York: Pantheon, 1984; Scruton, Roger. "Sartre's Paradox." In *Sexual Desire: A Moral Philosophy of the Erotic.* New York: Free Press, 1986, 120–25; Shestov, Lev [Yehuda Leib Shvartsman]. *Apofeoz bespochvennosti (Apotheosis of Groundlessness).* St. Petersburg, Russia: Obshestovenanya Polza, 1905. *All Things Are Possible.* Trans. S. S. Kotelianski. Foreword by D. H. Lawrence. London: Martin Secker, 1920. *All Things Are Possible and Penultimate Words and Other Essays.* Ed. Bernard Martin. Athens: Ohio University Press, 1977; Shestov, Lev [Yehuda Leib Shvartsman]. (1938) *Athens and Jerusalem.* Trans. Bernard Martin. Athens: Ohio University Press, 1966; Shestov, Lev [Yehuda Leib Schvartsman]. (1903) *Dostoevsky, Tolstoy, and Nietzsche: The Good in the Teaching of Tolstoy and Nietzsche: Philosophy and Preaching* and *Dostoevsky and Nietzsche: Tragic Philosophy.* Trans. Bernard Martin and Spencer Roberts. Ed. Bernard Martin. Athens: Ohio University Press, 1969; Simons, Margaret A. "Beauvoir and Sartre: The Philosophical Relationship." In H. V. Wenzel, ed., *Simone de Beauvoir: Witness to a Century. Yale French Studies,* no. 72 (1986), 165–79; Singer, Irving. (1958) "Ortega on Love." In *Explorations in Love and Sex.* Lanham, Md.: Rowman and Littlefield, 2001, 199–216; Singer, Irving. "Sartre and the Varieties of Existentialism." In *The Nature of Love,* vol. 3: *The Modern World.* Chicago,

Ill.: University of Chicago Press, 1987, 281–342; Solomon, Robert C. *Love: Emotion, Myth, and Metaphor*. Garden City, N.Y.: Anchor Press, 1981. Buffalo, N.Y.: Prometheus, 1990; Solomon, Robert C. *The Passions*. Garden City, N.Y.: Anchor/Doubleday, 1976; Solomon, Robert C. "Sexual Paradigms." *Journal of Philosophy* 71:11 (1974), 336–45. Reprinted in HS (81–90); POS1 (89–98); POS2 (53–62); POS3 (21–29); POS4 (21–29); Solomon, Robert C. "The Virtue of (Erotic) Love." In Peter A. French, Theodore E. Uehling, Jr., and Howard K. Wettstein, eds., *Ethical Theory: Character and Virtue*. *Midwest Studies in Philosophy* 13 (1988), 12–31. Reprinted in Robert C. Solomon and Kathleen Higgins, eds., *The Philosophy of (Erotic) Love*. Lawrence: University Press of Kansas, 1991, 492–518; STW (241–55); Solomon, Robert C. "The Virtues of a Passionate Life: Erotic Love and 'the Will to Power.'" *Social Philosophy and Policy* 15:1 (1998), 90–118; Solomon, Robert C., ed. (1974) *Existentialism*, 2nd ed. New York: Oxford University Press, 2004; Sontag, Susan. (1963) "Sartre's *Saint Genet*." In *Against Interpretation and Other Essays*. New York: Farrar, Straus and Giroux, 1966, 93–99; Spelman, Elizabeth V. (1988) "Simone de Beauvoir and Women: Just Who Does She Think 'We' Is? In Mary Lyndon Shanley and Carole Pateman, eds., *Feminist Interpretations and Political Theory*. University Park: Pennsylvania State University Press, 1991, 199–216; Taylor, Roger. "Sexual Experiences." *Proceedings of the Aristotelian Society* 68 (1967–1968), 87–104. Reprinted in POS1 (59–75); Todd, Olivier. *Albert Camus: A Life*. Trans. Benjamin Ivry. New York: Knopf, 1997. Reprinted, New York: Carroll and Graf, 2000; Vannoy, Russell. "The Structure of Sexual Perversity." In Alan Soble, ed., *Sex, Love, and Friendship*. Amsterdam, Holland: Rodopi, 1997, 359–73; Wall, Barbara E. *Love and Death in the Philosophy of Gabriel Marcel*. Washington, D.C.: University Press of America, 1977.

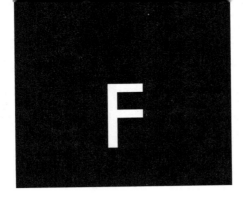

F

FANTASY. Sexual fantasy may be understood as a nonperceptual thought that is sexually arousing. Fantasy is similar to imagination; both are distinct from current perception, and both commonly do not depict true states of affairs. But fantasy scenarios need not be false. They might by chance correspond to an actual state of the world. Further, we often fantasize about experiences we have already had, so a fantasy might be historically true.

Sexual fantasy has three characteristic features: structure, control, and content. Regarding structure, there is a subject (the person entertaining the fantasy) and an object (the imagined scenario). There is also a relation between them, such that the subject takes sexual pleasure or interest in the object. (This distinguishes sexual fantasy from nonsexual fantasy.) The object is usually a mental state with quasi-perceptual (say, visual or olfactory) properties. A person fantasizing often experiences an imagined sexual event similarly to how the person would experience an actual sexual event. Supposing that fantasy includes this object is likely necessary to account for the fact that fantasies seem to be *about* something.

Sexual fantasies are typically under the control of the subject, who voluntarily arranges their occurrence and content. Of course, limits exist to the scenarios that sexually arouse or interest the subject; the voluntariness of fantasy does not mean we have *carte blanche* to fantasize sexually about any scenario, despite the fact that scenario events take place only mentally. One might argue that being voluntary is not essential to fantasy, since some people have fantasies that are beyond their control (as in obsessional ideation, in which thoughts race through one's head). Nevertheless, fantasy seems to be paradigmatically voluntary.

Fantasies also have semantic content; after all, the object is a scenario. These scenarios may be specific, in that they involve particular persons, acts, and emotions. They are also (and perhaps necessarily) vague, since many of the details of a scenario are often not filled in. Most often, the depicted scenario is a counterfactual event. That fantasies contain specific details, even if counterfactual, raises the question of how seriously we should take the scenario's propositional content. That X fantasizes (pleasurably) about raping a Y who enjoys (in the fantasy) being raped seems not to imply that X really believes that Y would actually enjoy being raped (let alone that all women enjoy being raped). So even if a sexual fantasy has misogynist psychological or social roots that are manifested in its volitional content, the fantasizer need not be misogynistic. In some cases, however, subjects may fantasize misogynist scenarios and genuinely agree with and endorse their content, rather than only engage in pretense, play, or simulation.

In exploring the moral status of fantasy and fantasizing, the distinction between intrinsic and extrinsic moral properties is important. An intrinsic property of something is a property it has in and of itself, while an extrinsic property is something it has in virtue of its relation to other things. A person having sexual fantasies could have many different extrinsic properties. For example, if a person allows his or her life to be consumed by sexual fantasies to the exclusion of family, friends, and work, such fantasies might be bad, and extrinsically so. On the other hand, if fantasies are employed to relax one's mind and encourage sleep, they are extrinsically good (*ceteris paribus*). In terms of having a multitude of possible consequences, sexual fantasies are similar to mental and physical states generally. What about the intrinsic moral properties of sexual fantasy? It can be argued that sexual fantasies, as deliberate mental acts, are wrong as a group in themselves. That would be the ultimate objection to sexual fantasies in terms of their intrinsic moral properties (see **Thomas Aquinas**, *Summa theologiae*, vol. 43, 2a2ae, ques. 154, art. 4). Maybe thinking about sex is *per se* morally objectionable. Alternatively, perhaps only some sexual fantasies are wrong in terms of their intrinsic properties.

In thinking about the morality of sexual fantasies, of obvious relevance is the classical dispute between consequentialist or teleological moral theories (e.g., the utilitarianism of John Stuart Mill [1806–1873]) and moral theories that are nonconsequentialist or deontological (e.g., the Natural Law ethics of Thomas Aquinas [1224/25–1274] and the Categorical Imperative of **Immanuel Kant** [1724–1804]).

On a consequentialist account, a person may engage in sexual fantasy if and only if doing so leads to the best overall results. Sexual fantasies often bring about short-term pleasure. If this pleasure is a good, fantasies are wrong only if they have bad effects that outweigh this value. This might happen in several (interrelated) ways. Perhaps **pornography** causes the subordination of or violence toward women (Langton, 293–330; **Catharine MacKinnon**, 21). Similar things might be true of sexual fantasies, even if not elicited by viewing pornography, especially fantasies that exhibit the **objectification** of women: those in which women are portrayed as being mere tools for men, as lacking autonomy, as being owned property, as fungible, and so forth (Nussbaum, 257). Perhaps sexual fantasies lead to changes in the subject in much the same way that violent pornography might shape a viewer's desires without his or her conscious assent (Scoccia, 790–92). Perhaps sexual fantasies defame women by asserting malicious falsehoods; for example, they enjoy being violated or exist only for men's sexual purposes (Hill, 43–52; Longino, 39–40). And perhaps fantasies, like pornography, lead to **masturbation** that might, when excessive, endanger one's sexual health or participation in healthy relationships. Consequentialist judgments about the morality of fantasy are sensitive to the truth-value of these claims. If they can be supported, they tend to make the consequentialist moral case against fantasy convincing, but otherwise fantasy is vindicated.

On a Kantian account, a person may engage in sexual fantasizing only if doing so does not treat a person, oneself or another, merely as a means. (See the Second Formulation of Kant's Categorical Imperative, Ak 4:429.) Sexual fantasy raises intriguing questions about what treating someone merely as a means is (see James, 53; Nozick, 32; Soble, 96; Stoltenberg, 41–44). Suppose Alice fantasizes about Betty, and Betty never finds out. Alice, in some sense, seems to be objectifying Betty; in some way, she seems to be using her. But, on the other hand, Alice does not touch Betty's body, and Betty, having no knowledge of the fantasy, is not affected by it. Perhaps Alice doesn't use *Betty* as a means to her sexual pleasure but only the *image* of Betty. This account is plausible, because subjects can have fantasies that are qualitatively identical to Alice's about Betty but do not correspond to any actual person. The question is thus suggested whether persons fantasize about simulations of events or counterfactual events. The simulation account explains an important pattern about fantasies, that persons often fantasize about acts of which they disapprove, such as **sadomasochism** (Bartky; Hopkins). The counterfactual account fits better with the introspective reports of many persons that they do fantasize about a counterfactual event, not its simulation (Corvino, 214–15). One possibility is that the ontological nature, as simulation or counterfactual event, of the object of fantasy varies between persons and perhaps for the same person at different times. The moral status of fantasies gets even more complex if their content is not within our control or consciously accessible (Neu, 147–48).

Sexual fantasies might also be bad on deontological grounds because they focus the subject on himself or herself and crowd out moral thoughts (Cherry, 131–32). Since the displacement occurs in all fantasizing, sexual or not, all fantasy would be morally wrong. To establish such a view, one must be able to argue that moral thoughts always take precedence over (or morally trump) the enjoyments of fantasy. Whether our moral duties are so demanding is not clear (James, 52).

Another interesting case is John's having sex with Jill while entertaining a sexual fantasy about a specific third party, about no one in particular, or even about Jill (see Neu, 139–43; Solomon, 344–45). John might very well in this case be treating Jill as a means to his own private pleasure (and this can happen even if he is not fantasizing). The resulting sex might be perverted since it lacks the mutual interpersonal awareness that on some accounts characterizes natural sex (Nagel, 44–48; Neu, 139–40). But what if John uses the fantasy so that he can share himself sexually with Jill, at least in part for her sake, because he finds her, for a variety of possible reasons, unattractive? That might count as either a decent consequentialist or deontological rationale for the fantasy. However, when such narrow conditions do not apply and private fantasies are inconsistent with a couple's mutually understood goal of sexual relations (say, the expression of **love** or appreciation), such fantasies may be wrong. But this is not to say that private fantasies during marital sex are wrong *qua* **adultery** (see Matt. 5:27–28) or that they are as wrong as adultery is.

Moral questions, of course, do not exhaust what is philosophically interesting about sexual fantasy. One question concerns why the experience of a fantasized activity sometimes does, but sometimes (more important) does not, bring us the joy we anticipated. Does reality not measure up to the fantasy because our fantasy was too specific, including too many unrealizable details? Or was it too vague, not including enough? Perhaps the mismatch between our sexual fantasies and subsequent reality is only a case of a more general human phenomenon: We tend to overestimate the value of what we (think we) want and do not yet have (see Hirschman, 21). Another question is about why we fantasize at all. The answer, that it brings us pleasure to do so, only skims the surface, for we still want to know why fantasizing bring us pleasure—and sometimes more pleasure than our current reality (as in the case of that well-known Everyman, Walter Mitty). The ordinary answer is that we sexually fantasize about something (or someone) because we desire it (or that person), but the relationship might be exactly the opposite: We desire something because we somehow already have, somewhere in our minds or brains, a fantasy about it (see Kay, 77).

See also Activity, Sexual; Adultery; Consequentialism; Cybersex; Desire, Sexual; Ethics, Sexual; Ethics, Virtue; Freud, Sigmund; Kant, Immanuel; Lacan, Jacques; Masturbation; Pornography; Sex Work

REFERENCES

Bartky, Sandra Lee. "Feminine Masochism and the Politics of Personal Transformation." *Women's Studies International Forum* 7:5 (1984), 323–34; Cherry, Christopher. "When Is Fantasising Morally Bad?" *Philosophical Investigations* 11:2 (1988), 112–32; Corvino, John. "Naughty Fantasies." *Southwest Philosophy Review* 18:1 (2002), 213–20; Hill, Judith. "Pornography and Degradation." *Hypatia* 2:2 (1987), 39–54; Hirschman, Albert O. "On Disappointment." In *Shifting Involvements:*

Private Interest and Public Action. Princeton, N.J.: Princeton University Press, 1982, 9–24; Hopkins, Patrick D. "Rethinking Sadomasochism: Feminism, Interpretation, and Simulation." *Hypatia* 9:1 (1994), 116–41; James, David. "An Ethics of Fantasy." *International Journal of Applied Philosophy* 8:1 (1993), 51–55; Kant, Immanuel. (1785) *Groundwork of the Metaphysic of Morals*. Trans. H. J. Paton. New York: Harper Torchbooks, 1964; Kay, Sarah. *Žižek: A Critical Introduction*. Cambridge, U.K.: Polity Press, 2003; Langton, Rae. "Speech Acts and Unspeakable Acts." *Philosophy and Public Affairs* 22:4 (1993), 293–330; Longino, Helen. "Pornography, Oppression, and Freedom: A Closer Look." In Laura Lederer, ed., *Take Back the Night: Women on Pornography*. New York: Morrow, 1980, 34–47; MacKinnon, Catherine A. *Only Words*. Cambridge, Mass.: Harvard University Press, 1993; Nagel, Thomas. (1969) "Sexual Perversion." In *Mortal Questions*. Cambridge: Cambridge University Press, 1979, 39–52; Neu, Jerome. "An Ethics of Fantasy?" *Journal of Theoretical and Philosophical Psychology* 22:2 (2002), 133–57; Nozick, Robert. *Anarchy, State, and Utopia*. New York: Basic Books, 1974; Nussbaum, Martha C. "Objectification." *Philosophy and Public Affairs* 24:4 (1995), 249–91; Scoccia, Danny. "Can Liberals Support a Ban on Violent Pornography?" *Ethics* 106:4 (1996), 776–99; Soble, Alan. *Sexual Investigations*. New York: New York University Press, 1996; Solomon, Robert C. "Sexual Paradigms." *Journal of Philosophy* 71:11 (1974), 336–45; Stoltenberg, John. *Refusing to Be a Man: Essays on Sex and Justice*. Portland, Ore.: Breitenbush Books, 1989; Thomas Aquinas. (1265–1273) *Summa theologiae*, 60 vols. Trans. Blackfriars. Cambridge, U.K.: Blackfriars, 1964–1976.

Stephen Kershnar

ADDITIONAL READING

Bartky, Sandra Lee. "Feminine Masochism and the Politics of Personal Transformation." *Women's Studies International Forum* 7:5 (1984), 323–34. Reprinted in *Femininity and Domination: Studies in the Phenomenology of Oppression*. New York: Routledge, 1990, 45–62; POS2 (219–42); Ben-Ze'ev, Aaron. "Online Imagination." In *Love Online: Emotions on the Internet*. Cambridge: Cambridge University Press, 2004, 78–94; Byrne, Donn. "The Imagery of Sex." In John Money and Herman Musaph, eds., *Handbook of Sexology*. Amsterdam, Holland: Excerpta Medica, 1977, 327–50; Card, Robert. "Intentions, the Nature of Fantasizing, and Naughty Fantasies." *Southwest Philosophy Review* 18:2 (2002), 159–61; Cowie, Elizabeth. "Pornography and Fantasy: Psychoanalytic Perspectives." In Lynne Segal and Mary McIntosh, eds., *Sex Exposed: Sexuality and the Pornography Debate*. New Brunswick, N.J.: Rutgers University Press, 1993, 132–52; Eisenstein, Zillah. *Global Obscenities: Patriarchy, Capitalism, and the Lure of Cyberfantasy*. New York: New York University Press, 1998; Friday, Nancy. *Men in Love*. New York: Dell, 1980; Friday, Nancy. *My Secret Garden: Women's Sexual Fantasies*. New York: Pocket Books, 1973; Grimshaw, Jean. "Ethics, Fantasy, and Self-Transformation." In A. Phillips Griffiths, ed., *Ethics* [*Philosophy* Supp. 35]. Cambridge: Cambridge University Press, 1993, 145–58. Reprinted in POS3 (175–87); Hartman, William E., and Marilyn A. Fithian. "Fantasies and Sex." In Vern L. Bullough and Bonnie Bullough, eds., *Human Sexuality: An Encyclopedia*. New York: Garland, 1994, 201–2; Hill, Judith M. "Pornography and Degradation." *Hypatia* 2:2 (1987), 39–54. Reprinted in Robert M. Baird and Stuart E. Rosenbaum, eds., *Pornography: Private Right or Public Menace?* rev. ed. Amherst, N.Y.: Prometheus, 1998, 100–113; Hopkins, Patrick D. "Rethinking Sadomasochism: Feminism, Interpretation, and Simulation." *Hypatia* 9:1 (1994), 116–41. Reprinted in POS3 (189–214); Hopkins, Patrick D. "Simulation and the Reproduction of Injustice: A Reply." *Hypatia* 10:2 (1995), 162–70; Kipnis, Laura. *Bound and Gagged: Pornography and the Politics of Fantasy in America*. New York: Grove, 1996; Langton, Rae. "Speech Acts and Unspeakable Acts." *Philosophy and Public Affairs* 22:4 (1993), 293–330. Reprinted in Susan Dwyer, ed., *The Problem of Pornography*. Belmont, Calif.: Wadsworth, 1985, 203–19; Longino, Helen. "Pornography, Oppression, and Freedom: A Closer Look." In Laura Lederer, ed., *Take Back the Night: Women on Pornography*. New York: Morrow, 1980, 34–47. Reprinted in Susan Dwyer, ed., *The Problem of Pornography*. Belmont, Calif.: Wadsworth, 1995, 34–47; Mann, Jay, and Natalie Shainess. "Sadistic Fantasies." *Medical Aspects of Human Sexuality* 8:2

(1974), 142–48; Martin, Mike W. (1989, 2001) "Fantasy." In *Everyday Morality: An Introduction to Applied Ethics*, 2nd ed. Belmont, Calif.: Wadsworth, 1995, 262–65, 370; Merkin, Daphne. "Eros Redux." *The New Yorker* (27 December 1993 and 3 January 1994), 154–59; Merkin, Daphne. "Unlikely Obsession." *The New Yorker* (26 February and 4 March 1996), 98–115; Montaigne, Michel. (1595) "Of the Power of the Imagination." In *The Complete Essays of Montaigne*. Trans. Donald M. Frame. Stanford, Calif.: Stanford University Press, 1958, 68–76; Nagel, Thomas. "Sexual Perversion." *Journal of Philosophy* 66:1 (1969), 5–17. Reprinted in P&S1 (247–60); POS1 (76–88). Reprinted, revised, in Thomas Nagel, *Mortal Questions*. Cambridge: Cambridge University Press, 1979, 39–52; and POS2 (39–51); POS3 (9–20); POS4 (9–20); STW (105–12); Neu, Jerome. "Fantasy and Memory: The Aetiological Role of Thoughts According to Freud." *International Journal of Psycho-Analysis* 54 (1973), 383–98; Neu, Jerome. "Freud and Perversion." In Jerome Neu, ed., *The Cambridge Companion to Freud*. Cambridge: Cambridge University Press, 1991, 175–208. Reprinted in *A Tear Is an Intellectual Thing: The Meanings of Emotion*. New York: Oxford University Press, 2000, 144–65; STW (87–104). Original publication in Earl E. Shelp, ed., *Sexuality and Medicine*, vol. 1: *Conceptual Roots*. Dordrecht, Holland: Reidel, 1987, 153–84; Nussbaum, Martha C. "Objectification." *Philosophy and Public Affairs* 24:4 (1995), 249–91. Reprinted in POS3 (283–321); POS4 (381–419). Reprinted, revised, in *Sex and Social Justice*. New York: Oxford University Press, 1999, 213–39; Petersen, Patricia. *Ethics and Sexual Fantasy*. Ph.D. dissertation. University of Queensland, 2000; Soble, Alan. "Pornography: Defamation and the Endorsement of Degradation." *Social Theory and Practice* 11:1 (1985), 61–87; Solomon, Robert C. "Sexual Paradigms." *Journal of Philosophy* 71:11 (1974), 336–45. Reprinted in HS (81–90); POS1 (89–98); POS2 (53–62); POS3 (21–29); POS4 (21–29); Sue, David. "Erotic Fantasies of College Students during Coitus." *Journal of Sex Research* 15:4 (1979), 299–305; Vadas, Melinda. "Reply to Patrick Hopkins." *Hypatia* 10:2 (1995), 159–61. Reprinted in POS3 (215–17); Žižek, Slavoj. *The Plague of Fantasies*. London: Verso, 1997.

FEMALE SEXUAL AGGRESSION. *See* Coercion (by Sexually Aggressive Women)

FEMINISM, FRENCH. French feminism arose with, and was influenced by, the same mid-twentieth-century events as French **poststructuralism**. The main writers, Simone de Beauvoir (1908–1986), Hélène Cixous, Luce Irigaray, Julia Kristeva, and Monique Wittig (1935–2003), pursued humans as divided by sex, culture, and **language**. A spectrum of French feminist writings can be found in *New French Feminisms* (edited by Marks and Courtivron), which includes writings by Annie Leclerc, Benoîte Groult, Claudine Hermann, Marguerite Duras (1914–1996), and others who are critical of Western masculinism and patriarchy. These writings propose new, alternative possibilities for women, relations between men and women, and future societies. The critique of the modern subject that pervades poststructuralism becomes a critique of the male subject, before and into modernity, and the ways in which male subjectivity is passed off as universal.

The characteristic writings of French feminism link issues of women, sexuality, pleasure, and bodies with writing itself, especially with unique and extraordinary forms of writing. Here the critical importance of Beauvoir plays a double role. In her novels, including *She Came to Stay* and *All Men Are Mortal*, Beauvoir explores being a woman and women's sexuality in traditional literary forms. In *The Second Sex*, "Must We Burn Sade?" and *The Coming of Age*, she presents critical sexual and social landscapes where new imaginations are essential. In returning to the **Marquis de Sade** (1740–1814) in the context of a feminist critique, she complicates relations between gender and sensibility, sexuality and violence, thought and pleasure, bondage and subordination. Sexual identity and gender are inseparable from sexual practices, and these cannot be circumscribed by social proprieties.

The famous question Beauvoir poses in *The Second Sex* is, "What is a woman?" From that moment, questions of human and gender identity, and of subjects and subjectivity, proliferated throughout social critique. Her answer is that "humanity is male and man defines woman not in herself but as relative to him: she is not regarded as an autonomous being" (xxii). French and other feminisms take their departure from this statement. It is more than a question of women's inequality, but of the framing of language and society in such a way that subordination and relativization represent the structure of society and thought. In male-dominated societies women are expected to live up to a male model, to care for and be subservient to men, and to be happy doing so. In other words, they lack full subjectivity. The modern subject is a male subject.

Julia Kristeva. Of the four writers discussed here—Cixous, Irigaray, Kristeva, Wittig— Kristeva is perhaps the most tenuously related to feminism and to the notion of writing in the feminine, though she wrote *Tales of Love*, which includes "Stabat Mater," both experiments in alternative writing. She was an active member of the French psychoanalytic school. Her career can be read as extended meditations on the role of the mother in psychoanalysis, a role that in **Jacques Lacan** (1901–1981) relates to the sexual identity of the subject, the pervasiveness of desire, the constitution of the subject by language, and the invisibility of the woman/mother.

Kristeva's most well known views on desire, language, and poetry are in her doctoral dissertation *Revolution in Poetic Language*, later expanded in *Desire in Language*, in which the symbolic (as in Lacan) represents the formed, determinate, significant side of language and consciousness, understood to emerge from the desiring, semiotic depths of language into poetry:

> Voice, hearing, and sight are the archaic dispositions where the earliest forms
> of discreteness emerge. The breast, given and withdrawn; lamplight capturing
> the gaze; intermittent sounds of voice of music . . . become a *there*, a place, a
> spot, a marker. The effect, which is dramatic, is no longer quiet but laughter.
> (*Desire*, 283)

The infant origin gives rise to an immense range of intense qualities that fall at the limits of what is considered public discourse: care, voice, music, laughter; poetry, desire, affect, **love**; melancholia, horror, abjection, strangeness, heterogeneity. All are sexual, desirous, deep, emergent, pervasive conditions of being human, understood through the infant-mother relation as underlying the formation of language and subjectivity. The indeterminate sides of life owe their existence to this primordial relation and signification. "[T]here is within poetic language (and therefore, although in a less pronounced manner, within any language) a *heterogeneousness* to meaning" (133). Her work explores this heterogeneity in language into remarkable places:

> A hymn to total giving to the other, such a love is also, and almost as explicitly,
> a hymn to the narcissistic power to which I may even sacrifice *it*, sacrifice *my-
> self*. (*Tales*, 1–2)

> A secret wound, often unknown to himself, drives the foreigner to wandering. . . .
> As far back as his memory can reach, it is delightfully bruised: misunderstood

> by a loved and yet absentminded mother, the exile is a stranger to his mother. (*Strangers to Ourselves*, 5)

> There looms, within abjection, one of those violent, dark revolts of being, directed against a threat that seems to emanate from an exorbitant outside or inside, ejected beyond the scope of the possible, the tolerable, the thinkable. (*Powers of Horror*, 1)

> The abject confronts us . . . with our earliest attempts to release the hold of *maternal* entity even before ex-isting outside of her, thanks to the autonomy of language. (*Powers*, 13)

These are heterogeneous, pervasive conditions of being, presences of desire. Here language and being, humanity and the world, are sexual and sexed in multiple senses of desire, corporeality, and pleasure—*jouissance* (a word from Sade and Lacan employed to mark unknown [woman's] sexual pleasures); of sex and gender, maternity and paternity, father and mother. Human beings are sexed beings, desiring and desired beings; the world is full of desire, of desired things, of heterogeneous conditions of desire and pleasure. Through abjection, Kristeva is able to evoke recurrent and pervasive elements of sexuality and bodies (odors, tastes, seepages, fluids, viscosity) in the registers of disgust and revulsion as well as joy.

Some of Kristeva's writings in the emergence of French feminism were influential, for example, "Stabat Mater," in which she raises the question of an unknown and perhaps impossible heretical ethics (*hérethique*, in the feminine), and "Women's Time" (1979), in which questions of feminism and feminist practice arise in linear time, while evoking through maternity and birth another time, another writing. Kristeva later became disenchanted with the feminist movement as a movement in lived, political time, as if to have lost the heterogeneity of infancy before symbolic time.

Hélène Cixous. Hélène Cixous is a remarkable writer for whom writing itself is both question and answer. In her hands, writing is the heterogeneous, that is, desire itself, transgressing itself. Transgression here pertains to any meaning of propriety, including violence, abjection, and cruelty, to relations between humans and animals, humans and eating, humans and things. Literature is a sexed, desirous writing in which the dark and light of desire coexist. Several of Cixous's writings are definitive of French feminism and of writing in the feminine (*L'écriture feminine*), including *The Newly Born Woman*, written with Catherine Clément, and "The Laugh of the Medusa."

In *Newly Born Woman*, Cixous and Clément engage in a dialogue situated between the cruelty toward women in European literature, sacrificial and redemptive, between traditional roles of women and the sense of alternative possibilities they evoke, and a new woman, new world, new sexualities, and *jouissances*. These include an affirmation of *"the other bisexuality"* as anything but neuter, "the location within oneself of the presence of both sexes . . . the multiplication of the effects of desire's inscription on every part of the body and the other body" (*Newly*, 85). This multiplication of desire inscribed on every part of multiple bodies expresses the theme of writing in the feminine, which has frequently been read as women's writing.

Such a reading can follow a brief encounter with the opening words of "The Laugh of the Medusa," which is among the most extravagant of Cixous's works:

> I shall speak about women's writing: about *what it will do*. Woman must write her self: must write about women and being women to writing, from which

they have been driven away as violently as from the bodies—for the same reasons, by the same law, with the same fatal goal. Woman must put herself into the text—as into the world and into history—by her own movement. . . . Write your self. Your body must be heard. (245, 250)

A critical question is how women's bodies, their breasts, vulvas, and vaginas, might be written, might transform writing. Cixous refuses that possibility. The bodies to be written do not precede the writing. "I refuse . . . to confuse the biological and the cultural" (245); "what I say has at least two sides and two aims: to break up, to destroy; and to foresee the unforeseeable, to project" (245); "writing is precisely *the very possibility of change*" (249).

Writing in the feminine presents at least two sides, to transform a world that oppresses women and to participate in the unforeseeable. Writing is the possibility of change, not the implementation of a goal. Sexuality ceases to be biological without becoming cultural:

It is impossible to *define* a feminine practice of writing, and this is an impossibility that will remain, for this practice can never be theorized, enclosed, coded—which doesn't mean that it doesn't exist. (264)

Such is the strength of women that, sweeping away syntax, breaking that famous thread (just a tiny little thread, they say) which acts for men as a surrogate umbilical cord . . . women will go right up to the impossible. (256)

It is impossible to define a feminine sexuality or a feminine sex. Sex, desire, and sexuality are transgressive in the sense of wrecking proprieties and of opening unknown improprieties.

Monique Wittig. Monique Wittig writes on sexuality and corporeality, in a lesbian register, including remarkable literary works and highly influential essays. In the essays, she comments on her lesbian writing, explaining that they are driven not only by lesbianism as a theme but by the struggle to make it visible where language and society are designed to make it invisible.

In a gendered language one cannot speak of women as the universal: The feminine plural, *elles*, does not mean *they* but means *the women. Elles* can mean *they* only in a world without men, something possible only in imagination and writing. Lesbianism is a fiction—except that some women are lesbians. This double gesture, between the impossibility and reality of lesbians and lesbianism, between heterosexuality, men and women, and lesbianism as an alternative, marks the gender in Wittig's writing.

The bar in the *j/e* of *The Lesbian Body* [*Le corps lesbien*] is a sign of excess. A sign that helps to imagine an excess of "I," an "I" exalted. "I" has become so powerful in *The Lesbian Body* that it can attack the order of heterosexuality in texts and assault the so-called love, the heroes of love, and lesbianize them, lesbianize the symbols, lesbianize the gods and the goddesses, lesbianize the men and the women. ("The Mark of Gender," *Straight*, 87)

Le corps lesbien has lesbianism as its theme, that is, a theme which cannot even be described as taboo, for it has no real existence in the history of literature. (*Lesbian*, 9)

Lesbianism, then, is both a lived alternative to heterosexual norms and something that exists only in its disappearance.

> I describe heterosexuality not as an institution but as a political regime which rests on the submission and the appropriation of women. . . . There is no escape (for there is no territory, no other side of the Mississippi, no Palestine, no Liberia for women). The only thing to do is to stand on one's own feet as a escapee, a fugitive slave, a lesbian. (*Straight*, xiii)

Wittig's essays are forceful critiques of heterosexual society that strive to define a universal that does not dominate the minority or the particular. Men and women exist in opposition under capitalism where neither is the universal, though it has been stolen by men.

> In the abstract, mankind, Man, is everybody—the Other, whatever its kind, is included. . . . It is part of our fight . . . to say that one out of two men is a woman, that the universal belongs to us although we have been robbed and despoiled at this level as well as at the political and economic ones. ("Homo Sum," *Straight*, 55–56)

> But for us there is no such thing as being-woman or being-man. "Man" and "woman" are political concepts of opposition, and the copula which dialectically unites them is, at the same time, the one which abolishes them. ("The Straight Mind," *Straight*, 29)

> Lesbians are not women. ("Straight Mind," 32)

The universal, then, is sexed and gendered, includes women and lesbians as full subjects, realities, and subjectivities, without being compared to men or to the masculine gender. "Men" and "women" exist in social systems of domination, where men dominate women and pass themselves off as the universal. The universal has no gender, but the female gender and lesbians are universal.

Luce Irigaray. Luce Irigaray remains perhaps most committed to the project of a French feminism. She fulfills her commitment across a remarkable spectrum of works, approaches, and writings. Her range is so great, her approaches frequently so disparate, that to assign her a position is difficult, even in a feminism whose position is multiplicity and alterity. Here are some of her presentations:

(1) A spectacular reading in *Speculum of the Other Woman* of **Sigmund Freud** (1856–1939) on "Femininity" and the Woman, linked with Lacan—she was originally a member of the French psychoanalytic school—under the figure of the speculum as a knowledge of women. "From the onset of the phallic phase, the *differences between the sexes are completely eclipsed by the agreements*. . . . THE LITTLE GIRL IS THEREFORE A LITTLE MAN" (25). *Speculum* also contains a penetrating reading of the cave passages in **Plato**'s (427–347 BCE) *Republic* (bk. 7, 514–17a) under the figure of the womb (*matrix, hystera*) and a number of essays about the "masculine" subject, feminine mystics, and a physics of fluidity. "Thus 'God' has created the soul to flare and flame in her desire," where the soul, *l'âme*, is feminine ("La Mystérique," *Speculum*, 197). Two of Irigaray's most prominent themes are present here: an ongoing engagement with traditional Western philosophy, read through the lenses of gender, sexual difference, and desire; and a vivid presentation of what it means that the world might be gendered, that sexual difference might be the first and most pervasive sense of alterity.

(2) An intense poetic reading in *This Sex Which Is Not One* of the sex of woman as not one, not the same, not in the shadow of the masculine universal—it is multiple, fluid, and indecipherable—yet the sex of woman is always in the context of the lived social conditions and experiences of women. One of her most famous and widely repeated figures—"When

our lips speak together"—appears in this book, a doubled and redoubled figure of lips, vulvas, language, speaking, collaboration, women together, lesbianism. "Kiss me. Two lips kissing two lips: openness is ours again. Our 'world.' And the passage from the inside out, from the outside in, the passage between us, is limitless" ("When Our Lips Speak Together," *This Sex*, 210).

(3) An exploration of sexual difference, in *An Ethics of Sexual Difference*, that begins with the famous question that defines our time:

> Sexual difference represents one of the questions or the question that is to be thought in our age. According to Heidegger, each age has one thought to think. One only. Sexual difference is probably the thought of our time. The thing of our time that, thought, will bring us "salvation" [<< *salut* >>]. (5)

It is the question of our time that defines who we are and our salvation, any possibility of a new world, a new ethics. This new ethics is also a poetics: "a new age of thought, art, poetry, and language: the creation of a new *poetics*" (5). It is also an ethics of love: "Sorcerer Love," a reading of Plato's *Symposium* (ca. 380 BCE); "Love of Self," readings of **René Descartes** (1596–1650) and **Baruch Spinoza** (1632–1677); "Love of Same, Love of Other"; and, finally "Love of the Other," readings of Maurice Merleau-Ponty (1908–1961) and **Emmanuel Levinas** (1906–1995). An ethics of sexual difference is a poetics, aesthetics, and erotics, new sexual relations between men and women, between the sexes.

(4) She reads a new love between men and women as addressing the alterity of the other that is central in Levinas's ethics, though she is critical of him on this point. "The function of the other sex as an alterity irreducible to myself eludes Levinas" ("Questions to Emmanuel Levinas," 180). Sometimes she understands sexual difference as so paradigmatic of alterity that she dismisses other human and social differences as minor even where they have experienced long histories of violence:

> Without doubt, the most appropriate content for the universal is sexual difference. Indeed, this content is both real and universal. Sexual differences is an immediate natural given and it is a real and irreducible component of the universal. The whole of human kind is composed of women and men and of nothing else. The problem of race is, in fact, a secondary problem. (*I Love*, 47)

(5) It is in sex and love that alterity appears; it is as love and sex that alterity works; desire is inseparable from alterity. In *I Love to You*, she defines a love *to* [*aimer à toi*] that is different from loves that impose and control:

> I love to you means I maintain a relation of indirection to you. I do not subjugate you or consume you. I respect you (as irreducible). I hail you: in you I hail. I praise you: in you I praise. I give you thanks: to you I give thanks for . . . I bless you, for . . . I speak to you, not just about something; rather, I speak *to* you, I tell you, not so much this or that, but rather tell to you. (109)

(6) Many of her later writings (*Elemental Passions* [1982], *Marine Lover of Friedrich Nietzsche* [1980]) are evocations of love and sexuality as alterity in an intensely poetic voice. Poetry appears throughout her work as the transformation called for in a new sexuality and a new salvation and in her emergent and imaginative relation to bodies and sexuality—a *poiêsis* of the body. (The "Irigarayan poetics of the body is not an expression of the body but a poiesis, a creation of the body"; Gallop, 94.) Through language, Irigaray creates a new sexed body, a new love, new sexual relations between men and women.

In these ways, the French feminists draw on critiques of language and bodies to engage in the critical double gesture in which women's worldwide subordination is linked with writing at the same time that writing opens the possibility of a new world for women and men.

See also Existentialism; Feminism, Lesbian; Freud, Sigmund; Lacan, Jacques; Language; Levinas, Emmanuel; Phenomenology; Poststructuralism; Psychology, Twentieth- and Twenty-First-Century; Queer Theory; Utopianism

REFERENCES

Beauvoir, Simone de. (1946) *All Men Are Mortal*. Trans. Euan Cameron. London: Virago, 1995; Beauvoir, Simone de. (1970) *The Coming of Age*. Trans. Patrick O'Brian. New York: Putnam, 1972; Beauvoir, Simone de. (1951–1952) "Must We Burn Sade?" Trans. Annette Michelson. In Austryn Wainhouse and Richard Seaver, comps., *The Marquis de Sade: The 120 Days of Sodom and Other Writings*. New York: Grove Press, 1966, 3–64; Beauvoir, Simone de. (1949) *The Second Sex*. Trans. Howard M. Parshley. New York: Knopf, 1971; Beauvoir, Simone de. (1943) *She Came to Stay*. Trans. Yvonne Moyse and Roger Senhouse. Cleveland, Ohio: World Publishing, 1945; Cixous, Hélène. (1975) "The Laugh of the Medusa." Trans. Keith Cohen and Paula Cohen. In Elaine Marks and Isabelle Courtivron, eds., *New French Feminisms: An Anthology*. New York: Schocken, 1981, 245–64; Cixous, Hélène, and Catherine Clément. *The Newly Born Woman*. Trans. Betsy Wing. Minneapolis: University of Minnesota Press, 1975; Gallop, Jane. *Thinking Through the Body*. New York: Columbia University Press, 1988; Irigaray, Luce. (1982) *Elemental Passions*. Trans. Joanne Collins and Judith Still. New York: Routledge, 1992; Irigaray, Luce. (1984) *An Ethics of Sexual Difference*. Trans. Carolyn Burke and Gillian C. Gill. Ithaca, N.Y.: Cornell University Press, 1993; Irigaray, Luce. (1992) *I Love to You: Sketch for a Felicity in History*. Trans. Alison Martin. New York: Routledge, 1996; Irigaray, Luce. (1980) *Marine Lover of Friedrich Nietzsche*. Trans. Gillian C. Gill. New York: Columbia University Press, 1991; Irigaray, Luce. "Questions to Emmanuel Levinas." In Margaret Whitford, trans. and ed., *The Irigaray Reader*. Oxford, U.K.: Blackwell, 1991, 178–89; Irigaray, Luce. (1974) *Speculum of the Other Woman*. Trans. Gillian C. Gill. Ithaca, N.Y.: Cornell University Press, 1985; Irigaray, Luce. (1977) *This Sex Which Is Not One*. Trans. Catherine Porter. Ithaca, N.Y.: Cornell University Press, 1985; Kristeva, Julia. (1980) *Desire in Language: A Semiotic Approach to Literature and Art*. Trans. Leon S. Roudiez. New York: Columbia University Press, 1980; Kristeva, Julia. (1980) *Powers of Horror: An Essay on Abjection*. Trans. Leon S. Roudiez. New York: Columbia University Press, 1982; Kristeva, Julia. (1974) *Revolution in Poetic Language*. Trans. Margaret Waller. New York: Columbia University Press, 1984; Kristeva, Julia. (1988) *Strangers to Ourselves*. Trans. Leon S. Roudiez. New York: Columbia University Press, 1991; Kristeva, Julia. (1983) *Tales of Love*. Trans. Leon S. Roudiez. New York: Columbia University Press, 1987; Kristeva, Julia. (1979) "Women's Time." In Toril Moi, ed., *The Kristeva Reader*. Trans. Alice Jardine and Harry Blake. New York: Columbia University Press, 1986, 187–213; Marks, Elaine, and Isabelle de Courtivron, eds. (1980) *New French Feminisms: An Anthology*. New York: Schocken, 1981; Plato. (ca. 375–370 BCE) *Republic*. Trans. G.M.A. Grube. Indianapolis, Ind.: Hackett, 1992; Plato. (ca. 380 BCE) *Symposium of Plato*. Trans. Tom Griffith (1986). Berkeley: University of California Press, 1989; Wittig, Monique. (1973) *The Lesbian Body [Le corps lesbien]*. Trans. David Le Vay. Boston, Mass.: Beacon Press, 1973; Wittig, Monique. *The Straight Mind and Other Essays*. Boston, Mass.: Beacon Press, 1992.

Stephen David Ross

ADDITIONAL READING

Allen, Jeffner, and Iris Marion Young, eds. *The Thinking Muse: Feminism and Modern French Philosophy*. Bloomington: Indiana University Press, 1989; Beauvoir, Simone de. (1947) *The Ethics of Ambiguity*. Trans. Bernard Frechtman. Secaucus, N.J.: Citadel Press/Philosophical Library, 1948; Blyth, Ian, and Susan Sellers. *Hélène Cixous: Live Theory*. New York: Continuum, 2004; Burke,

Carolyn. Review of *New French Feminisms: An Anthology*, ed. Elaine Marks and Isabelle de Courtivron. *Signs* 6:3 (1981), 515–17; Butler, Judith. *The Judith Butler Reader*. Ed. Sara Salih, with Judith Butler. Oxford, U.K.: Blackwell, 2004; Cixous, Hélène. *The Hélène Cixous Reader*. Ed. Susan Sellers. New York: Routledge, 1994; Cixous, Hélène, and Jacques Derrida. *Veils*. Trans. Geoffrey Bennington. Stanford, Calif.: Stanford University Press, 2001; Clément, Catherine. (1990) *Syncope: The Philosophy of Rapture*. Trans. Sally O'Driscoll and Deirdre M. Mahoney. Minneapolis: University of Minnesota Press, 1994; Deutscher, Penelope. *A Politics of Impossible Difference: The Later Work of Luce Irigaray*. Ithaca, N.Y.: Cornell University Press, 2002; Fraser, Nancy, and Sandra Lee Bartky, eds. *Revaluing French Feminism: Critical Essays on Difference, Agency, and Culture*. Bloomington: Indiana University Press, 1992; Gallop, Jane. *The Daughter's Seduction: Feminism and Psychoanalysis*. Ithaca, N.Y.: Cornell University Press, 1982; Grosz, Elizabeth. *Sexual Subversions: Three French Feminists*. Winchester, Mass.: Unwin Hyman, 1989; Heinämaa, Sara. "On Luce Irigaray's Inquiries into Intersubjectivity: Between the Feminine Body and Its Other." In Maria Cimitile and Elaine Miller, eds., *Returning to Irigaray*. Albany: State University of New York Press, 2005; Howells, Christina, ed. *French Women Philosophers: A Contemporary Reader*. New York: Routledge, 2003; Irigaray, Luce. *The Forgetting of Air in Martin Heidegger*. Trans. Mary Beth Mader. Austin: University of Texas Press, 1999; Irigaray, Luce. *The Irigaray Reader*. Trans. and ed. Margaret Whitford. Oxford, U.K.: Blackwell, 1991; Irigaray, Luce. *Sexes and Genealogies*. Trans. Gillian C. Gill. New York: Columbia University Press, 1993; Irigaray, Luce. (1984) "Sorcerer Love: A Reading of Plato's *Symposium*, Diotima's Speech." Trans. Eleanor H. Kuykendall. *Hypatia* 3:3 (1989), 32–44. Reprinted in Nancy Tuana, ed., *Feminist Interpretations of Plato*. University Park: Pennsylvania State University Press, 1994, 181–95; Kristeva, Julia. (1985) *In the Beginning Was Love: Psychoanalysis and Faith*. Trans. Arthur Goldhammer. New York: Columbia University Press, 1987; Kristeva, Julia. *The Kristeva Reader*. Ed. Toril Moi. Trans. Alice Jardine and Harry Blake. New York: Columbia University Press, 1986; Kristeva, Julia. (1979) "Women's Time." In Kelly Oliver, ed., *The Portable Kristeva*. New York: Columbia University Press, 1997, 349–68; Lechte, John, and Maria Margaroni. *Julia Kristeva: Live Theory*. New York: Continuum, 2004; Moi, Toril, ed. *French Feminist Thought: A Reader*. Oxford, U.K.: Blackwell, 1987; Nye, Andrea. "Irigaray and Diotima at Plato's Symposium." *Hypatia* 3:3 (1989), 46–61. Reprinted in Nancy Tuana, ed., *Feminist Interpretations of Plato*. University Park: Pennsylvania State University Press, 1994, 197–215; Oliver, Kelly, and Lisa Walsh, eds. *Contemporary French Feminism*. New York: Oxford University Press, 2004; Robinson, Hilary. "Whose Beauty? Women, Art, and Intersubjectivity in Luce Irigaray's Writings." In Peg Zeglin Brand, ed., *Beauty Matters*. Bloomington: Indiana University Press, 2000, 224–51; Schwarzer, Alice. *After* The Second Sex: *Conversations with Simone de Beauvoir*. Trans. Marianne Howarth. New York: Pantheon, 1984; Scott, Joan. *Only Paradoxes to Offer: French Feminists and the Rights of Man*. Cambridge, Mass.: Harvard University Press, 1996; Spelman, Elizabeth V. (1988) "Simone de Beauvoir and Women: Just Who Does She Think 'We' Is?" In Mary Lyndon Shanley and Carole Pateman, eds., *Feminist Interpretations and Political Theory*. University Park: Pennsylvania State University Press, 1991, 199–216.

FEMINISM, HISTORY OF. Women's sexuality has historically been conflated with procreation. In response to this traditional and widely entrenched equation, feminism and feminist philosophers have politicized the concepts and practices that surround female sexuality—chastity, **marriage**, reproduction, heterosexuality, **prostitution, sexual violence, incest, genital mutilation, abortion**, and many others—as one way for women to achieve equality. An important part of this equality is women's possessing both bodily integrity and sexual autonomy: They should be able to control their bodies, their sexuality, and when, how, and why they reproduce (if they reproduce). For the sake of this autonomy, feminism has focused on rejecting the patriarchal domination of women's sexuality in which women have submitted to marriage, reproduction, and raising children.

This theme slowly but gradually develops through the history of feminist thought, even though it is often hard to discern because women's voices have long been obscured. Women's writings about the family and the domestic sphere have been discounted as non-philosophical. But the message of much of women's philosophical writings is clear: Women should be equal to men, the patriarchal society that has limited and oppressed women must be dismantled, and women should be able to control their own sexuality.

Sappho (ca. 610–580 BCE), called "the Tenth Muse" by **Plato** (427–347 BCE; see Paton, 506; also Plato, *Phaedrus*, 235C), was a poet and teacher who wrote about sensual **love** between women (see her fragments in Lombardo). Her own sexuality was ambiguous. She did not limit her love to one sex, and legend has it that she committed suicide over a young ferryman. She married and had a daughter Cleis (see Hallett). Her school for young women, where they studied music and poetry and worshiped Aphrodite, was in Mytilene on the Isle of Lesbos. It was rumored that Mytilene was founded by legendary Amazons, independent women warriors who lived in an all-female society, using men only to reproduce and killing or giving away male babies. It is possible that Sappho's home on Lesbos led to "lesbian" becoming synonymous with female homosexuals. Natalie Barney (1876–1972), an American ex-patriot living in Paris, established Sappho as the proto-lesbian in her self-published lesbian love poems and in performing Sappho's work at her influential salon in Nevilly in the 1920s.

Beginning around 600 BCE with Theano of Crotona ("Theano I" [ca. 550 BCE]), a student and later the wife of Pythagoras (582–496 BCE), and lasting until 200 CE, there was a group of women Pythagoreans who believed that a woman's special virtue was temperance. Theano wrote that a wife was to have sex only with her husband, and all manner of sexual intercourse was pure if done to please her husband (Waithe, "Early Pythagoreans"). A woman was impure if she had sex with someone other than her husband. According to Theano, a wife's role was to maintain harmony and justice in her home, for domestic disorder would contribute to disorder in the public sphere. This idea was echoed by other Pythagoreans. Theano II (ca. 250–150 BCE) wrote to Nikostrate (ca. 240–160 BCE) that a wife must behave justly toward her husband even if he takes a courtesan (see Waithe, *History*, vol. 1, 43–47). Divorcing the unfaithful husband will lead either to a series of husbands (since not having a husband is for a woman an unbearable state) or to spinsterhood.

Julia Domna (170–217), a student of philosophy and, after marrying Septimius Severus (146–211) in 186, an empress of Rome, commanded Philostratus to compile a biography of Apollonius of Tyana. The interesting question was raised, while discussing chastity, whether eunuchs could have this virtue. No, was the answer. Their sexual **abstinence** was not of their own free will. The choice not to engage in **sexual activity**, not the inability to do so, makes chastity a virtue (see Waithe, *History*, vol. 1, 128–32).

The virtues of virginity and chastity were often valued over a married, sexually active life by social and religious norms (e.g., those of Christianity, as in **Augustine** [354–430]) as well as by early women philosophers. After her death, Makrina's (ca. 327–380) philosophy was transmitted by her brother Gregory of Nyssa (ca. 340–410) in *De vita Macrinae* (see Wolfskeel). Makrina led the life of a pure and chaste ascetic. Hypatia of Alexandria (ca. 355?–415), a pagan living during the early Christian period, was a teacher and renowned philosopher. She, too, was chaste and remained virginal. When one of her students sexually pursued her, she showed him rags stained with her menstrual blood and said, "This is what you love, young man, and it isn't beautiful!" which was enough to destroy his desire (according to Damascius [ca. 480–550]). In her philosophy, Hypatia was a Neo-Platonist who set forth Platonic ideals of civic virtue, goodness, and beauty. As a

Neo-Platonist, she removed all traces of Plato's passionate, desiring *eros* from her philoso-phy (hence her emphasis on chastity). Her death was violent and political, due in part to her being female and pagan in a Christian time. A group of monks, instigated by Cyril, bishop of Alexandria (d. 444), seized her and dragged her into a church, where they stripped, beat, and mutilated her (Dzielska, 66–100).

Many women medieval philosophers were mystics, such as (Saint) Hildegard of Bingen (1098–1179). In her moral writings she condemned **homosexuality** as a devilish **perver-sion**, yet in her medical writings, the *Causae et curae* (ca. 1155), she stated that a woman's sexual pleasure was not dependent "upon the touch of a man" (see Gössman, 50). *Causae* is an early positive view of human sexuality. Hildegard describes sexual pleasure from a woman's perspective and includes perhaps the first description of the female orgasm. Christine de Pisan (ca. 1364–1430) is considered the first European woman to discuss women's equality. Anticipating the thinking of the Enlightenment, she argued in *The Book of the City of Women* (1405) that removing women's oppression would improve society. She honored Joan of Arc with a poem, because Joan's victory was one for both France and women. St. Teresa of Avila (1515–1582) criticized Catholicism's view of chastity (see Feder et al., 188–89).

Women philosophers during the period 1600–1900 presented a diversity of views about sexuality, women, and men. Some believed that women's maternal instincts were natural and thus women were seen, consistently with the conventional view of the time, as limited by their sexual natures. Margaret Cavendish (1623–1673) saw masculine women as cor-rupt and imperfect (see Schiebinger). Christina, queen of Sweden (1626–1689), eschewed marriage and was perhaps a lesbian. She thought that the female sex was an embarrassment and an obstacle to virtue and merit (see Ackerman). Others, like Dutch philologist Anna Maria van Schurman (1607–1678), wrote that single women should be educated and that this education would not affect their traditional social roles (see Goreau). Still others, such as Damaris Cudworth Masham (1659–1708), took on the Church, contesting the idea that women's virtue depended on their chastity (see Frankel). Sor Juana Inés de la Cruz (1648–1695), who championed feminism in Mexico, exposed the sexual double standards in the cult of virginity. She was noted for her affairs with other nuns and the viceroy's wife. It was her lyric poetry criticizing the Church that led to the archbishop's silencing her (Franco; Merrim; Morkovsky).

Mary Astell (1666–1731), nicknamed the "Philosophical Lady," defended women's rights and equality in education. In *Some Reflections upon Marriage* (1700), she states that marriage should be between equals, and the man should not subject his wife to sexual slav-ery (see Smith). These ideas were echoed by Mary Wollstonecraft (1759–1797) and later by Harriet Taylor Mill (1807–1858). Wollstonecraft is considered the founder of modern feminism (see Lindemann). Her writings, including the famous *Vindication of the Rights of Woman* (1792), express her belief that women's sex and sexuality did not affect their in-tellectual abilities. Social differences, on her view—especially in lack of education for women—produced inequalities between men and women. Wollstonecraft based her ideas on Catherine Sawbridge Macaulay's (1731–1791) *Letters on Education* (1787), which crit-icized **Jean-Jacques Rousseau**'s (1712–1778) notion of the complementarity of the sexes (see Macaulay-Graham). Wollstonecraft asserted that to train women to think that their worth could be based only on the admiration of men is immoral. Wollstonecraft character-ized marriage as legal prostitution and linked male sexual passion with women's political subordination. She advocated that sexual passion between spouses should be transformed into **love** and affection, for as long as men were driven by their passions, women would be enslaved. Drawing on her own experience, she wrote *Mary, a Fiction* (1788), which chronicled a woman's devotion to another woman. Here Wollstonecraft coined the term "romantic friendship" for intense relationships between middle-class white women.

Harriet Taylor Mill's "Enfranchisement of Women" (1851) was more radical and influenced her husband's (John Stuart Mill [1806–1873]) later book *The Subjection of Women* (1869). Harriet argued that there should be no marriage laws; that the woman should take responsibility for her children (hence she need not keep having children to bind her husband to her); expounded on woman's equality within marriage; and defended no-fault divorce. Both Harriet and John were adamant about the rights of women to education, employment, and suffrage. But they differed on the wife's right to employment after marriage. Harriet was more radical for their time, since John believed that a wife who has had children could not devote sufficient time and energy to both child rearing and a job—she had to make a choice to do well at either endeavor. Harriet's defense of divorce was thematically consistent with other feminist writings critical of the idea (and social practice) that married women were the property of their husbands. Clarisse Coignet (1823–1918) argued, in *La Morale Indépendante dans Son Principe et Son Objet* (1869), that morality can transform women's roles so women are no longer the property of their husbands but can instead be respected for themselves. French socialist Flora Tristan (1803–1844), who baptised women "the proletariat of the proletariat" in her feminist tracts, called for women to have freedom in the choice of their husbands as well as the freedom of divorce and remarriage. She also sought equality and respect for unwed mothers (see Moon). Jenny Poinsard d'Héricourt (1809–1875) argued for the legalization of divorce in France. In *A Woman's Philosophy of Woman* (1860), she used her medical knowledge to refute the idea that menstruation proves women's inferiority.

First Wave feminism began in the nineteenth century and focused on women's social, political, and economic rights. The majority of the women in this movement were white and middle class. Although they believed that women were equal to men, women's maternal character and child-rearing abilities also made them different from men. Some believed that women's maternal role made them more virtuous than men. Julie Velten Favre (1834–1896), a French moral philosopher, glorified womanhood; women's virtue was to inculcate morality in others through precept and example (229–30). Others, by contrast, pushed to emancipate women from compulsory maternity. Margaret Fuller (1810–1850) relied on Transcendentalist philosophy in the first major American feminist manifesto, *Woman in the Nineteenth Century* (1845). Considered the first lesbian philosopher, Fuller advocated androgyny, claiming that there was no wholly masculine male nor wholly feminine female. At the same time, however, she believed that the majority of women would (still) mother, although women unfit for this role would be open to other work. Fuller felt that maternal or sex-specific functions did not limit women; rather, limitations were created by the lack of equal education (see Kornfeld).

From about 1880 to 1914, feminists attacked the sexual double standard (according to which men could be promiscuous, while women had to be virginal or monogamous) and tried to inject equality into sexual relations and relationships between men and women. To achieve this equality, women were not advised to be as promiscuous as men; rather, men were admonished to "control the beast within." In this way, feminists attempted to eradicate male sexual tyranny and give women bodily and sexual autonomy. They challenged the **sexual objectification** of women by politicizing sex, working through social purity/sex reform movements. These movements, which began in Great Britain and spread internationally, stressed women's domestic virtues and moral superiority. Men were condemned for their "indulgences, appetites, and vices," which obstructed "progress, harmony, and the social reconstruction of life" (Jeffreys, 6–9). Women, due to their maternal and domestic roles, were exalted. The social and political activities of these feminists centered on temperance, child abuse, prostitution, and stemming the exploitation of the female sex by men. The double standard that penalized adulterous women and judged prostitutes to be fallen women, while at the same time condoning male extramarital sexual relations, brought many suffragists into the social purity/sex reform movements. Middle-class feminists, though, had mixed feelings about both prostitution and the related right of working-class women to have autonomous control over their own sexuality.

The idea of protecting women and children from sexual abuse by males found its way into speeches on marriage reform and sexuality. American Lucinda B. Chandler (1829?–1906) wanted women to be able to exercise an effective reproductive choice as well as to possess their children (see Bland). Elizabeth Wolstenholme-Elmy (1834–1913), a founder of the Women's Franchise League (1889; Great Britain), wrote that women's political emancipation involved the recognition "that the slavery of sex is the root of all slavery" (see Jeffreys, 29–33). Her *Phases of Love* (1897) is about the ideal sexual relationship between men and women, which would include pleasurable, nonreproductive sexual activity and the freedom from unwanted marital sex. She wrote sexual education books for children in which she avoided stigmatizing the body. Her goal was to educate women to control their own bodies, their sexuality, and if, how, why, and when they reproduced. Wolstenholme-Elmy wrote *Phases* under the pseudonym "Ellis Ethelmer," which she also used for her *Westminster Review* article "Feminism" (1898), one of the earliest usages of that word in English (Delap, 626n.5).

These themes surrounding women's sexual autonomy were reiterated by other American and British suffragists. The sex reformists observed well the negative effects of male sexuality on women and thus sought to limit men's sexual access to women. One strategy was to encourage women to transcend concerns of the flesh. In 1898 Margaret Shurmer Sibthorp (ca. 1850–1930) wrote, "Sex is a *phase* which the spirit passes to gain experience and discipline" (Jeffreys, 41). These women rejected **contraception** because they felt that it led to more male sexual use of and tyranny over women, in that contraception weakens the bars to intercourse (see the similar arguments of contemporary feminist **Catharine MacKinnon**). By contrast, the family planning movement was supported by Emma Goldman (1869–1940) and Margaret Sanger (1879–1966), who thought contraception enabled women to control their reproduction and thus be better off both physically and economically. Other women took a completely different route: They were sexually active *outside* marriage. These 1890s feminists rejected marriage as part of the "free love" movement. Their goal was to counter the legal and social concept of women as the sexual property of their husbands, which made marital **rape** immune from prosecution, and to control access to their bodies even by the men they loved.

Victoria Woodhull (1838–1927) was an outspoken advocate of free love and women's suffrage. She delivered speeches and wrote about women's rights, economics, sexual relations, and spiritualism. Woodhull insisted that coitus between a woman and a man should occur only if and when the act was chosen unilaterally by the woman: "To woman, by nature, belongs the right of sexual determination. When the instinct is aroused in her, then and then only should commerce follow" (40; see **Andrea Dworkin** [1946–2005], *Intercourse*, 135–36; *Right-wing Women*, 60). In this arrangement, "woman rises from sexual slavery to sexual freedom, into the ownership and control of her sexual organs, and [the] man is obliged to respect this freedom." Although she speaks of this as a woman's "natural right," Woodhull also claims that sexual intercourse should be initiated by the woman and should occur only with a man she loves and desires (even if not a spouse), *because* coitus in these conditions would produce the most healthy offspring (37, 43). In this way, women can fulfill their maternal "divinity" (26).

Yet for Charlotte Perkins Gilman (1860–1935; author of *The Yellow Wallpaper* [1899]), views like Woodhull's were essentialist: They tethered women, through their capacity to give birth, to their biological nature. In *Women and Economics* (1898) Gilman condemned the Victorian image of the ideal woman: passive, pious, pure, submissive, domestic (see Cott). In contrast to the essentialism of some feminists, Gilman's **social constructionism** posited the social environment as that which determined gender roles. Further, Gilman critiqued the economic power men had over women and its effect on sexual relationships and marriage. In the absence of education and paid employment, women's only recourse was to use their sexuality: as a good woman in marriage (thereby also avoiding being ridiculed as a spinster) or as an outcast prostitute. Helena Swanwick (1914) held a quite opposite position. Noting the different roles of the male and the female in reproduction, she claimed (sounding nearly like a proponent of sociobiology) that these differences "produced differences in life, needs, and temperament" that made "men more concerned with property and women more concerned for the person" (49).

The late nineteenth century gave rise to **sexology** and a group of male sexologists for whom the study of homosexuality (or "sexual inversion") became important. In this setting, feminists such as Stella Browne (1880–1950) and Marie Stopes (1880–1958) promoted heterosexuality and stigmatized women's same-sex relationships (Lesbian History Group, 111), thereby building the foundation for "compulsory heterosexuality" (see Rich). Anna Rueling (1880–1953), the first known lesbian activist, united female homosexuality and the women's movement in her 1904 essay "What Interest Does the Women's Movement Have in the Homosexual Question?" Novelist Virginia Woolf (1882–1941), though chastely married to Leonard Woolf, wrote, "Women alone stir my imagination" (see Cook). She relied on women—her lover was Vita Sackville-West (1892–1962)—for her emotional and erotic life. Yet *A Room of One's Own* (1929) is a heterosexual feminist treatise, though Woolf does describe the ideal artist, the creative female, as androgynous (perhaps a code for lesbian).

Simone de Beauvoir (1908–1986), the French existentialist philosopher, is noted both for her book *The Second Sex* (1949) and her relationship with Jean-Paul Sartre (1905–1980). In *The Second Sex* Beauvoir proposes the idea of the social construction of women: "One is not born, but rather becomes, a woman" (267). Female biology does not make women; it is society that we should look at for the clues. In our society, woman is cast as a creature between male and eunuch. Men are subjects, but women, because of their sex-specific childbearing role, become objects, exploited by servicing men—for the purpose of pleasure or procreation—through their sexuality. Beauvoir's account of women as objects in patriarchal society set the stage for Betty Friedan's *The Feminine Mystique* (1963). In fact, Friedan dedicates her book—which is, in part, about women's isolation in the affluent 1950s suburban home—to Beauvoir. *The Feminine Mystique* was destined to become the cornerstone of Second Wave feminism.

See also Abstinence; Ethics, Professional Codes of; Ethics, Sexual; Existentialism; Feminism, French; Feminism, Lesbian; Feminism, Liberal; Feminism, Men's; Fichte, Johann Gottlieb; Friendship; Greek Sexuality and Philosophy, Ancient; Homosexuality and Science; Liberalism; MacKinnon, Catharine; Marriage; Queer Theory; Rousseau, Jean-Jacques; Schopenhauer, Arthur; Sex Education; Sexology; Singer, Irving; Wojtyła, Karol (Pope John Paul II)

REFERENCES

Ackerman, Susanna. "Kristina Wasa, Queen of Sweden." In Mary Ellen Waithe, ed., *A History of Women Philosophers*, vol. 3. Dordrecht, Holland: Kluwer, 1991, 21–40; Barney, Natalie. *A Perilous Advantage: The Best of Natalie Clifford Barney*. Ed. and trans. Anna Livia. Norwich, Vt.: New

Victoria Publishers, 1992; Beauvoir, Simone de. (1949) *The Second Sex*. Trans. Howard M. Parshley. New York: Knopf, 1953; Bland, Lucy. *Banishing the Beast: Sexuality and the Early Feminists*. New York: New Press, 1995; Coignet, Clarisse. *La Morale Indépendante dans Son Principe et Son Objet*. Paris: Bailliere, 1869; Cook, Blanche Wiesen. "Women Alone Stir My Imagination: Lesbianism and the Cultural Tradition." *Signs* 4:4 (1979), 718–39; Cott, Nancy F. "Passionlessness: An Interpretation of Victorian Sexual Ideology, 1790–1850." *Signs* 4:2 (1978), 219–36; Damascius. (ca. 529) *Life of Isadore*. Part translated as "The Life of Hypatia" by Jeremiah Reedy. In David Felder, ed., *Alexander 2: Cosmology, Philosophy, Myth, and Culture*. York Beach, Maine: Phanes Press, 1993. <www.cosmopolis.com/alexandria/hypatia-bio-suda.html> [accessed 19 October 2004]; Delap, Lucy. " 'Philosophical Vacuity and Political Ineptitude': *The Freewoman's* Critique of the Suffragette Movement." *Women's History Review* 11:4 (2002), 613–30; D'Héricourt, Jenny Poinsard. (1860) *A Woman's Philosophy of Woman, or Woman Enfranchised: An Answer to Michelet, Proudhon, Girardin, Legouve, Comte, and Other Modern Innovators*. New York: Carleton, 1864. Westport, Conn.: Hyperion Press, 1981; Dworkin, Andrea. *Intercourse*. New York: Free Press, 1987; Dworkin, Andrea. *Right-wing Women*. New York: Perigee, 1983; Dzielska, Maria. *Hypatia of Alexandria*. Cambridge, Mass.: Harvard University Press, 1995; Favre, Julie Velten. *La Morale de Socrate*. Paris: Alcan, 1888; Feder, Ellen K., Karmen MacKendrick, and Sybol S. Cook, eds. *A Passion for Wisdom: Readings in Western Philosophy on Love and Desire*. Upper Saddle River, N.J.: Prentice Hall, 2004; Franco, Jeran. *Plotting Women: Gender and Representation in Mexico*. New York: Columbia University Press, 1988; Frankel, Lois. "Damaris Cudworth Mashan." In Mary Ellen Waithe, ed., *A History of Women Philosophers*, vol. 3. Dordrecht, Holland: Kluwer, 1991, 73–86; Friedan, Betty. *The Feminine Mystique*. New York: Norton, 1963; Fuller, Margaret. (1845) *Woman in the Nineteenth Century: An Authoritative Text, Backgrounds, Criticism*. Ed. Larry J. Reynolds. New York: Norton, 1997; Gilman, Charlotte Perkins. (1898) *Women and Economics: A Study of the Economic Relation between Men and Women as a Factor in Social Evolution*. Introduction by Michael Kimmel and Amy Aronson. Berkeley: University of California Press, 1998; Gilman, Charlotte Perkins. (1899) *The Yellow Wall-Paper: A Sourcebook and Critical Edition*. Ed. Catherine J. Golden. New York: Routledge, 1994; Goreau, Angelina. *The Whole Duty of a Woman: Female Writers in 17th Century England*. Garden City, N.Y.: Dial Press, 1985; Gössman, Elisabeth. "Hildegard of Bingen." In Mary Ellen Waithe, ed., *A History of Women Philosophers*, vol. 2. Dordrecht, Holland: Kluwer, 1989, 27–66; Hallett, Judith P. "Sappho and Her Social Context: Sense and Sensuality." *Signs* 4:3 (1979), 447–64; Hildegard de Bingen. (ca. 1155) *On Natural Philosophy and Medicine: Selections from Cause et cure*. Trans. Margret Berger. Cambridge, U.K.: Brewer, 1999; Jeffreys, Sheila. (1985) *The Spinster and Her Enemies: Feminism and Sexuality, 1880–1930*. North Melbourne, Australia: Spinifex, 1997; Kornfeld, Eve. *Margaret Fuller: A Brief Biography with Documents*. New York: St. Martin's Press, 1996; Lesbian History Group. *Not a Passing Phase: Reclaiming Lesbians in History 1840–1985*. London: Women's Press, 1996; Lindemann, Kate. "Mary Wollstonecraft." In Mary Ellen Waithe, ed., *A History of Women Philosophers*, vol. 3. Dordrecht, Holland: Kluwer, 1991, 153–70; Macaulay-Graham, Catherine. *Letters on Education*. New York: Garland, 1974; MacKinnon, Catharine A. (1982) " 'More Than Simply a Magazine': *Playboy's* Money." In *Feminism Unmodified: Discourses on Life and Law*. Cambridge, Mass.: Harvard University Press, 1987, 134–45; MacKinnon, Catharine A. "Roe v. Wade: A Study in Male Ideology." In Jay Garfield and Patricia Hennessey, eds., *Abortion: Moral and Legal Perspectives*. Amherst: University of Massachusetts Press, 1984, 45–54; Merrim, Stephanie. *Early Modern Writing: Sor Juana Inez de la Cruz*. Nashville, Tenn.: Vanderbilt University Press, 1999; Mill, John Stuart, and Harriet Taylor Mill. *Essays on Sex Equality*. Ed. Alice S. Rossi. Chicago, Ill.: University of Chicago Press, 1970. ["Enfranchisement of Women" (1851), 91–121; *The Subjection of Women* (1869), 125–242]; Moon, S. Joan. "Feminism and Socialism: The Utopian Synthesis of Flora Tristan." In Marilyn A. Boxer and Jean H. Quataert, eds., *Socialist Women: European Socialist Feminism in the Nineteenth and Early Twentieth Centuries*. New York: Elsevier, 1978, 19–50; Morkovsky, Mary Christine. "Sor Juana Inés de la Cruz." In Mary Ellen Waithe, ed., *A History of Women Philosophers*, vol. 3. Dordrecht, Holland: Kluwer, 1991, 59–72; Paton, W. P., trans. "Epigram 16." In *The Greek Anthology*, book 3, vol. ix: *The Declamatory Epigrams*. Loeb Classical

Library. Cambridge, Mass.: Harvard University Press, 1917; Plato. (ca. 365 BCE) *Phaedrus*. In *The Collected Dialogues of Plato*. Ed. Edith Hamilton and Huntington Cairns. Trans. R. Hackforth. New York: Pantheon, 1961, 475–525; Rich, Adrienne. "Compulsory Heterosexuality and Lesbian Existence." *Signs* 5:4 (1980), 631–60; Rueling, Anna. (1904) "What Interest Does the Women's Movement Have in the Homosexual Question?" In Mark Blasius and Shane Phelan, eds., *We Are Everywhere*. New York: Routledge, 1997, 143–51; Sappho. *Poems and Fragments*. Trans. Stanley Lombardo. Ed. Susan Warden. Indianapolis, Ind.: Hackett, 2002; Schiebinger, Linda. "Margaret Cavendish, Duchess of New Castle." In Mary Ellen Waithe, ed., *A History of Women Philosophers*, vol. 3. Dordrecht, Holland: Kluwer, 1991, 1–20; Smith, Florence M. *Mary Astell*. New York: Columbia University Press, 1916; Stopes, Marie Carmichael. *Contraception (Birth Control): Its Theory, History, and Practice; a Manual for the Medical and Legal Professions*. London: J. Bale, 1923; Swanwick, Helena. *The Future of the Women's Movement*. London: G. Bell, 1914; Teresa of Avila (Saint). *The Wisdom of Teresa of Avila: Selections from the Interior Castle*. Trans. Otilio Rodríguez. New York: Paulist Press, 1997; Waithe, Mary Ellen. "Early Pythagoreans: Themstroclea, Theano, Arignote, Myia, and Damo." In Mary Ellen Waithe, ed., *A History of Women Philosophers*, vol. 1. Dordrecht, Holland: Martinus Nijhoff, 1987, 11–18; Waithe, Mary Ellen, ed. *A History of Women Philosophers*. Vol. 1: *Ancient Women Philosophers, 600 B.C.–500 A.D.* Dordrecht, Holland: Martinus Nijhoff, 1987. Vol. 2: *Medieval, Renaissance, and Enlightenment Women Philosophers, A.D. 500–1600*. Dordrecht, Holland: Kluwer, 1989. Vol. 3: *Modern Women Philosophers, 1600–1900*. Dordrecht, Holland: Kluwer, 1991. Vol. 4: *Contemporary Women Philosophers: 1900–Today*. Dordrecht, Holland: Kluwer, 1995; Wolfskeel, Cornelia W. "Makrina." In Mary Ellen Waithe, ed., *A History of Women Philosophers*, vol. 1. Dordrecht, Holland: Martinus Nijhoff, 1987, 139–68; Wollstonecraft, Mary. (1788, 1798) *Mary, a Fiction; and The Wrongs of Women*. Ed. Gary Kelly. New York: Oxford University Press, 1976; Wollstonecraft, Mary. (1792) *A Vindication of the Rights of Women*. Buffalo, N.Y.: Prometheus, 1989; Woodhull, Victoria C. (1874) "Tried as by Fire." In Madeleine B. Stern, ed., *The Victoria Woodhull Reader*. Weston, Mass.: M & S Press, 1974. [pages not consecutively numbered]; Woolf, Virginia. *A Room of One's Own*. New York: Harcourt, Brace, 1929.

JoAnne Myers

ADDITIONAL READING

Abbey, Ruth. "Odd Bedfellows: Nietzsche and Mill on Marriage." *History of European Ideas* 23:2–4 (1997), 81–104; Allen, Sister Prudence, R.S.M. *The Concept of Woman: The Aristotelian Revolution, 750 BC–1250 AD*. Grand Rapids, Mich.: Eerdmans, 1985; Atherton, Margaret. *Women Philosophers of the Early Modern Period*. Indianapolis, Ind.: Hackett, 1994; Bacchi, Carol Lee. *Same Difference: Feminism and Sexual Difference*. Boston, Mass.: Allen and Unwin, 1990; Barry, Kathleen. *Susan B. Anthony: A Biography of a Singular Feminist*. New York: New York University Press, 1988; Bell, Quentin. *Virginia Woolf*. New York: Harcourt Brace Jovanovich, 1972; Boles, Janet K., and Diane Long Hoeveler. (1996) *Historical Dictionary of Feminism*, 2nd ed. Lanham, Md.: Scarecrow Press, 2004; Broad, Jacqueline. *Women Philosophers of the Seventeenth Century*. Cambridge: Cambridge University Press, 2004; Cadden, Joan. "It Takes All Kinds: Sexuality and Gender Differences in Hildegard of Bingen's *Book of Compound Medicine*." *Traditio* 40 (1984), 149–74; Clark, Elizabeth A., and Herbert Richardson, eds. *Women and Religion: A Feminist Sourcebook of Christian Thought*, 1st ed. New York: Harper and Row, 1977. Revised and expanded ed., *Women and Religion: The Original Sourcebook of Women in Christian Thought*. San Francisco, Calif.: HarperCollins, 1996; Cott, Nancy F. *The Grounding of Modern Feminism*. New Haven, Conn.: Yale University Press, 1987; Cott, Nancy F. "Passionlessness: An Interpretation of Victorian Sexual Ideology, 1790–1850." *Signs* 4:2 (1978), 219–36. Reprinted in Nancy F. Cott and Elizabeth H. Pleck, eds., *A Heritage of Her Own: Toward a New Social History of the American Woman*. New York: Simon and Schuster, 1979, 162–81; DeSalvo, Louise, and Mitchell Leaska. *The Letters of Vita Sackville-West to Virginia Woolf*. New York: Morrow, 1985; Disse, Dorothy. "Other Women's Voices: Translations of Women's Writing before 1700" (1 June 2004). <home.infionline.net/~ddisse/index.html> [accessed 22 September 2004]; Duberman, Martin, Martha Vicinus, and George Chauncey, Jr., eds. *Hidden from History: Reclaiming the Gay and Lesbian Past*. New York: Meridian, 1990; Faderman, Lillian. *Surpassing the Love of Men: Romantic Friendship and Love between Women from the Renaissance to the Present*. New York: Morrow, 1981; Faderman, Lillian. *To Believe in Women: What Lesbians Have Done for America. A History*. Boston, Mass.: Houghton Mifflin, 1999; Falco, Maria J., ed. *Feminist Interpretations of Mary Wollstonecraft*. University Park: Pennsylvania State University Press, 1996; Gatens, Moira. "'The Oppressed State of My Sex': Wollstonecraft on Reason, Feeling, and Equality." In Mary Lyndon Shanley and Carole Pateman, eds., *Feminist Interpretations and Political Theory*. University Park: Pennsylvania State University Press, 1991, 112–28; Goldman, Emma. (1910) *Anarchism and Other Essays*. New York: Dover, 1969; Goldman, Emma. *Red Emma Speaks: An Emma Goldman Reader*. Ed. Alix Kate Shulman. New York: Schocken, 1983; Haaland, Bonnie. *Emma Goldman: Sexuality and the Impurity of the State*. New York: Black Rose Books, 1993; Hadewijch of Antwerp. [Selections] In Ellen K. Feder, Karmen MacKendrick, and Sybol S. Cook, eds., *A Passion for Wisdom: Readings in Western Philosophy on Love and Desire*. Upper Saddle River, N.J.: Prentice Hall, 2004, 158–71; Hayek, F. A. *John Stuart Mill and Harriet Taylor: Their Correspondence and Subsequent Marriage*. Chicago, Ill.: University of Chicago Press, 1951; Himmelfarb, Gertrude. *On Liberty and Liberalism: The Case of John Stuart Mill*. New York: Knopf, 1974; Honig, Bonnie, ed. *Feminist Interpretations of Hannah Arendt*. University Park: Pennsylvania State University Press, 1995; Jackson, Margaret. *The Real Facts of Life: Feminism and the Politics of Sexuality, 1850–1940*. Bristol, Pa.: Taylor and Francis, 1994; Jacobs, Jo Ellen. *The Voice of Harriet Taylor Mill*. Bloomington: Indiana University Press, 2004; Jeffreys, Sheila. *The Spinster and Her Enemies: Feminism and Sexuality, 1880–1930*. London: Pandora Press, 1985. North Melbourne, Australia: Spinifex, 1997; Kennedy, Ellen, and Susan Mendus, eds. *Women in Western Political Philosophy: Kant to Nietzsche*. New York: St. Martin's Press, 1987; Kent, Susan Kingsley. *Sex and Suffrage in Britain, 1860–1914*. Princeton, N.J.: Princeton University Press, 1987; Klein, Ellen Ruth. *Undressing Feminism*. St. Paul, Minn.: Paragon House, 2002; Myers, J. A. *The Historical Dictionary of the Lesbian Liberation Movement: Still the Rage*. Lanham, Md.: Rowman and Littlefield/Scarecrow, 2003; Nye, Andrea. *The Princess and the Philosopher: Letters of Elizabeth of the Palatine to René Descartes*. Lanham, Md.: Rowman and Littlefield, 1999; Offen, Karen. "A Nineteenth-Century French Feminist Rediscovered: Jenny P. d'Hericourt, 1809–1875." *Signs* 13:1 (1987), 144–58; Perrot, Michelle, ed. *Writing Women's History*. Trans. Felicia Pheasant. Oxford, U.K.: Blackwell, 1992; Rich, Adrienne. "Compulsory Heterosexuality and Lesbian Existence." *Signs* 5:4 (1980), 631–60. Reprinted in *Blood, Bread, and Poetry: Selected Prose 1979–1985*. New York: Norton, 1986, 23–75; and Henry Abelove, Michèle Aina Barale, and David M. Halperin, eds., *The Lesbian and Gay Studies Reader*. New York: Routledge, 1993, 227–54; Roe, Sue, and Susan Sellers. *The Cambridge Companion to Virginia Woolf*. Cambridge: Cambridge University Press, 2000; Rose, Phyllis. "Harriet Taylor and John Stuart Mill." In *Parallel Lives: Five Victorian Marriages*. New York: Knopf, 1984, 95–140; Rosen, Robyn. *Reproductive Health, Reproductive Rights: Reformers and the Politics of Maternal Welfare 1917–1940*. Columbus: Ohio State University Press, 2003; Rossi, Alice S., ed. *The Feminist Papers: From Adams to de Beauvoir*. New York: Columbia University Press, 1973; Schneir, Miriam, ed. *Feminism: The Essential Historical Writings*. New York: Random House, 1972; Schwarzer, Alice. *After The Second Sex: Conversations with Simone de Beauvoir*. Trans. Marianne Howarth. New York: Pantheon, 1984; Shanley, Mary Lyndon. "Marital Slavery and Friendship: John Stuart Mill's *The Subjection of Women*." *Political Theory* 9:2 (1981), 229–47. Reprinted in Mary Lyndon Shanley and Carole Pateman, eds., *Feminist Interpretations and Political Theory*. University Park: Pennsylvania State University Press, 1991, 164–80; Showalter, Elaine. *Sexual Anarchy: Gender and Culture at the Fin de Siècle*. New York: Viking, 1990; Simons, Margaret A., ed. *Feminist Interpretations of Simone de Beauvoir*. University Park: Pennsylvania State University Press, 1995; Stephen, James Fitzjames. (1873) "Equality." In *Liberty, Equality, Fraternity*. London: Cambridge University Press, 1967, 179–220; Stigers, Eva Stehle. "Romantic Sensuality, Poetic Sense: A Response to Hallett on Sappho." *Signs* 4:3 (1979), 465–71; Stopes, Marie Carmichael. (1928) *Enduring*

Passion: Further New Contributions to the Solution of Sex Difficulties, Being the Continuation of Married Love, 4th ed. New York: Putnam, 1931; Stove, David. "The Subjection of John Stuart Mill." *Philosophy* 68 (1993), 5–13; Todd, Janet. *Mary Wollstonecraft: A Revolutionary Life*. New York: Columbia University Press, 2000; Todd, Janet, ed. *The Collected Letters of Mary Wollstonecraft*. New York: Columbia University Press, 2004; Tomlin, Clare. *The Life and Death of Mary Wollstonecraft*. New York: Harcourt Brace Jovanovich, 1974; Wallace, Irving. "The Prostitute Who Ran for President" [Victoria Woodhull]. In *The Nympho and Other Maniacs*. New York: Simon and Schuster, 1971, 336–87; Warnock, Mary, ed. *Women Philosophers*. London: J. M. Dent, 1996; Winkler, John J. "Double Consciousness in Sappho's Lyrics." In *The Constraints of Desire: The Anthropology of Sex and Gender in Ancient Greece*. New York: Routledge, 1990, 162–87. Reprinted in Henry Abelove, Michèle Aina Barale, and David M. Halperin, eds., *The Lesbian and Gay Studies Reader*. New York: Routledge, 1993, 577–94; Witt, Charlotte. (2000) "Feminist History of Philosophy." In Edward N. Zalta, ed., *Stanford Encyclopedia of Philosophy*. <plato.stanford.edu/entries/feminism-femhist/> and <plato.stanford.edu/archives/win2000/entries/feminism-femhist/> [accessed 8 September 2004]. Supplement, "Bibliography of Feminist Philosophers." <plato.stanford.edu/entries/feminism-femhist/bib.html> [accessed 18 January 2005].

FEMINISM, LESBIAN. Lesbian feminist philosophy is concerned with the connections between lesbianism and **feminism** and between sexuality and gender within an oppressive sex/gender system (see Rubin, "Traffic"). However, there is no single lesbian feminist perspective about these connections. Two major themes in lesbian feminist philosophy are the nature, meaning, and possibility of women's sexual agency in a patriarchal society, and lesbianism as a feminist political choice. Other important topics include **pornography** and censorship, **sadomasochism**, **prostitution**, transsexual persons and women's space, separatism, butch and femme, **bisexuality**, monogamy, **marriage**, and motherhood. Lesbian feminist philosophy clearly covers a wide range of issues in the philosophy of sex.

To understand the variety of lesbian feminist philosophical positions on sexuality, one must understand the emergence of the lesbian feminist movement in the United States in the late 1960s and early 1970s. In response to the sexism manifested by men in gay left organizations and the sexism and homophobia exhibited in many antiracist, leftist organizations—in addition to the lesbian baiting of the National Organization for Women (NOW)—lesbian members of those organizations articulated specifically lesbian perspectives on oppression. In 1969, when Betty Friedan, president of NOW, called lesbians a " 'lavender menace' that would provide enemies with the ammunition to dismiss the women's movement as a bunch of man-hating dykes" (Rosen, 166), some lesbians in New York formed a group, the Radicalesbians, that characterized lesbianism as a political choice that was central to feminism (Radicalesbians, 19).

In 1970 the Radicalesbians wore "Lavender Menace" tee shirts to the Second Congress to Unite Women and took advantage of the open microphone to discuss lesbian politics. At this meeting, members of the group distributed "The Woman Identified Woman" (Rosen, 167–68). The first sentences of this essay famously defined "lesbian" as "the rage of all women condensed to the point of explosion" (Radicalesbians, 17). Radicalesbians called on feminists to examine the connections between heterosexuality (indeed, the categories "homosexual" and "heterosexual") and the patriarchal oppression of women and to embrace the unifying, radical potential of lesbianism in the feminist movement (18). They charged that those who were, at best, wary of and, at worst, hostile to a visible lesbian presence in the feminist movement were more concerned with achieving respectability for the movement than real liberation for women. They proclaimed, "Until women see in each other the possibility of primal commitment which includes sexual love, they will be denying themselves the love and value they readily accord to men, thus affirming their second-class status" (19).

Ten years later Adrienne Rich made similar points in "Compulsory Heterosexuality and Lesbian Existence." She expanded the meaning of "lesbian" to include all instances of woman-identified experience in a woman's life. These experiences were especially significant because they ran counter to a society structured in part by institutionalized compulsory heterosexuality that trained women to nourish primary attachments with men through a complex system of rewards and punishments. According to Rich, lesbian invisibility makes heterosexuality seem natural and helps mystify its compulsory nature. She defined woman-identified experiences as those in which women prioritized their relationships with other women, including mother-daughter relationships, "Boston marriages" (in the nineteenth century, romantic female friends who lived together), and **friendship**s between women. In advancing this broad concept of women-identified experiences, Rich strongly deemphasized genital sexuality in the lesbian continuum and the meaning of "lesbian."

Rich's essay had a continuing impact on feminist theories of sexuality. It was appropriately commemorated by a retrospective in a special issue of the *Journal of Women's History* in 2003 (see Rupp). The essay, however, has not been without its critics. Joan Nestle relates how she hated it the first time she read it because she perceived in it an "anti-sex stance" and gross generalizations about women and lesbians ("Wars," 51). Nestle was not alone in arguing that Rich did not leave any room to consider heterosexuality an authentic choice for women (English et al., 48). If heterosexuality is compulsory, are heterosexual women who initiate and enjoy sex with men patriarchal dupes? Nestle ties together social disapproval of lesbians and of promiscuous heterosexual women and imagines her mother's reply: "They called you freak and me whore and maybe they always will but we fight them the best when we keep on doing what they say we should not want or need for the joy we find in doing it. . . . Don't scream penis at me but help to change the world so no woman feels shame or fear because she likes to fuck" ("My Mother," 470). Further, Nestle rejects Rich's notion that lesbian **sexual desire**s and attitudes are radically different from those of gay men ("Wars," 51).

Other criticisms were that Rich's downplaying genital sexuality in defining "lesbian" left the expanded notion of "lesbian" nearly meaningless (Nestle, "Wars," 52; Califia, *Public*, xvii–xix). Another objection was that Rich's lesbian continuum includes women who are not dykes yet excludes women with so-called antifeminist sexual practices, such as butches, femmes, and sadomasochists (Califia, *Public*, xviii). Rich, along with other feminists opposed to pornography and sadomasochism, sought to "prettify sex," and efforts to "prettify sex" foster sexual shame rather than sexual liberation (Califia, *Public*, xxv–xxvi). Similarly, some who were opposed to Rich's exclusionary continuum denounced lesbian feminists who wanted to purge their own communities of what they labeled "male-identified" sexual practices like watching pornography and using dildos for penetration (Allison, 105–9, 122).

Mary Daly's elaboration of female "lustiness" (*Pure Lust*) is another noteworthy approach. She asserts that patriarchal culture is for women a death culture; women in this culture internalize attitudes and values that ultimately impede female bonding (xii). Feminism must reclaim lust from its phallic distortions. "Phallic lust" is characterized by obsession and aggression, both of which sustain a toxic, brutal environment for women and all living things (1). Female lustiness is, by contrast, the enthusiastic desire to connect with all of creation, the lustiness of a labrys-wielding "race of women" who defeat phallic lust and embrace "biophilic being" (2–4).

Daly's notion of a distinct female consciousness and affinity contributes to the theme of lesbian separatism, the view that women's freedom from oppression begins with their removing themselves from patriarchal culture and interpreting reality and making choices in woman- or lesbian-centered ways (Frye, "Reflections on Separatism," 96–97; Hoagland, 59–60). Women must create new meanings and values with other women and rid their minds of patriarchal presumptions that have made them reluctant or unable to resist oppression (Hoagland; Trebilcot). Women-only and women-centered spaces, in the form of coffeehouses, bookstores, and music festivals, have contributed to lesbian culture. According to separatists, the power of the powerful is established by their access to the labor, products, bodies, and minds of the powerless; the powerless begin to assert themselves as autonomous subjects when they deny this access (Frye, "Reflections," 103). The desire of some lesbian feminists to maintain women-only spaces has come into conflict with the desires of male-to-female transgendered or transsexual people to participate as women in these spaces. Jacqueline Anderson questions this participation and urges the development of an ethics formulated within the women's community to address this problem (146–49). For their part, transgendered people challenge the ethics and politics of women-born-women spaces on the grounds that, as Simone de Beauvoir (1908–1986) forcefully argued (*Second Sex*, 267), "One is not born, but rather becomes, a woman" (see Feinberg, 110).

Some lesbian feminists, questioning the privileges of heterosexual and bisexual women, have raised the question whether one must be a lesbian to be feminist (Echols, 239–40). Bisexual feminists assert that bisexuality is not automatically contrary to feminism; actually, bisexuality is critical for feminist and queer liberation because bisexuality more dramatically challenges the oppressive sex/gender system than do lesbianism and male **homosexuality** (Baker). Indeed, what might be suggested by bisexuality is that feminism must seek more than the liberation of women; it must seek the elimination of sex roles and the liberation of sexualities (Rubin, "Traffic," 52, 54; see Butler). Some feminists, however, have attempted to outline acceptable heterosexuality, one adopted only after serious consideration of nonheterosexual options and an examination of the role of compulsory heterosexuality in shaping sexual desire (Overall).

Marilyn Frye approaches this question by appealing to the early meaning of "virgin," a word that "did not originally mean a woman whose vagina was untouched by any penis, but a free woman, one not betrothed, not married, not bound to, not possessed by any man. It meant a female who is sexually and hence socially her own person" ("Willful Virgin," 133). Frye sketches the conditions a heterosexual woman would have to meet to be a virgin, and hence a feminist, such as not conforming to the norms of feminine appearance and behavior and refusing to marry and attend the weddings of friends and relatives. Frye remains doubtful about whether women can "fuck without losing [their] virginity" (136) and concludes that a woman must be "an undomesticated female, an impossible being," to be a feminist (136). Radically feminist lesbians are more likely to live virginity in this sense.

Another topic incisively discussed by Frye is how we should understand lesbian "sex," given that in our culture "having sex" is usually defined as penis-vagina intercourse (MacKinnon, 133; Sanders and Reinisch). Given that definition, it seems that lesbians (and gay men) could not "have sex." Definitions of "having sex" are important in many contexts, including the framing of legal statutes (prostitution, **rape**) and in social scientific studies of patterns of **sexual activity**—the frequency of sexual acts, the number of partners one has, and so forth. Frye wonders how lesbians are supposed to answer a survey question,

"How many times or how frequently do you have sex?" Criteria used by lesbians and gay males will have to be different from criteria standardly employed by heterosexuals, or a major change in how we conceive of "sex" must take place. In light of the penis-centered definition and nature of sexuality in patriarchy, Frye is not surprised by the purported relative infrequency of lesbian "sex" ("Lesbian 'Sex,' " 306, 313), the fact that surveys sometimes report that lesbians seem less interested in sex than other groups.

Another problem Frye raises is that lesbians do not talk enough about sexuality and, as a result, have not developed a vocabulary for describing what they do with each other when they "do it." They need to develop a **language** appropriate to the quality of their sexual experiences (314). Lesbian feminists have produced abundant literature about the impact on women's sexuality of classism, racism, sexism, anti-Semitism, **heterosexism**, homophobia, and ableism. Internalizing the messages and values of these social influences profoundly shapes what lesbians do in bed together and how they feel about doing it. For example, Audre Lorde argues that the power of the erotic has been denied to women in a patriarchal culture that conflates the erotic and the pornographic (*Sister Outsider*). Sarah Chin interprets Lorde's work as an experiment with ways to develop a new vocabulary for representing lesbian sexuality, a vocabulary that accentuates the sexual power of touch, not the (pornographic) sexual power of vision (182–83). Despite Lorde's criticisms of sadomasochism for its eroticization of power differentials, Chin claims that Lorde's emphasis on touch helps explain the erotic charge of sadomasochistic pornography. In this genre, the visible is "often an obstacle to the realities of desire," and participants must "locate their fantasy lives in the sensual world, disregarding what might otherwise be obvious" (182).

Indeed, sadomasochistic lesbians often describe their sexual activities as empowering, and they claim to experience no contradiction between practicing consensual sadomasochism and, at the same time, working to eliminate oppression. But some lesbian feminists claim, to the contrary, that sadomasochism lulls its practitioners into tolerating inequalities (Hoagland, 59). Claudia Card suggests that there are far more ethical issues surrounding sadomasochism (S/M) than have been so far addressed by proponents and opponents, issues concerning responsibilities between practitioners and responsibilities to nonparticipants who claim to be harmed by it (236). Critics of S/M should direct their energies at oppressive sexual norms and attitudes in society, because S/M itself is not the cause of oppression (236–37) but, likely, its result. For this reason Card thinks it possible that sadomasochism would not exist in a radically transformed world (237). Gayle Rubin makes a similar point about oppressive social norms and pornography when she denies that antipornography feminists are right to insist that pornography itself is the cause of violence against women (see English et al.).

Some lesbian feminists have also criticized butch/femme identities and relationships. In the early days of lesbian feminism there seemed to be two kinds of lesbians. On the one hand, some lesbian feminists understood lesbianism as a political choice. On the other, there were lesbians who came out in working-class bars, who came out into a world of butch and femme, and who were lesbian because they wanted and enjoyed having sex with other women. (See Hollibaugh and Moraga, "Rolling Around in Bed"; Lorde, *Zami*; Nestle, *Persistent Desire*. For the influence of classism on lesbian feminist responses to the butch/femme phenomenon, see Allison; Hollibaugh.) Femme lesbian feminists defend the eroticism of butch-femme difference and point out that a femme's dressing up for a butch is not the same as her dressing up for a man (Gomez, 101, 105). Honestly confronting lesbian desire requires acknowledging power as an inseparable part of sex, whether it be heterosexual, bisexual, gay male, or lesbian. The reluctance of some lesbian feminists to admit the role of power in bed underlies their hostility toward butches and femmes (Hollibaugh and Moraga, 397).

If lesbian sex already challenges standard definitions of sex, forcing any plausible definition to include much more than what patriarchy considers sex, disabled lesbian feminists also strive to expand the concept of sex and thereby reclaim their existence as sexual beings in a society that has traditionally denied sexuality to the disabled (Brownworth and Raffo; Califia, *Speaking*, 102–3; Franchild). Naomi Finkelstein writes about struggling with a disability that involves debilitating, chronic pain, yet wanting, as a butch, to please her femme. For Finkelstein, being disabled did not mean giving up her butchness. It meant transforming what it *is* to be butch, perceiving butch strength in surviving with her pain, and even "claiming a new masculinity" (313). Sharon Wachsler writes, similarly, about ways of transforming her femme identity in the face of being disabled. Having a **disability** that involves chemical sensitivities, Wachsler cannot utilize some of the accoutrements of lesbian femme identity (cosmetics and perfumes).

The "feminist sex wars," which stem from events surrounding a "Scholar and the Feminist IX" conference at Barnard College in April 1982, illustrate the variety of lesbian feminist approaches to sexuality. Conference organizers wanted to address both the pleasures and the dangers of female sexuality to broaden a feminist sexual dialogue that focused on women's victimization (Vance, 3). The conference was picketed by Women against Pornography, Women against Violence against Women, and the New York Radical Feminists, who objected to including in a feminist conference women who participated in and advocated what these groups called "anti-feminist" sexual practices ("Petition," 451). Protestors distributed a leaflet that named individual participants as morally unacceptable because they belonged to certain sexual groups ("Petition," 452). Eventually, the conference papers were published in Carole Vance's anthology *Pleasure and Danger*.

Antipornography feminists are inspired by **Catharine MacKinnon** and **Andrea Dworkin** (1946–2005), who argue that pornography is a form of violence against women. For MacKinnon, all forms of heterosexual sex in a pornography-saturated patriarchal society manifest the eroticization of dominance and hierarchy. MacKinnon has chastised the recognition of pleasure that emerged at Barnard:

> As if women under male supremacy have power to [negotiate sexual pleasure].
> As if "negotiation" is a form of freedom. As if pleasure and how to get it, rather than dominance and how to end it, is the "overall" issue sexuality presents feminism. As if women do just need a good fuck. (135)

Many feminists argue that pornography is not merely offensive. It harms and degrades women; it conditions men to view and treat women as sexual objects; and it impels both men and women to understand **objectification** as natural and inevitable (see Longino).

Sex radical feminists reply by pointing to a suspicious coalition between antipornography feminists and the Extreme Right in their common efforts to criminalize pornography, prostitution, and sadomasochism (see Williams). According to sex radicals, antipornography feminists adopt notions of permissible sexuality similar to those of their antifeminist enemies. Feminists opposed to pornography, nonmonogamy, prostitution, butch/femme, and sadomasochism contribute to the oppression of sexual minorities in patriarchal society. Furthermore, sex radicals question whether actions that target sex workers rather than seek to improve their working conditions are genuinely feminist (Califia, *Public*, 112; Query and Funari). Sex radical feminists are opposed to patriarchal violence against women; they believe, however, that feminists need to address this violence in sex-positive ways (English et al., 51).

The Kiss and Tell Collective tries to chart a middle ground, a move fueled by realizing that feminist efforts to curtail pornography often have the effect of endangering lesbian and gay sexual material (see Gilbert). Rather than concentrate exclusively on whether an image is harmful or pleasurable, they ask (17), "Is it possible to honour both the one woman's joy and the other woman's fear [of the same image]? Is it possible to admit the mutability of images without retreating to a position that says all images are neutral?" Chris Cuomo also searches for terrain between joy and fear, arguing that feminists should pay attention to the role of the unconscious in sexual desire: Sex is messy business, which makes it extremely difficult, if not impossible, to trace any connection between harm and intention (275). Cuomo urges a feminist ethics of sex that is both resistant and creative, that nurtures diversity as one of the strengths of feminism (285).

Lesbian feminists have not answered all the questions they have posed about sex. But provocative insights about the psychology and politics of sexuality have emerged from lesbian feminism, and no matter how internally divided, their discussions of sexuality have contributed substantially to the development of feminist theory and practice.

See also Abstinence; Activity, Sexual; Beauty; Bisexuality; Disability; Dworkin, Andrea; Dysfunction, Sexual; Feminism, French; Feminism, Liberal; Firestone, Shulamith; Friendship; Heterosexism; Judaism, Twentieth- and Twenty-First-Century; Language; Pornography; Queer Theory; Sadomasochism; Sex Work; Social Constructionism

REFERENCES

Allison, Dorothy. *Skin: Talking about Sex, Class, and Literature.* Ithaca, N.Y.: Firebrand, 1994; Anderson, Jacqueline. "Revolutionary Community." In Claudia Card, ed., *On Feminist Ethics and Politics.* Lawrence: University Press of Kansas, 1999, 140–49; Baker, Karin. "Bisexual Feminist Politics: Because Bisexuality Is Not Enough." In Elizabeth Reba Wise, ed., *Closer to Home: Bisexuality and Feminism.* Seattle, Wash.: Seal Press, 1992, 255–67; Beauvoir, Simone de. (1949) *The Second Sex.* Trans. Howard M. Parshley. New York: Knopf, 1953; Brownworth, Victoria A., and Susan Raffo, eds. *Restricted Access: Lesbians on Disability.* Seattle, Wash.: Seal Press, 1999; Butler, Judith. *Bodies That Matter: On the Discursive Limits of "Sex."* New York: Routledge, 1993; Califia, Pat. *Public Sex: The Culture of Radical Sex.* San Francisco, Calif.: Cleis Press, 1994; Califia, Pat. (Califia-Rice, Patrick) *Speaking Sex to Power: The Politics of Queer Sex.* San Francisco, Calif.: Cleis Press, 2002; Card, Claudia. *Lesbian Choices.* New York: Columbia University Press, 1995; Chin, Sarah. "Feeling Her Way: Audre Lorde and the Power of Touch." *GLQ: Journal of Lesbian and Gay Studies* 9:1–2 (2003), 181–204; Cuomo, Chris J. "Feminist Sex at Century's End: On Justice and Joy." In Claudia Card, ed., *On Feminist Ethics and Politics.* Lawrence: University Press of Kansas, 1999, 269–87; Daly, Mary. *Pure Lust: Elemental Feminist Philosophy.* Boston, Mass.: Beacon Press, 1984; Dworkin, Andrea. *Pornography: Men Possessing Women.* New York: Putnam, 1981; Echols, Alice. *Daring to Be Bad: Radical Feminism in America, 1967–1975.* Minneapolis: University of Minnesota Press, 1989; English, Deirdre, Amber Hollibaugh, and Gayle Rubin. "Talking Sex: A Conversation on Sexuality and Feminism." *Socialist Review* 11:4 (1981), 43–62; Feinberg, Leslie. *Transgender Warriors: Making History from Joan of Arc to Dennis Rodman.* Boston, Mass.: Beacon Press, 1996; Finkelstein, Naomi. "The Only Thing You Have to Do Is Live." *GLQ: Journal of Lesbian and Gay Studies* 9:1–2 (2003), 307–19; Franchild, Edwina. " 'You Do So Well': A Blind Lesbian Responds to Her Sighted Sisters." In Jeffner Allen, ed., *Lesbian Philosophies and Cultures.* Albany: State University of New York Press, 1990, 181–91; Frye, Marilyn. "Lesbian 'Sex.' " In Jeffner Allen, ed., *Lesbian Philosophies and Cultures.* Albany: State University of New York Press, 1990, 305–15; Frye, Marilyn. "Some Reflections on Separatism and Power." In *The Politics of Reality: Essays in Feminist Theory.* Freedom, Calif.: Crossing Press, 1983, 95–109; Frye, Marilyn. "Willful Virgin *or* Do You Have to Be a Lesbian to Be a Feminist?" In *Willful Virgin: Essays in Feminism, 1976–1992.* Freedom, Calif.: Crossing Press, 1992, 124–37; Gilbert, Harriet. "So Long as It's Not Sex and Violence: Andrea

Dworkin's *Mercy*." In Lynne Segal and Mary McIntosh, eds., *Sex Exposed: Sexuality and the Pornography Debate*. New Brunswick, N.J.: Rutgers University Press, 1993, 216–29; Gomez, Jewel L. "Femme Erotic Independence." In Sally R. Munt, ed., *Butch/Femme: Inside Lesbian Gender*. London: Cassell, 1998, 101–8; Hoagland, Sarah Lucia. *Lesbian Ethics: Toward New Value*. Palo Alto, Calif.: Institute for Lesbian Studies, 1988; Hollibaugh, Amber. *My Dangerous Desires: A Queer Girl Dreaming Her Way Home*. Durham, N.C.: Duke University Press, 2000; Hollibaugh, Amber, and Cherríe Moraga. "What We're Rolling Around in Bed With: Sexual Silences in Feminism." In Ann Snitow, Christine Stansell, and Sharon Thompson, eds., *Powers of Desire: The Politics of Sexuality*. New York: Monthly Review Press, 1983, 394–405; Kiss and Tell Collective (Persimmon Blackbridge, Lizard Jones, Susan Stewart). *Her Tongue on My Theory: Images, Essays, and Fantasies*. Vancouver, Can.: Press Gang Publishers, 1994; Longino, Helen. "Pornography, Oppression, and Freedom: A Closer Look." In Laura Lederer, ed., *Take Back the Night: Women on Pornography*. New York: Morrow, 1990, 40–54; Lorde, Audre. *Sister Outsider: Essays and Speeches*. Freedom, Calif.: Crossing Press, 1984; Lorde, Audre. *Zami: A New Spelling of My Name*. Freedom, Calif.: Crossing Press, 1982; MacKinnon, Catharine A. *Toward a Feminist Theory of the State*. Cambridge, Mass.: Harvard University Press, 1989; Moraga, Cherríe. *Loving in the War Years: Lo que nunca pasó por sus labios*. Boston, Mass.: South End Press, 1983; Nestle, Joan. "My Mother Liked to Fuck." In Ann Snitow, Christine Stansell, and Sharon Thompson, eds., *Powers of Desire: The Politics of Sexuality*. New York: Monthly Review Press, 1983, 468–70; Nestle, Joan. "Wars and Thinking." *Journal of Women's History* 15:3 (2003), 49–57; Nestle, Joan, ed. *The Persistent Desire: A Femme-Butch Reader*. Boston, Mass.: Alyson, 1992; Overall, Christine. "Heterosexuality and Feminist Theory." *Canadian Journal of Philosophy* 20:1 (1990), 1–17; "Petition in Support of the Scholar and Feminist IX Conference." [Signed by Henry Abelove et al.] In Carole S. Vance, ed., *Pleasure and Danger: Exploring Female Sexuality*. London: Routledge and Kegan Paul, 1984, 451–53; Query, Julia, and Vicky Funari, dirs. *Live Nude Girls Unite*. [film] 2000. Distributed by First Run Features; Radicalesbians. (1970) "The Woman Identified Woman." In Anne Koedt, Ellen Levine, and Anita Rapone, eds., *Radical Feminism*. [*Notes from the Second Year* and *Notes from the Third Year*] New York: Quadrangle Books, 1973, 240–45; Rich, Adrienne. "Compulsory Heterosexuality and Lesbian Existence." *Signs* 5:4 (1980), 631–60; Rosen, Ruth. *The World Split Open: How the Modern Women's Movement Changed America*. New York: Viking, 2000; Rubin, Gayle. (1975) "The Traffic in Women: Notes on the 'Political Economy' of Sex." In Linda Nicholson, ed., *The Second Wave: A Reader in Feminist Theory*. New York: Routledge, 1997, 27–62; Rupp, Leila J., ed. "Women's History in the New Millennium: Adrienne Rich's 'Compulsory Heterosexuality and Lesbian Existence'—A Retrospective." *Journal of Women's History* 15:3 (2003), 9–90; Sanders, Stephanie, and June Reinisch. "Would You Say You 'Had Sex' If . . . ?" *Journal of the American Medical Association* 281:3 (20 January 1999), 275–77; Trebilcot, Joyce. *Dyke Ideas: Process, Politics, and Daily Life*. Albany: State University of New York Press, 1994; Vance, Carole S., ed. *Pleasure and Danger: Exploring Female Sexuality*. London: Routledge and Kegan Paul, 1984; Wachsler, Sharon. "Still Femme." In Victoria A. Brownworth and Susan Raffo, eds., *Restricted Access: Lesbians on Disability*. Seattle, Wash.: Seal Press, 1999, 109–14; Williams, Linda. "Sexual Politics: Strange Bedfellows." *In These Times* (29 October–4 November 1986), 18–20.

Kim Q. Hall

ADDITIONAL READING

Allen, Jeffner, ed. *Lesbian Philosophies and Cultures*. Albany: State University of New York Press, 1990; Anzaldúa, Gloria, ed. *Making Face, Making Soul/Haciendo Caras: Creative and Critical Perspectives by Feminists of Color*. San Francisco, Calif.: Aunt Lute, 1990; Anzaldúa, Gloria, and Cherríe Moraga, eds. *This Bridge Called My Back: Writings by Radical Women of Color*. New York: Kitchen Table, 1981; Aptheker, Bettina. *Tapestries of Life: Women's Work, Women's Consciousness, and the Meaning of Daily Experience*. Amherst: University of Massachusetts Press, 1989; Bar On, Bat-Ami, and Ann Ferguson, eds. *Daring to Be Good: Essays in Feminist Ethico-Politics*. New York:

Routledge, 1998; Barrett, Michèle, and Anne Phillips, eds. *Destabilizing Theory: Contemporary Feminist Debates.* Stanford, Calif.: Stanford University Press, 1992; Beck, Evelyn Torton, ed. *Nice Jewish Girls: A Lesbian Anthology.* Trumansburg, N.Y.: Crossing Press, 1982; Blackwood, Evelyn, and Saskia Wieringa, eds. *Female Desires: Same-Sex Relations and Transgender Practices across Cultures.* New York: Columbia University Press, 1999; Bright, Susie. *The Sexual State of the Union.* New York: Simon and Schuster, 1997; Bright, Susie. *Susie Sexpert's Lesbian Sex World.* San Francisco, Calif.: Cleis, 1990; Brown, Jill. "The Daughter Is Mother of the Child: Cycles of Lesbian Sexuality." In Sue Cartledge and Joanna Ryan, eds., *Sex and Love: New Thoughts on Old Contradictions.* London: Women's Press, 1983, 75–88; Browne, Susan E., Debra Connors, and Nanci Stern, eds. *With the Power of Each Breath: A Disabled Women's Anthology.* Pittsburgh, Pa.: Cleis, 1985; Bunch, Charlotte. *Passionate Politics: Essays 1968–1986.* New York: St. Martin's Press, 1987; Butler, Heather. "What Do You Call a Lesbian with Long Fingers? The Development of Lesbian and Dyke Pornography." In Linda Williams, ed., *Porn Studies.* Durham, N.C.: Duke University Press, 2004, 167–97; Butler, Judith. *Gender Trouble: Feminism and the Subversion of Identity.* New York: Routledge, 1990; Butler, Judith. "Imitation and Gender Insubordination." In Diana Fuss, ed., *Inside/Out: Lesbian Theories, Gay Theories.* New York: Routledge, 1991, 13–31; Calhoun, Cheshire. *Feminism, the Family, and the Politics of the Closet: Lesbian and Gay Displacement.* New York: Oxford University Press, 2003; Califia, Pat. "Feminism and Sadomasochism." *Heresies* #12 ["Sex Issue"] 3:4 (1981), 30–34. Reprinted in *CoEvolution Quarterly* 33 (Spring 1982), 33–40; and Stevi Jackson and Sue Scott, eds., *Feminism and Sexuality: A Reader.* New York: Columbia University Press, 1996, 230–37; Card, Claudia. "Pluralist Lesbian Separatism." In Jeffner Allen, ed., *Lesbian Philosophies and Cultures.* Albany: State University of New York Press, 1990, 125–41; Card, Claudia. "Review Essay: Sadomasochism and Sexual Preference." *Journal of Social Philosophy* 15:2 (1984), 42–52; Card, Claudia, ed. *Adventures in Lesbian Philosophy.* Bloomington: Indiana University Press, 1994; Chauncey, George, Jr. (1983) "From Sexual Inversion to Homosexuality: The Changing Medical Conceptualization of Female Deviance." In Kathy Peiss and Christina Simmons, eds., *Passion and Power: Sexuality in History.* Philadelphia, Pa.: Temple University Press, 1989, 87–117; Cuomo, Chris J. *The Philosopher Queen: Feminist Essays on War, Love, and Knowledge.* Lanham, Md.: Rowman and Littlefield, 2002; Cuomo, Chris, and Kim Q. Hall, eds. *Whiteness: Feminist Philosophical Reflections.* Lanham, Md.: Rowman and Littlefield, 1999; Daly, Mary. *Beyond God the Father: Toward a Philosophy of Women's Liberation.* Boston, Mass.: Beacon Press, 1973; Daly, Mary. *Gyn/Ecology: The Metaethics of Radical Feminism.* Boston, Mass.: Beacon Press, 1978; De Lauretis, Teresa. *The Practice of Love: Lesbian Sexuality and Perverse Desire.* Bloomington: Indiana University Press, 1994; Dever, Carolyn. "Either/And: Lesbian Theories, Queer Theories." *GLQ: A Journal of Lesbian and Gay Studies* 5:3 (1999), 413–24. <muse.jhu.edu/demo/journal_of_lesbian_and_gay_studies/v005/5.3dever.html> [accessed 4 January 2005]; Duggan, Lisa. *Sapphic Slashers: Sex, Violence, and American Modernity.* Durham, N.C.: Duke University Press, 2000; Echols, Alice. "Cultural Feminism: Feminist Capitalism and the Anti-Pornography Movement." *Social Text* 7 (Spring–Summer 1983), 34–53; Esterberg, Kristin G. *Lesbian and Bisexual Identities: Constructing Communities, Constructing Selves.* Philadelphia, Pa.: Temple University Press, 1997; Faderman, Lillian. *Odd Girls and Twilight Lovers: A History of Lesbian Life in the Twentieth Century.* New York: Penguin, 1992; Faderman, Lillian. *Surpassing the Love of Men: Romantic Friendship and Love between Women from the Renaissance to the Present.* New York: Morrow, 1991; Feinberg, Leslie. *Trans Liberation: Beyond Pink or Blue.* Boston, Mass.: Beacon Press, 1998; Ferguson, Ann. *Blood at the Root: Motherhood, Sexuality, and Male Dominance.* London: Pandora, 1989; Ferguson, Ann. "Is There a Lesbian Culture?" In Jeffner Allen, ed., *Lesbian Philosophies and Cultures.* Albany: State University of New York Press, 1990, 63–88; Frye, Marilyn. "Lesbian 'Sex.'" In Jeffner Allen, ed., *Lesbian Philosophies and Cultures.* Albany: State University of New York Press, 1990, 305–15. Reprinted in *Willful Virgin: Essays in Feminism 1976–1992.* Freedom, Calif.: Crossing Press, 1992, 109–19; and Anne Minas, ed., *Gender Basics: Feminist Perspectives on Women and Men,* 1st ed. Belmont, Calif.: Wadsworth, 1993, 328–33; Gaard, Greta. "Anti-Lesbian Intellectual Harassment in the Academy." In VèVè Clark, Shirley Nelson Garner, Margaret Higonnet, and Ketu H. Katrak, eds., *Antifeminism in the*

Academy. New York: Routledge, 1996, 115–40; Griffin, Susan. *Rape: The Politics of Consciousness.* San Francisco, Calif.: Harper and Row, 1979; Grosz, Elizabeth, and Elspeth Probyn, eds. *Sexy Bodies: The Strange Carnalities of Feminism.* New York: Routledge, 1995; Hale, Jacob. "Are Lesbians Women?" *Hypatia* 11 (1996): 94–101; Hamblin, Angela. "Is Feminist Heterosexuality Possible?" In Sue Cartledge and Joanna Ryan, eds., *Sex and Love: New Thoughts on Old Contradictions.* London: Women's Press, 1983, 105–23; Hoagland, Sarah Lucia, and Julia Penelope, eds. *For Lesbians Only: A Separatist Anthology.* London: Onlywomen Press, 1988; Jay, Karla. "Radicalesbians." In Bonnie Zimmerman, ed., *Lesbian Histories and Cultures: An Encyclopedia.* New York: Garland, 2000, 635–36; Jeffreys, Sheila. *Anticlimax: A Feminist Perspective on the Sexual Revolution.* London: Women's Press, 1990. New York: New York University Press, 1991; Jeffreys, Sheila. *The Lesbian Heresy: A Feminist Perspective on the Lesbian Sexual Revolution.* North Melbourne, Australia: Spinifex, 1993; Jeffreys, Sheila. *Unpacking Queer Politics: A Lesbian Feminist Perspective.* Malden, Mass.: Blackwell, 2003; Jeffreys, Sheila, ed. *The Sexuality Debates.* New York: Routledge and Kegan Paul, 1987, 2001; Kennedy, Elizabeth Lapovsky, and Madeline D. Davis. *Boots of Leather, Slippers of Gold: The History of a Lesbian Community.* New York: Routledge, 1993; Kennedy, Elizabeth Lapovsky, and Madeline D. Davis. (1987) "The Reproduction of Butch-Fem Roles: A Social Constructionist Approach." In Kathy Peiss and Christina Simmons, eds., *Passion and Power: Sexuality in History.* Philadelphia, Pa.: Temple University Press, 1989, 241–56; LeMoncheck, Linda. *Loose Women, Lecherous Men: A Feminist Philosophy of Sex.* New York: Oxford University Press, 1997; Longino, Helen. "Pornography, Oppression, and Freedom: A Closer Look." In Laura Lederer, ed., *Take Back the Night: Women on Pornography.* New York: Morrow, 1990, 40–54. Reprinted in Susan Dwyer, ed., *The Problem of Pornography.* Belmont, Calif.: Wadsworth, 1995, 34–47; Lugones, María. "Purity, Impurity, and Separation." *Signs* 19:2 (1994), 458–79; Merck, Mandy. "The Feminist Ethics of Lesbian S/M." In *Perversions: Deviant Readings.* New York, Routledge, 1993, 236–66; Myers, J. A. *The Historical Dictionary of the Lesbian Liberation Movement: Still the Rage.* Lanham, Md.: Rowman and Littlefield/Scarecrow, 2003; Nestle, Joan. "Lesbians and Prostitutes: A Historical Sisterhood." In Frédérique Delacoste and Priscilla Alexander, eds., *Sex Work: Writings by Women in the Sex Industry,* 2nd ed. San Francisco, Calif.: Cleis Press, 1998, 247–63; Parks, Carlton W. "African American Lesbian and Gay Identities." In Timothy F. Murphy, ed., *Reader's Guide to Lesbian and Gay Studies.* Chicago, Ill.: Fitzroy Dearborn, 2000, 15–16; Phelan, Shane. *Getting Specific: Postmodern Lesbian Politics.* Minneapolis: University of Minnesota Press, 1994; Radicalesbians. (1970) "The Woman Identified Woman." In Anne Koedt, Ellen Levine, and Anita Rapone, eds., *Radical Feminism.* [*Notes from the Second Year* and *Notes from the Third Year*] New York: Quadrangle Books, 1973, 240–45. Reprinted in Sarah Lucia Hoagland and Julia Penelope, eds., *For Lesbians Only: A Separatist Anthology.* London: Onlywomen Press, 1988, 17–22; and Linda Nicholson, ed., *The Second Wave: A Reader in Feminist Theory.* New York: Routledge, 1997, 153–75. Online at Special Collections Library, Duke University, <scriptorium.lib.duke.edu/wlm/womid> [accessed 18 November 2004]; Rich, Adrienne. "Compulsory Heterosexuality and Lesbian Existence." *Signs* 5:4 (1980), 631–60. Reprinted in *Blood, Bread, and Poetry: Selected Prose 1979–1985.* New York: Norton, 1986, 23–75; in Ann Snitow, Christine Stansell, and Sharon Thompson, eds., *Powers of Desire: The Politics of Sexuality.* New York: Monthly Review Press, 1983, 177–205; and Henry Abelove, Michèle Aina Barale, and David M. Halperin, eds., *The Lesbian and Gay Studies Reader.* New York: Routledge, 1993, 227–54; Richardson, Diana. (1993) "Constructing Lesbian Sexualities." In Stevi Jackson and Sue Scott, eds., *Feminism and Sexuality: A Reader.* New York: Columbia University Press, 1996, 267–86; Robson, Ruthann. "Pedagogy, Jurisprudence, and Finger-Fucking: Lesbian Sex in a Law School Classroom." In Karla Jay, ed., *Lesbian Erotics.* New York: New York University Press, 1995, 28–39; Rubin, Gayle. "The Leather Menace: Comments on Politics and S/M." In Samois Collective, ed., *Coming to Power.* Palo Alto, Calif.: Up Press, 1981, 192–225; Rubin, Gayle. "Misguided, Dangerous, and Wrong: An Analysis of Anti-pornography Politics." In Alison Assiter and Avedon Carol, eds., *Bad Girls and Dirty Pictures.* London: Pluto Press, 1993, 18–40; Rubin, Gayle. [interviewed by Judith Butler] "Sexual Traffic." In Mandy Merck, Naomi Segal, and Elizabeth Wright, eds., *Coming Out of Feminism?* Oxford, U.K.: Blackwell, 1998, 36–73; Rubin, Gayle.

"Thinking Sex: Notes for a Radical Theory of the Politics of Sexuality." In Carole S. Vance, ed., *Pleasure and Danger: Exploring Female Sexuality*. London: Routledge and Kegan Paul, 1984, 267–319. Reprinted in Henry Abelove, Michèle Aina Barale, and David Halperin, eds., *The Lesbian and Gay Studies Reader*. New York: Routledge, 1993, 3–44; and Peter M. Nardi and Beth E. Schneider, eds., *Social Perspectives in Lesbian and Gay Studies*. New York: Routledge, 1998, 100–133; Rubin, Gayle. "The Traffic in Women: Notes on the 'Political Economy' of Sex." In Rayna Reiter, ed., *Toward an Anthropology of Women*. New York: Monthly Review Press, 1975, 157–210. Reprinted in Linda Nicholson, ed., *The Second Wave: A Reader in Feminist Theory*. New York: Routledge, 1997, 27–62; Segal, Lynne, and Mary McIntosh, eds. *Sex Exposed: Sexuality and the Pornography Debate*. New Brunswick, N.J.: Rutgers University Press, 1993; Smith, Barbara, and Beverly Smith. "Across the Kitchen Table: A Sister-to-Sister Dialogue." In Gloria Anzaldúa and Cherríe Moraga, eds., *This Bridge Called My Back: Writings by Radical Women of Color*. New York: Kitchen Table, 1981, 113–27; Snitow, Ann, Christine Stansell, and Sharon Thompson, eds. *Powers of Desire: The Politics of Sexuality*. New York: Monthly Review Press, 1983; Stein, Arlene, ed. *Sisters, Sexperts, and Queers: Beyond Lesbian Nation*. New York: Plume, 1993; Trujillo, Carla Mari, ed. *Chicana Lesbians: The Girls Our Mothers Warned Us About*. Berkeley, Calif.: Third Woman Press, 1991; Wittig, Monique. *The Lesbian Body*. Trans. David Le Vay. Boston, Mass.: Beacon Press, 1973; Young, Iris Marion. *Throwing Like a Girl and Other Essays in Feminist Philosophy and Social Theory*. Bloomington: Indiana University Press, 1990; Zimmerman, Bonnie, and Toni A. H. McNaron, eds. *The New Lesbian Studies: Into the Twenty-First Century*. New York: Feminist Press at CUNY, 1996; Zita, Jacquelyn N. *Body Talk: Philosophical Reflections on Sex and Gender*. New York: Columbia University Press, 1998.

FEMINISM, LIBERAL. Emphasizing equal individual rights and liberties for women and men and downplaying sexual differences, liberal feminism is the most widely accepted social and political philosophy among feminists. Liberal feminists defend the equal rationality of the sexes and emphasize the importance of structuring social, familial, and sexual roles in ways that promote women's autonomous self-fulfillment. They emphasize the similarities between men and women rather than the average differences between them, attribute most of the personality and character differences between the sexes to the social construction of gender, and tend to promote a single set of androgynous virtues for both women and men. While rejecting strong claims of sexual difference that might underwrite different and potentially hierarchical rights and social roles, liberal feminists otherwise avoid the promotion of particular conceptions of the good life for either men or women, instead defending a broad sphere of neutrality and **privacy** within which individuals may pursue forms of life most congenial to them. While liberal feminists acknowledge that some choices made by women are questionable because conditioned by sexist social practices, they also tend to avoid maternalism and any second-guessing of those choices made without coercion or threats. Fully informed and mentally competent adult women are assumed to be the final judges of their own best interests. Thus liberal feminists tend to resist legislative intervention that would gainsay the judgment of women.

The preeminence of this perspective owes much to the fact that it encompasses a wide range of related but distinct views that fit comfortably within the framework of political **liberalism**. It does not fundamentally challenge capitalism or heterosexuality; nor does it recommend separatism, as do more radical feminists. Instead, it aims to extend the full range of freedoms in a liberal democratic society to women, criticizing practices that deny women equal protection under the **law** as well as laws that *de facto* discriminate against women. Liberal feminists reject utopian visions of an ideal society in favor of one that eliminates coercion and promotes autonomous choices among all its citizens.

With regard to sexuality, liberal feminism maintains the tradition of liberalism, valuing personal privacy and autonomy in ways that appear, to some, to conflict with the goal of eradicating sexist norms. For example, liberal feminists tend to adopt a libertarian or public health approach regarding commercial **sexual activity**. Thus many liberal feminists reject calls to criminalize or even condemn **prostitution** and **pornography** when those who participate in their manufacture and consumption do so without coercion. They defend this position by citing privacy but also by invoking the inherent value of autonomous choice. Liberal feminists defend the liberty to decide on one's **sexual orientation**, partners, and practices as beyond the reach of law.

Liberal feminism has its roots in the writings of, among others, Mary Wollstonecraft (1759–1797), John Stuart Mill (1806–1873), and Harriet Taylor Mill (1807–1858). Many writers prior to Wollstonecraft, such as **Jean-Jacques Rousseau** (1712–1778), had explicitly argued that men and women were by nature not merely different in kind but different in "natural rank," with women being weaker physically, intellectually, and emotionally (358–61). Men were said to be more rational, women more emotional; their respective educations should reflect these differences. A few philosophers, such as John Locke (1632–1704), had argued that the sexes should receive the same education and that they shared equal rights and responsibilities with respect to their children (see *Some Thoughts*, 14; *Two Treatises*, 303). Nonetheless, these writers stopped short of defending complete sexual equality (either for social roles or legal rights), and putative sex differences have been, and in some parts of the world continue to be, the basis of laws denying women the right to retain property in **marriage** and the right to vote.

In *Vindication of the Rights of Woman*, Wollstonecraft wrote that many of the supposed differences between the sexes were either fabricated or exaggerated and therefore could not be used as the basis for differential rights and roles. Imposing different educational expectations on men and women was not only unjust but also counterproductive, tending to create less productive female citizens with "artificial, weak characters" (103). Both sexes, Wollstonecraft argued, have the capacity to reason; hence both should be educated as to enhance their rationality, which she defined as the ability to act as fully responsible moral agents. The realization of this ability would provide self-fulfillment for the moral agent and benefit society. On this account, women needed to become more rational, but there was no reason for men to cultivate their emotions.

John Stuart Mill echoed Wollstonecraft's sentiments in *The Subjection of Women* (1869). He described sex roles as a kind of caste system in which women were assigned lower status and restricted in what they were permitted to do simply because of their sex, even though there were no categorical differences between the sexes that could justify it. This not only stunted the moral development of women but also denied them the self-fulfillment that comes only with the freedom to pursue one's own good. Mill thought that when provided with the same educational and civic opportunities that men had, most women would choose to remain wives and mothers, improving domestic life for the family ("The Essay by John Stuart Mill" [on marriage and divorce; 1832], *Essays*, 76–77; see James Fitzjames Stephen's [1829–1894] reply to Mill, 180–98). Mill's future wife, Harriet Taylor [Mill], disagreed, arguing that women would choose to participate more fully in public life, going beyond simply voting and performing charity work. Women would choose to become the partners of men in productive industry and would have fewer children ("The Essay by Harriet Taylor" [on marriage and divorce; 1832], *Essays*, 84–86).

Feminists of all kinds continued to press for greater equality for women throughout the United States and Europe, culminating in the right to vote for Russian women in 1918, some British women in 1918, and all adult U.S. women in 1920. American liberal feminism experienced a resurgence in the middle of the twentieth century with the popular works of Betty Friedan, who was the first president of the National Organization for Women (NOW, 1966) and co-founder in 1971 of *Ms.* magazine with feminist activist and journalist Gloria Steinem. In *The Feminine Mystique* (1963), Friedan argued that women had a problem that "had no name" (15–32). Women in the United States had the right to vote and hold property and had achieved a significant degree of equal protection under the law. However, Friedan argued, they often led lives that were unfulfilling, if not stifling. They spent too much time polishing and organizing already clean and tidy homes, experiencing boredom and anxiety as a result. Friedan urged women, once their children were attending school, to seek employment that would challenge their capacities and provide personal satisfaction. Women could enjoy a family with children but needed to get involved in pursuits outside the domestic sphere as soon as possible by entering into public life and paid employment.

Friedan's early approach to the role of women in society is vulnerable to an objection that also plagues the views of Wollstonecraft and J. S. Mill: that this type of feminism is not about the liberation of women *per se* but only of middle- to upper-middle-class, heterosexual white women. As with the earliest forms of liberal feminism, Friedan made the mistake of supposing that all women faced the same form of sexual oppression. Friedan later came to accept that the feminism set forth in her early work reflected this bias, accepting the importance not only of class differences among women but also of sexuality as a feminist issue (see Tong, 26–35).

Following the work of feminists such as Friedan and Steinem, many obstacles to the full participation of women in public life were removed. Employment opportunities for women were widened, many discriminatory laws in the United States were abandoned, and sex-based employment discrimination was outlawed with Title VII of the Civil Rights Act (1964). Women began to feel that they could achieve things for themselves rather than simply for their families. The focus on women as equally entitled to autonomous self-fulfillment blended seamlessly with a burgeoning self-help movement emphasizing a more satisfying sexuality for women. Books like *Our Bodies, Ourselves* became popular as women rejected the idea of their sexuality as something mysterious and shameful. Sexuality was reconceived as aimed at personal satisfaction as much as, if not more than, reproduction. This led not only to greater awareness of the female body and sexual pleasure but also to increasing recognition for lesbian and bisexual women. But many feminists noticed that the liberal feminist goal of removing legal and social barriers to the full participation of women in education and employment did not completely address the issue of women's subordination. Two issues in particular remained to be addressed: the economic condition of women and the structure of the family. Liberal feminists took aim squarely at the nuclear family. Sex roles within the family had to become androgynous for the ideal of equality to be served, with neither parent assuming primary responsibility for rearing children and maintaining the home. "Mothers," wrote Virginia Held, "need not be the ones who *mother*" (243).

Unlike feminists who saw the family as little more than a source of oppression for women, Susan Moller Okin (1946–2004) argued that the traditional family in the West was unlikely to disappear and could be salvaged. What was necessary was an end to gender-structured marriage. Ideally, marriage should be reconceived as an equal partnership in which neither partner should leave the world of paid employment for the domestic sphere, which necessarily disadvantages the partner who maintains the home. Traditional marriage makes women vulnerable by channeling them into lower-paying, more flexible forms of employment before marriage, by reducing their negotiating power within marriage, and by impoverishing them in divorce. The expectation that women will be the primary caregivers for children and other dependents encourages women to make choices that militate against their own best interests; men are not similarly disadvantaged (134–69). Okin's argument exemplifies the liberal feminist commitment to justice, to the relative similarity between the sexes, and to equal concern and respect for men and women.

Okin's views in particular showcase a fundamental tension in liberal feminism. While she argues that the traditional family is *unjust*, she does not recommend that it be illegal or penalized. Instead, she proposes, for marriages where only one spouse has paid employment, that the income be divided in two by the employer and placed in separate accounts (181–82). The weakness and impracticality of this solution show how liberalism hamstrings itself when it takes on issues usually thought of as private—and therefore beyond the reach of justice (see Cohen). Injustice calls for institutional and legal remedy, but liberal feminism is loathe to address the problems of private life with public legal sanctions, which are regarded as a form of coercion in that realm.

Contemporary liberal feminists object to prostitution and pornography primarily because much of it involves coercion and choices that are not autonomous. In the 1980s, the issue of pornography became a central concern as some radical feminists argued that women participating in the manufacture of pornography and in prostitution were not, due to the background conditions of patriarchy, free to refuse. Legal scholar **Catharine MacKinnon** and feminist writer **Andrea Dworkin** (1946–2005) proposed legislation that would subject pornographers to civil lawsuits for the harm that pornography does (see their "model" ordinance in "Symposium," appendix). MacKinnon argued that violence was used in most cases to get women to participate in pornography and prostitution. Further, women's sexuality had been appropriated by men for their own purposes ("Men's power over women means that the way men see women defines who women can be"; 197), thereby robbing women of the autonomy necessary for their "yes" to be meaningful. MacKinnon also denied that pornography was speech, claiming instead that pornography *constituted* the subordination of women; as such, it should be legally actionable. Moreover, one cannot opt out of womanhood, despite liberal assertions that one can choose which aspects of one's historical, social, and familial inheritance to claim as one's own or reject. Other feminists, Carole Pateman for one, argued (*pace* liberal feminism) that prostitution was not the selling of sex but the selling of mastery. Prostitutes do not provide a service but sell their own subordination. The intimate bodily nature of prostitution makes it impossible that one is simply selling a service (*Contract*, 206–7). Thus radical feminists, in contrast to liberals, reject the possibility of "sound" prostitution, although many also reject its criminalization because doing so has harmful consequences (Pateman, "Defending Prostitution"; Shrage, 82–87).

Liberal feminists maintain that pornography is a form of expression that should be kept beyond the reach of governmental control. They have also pointed out that any violence and coercion involved in its production are already illegal. To insist that no woman in our society could freely **consent** to participate in the making of pornography (or in other sexual entertainment aimed at men) was "showing precisely the same disregard for women's autonomy and dignity that previous courts showed when they ruled that a woman's *nonconsent* to sexual intercourse did not mean that she had been raped" (Strossen, 189). Further, censorship would do nothing to stop discrimination against women and would only erode civil liberties. Martha Nussbaum has also argued that, in principle, a woman could sell her body for sex without being complicit in her own slavery. The intimate bodily nature of sexual interaction is not relevant to the issue of its justice; freedom from coercion is (285).

Still, many liberal feminists oppose prostitution and pornography. Many women who pose for pornography and engage in prostitution are violently forced or coerced into it. Gloria Steinem, in "The Real Linda Lovelace," documented a case of a woman compelled by her husband into performing sexually for the film *Deep Throat* (*Outrageous Acts*, 243–52). Childhood sexual abuse and later drug dependency and poverty are endemic among prostitutes and other sex workers (Illinois Coalition against Sexual Assault). However, for women who are not coerced and choose to engage in prostitution and pornography, liberals find themselves unable to criticize prostitution and tend to defend its decriminalization. Liberal feminists are, like radical feminists, usually opposed to the continued criminalization of these practices even in the case of nonviolent coercion (e.g., drug addiction), because criminalization tends to make prostitutes and other sex workers even worse off (Nussbaum, 297–98; Sample, 217). Showing that coercion has occurred is necessary but not sufficient for state intervention in commercial sexual activity; interference must also advance the interests of coerced agents.

Liberal feminists differ from "cultural feminists" and "sexual radicals" about sexuality. For cultural feminists, there are essential differences between men and women (whether cultural or biological); they advocate that women reject "male-identified" forms of life. Libertarian feminists or "sex radicals" do not (see Tong, 45–49). Cultural feminists insist that all current sexuality, be it heterosexual, gay, lesbian, or transgendered, is constituted and controlled by heterosexual men. Hence they reject sexualities that embody hierarchy and dominance and are promiscuous, seeking to empower women with a sexuality consistent with women's different nature. By contrast, sex radicals insist that "transgressive" forms of sexuality can be liberatory when practiced in a reflective way. Liberals insist that despite sexist social roles and norms, there remains a realm of autonomous choice with respect to one's sexuality: Women can to some degree choose their sexuality, at least in the sense that they can reject prevailing sexual norms when they reflect on them. Many liberal feminists also refuse to characterize promiscuity or **sadomasochism** as morally questionable, let alone degrading to women. Linda LeMoncheck, for example, suggests that we promote a "wide variety of sexual experiences, preferences, and desires. . . . [I]ndividual sexual needs . . . can be met with the active care and concern of a community of persons responsive to those needs" (*Loose Women*, 107). This is not to deny that some sexual practices are bad for or degrading to women. Indeed, LeMoncheck raises severe doubts about some consensual practices. When a woman consents to be treated as a dehumanized sex object in the prevailing cultural climate, that woman perpetuates a sexual norm that wrongly treats women as less than moral equals. Those who objectify women or acquiesce in their **objectification** violate the fundamental liberal feminist principle: Women and men are equally members of the moral community and deserve equal concern and respect (*Dehumanizing*, 24, 152–55).

The liberal principle of autonomy also extends to sexual orientation. Radical feminists have emphasized the extent to which every culture punishes women who violate social norms that insist that "normal" people must be heterosexual. Adrienne Rich observed in her famous 1980 essay that heterosexuality is compulsory for women. Compulsory heterosexuality is especially dangerous because it extends not simply to one's preference in sexual partners but to the wider forms of life that one may safely adopt: marriage (or at least cohabitation with a man), childbirth and child rearing, domesticity, and all the trappings of femininity that limit the freedom and power of women. Liberal feminists acknowledge that our culture enforces such norms but argue both that women are nonetheless free to reject the norms and that any legal arrangements that favor heterosexuality over other sexualities are unjust. Women who choose to enter heterosexual institutions (such as marriage) and who choose male sexual partners are not thereby participating in an injustice, unless they do so in a way that is prejudicial to other forms of sexual life (Colker, 146–47).

Liberal feminists generally defend the right to **abortion**. In 1972, Judith Jarvis Thomson published the most famous liberal feminist defense of abortion, "A Defense of Abortion." She appealed in part to a wide sphere of inviolable rights over one's life and liberty—rights that would trump the rights of a fetus, even if that fetus were regarded as a person with all the rights that personhood entails. Thomson argued that contemporary arguments against abortion typically took the point of view of the fetus and completely ignored the point of view of women who would be sustaining a fetus. This male bias against the perspective of women denigrates their personhood and interests.

Despite its widespread acceptance, liberal feminism has come under attack from both the Left and the Right. One criticism is that by emphasizing the equal rationality of women and men, liberal feminism tacitly relies on a sexist conception of the human person that is male-biased in its very notion of rationality (Jaggar, 44–45). Some have argued that the notion of objectivity, too, is a product of male bias (MacKinnon, 120–24). This may undermine the liberal feminist claim that individual women (as well as men) are in a position to distance themselves from their cultural inheritance and reject practices they find objectionable or freely adopt new, more congenial ones. In particular, the liberal feminist defense of pornography, prostitution, and sadomasochism, to the extent that these practices are freely chosen, may be weakened. If the idea of a rational, freely choosing agent reflects male bias, then the possibility of freely choosing one's sexuality and sexual practices under patriarchy is called into question. Others have argued that the liberal emphasis on instrumental rationality, in part in virtue of its emphasis on self-fulfillment, betrays a tacit commitment to (male) egoism as the standard of rationality, thereby downplaying (female) altruism and other-regarding actions (Elshtain, 374; Jaggar, 45). In this way liberalism might undermine its own effort to regard the differences between men and women as insignificant. Liberal feminists have responded by arguing that although there are strong obstacles to autonomous choice, they can sometimes be overcome, as the very existence of feminist resistance shows. Others have defended the notions of rationality and objectivity from the charge of male bias (for example, Haslanger, 239–42).

A second criticism, made by both some feminists and nonfeminists, is that the differences between men and women are greater than liberals acknowledge and that these differences should be taken into account to treat men and women fairly. The main point of Carol Gilligan's *In a Different Voice* (1982) was that women tend to respond to ethical quandaries differently than do men. And cultural feminists have argued that women have, in general, a completely different approach to living. Whether such differences are cultural/historical or biologically grounded, androgynous sex roles (as in, for example, the family) may be a poor fit for many men and women and hence not entirely desirable (Elshtain, 375; Fraser, 41–66). Liberal feminists nonetheless defend rational free agency as an androgynous ideal, arguing that many differences between the sexes are either a product of sexism or not sufficient to justify differential social roles. Women and men "are more than the sum of their sexual natures" (Groenhout, 73).

Ultimately, there are two fundamental tensions in liberal feminism. One is between the rejection of sexual difference and unequal treatment, on the one hand, and the commitment to improving the status of women, on the other. Critics of liberal feminism charge that by denying or ignoring the differences between the sexes, liberals are unable to advocate true sexual equality—which, in virtue of these differences, may not be best served or attained by identical treatment. Although many sexual differences may be a product of patriarchy, the androgynous ideal seems to disadvantage women if they do not adopt it as their own. Nancy Fraser notes that "equality strategies typically presuppose 'the male as norm,' thereby disadvantaging women and imposing a distorted standard on everyone" (44). Many women simply reject the role of primary breadwinner or public citizen as part of their core self, identifying instead as a private sphere nurturer. Liberal insistence only on equal protection under the law for women will not garner them equal concern and respect. Yet doing more than this seems to violate liberal neutrality.

The second tension is between the idea that women's sexual subordination is a kind of injustice and the idea that sexuality is located in a private realm of autonomous choice. Because liberals are committed to neutrality about specific forms of the good life for humans, they tend to reject any constraint on what happens "between consenting adults." Yet many women appear to agree to, or at least acquiesce in, relationships with men that are less than equal. Whether these relationships are institutionalized, as in marriage, or a template of patriarchal heterosexuality, as in sadomasochism and other relationships of sexual domination, they violate liberal ideals of equality and justice. Liberalism, however, relegates them to the realm of the private, beyond the reach of justice.

See also Aristotle; Coercion (by Sexually Aggressive Women); Consent; Feminism, History of; Feminism, Lesbian; Feminism, Men's; Genital Mutilation; Harassment, Sexual; Law, Sex and the; Liberalism; MacKinnon, Catharine; Marriage; Marxism; Paglia, Camille; Pornography; Privacy; Prostitution; Rape; Rape, Acquaintance and Date; Sex Work

REFERENCES

Boston Women's Health Book Collective. *Our Bodies, Ourselves.* New York: Simon and Schuster, 1973; Cohen, Joshua. "Okin on Justice, Gender, and the Family." *Canadian Journal of Philosophy* 22:2 (1992), 263–86; Colker, Ruth. "Feminism, Sexuality, and Authenticity." In Martha Fineman and Nancy Thomadsen, eds., *At the Boundaries of Law.* New York: Routledge, 1991, 135–47; Elshtain, Jean Bethke. (1982) "Antigone's Daughters." In Anne Phillips, ed., *Feminism and Politics.* Oxford, U.K.: Oxford University Press, 1998, 363–77; Fraser, Nancy. *Justice Interruptus: Critical Reflections on the "Postsocialist" Condition.* New York: Routledge, 1997; Friedan, Betty. *The Feminine Mystique.* New York: Norton, 1963; Gilligan, Carol. *In a Different Voice: Psychological Theory and Women's Development.* Cambridge, Mass.: Harvard University Press, 1982; Groenhout, Ruth E. "Essentialist Challenges to Liberal Feminism." *Social Theory and Practice* 28:1 (2002), 51–75; Haslanger, Sally. "On Being Objective and Being Objectified." In Louise Antony and Charlotte Witt, eds., *A Mind of One's Own: Feminist Essays on Reason and Objectivity.* Boulder, Colo.: Westview, 2002, 209–53; Held, Virginia. "The Obligations of Mothers and Fathers." In Mary Vetterling-Braggin, ed., *"Femininity," "Masculinity," and "Androgyny": A Modern Philosophical Discussion.* Totowa, N.J.: Rowman and Littlefield, 1982, 242–58; Illinois Coalition against Sexual Assault. "Prostitution." <www.icasa.org/uploads/prostitution.pdf> [accessed 12 October 2004]; Jaggar, Alison M. *Feminist Politics and Human Nature.* Totowa, N.J.: Rowman and Allanheld, 1983; LeMoncheck, Linda. *Dehumanizing Women: Treating Persons as Sex Objects.* Totowa, N.J.: Rowman and Allanheld, 1985; LeMoncheck, Linda. *Loose Women, Lecherous Men: A Feminist Philosophy of Sex.* New York: Oxford University Press, 1997; Locke, John. (1693) *Some Thoughts Concerning Education.* Ed. Ruth W. Grant and Nathan Tarcov. Indianapolis, Ind.: Hackett, 1996; Locke, John. (1689) *Two Treatises of Government.* Ed. Peter Laslett. Cambridge: Cambridge University Press, 1988; MacKinnon, Catharine A. *Toward a Feminist Theory of the State.* Cambridge, Mass.: Harvard

University Press, 1989; Mill, John Stuart, and Harriet Taylor Mill. *Essays on Sex Equality*. Ed. Alice S. Rossi. Chicago, Ill.: University of Chicago Press, 1970. [John Stuart Mill and Harriet Taylor, "Early Essays on Marriage and Divorce" (1832), 67–84 (John), 84–87 (Harriet); Harriet Taylor Mill, "Enfranchisement of Women" (1851), 91–121; John Stuart Mill, *The Subjection of Women* (1869), 125–242]; Nussbaum, Martha C. *Sex and Social Justice*. New York: Oxford University Press, 1999; Okin, Susan Moller. *Justice, Gender, and the Family*. New York: Basic Books, 1989; Pateman, Carole. "Defending Prostitution: Charges against Ericsson." *Ethics* 93:4 (1983), 561–65; Pateman, Carole. *The Sexual Contract*. Stanford, Calif.: Stanford University Press, 1988; Rich, Adrienne. "Compulsory Heterosexuality and Lesbian Existence." *Signs* 5:4 (1980), 631–60; Rousseau, Jean-Jacques. (1761) *Emile, or On Education*. Trans. Allan Bloom. New York: Basic Books, 1979; Sample, Ruth. "Sexual Exploitation and the Social Contract." *Canadian Journal of Philosophy*, "Feminist Moral Philosophy," supp. vol. 28 (2003), 189–217; Shrage, Laurie. *Moral Dilemmas of Feminism: Prostitution, Adultery, and Abortion*. New York: Routledge, 1994; Steinem, Gloria. *Outrageous Acts and Everyday Rebellions*. New York: Holt, Rinehart and Winston, 1983; Stephen, James Fitzjames. (1873) *Liberty, Equality, Fraternity*. London: Cambridge University Press, 1967; Strossen, Nadine. *Defending Pornography: Free Speech, Sex, and the Fight for Women's Rights*. New York: Scribner's, 1995; "Symposium on Pornography: Appendix." *New England Law Review* 20:4 (1984–1985), 759–77; Thomson, Judith Jarvis. "A Defense of Abortion." *Philosophy and Public Affairs* 1:1 (1972), 47–66; Tong, Rosemarie. (1989) *Feminist Thought: A More Comprehensive Introduction*, 2nd ed. Boulder, Colo.: Westview, 1998; Wollstonecraft, Mary. (1792) *A Vindication of the Rights of Woman*. Harmondsworth, U.K.: Penguin, 1975.

Ruth Sample

ADDITIONAL READING

Abbey, Ruth. "Odd Bedfellows: Nietzsche and Mill on Marriage." *History of European Ideas* 23:2–4 (1997), 81–104; Antony, Louise M., and Charlotte Witt, eds. *A Mind of One's Own: Feminist Essays on Reason and Objectivity*. Boulder, Colo.: Westview, 2002; Baehr, Amy R., ed. *Varieties of Liberal Feminism*. Lanham, Md.: Rowman and Littlefield, 2004; Boston Women's Health Collective. (1973) *Our Bodies, Ourselves for the New Century*, rev. and updated ed. New York: Touchstone, 1998; Burgess-Jackson, Keith. Review of *Loose Women, Lecherous Men: A Feminist Philosophy of Sex*, by Linda LeMoncheck. *Ethics* 110 (October 1999), 211–14; Butler, Melissa A. (1978) "Early Liberal Roots of Feminism: John Locke and the Attack on Patriarchy." In Mary Lyndon Shanley and Carole Pateman, eds., *Feminist Interpretations and Political Theory*. University Park: Pennsylvania State University Press, 1991, 74–94; Colker, Ruth. "Feminism, Sexuality, and Self: A Preliminary Inquiry into the Politics of Authenticity." *Boston University Law Review* 68:1 (1988), 217–64; Donner, Wendy. "John Stuart Mill's Liberal Feminism." *Philosophical Studies* 69 (1993), 155–66; Duggan, Lisa, and Nan D. Hunter. *Sex Wars: Sexual Dissent and Political Culture*. New York: Routledge, 1995; Echols, Alice. "Cultural Feminism: Feminist Capitalism and the Anti-Pornography Movement." *Social Text* 7 (Spring–Summer 1983), 34–53; Eisenstein, Zillah R. *The Radical Future of Liberal Feminism*. New York: Longman, 1981; Elshtain, Jean Bethke. "Nineteenth Century Liberal Sons: Jeremy Bentham and John Stuart Mill" and "Liberal Feminism: Why Can't a Woman Be More Like a Man?" In *Public Man, Private Woman: Women in Social and Political Thought*. Princeton, N.J.: Princeton University Press, 1981, 132–46, 228–55; Falco, Maria J., ed. *Feminist Interpretations of Mary Wollstonecraft*. University Park: Pennsylvania State University Press, 1996; Friedan, Betty. *The Second Stage*. New York: Summit Books, 1981; Garry, Ann. "Pornography and Respect for Women." *Social Theory and Practice* 4:4 (1978), 395–421. Reprinted in Sharon Bishop and Marjorie Weinzweig, eds., *Philosophy and Women*. Belmont, Calif.: Wadsworth, 1979, 128–39; Garry, Ann. "Sex (and Other) Objects." In Alan Soble, ed., *Sex, Love, and Friendship*. Amsterdam, Holland: Rodopi, 1997, 163–67; Garry, Ann. "Sex, Lies, and Pornography." In Hugh LaFollette, ed., *Ethics in Practice: An Anthology*, 2nd ed. Malden, Mass.: Blackwell, 2002, 344–55; Garry, Ann. "Why Are Love and Sex Philosophically Interesting?" *Metaphilosophy* 11:2 (1980), 165–77. Reprinted in POS2 (21–36);

SLF (39–50); Garry, Ann, and Marilyn Pearsall, eds. *Women, Knowledge, and Reality: Explorations in Feminist Philosophy*, 2nd ed. New York: Routledge, 1996; Gatens, Moira. " 'The Oppressed State of My Sex': Wollstonecraft on Reason, Feeling, and Equality." In Mary Lyndon Shanley and Carole Pateman, eds., *Feminist Interpretations and Political Theory*. University Park: Pennsylvania State University Press, 1991, 112–28; Gibson, Mary. "Rationality." *Philosophy and Public Affairs* 6:3 (1977), 193–225; Groenhout, Ruth. "Essentialist Challenges to Liberal Feminism." *Social Theory and Practice* 28:1 (2002), 51–75. Reprinted in Judith A. Boss, ed., *Analyzing Moral Issues*, 3rd ed. New York: McGraw Hill, 2005, 581–89; Haack, Susan. *Manifesto of a Passionate Moderate: Unfashionable Essays*. Chicago, Ill.: University of Chicago Press, 1998; Hekman, Susan J. "John Stuart Mill's *The Subjection of Women*: The Foundations of Liberal Feminism." *History of European Ideas* 15:4–6 (1992), 681–86; Jaggar, Alison M., ed. *Living with Contradictions: Controversies in Feminist Social Ethics*. Boulder, Colo.: Westview, 1994; Jaggar, Alison M., and Paula S. Rothenberg, eds. (1978, 1984) *Feminist Frameworks: Alternative Theoretical Accounts of the Relations between Women and Men*, 3rd ed. New York: McGraw-Hill, 1993; Klein, Ellen Ruth. *Undressing Feminism*. St. Paul, Minn.: Paragon House, 2002; Laden, Anthony Simon. "Radical Liberals, Reasonable Feminists: Reason, Power, and Objectivity in MacKinnon and Rawls." *Journal of Political Philosophy* 11:2 (2003), 133–52; Leidholdt, Dorchen, and Janice C. Raymond, eds. *The Sexual Liberals and the Attack on Feminism*. New York: Teachers College Press, 1990; Levinson, Nan. "Stalemate in the Sex Wars." [Review of *Sex Wars: Sexual Dissent and Political Culture*, by Lisa Duggan and Nan D. Hunter] *Women's Review of Books* 13:4 (1996), 14; MacKinnon, Catharine A. (1987, 1990) "Liberalism and the Death of Feminism." In *Women's Lives, Men's Laws*. Cambridge, Mass.: Harvard University Press, 2005, 259–68; Mendus, Susan. "Different Voices, Still Lives: Problems in the Ethics of Care." *Journal of Applied Philosophy* 10:1 (1993), 17–27; Mendus, Susan. *Feminism and Emotion: Readings in Moral and Political Philosophy*. New York: St. Martin's Press, 2000; Mendus, Susan, ed. *Justifying Toleration: Conceptual and Historical Perspectives*. Cambridge: Cambridge University Press, 1988; Mendus, Susan, and Jane Rendall, eds. *Sexuality and Subordination: Interdisciplinary Studies of Gender in the Nineteenth Century*. London: Routledge, 1989; Mitchell, Juliet. (1974) "Betty Friedan: The Freudian Mystique." In *Psychoanalysis and Feminism*. New York: Vintage, 1975, 319–27; Nussbaum, Martha C. *The Feminist Critique of Liberalism*. Lawrence: Philosophy Department, University of Kansas, 1997; Okin, Susan Moller. "John Stuart Mill, Liberal Feminist." In *Women in Western Political Thought*. Princeton, N.J.: Princeton University Press, 1979, 197–230; Radcliffe Richards, Janet. *The Sceptical Feminist: A Philosophical Inquiry*. London: Routledge and Kegan Paul, 1980; Reiman, Jeffrey. "Prostitution, Addiction, and the Ideology of Liberalism." *Contemporary Crises* 3 (1979), 53–68; Rich, Adrienne. "Compulsory Heterosexuality and Lesbian Existence." *Signs* 5:4 (1980), 631–60. Reprinted in *Blood, Bread, and Poetry: Selected Prose 1979–1985*. New York: Norton, 1986, 23–75; and Henry Abelove, Michèle Aina Barale, and David M. Halperin, eds., *The Lesbian and Gay Studies Reader*. New York: Routledge, 1993, 227–54; Ring, Jennifer. "Mill's *The Subjection of Women*: The Methodological Limits of Liberal Feminism." *Review of Politics* 47 (1985), 27–44; Russell, J. S. "Okin's Rawlsian Feminism? Justice in the Family and Another Liberalism." *Social Theory and Practice* 21:3 (1995), 397–426; Sample, Ruth. *Exploitation: What It Is and Why It's Wrong*. Lanham, Md.: Rowman and Littlefield, 2003; Schaeffer, Denise. "Feminism and Liberalism Reconsidered: The Case of Catharine MacKinnon." *American Political Science Review* 95:3 (2001), 699–708; Shanley, Mary Lyndon. "Marital Slavery and Friendship: John Stuart Mill's *The Subjection of Women*." *Political Theory* 9:2 (1981), 229–47. Reprinted in Mary Lyndon Shanley and Carole Pateman, eds., *Feminist Interpretations and Political Theory*. University Park: Pennsylvania State University Press, 1991, 164–80; Soble, Alan. "The Epistemology of the Natural and the Social in Mill's *The Subjection of Women*." *The Mill News Letter* 16:2 (1981), 3–9; Soble, Alan. Review of *Loose Women, Lecherous Men: A Feminist Philosophy of Sex*, by Linda LeMoncheck. *Teaching Philosophy* 22:2 (1999), 411–16; Tapper, Marion. "Can a Feminist Be a Liberal?" *Australasian Journal of Philosophy*, supp. to vol. 64 (1986), 37–47; Thomson, Judith Jarvis. "A Defense of Abortion." *Philosophy and Public Affairs* 1:1 (1971), 47–66. Reprinted in Robert M. Baird and Stuart E. Rosenbaum, eds., *The Ethics of Abortion: Pro-Life vs. Pro-Choice*, rev. ed. Buffalo,

N.Y.: Prometheus, 1993, 197–211; in Thomas A. Mappes and Jane S. Zembaty, eds., *Social Ethics*, 6th ed. New York: McGraw-Hill, 2002, 28–38; in Judith A. Boss, ed., *Analyzing Moral Issues*, 3rd ed. New York: McGraw Hill, 2005, 91–101; and P&S1 (305–23); P&S2 (210–17); P&S3 (231–45); Thomson, Judith Jarvis. "The Right to Privacy." *Philosophy and Public Affairs* 4:4 (1975), 295–314; Todd, Janet. *Mary Wollstonecraft: A Revolutionary Life*. New York: Columbia University Press, 2000; Todd, Janet, ed. *The Collected Letters of Mary Wollstonecraft*. New York: Columbia University Press, 2004; Tomlin, Clare. *The Life and Death of Mary Wollstonecraft*. New York: Harcourt Brace Jovanovich, 1974; Tong, Rosemarie. *Women, Sex, and the Law*. Totowa, N.J.: Rowman and Littlefield, 1984; West, Robin. "The Harms of Consensual Sex." *American Philosophical Association Newsletters* 94:2 (1995), 52–55. Reprinted in Thomas A. Mappes and Jane S. Zembaty, eds., *Social Ethics: Morality and Social Policy*, 6th ed. Boston, Mass.: McGraw-Hill, 2002, 184–88; and POS3 (263–68); POS4 (317–22).

FEMINISM, MEN'S. It is provocative and arguable that "Plato was the first feminist" (Lucas, 223; see Vlastos). What is well known is that **Plato** (427–347 BCE), in opposition to the beliefs of his ancient Greek culture, claimed that men and women were alike in intelligence and talent, that they should receive the same education, and that the City should be ruled equally by men and women guardians (*Republic*, bk. 5, 451–57). Even if we do not want to call Plato a "male feminist" *simpliciter*, he can still be seen, at least at this stage in his philosophical career, as a firm supporter of the major goals of one type of **feminism** and as someone who influenced many thinkers through Western history to take up the cause of women.

In the nineteenth century there were two prominent male figures who also championed women: liberal, utilitarian John Stuart Mill (1806–1873) and socialist Friedrich Engels (1820–1895). Mill, writing in an unreceptive Victorian age, began his famous *The Subjection of Women* with this announcement: "[T]he principle which regulates the existing social relations between the two sexes—the legal subordination of one sex to the other—is wrong . . . [and] ought to be replaced by a principle of perfect equality" (3). The relentless and powerful attack on male privilege that runs through *Subjection* seems to qualify Mill as a male feminist (see Susan Moller Okin [1946–2004], 197–230; Burgess-Jackson, "John Stuart Mill"), a judgment that would probably be endorsed by Harriet Taylor (1807–1858), the spouse with whom he had (for the time) a superlatively equal relationship. (Mill's sexual egalitarianism was rebutted, if not derided, by his contemporary James Fitzjames Stephen [1829–1894].)

Engels, although mostly concerned with the situation of the proletariat in an oppressive capitalist economic system, nonetheless recognized and railed against women's plight. Sounding much like many contemporary feminists, Engels declared that through the institution of **marriage** "the first class oppression [was] . . . that of the female sex by the male" (75). In capitalism, marriage degenerated "often enough into the crassest prostitution"; the married woman "only differs from the ordinary courtesan in that she does not let out her body on piece-work as a wage earner, but sells it once and for all into slavery" (82).

There was also, in the first half of the twentieth century, the British analytic philosopher **Bertrand Russell** (1872–1970). Russell was, during much of his life, known and derided as a feminist by his society, in part for renouncing the idea that men were superior to women. Russell, perhaps borrowing from Engels, prophetically—given developments in radical feminism later in the twentieth century—condemned the **sexual activity** engaged in by wives who were dependent economically on their spouses: "[T]he total amount of undesired sex endured by women is probably greater in marriage than in prostitution"

(153–55). But whether Russell fully deserves the label "male feminist" is clouded by his purported womanizing.

In the second half of the twentieth century, treatments of sexuality by heterosexual men taking an explicitly feminist perspective have been relatively few, yet they still have had an appreciable impact. Focus has been on what might be called historical analysis (e.g., Kimmel, *Manhood in America*) or on various aspects of sexuality, including homophobia (Kimmel, "Masculinity as Homophobia"), **pornography** (Brod; Stoltenberg), **rape** (Burgess-Jackson, "A Theory of Rape"; May and Strikwerda), **sexual harassment** (Hughes and May; McBride), linguistic practices (Baker), and **friendship** and intimacy (Strikwerda and May).

Male feminism has been substantially reactive, first responding to the burgeoning literature by women feminists and later replying to counterattacks by other males to feminist writings. It has also attempted to accommodate the research done by gay and transgendered scholars (Hale) and that emerging from varied ethnicities and cultures (see Schmitt). A significant amount of energy has been spent investigating, in support of women, what an appropriate male feminist standpoint or, alternatively, a supportive male profeminist voice might be (see Digby). Attention to feminist issues has been framed in terms of patriarchy, masculinity, and gender as a set of social practices. Stress has been placed on inequality, power relationships, and the relationship between them. Typical methodological approaches have been experiential and phenomenological, ethnographic, and philosophical.

A common theme in men's feminism is how men ought to act in response to oppressive, exploitative, and sexist social practices and institutions (for example, May's *Masculinity and Morality*). Given this emphasis on the social—for example, on historical and cultural variation in conceptions of masculinity, from the ancient Greeks and Romans to the twentieth-century West, and on the social construction of masculinity—there has been relatively little consideration of how the social and the biological intertwine in the formation and modification of sexuality. Among male feminists, there has been movement from assuming, simplistically, that sexuality is primarily biological to thinking that it is almost entirely a cultural phenomenon, or socially constructed, and then to an uneasiness with the latter type of explanation, without having yet developed a generally accepted account that is more than just a "both biology and culture" amalgam (Connell, *Gender*). Socially typical, as well as distorted, male adolescent sexual development is intensively studied (as in Messner), but articulation of what a mature, wholesome, nonsexist male feminist sexuality might be has been elusive. (But see some suggestions made by Fracher and Kimmel, who offer John Lennon [1940–1980], the onetime Beatle, cohort of Yoko Ono, and author/singer of "Imagine," as a model.)

Perhaps this lacuna is explicable, given that "man does not see the richness of his own sexuality and decrees that sex is woman" (Reynaud, 145). Male sexuality is analyzed in terms of power or potency, in effect reducing it to the vanishing point of the penis. This truncation in understanding is compounded when the penis and its associated apparatus are seen almost exclusively as biological entities. Robert Connell ("Psychoanalysis on Masculinity") provides a critical yet appreciative overview of psychoanalytical work on men's sexuality, but male feminists tend to eschew the psychological approaches of **Sigmund Freud** (1856–1939) and Carl Jung (1875–1961). One exception is the work of Victor Seidler. Consequently, the focus of men's feminism has remained on male sexuality as a form, expression, or manifestation of men's social power, rather than branching off into the study of the nature of male sexuality itself, as something worth examining at least partly independently of its social, cultural, or political meanings.

An overview of issues to be explored is provided by Michael Kimmel in his 2000 book *Gendered Society*. Kimmel points out that as friendship and **love** in the late twentieth century have become increasingly understood in terms of what had been previously and usually interpreted as a feminine ideal of intimacy, sexuality has nonetheless also become more "masculinized"—hence the preoccupation with such things as the number of sexual partners, the number of sex acts engaged in, the number of orgasms attained, the extent of one's sexual experimentation, and the like (see Whitehead; Whitehead and Barrett). Seidler attempts to develop an account of masculinity and sexuality through a personal and philosophical critique of rationalism in philosophy and social theory (*Rediscovering Masculinity*). He continued this project in later work, *Male Enough*, a critical appreciation of Robert Bly's mythopoetic masculinity (e.g., *Iron John*).

Men's feminism has investigated an increasing range of topics and provides fertile ground for future research. Laurence Thomas has given a sensitive account of male and female sensuality and sexuality and of the differences between them. Ronald Levant and Gary Brooks have collected a number of articles on male sexuality that examine "nonrelational sexuality," sexual relations without emotional intimacy or other social ties. Two essays that have begun to connect race and sexuality have been proffered by Jim Perkinson and Richard Schmitt. And in an essay by Lucy Candib and Schmitt, we find an empathetic analysis of how sexual potency and men's fears of losing it are linked to the male sense of identity.

See also Aristotle; Coercion (by Sexually Aggressive Women); Ethics, Sexual; Feminism, History of; Feminism, Liberal; Friendship; Greek Sexuality and Philosophy, Ancient; Harassment, Sexual; Language; Marxism; Plato; Pornography; Psychology, Evolutionary; Rape; Roman Sexuality and Philosophy, Ancient; Russell, Bertrand; Social Constructionism

REFERENCES

Baker, Robert B. (1975) " 'Pricks' and 'Chicks': A Plea for 'Persons.' " In Robert B. Baker, Kathleen J. Wininger, and Frederick A. Elliston, eds., *Philosophy and Sex*, 3rd ed. Amherst, N.Y.: Prometheus, 1998, 281–97; with " 'Pricks' and 'Chicks': A Postscript after Twenty-Five Years," 297–305; Bly, Robert. *Iron John: A Book about Men*. Reading, Mass.: Addison-Wesley, 1990; Brod, Harry. "Pornography and the Alienation of Male Sexuality." *Social Theory and Practice* 14:3 (1988), 265–84; Burgess-Jackson, Keith. "John Stuart Mill, Radical Feminist." *Social Theory and Practice* 21:3 (1995), 369–96; Burgess-Jackson, Keith. "A Theory of Rape." In Keith Burgess-Jackson, ed., *A Most Detestable Crime: New Philosophical Essays on Rape*. New York: Oxford University Press, 1999, 92–117; Candib, Lucy, and Richard Schmitt. "About Losing It: The Fear of Impotence." In Larry May, Robert Strikwerda, and Patrick D. Hopkins, eds., *Rethinking Masculinity: Philosophical Explorations in Light of Feminism*, 2nd ed. Lanham, Md.: Rowman and Littlefield, 1996, 211–34; Connell, Robert W. *Gender*. Cambridge, U.K.: Polity, 2002; Connell, Robert W. "Psychoanalysis on Masculinity." In Harry Brod and Michael Kauffman, eds., *Theorizing Masculinities*. Thousand Oaks, Calif.: Sage, 1994, 11–38; Digby, Tom, ed. *Men Doing Feminism*. New York: Routledge, 1998; Engels, Frederick. (1884) *The Origin of the Family, Private Property, and the State*. New York: International Publishers, 1942. Peking, China: Foreign Languages Press, 1978; Fracher, Jeffrey, and Michael S. Kimmel. (1989) "Hard Issues and Soft Spots: Counseling Men about Sexuality." In Michael S. Kimmel and Michael A. Messner, eds., *Men's Lives*, 3rd ed. Needham Heights, Mass.: Allyn and Bacon, 1995, 365–74; Hale, C. Jacob. "Tracing a Ghostly Memory in My Throat: Reflections on FTM Feminist Voice and Agency." In Tom Digby, ed., *Men Doing Feminism*. New York: Routledge, 1998, 99–129; Hughes, John C., and Larry May. "Sexual Harassment." *Social Theory and Practice* 6:3 (1980), 249–80; Kimmel, Michael S. *The Gendered Society*. New York: Oxford University Press, 2000; Kimmel, Michael S. *Manhood in America: A Cultural History*. New York: Free Press, 1996; Kimmel, Michael S. "Masculinity as Homophobia: Fear, Shame, and Silence in the Construction of Gender Identity." In Harry Brod and Michael Kauffman, eds., *Theorizing Masculinities*.

Thousand Oaks, Calif.: Sage, 1994, 119–41; Levant, Ronald F., and Gary R. Brooks, eds. *Men and Sex: New Psychological Perspectives.* New York: Wiley, 1997; Lucas, John. "Plato's Philosophy of Sex." In E. M. Craik, ed., *'Owls to Athens': Essays on Classical Subjects Presented to Sir Kenneth Dover.* Oxford, U.K.: Oxford University Press, 1990, 223–31; May, Larry. *Masculinity and Morality.* Ithaca, N.Y.: Cornell University Press, 1998; May, Larry, and Robert Strikwerda. "Men in Groups: Collective Responsibility for Rape." *Hypatia* 9:2 (1994), 134–51; McBride, William L. "Sexual Harassment, Seduction, and Mutual Respect: An Attempt at Sorting It Out." In Linda Fisher and Lester Embree, eds., *Feminist Phenomenology: Contributions to Phenomenology,* vol. 40. Dordrecht, Holland: Kluwer, 2000, 249–66; Messner, Michael A. *Power at Play: Sports and the Problem of Masculinity.* Boston, Mass.: Beacon Press, 1992; Mill, John Stuart. (1869) *The Subjection of Women.* Cambridge, Mass.: MIT Press, 1970; Okin, Susan Moller. *Women in Western Political Thought.* Princeton, N.J.: Princeton University Press, 1979; Perkinson, Jim. "The Body of White Space: Beyond Stiff Voices, Flaccid Feelings, and Silent Cells." In Nancy Tuana, William Cowling, Maurice Hamington, Greg Johnson, and Terrance MacMullan, eds., *Revealing Male Bodies.* Bloomington: Indiana University Press, 2003, 173–97; Plato. (ca. 375–370 BCE) *Republic.* Trans. G.M.A. Grube. Revised by C.D.C. Reeve. Indianapolis, Ind.: Hackett, 1992; Reynaud, Emmanuel. "Holy Virility: The Social Construction of Masculinity." In Peter F. Murphy, ed., *Feminism and Masculinities.* New York: Oxford University Press, 2004, 136–48; Russell, Bertrand. (1929) *Marriage and Morals.* New York: Liveright, 1970; Schmitt, Richard. "Large Propagators: Racism and the Domination of Women." In Nancy Tuana, William Cowling, Maurice Hamington, Greg Johnson, and Terrance MacMullan, eds., *Revealing Male Bodies.* Bloomington: Indiana University Press, 2003, 38–54; Seidler, Victor J. *Male Enough: Embodying Masculinities.* London: Sage, 1997; Seidler, Victor J. *Rediscovering Masculinity: Reason, Language, and Sexuality.* London: Routledge, 1989; Stephen, James Fitzjames. (1873) "Equality." In *Liberty, Equality, Fraternity.* London: Cambridge University Press, 1967, 179–220; Stoltenberg, John. *Refusing to Be a Man: Essays on Sex and Justice.* Portland, Ore.: Breitenbush Books, 1989; Strikwerda, Robert A., and Larry May. (1992) "Male Friendship and Intimacy." In Larry May, Robert Strikwerda, and Patrick D. Hopkins, eds., *Rethinking Masculinity: Philosophical Explorations in Light of Feminism,* 2nd ed. Lanham, Md.: Rowman and Littlefield, 1996, 79–94; Thomas, Laurence. "Erogenous Zones and Ambiguity: Sexuality and the Bodies of Men and Women." In Joseph A. Kuypers, ed., *Men and Power.* Amherst, N.Y.: Prometheus, 1999, 131–55; Vlastos, Gregory. (1989) "Was Plato a Feminist?" In Nancy Tuana, ed., *Feminist Interpretations of Plato.* University Park: Pennsylvania State University Press, 1994, 11–23; Whitehead, Stephen M. *Men and Masculinities: Key Themes and New Directions.* Cambridge, U.K.: Polity, 2002; Whitehead, Stephen, and Frank J. Barrett, eds. *The Masculinities Reader.* Cambridge, U.K.: Polity, 2001.

Robert A. Strikwerda

ADDITIONAL READING

Allen, Christine Garside. "Plato on Women." *Feminist Studies* 2:2–3 (1975), 1–8; Annas, Julia. "Mill and the Subjection of Women." *Philosophy* 52 (1977), 179–94; Baker, Robert B. " 'Pricks' and 'Chicks': A Plea for 'Persons.' " In Robert B. Baker and Frederick A. Elliston, eds., *Philosophy and Sex,* 1st ed. Buffalo, N.Y.: Prometheus, 1975, 45–64. Reprinted in P&S2 (249–67); and P&S3 (281–97), with " 'Pricks' and 'Chicks': A Postscript after Twenty-Five Years" (297–305); Bluestone, Natalie Harris. "Why Women Cannot Rule: Sexism in Plato Scholarship." *Philosophy of the Social Sciences* 18:1 (1988), 41–60. Reprinted in Nancy Tuana, ed., *Feminist Interpretations of Plato.* University Park: Pennsylvania State University Press, 1994, 109–30; Brod, Harry. "Pornography and the Alienation of Male Sexuality." *Social Theory and Practice* 14:3 (1988), 265–84. Reprinted in Larry May and Robert Strikwerda, eds., *Rethinking Masculinity: Philosophical Explorations in Light of Feminism,* 1st ed. Lanham, Md.: Rowman and Littlefield, 1992, 149–65; In Larry May, Robert Strikwerda, and Patrick D. Hopkins, eds., *Rethinking Masculinity: Philosophical Explorations in Light of Feminism,* 2nd ed. Lanham, Md.: Rowman and Littlefield, 1996, 237–53; POS2 (281–99); Brod, Harry, ed. *The Making of Masculinities: The New Men's Studies.* Boston, Mass.: Allen and Unwin,

1987; Brod, Harry, and Michael Kaufman, eds. *Theorizing Masculinities*. Thousand Oaks, Calif.: Sage, 1994; Burgess-Jackson, Keith. "The Backlash against Feminist Philosophy." In Anita M. Superson and Ann E. Cudd, eds., *Theorizing Backlash: Philosophical Reflections on the Resistance to Feminism*. Lanham, Md.: Rowman and Littlefield, 2002, 19–47; Burgess-Jackson, Keith. *Rape: A Philosophical Investigation*. Aldershot, U.K.: Dartmouth, 1996; Burgess-Jackson, Keith. Review of *Loose Women, Lecherous Men: A Feminist Philosophy of Sex*, by Linda LeMoncheck. *Ethics* 110 (October 1999), 211–14; Burgess-Jackson, Keith, ed. *A Most Detestable Crime: New Philosophical Essays on Rape*. New York: Oxford University Press, 1999; Connell, R. W. *Masculinities*. Berkeley: University of California Press, 1995; Connell, R. W., and G. W. Dowsett, eds. *Rethinking Sex: Social Theory and Sexuality Research*. Philadelphia, Pa.: Temple University Press, 1993; Davion, Victoria. "Rape, Group Responsibility, and Trust." *Hypatia* 10:2 (1995), 153–56; Ehrenreich, Barbara. *The Hearts of Men: American Dreams and the Flight from Commitment*. Garden City, N.Y.: Anchor/Doubleday, 1983; Faludi, Susan. *Stiffed: The Betrayal of the American Man*. New York: Morrow, 1999; Fasteau, Marc Feigen. *The Male Machine*. New York: Dell, 1975; Flood, Michael. (1992) "The Men's Bibliography" (20 September 2004). <mensbiblio.xyonline.net/> [accessed 25 May 2005]; Friedman, Marilyn, and Larry May. "Harming Women as a Group." *Social Theory and Practice* 11:2 (1985), 207–34; Goldrick-Jones, Amanda. *Men Who Believe in Feminism*. Westport, Conn.: Praeger, 2002; Goldstein, Leslie. "Mill, Marx, and Women's Liberation." *Journal of the History of Philosophy* 18 (1980), 319–34; Grady, Kathleen E., Robert Brannon, and Joseph H. Pleck. *The Male Sex Role: A Selected and Annotated Bibliography*. Rockville, Md.: U.S. Department of Health, Education, and Welfare, 1979; Hite, Shere. *The Hite Report on Male Sexuality*. New York: Knopf, 1981; Kimmel, Michael S. "Introduction: Guilty Pleasures—Pornography in Men's Lives." In Michael S. Kimmel, ed., *Men Confront Pornography*. New York: Crown, 1990, 1–22; Kimmel, Michael S., ed. *Men Confront Pornography*. New York: Crown, 1990; Kimmel, Michael, Jeff Hearn, and R. W. Connell, eds. *Handbook on Studies of Men and Masculinities*. Thousand Oaks, Calif.: Sage, 2004; Kimmel, Michael S., and Michael A. Messner, eds. *Men's Lives*, 1st ed. New York: Macmillan, 1989. 2nd ed. (1992) and 3rd ed. (1995), Needham Heights, Mass.: Allyn and Bacon; Komarovsky, Mirra. *Dilemmas of Masculinity: A Study of College Youth*. Lanham, Md.: Rowman and Littlefield, 2004; Kuypers, Joseph A., ed. *Men and Power*. Amherst, N.Y.: Prometheus, 1999; Lucas, John. "Plato's Philosophy of Sex." In E. M. Craink, ed., *'Owls to Athens': Essays on Classical Subjects Presented to Sir Kenneth Dover*. Oxford, U.K.: Oxford University Press, 1990, 223–31. <users.ox.ac.uk/~jrlucas/libeqsor/platsex.html> [accessed 14 October 2004]; Masson, Jeffrey Moussaieff. *A Dark Science: Women, Sexuality, and Psychiatry in the Nineteenth Century*. New York: Farrar, Straus and Giroux, 1986; May, Larry. *The Morality of Groups: Collective Responsibility, Group-Based Harm, and Corporate Rights*. Notre Dame: University of Notre Dame Press, 1987; May, Larry, and Edward Soule. "Sexual Harassment, Rape, and Criminal Sanctions." In Keith Burgess-Jackson, ed., *A Most Detestable Crime: New Philosophical Essays on Rape*. New York: Oxford University Press, 1999, 183–99; May, Larry, and Robert Strikwerda. "Men in Groups: Collective Responsibility for Rape." *Hypatia* 9:2 (1994), 134–51. Reprinted in P&S3 (594–610). Reprinted as "Rape and Collective Responsibility," in Larry May, *Masculinity and Morality*. Ithaca, N.Y.: Cornell University Press, 1998, 79–97. Revised version in Hugh LaFollette, ed., *Ethics in Practice: An Anthology*, 1st ed. Cambridge, Mass.: Blackwell, 1997, 418–28. 2nd ed., 2002, 418–27; May, Larry, and Robert Strikwerda. "Reply to Victoria Davion's Comments on May and Strikwerda." *Hypatia* 10 (Spring 1995), 157–58; May, Larry, and Robert Strikwerda, eds. *Rethinking Masculinity: Philosophical Explorations in Light of Feminism*, 1st ed. Lanham, Md.: Rowman and Littlefield, 1992; May, Larry, Robert Strikwerda, and Patrick D. Hopkins, eds. *Rethinking Masculinity: Philosophical Explorations in Light of Feminism*, 2nd ed. Lanham, Md.: Rowman and Littlefield, 1996; Messner, Michael A. *Politics of Masculinities: Men in Movements*. Lanham, Md.: AltaMira, 1997; Murphy, Peter F., ed. *Feminism and Masculinities*. New York: Oxford University Press, 2004; Okin, Susan Moller. "John Stuart Mill's Feminism: *The Subjection of Women* and the Improvement of Mankind." *New Zealand Journal of History* 7:2 (1973), 105–27; Okin, Susan Moller. "Plato" and "John Stuart Mill, Liberal Feminist." In *Women in Western Political Thought*. Princeton, N.J.: Princeton University Press, 1979, 15–70, 197–230; Pleck,

Joseph H. *The Myth of Masculinity*. Cambridge, Mass.: MIT Press, 1981; Pronger, Brian. "On Your Knees: Carnal Knowledge, Masculine Dissolution, Doing Feminism." In Tom Digby, ed., *Men Doing Feminism*. New York: Routledge, 1998, 69–79; Richards, David A. J. *Women, Gays, and the Constitution: The Grounds for Feminism and Gay Rights in Culture and Law*. Chicago, Ill.: University of Chicago Press, 1998; Roszak, Betty, and Theodore Roszak, eds. "Some Male Allies." Section of *Masculine/Feminine: Readings in Sexual Mythology and the Liberation of Women*. New York: Harper and Row, 1969, 51–104; Schulhofer, Stephen J. *Unwanted Sex: The Culture of Intimidation and the Failure of Law*. Cambridge, Mass.: Harvard University Press, 1998; Shanley, Mary Lyndon. "Marital Slavery and Friendship: John Stuart Mill's *The Subjection of Women*." *Political Theory* 9:2 (1981), 229–47. Reprinted in Mary Lyndon Shanley and Carole Pateman, eds., *Feminist Interpretations and Political Theory*. University Park: Pennsylvania State University Press, 1991, 164–80; Soble, Alan. "Male and Female Sexuality in Capitalism." In *Pornography: Marxism, Feminism, and the Future of Sexuality*. New Haven, Conn.: Yale University Press, 1986, 55–102; Soble, Alan. "Masturbation." *Pacific Philosophical Quarterly* 61:3 (1980), 233–44. Reprinted in HS (139–50). Revised as "Masturbation and Sexual Philosophy," POS2 (133–57). Revised again as "Masturbation," POS3 (67–85) and reprinted in David Benatar, ed., *Ethics for Everyday*. New York: McGraw-Hill, 2002, 180–96. Revised again as "Masturbation: Conceptual and Ethical Matters," POS4 (67–94); reprinted, abridged, as "Philosophies of Masturbation," in Martha Cornog, author and ed., *The Big Book of Masturbation: From Angst to Zeal*. San Francisco, Calif.: Down There Press, 2003, 149–66; Soble, Alan. "Men's Liberation." In *Sexual Investigations*. New York: New York University Press, 1996, 93–99; Soble, Alan. Review of *Loose Women, Lecherous Men: A Feminist Philosophy of Sex*, by Linda LeMoncheck. *Teaching Philosophy* 22:2 (1999), 411–16; Stoltenberg, John. "Refusing to Be a Man." In Jon Snodgrass, ed., *For Men against Sexism: A Book of Readings*. Albion, Calif.: Times Change Press, 1977, 36–40; Stove, David. "The Subjection of John Stuart Mill." *Philosophy* 68 (1993), 5–13; Strikwerda, Robert A., and Larry May. "Male Friendship and Intimacy." In Larry May and Robert Strikwerda, eds., *Rethinking Masculinity: Philosophical Explorations in Light of Feminism*, 1st ed. Lanham, Md.: Rowman and Littlefield, 1992, 95–110; and Larry May, Robert Strikwerda, and Patrick D. Hopkins, eds., *Rethinking Masculinity: Philosophical Explorations in Light of Feminism*, 2nd ed. Lanham, Md.: Rowman and Littlefield, 1996, 79–94; Superson, Anita M., and Ann E. Cudd, eds. *Theorizing Backlash: Philosophical Reflections on the Resistance to Feminism*. Lanham, Md.: Rowman and Littlefield, 2002; Tewksbury, Richard. "Male Strippers: Men Objectifying Men." In Christine L. Williams, ed., *Doing "Women's Work": Men in Nontraditional Occupations*. Newbury Park, Calif.: Sage, 1993, 168–81; Tuana, Nancy, William Cowling, Maurice Hamington, Greg Johnson, and Terrance MacMullan, eds. *Revealing Male Bodies*. Bloomington: Indiana University Press, 2003; Tucker, Scott. "Gender, Fucking, and Utopia: An Essay in Response to John Stoltenberg's *Refusing to Be a Man*." *Social Text*, no. 27 (1990), 3–34; Williams, Christine L., ed. *Doing "Women's Work": Men in Nontraditional Occupations*. Newbury Park, Calif.: Sage, 1993; Zilbergeld, Bernie. *The New Male Sexuality*. New York: Bantam, 1992.

FICHTE, JOHANN GOTTLIEB (1762–1814).

Johann Gottlieb Fichte, born to poor Saxon artisans, attended the University of Leipzig until his inattention to studies and apparently loose personal behavior cost him his scholarship in 1784, prior to completing his studies. He became a private tutor. Fichte first encountered the philosophy of **Immanuel Kant** (1724–1804) in 1790 through the study of his *Critique of Practical Reason* and traveled to Königsberg the next year to meet him. At Kant's suggestion, Fichte's *Attempt at a Critique of All Revelation* (1792) was published—inadvertently without the author's name—and a reviewer believed it was Kant's work. Kant's public correction of this error thrust Fichte into the forefront of post-Kantian German philosophy. (A full discussion of Fichte's early career can be found in La Vopa. For a summary, see Heinrich, 178–84.)

Securing a teaching appointment at Jena (after marriage in 1793), Fichte published his magnum opus, the *Wissenschaftslehre* (*The Science of Knowledge*; [*WL*]), in 1794. After a controversy over his supposed atheism (La Vopa, 368–424), Fichte in 1799 moved from Jena to Berlin, where his speculative system underwent a dramatic shift—partly in response to the philosophies of F.W.J. Schelling (1775–1854) and **G.W.F. Hegel** (1770–1831)—away from its earlier Kantianism toward an idealist version of Spinozism (Vater, 192, 195–96; Wright, 104), while his influence on the German philosophical scene steadily declined (Neuhouser, *Fichte's Theory*, 7–8). Fichte also exhibited an increasing interest during the Napoleonic era in German nationalism, in the rise of which he played a seminal role (see De Pascale; Engelbrecht). This interest can be seen in such later works as *Addresses to the German Nation* (1808). While an idealistic concern with intersubjectivity (or "interpersonality"), paired with a broadly Romantic notion of **love** (*Liebe*), runs throughout many of his later writings (see Gerten; Hunter), it is his discussion of sex, gender roles, and **marriage** in his *Grundlage des Naturrechts nach Principien der Wissenschaftslehre* (*Foundations of Natural Right*; [*GL*])—a discussion "largely ignored, perhaps for the reason that it is so odd" (Morrison, 179)—and its foundation in the first edition of *Wissenschaftslehre* that concern us here.

Fichte's philosophy of sex and marriage is deeply rooted in the idealistic "ontology of the human person" (Baumanns, 39) found in the *Wissenschaftslehre*. Against the transcendental idealism of Kant's *Critique of Pure Reason*, which firmly distinguished the independently existing object of knowledge (the "thing-in-itself"; *noumena*) from its appearance in consciousness (*phenomena*), Fichte argued that such an ontological divide could never be bridged, nor could it be made compatible with the ideal of radical freedom found in Kant's *Critique of Practical Reason*. In its place, Fichte proposed a monistic metaphysics in which the distinction between subject and object can be grounded in a more profound metaphysical unity. This ground of all Being, Fichte claimed, is nothing other than the "I" in its pure, self-positing activity (*WL*, 97), which both produces and transcends the subject-object distinction involved in all knowledge:

> We have unified the opposing self and not-self through the concept of divisibility. If we abstract from the specific content of the self and not-self . . . we obtain the logical proposition known hitherto as the *grounding* principle: A in part = ~ A, and vice versa. Every opposite is like its opponent in one respect, = X; and every like is opposed to its like in one respect, = X. Such a respect, = X, is called the ground, in the first case, of *conjunction*, and in the second of *distinction*. (*WL*, 110)

Scholars are still divided over the exact status of the external world in Fichte's system and the degree to which his system tends toward solipsism (see Breazeale; Findlay, 47–52; Neuhouser, *Fichte's Theory*, 66–116; Williams). These are interesting questions, but more important for grasping Fichte on sexuality is that "enunciated in this paragraph are what become two of the basic principles of German idealism: There is no distinction without a prior unity; no unity without a prior distinction" (Seidel, *Fichte's Wissenschaftslehre*, 70).

The implications of Fichte's metaphysics for understanding human sexuality are profound, and profoundly un-Kantian. For Kant, sex was ethically problematical; people experiencing **sexual desire** or engaged in **sexual activity** treated each other—autonomous and rational subjects—merely as means for their own sensual, bodily, gratification. The humanity of both parties is thereby demeaned (Kant, "Duties"; see Soble). Fichte, however, makes the biological complementarity and mutual desire of the sexes not a moral problem but a metaphysical necessity:

If nature were to be possible, the species had to have some organic existence other than its existence as a species; but it also had to exist as a species, so as to be able to reproduce itself. In order for this to be possible, the species-forming power had to be divided up and split into two perfectly matching halves, as it were, whose union alone would constitute a self-reproducing whole. (*GL*, 265)

The biological differences between the sexes thus become the epitome of Fichtean metaphysics. George Seidel expresses this theme very nicely (*Fichte's Wissenschaftslehre*, 74): "Difference always includes sameness. There can be a marital union or romantic love between a man and a woman because both alike are human beings. Nevertheless, the sameness also includes difference: although both the man and the woman are human beings, there is a difference between the two. *Vive la difference!*"

In determining this essential difference between the sexes, Fichte relies on a version of **Aristotle**'s (384–322 BCE) biology, wherein men are the "formal" cause of reproduction and women merely the "material" cause (*De generatione animalium*, I.20, 724a–729a; see Baker and Elliston, 24). Fichte writes: "The specific determination of this natural arrangement is that, in the satisfaction of the sexual drive or in the promotion of nature's end (in the actual act of procreation), the one sex is entirely active, the other entirely passive" (*GL*, 266). This passivity stands in stark contrast to Kant's insistence on the exclusive role of reason in constituting human nature: "The character of reason is absolute self-activity; mere passivity for its own sake contradicts reason and completely annuls it" (*GL*, 266).

This conflict between the (supposed) biological, sexual function of women and their rational nature as human beings admits three possible solutions:

Thus, either the second sex (even its potential) is non-rational, which contradicts our presupposition (namely, that they are supposed to be human beings); or else this potential, because of its peculiar nature, cannot be developed, which is self-contradictory . . . ; or finally, the second sex can never have the satisfaction of the sexual drive as an end. Reason and such an end completely annul each other. (*GL*, 266)

Since women are by nature both rational agents and passive recipients of a man's (active) sexual desire, Fichte is forced to redirect a woman's sexual *telos* away from reproduction, where she is merely a recipient, and toward romantic love, where she makes the possession and satisfaction of a man the end of her agency: "Her only need is to love and be loved. It is only in this way that the drive to surrender oneself acquires the character of freedom and activity, which it must have in order to be able to co-exist with reason. . . . This is also why, in sexual union, the woman is not in every sense a means for the man's end; she is the means for her own end, that of satisfying her heart" (*GL*, 269–70).

The institution of marriage, Fichte argues, is by nature (*GL*, 274) the only appropriate context for sexual activity (agreeing with Kant, but for different reasons), since it forces men to develop emotional bonds that can "ennoble" (*GL*, 284) the sexual drive while at the same time allowing women to cultivate the sort of exclusive relationship that is the presupposition of romantic love. In its absence, men behave as animals, driven solely by desire, while women are treated as the nonrational objects of male lust. Only within marriage, Fichte claims, is there "an external drive towards virtue. . . . There is no moral education of humankind, if it does not begin from this point" (*GL*, 273). Indeed, marriage constitutes the supreme human relationship since it reveals in its purest form the essentially social character (conceived ethically, not psychosocially; see Düsing) of human personality. He concludes, "The marriage relation is the most genuine mode of existence, as required by nature, for adult human beings of both sexes. It is only in this relation that all of the human faculties can develop" (*GL*, 274).

Fichte's vision of marriage and of the proper social roles for both sexes is quite foreign to modern, egalitarian sensibilities, unevenly combining, as it does, "the old theory of the natural inferiority of women with the Enlightenment's belief in the equality of men and women as essentially rational beings" (Heinz, 63). Since the rational fulfillment of woman comes in her complete loving submission to a man, Fichte argues that she naturally and properly surrenders all her rights to her husband. From the time of marriage, "the state from now on ceases to regard the wife as a juridically distinct person" (*GL*, 282). This dependence automatically disenfranchises her and bars her from public office (*GL*, 302). Fichte's subsequent discussion of marital right and the proper domestic arrangements within marriage shows no noticeable improvement in his view of women.

His willingness to collapse the woman's individuality into her husband's for the sake of her moral perfection arises in part from Fichte's distinction between morality and right (which roughly corresponds to Kant's distinction in the *Metaphysics of Morals* between the *Tugendlehre* and the *Rechtslehre*), that is, between the description of acts appropriate for individuals *qua* radically free rational agents (morality) and those choices that must be open to individuals *qua* self-determined, socially situated beings (rights). For Fichte, "rights, and the laws that safeguard them, concern only public life. These laws serve to keep the operation of individual wills from coming into conflict with each" (Morrison, 187). Thus, the moral end pursued by a rational being in marriage, such as the elevation of a woman through her free act of loving self-surrender, need not be matched by her legal rights—for example, the right to own and dispose of property—nor must the latter be deducible from the former. (For more on this distinction, see Neuhouser, "Fichte and the Relationship between Right and Morality.")

Since the moral end of marriage demands that it be entered into freely (*GL*, 275), the state does have a duty to regulate this institution and other family arrangements so as to ensure, as best it can, that women are not coerced into marriages against their will (*GL*, 274–78). This obligation extends to children not yet having reached the age of reason. Fichte argues that, beyond this concern, the state has no legitimate power to prohibit incestuous unions; they are obviously not prevented by nature and, in any case, they affect only households and not public order (*GL*, 279). Nor can the state licitly regulate the course of individual marriages since (he somewhat naively but consistently reasons, in a manner similar to Kant) "the two are one soul, and so the assumption is that they will not be at odds with one another or take each other to court, any more than a single individual would take himself to court" (*GL*, 281). Accordingly, Fichte places the question of nonmarital sex, and presumably also of sexual practices such as **homosexuality**, **bestiality**, and **masturbation**, largely outside the sphere of the law and within the moral or private realm. (For a discussion of the background and development of Fichte's political thought, see Perrinjaquet; Radrizzani; Schottky.) This libertarian attitude, as regards right, if not morality, extends also to **prostitution** and **adultery**, which the state should neither prohibit nor punish (*GL*, 287). However, Fichte curiously concedes that professional prostitutes can justly be expelled from the borders of the state due to insanity, if they admit to such a shameful profession, or due to vagrancy, if they refuse to disclose their source of income (*GL*, 289–90). Here Daniel Morrison's comment (see above) about the oddity of Fichte's philosophy of sex seems particularly apposite.

It is tempting, from the perspective of the twenty-first century, to dismiss Fichte's arguments and views about women, marriage, and sex as nothing more than justifications (or rationalizations) of the bourgeois, patriarchal morality of his era (La Vopa, 173). One need only consider his excusing men's adultery but not women's (*GL*, 284), a traditional piece of the sexual double standard; his specifying motherhood as a woman's primary and natural task (*GL*, 312); and his suggestion that women are naturally unsuited for abstract intellectual tasks (*GL*, 304). But Fichte's project is something more than male chauvinism (though it is that, at least in part). As Seidel points out, "Fichte is not entirely chauvinistic, for there is a surprising feminization of love in Fichte, even on the masculine side of romantic love. The element of surrender is not simply found in the role of the female" (*Knowledge*, 134). Further, Fichte's philosophy is not merely a biologically retrograde Aristotelianism, in which (as always happens in such systems) "procreation demands the sacrifice of women's humanity to their femininity" (Baker and Elliston, 27). Rather, Fichte attempts to situate human biology and human personality within a social framework that allows them to coexist, and to do so in such a way that the good of the species (survival through reproduction) neither entirely sacrifices nor is sacrificed to the free activity of rational agents, and in a manner that is compatible with the moral perfection of both partners in a marriage. "Individuals are not complete creatures [for Fichte]; neither male nor female is fully human. Each sex is a partial creature and each becomes most fully human only in marriage. . . . Nature split the species into two halves for more orderly procreation. And nature overcomes this split in marriage" (Morrison, 189). One cannot help notice here a theme from **Plato**'s (427–347 BCE) *Symposium*, the myth of Aristophanes (190e–193a), which can be found in Hegel, too.

Whether traditional, monogamous marriage constitutes the only social institution that can make possible the complete realization of human personality (an assumption that often underlies contemporary arguments for **same-sex marriage**) and whether the moral ends of marriage can be neatly separated from the legal rights of its contractors (the crux of much contemporary feminist social theory) are much debated questions. However, while Fichte's often reactionary attitude toward the ends and proper social outlets for the sexual impulse has seriously limited his influence on contemporary philosophical debates, his account of the person as both essentially rational and at the same time embodied and socially situated has attracted more than passing interest among contemporary philosophers (Heinz; Schell). This effort to connect human sexuality with the full development of the person, refusing to relegate it to a sinful or animal aspect of otherwise rational human existence, by itself makes Fichte's writings interesting for more than historical reasons.

See also Aristotle; Casual Sex; Dworkin, Andrea; Evolution; Existentialism; Feminism, French; Feminism, History of; Feminism, Lesbian; Feminism, Liberal; Feminism, Men's; Hegel, G.W.F.; Incest; Law, Sex and the; Liberalism; Marxism; Objectification, Sexual; Personification, Sexual; Phenomenology; Privacy; Schopenhauer, Arthur; Spinoza, Baruch; Westermarck, Edward

REFERENCES

Note: Volume numbers and inclusive page numbers, but not year dates, are provided for essays published in *Fichte-Studien*. Year dates are irregular. Aristotle. (ca. 340 BCE?) *De Partibus animalium* I and *De Generatione Animalium* I. Trans. David M. Balme. Oxford, U.K.: Clarendon Press, 1992; Baker, Robert B., and Frederick A. Elliston. "Introduction." In Robert B. Baker and Frederick A. Elliston, eds., *Philosophy and Sex*, 2nd ed. Buffalo, N.Y.: Prometheus, 1984, 11–36; Baumanns, Peter. *Fichtes ursprüngliches System: Sein Standort zwischen Kant und Hegel.* Stuttgart-Bad Cannstatt: Frommann-Holzboog, 1972; Breazeale, Daniel. "Check or Checkmate? The Finitude of the Fichtean

Self." In Karl Ameriks and Dieter Sturma, eds., *The Modern Subject: Conceptions of the Self in Classical German Philosophy*. Albany: State University of New York Press, 1995, 87–114; De Pascale, Carlo. "Der Primat Deutschlands bei Fichte." *Fichte-Studien* 3, 68–85; Düsing, Edith. "Individuelle und soziale Bildung der Ich-Identität. Fichtes Konzeption im Horizont moderner Alternativen." *Fichte-Studien* 11, 113–32; Engelbrecht, Helmuth Carol. (1933) *Johann Gottlieb Fichte: A Study of His Political Writings with Special Reference to His Nationalism*. New York: AMS Press, 1968; Fichte, Johann Gottlieb. (1808) *Addresses to the German Nation*. Ed. George Armstrong Kelly. Trans. R. F. Jones and G. H. Turnbull. New York: Harper and Row, 1968; Fichte, Johann Gottlieb. (1792) *Attempt at a Critique of All Revelation*. Trans. Garrett Green. Cambridge: Cambridge University Press, 1978; Fichte, Johann Gottlieb. (1797) *Foundations of Natural Right*. Trans. Michael Bauer. Cambridge: Cambridge University Press, 2000; Fichte, Johann Gottlieb. (1794, 1802) *Science of Knowledge with First and Second Introductions*. Trans. and ed. Peter Heath and John Lachs. New York: Appleton-Century-Crofts, 1970. Reprinted, corrected, as *The Science of Knowledge*. Cambridge: Cambridge University Press, 1982; Findlay, J. N. *Hegel: A Re-Examination*. New York: Collier, 1962; Gerten, Michael. "Das Verhältnis von Wissen, Moralität, und Liebe. Zum Philosophiebegriff des späten Fichte." *Fichte-Studien* 17, 299–318; Heinrich, Dieter. *Between Kant and Hegel: Lectures on German Idealism*. Ed. David S. Pacini. Cambridge, Mass.: Harvard University Press, 2003; Heinz, Marion. "Liebe und Ehe: Untersuchungen zu Fichtes Eherecht." *Fichte-Studien* 18, 49–63; Hunter, C. K. "The Problem of Fichte's Phenomenology of Love." *Idealistic Studies* 6:2 (1976), 178–90; Kant, Immanuel. (1788) *Critique of Practical Reason*. Trans. Mary Gregor. Cambridge: Cambridge University Press, 1997; Kant, Immanuel. (1781, 1787) *Critique of Pure Reason*. Trans. Lewis White Beck. Indianapolis, Ind.: Bobbs-Merrill, 1956; Kant, Immanuel. (ca. 1780) "Duties towards the Body in Respect of Sexual Impulse." In *Lectures on Ethics*. Trans. Louis Infield. Indianapolis, Ind.: Hackett, 1980, 162–71; Kant, Immanuel. (1797–1798) *The Metaphysics of Morals*. Trans. Mary Gregor. Cambridge: Cambridge University Press, 1991, 1996; La Vopa, Anthony J. *Fichte: The Self and the Calling of Philosophy, 1762–1799*. Cambridge: Cambridge University Press, 2001; Morrison, Daniel. "Women, Family, and the State in Fichte's Philosophy of Freedom." In Daniel Breazeale and Tom Rockmore, eds., *New Perspectives on Fichte*. Atlantic Highlands, N.J.: Humanities Press, 1996, 179–91; Neuhouser, Frederick. "Fichte and the Relationship between Right and Morality." In Daniel Breazeale and Tom Rockmore, eds., *Fichte: Historical Contexts/Contemporary Controversies*. Atlantic Highlands, N.J.: Humanities Press, 1994, 158–80; Neuhouser, Frederick. *Fichte's Theory of Subjectivity*. Cambridge: Cambridge University Press, 1990; Perrinjaquet, Alain. "Individuum und Gemeinschaft in der W[issenschafts]L[ehre] zwischen 1796 und 1800." *Fichte-Studien* 3, 7–28; Plato. (ca. 380 BCE) *The Symposium*. Trans. Christopher Gill. London: Penguin, 1999; Radrizzani, Ivan. "Fichte's Transcendental Philosophy and Political Praxis." In Daniel Breazeale and Tom Rockmore, eds., *New Perspectives on Fichte*. Atlantic Highlands, N.J.: Humanities Press, 1996, 193–212; Schell, Susan. " 'A Determined Stand': Freedom and Security in Fichte's Science of Right." *Polity* 25:1 (1991), 95–122; Schottky, Richard. "Staatliche Souveränität und individuelle Freiheit bei Rousseau, Kant und Fichte." *Fichte-Studien* 7, 119–42; Seidel, George J. *Fichte's Wissenschaftslehre of 1794: A Commentary on Part 1*. West Lafayette, Ind.: Purdue University Press, 1993; Seidel, George J. *Knowledge as Sexual Metaphor*. London: Associated University Presses, 2000; Soble, Alan. "Sexual Use and What to Do about It: Internalist and Externalist Sexual Ethics." *Essays in Philosophy* 2:2 (2001). <www.humboldt.edu/~essays/soble.html> [accessed 31 January 2005]; Vater, Michael G. "The *Wissenschaftslehre* of 1801–1802." In Daniel Breazeale and Tom Rockmore, eds., *Fichte: Historical Contexts/Contemporary Controversies*. Atlantic Highlands, N.J.: Humanities Press, 1994, 191–210; Williams, Robert R. "The Question of the Other in Fichte's Thought." In Daniel Breazeale and Tom Rockmore, eds., *Fichte: Historical Contexts/Contemporary Controversies*. Atlantic Highlands, N.J.: Humanities Press, 1994, 142–57; Wright, Walter E. "Reading the 1804 *Wissenschaftslehre*." In Daniel Breazeale and Tom Rockmore, eds., *New Perspectives on Fichte*. Atlantic Highlands, N.J.: Humanities Press, 1996, 95–106.

Lance Byron Richey

ADDITIONAL READING

Baker, Robert B., and Frederick A. Elliston. "Introduction." In Robert B. Baker and Frederick A. Elliston, eds., *Philosophy and Sex*, 1st ed. Buffalo, N.Y.: Prometheus, 1975, 1–28. Reprinted in P&S2 (11–36); P&S3 (17–40); Breazeale, Daniel, and Tom Rockmore, eds. *Fichte: Historical Contexts/Contemporary Controversies*. Atlantic Highlands, N.J.: Humanities Press, 1994; Breazeale, Daniel, and Tom Rockmore, eds. *New Perspectives on Fichte*. Atlantic Highlands, N.J.: Humanities Press, 1996; Fichte, Johann Gottlieb. *Fichte: Early Philosophical Writings*. Trans. Daniel Breazeale. Ithaca, N.Y.: Cornell University Press, 1988. Corrected paperback ed., 1993; Fichte, Johann Gottlieb. *J. G. Fichte-Gesamtausgabe der Bayerischen Akademie der Wissenschaften*. Ed. Reinhard Lauth, Hans Jacob, and Hans Gliwitzky. 34 vols. Stuttgart-Bad Cannstatt: Frommann-Holzboog, 1966– ; Hohler, T. P. "Fichte and the Problem of Finitude." *Southwestern Journal of Philosophy* 7:3 (1976), 15–33; Kant, Immanuel. (ca. 1780) "Duties towards the Body in Respect of Sexual Impulse." In *Lectures on Ethics*. Trans. Louis Infield. New York: Methuen, 1930. Indianapolis, Ind.: Hackett, 1980, 162–71. Reprinted in POS4 (199–205); STW (140–45); Kelly, George Armstrong. *Idealism, Politics, and History: Sources of Hegelian Thought*. Cambridge: Cambridge University Press, 1969; Lauth, Reinhard. "Le problème de l'interpersonalité chez J. G. Fichte." *Archives de Philosophie* 25 (1962), 325–44; Philonenko, Alexis. *La liberté humaine dans la philosophie de Fichte*. Paris: Vrin, 1966; Soble, Alan. "Sexual Use and What to Do about It: Internalist and Externalist Sexual Ethics." *Essays in Philosophy* 2:2 (2001). <www.humboldt.edu/~essays/soble.html> [accessed 31 January 2005]. Reprinted, revised, in POS4 (225–58); Turnbull, G. H. *The Educational Theory of J. G. Fichte: A Critical Account, Together with Translations*. London: University Press of Liverpool, 1926.

FINNIS, JOHN. *See* Natural Law (New)

FIRESTONE, SHULAMITH (1945–). Born into an Orthodox Jewish family in Ottawa, Shulamith Firestone attended the Art Institute of Chicago in the 1960s, where she was active in socialist Zionist politics and Students for a Democratic Society. Disillusioned with the New Left's failure to take women's issues seriously, she moved to New York City and became one of the most visible and outspoken figures in Second Wave American radical **feminism**. In 1967 she co-organized New York Radical Women, the city's first women's liberation group. Two years later she and Ellen Willis founded Redstockings and later, with Anne Koedt, the New York Radical Feminists. Firestone and Koedt assembled and edited the first substantial collections of radical feminist writings: *Notes from the First Year* (New York Radical Feminists, 1968), followed by, in 1970, *Notes from the Second Year* and, in 1971, *Notes from the Third Year* (Koedt et al., 1973).

Firestone is known for her remarkably brave, utopian, and frequently demonized manifesto *The Dialectic of Sex* (1970). *Dialectic* is an ambitious effort to synthesize Simone de Beauvoir's (1908–1986) sexual politics with **Sigmund Freud**'s (1856–1939) psychoanalysis and Karl Marx's (1818–1883) historical materialism to explain the persistence of patriarchy and develop a theory of feminist revolution. Following Beauvoir, Firestone argues that the material basis for women's oppression initially sprang from the reproductive differences between the sexes: Because women have the burden of carrying children, they were dependent on men for resources and protection. Shifting Marx's historical materialist method from economic class to "sex class," she argues that reproductive, rather than productive, relations are the primary forces driving history. Sex class, the division of society into two distinct biological classes for the purpose of reproduction, rather than economic class, is the master template for all social inequality. But Firestone is not a strict biological determinist. Reproductive biology might distinguish the sexes, but the socially constructed "sex-class system" reinforces and exaggerates the distinction through the family and the sexual division of labor.

Firestone is critical of the patriarchal family as a biological unit. Her analysis begins with a Freudian premise: The development of feminine behavior in girls and masculine behavior in boys is a result of children's perception of sexual differences between their parents. Unlike Freud, she analyzes these differences in political, not anatomical, terms. The Oedipus and Electra complexes, castration anxiety, and penis envy "can only make full sense in terms of power" (*Dialectic*, 47). Thus, on Firestone's reading of Freud, it is not the male organ that young girls envy; it is the privilege that accompanies it. For Firestone, childhood in general is a modern invention (see also Ariès; compare Acocella) that foments inequality by keeping children under the parental jurisdiction of the biological family for long periods of time.

Firestone's power-focused, gender-sensitive modifications of Freud and Marx naturally led her to challenge conventional assumptions about the family, childhood, sexuality, and romantic **love**. None of these institutions is free from the influence of the patriarchal biological family. The **incest** taboo, central to Freud's discussion of the development of male and female gender roles, is just an elaborate way of preserving power relations between father and mother and between parents and children. The sexual prohibitions against female sexual infidelity and **homosexuality** that result from the incest taboo exist because they suit the patriarchal need to control sexuality in ways that promote male dominance. In particular, homosexuals are in our present culture the "extreme casualties of the system of obstructed sexuality that develops in the family." Once the incest taboo is lifted a "healthy transexuality will be the norm" (*Dialectic*, 58).

Love between persons is, ideally, a mutual exchange of selves. The power imbalance of the sex-class system makes the mutual vulnerability needed for equal exchange between women and men impossible. Love and **marriage** have different meanings for men and women. To justify his descent into a lower caste, a man idealizes one woman above all others (*Dialectic*, 131–32). Men have difficulty loving because they fall in love with this idealized version. She is chosen because she most closely meets his needs for the ideal mother, housekeeper, cook, and companion. Women know the idealization they work hard to maintain is a lie. But this inauthenticity is necessary as long as women continue to be socially, economically, and psychologically dependent on men. Romantic love, then, is love corrupted by the sex-class system. A steady cultural diet of romance and the social pressure to be sexy and beautiful prevent women from seeing the real conditions of their sex class, so romanticism "is a cultural tool of male power" (*Dialectic*, 147). By focusing women's attention on male approval rather than their own desires and well-being, the culture of romance obscures the causes of women's oppression.

Because Firestone is not a strict biological determinist, on her view the biological providence of women's history need not shape their future. Nature produced the fundamental inequality between male and female, but a feminist cybernetic socialist revolution will liberate women and children by destroying the patriarchal family and the social and sexual order that supports it. Firestone's revolution goes deeper than modest liberal reforms to the sex/gender system. If basic differences in reproductive labor are the source of oppression, the revolution must be both biological and social. It will require elimination of "the sex *distinction* itself " so that "genital differences between human beings no longer matter" (*Dialectic*, 11). To accomplish this, Firestone advocates the abolition of the family, the automation of wage labor and household chores, and the technological liberation of women from their reproductive roles. Abolishing biologically based family units will end the incest taboo. With parent-child incest restrictions gone, the structures that narrowly mold sexuality into socially acceptable patterns will disappear, and women, children, and men will delight in an unlimited range of erotic behaviors. "Polymorphous perversity" (59) will eventually erode the strict division between masculine and feminine behaviors and, in time, people will pick and choose the gender traits that best suit them. A wide variety of androgynous expression awaits. The liberation of women and children also requires the extension of legal, sexual, and economic rights to children (239).

For the revolution to be complete, women must be liberated from their reproductive biology. Just as the elimination of economic class requires that workers revolt and seize control of the means of production, so women, as a sex class, must revolt and seize control of the means of reproduction (*Dialectic*, 206). Here Firestone proposes reliable **contraception**, kibbutz-style group parenting, and especially extrauterine gestation. Marge Piercy's novel *Woman on the Edge of Time* (1970) is an engaging fictionalized account of Firestone's utopia. (Extrauterine gestation had also been imagined less benignly in 1932 by Aldous Huxley [1894–1963] in *Brave New World*.)

Firestone's critics have almost univocally directed their comments at her condemnation of biological motherhood. For Elizabeth Spelman, Firestone's utopian solutions are oddly in step with Western patriarchal thinking. Firestone's description of pregnancy as deforming, painful, and barbaric, and her endorsement of artificial reproduction, frame liberatory projects so that dissociation from female bodily processes, and even heterosexual coitus itself, is the most direct route to women's freedom. (The confining effects of intercourse on women's sexual expression, and its role in the oppression of women, are explored in **Andrea Dworkin**'s [1946–2005] *Intercourse*.) Spelman coins the term "somatophobia," fear of and disdain for the body, to describe the philosophical tradition that privileges minds over bodies and culturally associates the body with all things feminine, female, or primitive (126–31).

Cultural feminists, who premise that women should reclaim all that is female or associated with "the feminine" as a source of power and celebration, wish Firestone had been more mindful about abandoning one of the few historic sources of women's power, *viz.*, their role in childbearing and child rearing. Adrienne Rich, for example, supports Firestone's account of how pernicious biological motherhood is under patriarchy but faults her for focusing on motherhood as a biological experience rather than a patriarchal institution. Nothing is inherently oppressive about pregnancy, childbirth, and child rearing. These practices become politically suspect only when obstetrics, gynecology, and child-rearing advice become the province of male experts and when women tie their sense of self exclusively to the sacrifices they make as mothers. Patriarchal expectations prevent women from reimagining the pains and pleasures of mothering in their own terms (174).

For Dworkin and Gena Corea, the shift from womb to laboratory is suspiciously in keeping with the pathologization and managed medical regulation of women's bodies. Dworkin claims that the methods used by infertility experts are a patriarchal attempt both to regulate the quality of children men are supposed to want and to alienate further women from their reproductive labor (*Right-wing Women*, 187–88). Corea is distrustful of the promises that egg and sperm donation, *in vitro* fertilization, and embryo transplant make to potential mothers and claims that male control of these technologies will be used to disempower women further (107–20).

Conservatives and moderate feminists have used Firestone's manifesto as convenient proof of the madness and impracticality of radical feminism. But to dismiss *Dialectic* as dated or naive is to forget the spirit of the era in which it was written. Firestone was shamelessly willing to dream, speculate, and make mistakes. For all its oversights, *Dialectic* is a fertile volume. Although not formally acknowledged, Firestone's revision of historical materialism most certainly provided inspiration for Nancy Hartsock's feminist standpoint theory. Firestone was one of the earliest thinkers to draw on Freud as a feminist resource. Her ability to see the liberatory potential of the reproductive technologies of her day foreshadows both the hopes and fears feminist bioethicists address today. Her attack on motherhood helped catalyze a lengthy philosophical debate. And her observations on the sexual politics of romance and the **beauty** culture remain salient. Firestone's *Dialectic* is valuable for the conversations she began.

See also Beauty; Dworkin, Andrea; Feminism, Lesbian; Freud, Sigmund; Freudian Left, The; Lacan, Jacques; MacKinnon, Catharine; Marxism; Reproductive Technology; Utopianism

REFERENCES

Acocella, Joan. "Little People." *The New Yorker* (18 and 25 August 2003), 138–42; Ariès, Philippe. *Centuries of Childhood: A Social History of Family Life*. Trans. Robert Baldick. New York: Knopf, 1962; Corea, Gena. *The Mother Machine: Reproduction Technologies from Artificial Insemination to Artificial Wombs*. New York: Harper and Row, 1985; Dworkin, Andrea. *Intercourse*. New York: Free Press, 1987; Dworkin, Andrea. *Right-wing Women*. New York: Coward-McCann, 1983; Firestone, Shulamith. *The Dialectic of Sex: The Case for Feminist Revolution*. New York: Bantam Books, 1970; Firestone, Shulamith, and Ellen Willis. (1969) "Redstockings Manifesto." In Miriam Schneir, ed., *Feminism in Our Time: The Essential Writings, World War II to the Present*. New York: Vintage Books, 1994, 125–29; Garner, Karen. "Shulamith Firestone." In Jennifer Scanlon, ed., *Significant Contemporary American Feminists: A Biographical Sketchbook*. Westport, Conn.: Greenwood Press, 1999, 98–103; Hartsock, Nancy C. M. "The Feminist Standpoint: Developing the Ground for a Specifically Feminist Historical Materialism." In Sandra Harding and Merrill B. Hintikka, eds., *Discovering Reality: Feminist Perspectives on Epistemology, Metaphysics, Methodology, and Philosophy of Science*. Dordrecht, Holland: Reidel, 1983, 283–311; Huxley, Aldous. (1932) *Brave New World*. New York: Harper Perennial, 1998; Koedt, Anne, Ellen Levine, and Anita Rapone, eds. *Radical Feminism*. New York: Quadrangle Books, 1973. [*Notes from the Second Year* and *Notes from the Third Year*]; New York Radical Women. *Notes from the First Year* (1968). Special Collections Library, Duke University. <scriptorium.lib.duke.edu/wlm/notes/> [accessed 18 November 2004]; Piercy, Marge. *Woman on the Edge of Time*. New York: Ballantine, 1997; Rich, Adrienne C. *Of Woman Born: Motherhood as Experience and Institution*. New York: Norton, 1995; Snitow, Anne. "Returning to the Well." [Review of *The Dialectic of Sex: The Case for Feminist Revolution*, by Shulamith Firestone] *Dissent* 41 (Fall 1994), 557–60; Spelman, Elizabeth. *The Inessential Woman: Problems of Exclusion in Feminist Thought*. Boston: Beacon Press, 1988.

Alison Bailey

ADDITIONAL READING

Dinnerstein, Dorothy. *The Mermaid and the Minotaur: Sexual Arrangements and Human Malaise*. New York: Harper and Row, 1976; Douglas, Carol Anne. *Love and Politics: Radical Feminist and Lesbian Theories*. San Francisco, Calif.: ism press, 1990; Echols, Alice. *Daring to Be Bad: Radical Feminism in America 1967–1975*. Minneapolis: University of Minnesota Press, 1989; Engels, Friedrich. *The Origin of the Family, Private Property, and the State*. New York: International Publishers, 1972; Ferguson, Ann. "On Conceiving Motherhood and Sexuality: A Feminist Materialist Approach." In Joyce Trebilcot, ed., *Mothering: Essays in Feminist Theory*. Savage, Md.: Rowman and Littlefield, 1983, 153–84; Firestone, Shulamith. *Airless Spaces (Native Agents)*. New York: Semiotext(e), 1998; Firestone, Shulamith. "Love in a Sexist Society." In Alan Soble, ed., *Eros, Agape, and Philia: Readings in the Philosophy of Love*, 2nd printing. St. Paul, Minn.: Paragon House, 1999,

29–39; Firestone, Shulamith, and Ellen Willis. (1969) "Redstockings Manifesto." In Miriam Schneir, ed., *Feminism in Our Time: The Essential Writings, World War II to the Present*. New York: Vintage Books, 1994, 125–29; and Betty Roszak and Theodore Roszak, eds., *Masculine/Feminine: Readings in Sexual Mythology and the Liberation of Women*. New York: Harper and Row, 1969, 272–74; Francoeur, Robert T. *Utopian Motherhood: New Trends in Human Reproduction*. Garden City, N.Y.: Doubleday, 1970; Hartsock, Nancy C. M. "The Feminist Standpoint: Developing the Ground for a Specifically Feminist Historical Materialism." In Sandra Harding and Merrill B. Hintikka, eds., *Discovering Reality: Feminist Perspectives on Epistemology, Metaphysics, Methodology, and Philosophy of Science*. Dordrecht, Holland: D. Reidel, 1983, 283–311. Reprinted in Nancy Tuana and Rosemarie Tong, eds., *Feminism and Philosophy: Essential Readings in Theory, Reinterpretation, and Application*. Boulder, Colo.: Westview, 1995, 69–90; Hartsock, Nancy C. M. *The Feminist Standpoint Reconsidered*. Boulder, Colo.: Westview, 1997; Hartsock, Nancy C. M. "Gender and Power: Masculinity, Violence, and Domination." In *Money, Sex, and Power: Toward a Feminist Historical Materialism*. New York: Longman, 1983, 155–85; Jaggar, Alison M. *Feminist Politics and Human Nature*. Totowa, N.J.: Rowman and Allanheld, 1983; Jordan, Bill. *Sex, Money, and Power: The Transformation of Collective Lives*. Malden, Mass.: Polity, 2004; Mitchell, Juliet. (1974) "Shulamith Firestone: Freud Feminized." In *Psychoanalysis and Feminism: Freud, Reich, Laing, and Women*. New York: Vintage, 1975, 346–50; O'Brien, Mary. *The Politics of Reproduction*. Boston, Mass.: Routledge and Kegan Paul, 1981; Rapaport, Elizabeth. "On the Future of Love: Rousseau and the Radical Feminists." *Philosophical Forum* 5:1–2 (1973–1974), 185–205. Reprinted in POS1 (369–88); Reed, Evelyn. "Women: Caste, Class, or Oppressed Sex?" In Alison M. Jaggar and Paula S. Rothenberg, eds., *Feminist Frameworks: Alternative Theoretical Accounts of the Relations between Women and Men*, 3rd ed. New York: McGraw-Hill, 1993, 170–73; Ruddick, Sara. *Maternal Thinking: Towards a Feminist Politics of Peace*. New York: Ballantine, 1989; Tong, Rosemarie. *Feminist Thought: A More Comprehensive Introduction*, 2nd ed. Boulder, Colo.: Westview, 1998; Trebilcot, Joyce, ed. *Mothering: Essays in Feminist Theory*. Savage, Md.: Rowman and Littlefield, 1983; Wajcman, Judy. *Technofeminism*. Malden, Mass.: Polity, 2004.

FLIRTING. Flirting is playful, yet a person can be said to flirt with disaster. It is allegedly semiserious but still might court danger. It is sexual and yet is not sex. It might be a prelude to **sexual activity** or an alternative to it. Flirting is thus essentially ambiguous. Therein may perhaps lie part of its morally problematic character.

Flirting is not sex, but it is sexualized behavior. Certainly someone has reason to resent his or her partner's flirting with another person, even if assured it was going nowhere. To flirt is best defined as engaging in behavior designed to arouse a sexual interest in another but not by means of unambiguous acts such as coitus and other physical intimacies. Flirtation proceeds subtly by looks, gestures, and words. These need not be sexually explicit. Indeed, the charm of flirtation consists in its uncertainty and ambiguity. Is she smiling because she finds me funny or because she finds me sexually attractive? Was his action in brushing lint from my coat that of a compulsive cleaner or a prospective lover? The flirt need not be sexually interested in the other, though he or she might be. Thus the flirt might intend to arouse a sexual interest that the flirt has no intention or wish to reciprocate. This is the allegedly morally irresponsible behavior of the coquette.

There is in much human sexual interaction an intriguing, mutually reinforcing interplay of sexual interest that is confirmed by psychological research. It is marvelously evoked in **Thomas Nagel**'s description of the escalating arousal of **sexual desire** between a man who observes a woman who in turn notices that she is being observed, the man in turn noticing that she notices his observing her, and so on. One of the points of this interaction is that rather than being attracted to another merely by virtue of their appearance, we are sexually interested in someone who is interested in us, and they are, in turn, interested in us because we are interested in them. Flirting can obviously play a role in this sophisticated interaction. At the same time, however, we should note that sexual interest can be aroused by the quite opposite strategy of consciously studied indifference (see Moulton, 537). Sometimes nothing is more challenging, and hence stimulating, than a person's showing no interest. But although indifference might be designed to arouse sexual interest, it would probably be an overextension of the word to call it flirting.

A range of behaviors, both verbal and nonverbal, comprise flirtation. Observers of human (and nonhuman) courtship are fond of documenting in great detail the many actions that constitute displays of sexual interest and sexual invitations. These include licking the lips, tilting the head, arching a leg, smiling, quick glances, firmly holding the other's eyes, and a brief touch—or a slightly too long handshake. Women who engage in these behaviors in dating contexts (e.g., a singles' bar) are apparently successful in soliciting interest from men: invitations to dance, initiations of intimate conversation, and so on. Flirting among humans can be interpreted in evolutionary terms as a mechanism for selecting the most appropriate reproductive mate, and it can be usefully compared with analogous behaviors of other animals. Yet flirting is not obviously a hardwired disposition. It certainly can be done unconsciously, even though it is most commonly consciously deliberate. There is evidence that young girls acquire flirting skills from each other that they practice among themselves (even if it has a cruder, brasher form than that of adult women). Someone might flirt without knowing that he or she is doing so. Indeed, someone might realize only belatedly that a behavior had disclosed a sexual interest in another.

An important dimension of flirtation is that it might be either an overture to sexual activity or an intrinsically enjoyable activity in its own right. Ms. Smith may happily flirt with Mr. Jones while having no intention to move on to sex with him, yet enjoy her flirtation anyway (as Jones might also). The problem is that flirting for its own sake could nevertheless be interpreted as an invitation to have sex. Very often flirtatious behavior is regarded as occupying the bottom rung of a ladder that ascends all the way: the look, the talk, the touch, the kiss, the sex. Ovid (43 BCE–17/18 CE) notoriously condemns "those who grab their kisses but not what follows" as deserving "to lose all they've gained" ("The Art of Love," stanzas 669–70).

Flirting *is* prior to sex, in the sense that it tends to be practiced between people who have not yet had sex. Those who are already sexually intimate can flirt, but flirting is largely the game of people new to one another. Still, it need not be a game whose planned or inevitable outcome is sex. Flirting, then, even as a purposive activity, is different from **seduction**, whose intended outcome is sex. It is also important to distinguish behavior that signals an interest in later having sex from behavior that directly signifies, by virtue of a convention or rule, **consent** to sex. Some philosophers (e.g., Husak and Thomas) have defended the existence of such conventions. There is, however, a critical reason for carefully disambiguating or clarifying a behavior's significance: the considerable evidence of a gender difference in how behaviors are understood (see Abbey; Bostwick and Deluica; Cahill; Kowalski; Muehlenhard and Schrag; Shotland and Craig). Men are, for example, consistently more likely than women to perceive a scenario or behavior as sexual. What a woman intends only as friendliness a man may be disposed to view as sexual interest. Men may regard as an expression of a willingness to have sex words and behaviors that are only to be taken as the negotiation of possible mutual attractiveness. The familiar schoolyard charge that a girl is a tease implies that she has refused to deliver what she initially promised. But no promise need be made either by displaying sexual interest or by inviting the other to show his interest.

Flirtation is obviously ambiguous. Is the behavior sexual or not? Is it an invitation to have sex or a playful sexual exercise not meant to go any further? Sociologist Georg Simmel (1858–1918) memorably defines flirting in terms of the play in **love** between having and not having. He further suggests a gender difference that rests on the traditional view that while it is the man who proposes, it is for the woman to dispose. The woman's power lies over whether to consent or refuse, but this power is possessed and exercised only *prior* to her decision. She might be sure of what she wants, but she outwardly conceals her resolve. By contrast, a man who does not much care whether the woman wants to have sex with him can easily and happily give himself up to the game of flirting.

Although (or even because) flirtation is ambiguous, its participants may employ it in a careful strategy of negotiation. "Flirting," according to psychoanalyst Adam Phillips, "creates the uncertainty it is also trying to control" (xviii). Flirtation is a negotiation that allows the partners to explore the extent of their own interest in the other and the other's interest in them, without any commitment to sexual activity. Hence writers on flirting often describe it not only in terms of ambiguity but in the **language** of playfulness and games. It is, moreover, a pleasurable playing. The pleasures of flirting are various: finding that another person is attracted to one; making the right moves in the game, and doing so skillfully; simply doing what is constitutive of flirting—conversing, touching, glancing, smiling. The hint of deferred sex can also be pleasurable. The negotiation of sexual interest or attraction through flirting is much more interesting and enjoyable than blunt inquiries or statements about the parties' sexual interest or availability.

Flirtation raises a number of moral concerns. One is that flirtation conforms to undesirable gender stereotypes: The aggressive, dominant male, explicit in his desires, responds to the coy, passive, and demure woman who, conventional morality demands, may only hint at what she might want. The psychological evidence, however, points in the opposite direction: Women can and do, deliberately and consciously, orchestrate their courtship of men. They might use coy glances, but they might also maintain direct eye contact and offer full, unabashed smiles. Indeed, women are more frequently the initiators of sexual interest than its targets (see Moore; Moore and Butler). The view that a woman's flirting is immodest and to be condemned as such plausibly rests on an old-fashioned and prejudicial understanding of gender roles.

A second concern is that flirtation can become **sexual harassment**. Moreover, in some cultural contexts publicly directing sexually colored remarks and gestures toward women can have serious consequences: the shaming of the woman and a provocation to violence on her behalf by her male protectors. This is the case with the prevalent practice of "Eve teasing" in India. Yet we can and should distinguish between benign, playful flirtation and hostile, misogynistic sexual harassment. Flirting is often described in honorific terms that imply innocent pleasure. Yet flirting can slide into something unwelcome and morally reprehensible. Some flirting could be an unwanted display of sexual interest, and the flirt becomes a leering sexual bully. Flirting, of course, might be mutual, but it can also be one-sided. Nevertheless, the person who finds the other's unreciprocated flirting tiresome, intrusive, or irritating need not always think of themselves as being harassed.

The playfulness of flirtation creates a third moral concern. The language of play can be pejorative, as when we speak of someone merely "toying" with another. Flirtation may occur in an asymmetrical situation in which one party controls, even manipulates, the desires of the other, or provokes the other's sexual interest while having no interest other than doing exactly that. Human interaction, especially sexual interaction, is of course marked by disappointed expectations and by failures to reciprocate declarations of desire or love. It could hardly be otherwise. But we should still condemn the heartless manipulator of emotions and recognize that sex represents one of the most notable domains for the exercise of such power (see Morgan). Is it in general wrong to give rise to expectations (of any sort) that one does not intend to satisfy? Probably, if the one who acts on the expectations is harmed by their disappointment and the other knew, or should have known, that this would be so. However, the question presupposes that flirtation is designed to and does give rise to the expectation that sex will ensue. But flirting is essentially about ambiguity and uncertainty. It is not a declaration of an intent to proceed to sex.

Fourth, flirting, it could be argued, represents a failure to make a choice, a retreat from the responsibility of being a free agent in control of one's sexuality. In a famous example of "bad faith," Jean-Paul Sartre (1905–1980) illustrates the phenomenon of refusing to acknowledge one's inescapable liberty. In the example, a woman knows full well the intentions of her suitor and seeks to disarm his behavior of its sexual purposes. Her efforts to do so climax with his taking her hand. Should she leave her hand where it is, she might be taken as consenting to engage herself with him sexually; should she take it away, she would bring to an end an enjoyable date. What she actually does is retain the hand holding but, to offset it, make herself all intellect, soul, and consciousness, divorced from her body. Thus her hand "rests inert between the warm hands of her companion—neither consenting nor resisting—a thing" (55–56). But the example need not be construed as a criticism of flirting for its inherent ambiguity. Sartre's woman is in bad faith for evading the sexual significance of her suitor's actions. The flirt, by contrast, is ordinarily aware of what she does; she does not evade; and the ambiguity she creates is suffered by the other. Sartre's woman is passive before the man's initiation of contact, while the flirt is active and enterprising. To suggest that ambiguous behavior is to be condemned for *being* ambiguous invites the response that much, if not all, of the performing arts (let alone stand-up comedy) is characterized by ambiguity and is meritorious precisely for that reason.

Flirting therefore escapes several charges of moral impropriety. Instead, it invites commendation for being an intriguing and enjoyable technique for exploring with others our own sexual desires and theirs, a technique that can do so on its own terms and without commitment.

See also Activity, Sexual; Casual Sex; Communication Model; Completeness, Sexual; Ethics, Sexual; Harassment, Sexual; Humor; Jealousy; Language; Nagel, Thomas; Psychology, Evolutionary; Rape, Acquaintance and Date; Seduction

REFERENCES

Abbey, Antonia. "Sex Differences in Attributions for Friendly Behavior: Do Males Misperceive Females' Friendliness?" *Journal of Personality and Social Psychology* 42:5 (1982), 830–38; Bostwick, Tracy D., and Janice L. Deluica. "Effects of Gender and Specific Dating Behaviors on Perceptions of Sex Willingness and Date Rape." *Journal of Social and Clinical Psychology* 11:1 (1992), 14–25; Cahill, Spencer E. "Cross-Sex Pseudocommunication." *Berkeley Journal of Sociology* 26 (1981), 75–88; Husak, Douglas N., and George C. Thomas III. "Date Rape, Social Convention, and Reasonable Mistakes." *Law and Philosophy* 11:1–2 (1992), 95–126; Kowalski, Robin M. "Inferring Sexual Interest from Behavioral Cues: Effect of Gender and Sexually Relevant Attitudes." *Sex Roles* 29:1–2 (1993), 13–36; Moore, Monica M. "Nonverbal Courtship Patterns in Women: Context and Consequences." *Etholology and Sociobiology* 1:3 (1995), 237–47; Moore, Monica M., and Diana L. Butler. "Predictive Aspects of Nonverbal Courtship Behavior in Women." *Semiotica* 76:3–4 (1989), 205–15; Morgan, Seiriol. "Dark Desires." *Ethical Theory and Moral Practice* 6:4 (2003), 377–410; Moulton, Janice. "Sexual Behavior: Another Position." *Journal of Philosophy* 73:16 (1976), 537–46; Muehlenhard, Charlene L., and Jennifer L. Schrag. "Nonviolent Sexual Coercion." In Andrea Parrot and Laurie

Bechhofer, eds., *Acquaintance Rape: The Hidden Crime*. New York: Wiley, 1991, 115–28; Nagel, Thomas. "Sexual Perversion." *Journal of Philosophy* 66:1 (1969), 5–17; Ovid. (1 BCE–1 CE) "The Art of Love." In *The Erotic Poems*. Trans. Peter Green. Harmondsworth, U.K.: Penguin, 1982, 166–238; Phillips, Adam. *On Flirtation*. London: Faber and Faber, 1994; Sartre, Jean-Paul. *Being and Nothingness: An Essay on Phenomenological Ontology*. Trans. Hazel E. Barnes. London: Methuen, 1957; Shotland, R. Lance, and Jane M. Craig. "Can Men and Women Differentiate between Friendly and Sexually Interested Behavior?" *Social Psychology Quarterly* 51:1 (1988), 66–73; Simmel, Georg. (1911) "Flirtation." In *On Women, Sexuality, and Love*. Trans. and ed. Guy Oakes. New Haven, Conn.: Yale University Press, 1984, 133–52.

David Archard

ADDITIONAL READING

Belliotti, Raymond. "A Philosophical Analysis of Sexual Ethics." *Journal of Social Philosophy* 10:3 (1979), 8–11; Ben-Ze'ev, Aaron. "Flirting On- and Offline." In *Love Online: Emotions on the Internet*. Cambridge: Cambridge University Press, 2004, 145–59; ChennaiOnline. "Eve Teasing—A Growing Menace." <www.chennaionline.com/society/eveteasing.asp> [accessed 7 May 2004]; Husak, Douglas N., and George C. Thomas III. "Date Rape, Social Convention, and Reasonable Mistakes." *Law and Philosophy* 11:1 (1992), 95–126. Reprinted, abridged, in Lori Gruen and George Panichas, eds., *Sex, Morality, and the Law*. New York: Routledge, 1997, 444–54; Lott, Deborah A., and Frank Veronsky. "The New Flirting Game." *Psychology Today* 32:1 (January–February 1999), 42–47. <www.psychologytoday.com/htdocs/prod/ptoarticle/pto-19990101-000034.asp> [accessed 11 May 2004]; Miller, Don. "To Seduce or to Flirt, That Is the Question." *Time and Society* 12:2–3 (2003), 281–91; Moulton, Janice. "Sexual Behavior: Another Position." *Journal of Philosophy* 73:16 (1976), 537–46. Reprinted in HS (91–100); POS1 (110–18); POS2 (63–71); POS3 (31–38); POS4 (31–38); Nagel, Thomas. "Sexual Perversion." *Journal of Philosophy* 66:1 (1969), 5–17. Reprinted, revised, in *Mortal Questions*. Cambridge: Cambridge University Press, 1979, 39–52; and P&S3 (326–36); POS2 (39–51); POS3 (9–20); POS4 (9–20); STW (105–12); Perper, Timothy, and David L. Weis. "Proceptive and Rejective Strategies of U.S. and Canadian College Women." *Journal of Sex Research* 23:4 (1987), 455–80; Portmann, John. "Chatting Is Not Cheating." In John Portmann, ed., *In Defense of Sin*. New York: Palgrave, 2001, 223–41; Rodgers, Joann Ellison, and Frank Veronsky. "Flirting Fascination." *Psychology Today* 32:1 (January–February 1999), 1–9. <www.psychologytoday .com/htdocs/prod/ptoarticle/pto-19990101-000033.asp> [accessed 11 May 2004]; Sabini, John, and Maury Silver. "Flirtation and Ambiguity." In *Moralities of Everyday Life*. Oxford, U.K.: Oxford University Press, 1982, 107–23; Soble, Alan. "Antioch's 'Sexual Offense Policy': A Philosophical Exploration." *Journal of Social Philosophy* 28:1 (1997), 22–36. Reprinted in Ellen K. Feder, Karmen MacKendrick, and Sybol S. Cook, eds., *A Passion for Wisdom: Readings in Western Philosophy on Love and Desire*. Upper Saddle River, N.J.: Prentice Hall, 2004, 742–54; David Boonin and Graham Oddie, eds., *What's Wrong? Applied Ethicists and Their Critics*. New York: Oxford University Press, 2005, 241–49; POS4 (323–40); Steindorff, Carrie M. "Communication and Sexuality." In Vern L. Bullough and Bonnie Bullough, eds., *Human Sexuality: An Encyclopedia*. New York: Garland, 1994, 131–35; Yelvington, Kevin. "Power/Flirting." *Journal of the Royal Anthropological Institute* 5:3 (1999), 457–59.

FOUCAULT, MICHEL (1926–1984). Michel Foucault, self-described historian of "systems of thought," is perhaps best represented not as a philosopher, historian, or literary critic (although his work is relevant to all) but as a public intellectual whose life work interrogated and altered guiding assumptions informing specific practices in the present by staging encounters with the past. Of particular interest to Foucault in the mid-1970s and early 1980s were the guiding assumptions informing theories and institutional practices associated with the emergence of modern "sexuality." His unfinished history of sexuality (*The History of Sexuality*, 3 vols., 1976–1984) has had profound influence on Anglo-American feminist studies, gender studies, and **queer theory**.

Born to an upper-middle-class family in the provincial French city of Poitiers, Foucault received his higher education in Paris, where he attended the elite École Normale Supérieure. He studied there with distinguished French existential-phenomenologist Maurice Merleau-Ponty (1908–1961) and met philosopher and historian of science George Canguilhem (1904–1995), who later served as the research director for his doctoral thesis *Folie et de'raison: Histoire de la folie à l'age classique*. Foucault received degrees in both philosophy (1948, 1952) and psychology (1949) as well as a diploma in psychopathology from the Institut de Psychologie at Paris (1952). In the 1950s and 1960s he taught philosophy and psychology in Paris and assumed academic posts in Sweden, Tunisia, and Germany. During this same period he published historical studies of madness (*Madness and Civilization*) and clinical medicine (*Birth of the Clinic*) as well as his magnum opus *The Order of Things*, a historical critique of the concept of "man" that serves as the foundation of the human sciences. In 1968 he was invited to develop a philosophy department at the experimental university in Vincennes, and the following year he was elected to the prestigious College de France, assuming the newly named chair of "history of systems of thought." He gave annual lectures on his research at the College de France and lectured throughout the world, including the United States, where he held a visiting professorship at the University of California, Berkeley, from 1983 until his AIDS (acquired immunodeficiency syndrome)-related death. An immensely erudite scholar and engaged political activist, Foucault's wide-ranging interests included not only philosophy, psychology, history of science, literature, music, and painting but also prison reform, sexual freedom, and political revolts throughout the world.

Foucault addressed sexuality as part of a larger "political history of the body" that commences explicitly with his *Discipline and Punish* (1975). In this genealogical history of the emergence of the "disciplines" (bodily practices and bodies of knowledge), Foucault isolated a distinctive set of modern techniques for regulating the body and society. Disciplinary power, which emerged in the seventeenth and early eighteenth century, does not entirely replace forms of sovereign or juridical power associated with legal prohibitions and the threat of violent punishment and death but underpins and gradually displaces them. It does so by legitimating with the imprimatur of science a panoply of normalizing techniques associated with the human sciences and their correlative institutions: prisons, schools, hospitals, and factories. Disciplinary power is a form of knowledge of and power over the gestures, capacities, predispositions, desires, habits, and behaviors of individual bodies. It both enhances the capacities of subjects, attaching them to particular identities and normative standards, while also rendering them more docile and reliable as citizens and workers. With the emergence of clinical examinations, the importation of religious confessional practices into the clinical context, and the development of more sophisticated techniques of observation and documentation, the lives of abnormal or "dangerous" individuals were increasingly scrutinized. Individuals became "cases" and were judged not only in terms of legal culpability, a practice associated with juridical power, but also in terms of their potential behaviors, their psychologies, and personalities. Thus medical and psychological expertise were rendered indispensable to legal judgment. Another distinguishing feature of disciplinary power is that individuals exercise it on themselves. Individuals ultimately learn to subject themselves to the norms and standards that emerge in this context. The soul (psyche) became "the prison of the body" (*Discipline*, 30).

An extension of ideas developed in *Discipline*, the first volume of his *History of Sexuality* was an experimental book intended as a preliminary sketch of the methods, key concepts, and issues he would take up in future volumes. Here Foucault introduced the term "biopower," an umbrella concept for two techniques of power: disciplinary power, which governed individual bodies, and "regulatory" power, which was inscribed in policies and strategies for governing populations. Regulatory or governmental power focused on the "species body," the substrate of human biological processes related to birth, death, health, and the longevity of the population. Whereas disciplinary power operated at the microlevel in the habits and gestures of individuals, regulatory power identified more global trends in the population that escape individual intention.

"Sexuality" assumed a particularly important role as a vehicle and target of biopower. According to Foucault, "Sexuality must not be thought of as a kind of natural given which power tries to hold in check. . . . It is the name that can be given to a historical construct" (*History*, vol. 1, 105). As an object of the human sciences and normalization, a vehicle for administering the health, education, and welfare of the population, and a target for interventions in family and individual lives by medical, psychiatric, and legal authorities, "sex" became an increasingly fruitful concept for controlling individuals and populations. To elaborate:

> The notion of "sex" made it possible to group together, in an artificial unity, anatomical elements, biological functions, conducts, sensations, and pleasures, and it enabled one to make use of this fictitious unity as a causal principle, an omnipresent meaning, a secret to be discovered everywhere. (*History*, vol. 1, 154–55)

In effect, "sex" was loaded with profound significance for both the individual and the society. This in part explains why **Sigmund Freud** (1856–1939; see *Civilization and Its Discontents*) and other social theorists linked the fate of civilization to repressing or sublimating human **sexual desire**.

Foucault emphasized the productive dimension of this new form of knowledge/power. Power does not simply repress sex, he claimed; rather, it operates through the production of the *dispositif* (apparatus or regime) of sexuality. "Apparatus" refers to a heterogeneous collection of elements, including discourses as well as nondiscursive practices. It links relations of power with bodies of knowledge. Moreover, it produces not only new ways of understanding sexuality and new techniques for controlling it but also sexual subjects. Queer theorist David Halperin has described the interiorization of sexuality as a process that "knits up desire, its objects, sexual behavior, gender identity, reproductive function, mental health, erotic sensibility, personal style, and degrees of normality or deviance into an individuating, normativizing feature of the personality called 'sexuality' " ("Forgetting Foucault," 25–26).

Psychiatry and **sexology** become linchpins of this new regime of sexuality. For example, relying on earlier sexological classificatory schemes, psychoanalytic accounts of psychosexual development isolated the numerous ways in which desire might go astray (for example, Freud's *Three Essays*). They established developmental norms, isolated multiple abnormal personages—the fetishist, the invert, the hysteric, to name only a few—and devised new corrective methods. **Perversion** was thereby incorporated into the individual, and in particular, the "homosexual" emerged as a particular type of individual. To be sure, sodomy predated the homosexual's arrival on the scene, and sexual morphologies as well as sexual subjectivities had previously been linked to sexual acts, but, as Halperin has argued, ancient and canonical codes did not link sodomy to "sexual identity" in the modern sense of the term ("Forgetting Foucault," 41–42). Foucault described our attachments to these new forms of sexual subjectivity, whether normal or abnormal, as part of an elaborate "government of individualization," a deployment of power that "applies itself to immediate everyday life which categorizes the individual, marks him by his own individuality, attaches him to his own identity, imposes a law of truth on him which he must recognize and which others have to recognize in him" ("Afterword: Subject and Power," 212). The relation of power to sex here is not principally repressive but productive. Individuals are repressed *through* an apparatus of sexuality that incites discourse about sex, produces desires and norms of psychosexual development, and thereby produces sexual subjects.

How to resist this insidious power is not obvious. What is clear is that if sex is an artifact of a regime of sexuality, and if power produces the idea of a true sex, then saying yes to sex, merely lifting repression or affirming one's sexual identity, is not saying no to power. Instead, it is merely a strategic move within the regime of sexuality. Foucault viewed demands by advocates of sexual revolution such as Wilhelm Reich (1897–1957) and Herbert Marcuse (1898–1979) to lift sexual repression and thereby unleash authentic human capacities and desires (and/or undermine capitalism) as "nothing more . . . than a tactical shift and reversal in the great deployment [*dispositif*] of sexuality" (*History*, vol. 1, 131). That the promises of such a revolution were not fulfilled despite a loosening of sexual mores in the 1970s and 1980s suggests that the "repressive hypothesis" did not capture all the modes of power over sex. In a similar vein, Foucault suggested that although movements for homosexual liberation may have succeeded in securing rights for some stigmatized sexual minorities, these movements remained tied to the regime of sexuality he was exposing, insofar as they preserved the idea of a "true sex."

Toward the end of the first volume of his *History*, Foucault famously declared that "the rallying point for the counterattack against the deployment of sexuality ought not to be sex-desire, but bodies and pleasures" (157). The regime of sexuality must be countered by strategies that might prefigure an alternative sexual economy, that is, "with the claims of bodies, pleasures, and knowledges, in their multiplicity and their possibility of resistance." Presumably this is not because "bodies and pleasures" represent the prediscursive fundamentals of any sexual economy, as some commentators have claimed (see Alcoff), but because the role they play has been less central to the modern normalizing regime of sexuality than have the concepts of "sex" and "desire."

Although in the early stages, Foucault intended to restrict his *History* to the modern regime of sexuality, he reconceived the project and shifted his focus to Greco-Roman and Christian problematizations of sex. In the second volume, *The Use of Pleasure*, he said that his aim in the later volumes would be to write a "genealogy" of the desiring subject, a study of "practices by which individuals were led to focus their attention on themselves, to decipher, recognize, and acknowledge themselves as subjects of desire" (5). To understand how modern persons come to experience themselves as subjects of a sexuality, as individuals whose sexual being harbored a profound truth about desire, Foucault deemed it essential to trace the process through which Western "man" had come to understand himself as a desiring subject, as a subject who experiences desire either as the sign of a lack in himself or as an ungovernable internal force. This marks a shift in his project from the study of power relations and the constitution of individuals within disciplinary apparatuses to the study of "ethics," that is, ways in which individuals relate to and transform themselves into moral agents.

Foucault's history of **ethics**—neither a history of people's actual behaviors nor a history of moral codes and laws—focuses on four aspects of the "self-relation": *ethical substance*, the prime material of our moral experience and the aspect of our selves that is subject to ethical judgment; *mode of subjection*, the way in which an individual establishes a relationship to moral authority; *technology of self*, the specific disciplines through which an individual transforms the self to become an ethical subject; and *telos*, the type of being to which one aspires in behaving ethically. Isolating this domain of ethical practices enabled Foucault to chart shifts in modes of subject formation that remain invisible if one studies only codes or behaviors. He explained his shift of focus:

> I wonder if our problem nowadays is not, in a way, similar to [the Greeks insofar as they did not relate ethics to science or law]. . . . [M]ost of us no longer believe that ethics is founded in religion, nor do we want a legal system to intervene in our moral, personal, private life. Recent liberation movements suffer from the fact that they cannot find any principle on which to base the elaboration of a new ethics. They need an ethics, but cannot find any other ethics than an ethics founded on so-called scientific knowledge of what the self is, what desire is, and so on. (*Essential Works* [*EW*], vol. 1, 343)

Disclosing ancient ethical practices might not only reveal the contingency of present practices but also suggest alternatives to present practices of ordering human sexual conduct, alternatives that are not linked to normalization. That the ancient Greeks did not regard constraints on sexuality as the bedrock of human civilization implies that civilization might well flourish without giving sexuality and its constraints such primacy. Moreover, Foucault suggested that to move beyond the regime of sexuality, we could make our bodies and pleasures the objects of creative and aesthetic practices of the self. Further, Foucault revealed not only discontinuities in modes of ethical subject formation in Western history; there were important continuities as well. Just as modern apparatuses of sexuality incorporated older techniques and practices of ethical subject formation and deployed them in new ways, so, he claimed, recent liberation movements might take up old practices in ways that resist current modes of subjection.

Although knowledge of the self played a central role in Greek ethics, Foucault emphasized that the Greeks subordinated the imperative to "know thyself" to the principle of *care* for the self. Care for the self was, he claimed, "one of the main rules for social and personal conduct and for the art of life" ("Technologies of the Self," *EW*, vol. 1, 226). Foucault lamented the decline of this broader, existential understanding of philosophy as a "way of life," which was eclipsed within post-Cartesian philosophies that subordinated concern for the self to the imperative of theoretical and scientific knowledge (Davidson, 195–202). This notion of care of the self—indeed, of treating the self as a work of art— was a strand of thought he attempted to resuscitate in some new form. Foucault laments that we moderns "have hardly any remnant of the idea in our society that the principal work of art which one must take care of, the main area to which one must apply aesthetic values, is oneself, one's life, one's existence" (*EW*, vol. 1, 271).

What distinguished ancient Greek sexual ethics from its later Christian and modern Western counterparts is not that they were more tolerant. Foucault never claimed to represent Greco-Roman antiquity as a "golden age" of sexual freedom. He recognized ancient elitism and sexism and pointed out that Greek and Roman canon law regarded acts "contrary to nature" as especially abominable. Moreover, significant overlap in prohibitive morality exists in Greco-Roman antiquity, the Christian middle ages, and the modern West, insofar as all three contain prohibitions against excessive **sexual activity**, extramarital sex, and homosexual relations. The Greco-Roman prohibitions against these acts were *juridical* and did not involve a medical disqualification of the homosexual as a pathological type. More important is that Greek sexual austerity was connected to a different form of ethical subjectivation than found in Christianity. For example, a central ethical task of a fourth-century (BCE) Greek citizen was to lead a beautiful life by learning techniques of self-mastery and regulating his pleasures, acts, and desires (*aphrodisia*). Doing so was also deemed essential for a man to be able to govern others. As Foucault described him, the ancient Greek citizen acted "to give to [his] life certain values (reproduce certain examples, leave behind . . . an exalted reputation, give the maximum possible brilliance to [his life]" (*EW*, vol. 1, 271). Although his project of self-mastery required knowledge of *aphrodisia* and the effects of particular bodily practices, he did not scrutinize his desires in a "search for their profound nature, their canonical forms, or their secret potential" (*Use of Pleasure*, 40). "[W]hat seems . . . to have formed the object of moral reflection for the Greeks in matters of sexual conduct was not exactly the act itself (considered in its different modalities), or desire (viewed from the standpoint of its origin or aim), or even pleasure (evaluated according to the different objects or practices that can cause it)." Instead, according to Foucault, "it was more the dynamics that joined all three in a circular fashion (the desire that leads to the act, that act that is linked to pleasure, and the pleasure that occasions desire). The ethical question that was raised was not: which desires? which acts? which pleasures? but rather: with what force is one transported . . . by the pleasures and desires . . . ?" (*Use of Pleasure*, 43).

In medieval Christian ethics one finds the self-relation dramatically restructured. The Christian of late antiquity experienced a new relationship to his sexual being. The ethical substance in this case was not pleasure but the flesh. Christianity replaced practices of self-creation with practices of self-analysis and self-renunciation. Whereas ancient Greeks exhibited a preoccupation with homosexual penetration insofar as it placed the receiver in a passive and hence feminine position, early Christians such as **Saint Augustine** (354–430) were more concerned with erection insofar as it represented the involuntary (and rebellious) movements of the flesh (Augustine, 14.15; Foucault, *EW*, vol. 1, 181–82). The persons and acts one desired became the *substance* of ethical preoccupation. Access to one's desires, to the truth about oneself, was provided through techniques of self-examination—for example, confessional practices and ascetic practices of self-renunciation whose purpose (*telos*) was to root out Satanic influences that might be lurking within the soul. Finally, the source of moral authority in this ethical system was divine law, not the desire for a beautiful existence. In the end, Christians replaced Greek self-control or self-mastery with self-purification, a constant struggle to rid themselves of impure thoughts (see Matt. 5:27–30) and, were it possible, not to desire at all. The self that emerged was a self that understood itself as dependent and fully aware of what it lacked in relation to the Divine. The form of ethical subjectivation is thus importantly different from its ancient Greek and Roman predecessors.

Through this genealogical inquiry Foucault hoped to do two things. First, he wanted to reveal the contingency of contemporary ethical self-understandings and loosen the grip of the discourses of desire and repression, the hermeneutics of the self, that has governed experiences of sexual subjects in the nineteenth and twentieth century. The relative influence of Christianity of course declined after the Enlightenment, yet practices of self-renunciation and self-deciphering (including Christian confessional practices) were incorporated into the modern disciplinary and juridical apparatus. Second, Foucault's point is not that such ethical techniques and practices are inherently oppressive, but they have been transformed, used for different purposes, and used in different ways throughout Western history. Modern individuals might also take them up in new ways and thereby resist current forms of subjection insofar as they are linked with normalization. Accordingly, he suggested that the task for homosexuals was not to liberate some intrinsic and fixed sexual desire but rather to *become* homosexual and to take advantage of their eccentric social locations as resources for experimenting and developing new forms of life. "To be 'gay,'" he declared, "is to try to define and develop a way of life" (*EW*, vol. 1, 138). In short, the focus of present homosexual activism might be self-creation, akin to that practiced by the ancient Greeks, and not simply self-acceptance or the affirmation of one's sexual identity. Rather than accept identities fashioned in the context of the regime of sexuality, individuals might experiment with possibilities of moving beyond sexuality altogether.

Foucault imagined a world in which human beings no longer felt compelled to decipher the deep meaning of sexual desires, feelings, and practices and to grant them profound significance. By revealing the contingency of this practice of the self, he hoped to create the intellectual space necessary for creating alternatives. He also urged sex radicals to move beyond the tendency to regard sexual transgression as the most heroic gestures in the struggle for sexual liberation. To transgress established mores is, in some sense, to depend on them. Part of his project in his later works, then, was to identify the systems of thought and the institutional practices that govern modern understandings of sexuality and of its liberation and to make their transformation possible. They should be changed because they are oppressive; they place unnecessary constraints on the freedom of individuals to develop their capacities for sexual and erotic pleasure, for "amorous and passionate relationships with others" (*EW*, vol. 1, 283).

Foucault's writings on sex and power have significantly influenced **feminism** and queer theory. Judith Butler, for example, has found Foucault's work especially useful for addressing the production of gendered identities within the context of patriarchal systems involving compulsory heterosexuality (see her *Gender Trouble*). But some feminists have criticized Foucault's history for its gender blindness and its failure to analyze the impact of the erasure of the feminine within androcentric culture (for example, Bartky). Queer theorists such as Gayle Rubin, David Halperin, and Timothy Dean have been interested in extending Foucault's insights about the production of normative gender and sexual identities to develop a radical account of sexual freedom as entailing resistance to normalization and assimilation. Rubin in particular has argued that sex has assumed too much moral significance in modern societies and that it is unjust to consider "perverts" more morally suspect on the basis of their sexual identities alone ("Thinking Sex"). Many queer theorists recommend moving beyond advancing gay and lesbian identity politics toward a more universalizing understanding of queerness as something that may be found across the homo/heterosexual divide and that can be used to open up other possible ways of being and being together with others. Moreover, Foucault's historicist approach to sexuality and sexual identity has encouraged some historians of sexuality to challenge historical accounts that presume that sexual identities such as **homosexuality** have always existed (see Halperin; Weeks). They have also been encouraged to provide accounts of the myriad specific forms of sexual subjectivity found throughout Western history instead of imposing modern categories onto the past.

See also Beauty; Boswell, John; Catholicism, History of; Freudian Left, The; Greek Sexuality and Philosophy, Ancient; Homosexuality and Science; Nietzsche, Friedrich; Phenomenology; Plato; Poststructuralism; Queer Theory; Roman Sexuality and Philosophy, Ancient; Sexology; Social Constructionism

REFERENCES

Alcoff, Linda Martín. "Dangerous Pleasures: Foucault and the Politics of Pedophilia." In Susan J. Hekman, ed., *Feminist Interpretations of Michel Foucault*. University Park: Pennsylvania State

University Press, 1996, 99–135; Augustine. (413–427) *The City of God*. Trans. Henry Bettenson. New York: Penguin, 1984; Bartky, Sandra Lee. "Foucault, Femininity, and the Modernization of Patriarchal Power." In Irene Diamond and Lee Quinby, eds., *Feminism and Foucault: Reflections on Resistance*. Boston, Mass.: Northeastern University Press, 1988, 61–86; Butler, Judith. *Gender Trouble: Feminism and the Subversion of Identity*. New York: Routledge, 1990; Davidson, Arnold I. "Introductory Remarks to Pierre Hadot." In Arnold I. Davidson, ed., *Foucault and His Interlocutors*. Chicago, Ill.: University of Chicago Press, 1997, 195–202; Dean, Timothy. *Beyond Sexuality*. Chicago, Ill.: University of Chicago Press, 2000; Foucault, Michel. "Afterword: The Subject and Power." In Hubert Dreyfus and Paul Rabinow, eds., *Michel Foucault: Beyond Structuralism and Hermeneutics*. Chicago, Ill.: University of Chicago Press, 1982, 208–26; Foucault, Michel. (1963) *The Birth of the Clinic: An Archaeology of Medical Perception*. Trans. A. M. Sheridan-Smith. New York: Vintage, 1975; Foucault, Michel. (1975) *Discipline and Punish: The Birth of the Prison*. Trans. Alan Sheridan. New York: Pantheon, 1977; Foucault, Michel. *The Essential Works of Michel Foucault, 1954–1984*, vol. 1: *Ethics: Subjectivity and Truth*. Ed. Paul Rabinow. Trans. Robert Hurley and others. New York: New Press, 1997; Foucault, Michel. (1976/1984/1984) *The History of Sexuality*. Vol. 1: *An Introduction*. Trans. Robert Hurley. New York: Vintage, 1978. Vol. 2: *The Use of Pleasure*. Trans. Robert Hurley. New York: Pantheon, 1985. Vol. 3: *The Care of the Self*. Trans. Robert Hurley. New York: Vintage, 1986; Foucault, Michel. (1961) *Madness and Civilization: A History of Insanity in the Age of Reason*. Trans. Richard Howard. New York: Random House, 1965; Foucault, Michel. (1966) *The Order of Things: An Archaeology of the Human Sciences*. New York: Pantheon, 1971; Freud, Sigmund. (1930) *Civilization and Its Discontents*. In *The Standard Edition of the Complete Psychological Works of Sigmund Freud*, vol. 21. Ed. and trans. James Strachey. London: Hogarth Press, 1953–1974, 57–145; Freud, Sigmund. (1905) *Three Essays on the Theory of Sexuality*. In *The Standard Edition of the Complete Psychological Works of Sigmund Freud*, vol. 7. Ed. and trans. James Strachey. London: Hogarth Press, 1953–1974, 125–245; Halperin, David M. "Forgetting Foucault." In *How to Do the History of Homosexuality*. Chicago, Ill.: University of Chicago Press, 2002, 24–47; Halperin, David M. *Saint Foucault: Towards a Gay Hagiography*. New York: Oxford University Press, 1995; Rubin, Gayle S. "Thinking Sex: Notes for a Radical Theory of the Politics of Sexuality." In Carole S. Vance, ed., *Pleasure and Danger: Exploring Female Sexuality*. London: Routledge and Kegan Paul, 1984, 267–319; Sawicki, Jana. *Disciplining Foucault: Feminism, Power, and the Body*. New York: Routledge, 1991; Weeks, Jeffrey. *Sexuality and Its Discontents: Meanings, Myths, and Modern Sexualities*. London: Routledge and Kegan Paul, 1985.

Jana Sawicki

ADDITIONAL READING

Babich, Babette E. "Nietzsche and Eros between the Devil and God's Deep Blue Sea: The Problem of the Artist as Actor—Jew—Woman." *Continental Philosophy Review* 33 (April 2000), 159–88; Bartky, Sandra Lee. "Foucault, Femininity, and the Modernization of Patriarchal Power." In Irene Diamond and Lee Quinby, eds., *Feminism and Foucault: Reflections on Resistance*. Boston, Mass.: Northeastern University Press, 1988, 61–86. Reprinted in *Femininity and Domination: Studies in the Phenomenology of Oppression*. New York: Routledge, 1990, 63–82; Baudrillard, Jean. (1977) *Forget Foucault*. Trans. Nicole Dufresne. New York: Semiotext(e), 1987; Bersani, Leo. "Foucault, Freud, Fantasy, and Power." *GLQ: A Journal of Lesbian and Gay Studies* 2:1–2 (1995), 11–33; Bersani, Leo. *Homos*. Cambridge, Mass.: Harvard University Press, 1995; Bouchard, Donald, ed. *Michel Foucault: Language, Counter-Memory, Practice. Selected Essays and Interviews*. Trans. Donald Bouchard and Sherry Simon. Ithaca, N.Y.: Cornell University Press, 1977; Breines, Paul. "Revisiting Marcuse with Foucault: *An Essay on Liberation* Meets *The History of Sexuality*." In John Bokina and Timothy J. Lukes, eds., *Marcuse: From the New Left to the Next Left*. Lawrence: University Press of Kansas, 1994, 27–40; Buhle, Mary Jo. *Feminism and Its Discontents: A Century of Struggle with Psychoanalysis*. Cambridge, Mass.: Harvard University Press, 1998; Butler, Judith. "Bodies and Pleasures, Revisited." In Dianna Taylor and Karen Vintges, eds., *Feminism and the Final Foucault*.

Urbana: University of Illinois Press, 2004, 183–94; Butler, Judith. *Bodies That Matter: On the Discursive Limits of Sex*. New York: Routledge, 1993; Butler, Judith. *The Psychic Life of Power: Theories in Subjection*. Stanford, Calif.: Stanford University Press, 1997; Cohen, Richard. "Merleau-Ponty, the Flesh, and Foucault." *Philosophy Today* 28 (Winter 1984), 329–38; Davidson, Arnold I. *The Emergence of Sexuality: Historical Epistemology and the Formation of Concepts*. Cambridge, Mass.: Harvard University Press, 2001; Dean, Carolyn J. "The Productive Hypothesis: Foucault, Gender, and the History of Sexuality." *History and Theory* 33:3 (1994), 271–96; Dean, Tim, and Christopher Lane, eds. *Homosexuality and Psychoanalysis*. Chicago, Ill.: University of Chicago Press, 2001; Diamond, Irene, and Lee Quinby, eds. *Foucault and Feminism: Reflections on Resistance*. Boston, Mass.: Northeastern University Press, 1988; Dollimore, Jonathan. *Sexual Dissidence: Augustine to Wilde, Freud to Foucault*. Oxford, U.K.: Clarendon Press, 1991; Earle, William. "Foucault's *The Use of Pleasure* as Philosophy." *Metaphilosophy* 20 (April 1989), 169–77; Feder, Ellen K. "Disciplining the Family: The Case of Gender Identity Disorder." *Philosophical Studies* 85:2–3 (1997), 195–211; Ferguson, Frances. *Pornography, the Theory: What Utilitarianism Did to Action*. Chicago, Ill.: University of Chicago Press, 2004; Flynn, Thomas R. "Truth and Subjectivation in the Later Foucault." *Journal of Philosophy* 82 (October 1985), 531–40; Foucault, Michel. *Abnormal: Lectures at the College de France, 1974–1975*. Trans. Graham Bruchell. Ed. Valerio Marchetti and Antonella Salomoni. English ed., Arnold I. Davidson. London: Verso, 2003; Foucault, Michel. *The Essential Foucault*. Ed. Paul Rabinow and Nikolas Rose. New York: New Press, 2003; Foucault, Michel. *The Essential Works of Michel Foucault, 1954–1984*, vol. 2: *Aesthetics, Method, and Epistemology*. Ed. James D. Faubion. Trans. Robert Hurley and others. New York: New Press, 1998; Foucault, Michel. *The Essential Works of Michel Foucault, 1954–1984*, vol. 3: *Power*. Ed. James D. Faubion. Trans. Robert Hurley and others. New York: New Press, 2000; Foucault, Michel. (1983) *Fearless Speech*. Six lectures [University of California, Berkeley] recorded, comp., and ed. Joseph Pearson. Los Angeles, Calif.: Semiotext(e), 2001. Available online as "Discourse and Truth: The Problematization of Parrhesia." <www.foucault.info/documents/parrhesia> [accessed 7 June 2005]; Foucault, Michel. (1978) *Herculine Barbin: Being the Recently Discovered Memoirs of a Nineteenth Century Hermaphrodite*. Trans. Richard McDougall. New York: Pantheon Books, 1980; Foucault, Michel. (1976/1984/1984) *The History of Sexuality*, 3 vols. Trans. Robert Hurley. New York: Vintage, 1988–1990; Foucault, Michel. "Power and Sex." In Lawrence D. Kritzman, ed., *Michel Foucault: Politics, Philosophy, Culture. Interviews and Other Writings, 1977–1984*. New York: Routledge, 1988, 110–24; Foucault, Michel. *Technologies of the Self: A Seminar with Michel Foucault*. Ed. Luther H. Martin, Huck Gutman, and Patrick H. Hutton. Amherst: University of Massachusetts Press, 1988; Franchi, Stefano. Review of *Fearless Speech*, by Michel Foucault. *Essays in Philosophy* 5:2 (2004). <www.humboldt.edu/~essays/franchirev.html> [accessed 4 June 2004]; Gearhart, Suzanne. "Foucault's Response to Freud: Sado-masochism and the Aestheticization of Power." *Style* 29 (Fall 1995), 389–403; Goldhill, Simon. *Foucault's Virginity: Ancient Erotic Fiction and the History of Sexuality*. Cambridge: Cambridge University Press, 1995; Gutting, Gary, ed. *The Cambridge Companion to Foucault*. Cambridge: Cambridge University Press, 1994. Updated and rev. ed., 2005; Hartsock, Nancy. "Foucault on Power: A Theory for Women?" In Linda J. Nicholson, ed., *Feminism/Postmodernism*. New York: Routledge, 1990, 157–75; Hekman, Susan J., ed. *Feminist Interpretations of Michel Foucault*. University Park: Pennsylvania State University Press, 1996; Hoy, David Couzens. *Critical Resistance: From Poststructuralism to Post-Critique*. Cambridge, Mass.: MIT Press, 2004; Hoy, David Couzens, ed. *Foucault: A Critical Reader*. Oxford, U.K.: Blackwell, 1986; Kimball, Roger. "The Perversions of Michel Foucault." [Review of *The Passion of Michel Foucault*, by James Miller] *The New Criterion* 11:7 (March 1993). *The New Criterion on line*, <www.newcriterion.com/archive/11/mar93/foucault.htm> [accessed 8 June 2005]; Knauft, Bruce M. "Foucault Meets South New Guinea: Knowledge, Power, Sexuality." *Ethos* 22:4 (1994), 391–438; Kritzman, Lawrence D., ed. *Michel Foucault. Politics, Philosophy, Culture: Interviews and Other Writings, 1977–1984*. New York: Routledge, 1988; Larmour, David H. J., Paul Allen Miller, and Charles Platter, eds. *Rethinking Sexuality: Foucault and Classical Antiquity*. Princeton, N.J.: Princeton University Press, 1997; Lloyd, G.E.R. "The Mind on Sex." [Review of *The Use of Pleasure*, by Michel Foucault] *New York Review of Books* (13 March 1986),

24–28; Lynch, Richard. "Michel Foucault's Shorter Works in English" [bibliography] (29 March 2004). <www.foucault.qut.edu.au/lynch.html> [accessed 9 September 2004]; Macey, David. *The Lives of Michel Foucault.* New York: Pantheon Books, 1994; MacIntyre, Alasdair. "Miller's Foucault, Foucault's Foucault." *Salmagundi* 97 (1993), 54–60; McNay, Lois. *Foucault and Feminism.* Cambridge, U.K.: Polity Press, 1992; McWhorter, Ladelle. *Bodies and Pleasures: Foucault and the Politics of Sexual Normalization.* Bloomington: Indiana University Press, 1999; McWhorter, Ladelle. "Foucault, Michel." In Timothy F. Murphy, ed., *Reader's Guide to Lesbian and Gay Studies.* Chicago, Ill.: Fitzroy Dearborn, 2000, 224–26; Miller, James. *The Passion of Michel Foucault.* New York: Simon and Schuster, 1993; Moss, Jeremy. *The Later Foucault: Politics and Philosophy.* Thousand Oaks, Calif.: Sage, 1998; Nehamas, Alexander. *The Art of Living: Socratic Reflections from Plato to Foucault.* Berkeley: University of California Press, 1998; Nehamas, Alexander. "Subject and Abject: The Examined Life of Michel Foucault." *The New Republic* (15 February 1993), 27–36; Plaza, Monique. "Our Damages and Their Compensation—Rape: The 'Will Not to Know' of Michel Foucault." *Feminist Issues* 1 (Summer 1981), 25–35; Rajchman, John. *Truth and Eros: Foucault, Lacan, and the Question of Ethics.* London: Routledge, 1991; Ramazanoglu, Caroline, ed. *Up against Foucault: Explorations of Some Tensions between Foucault and Feminism.* London: Routledge, 1993; Rubin, Gayle S. "Thinking Sex: Notes for a Radical Theory of the Politics of Sexuality." In Carole S. Vance, ed., *Pleasure and Danger: Exploring Female Sexuality.* London: Routledge and Kegan Paul, 1984, 267–319. Reprinted in Peter M. Nardi and Beth E. Schneider, eds., *Social Perspectives in Lesbian and Gay Studies.* New York: Routledge, 1998, 100–133; Ryan, Joanna. "Psychoanalysis and Women Loving Women." In Sue Cartledge and Joanna Ryan, eds., *Sex and Love: New Thoughts on Old Contradictions.* London: Women's Press, 1983, 196–209; Sawicki, Jana. (1986) "Foucault and Feminism: Toward a Politics of Difference." In Mary Lyndon Shanley and Carole Pateman, eds., *Feminist Interpretations and Political Theory.* University Park: Pennsylvania State University Press, 1991, 217–31; Sawicki, Jana. "Queering Foucault and the Subject of Feminism." In Gary Gutting, ed., *The Cambridge Companion to Michel Foucault,* updated and rev. ed. Cambridge: Cambridge University Press, 2005, 379–400; Shusterman, Richard. *Pragmatist Aesthetics: Living Beauty, Rethinking Art.* Oxford, U.K.: Blackwell, 1992; Shusterman, Richard. "The Self as a Work of Art." *Nation* (30 June 1997), 25–28; Singer, Linda. (posthumous) *Erotic Welfare: Sexual Theory and Politics in the Age of Epidemic.* Ed. Judith Butler and Maureen MacGrogan. New York: Routledge, 1993; Smart, Barry. "On the Subjects of Sexuality, Ethics, and Politics in the Work of Foucault." *boundary 2* 18:1 (1991), 201–25; Soper, Kate. "Ruling Passion Strong in Death." *Radical Philosophy* 66 (Spring 1994), 44–46; Steiner, George. "Power Play." *The New Yorker* (17 March 1986), 105–9; Stoler, Ann Laura. *Race and the Education of Desire: Foucault's History of Sexuality and the Colonial Order of Things.* Durham, N.C.: Duke University Press, 1995; Thacker, Andrew. "Foucault's Aesthetics of Existence." *Radical Philosophy* 63 (Spring 1993), 13–21; Veyne, Paul. "The Final Foucault and His Ethics." Trans. Catherine Porter and Arnold I. Davidson. *Critical Inquiry* 20 (Autumn 1993), 1–9; Weeks, Jeffrey. "Foucault for Historians." In *Making Sexual History.* Oxford, U.K.: Blackwell, 1999, 106–22.

FRENCH FEMINISM. *See* Feminism, French

FREUD, SIGMUND (1856–1939). The twentieth century saw perhaps no more influential thinker on sexuality than Sigmund Freud. While many aspects of his theory have entered the vernacular (Oedipus complex, penis envy, castration anxiety) and have left an indelible mark on how we think about sexuality, the status of Freud's theory is still contested, and his reputation continues to undergo periodic rises and falls. Detractors from different orientations argue that Freud's theories condone everything from the oppression of women and sexual minorities to sexual licentiousness and immorality. In his own day,

Freud's view that sexuality was intrinsically "perverse" was provocative, insightful, and in some ways progressive.

Freud was born in the small town Freiburg (Příbor) in Moravia, an area of the Austro-Hungarian empire that eventually became, in 1993, the Czech Republic. His family moved to Vienna when he was four, and Freud spent most of his life there. A Jew, although never religious, he was compelled to seek exile in England in 1938 after Germany's annexation of Austria. He died in London from cancer (he had developed tumors on the palate, perhaps from smoking cigars, by 1917). As a young man, Freud studied medicine at the University of Vienna and in 1885 went to Paris for an internship under Jean-Martin Charcot (1825–1893), a leading researcher on hysteria. Charcot had been using, with success, hypnosis in the treatment of hysterics, and Freud's experience with Charcot led him to turn his studies to psychology. Returning to Vienna a year later, Freud established a private practice and replaced the use of hypnotism with the "free association" technique, establishing the basis for what would become psychoanalytic theory and practice.

The importance of sexuality for Freud's work is already present in his claim in the early *Studies on Hysteria* (1895), written with Josef Breuer (1842–1925), that the symptoms of hysteria are sexual in nature even when they do not appear to be overtly sexual. Hysterical patients often suffered from choking or coughing fits, fainting spells, or false paralyses—all symptoms without an underlying organic disturbance. A hysterical paralysis would not follow the neurological paths of a true paralysis, and hysterical coughing was not accompanied by any virus or infection. To support his view that in these cases *"the patient's symptoms constitute his sexual activity"* Freud pointed to the mechanism of repression ("My Views," 278). The free association technique encouraged patients to say whatever came into their minds, however nonsensical or irrelevant it might seem. This technique unearthed long repressed ideas and memories, generally with an overtly sexual content, that were associated with the hysteric's symptoms. Reconnecting these sexual ideas to the symptom led, in many cases, to the dissolution of the symptom. Freud hypothesized, then, that while the ideas and memories associated with sexuality can be repressed, the affects associated with sexuality cannot be. These affects are forced to express themselves in a distorted form, in the form of a hysterical symptom with no apparent link to the repressed ideas.

Freud came to the view that sexuality is at work in hysteria early in his career but still did not have a theory that accounted for the cause of the dissociation between sexuality as an affect and the ideas associated with it. For several years in the 1890s, Freud held that hysteria was caused by a traumatic encounter with sexuality in childhood, through abuse or molestation. He held that this early traumatic encounter with sexuality would create incompatible ideas for the child about the molester (such as feelings of hostility or betrayal toward a previously beloved family member). The incompatibility of the new ideas associated with the seducer would lead to a repression of the **seduction**. This view, the "seduction theory," assumed that sexuality is not naturally present in childhood; its presence was understood to be due to the actions of an adult or older child. The seduction theory required that anyone suffering from hysterical symptoms in adulthood must have been a victim of sexual abuse in the past. This became harder and harder for Freud to maintain, and he eventually came to feel that the condition of hysteria was far more widespread than could be accounted for by the seduction theory. Thus, he abandoned this theory of hysteria in favor of a new one that placed the cause of hysteria no longer in a traumatic sexual event but in "normal" infantile sexuality. His rejection of the seduction theory has been criticized by some who accuse Freud of neglecting the fact of child sexual abuse even when he had evidence to the contrary (see Masson). Others have written that this criticism does not withstand scrutiny (see Crews et al. for discussion). Some neuroses were clearly caused by sexual abuse, Freud felt. Others were not, and for some of these cases Freud argued that the memories his patients had of sexual abuse were actually fantasies. The hysterical symptoms in these cases were formed because of the repression of these sexual fantasies, which contained sexual ideas concerning family members or other important childhood figures.

The view that sexuality is already present in the infancy and childhood of both neurotic and healthy individuals became a central tenet of psychoanalytic theory, and the events that occurred during the course of the development of infantile sexuality through adulthood were seen to prescribe "the direction that will be taken by later sexual life after maturity" ("My Views," 274). To paraphrase poet William Wordsworth (1770–1850), the child is the father of the adult: The contingencies of infantile sexuality laid the groundwork for the sexual behaviors of adulthood.

Infantile sexuality appears in three main stages, each centered on different parts of the body, called the erotogenic zones, which act as sources of stimulation: the oral, anal, and genital zones. These are not the only erotogenic zones, but they are the central ones. Indeed, Freud claimed that any part of the body could serve as an erotogenic zone. The symptoms of hysteria showed this. Parts of the body not normally associated with sexuality become in hysteria areas of **sexual activity**: The throat in hysterical choking, the lungs in hysterical coughing, the limbs of the body in hysterical paralysis are all cases in which parts of the hysteric's body became sexualized.

To pinpoint the nature of sexuality (infantile and adult; normal, neurotic, and perverse) Freud distinguished stimuli that originate from an organism's external world from stimuli that originate from within an organism. Examples of the latter would be hunger and thirst but also the kinds of instincts that Freud would call sexual drives. (The standard translations of Freud render the *Trieb* as "instinct," but more recent translations and many psychoanalysts and scholars prefer "drive," to avoid confusion with what are commonly called instincts, as well as to avoid confusion with the German cognate *Instinkt*.) Organisms deal with stimuli coming from the external world by means of instantaneous reactions; for example, a contraction of the pupil in response to a bright light, or running away from a threatening situation. Instincts like hunger and thirst are sources of stimulation coming from inside the organism, and the fact that "no flight can avail" against such stimuli forces the organism to adopt other methods to deal with the stimulation ("Instincts and Their Vicissitudes," 118).

All instincts are sources of stimulation coming from within an organism, and sexual drives could be considered a special set of such instincts. Freud felt that this difference needed to be reinforced by a terminological distinction. "Libido" is Freud's word for the quantity of energy associated with a sexual drive. This quantity can appear in different forms and be put to a variety of uses, but whatever its form and whatever its use, the presence of this type of stimulation qualifies as sexual. To make an analogy: If sexuality is thought of as an organ, libido could be thought of as the substance that the organ secretes. This substance can appear in greater or lesser quantities, and it can take on a variety of different forms (symptoms, sexual acts, fantasies, dreams).

With the *Three Essays on the Theory of Sexuality* (1905) Freud aimed in part to criticize a view of sexuality according to which it first appears only in puberty and in only one particular form: an attraction to members of the opposite sex for the purpose of reproduction. Freud felt that this was an idealized and limited view of sexuality and argued that what we call sexuality in adulthood (coitus) is but one particular form in which sexuality appears: It cannot claim to be more natural, nor can it claim to be a developmental inevitability. This was also true of heterosexuality: "[F]rom the point of view of psycho-analysis the exclusive sexual interest felt by men for women is also a problem that needs elucidating and is not a self-evident fact" (*Three Essays*, 146; note added in 1915). To support his view, Freud distinguishes between sexual aims and sexual objects. Freud claimed that the aim of any instinct "is in every instance satisfaction, which can only be obtained by removing the state of stimulation at the source of the instinct" ("Instincts," 122). According to Freud, the purpose of the nervous system of any organism is to reduce the amount of stimulation within the organism "to the lowest possible level" (120). This rule, called the pleasure principle, is applied to sources of stimulation from both inside and outside the organism. Whatever the source of the stimulation, a feeling of pleasure is brought about when the quantity of stimulation in an organism is lessened, and a feeling of displeasure occurs when there is an increase in stimulation. While all instincts share the same aim, the ways in which instincts obtain satisfaction differ, and this is where the status of an instinct's object becomes important. The object of an instinct is what an instinct uses to achieve its aim. Hunger requires food, thirst requires liquid, and both hunger and thirst are satisfied by incorporating things from the external world into the body. In the case of these instincts, there is a close link between the aim and the object: Special sorts of objects are required for the instinct's satisfaction. In the case of sexual drives, however, Freud claimed that the aim and the object are merely "soldered together" and are in principle independent of each other (*Three Essays*, 148). The object a sexual drive uses to obtain satisfaction may be anything from an inanimate object (fetishism) to another species (**bestiality**); from another person or a part of that person's body to one's own body. Freud argued that it is even possible for an organism to obtain satisfaction for its instincts by merely hallucinating or imagining the presence of its object. Thus, the object of a sexual drive may in some instances be entirely phantasmatic. This idea played an important role in Freud's theory of dreams and **fantasy** (including daydreams): Experiencing thirst while sleeping, a person may dream about drinking, thereby temporarily alleviating the thirst instinct while also being able to fulfill the simultaneous wish to stay asleep. While "hallucinations" only temporarily alleviate instincts such as hunger or thirst before the need to eat and drink becomes too strong, the aim of sexual drives can be fully attained by such means.

The loose connection between the aim and object of sexual drives permits sexual drives to be sublimated. Sublimation occurs when a drive does not achieve the aim of satisfaction through its normal channels and its normal objects but through objects and actions that are devoid of any overt sexual significance, such as artistic activities, religious practices, and other behaviors.

Freud's theory of sexuality thus stretches the concept of sexuality beyond its conventional use. This stretching made Freud vulnerable to one persistent objection, that he advocates pansexualism. Pansexualism holds that all human desires and actions boil down to the satisfaction of sexual drives: Psychoanalysis would, on this view, reduce everything to sex. Freud argued that while the importance of sexuality as a contributing factor to the neuroses, psychoses, and perversions cannot be neglected and must be upheld by any theory calling itself psychoanalytic, psychoanalysis does not claim that sexuality is the exclusive source or purpose of all human actions, desires, and interests. Nor does it claim that it is the exclusive cause of psychological troubles, although psychoanalysis does claim that sexuality is a factor in more psychological problems and more types of human behavior than is generally believed. To those who continued to object to his extension of sexuality, Freud pointed out that his view had precedent in "the Eros of the divine Plato," which was also not restricted to adult, heterosexual coitus (*Three Essays*, 134).

Freud's "On Narcissism" (1914) added to the pansexualist controversy. Prior to this paper, Freud held that there were two basic orders of drives: sexual drives as well as "ego" drives. The latter serve the interest of self-preservation yet are also the source of affectionate feelings toward others ("Universal Tendency," 180). In "On Narcissism," Freud argued that a child's ego is first formed as an object by his or her sexual drives. This makes narcissism an extension of the autoeroticism that Freud held to be one of the main characteristics of infantile sexuality. The implication, then, is that the affectionate and self-interested drives that Freud claimed originate from the ego are actually just a subset of the sexual drives, since they come from an "object," albeit an internal object, that was created by the investment of the sexual drives. Many of Freud's colleagues felt that this brought Freud's theory closer to pansexualism (Jones, *Life and Work*, 303).

Narcissism, for Freud, is an extension of the early autoerotic activities of childhood. Autoeroticism is but one of two major characteristics of infantile sexuality. The other one is that this sexuality attaches to activities involved in the satisfaction of the infant's organic needs. Freud takes sensual sucking to be the infant's earliest sexual activity. Sucking is necessary for the infant to obtain nourishment, and while the satisfaction of the hunger instinct occurs by taking in objects (milk) from the external world, the activity of sucking on its own provides satisfaction that Freud dubs sexual: In sensual sucking "the need for repeating the sexual satisfaction now becomes detached from the need for taking nourishment" (*Three Essays*, 182). This pursuit of sexual satisfaction in sucking, divorced from biological needs yet using the avenues the body employs in meeting its needs, is typical of the perverse kernel of sexuality. The child can find any number of substitutes (a thumb, a pacifier) to obtain this satisfaction, and what makes it a sexual satisfaction is its independence from hunger or any other instinct.

The infant's next source of sexual satisfaction comes from the anal zone. Again, this is a zone of the body that, like the lips and mouth, plays an important role in the infant's ability to fulfill its biological needs. Just as was the case for the mouth and lips in hunger, the anal zone provides a sexual satisfaction on top of the satisfaction of the needs relieved through that zone. This satisfaction can also be repeated in separation from any need: through stimulation from rubbing or the intentional release and retention of the contents of the bowels.

Oral and anal sexuality show that infants engage in autoerotic activity even before their genitals are of any real interest to them. So Freud remarks that the genitals are not at all the original or oldest sources of sexual stimulation. The genitals become objects of interest to boys and girls in association with the need to urinate, and the conditions in which the genitals become an erotogenic zone and a center of autoerotic activity are similar to the conditions seen in the two previous zones. Freud also argues, however, that once an infant is familiar with the autoerotic activity available from oral sexuality, the genitals will be found to provide a particularly acute source of autoerotic pleasure.

Freud's description of the three initial stages of infantile sexuality suggests that the sex of the infant does not make any difference for either the nature or the development of sexuality up to the genital stage. Freud pointed out that around age four an important modification occurs in genital sexuality, and at this point whether the child is male or female is important. This second genital stage is a critical stage in the development of sexuality, for it is a stage at which the autoerotic behavior that characterizes infantile sexuality changes back into a form of sexuality that seeks satisfaction from objects in the external world. Initially, before it became autoerotic, the oral drive did have an object: the breast. This return to an object, in what Freud calls an "object-choice," is now accompanied by drives coming from the ego: the drives that are involved in **love** for others. Yet the objects sought by the sexual drives in this second genital phase are repetitions of the initial sexual object: "There are thus good reasons why a child sucking at his mother's breast has become the prototype of every relation of love. The finding of an object is in fact a refinding of it" (*Three Essays*, 222). With the convergence of ego-drives and sexual drives upon the same external object, which is a repetition of the original object, the stage is set for the Oedipus complex.

First mentioned in his *The Interpretation of Dreams* (1900), the Oedipus complex is one of Freud's most significant theoretical legacies (see also *The Ego and the Id*, chap. 3). Freud argued that both boys and girls go through a period during the second phase of genital sexuality that deserved to be compared to the situation of the Greek hero. Sophocles's (495–405 BCE) *Oedipus Rex* tells of an Oedipus who murdered his father and took his mother as his wife. The Freudian Oedipus complex is not a literal repetition of this scenario; however, the Oedipus complex involves more than mere wishing and hidden desires. Freud pointed out how a young boy "may show the most undisguised sexual curiosity about his mother, he may insist upon sleeping beside her at night, he may force his presence on her while she is dressing or may even make actual attempts at seducing her" (*Introductory Lectures on Psycho-Analysis*, 333). While a boy of four or five would not aspire to coitus, having no idea about it, he may seek out his mother as a source of genital arousal (in exhibitionism, incidental contact during washing, and so forth).

For a time Freud held that girls go through an Oedipus complex, too, simply with the genders reversed: love for the father and rivalry with the mother. He later argued that the situation was more complicated than that. Both boys and girls, Freud claimed, enter the Oedipus complex under the same conditions: with the mother as the primary object and the father as a rival. For boys, the penis remains the primary erotogenic zone before, during, and after the Oedipus complex. Yet for girls both the object and the source of the sexual drive changes: The object changes from mother to father, and the source of stimulation changes from the clitoris to the vagina. Thus, the Oedipus complex for girls is the structure in which girls attain femininity. Femininity is seen by Freud as an accomplishment because he saw the autoerotic activity of girls prior to the Oedipus complex as basically masculine. Clitoral **masturbation** is the primary sexual activity during a girl's genital phase, and Freud did not believe that this activity differed in kind from the masturbatory activity of boys. Both could be called "phallic" and "masculine" since they are primarily characterized by an activity centered on the genitals. Thus, Freud claimed that libido is essentially masculine in nature, even in the case of female sexuality, insofar as it is primarily active. Yet feminine sexuality becomes different in kind from masculine sexuality when it has a "passive aim." The shift from masculine libidinal activity to feminine occurs when the vagina replaces the clitoris as a girl's primary source of sexual stimulation ("Female Sexuality," 228). This is, not surprisingly, one of the more controversial aspects of Freud's theory of sexuality, and it was contested even in his lifetime by psychoanalysts such as Ernest Jones (1869–1958; *Papers on Psychoanalysis*, 438 ff.) and Karen Horney (1885–1952; *Feminine Psychology*, 37–53).

Freud also held that both boys and girls experience a castration complex. Interestingly, however, for boys the castration complex occurs after the Oedipus complex, whereas girls enter Oedipus with a castration complex already in place. The castration complex is characterized, for boys, by an anxiety over the loss of the penis. During the Oedipus complex, the boy fears that he may be punished with castration by his father or a similar authority figure for his feelings toward his mother. This leads to a repression or destruction of the

Oedipus complex, yet the feelings aroused in him later by other women in adulthood will echo the feelings he initially had for his mother. This makes the romantic life of adulthood a difficult libidinal challenge, since it will always run up against what Freud referred to as the "rock of castration": a fear of punishment for breaking the **incest** taboo ("Analysis Terminable," 252). Castration anxiety, Freud argued, could account for such phenomena as psychical impotence (for example, an inability to have sex with one's wife or partner but concurrent with an ability to have sex with anyone else) and some men's overestimation of certain women as pure, unstained love objects and simultaneous devaluation of the women with whom they have sex. In "Universal Tendency" (186), Freud offers the following sobering advice: "[I]t sounds not only disagreeable but also paradoxical, yet it must nevertheless be said that anyone who is to be really free and happy in love must have surmounted his respect for women and have come to terms with the idea of incest with his mother or sister."

Since girls enter the Oedipus complex with a castration complex already in place, it cannot be said that girls fear castration: Rather, what they fear during and after Oedipus is a loss of love from their mothers as punishment for their incestuous desires. This difference is due in part to the fact that girls do not interpret sexual difference the same as boys do. Boys tend not to believe their eyes when confronted with the anatomical difference between boys and girls and hold on to the belief that girls have penises for as long as possible. When this is no longer possible, boys frequently believe that girls used to have penises but have lost them (are castrated) and that this loss was due to a punishment. (Freud felt that this accounts for why many men hold women to be inferior beings in adulthood.) Girls are less inclined to interpret sexual difference in this way, and at any rate, they do not experience castration anxiety when confronted with the anatomical difference: Freud argued that they experience themselves as already castrated. Freud writes that along with this "they are overcome by envy for the penis—an envy culminating in the wish . . . to be boys themselves" (*Three Essays*, 195).

Given this primary childhood wish to be a boy and have a penis, Freud discerned three distinct lines of development for girls, only one of which would result in "normal" womanhood. One line results in sexual inhibition (a general lack of interest in sex and sexual satisfaction). This is a response to penis envy in which a woman renounces sexual satisfaction altogether to avoid being reminded of her castration: any sexual satisfaction would evoke the disappointment she felt as a girl at the difference between her clitoris and a penis. Another option is what Freud calls the "masculinity complex," in which the girl "clings to her clitoridal activity" and identifies either with her father or mother, whom she continues to believe, unconsciously, is not castrated (thus, Freud calls this a "phallic" mother; *New Introductory Lectures*, 130). In this position, a girl acts as if her wish to be a boy and have a penis has already been fulfilled. The last possibility is what Freud refers to as "normal femininity," in which the wish for a penis is replaced by a wish for a baby. This wish for a baby is an important factor in the girl's entry into the Oedipus complex. In the feminine Oedipus complex, instead of remaining with the wish to have a penis, the girl wishes for a child from her father and experiences her mother as a rival for her father's love (*New Introductory Lectures*, 128).

Freud held that after the Oedipus complex, children entered a latency period, which lasts from the age of six or seven to puberty. This period is characterized by a general repression of the autoerotic activity of early childhood, and it is during this period that what Freud called infantile amnesia occurs: our inability to remember much of anything about the sexual life and the sexual fantasies of early childhood. Sexuality and fantasy life awaken once again with the onset of puberty, which can lead to a revival of the Oedipus complex.

Freud's view of female sexuality has been roundly criticized for its phallocentrism by feminist writers interested in and even attracted to, yet also critical of, other aspects of

Freud's theory (see, for example, Nancy Chodorow, Jane Gallop, Evelyn Fox Keller, and Juliet Mitchell). His views on **sexual perversion** and **homosexuality** also continue to be the subject of lively debate. Freud's use of the term "perverse" was not meant to imply any devaluation or ethical dismissal of the actions in perversion, yet Freud's views on perversion seem to suggest that people whose sole sexual activities are "perverse" are psychologically immature. Freud did claim that "the extraordinarily wide dissemination of the perversions forces us to suppose that the disposition to perversions is itself of no great rarity but must form a part of what passes as the normal constitution" (*Three Essays*, 171). Passages like this suggest that for Freud the difference between perversion and normalcy is not all that great (for discussion, see Neu); indeed, perverse sexuality exemplifies the crucial distinction between the sexual aim and the sexual object. Freud even claimed that in a certain sense homosexuality was universal, insofar as everyone makes unconscious homosexual "object-choices." These are present in **friendship**s for members of the same sex or in identifications with same-sex figures (parents, teachers, peers, and role models) throughout life (*Three Essays*, 144n.1). This type of universal homosexuality is, however, significantly different from what we ordinarily call homosexuality, which is defined by specific sexual practices. For many, Freud's definition of sexual perversion in terms of nonprocreative, infantile forms of sexuality continues to suggest that even though perversion is also a component of normal sexuality, nevertheless normal sexuality may mark a progression away from an exclusive practice of perverse sexuality. Still, Freud was far from seeing homosexuality as immoral. In a famous letter to a concerned mother who wrote to Freud about her son's homosexuality, Freud sought to assuage her concerns and at the same time managed to put his views on homosexuality quite clearly:

> Homosexuality is assuredly no advantage, but it is nothing to be ashamed of, no vice, no degradation; it cannot be classified as an illness; we consider it to be a variation of the sexual function, produced by a certain arrest of sexual development. Many highly respectable individuals of ancient and modern times have been homosexuals, several of the greatest men among them. (Plato, Michelangelo, Leonardo da Vinci, etc.) It is a great injustice to persecute homosexuality as a crime—and a cruelty, too. (Letter 277 [9 April 1935], Ernst Freud, *Letters of Sigmund Freud*, 423)

Freud is widely credited with having changed the way we think about sexuality. Starting with the basic idea that hysterical symptoms were actually forms of sexual activity, Freud was led to understand human beings as fundamentally sexual creatures, beginning at birth. Central to Freud's theory of sexuality is the view that sexuality is defined neither by genital activity nor by the aim of reproduction. It appears initially in the form of oral activity and becomes autoerotic with the infant's ability to find a satisfaction in sucking that is detached from the need for food. The fact that sexuality later becomes an activity that is not primarily autoerotic is seen by Freud to be an accomplishment and not at all an inevitable one. It is an incredibly fragile accomplishment, and sexuality is always inclined to regress or fixate on its earlier forms. Whether Freud held that adult heterosexual coitus is somehow developmentally superior to forms of infantile sexuality and the perversions, he lends to sexuality an intrinsically perverse core.

See also African Philosophy; Arts, Sex and the; Bisexuality; Ellis, Havelock; Firestone, Shulamith; Freudian Left, The; Kolnai, Aurel; Lacan, Jacques; Leibniz, Gottfried; Paraphilia; Perversion, Sexual; Poststructuralism; Psychology, Twentieth- and Twenty-First-Century; Schopenhauer, Arthur; Sexology; Sherfey, Mary Jane; Singer, Irving; Spinoza, Baruch; Westermarck, Edward

REFERENCES

Chodorow, Nancy. *The Reproduction of Mothering: Psychoanalysis and the Sociology of Gender.* Berkeley: University of California Press, 1978; Crews, Frederick C., and 18 others. *The Memory Wars: Freud's Legacy in Dispute.* New York: A New York Review Book, 1995; Freud, Ernst L., ed. *Letters of Sigmund Freud.* New York: Basic Books, 1960; Freud, Sigmund. The following works by Freud are in *The Standard Edition of the Complete Psychological Works of Sigmund Freud,* 24 vols. Trans. and ed. James Strachey. London: Hogarth Press, 1953–1974; Freud, Sigmund. (1937) "Analysis Terminable and Interminable." Vol. 23 (1937–1939), 211–54; Freud, Sigmund. (1923) *The Ego and the Id.* Vol. 19 (1923–1925), 3–66; Freud, Sigmund. (1931) "Female Sexuality." Vol. 21 (1927–1931), 223–43; Freud, Sigmund. (1915) "Instincts and Their Vicissitudes." Vol. 14 (1914–1916), 111–40; Freud, Sigmund. (1900) *The Interpretation of Dreams.* Vol. 5 (1900–1901), 339–627; Freud, Sigmund. *Introductory Lectures on Psycho-Analysis* (Part III). Vol. 16 (1916–1917); Freud, Sigmund. (1905 [1906]) "My Views on the Part Played by Sexuality in the Aetiology of the Neuroses." Vol. 7 (1901–1905), 271–79; Freud, Sigmund. (1933) *New Introductory Lectures on Psycho-Analysis.* Vol. 22 (1932–1936), 3–182; Freud, Sigmund. (1914) "On Narcissism." Vol. 14 (1914–1916), 67–102; Freud, Sigmund. (1912) "On the Universal Tendency to Debasement in the Sphere of Love." Vol. 11 (1910), 179–90; Freud, Sigmund. (1895) *Studies on Hysteria.* Vol. 2 (1893–1895), 1–335; Freud, Sigmund. (1905) *Three Essays on the Theory of Sexuality.* Vol. 7 (1901–1905), 125–245; Gallop, Jane. *The Daughter's Seduction: Feminism and Psychoanalysis.* Ithaca, N.Y.: Cornell University Press, 1982; Horney, Karen. *Feminine Psychology.* New York: Norton, 1937; Jones, Ernest. *The Life and Work of Sigmund Freud,* vol. 2. New York: Basic Books, 1955; Jones, Ernest. *Papers on Psychoanalysis.* Boston, Mass.: Beacon Press, 1948; Keller, Evelyn Fox. *Reflections on Gender and Science.* New Haven, Conn.: Yale University Press, 1985; Masson, Jeffrey Moussaieff. *The Assault on Truth: Freud's Suppression of the Seduction Theory.* New York: Farrar, Straus and Giroux, 1984; Mitchell, Juliet. *Psychoanalysis and Feminism: Freud, Reich, Laing, and Women.* New York: Vintage, 1975; Neu, Jerome. "Freud and Perversion." In Jerome Neu, ed., *The Cambridge Companion to Freud.* Cambridge: Cambridge University Press, 1991, 175–208.

Ed Pluth

ADDITIONAL READING

Abelove, Henry. "Freud, Male Homosexuality, and the Americans." In Henry Abelove, Michèle Aina Barale, and David M. Halperin, eds., *The Lesbian and Gay Studies Reader.* New York: Routledge, 1993, 381–93; Althusser, Louis. *Writings on Psychoanalysis: Freud and Lacan.* New York: Columbia University Press, 1996; Andreas-Salomé, Lou. *The Freud Journal of Lou Andreas-Salomé.* Trans. Stanley A. Leavy. New York: Basic Books, 1964; Balbus, Isaac D. *Marxism and Domination: A Neo-Hegelian, Feminist, Psychoanalytic Theory of Sexual, Political, and Technological Liberation.* Princeton, N.J.: Princeton University Press, 1982; Benjamin, Jessica. *The Bonds of Love: Psychoanalysis, Feminism, and the Problem of Domination.* New York: Pantheon, 1988; Bergmann, Martin S. *The Anatomy of Loving: The Story of Man's Quest to Know What Love Is.* New York: Columbia University Press, 1987; Bergo, Bettina. "Freud's Debt to Philosophy and His Copernican Revolution." In Jennifer Radden, ed., *The Philosophy of Psychiatry: A Companion.* New York: Oxford University Press, 2004, 338–50; Bersani, Leo. *Baudelaire and Freud.* Berkeley: University of California Press, 1977; Bersani, Leo. "Foucault, Freud, Fantasy, and Power." *GLQ: A Journal of Lesbian and Gay Studies* 2:1–2 (1995), 11–33; Bersani, Leo. *The Freudian Body: Psychoanalysis and Art.* New York: Columbia University Press, 1986; Bilsker, Richard. "Freud and Schopenhauer: Consciousness, the Unconscious, and the Drive towards Death." *Idealistic Studies* 27:1–2 (1997), 79–90; Boothby, Richard. *Freud as Philosopher: Metapsychology after Lacan.* New York: Routledge, 2000; Brecher, Edward M. "The Child as Father of the Man." In *The Sex Researchers.* Boston, Mass.: Little, Brown, 1969, 61–81; Brennan, Teresa. *The Interpretation of the Flesh: Freud and Femininity.* New York: Routledge, 1992; Brown, Norman O. *Life against Death: The Psychoanalytic Meaning of History.*

Middletown, Conn.: Wesleyan University Press, 1959; Buhle, Mary Jo. *Feminism and Its Discontents: A Century of Struggle with Psychoanalysis*. Cambridge, Mass.: Harvard University Press, 1998; Buller, David J. "DeFreuding Evolutionary Psychology." In V. Gray Hardcastle, ed., *Where Biology Meets Psychology: Philosophical Essays*. Cambridge, Mass.: MIT Press, 1999, 99–114; Butler, Clark. "Hegel and Freud: A Comparison." *Philosophy and Phenomenological Research* 36:4 (1976), 506–22; Carr, David. "Freud and Sexual Ethics." *Philosophy* 62:241 (1987), 361–73; Cavell, Marcia. *The Psychoanalytic Mind: From Freud to Philosophy*. Cambridge, Mass.: Harvard University Press, 1993; Chodorow, Nancy J. *Femininities, Masculinities, Sexualities: Freud and Beyond*. Lexington: University Press of Kentucky, 1994; Chodorow, Nancy J. *Feminism and Psychoanalytic Theory*. New Haven, Conn.: Yale University Press, 1989; Chodorow, Nancy J. (1978) *The Reproduction of Mothering: Psychoanalysis and the Sociology of Gender*. With a new preface. Berkeley: University of California Press, 1999; Cohen, Robert S., and Larry Laudan, eds. *Physics, Philosophy, and Psychoanalysis: Essays in Honor of Adolf Grünbaum*. Boston, Mass.: Reidel, 1983; Connell, Robert W. "Psychoanalysis on Masculinity." In Harry Brod and Michael Kauffman, eds., *Theorizing Masculinities*. Thousand Oaks, Calif.: Sage, 1994, 11–38; Crews, Frederick C. *Unauthorized Freud: Doubters Confront a Legend*. New York: Viking, 1998; de Sousa, Ronald. "Norms and the Normal." In Richard Wollheim, ed., *Freud: A Collection of Critical Essays*. Garden City, N.Y.: Anchor Books, 1974, 196–221; Dean, Tim, and Christopher Lane, eds. *Homosexuality and Psychoanalysis*. Chicago, Ill.: University of Chicago Press, 2001; Derrida, Jacques. (1980) *The Post Card: From Socrates to Freud and Beyond*. Trans. Alan Bass. Chicago, Ill.: University of Chicago Press, 1987; Dickason, Anne. "Anatomy Is Destiny: The Role of Biology in Plato's Views of Women." *Philosophical Forum* 5:1–2 (1973–1974), 45–53; Dollimore, Jonathan. *Sexual Dissidence: Augustine to Wilde, Freud to Foucault*. Oxford, U.K.: Clarendon Press, 1991; Drassinower, Abraham. *Freud's Theory of Culture: Eros, Loss, and Politics*. Lanham, Md.: Rowman and Littlefield, 2003; duBois, Page. *Sowing the Body: Psychoanalysis and Ancient Representations of Women*. Chicago, Ill.: University of Chicago Press, 1988; Elshtain, Jean Bethke. "Psychoanalytic Feminism: Gender, Identity, and Politics." In *Public Man, Private Woman: Women in Social and Political Thought*. Princeton, N.J.: Princeton University Press, 1981, 285–97; Feldstein, Richard, and Judith Roof, eds. *Feminism and Psychoanalysis*. Ithaca, N.Y.: Cornell University Press, 1989; Flanagan, Owen J., Jr. "Freud: Masculinity, Femininity, and the Philosophy of Mind." In Mary Vetterling-Braggin, ed., *"Femininity," "Masculinity," and "Androgyny": A Modern Philosophical Discussion*. Totowa, N.J.: Littlefield, Adams, 1982, 60–76; Fóti, Véronique M. "Thought, Affect, Drive, and Pathogenesis in Spinoza and Freud." *History of European Ideas* 3:2 (1982), 221–36. Reprinted in Genevieve Lloyd, ed., *Spinoza: Critical Assessments*, vol. 4. London: Routledge, 2001, 289–305; Freeman, Lucy. *The Story of Anna O*. New York: Walker, 1972; Freud, Sigmund. *Sexuality and the Psychology of Love*. Ed. Philip Rieff. New York: Collier, 1963; Freud, Sigmund. (1905) *Three Essays on the Theory of Sexuality*. Trans. James Strachey. New York: Basic Books, 1975; Freud, Sigmund. (1913) *Totem and Taboo*. In *The Standard Edition of the Complete Psychological Works of Sigmund Freud*, vol. 13. Trans. James Strachey. London: Hogarth Press, 1953–1974, ix–161; Fromm, Erich. *The Crisis of Psychoanalysis: Essays on Freud, Marx, and Social Psychology*. Greenwich, Conn.: Fawcett, 1971; Frosh, Steven. (1987) *The Politics of Psychoanalysis: An Introduction to Freudian and Post-Freudian Theory*, 2nd ed. New York: New York University Press, 1999; Gardner, Sebastian. *Irrationality and the Philosophy of Psychoanalysis*. Cambridge: Cambridge University Press, 1993; Gay, Peter. *Freud: A Life for Our Time*. New York: Norton, 1988; Gay, Volney P. *Freud on Sublimation: Reconsiderations*. Albany: State University of New York Press, 1992; Gay, Volney P. *Reading Freud: Psychoanalysis, Neurosis, and Religion*. Chico, Calif.: Scholars Press, 1983; Gearhart, Suzanne. "Foucault's Response to Freud: Sadomasochism and the Aestheticization of Power." *Style* 29 (Fall 1995), 389–403; Grünbaum, Adolf. *The Foundations of Psychoanalysis: A Philosophical Critique*. Berkeley: University of California Press, 1984; Gupta, R. K. "Freud and Schopenhauer." *Journal of the History of Ideas* 36:4 (1975), 721–28; Hannan, Barbara. "Love and Human Bondage in Maugham, Spinoza, and Freud." In Roger E. Lamb, ed., *Love Analyzed*. Boulder, Colo.: Westview, 1997, 93–106; Hessing, Siegfried. "Freud's Relation with Spinoza." In Siegfried Hessing, ed., *Speculum Spinozanum: 1677–1977*. London:

Routledge and Kegan Paul, 1977, 224–39; Hook, Sidney, ed. (1959) *Psychoanalysis, Scientific Method, and Philosophy*. New Brunswick, N.J.: Transaction, 1990; Horowitz, Gad. *Repression. Basic and Surplus Repression in Psychoanalytic Theory: Freud, Reich, and Marcuse*. Toronto, Can.: University of Toronto Press, 1977; Hutcheon, Pat Duffy. "Through a Glass Darkly: Freud's Concept of Love." In David Goicoechea, ed., *The Nature and Pursuit of Love: The Philosophy of Irving Singer*. Amherst, N.Y.: Prometheus, 1995, 183–95; Jacoby, Russell. (1983) *The Repression of Psychoanalysis: Otto Fenichel and the Political Freudians*. Chicago, Ill.: University of Chicago Press, 1986; Kaplan, Alan. "Spinoza and Freud." *Spinoza Studies* (Haifa) (1978), 85–110; Kofman, Sarah. (1980) *The Enigma of Woman: Woman in Freud's Writings*. Trans. Catharine Porter. Ithaca, N.Y.: Cornell University Press, 1985; Kovel, Joel. *The Age of Desire: Reflections of a Radical Psychoanalyst*. New York: Pantheon, 1981; Kristeva, Julia. (1985) *In the Beginning Was Love: Psychoanalysis and Faith*. Trans. Arthur Goldhammer. New York: Columbia University Press, 1987; Laplanche, Jean. *Life and Death in Psycho-analysis*. Trans. Jeffrey Mehlman. Baltimore, Md.: Johns Hopkins University Press, 1976; Levine, Michael P. "Etiology of Emotion and Ossification of Self: You Can't Change People Because People Don't Change." In Man Cheung Chung, ed., *Psychoanalytic Knowledge and the Nature of Mind*. London: Palgrave, 2003, 96–119; Levine, Michael P. "A Fun Night Out: Horror and Other Pleasures of the Cinema." In Steven Schneider, ed., *The Horror Film and Psychoanalysis: Freud's Worst Nightmares*. Cambridge: Cambridge University Press, 2004, 35–54. Prepublished in *Senses of Cinema* (15 January 2001). <www.sensesofcinema.com/contents/01/15/horror_fun.html> [accessed 20 September 2004]; Levine, Michael P., ed. *The Analytic Freud: Philosophy and Psychoanalysis*. New York: Routledge, 2000; Lorber, Judith, Rose Laub Coser, Alice S. Rossi, and Nancy Chodorow. "On *The Reproduction of Mothering*: A Methodological Debate." *Signs* 6:3 (1981), 482–514; Marcus, Steven. (1966) "A Child Is Being Beaten." In *The Other Victorians: A Study of Sexuality and Pornography in Mid-Nineteenth-Century England*. New York: Bantam, 1977, 255–68; Marcuse, Herbert. (1955) *Eros and Civilization: A Philosophical Inquiry into Freud*. Boston, Mass.: Beacon Press, 1966; Mead, Margaret. "On Freud's View of Female Psychology." In Jean Strouse, ed., *Women and Analysis: Dialogues on Psychoanalytic Views of Femininity*. New York: Grossman, 1974, 95–106; Miller, Jean Baker, ed. *Psychoanalysis and Women*. Baltimore, Md.: Penguin, 1973; Miller, William Ian. *The Anatomy of Disgust*. Cambridge, Mass.: Harvard University Press, 1997; Mitchell, Juliet. "On Freud and the Distinction between the Sexes." In Jean Strouse, ed., *Women and Analysis: Dialogues on Psychoanalytic Views of Femininity*. New York: Grossman, 1974, 27–36; Morgan, Douglas N. *Love: Plato, the Bible, and Freud*. Englewood Cliffs, N.J.: Prentice-Hall, 1964; Murphy, Timothy F. "Freud, Sigmund." In Timothy F. Murphy, ed., *Reader's Guide to Lesbian and Gay Studies*. Chicago, Ill.: Fitzroy Dearborn, 2000, 233–34; Nails, Debra. "Conatus versus Eros/Thanatos: On the Principles of Spinoza and Freud." *Dialogue* (PST) 21:2–3 (1979), 33–40; Neu, Jerome. *Emotion, Thought, and Therapy: A Study of Hume and Spinoza and the Relationship of Philosophical Theories of the Emotions to Psychological Theories of Therapy*. London: Routledge and Kegan Paul, 1977; Neu, Jerome. "Fantasy and Memory: The Aetiological Role of Thoughts According to Freud." *International Journal of Psycho-Analysis* 54 (1973), 383–98; Neu, Jerome. "Freud and Perversion." In Jerome Neu, ed., *The Cambridge Companion to Freud*. Cambridge: Cambridge University Press, 1991, 175–208. Reprinted in *A Tear Is an Intellectual Thing: The Meanings of Emotion*. New York: Oxford University Press, 2000, 144–65; STW (87–104). Original publication in Earl E. Shelp, ed., *Sexuality and Medicine*, vol. 1: *Conceptual Roots*. Dordrecht, Holland: Reidel, 1987, 153–84; Neu, Jerome. "Genetic Explanation in *Totem and Taboo*." In Richard Wollheim, ed., *Freud: A Collection of Critical Essays*. Garden City, N.Y.: Doubleday/Anchor, 1974, 366–97; Neu, Jerome, ed. *The Cambridge Companion to Freud*. Cambridge: Cambridge University Press, 1991; Nussbaum, Martha C. "Foul Play." [Review of *The Anatomy of Disgust*, by William Ian Miller] *The New Republic* (17 November 1997), 32–38; Oring, Elliot. *The Jokes of Sigmund Freud: A Study in Humor and Jewish Identity*. Philadelphia: University of Pennsylvania Press, 1984; Phillips, Adam. *On Flirtation*. London: Faber and Faber, 1994; Phillips, Adam. *Promises, Promises: Essays on Psychoanalysis and Literature*. New York: Basic Books, 2001; Prose, Francine. "Lou Andreas-Salomé." In *The Lives of the Muses: Nine Women and the Artists They Inspired*. New York: HarperCollins,

2002, 139–85; Rice, Lee C. "Freud, Sartre, Spinoza: The Problematic of the Unconscious." *Giornale di Metafisica* 17:1 (1995), 87–106; Ricoeur, Paul. *Freud and Philosophy: An Essay on Interpretation.* Trans. Denis Savage. New Haven, Conn.: Yale University Press, 1970; Rieff, Philip. *Freud: The Mind of the Moralist.* New York: Viking, 1959; Rieff, Philip. *The Triumph of the Therapeutic: Uses of Faith after Freud.* New York: Harper and Row, 1966; Ritvo, Lucille. *Darwin's Influence on Freud: A Tale of Two Sciences.* New Haven, Conn.: Yale University Press, 1990; Robinson, Paul. *Freud and His Critics.* Berkeley: University of California Press, 1993; Rycroft, Charles. (1968) *A Critical Dictionary of Psychoanalysis*, 2nd ed. London: Penguin, 1995; Santas, Gerasimos. *Plato and Freud: Two Theories of Love.* Oxford, U.K.: Blackwell, 1988; Sartre, Jean-Paul. *Existential Psychoanalysis.* Trans. Hazel E. Barnes. Washington, D.C.: Regnery, 1962; Seidenberg, Robert. (1970) "Is Anatomy Destiny?" In Jean Baker Miller, ed., *Psychoanalysis and Women.* Baltimore, Md.: Penguin, 1973, 306–29; Sherfey, Mary Jane. "The Evolution and Nature of Female Sexuality in Relation to Psychoanalytic Theory." *Journal of the American Psychoanalytic Association* 14:1 (1966), 28–128; Shulgasser, Mark. "Sigmund Freud—Pisces?" *Astrological Journal* 42:2 (2000), 19–25; Singer, Irving. "Freud." In *The Nature of Love*, vol. 3: *The Modern World.* Chicago, Ill.: University of Chicago Press, 1987, 97–158; Spain, David H. "The Westermarck-Freud Incest-Theory Debate: An Evaluation and Reformulation." *Current Anthropology* 28:5 (1987), 623–45; Stoller, Robert J. "Impact of New Advances in Sex Research on Psychoanalytic Theory." In *Perversion: The Erotic Form of Hatred.* New York: Dell, 1975, 12–45; Strouse, Jean, ed. *Women and Analysis: Dialogues on Psychoanalytic Views of Femininity.* New York: Grossman, 1974; Sulloway, Frank J. *Freud, Biologist of the Mind: Beyond the Psychoanalytic Legend.* New York: Basic Books, 1979; Thornton, Stephen P. (2001) "Sigmund Freud (1856–1939)." In James Fieser, ed., *The Internet Encyclopedia of Philosophy.* <www.utm.edu/research/iep/f/freud.htm> [accessed 27 October 2004]; Trupp, Michael S. *On Freud.* Belmont, Calif.: Wadsworth, 2000; Van Herik, Judith. *Freud on Femininity and Faith.* Berkeley: University of California Press, 1982; Weeks, Jeffrey. *Sexuality and Its Discontents: Meanings, Myths, and Modern Sexualities.* London: Routledge and Kegan Paul, 1985; Westermarck, Edward. (1934) "The Oedipus Complex." In *Three Essays on Sex and Marriage.* London: Macmillan, 1934, 1–123; Wollheim, Richard. *Sigmund Freud.* New York: Viking, 1971; Wollheim, Richard, ed. *Freud: A Collection of Critical Essays.* Garden City, N.Y.: Anchor Books, 1974; Wortis, Joseph. *Fragments of an Analysis with Freud.* New York: Simon and Schuster, 1954; Wright, Elizabeth, ed. *Feminism and Psychoanalysis: A Critical Dictionary.* Oxford, U.K.: Oxford University Press, 1992; Young, Christopher, and Andrew Brook. "Schopenhauer and Freud." *International Journal of Psychoanalysis* 75 (1994), 101–18. <www.carleton.ca/~abrook/SCHOPENY.htm> [accessed 18 October 2004].

FREUDIAN LEFT, THE. In the "Preface" to Gilles Deleuze (1925–1995) and Félix Guattari's (1930–1992) influential *Anti-Oedipus*, **Michel Foucault** (1926–1984) offers the following reflections:

> During the years 1945–1965 (I am referring to Europe), there was a certain way of thinking correctly, a certain style of political discourse, a certain ethics of the intellectual. One had to be on familiar terms with Marx, not let one's dreams stray too far from Freud. (xi)

For many on the Left, disillusioned by the sudden rise of both fascism and totalitarian regimes in Europe and the Soviet Union, **Marxism** still represented the way forward, even if it needed to be supplemented with psychological categories so as to explain these developments. Wilhelm Reich (1897–1957), himself a pupil of **Sigmund Freud** (1856–1939), could write as early as 1934 that "when I was studying Marx, it seemed to me that Marx does not answer the question of the origin of man's inner contradictions" (*Sex-Pol*, 39n.40). And there we have the research agenda for what Paul Robinson termed "The Freudian

Left"—namely, the attempts by theoreticians Herbert Marcuse (1898–1979), Norman O. Brown (1913–2002), and Reich both to extend Freud's psychosocial analyses—as found in his later works *Future of an Illusion* (1927) and *Civilization and Its Discontents* (1930)—and to explain how orthodox Marxism left the totalitarian personality anomalous. In contrast to the conservative neo-Freudian "revisionists" (for example, Alfred Adler [1870–1937], Karen Horney [1885–1952], and Erich Fromm [1900–1980]), who came to dominate psychoanalysis in the Anglo-American world and for whom the goal of therapy was adjustment to social reality (of whatever degree of irrationality; see Jacoby), the Freudian Left would press a cornerstone of Freudian psychoanalysis, *viz.*, that the wages of civilization are neuroses, and offer up not only the most radical critique of Western liberalism of the last century but also a bold and positive vision of human liberation. In doing so, the Freudian Left lay the groundwork for postmodernist theoreticians such as Foucault and **Jacques Lacan** (1901–1981) and served as a lighthouse for many of the key constituencies—students, homosexuals, greens, women—of the New Left.

If the historical catalyst for this Freud-Marx confluence is clear enough (see Martin Jay for the details), understanding the deeper, philosophical rationale for this most unlikely of partnerships requires an examination of the humanism of Karl Marx (1818–1883) as well as Freud's own views of the origins of man's inner contradictions. For, *prima facie*, the two thinkers are absolute antipodes (see Balbus; Lichtman). Marx is the dialectical, utopian socialist; Freud is the dualistic, pessimistic elitist, whose *massenpsychologie* (in, say, *Totem and Taboo*) is full of disdain for the ordinary man. Philip Rieff, one of the conservative interpreters of Freud, summarizes their division sharply: "For Marx, the past is pregnant with the future, with the proletariat as the midwife of change. For Freud, the future is pregnant with the past, a burden of which only the physician, and luck, can deliver us" (215). And Deleuze thinks that reconciling two economies, Marx's political economy and Freud's libidinal economy, is misconceived from the very start, for "there is but one economy. . . . It is economy itself that is political economy and desiring economy" (276). That Freud remained a stalwart bourgeois liberal, declaring that communism's "psychological premises" were "an untenable illusion" (*Civilization*, 113), must be put alongside his later focus on the instincts and their "vicissitudes" within social settings. Despite this, many have questioned whether his medical agenda and universal biological instincts are compatible with the historical materialist reading Reich claims for him. It was Reich, for whom "the Oedipal relationship is not a biological but a social phenomenon" (*Sex-Pol*, 82), who first and foremost historicizes psychoanalysis, even asserting that "psychoanalysis fully confirms Marx's dictum that social being determines consciousness" (39). Abraham Drassinower approves the Reichian synthesis, identifying the "forgotten claims of Eros" as the libidinal ties that bind communities in **G.W.F. Hegel**'s (1770–1831) own "dialectic of recognition" (53).

In any case, neither Marx nor Freud survives fully intact in Marcuse, Reich, or Brown, though all three were self-conscious of remaining true to both. Reich provides the most explicit statement of the Freudian Left's most obvious departure from orthodox Marxism:

> An effective policy, whose ultimate goal is the achievement of socialism and the establishment of the rule of labor over capital, must not only be based on a recognition of those movements and changes which occur objectively and independently of our will as a result of the development of the productive forces. This policy must also, simultaneously, and on the same level, take account of what happens "in people's heads," i.e., in the psychical structures of the human beings who are subjected to these processes and who actually carry them out. (*Sex-Pol*, 284)

Reich's relationship to Freud is equally troubled. He would agree with Marcuse's melioristic criticism:

> In Freud's theory, freedom from repression is a matter of the unconscious, of the subhistorical and even subhuman past, of primal biological and mental processes; consequently, the idea of a non-repressive reality principle is a matter of retrogression. That such a principle could itself become a historical reality, a matter of developing consciousness, that the images of phantasy could refer to the unconquered future of mankind rather than to its (badly) conquered past—all this seemed to Freud at best a nice utopia. (*Eros*, 147)

Brown, however, locates a deeper affinity between Freud and his Marxist psychologists. What makes Freud so amenable to Critical Theory, the Frankfurt School, and twentieth-century Marxists is the role of the negative, of tension, of contradiction and resolution, in mapping "man's inner contradictions." As Brown writes:

> The Freudian revolution is that radical revision of traditional theories of human nature and human society which becomes necessary if repression is recognized as a fact. In the new Freudian perspective, the essence of society is repression of the individual, and the essence of the individual is repression of himself. (*Life*, 3)

For the philosophy of sex, the relevant point of contact for Marx and Freud is alienation; both saw social forces as essentially stripping man of his power and conceived of the practical recovery of this power and freedom through "consciousness-raising" as the goal of their respective programs. Demystifying the historical forces responsible for material production (for Marx) and revealing the repressed contents of the unconscious (for Freud) were meant to decrease the irrationality of existence and to liberate mankind. Alienated labor within capitalist political economy was for Marx, in the *Manuscripts of 1844*, and for Marx and Friedrich Engels (1820–1895), in *The German Ideology*, the crucial nexus of this loss of power:

> This crystallization of social activity, this consolidation of what we ourselves produce into an objective power above us, growing out of our control, thwarting our expectations, bringing to naught our calculations, is one of the chief factors in historical development up till now. . . . The social power, i.e., the multiplied productive force . . . appears to these individuals, since their cooperation is not voluntary but natural, not as their united power, but as an alien force existing outside them, of the origin and end of which they are ignorant, which they thus cannot control, which, on the contrary, passes through a peculiar series of phases and stages independent of the will and the action of man, nay even being the prime governor of these. (*German Ideology*, 254–55)

From this perspective, Freud's notion of a dynamic superego is a theory of ideology. The boy (Freud superimposes this on the girl) identifies first with his father and develops an object-cathexis for his mother, who becomes (as the boy receives less of her affection) a competitor. Eros is then sublimated (displaying its flexibility—the key Freudian insight taken up by Reich, Marcuse, and Brown) and the child intensifies his identification with the father figure, and hence to authority, and to society (internalized as "conscience") as a whole. Identity formation, the culmination of the Oedipal complex, can be seen as the result of an individuality repressed by societal demands. (So Marcuse: "[A]ccording to Freud, the history of man is the history of his repression"; *Eros*, 11.)

The particularly sexual form that this repression takes recasts Freud's shadow over the Left in the 1960s. Whereas many of Freud's successors within psychoanalysis—Adler, Horney, Fromm, and so on—downplayed his theories of sexuality and dismissed his early claim that all neuroses spring from (anxiety over) sexual needs, Reich, Brown, and Marcuse elevate the libido and the body: They are the focus of social repression and hence of man's liberation. However, the theories of repression developed by Marcuse, Reich, and Brown differ greatly. Further, the nature of the envisioned liberation varies: For Reich, its axis is the libido in strictly mechanical and genital "orgiastic" terms; for Marcuse, sexual "phantasy" and polymorphous perversity take center stage; while Brown came to think of sex in almost mystical categories, like William Blake (1757–1827). Still, the liberating potential of the erotic unites the three as Freudian revolutionaries; it also unites them in a project explicitly renunciated by Freud—the possibility of a society and human life free of repression.

For Reich, all neuroses and illness resulted from incomplete or failed orgiastic release, which he conceived of a biological force: "Cosmic Orgone Energy." The healthy resolution of the Oedipal conflict led normally to heterosexual genitality, which Reich saw as distorted or repressed only by economic conditions and social forces, including the family. Reich stands apart from Freud (and Marcuse) in rejecting the conciliatory thesis that some residual repression and sublimation were required for civilization. His two main works in this context, *Mass Psychology of Fascism* and *Sexual Revolution*, were hugely influential in searching for the origins of Nazism and Stalinism (respectively) in the submissive character structure produced by bourgeois families, their authoritarian father figures, and attendant sexual repression. Gad Horowitz emphasizes the originality and daring of Reich's break from Freud, especially his denial of the irrevocability and hence ahistoricity of social repression (see *Repression*, chap. 5). Reich claimed that sublimation (and the death drive, *thanatos*, itself) was merely historically contingent on the form that society, and the family within it, took. Horowitz does take Reich to task for upholding "the frustration of the non-incestuous genital sexuality of oedipal children" to be the only source of repression (129). In general, however, Reich's historicism is the *sine qua non* of the Freudian Left, since only then can we say that the importance of psychoanalysis lies in making its central object of study the nature and genesis of the "head and heart" of the socialized human being (Fromm, 155).

The body was also the nexus of repression for Brown; his "eschatology of immanence" (Susan Sontag's memorable phrase; 262) foreshadows the postmodernism of many from Deleuze to Luce Irigaray:

> With the whole world still in the bourgeois stage of competitive development and war, the thing to remember about Marx is that he was able to look beyond this world to another possible world, of union, communion, communism. . . . And after Freud, we have to add that there is also a sexual revolution; which is not to be found in the bourgeois cycle of repression and promiscuity, but in the transformation of the human body, and abolition of genital organization. ("Reply," 246)

Brown is at pains to point out that the most basic of Freud's speculations demand not only a science of culture but also a revolution:

> In a neurosis, according to Freud, the ego accepts reality and its energy is directed against the id. . . . In a psychosis the ego is overwhelmed by the id, severs

its connection with reality, and proceeds to create for itself a new outer and inner world. The healthy reaction, according to Freud, like a neurosis, does not ignore reality; like a psychosis it creates a new world, but, unlike psychosis, it creates a new world in the real world; that is, it changes reality. (*Life*, 154)

For Brown, the most Freudian of our triumvirate, sublimation (the result of repression) is essentially desexualization wherein the ego, incapable of accepting its own negation in death, dilutes its life and connects its "higher sublimations" (socially accepted transferences of erosic energy such as work and industry) to lower regions of the body in what Brown terms a "dialectical affirmation-by-negation" (*Life*, 161). If the simplest example of such sublimation-as-desexualizing is infantile thumb-sucking, the "most paradoxical" is anality: "It is by being the negation of excrement that money is excrement; and it is by being the negation of the body (the soul) that the ego remains a body-ego" (161). Brown therefore winds up *Life against Death*, his *magnum opus*, with an astonishing deconstruction of "the excremental vision" in Western literature and philosophy, a discussion ranging from Martin Luther's (1483–1546) eschatology to George Berkeley's (1685–1753) tarwater and **Immanuel Kant**'s (1724–1804) "categories of repression." The larger point is that the symbolized and sublimated manipulation of excrement is the root of human reason, "progress," and aggression.

Marcuse came to Freud only after a thorough dose of Hegel, Wilhelm Dilthey (1833–1911), Marx, and **Martin Heidegger** (1889–1976). In his role as the major theoretician and philosopher of the Institute for Social Research (beginning in Frankfurt, Germany), Marcuse reviewed the first English translation of Marx's *Economic and Philosophic Manuscripts of 1844*. This work first reveals Marcuse's (but also Marx's) *idée fixe*: labor as an ontological category. Marcuse is out to uncover Marx as a philosopher, not an economist, and as a humanist-existentialist, not a determinist: "[T]he crude communism which he [Marx] opposed . . . exists on the same level as capitalism—but it is precisely that level which Marx wants to abolish" ("Foundations," 9). It also reveals a contradiction, though some might call it a dialectical movement, that asserts work to be an ontological category, hence a universal necessity, at the same time it is considered, as is *"ananke"* (scarcity) and the struggle for existence, a historical contingency, to be overcome by a new kind of man. This tension turns on the related notions of alienation, **objectification**, and reification, and concerns the relationship between consciousness or culture and nature. We could locate it here:

> The objective world, as the necessary objectivity of man, through the appropriation and supersession of which his human essence is first "produced" and "confirmed," is part of man himself. It *is* real objectivity only for self-realizing man, it is the "self-objectification" of man, of human objectification. But this same objective world, since it is real objectivity, can appear as a precondition of his being which does *not* belong to his being, is beyond his control, and is "overpowering." ("Foundations," 18)

From Hegel, Marcuse inherits the liberal notion that freedom derives from our recognizing that the source of culture, morality, and sexuality is human consciousness itself: Self-realization, as in Freud, amounts to a cure, as it also results in new forms of culture, politics, morality, and sexuality. (The optimistic strand is subjected to an unfortunately well-known criticism, as being inherently un-Freudian and anti-Marxist, by Alasdair MacIntyre [70, 80 ff.], which in turn is properly lambasted by W. Mark Cobb [165 ff.].) This ambivalence—man's artistic and intellectual creations are an appropriation of nature and hence possibly signify a liberation to our true nature but at the same time express a domination of nature, and in that case represent the continued repression of instinct, feeling, and true need—is recast by Marcuse into a critique of contemporary "affluent society" and its military-industrial-technological basis. The critique is one that also argues for the "emergence of a new Reality Principle: under which a new sensibility and a desublimated scientific intelligence would combine in the creation of an *aesthetic ethos*" (*Essay*, 24). This ambivalence can be found in Marcuse's later, utopian/dystopian writings. By 1969 he could urge the New Left to move "from Marx to Fourier . . . from realism to surrealism" (*Essay*, 22).

The "aesthetic dimension" is intended to resolve this tension in Marcuse, if only in the most abstract terms. (Reitz's influential *Art, Alienation, and the Humanities* opened up this line of Marcusean scholarship.) Recall Kant's understanding of aesthetic judgment as contrasted with the intellect. "Sinnlichkeit" or "sensuousness" was seen as the realm of lawless freedom and as the central mental faculty through which, writes Marcuse, "nature becomes susceptible to freedom, necessity to autonomy" (*Eros*, 174). Orpheus, the original representative of polymorphous perversity, now can achieve "the erotic reconciliation (union) of man and nature in the aesthetic attitude, where order is beauty and work is play" (176). Reason and intellect (and the performance principle itself) are increasingly described by Marcuse as repressive and ideological, as they often are in Brown. The reeroticization of the natural world would make it an object of contemplation and would transform work into "*display*—the free manifestation of potentialities" (190). (The continued emphasis on labor is significant; it answers the charge that aesthetic, imaginative liberation is too superficial and merely a philosophical gloss on the irony, playfulness, and nihilism of twentieth-century modernism. Marcuse disavows hippies and beatniks as the revolutionary subject; the working class remains its locus. See *Five Lectures*, 69.) Liberation, or at least nonrepressive desublimation, would not result in sexual libertinism (as, similarly, liberation in Brown does not mean promiscuity) but the spread "from sexuality constrained under genital supremacy to eroticisation of the entire personality" (*Eros*, 201). In any case, most of Marcuse's optimism would flip over into pessimism by the time of *One-Dimensional Man* (ODM). Its bleak picture of the advanced technology, managerial prowess, and wealth of late capitalist America would be Marcuse's greatest legacy as a public intellectual.

ODM, arguably Marcuse's least coherent yet most well-known work, remains famous for its vision of a hyperinstrumentalized sexuality, where the sexual freedom visible in contemporary youth culture masks a deeper, invidious form of managerial control. Kevin Floyd finds in ODM "an argument for its status [i.e., of the homosexual strain in New Left activism] as a direct affront to the bourgeois democratic state and to a normalized, phobically heterosexist culture" (105). At the same time, however, he notes the "nostalgic puritanism" of this often-quoted passage from ODM:

> Compare lovemaking in a meadow and in an automobile, on a lover's walk outside the town walls and on a Manhattan street. In the former cases, the environment partakes of and invites libidinal cathexis and tends to be eroticized. Libido transcends beyond the immediate erotogenic zones—a process of nonrepressive sublimation. In contrast, a mechanized environment seems to block such self-transcendence of the libido. Impelled in the struggle to extend the field of erotic gratification, libido becomes less "polymorphous," less capable of eroticism beyond localized sexuality, and the *latter* is intensified. (73)

Perhaps what Floyd (or any other member of "the homosexual strain in New Left activism") might sense here is a veiled critique of the urban gay male community, whose members commonly use the sex toys, slings, lotions, and poppers made possible by technology and are more likely to engage in sex in bathrooms, bathhouses, basements, deserted alleys and hallways, SUVs, and vans than in the flower fields of D. H. Lawrence's (1885–1930) *Women in Love* and, further, are more likely to do so (or not to mind doing so) than their heterosexual **casual sex** counterparts (or "feminine" men and women, for that matter).

In criticism of the Freudian left, recall Emile Durkheim's (1858–1917) famous dictum: "Whenever a social phenomenon is directly explained by a psychological phenomenon, we may be sure that the explanation is false" (128). That is, the romantic and idealistic (Hegelian) dimensions of this liberatory program hardly survive the postmodern deconstruction of this area of thought. The critique of late capitalism in terms of rampant narcissism, the authoritarian personality, or the fascist character structure is perhaps too dependent on presupposing the reality of an unrepressed, "natural" self—an imaginary Thomas Hobbesian (1588–1679) or John Rawlsian (1921–2002) state of nature—to remain unscathed by the challenge of the students and successors of Jacques Derrida (1930–2004), Lacan, and Stanley Fish (see, for example, Butler, 98 ff.; Žižek, 12 ff.). If, as Foucault argues, the self is a cultural construction, if sex is an "imaginary point," and if even the notion of "repression" must be counted among those "juridical practices" responsible for the production, organization, and fabrication of self and sexuality (*History*, 81 ff.), then Marcuse's "great refusal," Brown's resexualization, and Reich's vegetotherapy, like Marx's "species being," resolve themselves into, at best, tactical or rhetorical maneuvers. (Whether *modus ponens* is the right operation here, or *modus tollens*, is not clear.) Further, that the Freudian Left, and Marcuse in particular, ignore Freudian clinical observations makes that approach "ahistorical to a degree which Freud's [model] actually is not" (Weeks, 168). Douglas Kellner, while generally positive, voices a similar critique, calling Marcuse's ODM a "historical synoptic" that "pictures the development of industrial society as a successful attempt on the part of corporate capitalism to dominate totally its helpless and passive victims" (273). Here Kellner sounds, uncannily, much like those liberal feminists who criticize "victim feminism," which portrays patriarchy as totally dominating resourceless female victims. He quickly adds, however, that Marcuse's writings serve as a good "barometer" of social criticism and that his later, post-1965 writings reflect the turn seen especially in France, following Foucault and Pierre Bourdieu (1930–2002), toward more pluralistic and localized (poststructuralist) analyses of agency and resistance movements and away from the amorphous enemy, advanced capitalism. Both Paul Breines (48 ff.) and W. Mark Cobb (181) argue that Marcuse foreshadows this very feature (among others) of Foucault's thought.

Its biologism and essentialism, not to mention the phallocentrism and **heterosexism** (of Reich alone), make the Freudian Left less attractive than these subsequent analyses to certain sensibilities, but it still pays us to attend to the more positive, universal, and hence modernist picture of man and man's liberation that is the Freudian Left's latest incarnation of the Enlightenment tradition.

See also Feminism, French; Firestone, Shulamith; Freud, Sigmund; Heidegger, Martin; Lacan, Jacques; MacKinnon, Catharine; Marxism; Mead, Margaret; Objectification, Sexual; Paglia, Camille; Poststructuralism; Psychology, Twentieth- and Twenty-First-Century; Utopianism

REFERENCES

Balbus, Isaac D. *Marxism and Domination: A Neo-Hegelian, Feminist, Psychoanalytic Theory of Sexual, Political, and Technological Liberation.* Princeton, N.J.: Princeton University Press, 1982;

Breines, Paul. "Revisiting Marcuse with Foucault: *An Essay on Liberation* Meets *The History of Sexuality.*" In John Bokina and Timothy J. Lukes, eds., *Marcuse: From the New Left to the Next Left.* Lawrence: University Press of Kansas, 1994, 27–40; Brown, Norman O. *Life against Death: The Psychoanalytic Meaning of History.* Middletown, Conn.: Wesleyan University Press, 1959; Brown, Norman O. "A Reply to Marcuse." In Herbert Marcuse, *Negations: Essays in Critical Theory.* Trans. Jeremy Shapiro. Boston, Mass.: Beacon Press, 1968, 227–48; Butler, Judith. *The Psychic Life of Power: Theories in Subjection.* Stanford, Calif.: Stanford University Press, 1997; Cobb, W. Mark. "Diatribes and Distortions: Marcuse's Academic Reception." In John Abromeit and W. Mark Cobb, eds., *Herbert Marcuse: A Critical Reader.* New York: Routledge, 2004, 163–87; Deleuze, Gilles. (1973) "Five Propositions on Psychoanalysis." In *Desert Islands and Other Texts 1953–1974.* Trans. Michael Taormina. Los Angeles, Calif.: Semiotext(e), 2004, 274–80; Drassinower, Abraham. *Freud's Theory of Culture: Eros, Loss, and Politics.* Lanham, Md.: Rowman and Littlefield, 2003; Durkheim, Emile. (1901) *The Rules of Sociological Method.* Trans. W. D. Halls. Introduction and selection by Steven Lukes. New York: Free Press, 1982; Floyd, Kevin. "Rethinking Reification: Marcuse, Psychoanalysis, and Gay Liberation." *Social Text* 19:1 (2001), 103–28; Foucault, Michel. (1976) *The History of Sexuality,* vol. 1: *An Introduction.* Trans. Robert Hurley. New York: Vintage, 1978; Foucault, Michel. (1972) "Preface." In Gilles Deleuze and Félix Guattari, *Anti-Oedipus: Capitalism and Schizophrenia.* Trans. Robert Hurley, Mark Seem, and Helen R. Lane. Minneapolis: University of Minnesota Press, 1983, xi–xiv; Freud, Sigmund. (1930) *Civilization and Its Discontents.* In *The Standard Edition of the Complete Psychological Works of Sigmund Freud,* vol. 21. Trans. James Strachey. London: Hogarth Press, 1953–1974, 64–145; Freud, Sigmund. (1927) *Future of an Illusion.* In *The Standard Edition of the Complete Psychological Works of Sigmund Freud,* vol. 21. Trans. James Strachey. London: Hogarth Press, 1953–1974, 1–56; Freud, Sigmund. (1913) *Totem and Taboo.* In *The Standard Edition of the Complete Psychological Works of Sigmund Freud,* vol. 13. Trans. James Strachey. London: Hogarth Press, 1953–1974, ix–161; Fromm, Erich. (1932) "The Method and Function of an Analytic Social Psychology: Notes on Psychoanalysis and Historical Materialism." In *The Crisis of Psychoanalysis: Essays on Freud, Marx, and Social Psychology.* Greenwich, Conn.: Fawcett, 1971, 138–62; Horowitz, Gad. *Repression. Basic and Surplus Repression in Psychoanalytic Theory: Freud, Reich, and Marcuse.* Toronto, Can.: University of Toronto Press, 1977; Jacoby, Russell. *Social Amnesia: A Critique of Conformist Psychology from Adler to Laing.* Boston, Mass.: Beacon Press, 1975. With a new introduction, New Brunswick, N.J.: Transaction, 1996; Jay, Martin. *The Dialectical Imagination: A History of the Frankfurt School and the Institute of Social Research 1923–1950.* Boston, Mass.: Little, Brown, 1973; Kellner, Douglas. *Herbert Marcuse and the Crisis of Marxism.* Berkeley: University of California Press, 1984; Lichtman, Richard. *The Production of Desire: The Integration of Psychoanalysis into Marxist Theory.* New York: Free Press, 1982; MacIntyre, Alasdair. *Herbert Marcuse: An Exposition and a Polemic.* New York: Viking, 1970; Marcuse, Herbert. (1955) *Eros and Civilization: A Philosophical Inquiry into Freud.* Boston, Mass.: Beacon Press, 1966; Marcuse, Herbert. *An Essay on Liberation.* Boston, Mass.: Beacon Press, 1969; Marcuse, Herbert. *Five Lectures.* Boston, Mass.: Beacon Press, 1970; Marcuse, Herbert. (1932) "The Foundations of Historical Materialism." In *Studies in Critical Philosophy.* Trans. Joris De Bres. London: NLB, 1972, 1–49; Marcuse, Herbert. *One-Dimensional Man: Studies in the Ideology of Advanced Industrial Society.* Boston, Mass.: Beacon Press, 1964; Marx, Karl. *The Economic and Philosophic Manuscripts of 1844.* Trans. Martin Milligan. Ed. Dirk Struik. New York: International Publishers, 1964; Marx, Karl, and Friedrich Engels. (1845–1846) *The German Ideology.* In Lewis S. Feuer, ed., *Basic Writings on Politics and Philosophy.* New York: Doubleday, 1959, 246–62; Reich, Wilhelm. (1946) *The Mass Psychology of Fascism.* Trans. Vincent Carfagno. New York: Farrar, Straus and Giroux, 1970; Reich, Wilhelm. *Sex-Pol: Essays 1929–1934.* Ed. Lee Baxandall. Trans. Anna Bostock, Tom DuBose, and Lee Baxandall. New York: Random House, 1972. New York: Columbia University Press, 1994; Reich, Wilhelm. (1945) *Sexual Revolution: Toward a Self-Governing Character Structure.* Trans. Theodore P. Wolfe. New York: Farrar, Straus and Giroux, 1970; Reitz, Charles. *Art, Alienation, and the Humanities: A Critical Engagement with Herbert Marcuse.* Albany: State University of New York Press, 2000; Rieff, Philip. *Freud: The Mind of the*

Moralist. New York: Viking, 1959; Robinson, Paul. *The Freudian Left: Wilhelm Reich, Geza Roheim, Herbert Marcuse*. New York: Harper and Row, 1969; Sontag, Susan. (1961) "Psychoanalysis and Norman O. Brown's *Life against Death*." In *Against Interpretation and Other Essays*. New York: Farrar, Straus and Giroux, 1966, 256–62. Garden City, N.Y.: Anchor/Doubleday, 1990; Weeks, Jeffrey. *Sexuality and Its Discontents: Meanings, Myths, and Modern Sexualities*. London: Routledge and Kegan Paul, 1985; Žižek, Slavoj. "The Deadlock of 'Repressive Desublimation.' " In *The Metastases of Enjoyment: Six Essays on Women and Causality*. London: Verso, 1994, 7–28.

Nicholas P. Power

ADDITIONAL READING

Abromeit, John, and W. Mark Cobb, eds. *Herbert Marcuse: A Critical Reader*. New York: Routledge, 2004; Adorno, Theodor W. "On Kierkegaard's Doctrine of Love." *Studies in Philosophy and Social Science* 8 (1940), 413–29; Bokina, John, and Timothy J. Lukes, eds. *Marcuse: From the New Left to the Next Left*. Lawrence: University Press of Kansas, 1994; Breines, Paul, ed. *Critical Interruptions: New Left Perspectives on Herbert Marcuse*. New York: Herder and Herder, 1970; Brod, Harry. "Pornography and the Alienation of Male Sexuality." *Social Theory and Practice* 14:3 (1988), 265–84. Reprinted in Larry May, Robert Strikwerda, and Patrick D. Hopkins, eds., *Rethinking Masculinity: Philosophical Explorations in Light of Feminism*, 2nd ed. Lanham, Md.: Rowman and Littlefield, 1996, 237–53; POS2 (281–99); Brown, Norman O. *Love's Body*. New York: Vintage, 1966; Chesser, Eustace. *Reich and Sexual Freedom*. London: Vision Press, 1972; Davis, Angela. "Marcuse's Legacies." In John Abromeit and W. Mark Cobb, eds., *Herbert Marcuse: A Critical Reader*. New York: Routledge, 2004, 43–50; Fromm, Erich. "Foreword." In Edward Bellamy, *Looking Backward: 2000–1887*. New York: New American Library, 1960, v–xx; Frosh, Steven. (1987) *The Politics of Psychoanalysis: An Introduction to Freudian and Post-Freudian Theory*, 2nd ed. New York: New York University Press, 1999; Gendron, Bernard. "Sexual Alienation." In *Technology and the Human Condition*. New York: St. Martin's Press, 1977, 114–33. Reprinted in POS1 (281–98); Green, Andre. "Sexuality and Ideology in Marx and Freud." *Human Context* 6 (1974), 362–84; Horkheimer, Max, and Theodor Adorno. (1944) *Dialectic of Enlightenment*. Trans. John Cumming. New York: Continuum, 1990; Jacoby, Russell. (1983) *The Repression of Psychoanalysis: Otto Fenichel and the Political Freudians*. Chicago, Ill.: University of Chicago Press, 1986; Kimball, Roger. "The Perversions of Michel Foucault." *The New Criterion* 11:7 (March 1993). <www.newcriterion.com/archive/11/mar93/foucault.htm> [accessed 8 June 2005]; King, Richard. *The Party of Eros*. Chapel Hill: University of North Carolina Press, 1971; Kipnis, Laura. "Adultery." *Critical Inquiry* 24:2 (1998), 289–327; Kovel, Joel. *The Age of Desire: Reflections of a Radical Psychoanalyst*. New York: Pantheon, 1981; Laplanche, Jean. *Life and Death in Psychoanalysis*. Trans. Jeffrey Mehlman. Baltimore, Md.: Johns Hopkins University Press, 1976; Lewin, Ralph A. *Merde: Excursions in Scientific, Cultural, and Sociohistorical Coprology*. New York: Random House, 1999; Marcuse, Herbert. "Love Mystified: A Critique of Norman O. Brown." In *Negations: Essays in Critical Theory*. Trans. Jeremy Shapiro. Boston, Mass.: Beacon Press, 1968, 227–43; Marx, Karl, and Friedrich Engels. *The German Ideology*. Ed. C. J. Arthur. New York: International Publishers, 1981; Mitchell, Juliet. "On Freud and the Distinction between the Sexes." In Jean Strouse, ed., *Women and Analysis: Dialogues on Psychoanalytic Views of Femininity*. New York: Grossman, 1974, 27–36; Mitchell, Juliet. *Psychoanalysis and Feminism: Freud, Reich, Laing, and Women*. New York: Vintage, 1975; Ollman, Bertell. (1971) *Alienation: Marx's Conception of Man in Capitalistic Society*, 2nd ed. Cambridge: Cambridge University Press, 1976; Ollman, Bertell. *Social and Sexual Revolution: Essays on Marx and Reich*. Boston, Mass.: South End Press, 1979; Pippin, Robert, Andrew Feenberg, and Charles P. Webel, eds. *Marcuse: Critical Theory and the Promise of Utopia*. South Hadley, Mass.: Bergin and Harvey, 1988; Press, Howard. "The Marxism and Anti-Marxism of Wilhelm Reich." *Telos*, no. 6 (1971), 65–82; Reich, Wilhelm. (1942) *The Discovery of the Orgone*, vol. 1: *The Function of the Orgasm. The Sex-Economic Problems of Biological Energy*. Trans. Vincent R. Carfagno. Oxford, U.K.: Touchstone, 1973; Reich, Wilhelm. (1930) *The Sexual Revolution: Toward a Self-Governing Character*

Structure, 4th ed., rev. [*Die Sexualität im Kulturkampf*]. Trans. Theodore P. Wolfe. New York: Noonday, 1969; Reiche, Reimut. *Sexuality and the Class Struggle*. Trans. S. Bennett. New York: Praeger, 1971; Robinson, Paul. *The Modernization of Sex: Havelock Ellis, Alfred Kinsey, William Masters and Virginia Johnson*. New York: Harper and Row, 1976; Roszak, Theodore. *The Making of a Counter Culture: Reflections on the Technocratic Society and Its Youthful Opposition*. Garden City, N.Y.: Doubleday, 1969; Schneider, Michael. (1973) *Neurosis and Civilization: A Marxist/Freudian Synthesis*. Trans. Michael Roloff. New York: Seabury Press, 1975; Slater, Philip E. *The Origin and Significance of the Frankfurt School*. London: Routledge and Kegan Paul, 1977; Slater, Philip E. (1970) *The Pursuit of Loneliness: American Culture at the Breaking Point*. Boston, Mass.: Beacon Press, 1990; Soble, Alan. "The Freudo-Marxism of Wilhelm Reich" and "The Agnosticism of Marcuse." In *Pornography: Marxism, Feminism, and the Future of Sexuality*. New Haven, Conn.: Yale University Press, 1986, 10–37, 49–53.

FRIENDSHIP. In Western culture, the ideal **marriage** has often been seen as at once a "perfect" lifelong friendship between a woman and a man and as a union motivated by eros or sexual **love**. Philosophers both past and present, from **Aristotle** (384–322 BCE) and Cicero (106–43 BCE) to Michel Montaigne (1533–1592) and many contemporary philosophers (see Badhwar, *Friendship*; Pakaluk) have articulated an understanding of perfect friendship as an intimate relationship grounded in shared values and virtues and marked by equal and reciprocal love, respect, concern, and pleasure. Many philosophers have thought of eros also as having these features, insofar as it is an intimate love between two equals. But what is central to eros is sexuality. **Irving Singer** captures a common reflective understanding of eros when he characterizes it as mutual desire for sexual and psychological union and for sensual pleasures (64, 66). When people wonder, then, whether it is possible to have erotic love and friendship for or with the same person, what they want to know is whether eros, with its characteristic attitudes—its desires, feelings, and perceptions—is compatible with friendship, with *its* characteristic attitudes, or at odds with it.

Philosophical views about friendship and eros, their similarities and differences, and the relationship between them are varied and have given rise to a number of different traditions in the history of philosophy. **Plato** (427–347 BCE), for example, argued that both friendship and eros were actually confused gropings for (the Forms of) **Beauty** or the Good (*Lysis*, 249d; *Symposium*, 210–12b). And **Sigmund Freud** (1856–1939), in his provocative *Civilization and Its Discontents*, proposed that friendship and other "higher" loves (especially Christian neighbor love) were merely forms of "aim-inhibited" eros (or libido), the product of the "repression" of the sexual instinct.

C. S. Lewis (1898–1963) famously proposed that the crucial difference between friendship and erotic love was that lovers are characteristically "face to face, absorbed in each other." By contrast, friends are characteristically "side by side, absorbed in some common interest" (91). But this difference, says Lewis, does not imply that eros and friendship are incompatible; indeed, friendship between men and women often leads to erotic love and conversely (91, 98–99). Lovers may experience their mutual absorption as the fulfillment of a desire to (re)unite with their "other half," as in the myth narrated by Aristophanes in Plato's *Symposium* (189a–93d). Alternatively, it may be that "falling in love, including love at first sight, is a kind of . . . reaching . . . for one's future and better self" (Solomon, 146). In the account developed by Robert Nozick (1938–2002), what is essential to romantic love is the desire to create a new entity, "a *we*"; the actual creation of this "we" is not essential, because the love might not be reciprocated (70). But when it is, Mark Fisher holds, lovers think so much in terms of "us" rather than "I" that they "perceive, feel and act as a single person [in that] . . . neither can say who originated" the perception, feeling, or act (28).

Eros is an I-thou relationship (Scruton, 231) in which imagination and **fantasy** play a large role, creating for the lovers their own private world (Solomon, 162). By contrast, fantasy plays only a small role in the world that adult friends create together, and the desire for identification with a friend typically falls short of the desire for creating a new joint identity. Only "typically," however, for a friendship, too, can be a bond of intense identification, an I-thou affair of the soul. Montaigne describes his friendship with Étienne de La Böetie as a matter of souls being "mingled and confounded" to form a seamless unity (211–12). Each was brought to "plunge" his "will" into the other's and "lose itself," so that "nothing was his or mine." So intense a union leaves no room for any other intimate friendships; for Montaigne, perfect friendship is, like eros, exclusive. Even marital friendship cannot measure up to perfect friendship, because women seem unable to respond to the "familiarity and mutual confidence" (210) of perfect friendship. (Gilbert Meilaender suggests a different sort of obstacle to friendship between men and women: A friend is another self, but men and women have substantially different selves.)

Montaigne was not alone in enjoying a passionate same-sex friendship. Much of the poetry of Katherine Philips (1631–1664) celebrates these friendships (see "To Mrs. Mary Awbrey" [1664]; Welty and Sharp, 152). Indeed, passionate or "romantic" same-sex friendships were widely accepted in Europe and America until the eighteenth century for men and until the late nineteenth century for women (see Faderman). They were also celebrated in Native American, Polynesian, African, and Asian cultures (see Brain). Romantic friendships share with erotic love the intense emotional focus of the two on each other, their desire for psychological union, the enchantment, the physical tenderness, and, typically, exclusivity. What distinguishes them from eros, then, seems to be simply the absence of the desire for sexual union.

But are same-sex romantic friendships simply expressions of repressed (or not consciously admitted or acknowledged) **homosexuality**? For some, Montaigne's judgment that homosexuality was "abhorrent" (211) will perversely serve as evidence for repression; but that move makes the "repression" thesis unfalsifiable. Further, even if romantic friendships are expressions of repressed homosexuality, the fact that even cultures that openly *accept* homosexuality celebrate these friendships largely undercuts the "repression" thesis (see the Web site "Celebratefriendship"). Moreover, given that the desire for sexual contact can exist without the desire for psychological intimacy, there is little reason to deny that the desire for psychological intimacy can exist without **sexual desire**. The variety of desires for physical and psychological intimacy may have the same autonomy relative to each other as the variety of desires for food or drink.

Just as the desires for sexual union and sensual pleasures seem to be the features that differentiate eros from romantic friendship, so physical tenderness and intensity of feeling seem to be the features that differentiate romantic from nonromantic friendships. All the other features of romantic friendship, in different combinations of intensity or scope, may be present in nonromantic friendship as well. A friend, says Aristotle, is "another self," a "mirror" in whom we can observe our own souls (*Nicomachean Ethics* [*NE*] 1169b28–1170a4, 1170b1–14). Friendship, says **Immanuel Kant** (1724–1804), is "the union of two persons through equal mutual love and respect" and is, indeed, "the most intimate union of love with respect" (*Metaphysics of Morals*, Ak 6:469). The love of which Kant speaks is "practical" love or beneficence, and the intimacy comes from the mutual self-disclosure of two equals. This intimacy approaches the merging of two into one, but it must be limited by each person respecting the other's autonomy (*Metaphysics*, Ak 6:471). Simone Weil (1909–1943) also emphasizes respect for autonomy in genuine friendship: "[E]ach wishes to preserve the faculty of free consent both in himself and in the other" and does so by preserving "a certain distance" from the friend, even though the friend is "as necessary to him as food" ("Friendship" [1951]; Welty and Sharp, 526).

If it is true that perfect friendship includes respect of a sort that requires an autonomy-preserving distance, then literal psychological union, in which two selves are replaced by a new joint self, is incompatible with perfect friendship. So, if this sort of union is characteristic of eros and romantic friendship, as Montaigne, Nozick, and others hold, then eros and romantic friendship are incompatible with perfect friendship. It might also be argued that the obliteration of the self-other distinction in literal psychological union is incompatible with "robust" (Aristotelean or Kantian) concern for each other's well-being, and thus with friendship, because robust concern entails the possibility of genuinely sacrificing one's *own* good for the other's sake (see Soble). Further, the obliteration of the self's boundaries in union may be incompatible with a chief epistemic value of intimate love: insight into ourselves and others. This insight requires that friends and lovers affirm each other's conceptions of themselves and the world only insofar as these conceptions are veridical and that they challenge, or at least not endorse, them if they are false or inadequate (Badhwar, "Love"). But only friends and lovers with distinct, autonomous selves have the distance and objectivity necessary for this epistemic virtue. Those who lose their independent perspectives confirm each other's blind spots and self-deceptions and become, not mirrors that *reflect* each other's souls, but mirrors of *distortion*. The idea of union in eros or friendship, however, is not always the idea of a literal psychological union but, rather, the idea of a fundamental emotional, moral, and intellectual affinity, a passion for "the same truth" (Lewis, 96, 97). In intense emotional moments, this affinity may lead to a sense of oneness, but such moments are *only* moments in the separate existence of two selves. In such relationships, neither robust concern nor epistemic virtue is threatened.

Minus the idea of literal psychological union, then, erotic love, passionate friendship, and friendship may be seen as lying on a continuum of psychological intimacy. Why, then, have eros and friendship sometimes been seen as necessarily incompatible? One reason stems from the idea that eros is essentially *exclusive* and *jealous*, while friendship is essentially inclusive or, at least, plural (Lewis, 91–92; Meilaender, 187; see also Aristotle, *NE* 1171a9). The worry this raises is that eros must lead to a desire to control and constrain the other that is incompatible with respect for the other's freedom and separateness and, thus, with friendship. John McMurtry, however, rejects the idea that "sex-love" (as he calls it) is necessarily exclusive and jealous. He observes, along with others (LaFollette, 179–80; Thomas, 125), that **jealousy** and the desire for exclusivity can afflict both sex-love and friendship but argues that in both they are signs of immaturity and insecurity (178–80). Inclusivity and the absence of jealousy are essential for good friendship and good sex-love, for the good "is *what enables a more inclusive range of being* . . . of thought, of experience, or of action" (174). To transcend the "win-or-lose" structure of exclusive sex-love, to overcome jealousy (with its attendant cruelties, hatreds, and suspicions), we must reconceptualize sex-love as a form of friendship and share our erotic lives with a wider circle of friends (181). Since we are "open elective space[s]" who make our own identities (169), it is up to us to effect this change.

Is this view too optimistic? Jo-Ann Pilardi complains that it ignores the psychoanalytic insights that "a person is a space of *conflicting* needs" and our rational choices are limited by unconscious processes (187). Moreover, Pilardi observes, the desire for exclusivity might be an expression not of jealousy but of the choice to hold someone as special and thus *create* love. Pilardi apparently grants, however, that insecurity and jealousy are irrational, suggesting that they are somehow linked to patriarchy. But this may be challenged by the following argument. All love requires the investment of two scarce resources: time and attention. Other things being equal, then, a new love interest must divert some of these resources from the old love interest to itself. This fact of our psychological economy is independent of patriarchy but sufficient for creating a perfectly justified insecurity and jealousy. For "the heart of jealousy" is the loss of affection, and focused attention is central to affection (Neu, 70). If so, then overcoming patriarchy will not eliminate jealousy. Indeed, jealousy, exhibited even by babies—not to mention dogs—may be nature's way of constraining the promiscuous exercise of our capacity for love and hence a condition of the very possibility of intimate love. All love is exclusive and jealous and desirous of constraining the other's freedom to some extent without, thereby, being incompatible with respect for the other's separateness and freedom. Eros is typically more frequently or more intensely jealous than friendship, because it involves a greater range of passions and vulnerabilities and, thus, needs more focused attention to flourish. For this reason, eros is also more prone than friendship to irrational jealousy. The tensions within eros tend to be greater than within friendship, but that does not make eros incompatible with friendship.

But there are other reasons for thinking that eros and friendship are necessarily incompatible. One stems from the all too widely held view that lust is an appetite that reduces the other person to a mere object for one's enjoyment (see, for example, Kant, *Lectures*, 163–64). By contrast, perfect friendship is "the most intimate union of love with respect" (Kant, *Metaphysics*, Ak 6:469). In objectifying the other, lust violates the requirements of love, equality, and reciprocity and thus seems incompatible with friendship. Marriage, however, redeems sexual love, because it makes of two people "a unity of will" in which both have rights over each other (*Lectures*, 167). Marriage, and only marriage, gives the individual "practical recognition" that she is fundamentally "an object of respect" rather than "an object of sensual enjoyment" (Denis, 11). So marriage makes friendship between the spouses possible. Even so, because marriage is based on lust and women are inferior to men, according to Kant, marital friendship is less intimate and less moral than perfect friendship.

Lara Denis argues, however, that even if we grant that eros is an objectifying appetite, so long as we reject Kant's view of women, this conclusion does not follow. For a particular marriage might be based on mutual love and respect, with erotic desire playing only a small role in it (17). Denis may be right about this. But the problem remains that Kant's view of lust as an objectifying appetite makes eros as such incompatible with friendship. Aristotle provides a deeper understanding of what makes sexual desire objectifying or otherwise inappropriate by distinguishing between the refined appetites and pleasures of the temperate man and the gross appetites and pleasures of the intemperate man (*NE* 3.10–12). Just as the intemperate man is insensitive to the flavors and textures of food, enjoying only the feeling of food going down his throat, so (Aristotle suggests by analogy) he is insensitive to the sensual and aesthetic pleasures of sex, enjoying only the relief of tension. Someone who treats his sexual partner as a mere object lacks the self-awareness and other-awareness necessary for such sensitivity and, therefore, counts as intemperate. It is intemperate sexual appetite, then, that is incompatible with perfect marital friendship, not sexual appetite as such. Nor is women's alleged moral and intellectual inferiority incompatible with marital friendship, says Aristotle, because a couple can achieve "proportional" equality through the wife's loving the more worthy husband more than she is loved by him (*NE* 8.7).

In rejecting the idea that sexuality necessarily objectifies, **Roger Scruton** turns Kant on his head: [I]t is "only in erotic love," he says, that persons gain "a full understanding of what it is . . . to be 'ends in themselves' " and "centers of value" (251). This "only" seems hyperbolic; but we can agree with Nathaniel Branden that in good sex we have the most vivid, direct, and intense experience of being ends in ourselves and centers of value, because sexual pleasure, alone among pleasures, integrates mind and body and makes us "visible" to ourselves in our totality (85–88). This visibility comes from the other's responses to us and to the world, responses that also (one might add) make the other more visible to us. Visibility is enhanced when good sex is part of a relationship with a high degree of reciprocity, equality, and intersubjectivity, for such a relationship involves more of the self. The surprising conclusion, on such an account, is that at their best, eros and friendship, rather than being incompatible, reinforce each other. Let us not, however, be complacent, for Scruton may have a point when he states:

> Love has a tendency to grow with time, while desire has a tendency to wither. . . . Eventually desire is replaced by a love which is no longer erotic, but based in trust and companionship. . . . The problem is, how to shut out the third party[,] . . . how to prevent the calm love of nuptial union from being shattered by the turbulence of a new desire. (244)

See also Augustine (Saint); Bestiality; Bisexuality; Ethics, Virtue; Feminism, Lesbian; Firestone, Shulamith; Jealousy; Kant, Immanuel; Leibniz, Gottfried; Love; Marriage; Objectification, Sexual; Paul (Saint); Plato

REFERENCES

Aristotle. (ca. 325 BCE?) *Nicomachean Ethics*. Trans. Terence Irwin. Indianapolis, Ind.: Hackett, 1985; Badhwar, Neera K. "Love." In Hugh LaFollette, ed., *The Oxford Handbook of Practical Ethics*. Oxford, U.K.: Oxford University Press, 2003, 42–69; Badhwar, Neera K., ed. *Friendship: A Philosophical Reader*. Ithaca, N.Y.: Cornell University Press, 1993; Brain, Robert. *Friends and Lovers*. New York: Basic Books, 1976; Branden, Nathaniel. *The Psychology of Romantic Love*. New York: Bantam, 1980; Celebratefriendship. (Web site) <www.celebratefriendship.org> [accessed 20 October 2004]; Cicero, Marcus Tullius. (ca. 44 BCE) *De amicitia*. Trans. W. A. Falconer. Loeb Classical Library. London: W. Heinemann, 1923; Denis, Lara. "From Friendship to Marriage: Revising Kant." *Philosophy and Phenomenological Research* 63:1 (2001), 1–28; Faderman, Lillian. *Surpassing the Love of Men: Romantic Friendship and Love between Women from the Renaissance to the Present*. New York: Morrow, 1981; Fisher, Mark. *Personal Love*. London: Duckworth, 1990; Freud, Sigmund. (1930) *Civilization and Its Discontents*. In *The Standard Edition of the Complete Psychological Works of Sigmund Freud*, vol. 21. Trans. James Strachey. London: Hogarth Press, 1953–1974, 57–145; Kant, Immanuel. (ca. 1780) *Lectures on Ethics*. Trans. Louis Infield. New York: Harper and Row, 1963; Kant, Immanuel. (1797) *The Metaphysics of Morals*. Trans. Mary Gregor. New York: Cambridge University Press, 1996; LaFollette, Hugh. *Personal Relationships: Love, Identity, and Morality*. Oxford, U.K.: Blackwell, 1996; Lewis, C. S. (1960) *The Four Loves*. San Diego, Calif.: Harcourt Brace Jovanovich, 1988; McMurtry, John. "Sex, Love, and Friendship." In Alan Soble, ed., *Sex, Love, and Friendship*. Amsterdam, Holland: Rodopi, 1997, 169–83; Meilaender, Gilbert. "When Harry and Sally Read the *Nicomachean Ethics*: Friendship between Men and Women." In Leroy S. Rouner, ed., *The Changing Face of Friendship*. Notre Dame, Ind.: University of Notre Dame Press, 1994, 183–96; Montaigne, Michel. (1580–1595) "On Affectionate Relationships." In *The Essays of Michel de Montaigne*. Trans. M. A. Screech. New York: Penguin, 1987, 205–19; Neu, Jerome. *A Tear Is an Intellectual Thing*. New York: Oxford University Press, 2000; Nozick, Robert. "Love's Bond." In *The Examined Life*. New York: Simon and Schuster, 1989,

68–86; Pakaluk, Michael, ed. *Other Selves: Philosophers on Friendship*. Indianapolis, Ind.: Hackett, 1991; Pilardi, Jo-Ann. "Why Should We Exclude Exclusivity?" In Alan Soble, ed., *Sex, Love, and Friendship*. Amsterdam, Holland: Rodopi, 1997, 185–89; Plato. (ca. 392 BCE) *Lysis*. Trans. Stanley Lombardo. In John Cooper, ed., and D. S. Hutchinson, assoc. ed., *Plato: Complete Works*. Indianapolis, Ind.: Hackett, 1997, 687–707; Plato. (ca. 380 BCE) *Symposium*. Trans. Alexander Nehamas and Paul Woodruff. Indianapolis, Ind.: Hackett, 1989; Scruton, Roger. *Sexual Desire: A Moral Philosophy of the Erotic*. New York: Free Press, 1986; Singer, Irving. *The Pursuit of Love*. Baltimore, Md.: Johns Hopkins University Press, 1994; Soble, Alan. "Union, Autonomy, and Concern." In Roger E. Lamb, ed., *Love Analyzed*. Boulder, Colo.: Westview, 1997, 65–92; Solomon, Robert C. *About Love: Reinventing Romance for Our Times*. New York: Simon and Schuster, 1988; Thomas, Laurence M. *Living Morally: A Psychology of Moral Character*. Philadelphia, Pa.: Temple University Press, 1989; Welty, Eudora, and Ronald A. Sharp, eds. *The Norton Book of Friendship*. New York: Norton, 1991.

Neera K. Badhwar

ADDITIONAL READING

Aelred of Rievaulx. (1148) *De Spiritali Amicitia*. Trans. Mary Eugenia Laker. *Cistercian Fathers Series*, vol. 5. Kalamazoo, Mich.: Cistercian Publications, 1974; Annas, Julia. "Plato and Aristotle on Friendship and Altruism." *Mind* 86 (October 1977), 532–54; Badhwar, Neera. "Friends as Ends in Themselves." *Philosophy and Phenomenological Research* 48:1 (1987), 1–23. Reprinted, revised, in Alan Soble, ed., *Eros, Agape, and Philia: Readings in the Philosophy of Love*. New York: Paragon House, 1989, 165–86; SLF (333–52); Badhwar, Neera. "The Nature and Significance of Friendship." In Neera Badhwar, ed., *Friendship: A Philosophical Reader*. Ithaca, N.Y.: Cornell University Press, 1993, 1–37; Baumgarte, Roger. "Cross-Gender Friendship: The Troublesome Relationship." In Robin Goodwin and Duncan Cramer, eds., *Inappropriate Relationships: The Unconventional, the Disapproved, and the Forbidden*. Mahwah, N.J.: Erlbaum, 2002, 103–24; Bloom, Allan. *Love and Friendship*. New York: Simon and Schuster, 1993; Blum, Lawrence. *Friendship, Altruism, and Morality*. London: Routledge and Kegan Paul, 1980; Bushnell, Dana E. "Love without Sex." *Philosophy and Theology* 1:4 (1987), 369–73. Reprinted in SLF (381–83); Caraway, Carol. "Romantic Love: A Patchwork." *Philosophy and Theology* 2:1 (1987), 76–96. Reprinted in SLF (403–19); Caraway, Carol. "Romantic Love: Neither Sexist Nor Heterosexist." *Philosophy and Theology* 1:4 (1987), 361–68. Reprinted in SLF (375–79); Conlon, James. "Why Lovers Can't Be Friends." In Robert M. Stewart, ed., *Philosophical Perspectives on Sex and Love*. New York: Oxford University Press, 1995, 295–99; Cooper, John. "Aristotle on Friendship." In Amélie Oksenberg Rorty, ed., *Essays on Aristotle's Ethics*. Berkeley: University of California Press, 1980, 301–40; Delaney, Neil. "Romantic Love and Loving Commitment: Articulating a Modern Ideal." *American Philosophical Quarterly* 33:4 (1996), 339–56; Denizet-Lewis, Benoit. "Friends, Friends with Benefits, and the Benefits of the Local Mall." *New York Times Magazine* (30 May 2004), 30, 35, 54–59; Farrell, Daniel M. "Jealousy." *Philosophical Review* 89:4 (October 1980), 527–59; Farrell, Daniel M. "Jealousy and Desire." In Roger E. Lamb, ed., *Love Analyzed*. Boulder, Colo.: Westview, 1997, 165–88; Friedman, Marilyn. "Feminism and Modern Friendship: Dislocating the Community." *Ethics* 99:2 (1989), 275–90; Friedman, Marilyn. *What Are Friends For?* Ithaca, N.Y.: Cornell University Press, 1993; Gaylin, Willard. *Rediscovering Love*. New York: Viking Penguin, 1985; Gilbert, Paul. "Loving Friends." In *Human Relationships: A Philosophical Introduction*. Oxford, U.K.: Blackwell, 1991, 56–79; Golash, Deirdre. "Power, Sex, and Friendship in Academia." *Essays in Philosophy* 2:2 (2001). <www.humboldt.edu/~essays/golash.html> [accessed 3 June 2005]; Gooch, Paul. "A Mind to Love: Friends and Lovers in Ancient Greek Philosophy." In David Goicoechea, ed., *The Nature and Pursuit of Love: The Philosophy of Irving Singer*. Amherst, N.Y.: Prometheus, 1995, 83–97; Hatfield, Elaine, and Richard Rapson. *Love, Sex, and Intimacy*. New York: HarperCollins, 1993; Hauerwas, Stanley. "Gay Friendship: A Thought Experiment in Catholic Moral Theology." In

Eugene F. Rogers, Jr., ed., *Theology and Sexuality: Classic and Contemporary Readings*. Oxford, U.K.: Blackwell, 2002, 289–305; Jeffreys, Sheila. (1985) "Women's Friendships and Lesbianism." In Stevi Jackson and Sue Scott, eds., *Feminism and Sexuality: A Reader*. New York: Columbia University Press, 1996, 46–56; Jollimore, Troy. *Friendship and Agent-Relative Morality*. New York: Garland, 2001; Kimmel, Michael S., and Michael A. Messner, eds. "Men with Men: Friendships and Fears." Part Seven of *Men's Lives*, 3rd ed. Needham Heights, Mass.: Allyn and Bacon, 1995, 323–61; Kooper, Erik. "Loving the Unequal Equal: Medieval Theologians and Marital Affection." In Robert R. Edwards and Stephen Spector, eds., *The Olde Daunce: Love, Friendship, Sex, and Marriage in the Medieval World*. Albany: State University of New York Press, 1991, 44–56; Kuefler, Mathew. "Male Friendship and the Suspicion of Sodomy in Twelfth-Century France." In Carol B. Pasternack and Sharon Farmer, eds., *Difference and Genders in the Middle Ages*. Minneapolis: University of Minnesota Press, 2003, 145–81; Kupfer, Joseph. "Can Parents and Children Be Friends?" *American Philosophical Quarterly* 27 (1990), 15–26; Lesser, A. H. "Love and Lust." *Journal of Value Inquiry* 14:1 (1980), 51–54; McEvoy, James. "Friendship within Marriage: A Philosophical Essay." In Luke Gormally, ed., *Moral Truth and Moral Tradition: Essays in Honour of Peter Geach and Elizabeth Anscombe*. Dublin, Ire.: Four Courts Press, 1994, 194–202; Merino, Noël. "The Problem with 'We': Rethinking Joint Identity in Romantic Love." *Journal of Social Philosophy* 35:1 (2004), 123–32; Millgram, Elijah. "Aristotle on Making Other Selves." *Canadian Journal of Philosophy* 17:2 (1987), 361–76; Millgram, Elijah. "Kantian Crystallization." *Ethics* 114:3 (2004), 511–13; Mondschein, Ken. "Surpassing the Love of Women: Male Homosexuality in the Pre-Modern World." *Renaissance* 9:6, no. 40 (2004), 43–50; Peters, F. E. "érōs: *desire, love*." In *Greek Philosophical Terms: A Historical Lexicon*. New York: New York University Press, 1967, 62–66; Price, A. W. *Love and Friendship in Plato and Aristotle*. Oxford, U.K.: Clarendon Press, 1989; Principe, Walter. "Loving Friendship According to Thomas Aquinas." In David Goicoechea, ed., *The Nature and Pursuit of Love: The Philosophy of Irving Singer*. Amherst, N.Y.: Prometheus, 1995, 128–41; Raymond, Janice G. *A Passion for Friends: Toward a Philosophy of Female Affection*. Boston, Mass.: Beacon Press, 1986; Reeve, C.D.C. "Plato on Eros and Friendship." In Edward Zalta, ed., *Stanford Encyclopedia of Philosophy*. <plato.stanford.edu/entries/plato-friendship> [accessed 2 February 2005]; Rogers, Kelly. "Aristotle on Loving Another for His Own Sake." *Phronesis* 39:3 (1994), 291–302; Rosenberg, Miles. "Friendship." In Timothy F. Murphy, ed., *Reader's Guide to Lesbian and Gay Studies*. Chicago, Ill.: Fitzroy Dearborn, 2000, 234–36; Ryan, Joanna. "Psychoanalysis and Women Loving Women." In Sue Cartledge and Joanna Ryan, eds., *Sex and Love: New Thoughts on Old Contradictions*. London: Women's Press, 1983, 196–209; Schlabach, Gerald W. "Friendship as Adultery: Social Reality and Sexual Metaphor in Augustine's Doctrine of Original Sin." *Augustinian Studies* 23 (1992), 125–47; Shanley, Mary Lyndon. "Marital Slavery and Friendship: John Stuart Mill's *The Subjection of Women*." *Political Theory* 9:2 (1981), 229–47. Reprinted in Mary Lyndon Shanley and Carole Pateman, eds., *Feminist Interpretations and Political Theory*. University Park: Pennsylvania State University Press, 1991, 164–80; Sherman, Nancy. "Aristotle on Friendship and the Shared Life." *Philosophy and Phenomenological Research* 47:4 (1987), 589–613; Smith-Rosenberg, Caroll. "The Female World of Love and Ritual: Relations between Women in Nineteenth-Century America." *Signs* 1:1 (1975), 1–29. Reprinted in Nancy F. Cott and Elizabeth H. Pleck, eds., *A Heritage of Her Own: Toward a New Social History of the American Woman*. New York: Simon and Schuster, 1979, 311–42; Soble, Alan. "A Lakoma." [Reply to John McMurtry, "Sex, Love, and Friendship"] In *Sex, Love, and Friendship*. Amsterdam, Holland: Rodopi, 1997, 191–97; Soble, Alan. "The Unity of Romantic Love." *Philosophy and Theology* 1:4 (1987), 374–97. Reprinted in SLF (385–401); Stafford, J. Martin. "On Distinguishing between Love and Lust." *Journal of Value Inquiry* 11:4 (1977), 292–303. Reprinted in *Essays on Sexuality and Ethics*. Solihull, U.K.: Ismeron, 1995, 53–64; Strikwerda, Robert A., and Larry May. (1992) "Male Friendship and Intimacy." In Larry May and Robert Strikwerda, eds., *Rethinking Masculinity: Philosophical Explorations in Light of Feminism*, 1st ed. Lanham, Md.: Rowman and Littlefield, 1992, 95–110; and Larry May, Robert Strikwerda, and Patrick D. Hopkins, eds., *Rethinking Masculinity: Philosophical Explorations in Light of Feminism*, 2nd ed. Lanham, Md.: Rowman and Littlefield, 1996, 79–94; Sullivan, Andrew. *Love Undetectable:*

Reflections on Friendship, Sex, and Survival. New York: Knopf, 1998; Vacek, Edward Collins. *Love, Human and Divine: The Heart of Christian Ethics.* Washington, D.C.: Georgetown University Press, 1994; Velleman, David. "Love as a Moral Emotion." *Ethics* 109:4 (1999), 338–74; Walker, A.D.M. "Aristotle's Account of Friendship in the *Nicomachean Ethics.*" *Phronesis* 24:2 (1979), 180–96; Williams, Clifford, ed. *On Love and Friendship: Philosophical Readings.* Boston, Mass.: Jones and Bartlett, 1995.

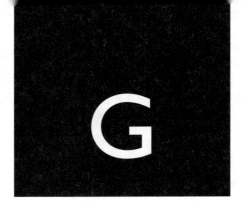

GENITAL MUTILATION. The expression "genital mutilation" is most frequently used to refer to various forms of female circumcision (e.g., clitoridectomy and infibulation), though it may also include penile subincision (as in some Australian aborigines imitating women's experience of menstruation and childbirth; see Gross), castration (surgical or chemical), and removal of the penile foreskin (male circumcision; see Graber).

Genital surgeries, which have been practiced by diverse ethnic and religious groups around the world for thousands of years, have been increasingly questioned in the West as its concept of the human self has come to stress individual autonomy. Related shifts toward recognizing the rights of women and children and toward the democratization of political and social authority have also contributed to the (re)interpretation of some traditional surgeries as unacceptable genital mutilation. In virtue of the emphasis on autonomy and rights, we find considerably more objection to the mutilation of the body done for a communal purpose, for example, ethnic identification, than to mutilation done out of personal desire: tattoos, the piercing of nipples, tongues, navels, foreskins, and labia, especially among the young, as well as breast augmentation, face lifts, nose jobs, liposuction, and penile implants. It is debatable, and of course difficult to decide, whether or to what extent these latter mutilating practices are done out of an individual's autonomous choice as opposed to being socially contrived or ethnically or culturally generated.

While some defenders of female circumcision reject all criticisms of the practice, arguing that persons outside a culture that practices female circumcision have no standing to object to that culture's practices (see Bradford and McClure), others argue, at the other end of the spectrum, that all surgical interventions on female genitalia are unacceptable mutilation that wrongly presuppose the inadequacy of the female genitalia in nature (see Gruenbaum). A middle position claims that cultures may mark the bodies of their members as long as the members **consent** to the interventions, the markings are not detrimental to the health or welfare of those marked (through, for example, antiseptic and anaesthetic procedures), and the markings do not convey a status inconsistent with human equality and rights. This position would allow some female circumcision: that in which "cutting" is symbolic (the Indonesian Maduranese practice of rubbing spices on the clitoris in the circumcision ceremony) and that in which the cutting is limited to the excision of the clitoral hood (in analogy with the removal of the foreskin from the penis). But it would condemn clitoridectomy and infibulation. In Africa, over 80 percent of all female circumcisions include at least clitoridectomy, and excision of only the clitoral hood is the rarest form. In other areas of the world, especially Asia, the milder forms of female circumcision prevail and receive little attention. Much of the international focus has been on Africa, especially after the condemnation of female genital mutilation by the United Nations Fourth World Conference on Women (1995), which followed the lead of the Organization of African Unity (1990).

Between 80 and 125 million living women have undergone female circumcision, most of them receiving serious levels of excision. Though the last clitoridectomies in the United States were performed in the 1930s (to "cure" **masturbation**), over 168,000 immigrant women in the States today have experienced clitoridectomy or infibulation and are treated by gynecologists and family doctors who have no training in the medical problems involved in these circumcisions (U.S. Department of State). Some have suggested that the practice should be specifically criminalized in the United States as it is in France (Gillette-Frenoy). A few African women have made successful claims for asylum in the United States on the grounds that if they could not flee their homes, they would be subject to severe danger to health and life from forced circumcision (Armstrong).

Some defenses of female circumcision, even those associated with African Islamic and African tribal religious practice (see Ishaq), have been dismissed as being scientifically ignorant and incompatible with women's rights and dignity. The folk belief that uncircumcised vulvas have odorous labia that grow down to a woman's knees, and the notions that uncircumcised women cannot become pregnant, deliver their infants safely, or have male children, are seen as ridiculous superstitions by societies that do not circumcise women. (This is also how Western societies view the Sambian belief that young boys must ingest semen—by fellating older males—to attain adult procreative capacity; see **Gilbert Herdt**.) Claims that clitoridectomy and infibulation are necessary to protect women from their own inclinations toward lust or **adultery**, or that infibulation increases a husband's pleasure by ensuring a tight vaginal opening, are similarly dismissed for assuming that women are the possessions of men, that women are especially liable to sexual transgression, or that (to mention just one more piece of the patriarchal *ethos*) women are not entitled to sexual pleasure.

The lack of organized movements against or systematic objections to piercing, tattooing, and much cosmetic plastic surgery, despite the health risks involved (bacterial and viral infections, including HIV/AIDS [human immunodeficiency virus/acquired immunodeficiency syndrome]; anaesthesia accidents) suggests that a central problem with genital mutilation is the fact that most affected females are circumcised young, that is, not given a genuine choice. Some children are physically coerced into circumcision the way children elsewhere are coerced into immunizations or dental care. However, in the case of genital mutilation the common justification for coercing children, that the procedure is medically necessary or therapeutic, is much more difficult to sustain. (Note that whether surgery on intersexed—and nonconsenting—children, which excises or constructs genital tissue, is always justifiable as therapeutic is unclear; see Feder.) But if choice or consent is the issue, would the moral objection to genital mutilation evaporate were, say, girls aged around sixteen to choose clitoridectomy? Surely at that age girls can freely choose to do many things: what to eat, what to read, and so forth. But at what age, with respect to *this* kind of decision in particular, should a person's consent be respected? If genuine consent is necessary, because genital surgery involves serious risks to health and welfare, perhaps only adults, who are better able to weigh the risks, could consent to genital surgery. An interesting parallel question arises about convicted adult sex offenders who opt for surgical or chemical castration as a condition for parole. Is this choice free, or is it coerced by the promise of parole?

In Africa, as in other areas of the world where female genital mutilation is common, it is women—mothers and grandmothers—who insist on and arrange female circumcision. Though the ultimate beneficiaries are men, whose control of women's sexuality is enhanced, women carry out the surgeries. These women explain that they do it, despite its pains and risks, out of **love** and concern for their daughters, who would be unmarriageable without circumcision. Unmarried women in many African societies not only lack access to basic resources but also exist at the periphery of society, without standing. Mothers and grandmothers have some self-interest as well, even if this is not their primary motive, since their own social standing is tied in part to that of their daughters and granddaughters; further, they want to become grandmothers and great-grandmothers through the daughter's children (Hayes; Walley).

For decades, governments in Africa have tried through the law to end genital mutilation, but since they are reluctant to punish parents, they have made little headway (Kouba; Thomas). Parents who do not circumcise a daughter in a society practicing female circumcision condemn that daughter to be unmarried or at least drastically lowers her bride price and her value to a husband's family. Few families arrange, or allow their son to arrange, **marriage** to an uncircumcised girl when circumcised girls are available. Hence renunciation of the practice by one set of parents depends on group renunciation (Olayinko). Eradication programs in Ghana, Senegal, and Sudan involving a number of adjacent villages, within which religious leaders, medical providers, civil authorities, circumcisers, women's organizations, and tribal elders were targeted by an extended information campaign, have proved successful. Health officials displayed films of women in labor bleeding to death from torn scar tissue and of infected vulvas filled with pockets of urine and menstrual blood; they also explained higher rates of HIV transmission to circumcised women. Men and women testified to infibulated women's discomfort during coitus; women with clitoridectomies testified to impaired ability to enjoy sex; husbands testified to their own sadness at being unable to bring their wives sexual pleasure and to their own suffering at causing their wives pain and danger to have children. At the end of such campaigns, many villages collectively decide to abolish female circumcision. Their decision is publicized by newspapers, radio, and television, and the movement spreads. African experience indicates that reform can occur only when the changes are embraced by enough people to lower significantly the social costs for individuals who do not comply with traditional practices.

See also African Philosophy; Beauty; Chinese Philosophy; Consent; Dworkin, Andrea; Ethics, Sexual; Feminism, Liberal; Herdt, Gilbert; Intersexuality; Islam; Money, John; Pedophilia; Violence, Sexual

REFERENCES

Armstrong, Patricia A. "Female Genital Mutilation: The Move toward Recognition of Violence against Women as a Basis for Asylum in the United States." *Maryland Journal of International Law and Trade* 21 (Spring 1997), 95–122; Bradford, Qiana, and Kimberly McClure. "Case Study on the Role and Relevance of Human Rights Language in Combating Female Genital Mutilation in Egypt." *Harvard Journal of African American Public Policy* 9 (Summer 2003), 151–86; Feder, Ellen K. " 'Doctors' Orders': Parents and Intersexed Children." In Eva Feder Kittay and Ellen K. Feder, eds., *The Subject of Care: Feminist Perspectives on Dependency.* Lanham, Md.: Rowman and Littlefield, 2002, 294–320; Gillette-Frenoy, Isabelle. "The Practice of Clitoridectomy in France." *Ethnographie* 88:2 (1992), 5–6, 21–50; Graber, Robert Bates. "A Psychocultural Theory of Male Genital Mutilation." *Journal of Psychoanalytic Anthropology* 4:4 (1981), 413–34; Gross, Rita. "Menstruation and Childbirth as Ritual and Religious Experience among Native Australians." In Nancy A. Falk and Rita M. Gross, eds., *Unspoken Worlds: Women's Religious Lives.* Belmont, Calif.: Wadsworth, 2002, 301–10; Gruenbaum, Ellen. "Cultural Debate over Female Circumcision: The Sudanese Are Arguing This One Out for Themselves." *Medical Anthropology Quarterly* 10:4 (1996), 455–75; Hayes, Rose O. "Female Genital Mutilation, Fertility Control, Women's Roles, and the Patrilineage in Modern Sudan: A Functional Analysis." *American Ethnologist* 2:4 (1975), 619–33; Herdt, Gilbert. *Sambia*

Sexual Culture: Essays from the Field. Chicago, Ill.: University of Chicago Press, 1999; Ishaq, Farid. *Islam and Pluralism: An Islamic Perspective on Interreligious Solidarity against Oppression*. Oxford, U.K.: Oneworld, 1997; Kouba, Leonard J. "Female Circumcision in Africa: An Overview." *African Studies Review* 28:1 (1985), 95–110; Olayinko, Kaso-Thomas. *The Circumcision of Women: A Strategy for Eradication*. London: Zed Books, 1987; Thomas, Lynn M. "Imperial Concerns and 'Women's Affairs': State Efforts to Regulate Clitoridectomy and Eradicate Abortion in Meru, Kenya, c. 1910–1950." *Journal of African History* 39:1 (1998), 121–45; United States Department of State, Under Secretary for Global Affairs. "Female Genital Mutilation (FGM) or Female Genital Cutting (FGC): Individual Country Reports." U.S. Dept. of State (1 June 2001). <www.state.gov/g/wi/rls/rep/crfgm/> [accessed 3 April 2004]; Walley, Christine J. "Searching for 'Voices': Feminism, Anthropology, and the Global Debate over Female Genital Operations." *Cultural Anthropology* 12:3 (1997), 405–38.

Christine E. Gudorf

ADDITIONAL READING

Ahmad, Imad-ad-Dean. *Female Genital Mutilation: An Islamic Perspective*. Bethesda, Md.: Minaret of Freedom Institute, Pamphlet no. 1 (2000). <www.minaret.org/fgm-pamphlet.htm> [accessed 8 June 2005]; Al-Sabbagh, Muhammed Lufti. *Islamic Ruling on Male and Female Circumcision*. Alexandria, Egypt: World Health Organization, 1992; Avedon, Richard. "Revelations: A Work in Progress." [photographs] *The New Yorker* (29 November 1999), 92–108, 141; Bartels, Edien. "Medical Ethics and Rites Involving Blood." *Anthropology and Medicine* 10:1 (2003), 105–14; Bordo, Susan. *Unbearable Weight: Feminism, Western Culture, and the Body*. Berkeley: University of California Press, 1993; Caldwell, John C. "Female Genital Mutilation: Conditions of Decline." *Population Research and Policy Review* 19:3 (2000), 233–54; Center for Reproductive Law and Policy (now Center for Reproductive Rights). *Adolescent Reproductive Rights: Laws and Policies to Improve Their Health and Lives*. New York: Author, 1999; Cohen, Lawrence. "The Pleasures of Castration: The Postoperative Status of Hijras, Jankhas, and Academics." In Paul R. Abramson and Steven D. Pinkerton, eds., *Sexual Nature Sexual Culture*. Chicago, Ill.: University of Chicago Press, 1995, 276–304; DeMello, Margo. *Bodies of Inscription: A Cultural History of the Modern Tattoo Community*. Durham, N.C.: Duke University Press, 2000; Feder, Ellen K. " 'Doctors' Orders': Parents and Intersexed Children." In Eva Feder Kittay and Ellen K. Feder, eds., *The Subject of Care: Feminist Perspectives on Dependency*. Lanham, Md.: Rowman and Littlefield, 2002, 294–320. <www.bodieslikeours.org/research-and-studies/feder-docsorders-2.html> and <www.bodieslikeours.org/respdf/Feder2002.pdf> [accessed 16 February 2005]; Filan, Kevin. "Criminals, Slaves, and Opera Stars: The Victims of Castration." *Renaissance* 9:6, no. 40 (2004), 55–58; Gruenbaum, Ellen. *The Female Circumcision Controversy: An Anthropological Perspective*. Philadelphia: University of Pennsylvania Press, 2001; Gruenbaum, Ellen. "Women's Rights and Cultural Self-Determination in the Female Genital Mutilation Controversy." *Anthropology Newsletter* (May 1995), 14–15; Gudorf, Christine E. "The Erosion of Sexual Dimorphism: Challenges to Religion and Religious Ethics." *Journal of the American Academy of Religion* 69:4 (2001), 863–91; Hosken, Fran P. "Female Genital Mutilation: Strategies for Eradication." International Symposium on Circumcision (1–2 March 1989), Anaheim, Calif. <www.nocirc.org/symposia/first/hosken.html> [accessed 26 May 2004]; Kessler, Suzanne J. "Evaluating Genital Surgery." In *Lessons from the Intersexed*. New Brunswick, N.J.: Rutgers University Press, 1998, 52–76; Ko, Dorothy. "The Body as Attire: The Shifting Meanings of Footbinding in Seventeenth-Century China." *Journal of Women's History* 8:4 (1997), 8–27; Kopelman, Loretta M. "Female Circumcision and Genital Mutilation." In Ruth Chadwick, ed., *Encyclopedia of Applied Ethics*, vol. 2. San Diego, Calif.: Academic Press, 1998, 249–59; Levy, Howard S. *The Lotus Lovers: The Complete History of the Curious Erotic Custom of Footbinding in China*. Buffalo, N.Y.: Prometheus, 1992; Lightfoot-Klein, Hanny. *Prisoners of Ritual: An Odyssey into Female Circumcision in Africa*. New York: Harrington Park Press, 1989; Meyers, Diana Tietjens. "Feminism and Women's Autonomy: The Challenge of Female Genital Cutting." *Metaphilosophy* 31:5 (2000), 469–91; Money, John. "The Skoptic Syndrome: Castration and Genital Mutilation." In *The Adam Principle. Genes, Genitals, Hormones, &*

Gender: Selected Readings in Sexology. Buffalo, N.Y.: Prometheus, 1993, 343–53; Money, John. "Three Cases of Genital Self-Surgery and Their Relationship to Transexualism." In *The Adam Principle. Genes, Genitals, Hormones, & Gender: Selected Readings in Sexology.* Buffalo, N.Y.: Prometheus, 1993, 326–34; Myers, James. "Nonmainstream Body Modification: Genital Piercing, Branding, Burning, and Cutting." *Journal of Contemporary Ethnography* 21:3 (1992), 267–306. Reprinted in Thomas S. Weinberg, ed., *S&M: Studies in Dominance and Submission.* Amherst, N.Y.: Prometheus, 1995, 151–91; Nanda, Serena. (1990) *Neither Man nor Woman: The Hijras of India,* 2nd ed. Belmont, Calif.: Wadsworth, 1998; Parker, Melissa. "Rethinking Female Circumcision." *Africa* 65:4 (1995), 506–23; Sanders, Clinton R. *Customizing the Body: The Art and Culture of Tattooing.* Philadelphia, Pa.: Temple University Press, 1989; Toubia, Nahid F. "Social and Political Implications of Female Circumcision: The Case of the Sudan." In Elizabeth Warnock Fernea, ed., *Women and the Family in the Middle East.* Austin: University of Texas Press, 1985, 148–59; Tuzin, Donald. "Discourse, Intercourse, and the Excluded Middle." In Paul R. Abramson and Steven D. Pinkerton, eds., *Sexual Nature Sexual Culture.* Chicago, Ill.: University of Chicago Press, 1995, 257–75; Walker, Alice, and Pratibha Parmar. *Warrior Marks: Female Genital Mutilation and the Sexual Blinding of Women.* New York: Harcourt Brace, 1993; Wassef, Nadia. "Masculinities and Mutilations: Female Genital Mutilation in Egypt." *Middle Eastern Women's Studies Review* 13:2 (1998), 1–4.

GNOSTICISM. "Gnosticism" is used to refer to certain groups within the early church that emphasized *gnosis* (Greek, knowledge) as the means of salvation. This knowledge concerned the nature of the universe, which was understood dualistically as an opposition between matter and spirit. Something had gone awry so that originally pure spirits had become trapped in a created material world that was the source of evil and corruption. The goal of gnosis was to restore the spirits to their original position and state. Understood this way, the Gnostic concept of salvation was both strikingly different from and in some ways parallel to that of early Christianity.

Especially characteristic of the Gnostic viewpoint was the radical (though, given its suppositions, logical) conclusion that since the material world was the source of evil, it could not have been created by the highest and only true God. Rather, it was the product of a lesser being, a demiurge often called "Ialdabaoth," who in ignorance thought *he* was God. Moreover, since the Old Testament begins with the creation of the material world, the Old Testament God could only be Ialdabaoth. As a result, the early chapters of Genesis figure very large in extant Gnostic literature.

A redeemer figure was usually the mediator of gnosis to the spirits trapped in the material world. In many texts this mediator was Christ, but others mention Melchizedek and Seth (both identified with Christ). Seth was of particular interest as the son born to Adam and Eve after Cain slew Abel. Seth was a new beginning, the hope of better things, and identified as the progenitor of the Gnostic race. Indeed, "seed of Seth" and "race of Seth" are frequently found in Gnostic works as terms of self-reference. Another revealer figure in certain Gnostic writings is the serpent. Reversing the usual Christian view, some Gnostic groups believed that the serpent was good: He encouraged Adam and Eve to partake of the tree of knowledge. Moreover, the serpent's statement that God did not want humans to have this knowledge revealed to them that this God was jealous and not the supreme God at all.

Melchizedekians, Sethians, and Ophites (from the Greek *ophis,* serpent) appear in the lists of Gnostic groups described by their Christian opponents. Other Gnostic groups were sometimes named after prominent teachers: Valentinus (ca. 100–ca. 175), Basilides (second century), Satornil (or Saturninus; late first century), Cerinthus (first half of second century), Carpocrates (second century). These Gnostic groups agreed on certain issues, such as the creation of the world by an evil God, but they had a stunning variety of speculations about precisely how the material world came into existence. On other matters of belief and practice there seems to have been little agreement. With regard to **sexual ethics** there was a range of attitudes, including advocacy of complete abstention, moderation in monogamous relationships, ritualized sex, and free enjoyment of sensual pleasures. Because differences abound, some scholars have questioned the suitability of uniting all the groups under the single term "Gnosticism" (see Williams). The ancient sources do not use the word, which dates from the eighteenth century. And though "Gnostics" is used by the church fathers to refer to certain groups, it is very seldom used to refer to the entire range of groups that moderns include under that rubric. Further complicating the issue is the fact that some writers used "Gnostic" to refer to Christians who had a more advanced understanding of the philosophical principles underlying their faith (for example, Clement of Alexandria [ca. 150–215], *Stromateis* [ca. 200], bk. 7). Caution must be used not to be led astray by our own categories. Still, there is reason to use "Gnostic" to denote the variety of groups flourishing from the second to the fourth century that held some common views (radical dualism between spirit and matter; gnosis as the key to transcending the material plane) and in some instances were related to each other, in that one group arose from another.

The Neo-Platonist philosopher Plotinus (205–269) wrote a work against Gnosticism in which he claimed that whatever truth it contained had been derived from **Plato** (427–347 BCE), but much error had been mixed in from elsewhere (*Enneads* 2.9). Some early Christian writers—Irenaeus (130–ca. 202; *Adversus haereses* 2.14); Tertullian (ca. 160–240; *De praescriptione haereticorum* 7.30)—likewise suggested origins in pagan philosophy. Hippolytus (ca. 170–236) claimed that certain elements were derived from astrology and Greek mystery religions (*Refutatio omnium haeresium*, prae. 8). While acknowledging these influences, Christian writers traced Gnosticism back to the archheretic Simon Magus (first century), a Samaritan. A Jewish origin is commonly urged on the grounds that similar ideology, motifs, and interpretations appear in Gnostic texts and contemporary and later Jewish writings. Some have gone so far as to claim that a pre-Christian Gnosticism had developed out of **Judaism** (see Rudolph, 277–82). However, there is one fundamental difference between Judaism and Gnosticism: For Gnostics, but not Jews, the Old Testament was important primarily as a description of the source of humanity's problems, not their solution.

Information about Gnostic practices and beliefs comes from two sources. The first are Christian writings, the works of Irenaeus, Tertullian, Hippolytus, and Epiphanius (ca. 315–403). The second is an entire library of Gnostic literature, discovered in 1945 at Nag Hammadi (Egypt), which consists of fifty-two works in thirteen codices that date to the fourth century. One problem is how reliable the testimony of church writers is—writers who, at best, may have misunderstood the groups they describe and, at worst, may have exaggerated to bolster their accusations of the groups' heresies. This problem is exacerbated by the fact that the church writers sometimes provide exactly the information missing from Nag Hammadi documents: accounts about specific teachers, relationships between groups, and more important, details about Gnostic practices. Thus much care is needed in evaluating the evidence.

A prominent aspect of Gnosticism is its speculation about the origin and nature of the material world and humankind, speculation involving at some level a retelling of Genesis. What is fascinating is that representations of gender are thickly interwoven into the basic fabric of the story, and interwoven in ways that are only tangential to matters found in the

Genesis account. Although there is an astonishing variety of tellings of the creation story, one that seems to have been particularly important for Gnostics is the *Apocryphon of John*. This work is preserved in the Nag Hammadi codices and is also found in the Berlin Codex that was discovered in Egypt in 1896. In addition, Irenaeus gives a summary of this work in *Adversus haereses*, so it is one of the few points where we can measure the accuracy of a report in a non-Gnostic writer against an actual Gnostic text.

According to the *Apocryphon of John*, the monad or unity that is the supreme God and Parent (or Father) of the entirety (that is, everything else) exists alone, at first. The Parent's thought takes form as an emanation or aeon known as Forethought or Barbelo. Barbelo becomes the womb for the rest of the spiritual universe. In the *Apocryphon*, Barbelo is given a series of attributes or names, including "the mother-father, the first human being, the holy spirit, the thrice-male, the three powers, the thrice androgynous name" (*Apoc. Jn.* 5:5–6). The collocation of titles that seem to transcend gender is typical of many Gnostic texts.

From Barbelo came forth other emanations, by the consent of the Parent, and are given names that are also attributes, such as "prior acquaintance," "incorruptibility," "eternal life," and "truth." These four emanations together with Barbelo are called "the androgynous quintet of aeons." Next, Barbelo conceives by a glance from the Parent and brings forth the only begotten, also called "Christ." The process that produces the only-begotten is different; the Parent was not involved in the creation of the other emanations—they were not begotten but just appeared. From Christ come forth further emanations, twelve in number. The last of these is Sophia (Wisdom). Next comes the perfect human being, Geradamas. At this point all the emanations glorify the invisible spirit, the Parent. But now something goes awry, and Sophia conceives a thought without the consent of "her maleness" (the virgin spirit). This thought becomes realized, and she names it "Ialdabaoth." Ialdabaoth is without sense and impious but has somehow taken power from his mother and brings forth his own emanations, "authorities," and then claims to be the only god. He and his authorities create Adam after the image of Geradamas that they had seen reflected in the waters of the heavens.

At this point Sophia grieves at the events that have transpired and entreats Barbelo for help. Barbelo sends Christ, who induces Ialdabaoth to blow on Adam, and in so doing the power he had stolen from his mother flees and passes to Adam. In this way Adam becomes a spiritual being, superior even to Ialdabaoth and his authorities. Out of jealousy, Ialdabaoth and the authorities cast Adam into the lowest part of the material world. But Afterthought (also called "Life" and related to or identical with Sophia) descends and dwells within Adam to teach him both about his true origin and how to ascend back to the world above. Ialdabaoth tries to take back his power from Adam, but in the end winds up only creating woman, who also now has the same spiritual nature as Adam. Placed in the Garden, it is Christ who causes the man and woman to eat from the tree of knowledge.

One can immediately see in this story that the categories of male and female were fecund in the minds of Gnostic writers. The distinction between them is used to express the fundamental duality of the created universe. Yet, at the same time, this duality is secondary, and at the highest level of existence, that of Barbelo, such dualities are transcended.

A very important female figure in the *Apocryphon* is Sophia. But is she villain or heroine? It is her act that leads to the creation of the material world and the entrapment of spirit within it; but she instigates the events that correct the mistake, and her repentance and restoration become the model for that of humans. Such ambiguities exist in other Nag Hammadi documents. Consider the Gnostic Gospel of Thomas, logion 22:

Jesus saw some little ones nursing. He said to his disciples, "What these little ones who are nursing resemble is those who enter the kingdom." They said to him, "So shall we enter the kingdom by being little ones?" Jesus said to them, "When you (pl.) make the two one and make the inside like the outside and the outside like the inside and the above like the below, and that you might make the male and female be one and the same, so that the male might not be male nor the female be female, when you make eyes in place of an eye and a hand in place of a hand and a foot in place of a foot, an image in place of an image—then you will enter [the kingdom]." (Layton's translation, 384)

Reunification of male and female is presented here as the key to "entering the kingdom." This passage seems to assert the equality of male and female or, better, indicates a deeper unity where gender is transcended. But logion 114, an exchange between Jesus and Peter, contradicts this idea:

Simon Peter said to them, "Mary should leave us, for females are not worthy of life." Jesus said, "See, I am going to attract her to make her male so that she too might become a living spirit that resembles you males. For every female (element) that makes itself male will enter the kingdom of heavens." (Layton, 399)

Similar statements about the need for the female to become male occur in other Gnostic texts.

What view of gender is in the cosmic pattern of fall and redemption in the *Apocryphon*? Some scholars point out that in both the upper and lower realms, trouble occurs when the female power (Barbelo, Sophia) creates without the involvement or guidance of a male power. The goal of salvation is the restoration of the female to the male, as the Gospel of Thomas hints. But other scholars argue that the androgynous nature of the Parent and Barbelo and the fact that female figures play a large role in the restoration of things indicate a Gnostic willingness to part with the typical Greco-Roman views of gender. Did this open up new possibilities for women in Gnostic circles? A direct piece of evidence for women's participation in Gnostic groups is the third-century burial inscription of Flavia Sophe found in Rome:

You, who did yearn for the paternal light,
Sister, spouse, my Sophē,
Anointed in the baths of Christ with everlasting, holy oil,
Hasten to gaze at the divine features of the aeons,
The great Angel of the great council (i.e. the Redeemer),
The true Son;
You entered the bridal chamber and deathless ascended
To the bosom of the Father. (Rudolph's translation, 212)

"Gaze at . . . the aeons" and "entered the bridal chamber" indicate that Flavia was a Gnostic. Written in Greek, the style of the inscription shows that she was fairly well-to-do.

From the testimony of church fathers it seems that women were occasionally involved in the founding of Gnostic groups. One group, active in Rome during the time of Bishop Anicetus (ca. 155–160), followed Marcellina. Origen (ca. 185–251), in his work against the pagan critic Celsus (late second century), says that Celsus knew not only Marcellina but also "Harpocratians who follow Salome, and others who follow Mariamme, and others who follow Martha" (*Contra Celsus* 5.62). While these women are otherwise unknown, some scholars suggest that Mariamme should be identified with Mary Magdalene and that all three women were not contemporaries of Marcellina but figures from the New Testament. Another woman, Helena, was not said to have started her own group but to have been associated with a man who did. She was the partner of Simon Magus, the father of all heresies, according to the patristic writers. Helena was a former prostitute from Tyre who was said to have accompanied Simon during the rule of the Emperor Claudius (41–54). Simon claimed that he was the first god and that Helena was his first thought (Greek, *ennoia*) and the mother of all else. She had created angels and powers, who created the world and then rebelled against her. Taking her captive, they imprisoned her in various bodies, including that of Helen of Troy, and she eventually ended up in the brothel where Simon found her. Simon had descended to earth in disguise to rescue her. Origen states that there are some Simonians "who reverence as teacher Helena" (*Contra Celsus* 5.62). Whatever one makes of the historical accuracy of Simon and Helena as the source of Gnosticism, if the tradition was accepted in Gnostic circles, that at least shows they were willing to entertain the idea that Gnostic mythology could be associated with individual women and that women could act as teachers.

Information about Gnostic sexual practices comes from the heresiologists, who criticize Gnosticism severely and go into far greater detail about its sexual excess than its asceticism. Scholars have tended to discount much of this ancient criticism as pure fabrication, exaggeration, or misunderstanding of Gnostic metaphors. Some scholars have suggested that church writers cleverly used against the Gnostics the same, and equally wrong, charges that had been used against them by pagan critics. But Stephen Benko has boldly proposed that some pagan critics may actually have had Gnostic excess in mind when they accused Christians of licentiousness (67–73). Unfortunately, extant Gnostic texts do not tell us much about their sexual practices. What the texts do say about sexuality is usually metaphorical and describes Gnostic speculation about how the universe was created.

In discussing the issue of ethics, Bentley Layton writes that

> the classic gnostic scriptures almost never . . . draw explicit conclusions about the way that gnostics should . . . behave. This is understandable, for the literary form of the gnostic scriptures provides almost no occasion for ethical conclusions to be drawn. To some extent, such ethical conclusions may have seemed too obvious to state; for, to many thinkers in the second century . . . the acceptance of a split between body and soul implied that the best mode of life was continence, so as to minimize the body's adverse influence upon the soul. (199)

Consider, as an example, the *Apocryphon*. Here the first sexual act was not between Adam and Eve but between Ialdabaoth and Eve. Ialdabaoth beheld Eve standing with Adam and "became filled with lack of acquaintance . . . defiled her and begot on her two sons" (24:12–15). These two sons are later identified as Cain and Abel. The *Apocryphon* generalizes from this first sexual act:

> And to the present day sexual intercourse, which originated from the first ruler [Ialdabaoth], has remained. And in the female who belonged to Adam it sowed a seed of desire; and by sexual intercourse it raised up birth in the image of bodies. (24:26–30)

But is there a moral lesson to be learned from this? Later, the text describes those who will attain salvation as "being anxious for nothing except incorruptibility alone; meditating on it thenceforth without anger, envy, grudging, desire, or insatiableness as regards the entirety; restrained by nothing but the subsistent entity of the flesh, which they wear, awaiting the time when they will be visited by those beings who take away" (25:29–26:1).

On the basis, apparently, of passages like this, Kurt Rudolph argues that asceticism was the most characteristic approach of Gnostics and that "the overwhelming majority of the sources give unequivocal support to this aspect of Gnostic morality" (257). Granting this, it is nonetheless possible that, despite Gnostic asceticism, while a person remained in the flesh **sexual activity** was allowed in certain circumstances such as **marriage**.

Here and there mention is made of something called "spiritual marriage" in connection with Gnosticism. The theme of marriage is especially prominent in the Gospel of Philip, a Nag Hammadi text (in Robinson) commonly attributed to the Valentinian branch of Gnosticism and perhaps dating to the second half of the third century. About this gospel, Wesley Isenberg writes (313): "The primary interest of *Gos. Phil.* is the restoration of Adam's original androgynous nature. . . . The reunion can be effected in the sacramental bridal chamber (70:17–22), where 'mysteries of truth' are revealed in type and image (84:20–21; 85:14–19)." A clear statement of this theme is in Gospel of Philip 70:9–23:

> If the woman had not separated from the man, she should not die with the man. His separation became the beginning of death. Because of this Christ came to repair the separation which was from the beginning and again unite the two, and to give life to those who died as a result of the separation and unite them. But the woman is united to her husband in the bridal chamber. Indeed those who have united in the bridal chamber will no longer be separated. Thus Eve separated from Adam because it was not in the bridal chamber that she united with him. (Isenberg's translation, in Robinson, 151–52)

Moreover, that the bridal chamber was part of a system of rites seems warranted from Gospel of Philip 67:27–30: "The Lord did everything in a mystery, a baptism and a chrism and a eucharist and a redemption and a bridal chamber." But of what this rite consisted is difficult to say. Michael Williams argues that the idea here is a marriage between a man and woman who would live together but remain celibate. This type of marriage would then be identical to the celibate marriages known in the wider church among ascetically minded Christians. In support of this interpretation, Williams cites Gospel of Philip 81:34–82:10, where the sexual intercourse of "defiled marriage" is contrasted with undefiled marriage (148–49). The latter "is not fleshly but pure. It belongs not to desire but to the will. It belongs not to the darkness or the night but to the day and the light." If sexual intercourse characterizes defiled marriage, then celibacy likely characterizes undefiled marriage.

However, the more usual interpretation (see Grant; Rudolph, 245–46) is that the bridal chamber is an initiation ceremony symbolizing the new member's entry into the heavenly realms of the emanations (the pleroma). This reading understands passages like Gospel of Philip 81:34–82:10 not to be contrasting sexual marriage with celibate marriage but an earthly experience with a spiritual one. Indeed, spiritual marriage is basic to Gnosticism: "If anyone becomes a son of the bridal chamber, he will receive the light" (Gos. Phil. 86:4–5). Here "light" refers to Gnostic insight and freedom from the powers that rule the material realm: "The powers do not see those who are clothed in the perfect light, and consequently are not able to detain them. One will clothe himself in this light sacramentally in the union" (Gos. Phil. 70:5–9).

Two more aspects of the bridal chamber should be mentioned. First, while the idea of entering the bridal chamber is related to being freed from the powers, another way of expressing this idea has to do with angels and demons. Gospel of Philip 65:1–26 refers to male and female evil spirits as sexual predators that attack women and men, respectively, to have intercourse with them. The only way to escape the evil spirits is for the human to be joined, in the bridal chamber, with an angel of the opposite sex. In this way the evil spirits cannot overpower the human soul. Second, there is the question of how the bridal chamber ceremony relates to the kiss that appears in passages such as Gospel of Philip 59:2–3: "For it is by a kiss that the perfect conceive and give birth. For this reason we also kiss one another. We receive conception from the grace which is in one another." In an intriguing (but damaged) passage, reference is also made to Jesus's kissing Mary Magdalene: "And the companion of the [. . .] Mary Magdalene [. . . loved] her more than [all] the disciples [and used to] kiss her [often] on her [. . .]" (Gos. Phil. 63:33–36; Isenberg). A parallel in Gospel of Philip 58–59 indicates that the kiss was on her mouth. Robert Grant accepts that the kiss was part of the marriage ceremony (139); Rudolph denies it (245).

Valentinian practices are also mentioned by church writers. Clement of Alexandria says that Valentinians approved of marriage and that they held this view based on the pairings of the emanations in the pleroma (*Strom.* 3.1). Williams, even though he favors the notion that the marriage mentioned in Gospel of Philip is chaste or celibate, believes that Clement is speaking here of a Valentinian marriage that involved sexual intercourse and procreation (152).

The bridal chamber ritual is described by Irenaeus: "Some of them (Valentinians) prepare a 'bridal chamber' and perform a mystic rite (mystagogia), with certain invocations, for those who are being consecrated (or perfected), and they claim that what they are effecting is a 'spiritual marriage,' after the image of the conjunctions (syzygies)" (*Adv. haer.* 1.21.3; Rudolph's translation, 245). Earlier in *Adversus haereses* Irenaeus mentions a late-second-century Valentinian leader, Marcus, who engaged in the bridal chamber ceremony this way:

> He is especially concerned about women, and those who are well-dressed and clothed in purple and of great wealth, whom he often attempts to seduce. Flatteringly he says to them: "If you want to partake of my Grace (*Charis*) because the Father of all sees your angel in his presence . . . it behooves us to be united. First receive Grace from me and through me. Adorn yourself as a bride awaiting her bridegroom that you may be what I am, and I may be what you are. Put the 'seed' of light in your bridal chamber. Take from me the bridegroom. Receive him and be received in him. Look, Grace is descending upon you. Open your mouth and prophesy." . . . From now on she considers herself a prophetess and thanks Marcus for having given her of his Charis. She tries to reward him not only by the gift of her possessions—in this manner he has amassed a fortune—but by sharing her body, desiring to unite herself with him in every way so that she may become one with him. (*Adv. haer.* 1.13.3; McGuire's translation, 263)

Whether this report is an aberration, exaggeration, or outright falsehood has been much debated. At least one may note that patristic reports about Valentinians are not unrelentingly negative. But reports about the Carpocratians were. Clement of Alexandria charges them with libertinism, says that they consider wives to be common property, and states that they have "love feasts" at which they sate themselves with food and then have intercourse with any women they want (*Strom.* 3.6–10). Irenaeus also accuses Carpocratians of engaging in indiscriminate sex and practicing multiple marriages (*Adv. haer.* 1.28.2). Note that

Carpocrates held the view that good and evil are only human categories and that *both* must be experienced to end the cycle of reincarnation. Other groups that supposedly practiced "free love" were the Simonians and Ophites.

The most extravagant reports of all are those of Epiphanius of Salamis concerning a group known variously as the Phibionites, Borborites, or Stratiotics. Epiphanius claims to have had personal knowledge of this group; when he was a young man, some women members enticed him to join, though he was able to escape. This group held their women in common, engaged in sex freely, and practiced *coitus interruptus*. The main goal of the latter was to bring forth semen, which was then offered heavenward by the man and woman and then eaten by them. The same was done with female menses. These offerings were accompanied by prayers in which the Phibionites—in imitation of the eucharist formula—referred to the semen as the body of Christ and the menstrual blood as the blood of Christ. Epiphanius states that the rationale for all this was "the necessity of collecting, from out of the power within bodies, the parts plundered from the superior mother by the ruler who made the world and by the others in its company—gods, angels, demons—by means of emissions of males and females" (*Panarion* 26.1.9; Layton's translation, 204). The shortcutting of the normal result of sexual intercourse aided in the return of spiritual matter to the heavenly spheres. Moreover, if *coitus interruptus* failed and the man ejaculated, causing pregnancy, the Phibionites would induce an **abortion**, grind up the fetus, mix it with spices and aromatics, and eat it.

The warrant for these practices came from certain books they possessed. Epiphanius mentions one of these, *Greater Questions of Mary*, which contained a narrative in which Jesus took Mary to a mountain, produced a woman from his side, and began to have sexual relations with her. When the semen was produced, he partook of it and said, "We must act thus so that we might live" (*Panarion* 26.8.2). In this way the Phibionites, perhaps as the Gospel of Philip relates its story about Jesus's kissing Mary, sought to base their practices in the acts of Jesus. Another unusual feature of Phibionite practice was that some of their members, after having their fill of sex with women, turned to one another and practiced homosexual acts along with **masturbation** (*Panarion* 26.11.1–8). The goal was the same as their *coitus interruptus*. Epiphanius also mentions that there were actually among these Gnostics a group of individuals designated Levites who did not have sexual intercourse with females at all but only with other males. These Levites were held in great honor among them (*Panarion* 26.13.1). These practices seem to stand in contrast with the usual Gnostic emphasis on male-female pairings.

Can any of this be believed? There is nothing in the Nag Hammadi texts similar to what Epiphanius wrote. Still, two considerations keep the question open. First, Epiphanius refers to his own acquaintance with certain members of the group, so that his knowledge, in this case, was supposedly firsthand. Second, such practices are alluded to in two late Gnostic works, the second book of *Jeu* and the *Pistis Sophia*, which curses in the name of Jesus those "who take male semen and female menstrual blood and make it into a lentil dish and eat it" (*Pistis Sophia* 251:14–19; Rudolph's translation, 250).

See also Abstinence; Augustine (Saint); Catholicism, History of; Hinduism; Judaism, History of; Manichaeism; Paul (Saint); Social Constructionism; Tantrism; Utopianism

REFERENCES

Benko, Stephen. *Pagan Rome and the Early Christians*. Bloomington: Indiana University Press, 1984; Grant, Robert. "The Mystery of Marriage in the Gospel of Philip." *Vigiliae Christianae* 15:3 (1961), 129–40; Isenberg, Wesley W. "Philip, Gospel of." In David N. Freedman, ed., *The Anchor*

Bible Dictionary, vol. 5. New York: Doubleday, 1992, 312–13; Layton, Bentley. *The Gnostic Scriptures: Ancient Wisdom for the New Age*. New York: Doubleday, 1987; McGuire, Anne. "Women, Gender, and Gnosis in Gnostic Texts and Traditions." In Ross Shepard Kraemer and Mary Rose D'Angelo, eds., *Women and Christian Origins*. Oxford, U.K.: Oxford University Press, 1999; Origen. *Contra Celcum*. Trans. Henry Chadwick. Cambridge: Cambridge University Press, 1953, 1965, 1980; Origen. *Contra Celcus*, bk. 5. The Gnostic Society Library. <www.gnosis.org/library/orig_cc5.htm> [accessed 25 May 2005]; Robinson, James, ed. *The Nag Hammadi Library in English*, rev. ed. San Francisco, Calif.: Harper and Row, 1988; Rudolph, Kurt. *Gnosis: The Nature and History of Gnosticism*. San Francisco, Calif.: Harper and Row, 1987; Williams, Michael. *Rethinking Gnosticism: An Argument for Dismantling a Dubious Category*. Princeton, N.J.: Princeton University Press, 1996.

Erik W. Larson

ADDITIONAL READING

Buckley, Jorunn Jacobsen. *Female Fault and Fulfillment in Gnosticism*. Chapel Hill, N.C.: University of North Carolina Press, 1986; Brown, Peter. *The Body and Society: Men, Women, and Sexual Renunciation in Early Christianity*. New York: Columbia University Press, 1988; Clark, Elizabeth A. *Clement's Use of Aristotle: The Aristotelian Contribution to Clement of Alexandria's Refutation of Gnosticism*. New York: Mellen Press, 1977; Davis, Murray. *Smut: Erotic Reality/Obscene Ideology*. Chicago, Ill.: University of Chicago Press, 1983; The Gnostic Archive. (Web site) <www.gnosis.org> [accessed 25 May 2005]; Hoeller, Stephan A. "Valentinus: A Gnostic for All Seasons." <www.gnosis.org/valentinus.htm> [accessed 3 March 2005]; King, Karen L. Review of *Female Fault and Fulfillment in Gnosticism*, by Jorunn Jacobsen Buckley. *Signs* 13:4 (1988), 878–79; King, Karen L. *What Is Gnosticism?* Cambridge, Mass.: Harvard University Press, 2003; King, Karen, ed. *Images of the Feminine in Gnosticism*. Studies in Antiquity and Christianity, 4. Philadelphia, Pa.: Fortress Press, 1988. Harrisburg, Pa.: Trinity Press, 2000; Origen. *Contra Celcus*. In *Ante-Nicene Fathers*, vol. 4. Christian Classics Ethereal Library. <www.ccel.org/fathers2/ANF-04/TOC.htm> [accessed 25 May 2005]; Pagels, Elaine. *The Gnostic Gospels*. New York: Random House, 1979. New York: Vintage, 1989; Pearson, Birger. *Gnosticism, Judaism, and Egyptian Christianity*. Studies in Antiquity and Christianity, 5. Minneapolis, Minn.: Fortress Press, 1990; Pearson, Birger. "The Other Christians." [Review of *Beyond Belief: The Secret Gospel of Thomas*, by Elaine Pagels] *New York Review of Books* (23 October 2003), 12–15; Perkins, Pheme. *Gnosticism and the New Testament*. Minneapolis, Minn.: Fortress Press, 1993; Shattuck, Roger. *Forbidden Knowledge: From Prometheus to Pornography*. San Diego, Calif.: Harcourt Brace, 1996; Yamauchi, Edwin M. *Gnostic Ethics and Mandaean Origins*. Harvard Theological Studies XXIV. Cambridge, Mass.: Harvard University Press, 1970; Yamauchi, Edwin M. (1973) *Pre-Christian Gnosticism: A Survey of the Proposed Evidences*, 2nd ed. Grand Rapids, Mich.: Baker Book House, 1983.

GREEK SEXUALITY AND PHILOSOPHY, ANCIENT. The modern study of sexuality in the ancient Greco-Roman world has been closely tied up with contemporary **feminism** (Keuls; Pomeroy) and the growing interest in same-sex relationships (Halperin). Scholars during the past thirty years have seen Greco-Roman antiquity as either a negative or positive paradigm, and the study of the Classical past has challenged modern classifications of sexual conduct by pointing toward a different system of categories in the ancient world. Though there were various studies of ancient sexuality prior to the last generation, these studies have by and large been superseded by more modern research. Some more technical investigations from prior to that period are still useful (e.g., Vorberg, *Glossarium Eroticum*, [1932]). One major inspiration for modern scholarship has been **Michel Foucault**'s (1926–1984) unfinished work *The History of Sexuality*, which covers ancient Greece and Rome, but as always with Foucault's work, both his method and results have been disputed.

Sex was not a main concern for most philosophers in antiquity. The attitudes expressed by those who did discuss **love** and sex, notably **Plato** (427–347 BCE) and **Aristotle** (384–322 BCE), were not necessarily typical for the societies in which they lived, since their attitudes differ from views of sex provided by other literary and historical sources from their contemporary society. One major problem in the study of sexuality in the ancient world is that almost all our sources were written or created by men, and we know about female sexuality only from a male point of view. The one major exception are the scanty remains of the lyric poet Sappho (ca. 610–580 BCE; see below).

The goddess of Love in ancient Greece was Aphrodite, but she had at her side a more primeval divine force, Eros, who in one of the earliest pieces of Greek poetry, Hesiod's (ca. 700 BCE) *Theogony*, is among the first divinities in the development of the world. Eros is described as being "the most beautiful of the immortal gods, who in every man and in every god softens the limbs and overpowers the mind and prudent determination" (*Theogony*, lines 120–22). This characterization of Eros (the term is used both about the god and about **sexual desire** in general) is typical of the Greeks' attitude toward sex: Eros is a fundamental force in human life, he/it is irresistible on a physical level, and he/it prevents those attacked from using their rational mind in the proper way. The fifth-century BCE Sophist Prodicus said that "desire doubled is eros, eros doubled is madness" (fragment DK 84, B 7; Dillon and Gergel). Aristotle's successor, Theophrastus (ca. 370–285 BCE), defined eros as "an excess of irrational desire" (frag. 557). Eros is often described as being equipped with bow and arrow, an image that means little to us today but in fact tells us that the ancients considered eros very dangerous: An arrow can hit us from afar when we least expect it and inflict a most painful wound. It is important to understand that falling in love in most ancient Greek literature is not described as a wonderful experience but as something that is painful and disturbing, because it makes us behave erratically. Hence, whenever a person is overcome by eros, it means that he or she behaves in a way that is beyond (rational) control. In Homer's (ca. 700 BCE) *Iliad* (bk. 14, lines 216–17), Hera borrows from Aphrodite her breastband with "love, desire and sweet talk that steals the mind away even from the thoughtful" and seduces her husband Zeus so that he neglects to support the Trojans. In Euripides's (ca. 485–406 BCE) tragedy *Hippolytos* Phaedra is devastated by eros for her own stepson and commits suicide when her feelings are not returned. And in the Sophist Gorgias's (ca. 480–390 BCE) defense of the mythical Helena who was accused of eloping with Prince Paris to Troy and thus causing the Trojan War, she is claimed to be innocent because it is impossible to resist eros (DK 82, B 11, §15; Dillon and Gergel).

The ancient Greeks were not afraid of love and sex. The Cynic philosophers in the third century BCE may have shocked their contemporaries by having sexual intercourse and masturbating in public, but these acts were not shameful as such. Hence, sexual topics can turn up in both literature and pictorial art without causing embarrassment. It is often difficult to decide to what extent the many erotic scenes on Greek vases or allusions to sex in Aristophanes's (ca. 445–385 BCE) comedies express moments of Greek daily life or are the result of male fantasies (many sexual pictures occur on utensils used for symposia where only men participated), but they are vivid and direct. Furthermore, all Greek streets were adorned with herms, that is, statues with a bust of a male figure on top of a square pillar with male sexual organs, often erect. Much Greek art showed naked male and female figures, and Greek men exercised in the palaestra naked, though women generally must have been excluded from athletic events. The ubiquity of sexual representations is part of the explanation that sexual phenomena play so important a role in Aristophanes's comedies (performed 425–385 BCE). Not only are the plays full of obscene jokes, but sex is also something the characters on the stage, both male and female, talk about. The plot of one renowned play, *Lysistrata*, is built around the idea that the women, tired of the endless Peloponnesian War for erotic as well as other reasons (they are no longer able to import good leather dildos!), engage in a sex strike, thus forcing the men to give up war. Needless to say, both men and women in the play suffer from sexual deprivation. Only Victorian attitudes towards sex have provoked the belief that women were not present at the dramatic performances, which were the most attended public events of the year in ancient Athens.

Even though the *Lysistrata*, along with other kinds of evidence, provides testimony that women were not powerless in a Greek city-state, there can be no doubt that the position of women was inferior to that of men in ancient Greece. Only men counted as citizens and could participate in public life. Men ran the administration of the cities and defended the state in military conflicts, while in both their childhood and adult life women seem to have been confined to living within the walls of the private house, at least if they belonged to the wealthier families (Pomeroy). This situation is most vividly described in Xenophon's (ca. 428–354 BCE) dialogue *Oikonomikos* (*Essay on How to Run Your House*), written in the middle of the fourth century BCE. There we meet an Athenian male who describes his view of his household and the role of his wife who is much younger than he is. She was expected to take care of the home and make sure that what he brought in from his outside activities was well taken care of. Xenophon's text as well as other evidence attest that men in general were mature and sexually experienced when they married, while their brides were in their mid-teens and moved directly from the protection of their parents' house into their spouse's home.

The dominance of men in society gave many more sexual opportunities to men than to women. Elite men spent much time together with other men, while women of the same social standing as the men were secluded from male company, and men formed emotional relationships with other men, in particular younger men. It is mistaken to claim that **homosexuality** was more common or more accepted in the ancient world than in modern times, but it is undeniable that most Greek men at least in part of their lives had both same-sex and heterosexual relationships at one and the same time. It was part of the traditional upbringing, in particular in Athens, that a mature man functioned as an educator and lover (usually called *erastes* = lover) of a younger man (called *eromenos* = beloved), as a role model, so to speak, but it is also clear that this relationship often also had a physical component (see Dover). This situation is documented not only in literary sources but also in Attic vase paintings. In Plato's dialogue *Symposium*, for example, the young and beautiful Alcibiades expresses consternation over the fact that he was unable to have a physical relationship with Socrates (469–399 BCE), who had expressed his love for his young friend (217b–219e). Socrates's self-control and love of the ideal made him neglect the physical **beauty** of young males, since it is so transient. "Platonic love" is exactly what the expression implies: a specific feature in the philosophy of Plato, not something that was common in real life among men in ancient Greece.

In many ways the most important sexual distinction in ancient Greece was not between same-sex and heterosexual relations but between being the active and the passive partner in a relationship, whatever the gender of the partners. (Greek had no terms corresponding to our words "heterosexual," "homosexual," or "bisexual.") Mutual affections may have existed, but sex and love were in general perceived as something that took place between an active partner who occupied a more powerful position, whether by age, social status, or gender, and a receiving partner, whether younger, female, or of slave status. In the case of women and slaves, this inequity was unproblematic: Men had every right to behave as they found stimulating, provided that they did not approach married women. In case of men who were citizens, sex was not without complications: A young man was not supposed to give in to a lover without resistance (see *Symp.* 184a), and too much willingness to submit to being passive and being penetrated was considered unacceptable and unmanly. In same-sex male relationships, intercrural intercourse seems to have been more common than anal penetration; in pictorial representations the person who is the object of someone's sexual attention is never shown as being sexually stimulated (that is, with an erection) or enjoying the sexual act. Exclusively homosexual relationships were not highly estimated. In pictorial representations of sexual intercourse, both heterosexual and same-sex, the standing position seems to be more common than any other, and heterosexual intercourse is often from behind. Anal intercourse seems to have been common, but we find no explanation of this preference. One possible explanation is it was one of the few effective methods of preventing pregnancy.

One aspect of the lower estimate of women's abilities was that they were considered to be less rational and less capable of controlling themselves than men (see Aristotle, *Politics*, 1.12–13 [1259a35–1260a30]). Many Greek texts express a powerful fear that female sexuality is dangerous and overwhelming. According to one early text (Hesiod, *Melampodia*, frag. 3; in Evelyn-White), there was a dispute between Zeus and Hera about whether men or women enjoyed sex the most; it was decided that women enjoy sex much more than men. This was one reason why female sexuality had to be controlled. Another reason was that it was important to establish the paternity of children so that it could be ensured that only legitimate children got the opportunity to enjoy the rights of inheritance and citizenship. It was not necessary to control male sexuality the same way since only children of a legitimate wife had these rights. This is the context in which we must understand a famous remark by an unknown orator in a lawsuit (343–340 BCE) against a prostitute: "This is what it means to set up a household with a woman, with whom one has children, and one introduces the sons to the clan and deme, and betroths daughters to men as one's own. Courtesans we have for pleasure, concubines to daily care of our bodies, and wives to bear legitimate children and to be the trusty guardian at home" (Demosthenes [384–322 BCE] or Apollodoros [394–after 343 BCE]; oration 59, §122, *Against Neaira*). As long as it did not involve citizens and their spouses, **prostitution** was an accepted profession, and in all Greek cities there were slaves and foreigners to serve this function. Interaction with prostitutes of both sexes was not problematic for men, but it was illegal for persons of citizen status to offer their sexual services for money. In *Against Timarchos* (346 BCE), Aeschines (ca. 390–322 BCE) offers a picture of the many sexual opportunities men had, provided they did not prostitute themselves.

The modern term "lesbianism" goes back to a Greek term meaning "to act like women from Lesbos," which refers to oral sex but not necessarily sex between two women. But it is much harder to describe same-sex relations between women in Greek antiquity than between men. There is no reason to deny that Sappho wrote poetry to and about women on the island of Lesbos around 600 BCE, and it is obvious that Sappho expresses more mutual feelings of sex and love than most male poets did, but it is impossible to give a clear description of the physical aspects of her relationship to other women. It is, however, clear that she describes eros as having the same irresistible force when love is between two women as between a man and a woman. One of the longest texts by Sappho describes her feelings when she is forced to look at a female friend sitting next to a man: "one glance at you and I can't get any words out, my voice cracks, a thin flame pours down my body, I tremble all over, turn paler than grass" (Lombardo, frag. 20; Campbell, frag. 31). Some modern feminist scholars interpret the last statement differently, "I become more moist than grass," and find in it a description of an orgasm. If so, this is the most intimate detail we find about female sexuality in ancient literature (Snyder, 33). There is, however, very little pictorial evidence for same-sex situations involving women, something significant when we consider how common erotic motifs were. Same-sex relations between women were part of life behind the wall of the private house and thus not part of male-oriented art and literature. However, the notion of same-sex relations among women was well known among the Greeks.

In Sparta, which was an even more militaristic society than Athens, private life was more limited than in Athens, and same-sex relationships between both men and women seem to have been the norm. This was because Spartan society to a great extent was built as a military organization in which the family was less important as a social unit than in Athens. Most ancient sources on Spartan life, however, were written long after the Spartan state ceased to exist and may therefore be the result of male fantasies rather than historical facts. We know little about sexuality outside Athens and Sparta.

Few Greek philosophers discussed sex, and when they did, it was often in the context of life in an ideal society (see Plato and Aristotle, and below); hence their testimony must often be considered normative rather than descriptive. The Presocratic philosopher Empedocles (ca. 490–430 BCE) developed a philosophy in which the driving forces of the world were Love and Strife, but his Love appears to have little to do with eros (sex) as the Greeks described it in the divine and human world. Empedocles calls his Love *Philotes*, a word that can cover all aspects of love from sexual desire to friendly feelings.

From some time in the fourth century BCE the Greek attitude toward sex seems to have changed. Sexuality plays no role in the comedies of Menander (341–ca. 290 BCE) from around 300 BCE, and the absence of obscene jokes is in marked contrast to earlier comedy. **Marriage** contracts from Hellenistic Egypt indicate that marital fidelity from both parties was now generally expected. The concept of "romantic love" becomes more common in literary texts: Several of Menander's comedies involve the complications arising from love and sex between young people before marriage, a topic that is absent from earlier literature. Depictions of sexuality generally disappear from Greek art, although Roman art displays many sexual themes; it is, however, significant that sexual situations in art now were limited to individual couples.

In this period we find sex discussed by both Epicurean and Stoic philosophers in particular in connection with their discussion of the life of the ideal philosopher (the Wise Man), who in both schools is a person who lives a life that is radically different from the lives of ordinary men. In both schools it seems to have been accepted that sex need not be part of the ideal life, though Epicurus (341–270 BCE) was more concerned that it might also bring harm to the Wise: "Eros is an intense desire for intercourse, accompanied by agony and distraction" (frag. 483; Nussbaum, 149–53). For the Stoics sex was one of the so-called indifferent elements in life that have no moral significance. The Stoic Wise Man is encouraged to eliminate passions from his life, but he may have sexual relations with both women and men; erotic love could be defined as an effort to form a **friendship** due to the perceived beauty of young men in their prime. This seems to be a continuation of the earlier Athenian custom, but as it is part of the Stoic utopian city, we do not know to what extent it reflects historical reality. At the same time, the Stoics seem to have advocated a communistic society (Zeno and others; see Schofield, 22–56) not unlike Plato's ideal city in which all men could have sex with all women, and all children were considered common to the older generations (*Republic*, bk. 5). The Stoics thought that men and women had the same possibilities of becoming wise and hence could live together in a perfectly good society; nevertheless, they seem to have been more concerned with love and sex between men.

See also Aristotle; Beauty; Bestiality; Boswell, John; Chinese Philosophy; Feminism, Lesbian; Foucault, Michel; Humor; Orientation, Sexual; Plato; Pornography; Roman Sexuality and Philosophy, Ancient; Social Constructionism

REFERENCES

Aeschines. *Against Timarchos*. Trans. Nick Fisher. Oxford, U.K.: Oxford University Press, 2001; Aristophanes. *Aristophanes*, vols. 1–3. Trans. and ed. Jeffrey Henderson. Loeb Classical Library. Cambridge, Mass.: Harvard University Press, 1998–2002; Aristotle. (330 BCE) *Politics* and *Poetics*. Trans. Benjamin Jowett. Cleveland, Ohio: Fine Editions Press, 1952; Campbell, David. *Greek Lyric*, vol. 1: *Sappho and Alcaeus*. Cambridge, Mass.: Harvard University Press, 1982; Cantarella, Eva. *Bisexuality in the Ancient World*. Trans. Cormac Ó Cuilleanáin. New Haven, Conn.: Yale University Press, 1992; Demosthenes. *Private Orations L-LVIII and In Neaeram LIX*. Trans. Augustus T. Murray. Loeb Classical Library. Cambridge, Mass: Harvard University Press, 1939; Dillon, John, and Tania Gergel, trans. *The Greek Sophists*. London: Penguin, 2003; Dover, Kenneth. (1978) *Greek Homosexuality*. Updated and with a New Postscript. Cambridge, Mass.: Harvard University Press, 1989; Empedocles. *The Poems of Empedocles*, rev. ed. Trans. Brad Inwood. Toronto, Can.: University of Toronto Press, 2001; Euripides. (427 BCE) *Hippolytos*. In *Euripides*, vol. 2. Ed. David Kovacs. Loeb Classical Library. Cambridge, Mass.: Harvard University Press, 1995; Foucault, Michel. (1976/1984/1984) *The History of Sexuality*. Vol. 1: *An Introduction*. Trans. Robert Hurley. New York: Vintage, 1978. Vol. 2: *The Use of Pleasure*. Trans. Robert Hurley. New York: Pantheon, 1985. Vol. 3: *The Care of the Self*. Trans. Robert Hurley. New York: Vintage, 1986; Halperin, David. *One Hundred Years of Homosexuality: And Other Essays on Greek Love*. New York: Routledge, 1990; Hesiod. *The Homeric Hymns and Homerica*. Trans. Hugh G. Evelyn-White. Loeb Classical Library. Cambridge, Mass.: Harvard University Press, 1914; Hesiod. (ca. 700 BCE) *Theogony* and *Works and Days*. Trans. Martin L. West. New York: Oxford University Press, 1999; Homer. (ca. 700 BCE) *The Iliad*. Trans. Robert Fagles. New York: Penguin, 1990; Keuls, Eva. *The Reign of the Phallus: Sexual Politics in Ancient Athens*. New York: Harper and Row, 1985; Menander. *Menander*, vols. 1–3. Trans. and ed. W. G. Arnott. Loeb Classical Library. Cambridge, Mass.: Harvard University Press, 1979–2000; Nussbaum, Martha C. *The Therapy of Desire: Theory and Practice in Hellenistic Ethics*. Princeton, N.J.: Princeton University Press, 1994; Plato. (ca. 375–370 BCE) *Republic*. Trans. G.M.A. Grube. Indianapolis, Ind.: Hackett, 1992; Plato. (ca. 380 BCE) *Symposium of Plato*. Trans. Tom Griffith (1986). Berkeley: University of California Press, 1989; Pomeroy, Sarah. B. *Goddesses, Whores, Wives, and Slaves: Women in Classical Antiquity*. New York: Schocken, 1975; Sappho. *Poems and Fragments*. Trans. Stanley Lombardo. Ed. Susan Warden. Indianapolis, Ind.: Hackett, 2002; Schofield, Malcolm. *The Stoic Idea of the City*. Cambridge: Cambridge University Press, 1991; Snyder, Jane M. *Lesbian Desire in the Lyrics of Sappho*. New York: Columbia University Press, 1997; Theophrastus. *Theophrastus of Eresus: Sources for His Life, Writings, Thought, and Influence*. Trans. and ed. W. W. Fortenbaugh, Pamela M. Huby, Robert W. Sharples, and Dimitri Gutas. Leiden, Holland: Brill, 1992; Vorberg, Gaston. *Glossarium Eroticum*. Stuttgart, Ger.: Puttmann, 1932; Xenophon. (370–360 BCE) *Oeconomicus: A Social and Historical Commentary*. Trans. Sarah B. Pomeroy. Oxford, U.K.: Oxford University Press, 1994.

Jørgen Mejer

ADDITIONAL READING

Aeschines. *Speeches*. Trans. Charles Darwin Adams. Loeb Classical Library. Cambridge, Mass.: Harvard University Press, 1919; Allen, Prudence. *The Concept of Woman: The Aristotelian Revolution*. Grand Rapids, Mich.: Eerdmans, 1997; Annas, Julia. *The Morality of Happiness*. Oxford, U.K.: Oxford University Press, 1993; Arthur-Katz, Marilyn. "Sexuality and the Body in Ancient Greece."

Mètis 4 (1989), 155–89; Blayney, Jan. "Theories of Conception in the Ancient World." In Beryl Rawson, ed., *The Family in Ancient Rome: New Perspectives*. Ithaca, N.Y.: Cornell University Press, 1986, 230–39; Boardman, John, and Eugenio la Rocca. *Eros in Greece*. New York: Erotic Art Society, 1975; Brendel, Otto J. "The Scope and Temperament of Erotic Art in the Graeco-Roman World." In Theodore Bowie and Cornelia V. Christenson, eds., *Studies in Erotic Art*. New York: Basic Books, 1970, 3–107; Brisson, Luc. *Sexual Ambivalence: Androgyny and Hermaphrodism in Graeco-Roman Antiquity*. Trans. Janet Lloyd. Berkeley: University of California Press, 2002; Buffière, Felix. *Eros adolescent, la pédérastie dans la Grèce antique*. Paris: Les belles letters, 1980; Cantarella, Eva. (1981) *Pandora's Daughters: The Role and Status of Women in Greek and Roman Antiquity*. Trans. Mauren K. Fant. Baltimore, Md.: Johns Hopkins University Press, 1987; Cohen, David. "Consent and Sexual Relations in Classical Athens." In Angeliki E. Laiou, ed., *Consent and Coercion to Sex and Marriage in Ancient and Medieval Societies*. Washington, D.C.: Dumbarton Oaks, 1993, 5–16; Cohen, David. *Law, Sexuality, and Society: The Enforcement of Morals in Classical Athens*. Cambridge: Cambridge University Press, 1991; Cole, Eve Browning. "Sappho." In Timothy F. Murphy, ed., *Reader's Guide to Lesbian and Gay Studies*. Chicago, Ill.: Fitzroy Dearborn, 2000, 528–29; Davidson, James. *Courtesans and Fishcakes: The Consuming Passions of Classical Athens*. London: HarperCollins, 1997; Demosthenes. "Speech 59" [*Apollodoros against Neaera*]. Tuft University's Perseus Web site. <www.perseus.tufts.edu/cgi-bin/ptext?lookup=Dem.+59+1> [accessed September 8, 2004]; Demosthenes. *Speeches 50–59*. Trans. Victor Bers. Austin: University of Texas Press, 2003; Dierichs, Angelika. *Erotik in der Kunst Griechenlands*. Zürich, Switz.: Raggi-Verl, 1988; Doniger, Wendy. *Splitting the Difference: Gender and Myth in Ancient Greece and India*. Chicago, Ill.: University of Chicago Press, 1999; Dover, Kenneth J. *Greek Popular Morality*. Oxford, U.K.: Oxford University Press, 1974; duBois, Page. *Sowing the Body: Psychoanalysis and Ancient Representations of Women*. Chicago, Ill.: University of Chicago Press, 1988; Dynes, Wayne R., and Stephen Donaldson, eds. *Homosexuality in the Ancient World*. New York: Garland, 1982; Engels, Frederick. (1884) "The Greek Gens" and "The Rise of the Athenian State." In *The Origin of the Family, Private Property, and the State*. Peking, China: Foreign Language Press, 1978, 117–27, 128–41; Empedocles (of Acragas). [Fragments] In G. S. Kirk and J. E. Raven, *The Presocratic Philosophers: A Critical History with a Selection of Texts*. Cambridge: Cambridge University Press, 1971, 320–61; Flacelière, Robert. (1960) *Love in Ancient Greece*. Trans. James Cleugh. New York: Crown, 1962; Garrison, David H. *Sexual Culture in Ancient Greece*. Norman: University of Oklahoma Press, 2000; Goldhill, Simon. *Foucault's Virginity: Ancient Erotic Fiction and the History of Sexuality*. Cambridge: Cambridge University Press, 1995; Goldhill, Simon. *Love, Sex, and Tragedy: How the Ancient World Shapes Our Lives*. Chicago, Ill.: University of Chicago Press, 2004; Gooch, Paul. "A Mind to Love: Friends and Lovers in Ancient Greek Philosophy." In David Goicoechea, ed., *The Nature and Pursuit of Love: The Philosophy of Irving Singer*. Amherst, N.Y.: Prometheus, 1995, 83–97; Goodman, Martin, ed. *Jews in a Graeco-Roman World*. Oxford, U.K.: Clarendon Press, 1999; Green, Peter. "Sex and Classical Literature." In *Classical Bearings: Interpreting Ancient History and Culture*. New York: Thames and Hudson, 1989, 130–51; Greene, Ellen, ed. *Reading Sappho: Contemporary Approaches*. Berkeley: University of California Press, 1996; Greene, Ellen, ed. *Re-Reading Sappho: Reception and Transmission*. Berkeley: University of California Press, 1996; Griffin, Jasper. "The Love That Dared to Speak Its Name." [Review of *Bisexuality in the Ancient World*, by Eva Cantarella] *New York Review of Books* (22 October 1992), 30–32; Gross, Nicolas P. *Amatory Persuasion in Antiquity: Studies in Theory and Practice*. Chap. 1: "Love and Persuasion: Ancient Sources," 15–31; Chap. 2: "The Rhetoric of Seduction," 32–68. Newark: University of Delaware Press; Cranbury, N.J.: Associated University Presses, 1985; Hallett, Judith P. "Sappho and Her Social Context: Sense and Sensuality." *Signs* 4:3 (1979), 447–64; Halperin, David. "Sex before Sexuality: Pederasty, Politics, and Power in Classical Athens." In Martin Duberman, Martha Vicinus, and George Chauncey, Jr., eds., *Hidden from History: Reclaiming the Gay and Lesbian Past*. New York: New American Library, 1989, 37–53; Halperin, David, John J. Winkler, and Froma I. Zeitlin, eds. *Before Sexuality: The Construction of Erotic Experience in the Ancient Greek World*. Princeton, N.J.: Princeton University Press, 1990; Hamel, Debra. *Trying Neaira: The True Story of a Courtesan's*

Scandalous Life in Ancient Greece. New Haven, Conn.: Yale University Press, 2003; Hawkes, Gail. *Sex and Pleasure in Western Culture*. Malden, Mass.: Polity, 2004; Henderson, Jeffrey. "Greek Attitudes toward Sex." In Michael Grant and Rachel Kitzinger, eds., *Civilization of the Ancient Mediterranean: Greece and Rome*, vol. 2. New York: Scribner's, 1988, 1249–63; Henderson, Jeffrey. (1975) *The Maculate Muse: Obscene Language in Attic Comedy*, 2nd ed. New York: Oxford University Press, 1991; Hesiod. *The Poems of Hesiod*. Trans. R. Frazer. Norman: University of Oklahoma Press, 1983; Hubbard, Thomas K. *Homosexuality in Greece and Rome: A Sourcebook of Basic Documents*. Berkeley: University of California Press, 2003; Irwin, T. H. "Happiness, Virtue, and Morality." *Ethics* 105 (October 1994), 153–77; Johns, Catharine. *Sex or Symbol? Erotic Images of Greece and Rome*. Austin: University of Texas Press, 1982; Kampen, Nathalie. *Sexuality in Ancient Art*. Cambridge: Cambridge University Press, 1996; Kilmer, Martin F. *Greek Erotica on Attic Red-figures Vases*. London: Duckworth, 1993; Koloski-Ostrow, Ann O., and Claire L. Lyons. *Naked Truth: Women, Sexuality, and Gender in Classical Art and Archaeology*. New York: Routledge, 1997; Konstan, David. *Sexual Symmetry: Love in the Ancient Novel and Related Genres*. Princeton, N.J.: Princeton University Press, 1994; Konstan, David, and Martha C. Nussbaum, eds. "The Construction of Sexuality in the Classical World." *differences: A Journal of Feminist Cultural Studies* [special issue] 2:1 (1990); Konstan, David, and N. Keith Rutter, eds. *Envy, Spite, and Jealousy: The Rivalrous Emotions in Ancient Greece*. Edinburgh, Scot.: Edinburgh University Press, 2003; Laqueur, Thomas. *Making Sex: Body and Gender from the Greeks to Freud*. Cambridge, Mass.: Harvard University Press, 1990; Larmour, David H. J., Paul Allen Miller, and Charles Platter, eds. *Rethinking Sexuality: Foucault and Classical Antiquity*. Princeton, N.J.: Princeton University Press, 1997; Lefkowitz, Mary R. "Seduction and Rape in Greek Myth." In Angeliki E. Laiou, ed., *Consent and Coercion to Sex and Marriage in Ancient and Medieval Societies*. Washington, D.C.: Dumbarton Oaks, 1993, 17–37; Louden, Robert B., and Paul Schollmeier, eds. *The Greeks and Us: Essays in Honor of Arthur W. H. Adkins*. Chicago, Ill.: University of Chicago Press, 1996; Marcadé, Jean. *Eros kalos: Essay on Erotic Elements in Greek Art*. Geneva, Switz.: Nagel, 1962; McClure, Laura K., ed. *Sexuality and Gender in the Classical World: Readings and Sources*. Malden, Mass.: Blackwell, 2002; Nussbaum, Martha C. *The Fragility of Goodness: Luck and Ethics in Greek Tragedy and Philosophy*. Cambridge: Cambridge University Press, 1986; Nussbaum, Martha C. "Platonic Love and Colorado Law: The Relevance of Ancient Greek Norms to Modern Sexual Controversies." *Virginia Law Review* 80:7 (1994), 1515–1651. Shorter versions reprinted in *Sex and Social Justice*. New York: Oxford University Press, 1999, 299–331; and Robert B. Louden and Paul Schollmeier, eds., *The Greeks and Us: Essays in Honor of Arthur W. H. Adkins*. Chicago, Ill.: University of Chicago Press, 1996, 168–218; Nussbaum, Martha C., and Juha Sihvola, eds. *The Sleep of Reason: Erotic Experience and Sexual Ethics in Ancient Greece and Rome*. Chicago, Ill.: University of Chicago Press, 2002; Osborne, Catherine. *Eros Unveiled: Plato and the God of Love*. Oxford, U.K.: Clarendon Press, 1994; Paglia, Camille. (1991) "Junk Bonds and Corporate Raiders: Academe in the House of the Wolf." In *Sex, Art, and American Culture: Essays*. New York: Vintage, 1992, 170–248; Patzer, Harald. *Die griechische Knabenliebe*. Wiesbaden, Ger.: F. Steiner, 1982; Percy, William A. *Pederasty and Pedagogy in Archaic Greece*. Urbana: University of Illinois Press, 1996; Peters, F. E. *Greek Philosophical Terms: A Historical Lexicon*. New York: New York University Press, 1967, 62–66; Rabinowitz, Nancy S., and Lisa Auanger, eds. *Among Women: From the Homosexual to the Homoerotic in the Ancient World*. Austin: University of Texas Press, 2002; Rabinowitz, Nancy, and Amy Richlin, eds. *Feminist Theory and the Classics*. New York: Routledge, 1993; Reinberg, Catherine. *Ehe, Hetärentum, und Knabenliebe im antiken Griechenland*. Munich, Ger.: C. H. Beck, 1989; Richlin, Amy, ed. *Pornography and Representation in Greece and Rome*. New York: Oxford University Press, 1992; Sappho. [Selected fragments] In Ellen K. Feder, Karmen MacKendrick, and Sybol S. Cook, eds., *A Passion for Wisdom: Readings in Western Philosophy on Love and Desire*. Upper Saddle River, N.J.: Prentice Hall, 2004, 1–10; Siems, Andreas K., ed. *Sex und Erotik in der Antike*. Darmstadt, Ger.: Wissenschaftliches Buchgesellschaft, 1988; Skinner, Marilyn B. "Women and Language in Archaic Greece, or, Why Is Sappho a Woman?" In Nancy Rabinowitz and Amy Richlin, eds., *Feminist Theory and the Classics*. New York: Routledge, 1993, 125–44; Slater, Philip E. *The Glory of Hera: Greek*

Mythology and the Greek Family. Boston, Mass.: Beacon Press, 1968; Smith, Mark. "Ancient Bisexuality and the Interpretation of Romans 1:26–27." *Journal of the American Academy of Religion* 64:2 (1996), 223–56; Stigers, Eva Stehle. "Romantic Sensuality, Poetic Sense: A Response to Hallett on Sappho." *Signs* 4:3 (1979), 465–71; Stone, Lawrence. "Sex in the West." *The New Republic* (8 July 1985), 25–37; Thornton, Bruce S. *Eros: The Myth of Ancient Greek Sexuality.* Boulder, Colo.: Westview, 1997; Thornton, Bruce S. "Social Constructionism and Ancient Greek Sex." *Helios* 18 (1991), 181–93; Vanita, Ruth. *Sappho and the Virgin Mary: Same-Sex Love and the English Literary Imagination.* New York: Columbia University Press, 1996; Winkler, John J. *The Constraints of Desire: The Anthropology of Sex and Gender in Ancient Greece.* New York: Routledge, 1990; Winkler, John J. "Double Consciousness in Sappho's Lyrics." In *The Constraints of Desire: The Anthropology of Sex and Gender in Ancient Greece.* New York: Routledge, 1990, 162–87. Reprinted in Henry Abelove, Michèle Aina Barale, and David M. Halperin, eds., *The Lesbian and Gay Studies Reader.* New York: Routledge, 1993, 577–94.

GRISEZ, GERMAIN. *See* Natural Law (New)

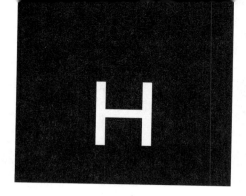

HARASSMENT, SEXUAL.

HARASSMENT, SEXUAL. The concept of sexual harassment was first articulated in the mid-1970s, in the context of feminist efforts to expand antidiscrimination law, and it evolved through legal developments resulting from the success of those efforts. Since 1980, the most frequently used definition of sexual harassment is that formulated by the U.S. Equal Employment Opportunity Commission:

> Unwelcome sexual advances, requests for sexual favors, and other verbal or physical conduct of a sexual nature constitute sexual harassment when (1) submission to such conduct is made either explicitly or implicitly a term or condition of an individual's employment, (2) submission to or rejection of such conduct by an individual is used as the basis for employment decisions affecting such individual, or (3) such conduct has the purpose or effect of unreasonably interfering with an individual's work performance or creating an intimidating, hostile, or offensive working environment. (29 *Code of Federal Regulations*, §1604.11 [a])

The conduct covered by elements (1) and (2) of this definition is usually referred to as *quid pro quo* sexual harassment, while the conduct covered by element (3) is usually referred to as *hostile-environment* sexual harassment. The definition, by its own terms, applies only to harassment in employment, but it can be, and has been, adapted to other settings (for example, education). It must be noted that "sexual harassment" is a technical term whose meaning is not a straightforward combination of the meanings of "sexual" and "harassment." Sexual harassment is not always harassment in the everyday sense of the word "harassment."

At the core of feminist arguments for the creation and development of the law of sexual harassment was the claim that such conduct constituted discrimination on the basis of sex. As discrimination on the basis of sex was already legally prohibited at the time (most notably by the federal Civil Rights Act of 1964), it followed that there was no need for the enactment of new statutes aimed at sexual harassment. The feminist arguments were, therefore, "addressed" not to legislatures but to the courts; their principal contention was that courts should treat sexual harassment as violating already existing antidiscrimination statutes. When legal practitioners inspired by **feminism** advanced such arguments in actual litigation, the arguments were at first rejected outright by the courts. In April 1976, however, in *Williams v. Saxbe*, one federal district court did accept the argument that the kind of conduct that later came to be known as sexual harassment constituted discrimination on the basis of sex. In the years that followed, a number of other courts, including some appellate courts, accepted the argument, and by 1980 the law of sexual harassment could be regarded as an emerging area of litigation within antidiscrimination law. In that year, the Equal Employment Opportunity Commission issued the document that came to be known as the "Guidelines on Sexual Harassment," which defined sexual harassment and declared it to be a form of discrimination on the basis of sex. Such guidelines issued by administrative agencies do not have the force of law on their own, but they often influence the courts and so become part of the law by being cited in judicial opinions. The "Guidelines on Sexual Harassment" thereby gave further impetus to sexual harassment litigation and to the strengthening of the law in that area.

In 1986, the Supreme Court decided its first sexual harassment case, *Meritor Savings Bank v. Vinson*. In *Meritor* the Court, by and large, endorsed the developments of the law that had been occurring in the lower courts during the preceding ten years. The idea that sexual harassment is a form of sex discrimination thus became firmly entrenched in U.S. law. The Supreme Court, however, did not play a very active role in giving direction to the law of sexual harassment until relatively late in its development: *Meritor* and *Harris v. Forklift Systems* (1993) were its only two decisions in this area prior to 1998, the year in which it decided four sexual harassment cases.

As a result of these developments in federal law, prohibitions of sexual harassment started appearing in the laws of the individual states within the United States and in the laws of other countries. While the sexual harassment laws of different jurisdictions differ in detail, they are, throughout the developed countries of the English-speaking world, modeled after federal U.S. law. Most of the general theoretical issues that can be raised about the federal law on sexual harassment are thus relevant to the laws in these other jurisdictions. More recently, terms that are direct translations of "sexual harassment" were introduced into some legal systems outside the English-speaking world. The sexual harassment laws of these countries are often very different from their counterparts in English-speaking countries, and theoretical discussions of U.S. law have only limited relevance to them.

The first sexual harassment cases concerned harassment in employment. Later, the law against sexual harassment was extended to other settings: education, professional services, and the provision of housing. The law regarding sexual harassment in employment still remains far more developed than the laws about sexual harassment in other settings, and the courts dealing with the cases that concern sexual harassment outside employment often "borrow" from the employment-related precedents. The laws regarding harassment in the various settings are thus interconnected. For this reason, many theoretical questions that can be raised about sexual harassment in one setting are relevant to sexual harassment in other settings.

The most influential of all writings on sexual harassment is undoubtedly **Catharine MacKinnon**'s *Sexual Harassment of Working Women*. The book appeared in 1979, but the ideas it contains were informally circulated and discussed for some time before the book's publication. It is largely due to the influence of MacKinnon's arguments, presented in that book, on other legal scholars and legal practitioners, that the law of sexual harassment developed the way it did. Indeed, many regard MacKinnon as *the* ultimate creator of the law of sexual harassment. In influencing the course of sexual harassment law, MacKinnon was far more successful than she was in her attempts to change the legal treatment of **pornography**. (At least in the United States, antipornography ordinances based on MacKinnon's approach to pornography did not survive judicial scrutiny. See *American Booksellers Association, Inc. v. Hudnut*.)

Sexual Harassment of Working Women contains two principal arguments that sexual harassment is sex discrimination. One argument MacKinnon calls the "differences argument." It points out that an individual subjected to sexual harassment would not have been subjected to it if the individual had been of a different sex: A women sexually harassed by a heterosexual man would not have been subjected to that harassment had she not been a women. According to the argument, this entails that, in being subjected to harassment, she was discriminated against on the basis of sex (192–208). The other argument is the "inequality argument," which claims that sexual harassment is discriminatory because it exemplifies and strengthens a pattern of inequality between men and women that pervades most societies (174–92).

The arguments are very different. In the inequality argument the discriminatory character of a particular act of sexual harassment depends on certain features of the society in which it takes place; what makes that act discriminatory could not be understood if one were to examine the act in isolation. On the other hand, in the differences argument the discriminatory character of a particular act of sexual harassment can be found within the act itself, without considering the social setting in which it takes place. The inequality argument assumes certain theories about the society as a whole and about human sexuality, which are, in some of their aspects, controversial; the differences argument has far fewer general theoretical commitments. Moreover, the inequality argument implies that sexual harassment of women by men needs to be analyzed very differently from sexual harassment of men by women; the differences argument implies that the two types are much more similar. MacKinnon has greater sympathy for the inequality argument. But she develops both in her book at considerable length without making it clear how the two are supposed to fit together.

Both arguments have been widely influential, but in different arenas. The acceptance by the courts of the idea that sexual harassment is a form of discrimination on the basis of sex was largely due to the differences argument; there is very little in the judicial opinions on sexual harassment that reflects the inequality argument. The nonlegal literature, both popular and scholarly, that supports the fight against sexual harassment is, on the other hand, mostly informed by the inequality argument. This prevalence of the inequality argument in the nonlegal literature is sometimes a source of misunderstandings of the law and of insufficient appreciation of the role of the differences argument in its development. Many people who support the law of sexual harassment do so on the basis of some version of the inequality argument that they find in the nonlegal literature, even though the law that they support itself embodies the differences argument.

After MacKinnon's *Sexual Harassment*, the development of the law of sexual harassment was accompanied by a proliferation of other literature on the topic. Much of it consists of popular materials that inform the public about the law without examining it critically, offer advice on how to deal with sexual harassment, or report on specific incidents of sexual harassment and responses to them. In the literature that examines the topic more systematically, the dominant materials are those reporting the results of empirical, mostly psychological, research into the phenomenon of sexual harassment, and those in which contributors to law reviews analyze the details of the law and its application. The articles in law reviews often contain criticisms of the law, but most of the criticisms are narrowly aimed at its specific aspects; critical examination of the law as a whole and its foundations is relatively rare.

Among the books that support the fight against sexual harassment, particularly influential have been Billie Wright Dziech and Linda Weiner's *The Lecherous Professor* (1984) and a collection of essays edited by Michelle Paludi, *Ivory Power: Sexual Harassment on Campus* (1990). Both deal with sexual harassment in higher education.

In the early years of the development of sexual harassment law, almost all the published commentary on it was favorable. Before the 1990s, there was relatively little public debate about sexual harassment and almost no systematic published criticism of the fight against it. Only in the fall of 1991, by which time sexual harassment law was well established, was impetus given to public debate about it by allegations issuing from the law professor Anita Hill that Clarence Thomas, a Supreme Court justice nominee, had years earlier engaged in sexual harassment. Similar impetus to the public debate was later provided by the allegations (and protracted legal proceedings based on them) that President William Clinton, when he had been governor of Arkansas, had sexually harassed a low-level state employee (Paula Jones). Two books written for a wide audience and published in the mid-1990s articulated the dissatisfaction that many felt about the fight against sexual harassment and contributed to the public debate: Katie Roiphe's *The Morning After* (1993) and Rene Denfeld's *The New Victorians* (1995).

Writings on sexual harassment by scholars whose background is in philosophy have been relatively sparse. Fewer philosophical publications appeared on this topic than on comparable issues in applied ethics. Two early philosophical discussions of sexual harassment focused on *quid pro quo* harassment: One essay by John Hughes and Larry May (1980) and another by Nancy Tuana (1988) grappled with the question of what makes sexual harassment wrong in cases in which it involves an offer of (what appears to be) more favorable treatment than one would otherwise be entitled to, in exchange for sexual favors.

Most of the philosophical writings on sexual harassment are, however, devoted to the analysis of the concept. Such articles usually aim at capturing some theoretically illuminating and morally significant concept that could aptly be expressed by the phrase "sexual harassment"; they are generally not concerned with how the concept of sexual harassment actually functions in the law. For example, Susan Dodds and her colleagues offered, as the definition of sexual harassment, "the behavior which is typically associated with a mental state representing an attitude which seeks sexual ends without any concern for the person from whom those ends are sought, and which typically produces an unwanted and unpleasant response in the person who is the object of the behavior" (120). They expressly reject (113–14) the view that the wrong of sexual harassment is a wrong of discrimination (which view had played a crucial role in the development of sexual harassment law). Anita Superson, on the other hand, defined sexual harassment as "any behavior (verbal or physical) caused by a person, A, in the dominant class directed at another, B, in the subjugated class, that expresses and perpetuates the attitude that B or members of B's sex is/are inferior because of their sex, thereby causing harm to either B and/or members of B's sex" (46). Jan Crosthwaite and Graham Priest similarly defined harassment as "any form of sexual behaviour by members of a dominant gender group towards members of a subordinate gender group whose typical effect is to cause members of the subordinate group to experience their powerlessness as a member of that group" (72). Both Superson's and Crosthwaite and Priest's analyses attempt to establish a conceptual connection between sexual harassment and existing relationships of dominance and in that respect fit well with MacKinnon's inequality argument.

Probably the strongest justification of the sexual harassment law in the philosophical literature is Andrew Altman's. Altman takes MacKinnon's views as his starting point, but he refines them in a way that better satisfies the standards of argumentation that characterize analytic philosophy and modifies them in a way that enables him to avoid committing himself to some of the most controversial aspects of MacKinnon's position.

Philosophers have also criticized the fight against sexual harassment. For example, Ellen Frankel Paul argues that the prohibition of sexual harassment is not consistent with the framework of antidiscrimination law and that, to the extent that such conduct deserves to be legally prohibited, it would be better to deal with it within the law of torts. F. M. Christensen has provided a condensed formulation of a wide array of different arguments that the fight against sexual harassment is unjustified. But the controversial issues surrounding sexual harassment have not yet received as much discussion as they warrant. There are at least six important issues that have been touched on in the philosophical literature but need further discussion.

The first is whether "sexual harassment" is a morally significant concept, that is, whether sexual harassment *as a distinct type of conduct* is morally wrong. The issue arises because sexual harassment overlaps with many kinds of conduct that have been long and widely regarded as morally wrong, such as **adultery**, promiscuity, and abuse of institutional power. It is thus possible to regard many individual acts of sexual harassment as wrong on grounds that have nothing to do with their being acts of sexual harassment. To think about sexual harassment clearly, one must keep one's moral judgments about sexual harassment as such distinct from judgments about kinds of conduct with which it happens to overlap. Once these distinctions are made, it becomes debatable whether there is any moral judgment left to make about sexual harassment itself—that is, whether the wrongness of sexual harassment is exhausted by the wrongness of other kinds of conduct it often includes or involves.

A vivid challenge to the widespread belief that "sexual harassment" is a morally significant concept has been made by Christensen, who has argued that the introduction of that concept is analogous to somebody's introducing

> the notion of "automobile harassment," meant to include shooting at someone from a car, speeding dangerously past in or running someone down with a car, insulting someone from a car, and waving at someone who doesn't want to be waved at from a car. Such a category would be very suspicious: (1) It lumps together serious crimes, minor offenses, and actions that are arguably not wrong at all. (2) What the actions do have in common—the fact that they all involve a car—is irrelevant to what it is about each action that makes it wrong. Confronted with such an artificial concept, one would wonder what irrationality or hidden agenda had led to that lumping together. (1)

The second issue, a special version of the first, is whether sexual harassment is a form of discrimination on the basis of sex, which thesis has played a crucial role in the creation of sexual harassment law. The thesis is problematic because the wrong of discrimination is, by definition, a comparative wrong (it is a wrong because it puts somebody, say women, in a different position than somebody else, say men), while the wrong of sexual harassment strikes many people as a noncomparative wrong (as something wrong regardless of how other people are treated). One way to understand this issue is to consider a bisexual person who harasses men and women to the same extent. This harasser does not choose on the basis of sex to whom to direct such conduct; on the differences argument, then, no sex discrimination is involved. Because the law is based on the differences argument, the law does not apply to the conduct of such a harasser. So far as the law is concerned, the conduct simply is not sexual harassment, even though it may be quite similar to the heterosexual and homosexual harassment that are prohibited by the law. That the law has this implication, and that the implication is odd, has been acknowledged by courts and commentators. There is, however, a great deal of disagreement as to what follows from this odd aspect of the law. Some believe that it is a detail of no great significance, since such cases are rare. Others argue that bisexual harasser cases, regardless of how rare they are, cast doubt on the justifiability of treating sexual harassment as a form of sex discrimination and thus threaten the very basis of harassment law. It is also possible to argue that the problem of bisexual harassers shows that the differences argument is mistaken and that sexual harassment law should be based on the inequality argument instead. This response, however, opens various further issues about the theoretical assumptions of the inequality argument and, in any event, will not help justify the law in its present form, given that it embodies the differences argument.

The prohibitions of sexual harassment, on their face, seem to be prohibitions of only one particular type of sexual conduct and to leave the rest of human sexuality untouched. The third controversial issue is whether that appearance is misleading. It has been argued that, in their actual operation, the prohibitions of sexual harassment end up being prohibitions of all sexual conduct within the settings to which they apply, such as employment and education (Hajdin, 42–101). This is because it is practically impossible to determine whether a particular act of a sexual nature will have the defining characteristics of sexual harassment (e.g., unwelcomeness and offensiveness) ahead of performing it; almost any act of a sexual nature may *turn out* to have these characteristics (even if well intended and expressly consented to). It has also been argued that the ideological basis of the fight to eradicate sexual harassment is a general hostility to sexuality in its heterosexual form. (Daphne Patai has provided the most developed version of this line of argument.) These two arguments present the defenders of the prohibitions of sexual harassment with the choice of either trying to modify their position so as to prevent it from having such implications for human sexuality as a whole or, alternatively, of openly acknowledging that the fight against sexual harassment is a part of a general fight to limit sexual freedom. The latter route is more likely to lead to a theoretically coherent position, but it will be plausible only under certain very controversial assumptions.

Some institutions of higher education have enacted explicit general prohibitions of sexual (and otherwise romantic) relationships between faculty and students. While these prohibitions do not use the term "sexual harassment" and are thus, on their face, independent of the prohibitions of sexual harassment, their enactment is viewed by some as a further step in the implementation of the same ideology that drives the fight against sexual harassment and as a proof that the ideology is generally hostile to (or suspicious of) sexuality. Some debates over the prohibition of faculty-student relationships are thus extensions of the debates over sexual harassment. But, on the other hand, the prohibitions of faculty-student relationships may be regarded as a manifestation of a general concern about conflicts of interests whose theoretical roots are independent of the theoretical roots of the fight against sexual harassment.

An important consequence of the fact that the law of sexual harassment developed under the umbrella of antidiscrimination law is that the law requires employers to ensure that there is no sexual harassment of their employees; it similarly requires educational institutions to ensure that no sexual harassment of students takes place. Employers and educational institutions comply with that requirement by enacting and enforcing regulations of their own that prohibit individuals under their control from engaging in sexual harassment. The law against sexual harassment is thereby a mechanism by which the state regulates conduct of individuals through intermediaries. The fourth issue regarding sexual harassment is whether the state's regulation of individual conduct through intermediaries is compatible with the political and legal traditions of Western societies. The issue arises because even though the intermediaries' enactment and enforcement of their regulations, which ultimately govern the conduct of individuals, are prompted by the state, they are not subject to the political and legal constraints that otherwise govern the state's regulation of individual conduct. For example, when employers investigate allegations of sexual harassment, they normally do not provide the accused with the due-process safeguards that the state would have to provide if it investigated them directly.

The notion of sexual harassment covers, among other things, certain kinds of speech. This gives rise to the fifth controversial issue: Can the prohibition of such speech be made consistent with a general commitment to the freedom of speech? For some kinds of harassing speech, the consistency is probably not too difficult to achieve. Uttering certain words as part of an act of *quid pro quo* harassment can be convincingly analogized to uttering the words that constitute extortion of bribery. Most people would agree that the prohibitions of extortion and bribery are consistent with respecting freedom of speech; the same, following this analogy, can be said of *quid pro quo* harassment. But the notion of sexual harassment also covers speech of very different kinds. Expressing certain viewpoints on the differences between men and women, on the proper role of women, or the suitability of women for particular occupations can create an "an intimidating, hostile, or offensive working environment" for women and thus constitute sexual harassment. Such views may well be false or repugnant to most people, but the principle of freedom of speech is normally understood to entail that speech may not be prohibited on the ground that it is false or repugnant to the majority. Legal scholar Kingsley Browne was the first to articulate this problem; he argued that the law was unconstitutional, insofar as it prohibited such speech. The problem has subsequently been the subject matter of some debate in law reviews, but it has not received as much attention from philosophers as it deserves.

Sexual harassment has been the topic of a great deal of empirical research, and the results of that research are often used to support the fight against sexual harassment. Empirical studies of sexual harassment are frequently invoked in the context of the inequality argument, as proofs of the connection between sexual harassment and the overall inequality between men and women. Research results are also used to show that sexual harassment is a problem of considerable magnitude and causes much harm and is therefore a problem to which substantial resources should be devoted. Whether the empirical research really supports such conclusions is not a purely scientific question; the question involves philosophical scrutiny of the research. Hence the sixth controversial issue regarding sexual harassment: whether the research is biased because scientists have been (consciously or unconsciously) avoiding investigating aspects of sexual harassment that might cast doubt on their preexisting feminist convictions (see Landau).

See also Coercion (by Sexually Aggressive Women); Communication Model; Consent; Ethics, Professional Codes of; Ethics, Sexual; Flirting; Humor; Language; Military, Sex and the; Rape; Rape, Acquaintance and Date; Seduction; Violence, Sexual

REFERENCES

Altman, Andrew. "Making Sense of Sexual Harassment Law." *Philosophy and Public Affairs* 25:1 (1996), 36–64; *American Booksellers Association, Inc. v. Hudnut.* 771 F.2d 323 (1985); Browne, Kingsley R. "Title VII as Censorship: Hostile-Environment Harassment and the First Amendment." *Ohio State Law Journal* 52:2 (1991), 481–550; Christensen, F[errel] M. " 'Sexual Harassment' Must Be Eliminated." *Public Affairs Quarterly* 8:1 (1994), 1–17; "Code of Federal Regulations (CFR): Main Page." <www.gpoaccess.gov/cfr/index.html> [search "29cfr1604.11"; accessed 9 June 2005]; Crosthwaite, Jan, and Graham Priest. "The Definition of Sexual Harassment." *Australasian Journal of Philosophy* 74:1 (1996), 66–82; Denfeld, Rene. *The New Victorians: A Young Women's Challenge to the Old Feminist Order.* New York: Warner Books, 1995; Dodds, Susan M., Lucy Frost, Robert Pargetter, and Elizabeth W. Prior. "Sexual Harassment." *Social Theory and Practice* 14:2 (1988),

111–30; Dziech, Billie Wright, and Linda Weiner. (1984) *The Lecherous Professor: Sexual Harassment on Campus*, 2nd ed. Urbana: University of Illinois Press, 1990; Hajdin, Mane. *The Law of Sexual Harassment: A Critique*. Selinsgrove, Pa.: Susquehanna University Press, 2002; *Harris v. Forklift Systems, Inc.* 510 U.S. 17, 114 S.Ct. 367, 126 L.Ed. 2d 295 (1993); Hughes, John C., and Larry May. "Sexual Harassment." *Social Theory and Practice* 6:3 (1980), 249–80; Landau, Iddo. "Is Sexual Harassment Research Biased?" *Public Affairs Quarterly* 13:3 (1999), 241–54; MacKinnon, Catharine A. *Sexual Harassment of Working Women: A Case of Sex Discrimination*. New Haven, Conn.: Yale University Press, 1979; *Meritor Savings Bank v. Vinson*. 477 U.S. 57, 106 S.Ct. 2399, 91 L.Ed. 2d 49 (1986); Paludi, Michele A., ed. *Ivory Power: Sexual Harassment on Campus*. Albany: State University of New York Press, 1990; Patai, Daphne. *Heterophobia: Sexual Harassment and the Future of Feminism*. Lanham, Md.: Rowman and Littlefield, 1998; Paul, Ellen Frankel. "Sexual Harassment as Discrimination: A Defective Paradigm." *Yale Law and Policy Review* 8:2 (1990), 333–65; Roiphe, Katie. *The Morning After: Sex, Fear, and Feminism on Campus*. Boston, Mass.: Little, Brown, 1993; Superson, Anita M. "A Feminist Definition of Sexual Harassment." *Journal of Social Philosophy* 24:1 (1993), 46–64; Tuana, Nancy. "Sexual Harassment: Offers and Coercion." *Journal of Social Philosophy* 19:2 (1988), 30–42; *Williams v. Saxbe*. 413 F. Supp. 654 (1976).

Mane Hajdin

ADDITIONAL READING

Adam, Alison. "Cyberstalking and Internet Pornography: Gender and the Gaze." *Ethics and Information Technology* 4:2 (2002), 133–42; Altman, Andrew. "Making Sense of Sexual Harassment Law." *Philosophy and Public Affairs* 25:1 (1996), 36–64. Reprinted in William H. Shaw and Vincent Barry, eds., *Moral Issues in Business*, 8th ed. Belmont, Calif.: Wadsworth, 2001, 463–70; HS (403–31); Altman, Andrew. "Speech Codes and Expressive Harm." In Hugh LaFollette, ed., *Ethics in Practice: An Anthology*, 2nd ed. Malden, Mass.: Blackwell, 2002, 376–85; Beidler, Peter G., and Rosemarie Tong. "Love in the Classroom." *Journal on Excellence in College Teaching* 2:1 (1991), 53–70; Benedet, Janine. "Pornography as Sexual Harassment in Canada." In Catharine A. MacKinnon and Reva B. Siegel, eds., *Directions in Sexual Harassment Law*. New Haven, Conn.: Yale University Press, 2004, 417–36; Bernstein, Anita. "Treating Sexual Harassment with Respect." *Harvard Law Review* 111:2 (1997), 445–527; Bowman, Cynthia Grant. "Street Harassment and the Informal Ghettoization of Women." *Harvard Law Review* 106:3 (1993), 517–80; Brewis, Joanna, and Stephen Linstead. "Sexual Harassment." In *Sex, Work and Sex Work: Eroticizing Organization*. London: Routledge, 2000, 71–97; *Burlington Industries, Inc. v. Ellerth*. 524 U.S. 742, 118 S.Ct. 2257, 141 L.Ed. 2d 633 (1998); Christensen, F[errel] M. " 'Sexual Harassment' Must Be Eliminated." *Public Affairs Quarterly* 8:1 (1994), 1–17. Reprinted in Diane Michelfelder Wilcox and William H. Wilcox, eds., *Applied Ethics in American Society*. Fort Worth, Tex.: Harcourt Brace, 1997, 706–15; Cochran, Augustus B., III. *Sexual Harassment and the Law: The Mechelle Vinson Case*. Lawrence: University Press of Kansas, 2004; Cohen, Lloyd R. "On Harassment." *Academic Questions* 3:2 (1990), 23–35; Cornell, Drucilla. *The Imaginary Domain: Abortion, Pornography, and Sexual Harassment*. New York: Routledge, 1995; Crosthwaite, Jan, and Christine Swanton. "On the Nature of Sexual Harassment." *Australasian Journal of Philosophy* 64, supp. (June 1986), 91–106. Reprinted in HS (345–60); Crouch, Margaret A. *Thinking about Sexual Harassment: A Guide for the Perplexed*. New York: Oxford University Press, 2001; Dalmiya, Vrinda. "Why Is Sexual Harassment Wrong?" *Journal of Social Philosophy* 30:1 (1999), 46–64; *Davis v. Monroe County Board of Education*. 526 U.S. 629, 119 S.Ct. 1661, 143 L.Ed. 2d 839 (1999); DeBruin, Debra A. "A Critique of Superson's Feminist Definition of Sexual Harassment." *Journal of Social Philosophy* 29:1 (1998), 49–62; Dershowitz, Alan M. "The Talmud as Sexual Harassment." In *The Abuse Excuse and Other Cop-outs, Sob Stories, and Evasions of Responsibility*. Boston, Mass.: Little, Brown, 1994, 251–54; Dixon, Nicholas. "The Morality of Intimate Faculty-Student Relationships." *The Monist* 79:4 (1996), 521–26; Dodds, Susan M., Lucy Frost, Robert Pargetter, and Elizabeth W. Prior. "Sexual Harassment." *Social Theory and Practice* 14:2 (1988), 111–30. Reprinted in Thomas I. White, ed., *Business*

Ethics: A Philosophical Reader. New York: Macmillan, 1993, 674–86; and Lawrence M. Hinman, ed., *Contemporary Moral Issues: Diversity and Consensus.* Upper Saddle River, N.J.: Prentice Hall, 1996, 290–302; Dollar, Katherine, Andrea Perry, Mary Fromouth, and Aimee Holt. "Influence of Gender Roles on Perceptions of Teacher/Adolescent Student Sexual Relations." *Sex Roles* 50:1–2 (2004), 91–101; *Ellison v. Brady.* 924 F.2d 872 (1991); Epstein, Deborah. "Can a 'Dumb Ass Woman' Achieve Equality in the Workplace? Running the Gauntlet of Hostile Environment Harassing Speech." *Georgetown Law Journal* 84:3 (1996), 399–451; Epstein, Deborah. "Free Speech at Work: Verbal Harassment as Gender-Based Discriminatory (Mis)treatment." *Georgetown Law Journal* 85:3 (1997), 649–66; *Faragher v. City of Boca Raton.* 524 U.S. 775, 118 S.Ct. 2275, 141 L.Ed. 2d 662 (1998); Farley, Lin. *Sexual Shakedown: The Sexual Harassment of Women on the Job.* New York: McGraw-Hill, 1978; Feary, Vaughana Macy. "Sexual Harassment: Why the Corporate World Still Doesn't 'Get It.' " *Journal of Business Ethics* 13:8 (1994), 649–62. Reprinted in Edmund Wall, ed., *Sexual Harassment: Confrontations and Decisions,* rev. ed. Buffalo, N.Y.: Prometheus, 2000, 78–98; Francis, Leslie P. *Sexual Harassment as an Ethical Issue in Academic Life.* Lanham, Md.: Rowman and Littlefield, 2001; Francis, Leslie P. "Sexual Harassment: Developments in Philosophy and Law." *American Philosophical Association Newsletters. Newsletter on Philosophy and Law* 02:1 (Fall 2002), 158–61; Franke, Katherine M. "What's Wrong with Sexual Harassment?" *Stanford Law Review* 49:4 (1997), 691–772; Gaard, Greta. "Anti-Lesbian Intellectual Harassment in the Academy." In VèVè Clark, Shirley Nelson Garner, Margaret Higonnet, and Ketu H. Katrak, eds., *Antifeminism in the Academy.* New York: Routledge, 1996, 115–40; Gallop, Jane. *Feminist Accused of Sexual Harassment.* Durham, N.C.: Duke University Press, 1997; *Gebser v. Lago Vista Independent School District.* 524 U.S. 274, 118 S.Ct. 1989, 141 L.Ed. 2d 277 (1998); Gerdes, Louise I., ed. *Sexual Harassment.* San Diego, Calif.: Greenhaven, 1999; Golash, Deirdre. "Power, Sex, and Friendship in Academia." *Essays in Philosophy* 2:2 (2001). <www.humboldt.edu/~essays/golash.html> [accessed 3 June 2005]; Greve, Michael S. "Sexual Harassment: Telling the Other Victims' Story." *Northern Kentucky University Law Review* 23:3 (1996), 523–41; Griffith, Stephen. "Sexual Harassment and the Rights of the Accused." *Public Affairs Quarterly* 13:1 (1999), 43–71; Gutek, Barbara A. *Sex and the Workplace: The Impact of Sexual Behavior and Sexual Harassment on Women, Men, and Organizations.* San Francisco, Calif.: Jossey-Bass, 1985; Hajdin, Mane. "Sexual Harassment and Negligence." *Journal of Social Philosophy* 28:1 (1997), 37–53; Hajdin, Mane. "Sexual Harassment in the Law: The Demarcation Problem." *Journal of Social Philosophy* 25:3 (1994), 102–22. Reprinted in HS (361–81). Revised and reprinted in POS3 (229–48); POS4 (283–302); Hitt, Jack, Joan Blythe, John Boswell, Leon Botstein, and William Kerrigan. "New Rules about Sex on Campus." *Harper's Magazine* (September 1993), 33–42. Reprinted as "Student-Professor Sexual Relations: A Forum Discussion." In Bruno Leone and Katie de Koster, eds., *Rape on Campus.* San Diego, Calif.: Greenhaven, 1995, 87–98; Holmes, Robert L. "Sexual Harassment and the University." *The Monist* 79:4 (1996), 499–518. Reprinted, abridged, in Leslie P. Francis, *Sexual Harassment as an Ethical Issue in Academic Life.* Lanham, Md.: Rowman and Littlefield, 2001, 183–90; Hunter, Nan D. *The Power of Procedure: The Litigation of Jones v. Clinton.* New York: Aspen Law and Business, 2002; Jenness, Valerie. "Feminism, Sexual Harassment, and the Atypical Case" [Review of *Feminist Accused of Sexual Harassment,* by Jane Gallop]. In Barry M. Dank and Roberto Refinetti, eds., *Sex Work and Sex Workers.* New Brunswick, N.J.: Transaction Publishers, 1999, 191–200; Kaplan, Leonard V., and Beverly I. Moran, eds. *Aftermath: The Clinton Impeachment and the Presidency in the Age of Political Spectacle.* New York: New York University Press, 2001; Kenrick, Douglas T., Melanie R. Trost, and Virgil L. Sheets. "Power, Harassment, and Trophy Mates: The Feminist Advantages of an Evolutionary Perspective." In David M. Buss and Neil M. Malamuth, eds., *Sex, Power, Conflict: Evolutionary and Feminist Perspectives.* New York: Oxford University Press, 1996, 29–53; Kipnis, Laura. "The Anxiety of (Sexual) Influence: Are Onetime 'Unwanted Advances' Really a Feminist Issue?" <slate.msn.com/id/2097411/> [accessed 28 June 2004]; Klein, Ellen Ruth. "Sex with the Teacher?" *The Philosophers' Magazine Online,* no. 27 (3rd Q. 2004). <www.philosophersmag.com/article.php?id=728> [accessed 13 September 2004]; Kors, Alan Charles, and Harvey A. Silverglate. *The Shadow University: The Betrayal of Liberty on America's Campuses.* New York: Free

Press, 1998; Landau, Iddo. "On the Definition of Sexual Harassment." *Australasian Journal of Philosophy* 77:2 (1999), 216–23; Landau, Iddo. "Sexual Harassment and the 'Repetition Requirement.'" *Philosophy of the Social Sciences* 34:2 (2004), 79–83; Landau, Iddo. "Sexual Harassment as 'Wrongful Communication.'" *Philosophy of the Social Sciences* 33:2 (2003), 225–34; LeMoncheck, Linda, and Mane Hajdin. *Sexual Harassment: A Debate*. Lanham, Md.: Rowman and Littlefield, 1997; LeMoncheck, Linda, and James P. Sterba, eds. *Sexual Harassment: Issues and Answers*. New York: Oxford University Press, 2001; MacKinnon, Catharine A. "The Logic of Experience: Reflections on the Development of Sexual Harassment Law." *Georgetown Law Journal* 90:3 (2002), 813–33; MacKinnon, Catharine A. (1986) "Sexual Harassment: Its First Decade in Court." In *Feminism Unmodified: Discourses on Life and Law*. Cambridge, Mass.: Harvard University Press, 1987, 103–16; MacKinnon, Catharine A. *Women's Lives, Men's Laws*. Cambridge, Mass.: Harvard University Press, 2005; MacKinnon, Catharine A., and Reva B. Siegel, eds. *Directions in Sexual Harassment Law*. New Haven, Conn.: Yale University Press, 2004; Mappes, Thomas A. (1985) "Sexual Morality and the Concept of Using Another Person." In Thomas A. Mappes and Jane S. Zembaty, eds., *Social Ethics: Morality and Social Policy*, 4th ed. New York: McGraw-Hill, 1992, 203–16. 5th ed., 1997, 163–76. 6th ed., 2002, 170–83. Reprinted in POS4 (207–23); May, Larry, and Edward Soule. "Sexual Harassment, Rape, and Criminal Sanctions." In Keith Burgess-Jackson, ed., *A Most Detestable Crime: New Philosophical Essays on Rape*. New York: Oxford University Press, 1999, 183–99; McBride, William L. "Sexual Harassment, Seduction, and Mutual Respect: An Attempt at Sorting It Out." In Linda Fisher and Lester Embree, eds., *Feminist Phenomenology: Contributions to Phenomenology*, vol. 40. Dordrecht, Holland: Kluwer, 2000, 249–66; Menard, Kim, Gordon Nagayama Hall, Amber Phung, Marian Gherbial, and Lynette Martin. "Gender Differences in Sexual Harassment and Coercion in College Students." *Journal of Interpersonal Violence* 18:10 (2003), 1222–39; Nehring, Cristina. "The Higher Yearning—Sexual Harassment." *Harper's Magazine* (September 2001). <www.findarticles.com/p/articles/mi_m1111/is_1816_303/ai_77702892> [accessed 14 October 2004]; Nelson, Terri Spahr. *For Love of Country: Confronting Rape and Sexual Harassment in the U.S. Military*. Binghamton, N.Y.: Haworth Maltreatment and Trauma Press, 2002; Nussbaum, Martha C. "'Don't Smile So Much': Philosophy and Women in the 1970s." In Linda Martín Alcoff, ed., *Singing in the Fire: Stories of Women in Philosophy*. Lanham, Md.: Rowman and Littlefield, 2003, 93–108; O'Donohue, William, ed. *Sexual Harassment: Theory, Research, and Treatment*. Boston, Mass.: Allyn and Bacon, 1997; *Oncale v. Sundowner Offshore Services, Inc.* 523 U.S. 75, 118 S.Ct 998, 140 L.Ed. 2d 201 (1998); Paludi, Michele A., ed. *Sexual Harassment on College Campuses: Abusing the Ivory Power*. Albany: State University of New York Press, 1996. (Rev. ed. of *Ivory Power: Sexual Harassment on Campus*); Patai, Daphne. "Women on Top" [Review essay] *Academic Questions* 16:2 (2003), 70–82; Patai, Daphne, and Noretta Koertge. *Professing Feminism: Cautionary Tales from the Strange World of Women's Studies*. New York: Basic Books, 1994. *Professing Feminism: Education and Indoctrination in Women's Studies*, new and expanded ed. Lanham, Md.: Lexington, 2003; Paul, Ellen Frankel. "Sexual Harassment." In Ruth Chadwick, ed., *Encyclopedia of Applied Ethics*, vol. 4. San Diego, Calif.: Academic Press, 1998, 83–100; Paul, Ellen Frankel. "Sexual Harassment as Discrimination: A Defective Paradigm." *Yale Law and Policy Review* 8:2 (1990), 333–65. Reprinted, abridged, in Leslie P. Francis, *Sexual Harassment as an Ethical Issue in Academic Life*. Lanham, Md.: Rowman and Littlefield, 2001, 164–74; Paulson, Amanda. "Student/Teacher Romances: Off Limits." *Christian Science Monitor* (17 February 2004). <www.csmonitor.com/2004/0217/p11s02-legn.html> [accessed 20 February 2004]; Primoratz, Igor. "Sexual Harassment and Rape." In *Ethics and Sex*. London: Routledge, 1999, 144–66; Rapaport, Elizabeth. "Sex and Politics at the Close of the Twentieth Century: A Feminist Looks Back at the Clinton Impeachment and the Thomas Confirmation Hearings." In Leonard V. Kaplan and Beverly I. Moran, eds., *Aftermath: The Clinton Impeachment and the Presidency in the Age of Political Spectacle*. New York: New York University Press, 2001, 22–33; Roberts, Melinda A. "Sexual Harassment, the Acquiescent Plaintiff, and the 'Unwelcomeness' Requirement." In Dana E. Bushnell, ed., *"Nagging Questions": Feminist Ethics in Everyday Life*. Lanham, Md.: Rowman and Littlefield, 1995, 105–21; Sandler, Bernice R., and Robert J. Shoop. *Sexual Harassment on Campus: A Guide for Administrators, Faculty, and Students*.

Boston, Mass.: Allyn and Bacon, 1997; Schulhofer, Stephen J. *Unwanted Sex: The Culture of Intimidation and the Failure of Law*. Cambridge, Mass.: Harvard University Press, 1998; Soble, Alan. "Antioch's 'Sexual Offense Policy': A Philosophical Exploration." *Journal of Social Philosophy* 28:1 (1997), 22–36. Reprinted in Ellen K. Feder, Karmen MacKendrick, and Sybol S. Cook, eds., *A Passion for Wisdom: Readings in Western Philosophy on Love and Desire*. Upper Saddle River, N.J.: Prentice Hall, 2004, 742–54; in David Boonin and Graham Oddie, eds., *What's Wrong? Applied Ethicists and Their Critics*. New York: Oxford University Press, 2005, 241–49; POS4 (323–40); Studd, Michael V. "Sexual Harassment." In David M. Buss and Neil M. Malamuth, eds., *Sex, Power, Conflict: Evolutionary and Feminist Perspectives*. New York: Oxford University Press, 1996, 54–89; Superson, Anita M. "Amorous Relationships between Faculty and Students." *Southern Journal of Philosophy* 39:3 (2001), 419–40; Superson, Anita M. "A Feminist Definition of Sexual Harassment." *Journal of Social Philosophy* 24:1 (1993), 46–64. Reprinted in Hugh LaFollette, ed., *Ethics in Practice: An Anthology*, 2nd ed. Malden, Mass.: Blackwell, 2002, 400–409; in Diane Michelfelder Wilcox and William H. Wilcox, eds., *Applied Ethics in American Society*. Fort Worth, Tex.: Harcourt Brace, 1997, 698–705; HS (383–401); Thomas, Alison M., and Celia Kitzinger, eds. *Sexual Harassment: Contemporary Feminist Perspectives*. Buckingham, U.K.: Open University Press, 1997; Tong, Rosemarie. "Sexual Harassment." In *Women, Sex, and the Law*. Totowa, N.J.: Rowman and Allanheld, 1984, 65–89; Volokh, Eugene. "Freedom of Speech and Workplace Harassment." *UCLA Law Review* 39:6 (1992), 1791–1872; Volokh, Eugene. "What Speech Does 'Hostile Work Environment' Harassment Law Restrict?" *Georgetown Law Journal* 85:3 (1997), 627–48; Wall, Edmund. "The Definition of Sexual Harassment." *Public Affairs Quarterly* 5:4 (1991), 371–85. Reprinted, revised, in Edmund Wall, ed., *Sexual Harassment: Confrontations and Decisions*, rev. ed. Amherst, N.Y.: Prometheus, 2000, 63–77; Wall, Edmund. "Sexual Harassment and Wrongful Communication." In Edmund Wall, ed., *Sexual Harassment: Confrontations and Decisions*, rev. ed. Amherst, N.Y.: Prometheus, 2000, 99–111; Wall, Edmund, ed. *Sexual Harassment: Confrontations and Decisions*, 1st ed. Buffalo, N.Y.: Prometheus, 1992. Revised ed., Amherst, N.Y.: Prometheus, 2000; Weinstein, James. *Hate Speech, Pornography, and the Radical Attack on Free Speech Doctrine*. Boulder, Colo.: Westview, 1999; Weisberg, D. Kelly, ed. "Sexual Harassment." Section of *Applications of Feminist Legal Theory to Women's Lives: Sex, Violence, Work, and Reproduction*. Philadelphia, Pa.: Temple University Press, 1996, 725–859; Welsh, Sandy. "Gender and Sexual Harassment." *Annual Review of Sociology* 25 (1999), 169–90; West, Robin. "Unwelcome Sex: Toward a Harm-Based Analysis." In Catherine A. MacKinnon and Reva B. Siegel, eds., *Directions in Sexual Harassment Law*. New Haven, Conn.: Yale University Press, 2004, 138–52; Williams, Christine, Patti Giuffre, and Kirsten Dellinger. "Sexuality in the Workplace: Organizational Control, Sexual Harassment, and the Pursuit of Pleasure." *Annual Review of Sociology* 25 (1999), 73–93; Wilson, Fiona. "The Social Construction of Sexual Harassment and Assault of University Students." *Journal of Gender Studies* 9:2 (2000), 171–88.

HEGEL, G.W.F. (1770–1831).

Georg Wilhelm Friedrich Hegel was born in Stuttgart, Germany. After attending seminary in Tübingen, where he became friends with Friedrich Hölderin (1770–1843) and Friedrich Wilhelm Joseph von Schelling (1775–1854), Hegel spent twenty years in a variety of academic posts (including Jena) before gaining professorships in Heidelberg (1816) and Berlin (1818). Like **Immanuel Kant** (1724–1804), Hegel was a system-builder, developing a philosophy that incorporated science, metaphysics, ethics, and world history.

In Hegel's view, the task of philosophy is to reveal the inner rationality of the world. By showing that the world operates in accordance with reason, philosophy reconciles us to aspects of it that would otherwise seem alien. Philosophy's role is not to give "instructions on how the world ought to be" (*Elements of the Philosophy of Right*, 23). Philosophy cannot prescribe; it can only explain developments that have already attained completion: "[T]he owl of Minerva begins its flight only with the onset of dusk" (*Right*, 23). There are long-standing debates over the political implications of Hegel's thesis, "What is rational is actual; and what is actual is rational" (*Right*, 20). While Hegel's claim that the world is rational apparently endorses whatever institutions exist, writers such as Allen Wood argue that his view implies that existing institutions may fail to actualize their inner rationality, thus allowing that existing institutions may be reformed (10–11).

Hegel couches his philosophy in dialectical terms. The Hegelian dialectic both generates and resolves contradictions—it is at once the sole adequate method of philosophy and a thesis about how the world works. Hegel holds that any concept must be limited, since its content must exclude some other content. This limitation creates an opposition, so that concepts produce their own opposites. The dialectic reconciles these opposites into a higher-level concept containing both. Not surprisingly, Hegel explains the rationality of sex, **love**, and **marriage** in dialectical terms. In his view, mammalian reproduction, human sexual love, and the institution of marriage all exhibit the same rational structure.

Hegel attempted to show the rationality of the natural world by explaining physics, chemistry, and biology in dialectical terms. In a dubious argument, he attempts to give an account of reproductive biology, beginning with the claim that males and females are complementarily incomplete. Mammalian reproduction, in Hegel's dialectical biology, resolves the incompleteness through the union of these opposites into a more complete whole. Male and female genitals, according to Hegel, share the same type, but each sex is more developed where the other is lacking: "[T]he uterus in the male is reduced to a mere gland [the prostate], while . . . the male testicle in the female remains enclosed within the ovary" (*Philosophy of Nature*, par. 368A [A = addition]). As in **Aristotle**'s (384–322 BCE) account of reproduction (*Generation of Animals*, bk. 1, chap. 21), Hegel identifies the male role as active, the female as passive (*Nature*, par. 368A; *Jenaer Systementwürfe III*, 158–63).

The sex drive is a desire to overcome these anatomical differences. In sexual relations, the pair find themselves in each other by acquiring the deficient parts of themselves that the other has. (Note the resemblance to Aristophanes's story in **Plato**'s [427–347 BCE] *Symposium*, 190e–193a.) In this union, species members feel their connection to the species, thereby transcending their individual limits. In a formidably abstract discussion of sexual experience, Hegel writes, "This feeling of universality [of connection with the species] is the supreme moment of the animal's capabilities" (*Nature*, par. 368A). Hegel also links sexual difference with disease and death, which he sees as resulting from an overstimulation of the gendered elements within a single organism (*Nature*, par. 371; Pillow, 84–85). While Hegel's philosophy of nature seems less relevant today than other aspects of his thought, his view that sexual difference is not a brute biological fact but a self-generating opposition animated by reason (hence subject to rational explication) is striking.

Hegel's more enduring contribution to the philosophy of sex concerns the uniquely human activities of love and marriage. For Hegel, an individual's self-consciousness depends on being acknowledged by others. His famous discussion of this idea involves, ironically, not love but mortal combat. In his parable of the master and slave, two men, gaining recognition of their personhood from each other, engage in a struggle to the death to secure this recognition. One man, preferring life to honor, eventually yields and is enslaved. Paradoxically, the slave now finds a sense of self in his labor, but the master cannot secure acknowledgment from the slave, since the slave is no longer his equal (*Phenomenology of Spirit*, pars. 178–96). In the modern world, freedom is achieved by overcoming the artificial separation of self from the world—yet another dialectical progression—to achieve stable recognition of personhood. One aspect of this is the reconciliation of the individual and society. Male citizens overcome their isolated individuality through a relationship of trust and unity with other fellow citizens. But the model for, and the first stage of, this relationship of trust is married sexual love. Hegel incorporates the family into his political philosophy to an unusual degree, particularly in his attention to how the family prepares male citizens for participation in public life and contributes to their distinctly modern sense of subjective freedom (see Pateman; Siebert; Westphal).

Sexual love allows for stable mutual recognition by a dialectical transcendence of mutual limitation. Love both engenders and cures a feeling of incompleteness. In the first stage, lovers feel "deficient and incomplete" on their own. In the second stage, they "gain recognition" in each other. Love "is therefore the most immense contradiction" (*Right*, par. 158A). As Kant does (*Lectures*, Ak 27:386–89), Hegel holds that lovers give their whole selves to each other. "What in the first instance is most the individual's own [the body] is united into the whole in the lovers' touch and contact; consciousness of a separate self disappears, and all distinction between the lovers is annulled" ("Love," 307; see Soble, 69–70). For Hegel, the loss of individuality leads to a transformation Kant did not envision: "[T]he *union* of the natural sexes . . . is transformed into a *spiritual* union" (*Right*, par. 161). Lovers then overcome their isolated subjectivities and gain a deeper sense of self: "Love means in general the consciousness of my unity with another, so that I am not isolated on my own, but gain my self-consciousness only through the renunciation of my independent existence and through knowing myself as the unity of myself with another and the other with me" (*Right*, par. 158A; see *Aesthetics*, 562–63). When lovers become spouses, they surrender their independent personalities to take on identities as family members. Hegel argues that this ethical union may be achieved only in marriage.

Accordingly, Hegel excoriated sexual liberals who defended free love and who dismissed marriage as eliminating passion. In 1799, Friedrich von Schlegel published the (apparently autobiographical) novel *Lucinde*, which contained a radical theory of sex, love, and marriage. It argued, as Hegel put it, that "the marriage ceremony is superfluous and a formality which could be dispensed with, on the grounds that love is the substantial element and that its value may even be diminished by this celebration." Schlegel's view that sex "prove[s] the freedom and intensity of love" is, says Hegel, just the argument used by seducers! (*Right*, par. 164A). Hegel's point against Schlegel is that women, whose vocation is marriage, will be ruined by extramarital sex. His more intriguing argument is that marriage is both liberation and an ethical duty, because ethical love, which is distinct from passionate love and can exist only in marriage, is an important step in the realization of freedom: "Marriage should not be disrupted by passion, for the latter is subordinate to it" (*Right*, par. 163A). In Hegel's theory, the emancipatory power of ethical love depends on its formalization as marriage. First, marriage provides publicly recognized roles that confer an identity on the individual. Second, the responsibilities of marriage tame disruptive desires. Third, marriage unites the spouses in a relationship transcending self-interest and freeing them from isolation. (Siebert exhaustively documents Hegel's idea that marriage is a step in human freedom.) Each of these elements is important in the context of Hegel's political philosophy.

Hegel's political philosophy explains the inner rationality of laws and social institutions, such as marriage. These institutions serve reason by creating conditions in which human freedom can be realized. This freedom, properly understood, is not simply an absence of restraint allowing the pursuit of every passing urge. Hegel's theory of freedom involves the "purification of the drives" and their ordering into a "rational system" (*Right*, par. 19). Freedom, then, is a state in which the individual's desires reflect his or her identity and fit into a system that harmonizes the desires of all members of society. This process takes place in ethical life, which consists in social customs and institutions: family, civil society, and the state. Individuals achieve freedom through the social roles they take on in these spheres.

Marriage shapes desire by making sex subordinate in an ethical relationship, that is, a relationship of trust and mutual identification structured by socially recognized roles. Hegel criticizes attempts to reduce marriage to its "physical aspect or natural character" as a "sexual relationship" for reproduction (*Right*, par. 161A). In marriage,

> the natural drive is reduced to the modality of a moment of nature which is destined to be extinguished in its very satisfaction, while the spiritual bond asserts *its rights* as the substantial factor and thereby stands out as indissoluble *in itself* and exalted above the contingency of the passions and of particular transient caprice. (*Right*, par. 163)

Marriage, unlike the sex drive, is not vulnerable to passing fancies or shifting moods. In contrast with the natural drive, marriage is a *spiritual* phenomenon (a Hegelian term of art). As a publicly recognized institution, marriage represents the spirit of a community, as that is manifest in its customs and institutions. In turn, public recognition of individual marriages strengthens their ethical bond. For the spouses, marriage provides a role in which they gain the self-definition required for freedom.

Further, as a relationship of love and trust, marriage allows the transcendence of isolated individuality. In Hegel's view, marriage originates in a contract only *"in order to supersede"* the individualistic standpoint of contract (*Right*, par. 163). Hegel castigates Kant for viewing marriage as essentially contractual, a "disgraceful" idea that wrongly depicts marriage as self-interested and debases it to a contract of mutual use (*Right*, pars. 75, 161A). Ethical union, in contrast, transcends individual self-interest. The identification among individuals experienced in relationships of love or trust is incompatible with the contract model (see de Laurentiis; Pateman). While Hegel conceded that divorce must be legally permitted, marriage is essentially an indissoluble union (*Right*, pars. 163A, 176A).

Hegel's theory of sexual difference seems to underlie his view of ethical union as achieving unity in difference. The sexual roles Hegel assigns in marriage are derived from his logic, and these interdependent roles are necessary for ethical union (Halper). In the human realm, Hegel extends his view of sexual difference by associating men with the "particular," having an individual identity, and women with the "universal," defined by community (*Phenomenology*, par. 457; *Right*, pars. 165–66). Infamously, he likens men to animals and women to plants (*Right*, par. 166A). Hegel also argues that since marriage unites difference, it must not take place between *"naturally identical"* blood relations: "Familiarity, acquaintance, and the habit of shared relations should not be present before marriage: they should be discovered only within it" (*Right*, par. 168).

Hegel's philosophy has had great influence, often being transformed in the process. His early followers included the "Young Hegelians" (Berlin, 47–60), among them Karl Marx (1818–1883) and Friedrich Engels (1820–1895). Marx, influenced by Ludwig Feuerbach (1804–1872), "turned Hegel on his head." In opposition to Hegel's statement of the task of philosophy (*Right*, 23), Marx wrote in his "Theses on Feuerbach" that "the philosophers have only *interpreted* the world, in various ways; the point, however, is to *change* it" (145). Hegel also influenced existentialist philosophers, notably **Søren Kierkegaard** (1813–1855), whose Judge William echoes Hegel's defense of marriage (*Either/Or*, vol. II, 5–157; see Thulstrup, 322–28). Hegel has also provoked response from postmodernist thinkers such as Luce Irigaray, Jacques Derrida, and Judith Butler. Butler's *Subjects of Desire* traces the evolution of Hegel's account of desire through **Jacques Lacan** (1901–1981), Jean-Paul Sartre (1905–1980), and **Michel Foucault** (1926–1984).

In *The Second Sex*, Simone de Beauvoir (1908–1986) paid serious attention to Hegel's theory of sexual difference and his seemingly ludicrous theorizing about the genitals. She thought that Hegel's dialectical explanation of sexuality and the nature of the sexes contained a valuable insight. "Man gives significance to the sexes and their relations through sexual activity" (7)—a point made much later by **Catharine MacKinnon** in her critique of sexuality (*Feminism Unmodified*, 46–62). But, Beauvoir continues, Hegel was mistaken to argue from socially given significance to necessity. Whereas Hegel claimed that sexual difference followed an inner rationality and hence was part of the necessary structure of the world, Beauvoir proposed that this inner rationality was the product of social construction. Beauvoir also suggested, controversially, that Hegel's master-slave parable applied better to relationships between men and women than between men. Later feminists, such as Irigaray, Rosalyn Diprose, Patricia Mills, and Kimberly Hutchings, also took interest in Hegel, not only in his theory of sexual difference but also in his discussion of the Greek tragic heroine Antigone (*Phenomenology*, pars. 437, 470; *Right*, par. 166). Hegel has also influenced British analytic philosophy of sex: **Roger Scruton** echoes Hegel in his account of erotic love as intensifying self-consciousness and his defense of marriage as strengthening the merely private bond between lovers (337, 357).

Hegel says little about **homosexuality**. Some recent commentators have suggested that his conception of ethical love and marriage can be extended to same-sex unions (Knowles, 251; Nicolacopoulos and Vassilacopoulos, 164–66; Winfield, chap. 4). But Kirk Pillow argues that, for Hegel, homosexual desire is not merely unnatural, as in Kant (*Lectures*, Ak 27:390–92), but "logically incoherent," since **sexual desire** essentially aims to "unify opposed anatomies" (86). So, Pillow concludes, Hegel's system is heterosexist. Nonetheless, Hegel offers a rich, subtle, and coherent picture of love and sexuality.

See also Bataille, Georges; Desire, Sexual; Existentialism; Feminism, French; Fichte, Johann Gottlieb; Heterosexism; Homosexuality, Ethics of; Kant, Immanuel; Kierkegaard, Søren; Lacan, Jacques; Love; MacKinnon, Catharine; Marriage; Marxism; Phenomenology; Poststructuralism

REFERENCES

Aristotle. (ca. 340 BCE?) *Generation of Animals*. Trans. Arthur L. Peck. Cambridge, Mass.: Harvard University Press, 1979; Beauvoir, Simone de. (1949) *The Second Sex*. Trans. Howard M. Parshley. New York: Vintage, 1989; Berlin, Isaiah. (1939) "The Young Hegelians." In *Karl Marx: His Life and Environment*, 4th ed. Oxford, U.K.: Oxford University Press, 1978, 47–60; Butler, Judith. *Subjects of Desire: Hegelian Reflections in Twentieth-Century France*. New York: Columbia University Press, 1999; De Laurentiis, Allegra. "Kant's Shameful Proposition: A Hegel-Inspired Criticism of Kant's Theory of Domestic Right." *International Philosophical Quarterly* 40:3 (2000), 297–312; Halper, Edward. "Hegel's Family Values." *Review of Metaphysics* 54:4 (2001), 815–58; Hegel, G.W.F. (1821) *Elements of the Philosophy of Right*. Ed. Allen W. Wood. Trans. Hugh B. Nisbet. Cambridge: Cambridge University Press, 1995; Hegel, G.W.F. (1823–1829) *Hegel's Aesthetics: Lectures on Fine Art*. Trans. Thomas M. Knox. Oxford, U.K.: Oxford University Press, 1975; Hegel, G.W.F. (1830) *Hegel's Philosophy of Nature*, vol. 3: *Organics*. Ed. and trans. Michael J. Petry. London: Allen and Unwin, 1970; Hegel, G.W.F. (1804–1805) *Jenaer Systementwürfe III*. Ed. Rolf-Peter Horstmann. Hamburg, Ger.: Felix Meiner Verlag, 1987; Hegel, G.W.F. (1797–1798) "Love." In *On Christianity: Early Theological Writings*. Trans. Thomas M. Knox and Richard Kroner. New York: Harper Torchbooks, 1961, 302–8; Hegel, G.W.F. (1807) *Phenomenology of Spirit*. Trans. Arnold V. Miller. Oxford, U.K.: Clarendon Press, 1977; Kant, Immanuel. (ca. 1762–1794) *Lectures on Ethics*. Trans. Peter

Heath. Ed. Peter Heath and Jerome B. Schneewind. Cambridge: Cambridge University Press, 1997; Kierkegaard, Søren. (1843) *Either/Or*, 2 vols. Trans. Walter Lowrie. Princeton, N.J.: Princeton University Press, 1954; Knowles, Dudley. *Hegel and the Philosophy of Right*. London: Routledge, 2002; MacKinnon, Catharine A. *Feminism Unmodified: Discourses on Life and Law*. Cambridge, Mass.: Harvard University Press, 1987; Marx, Karl. (1845) "Theses on Feuerbach." In Robert Tucker, ed., *The Marx-Engels Reader*, 2nd ed. New York: Norton, 1978, 143–45; Nicolacopoulos, Toula, and George Vassilacopoulos. *Hegel and the Logical Structure of Love: An Essay on Sexualities, Family, and the Law*. Aldershot, U.K.: Ashgate, 1999; Pateman, Carole. "Hegel, Marriage, and the Standpoint of Contract." In Patricia J. Mills, ed., *Feminist Interpretations of G.W.F. Hegel*. University Park: Pennsylvania State University Press, 1996, 209–23; Pillow, Kirk. "Hegel and Homosexuality." *Philosophy Today: SPEP Supplement* 16:5 (2002), 75–91; Plato. (ca. 380 BCE) *The Symposium*. Trans. Christopher Gill. London: Penguin, 1999; Scruton, Roger. *Sexual Desire: A Moral Philosophy of the Erotic*. New York: Free Press, 1986; Siebert, Rudolf. "Hegel's Concept of Marriage and Family: The Origin of Subjective Freedom." In Donald P. Verene, ed., *Hegel's Social and Political Thought: The Philosophy of Objective Spirit*. Atlantic Highlands, N.J.: Humanities Press, 1980, 177–214; Soble, Alan. "Union, Autonomy, and Concern." In Roger Lamb, ed., *Love Analyzed*. Boulder, Colo.: Westview, 1997, 65–92; Thulstrup, Niels. *Kierkegaard's Relation to Hegel*. Trans. George L. Stengren. Princeton, N.J.: Princeton University Press, 1980; Von Schlegel, Friedrich. (1799) *Friedrich Schlegel's "Lucinde" and the Fragments*. Ed. and trans. Peter Firchow. Minneapolis: University of Minnesota Press, 1971; Westphal, Merold. "Hegel's Radical Idealism: Family and State as Ethical Communities." In Zbigniew A. Pelczynski, ed., *The State and Civil Society: Studies in Hegel's Political Philosophy*. Cambridge: Cambridge University Press, 1984, 77–92; Winfield, Richard Dean. *The Just Family*. Albany: State University of New York Press, 1998; Wood, Allen W. *Hegel's Ethical Thought*. Cambridge: Cambridge University Press, 1990.

Elizabeth Brake

ADDITIONAL READING

Avineri, Shlomo. *Hegel's Theory of the Modern State*. Cambridge: Cambridge University Press, 1972; Benhabib, Seyla. "On Hegel, Women, and Irony." In Mary Lyndon Shanley and Carole Pateman, eds., *Feminist Interpretation and Political Theory*. University Park: Pennsylvania State University Press, 1991, 129–45; Benjamin, Jessica. "Master and Slave: The Fantasy of Erotic Domination." In Ann Snitow, Christine Stansell, and Sharon Thompson, eds., *Powers of Desire: The Politics of Sexuality*. New York: Monthly Review Press, 1983, 280–99; Blum, Lawrence. "Kant's and Hegel's Moral Rationalism: A Feminist Perspective." *Canadian Journal of Philosophy* 12 (June 1982), 287–302; Brake, Elizabeth. "Love's Paradox: Making Sense of Hegel on Marriage." In Stella Stanford and Alison Stone, eds., *Hegel and Feminism, Women's Philosophy Review*, Special Issue no. 22 (Autumn, 1999), 80–104; Butler, Clark. "Hegel and Freud: A Comparison." *Philosophy and Phenomenological Research* 36:4 (1976), 506–22; Butler, Judith. *Antigone's Claim*. New York: Columbia University Press, 2000; Cullen, Bernard. *Hegel's Social and Political Thought: An Introduction*. Dublin, Ire.: Gill and Macmillan, 1979; Derrida, Jacques. *Glas*. Trans. John P. Leavey, Jr., and Richard Rand. Lincoln: University of Nebraska Press, 1986; Diprose, Rosalyn. *The Bodies of Women*. London: Routledge, 1994; Engels, Friedrich. (1884) *The Origin of the Family, Private Property, and the State, in the Light of the Researches of Lewis H. Morgan*. New York: International, 1972; Fromm, Erich. (1956) *The Art of Loving*. New York: Harper Perennial Library, 1974; Harris, Henry S. *Hegel's Development: Toward the Sunlight 1770–1801*. Oxford, U.K.: Clarendon Press, 1972; Hegel, G.W.F. (1821) *Hegel's Philosophy of Right*. Trans. Thomas M. Knox. Oxford, U.K.: Oxford University Press, 1942; Hegel, G.W.F. (1802–1804) *System of Ethical Life and First Philosophy of Spirit*. Ed. and trans. Henry S. Harris and Thomas M. Knox. Albany: State University of New York Press, 1979; Hutchings, Kimberly. *Hegel and Feminist Philosophy*. Cambridge, U.K.: Polity Press, 2003; Inwood, Michael. *A Hegel Dictionary*. Oxford, U.K.: Blackwell, 1992; Irigaray, Luce. "The Eternal Irony of the Community." In *Speculum of the Other Woman*. Trans. Gillian C.

Gill. Ithaca, N.Y.: Cornell University Press, 1985, 214–26. Reprinted in Patricia J. Mills, ed., *Feminist Interpretations of G.W.F. Hegel*. University Park: Pennsylvania State University Press, 1996, 45–57; Jung, Patricia, and Ralph Smith. *Heterosexism: An Ethical Challenge*. Albany: State University of New York Press, 1993; Kant, Immanuel. (ca. 1780) *Lectures on Ethics*. Trans. Louis Infield. Indianapolis, Ind.: Hackett, 1963; Koppelman, Andrew. "Sex Equality and/or the Family: From Bloom vs. Okin to Rousseau vs. Hegel." *Yale Journal of Law and the Humanities* 4 (Summer 1992), 399–432; Krell, David Farrell. *Contagion: Sexuality, Disease, and Death in German Idealism and Romanticism*. Bloomington: Indiana University Press, 1998; Krell, David Farrell. "Lucinde's Shame: Hegel, Sensuous Woman, and the Law." *Cardozo Law Review* 10:5–6 (1989), 1673–86. Reprinted in Patricia J. Mills, ed., *Feminist Interpretations of G.W.F. Hegel*. University Park: Pennsylvania State University Press, 1996, 89–107; Krell, David Farrell. "Pitch: Genitality/Excrementality from Hegel to Crazy Jane." *boundary 2* 12:2 (1984), 113–41; Liehu, Heidi. *Søren Kierkegaard's Theory of Stages and Its Relation to Hegel*. Helsinki: Philosophical Society of Finland, 1990; McLellan, David, ed. (1977) *Karl Marx: Selected Writings*, 2nd ed. Oxford, U.K.: Oxford University Press, 2000; Mills, Patricia Jagentowicz, ed. *Feminist Interpretations of G.W.F. Hegel*. University Park: Pennsylvania State University Press, 1996; Nozick, Robert. "Love's Bond." In *The Examined Life*. New York: Simon and Schuster, 1989, 68–86. Reprinted in STW (231–40); Olsen, Frances. "Hegel, Sexual Ethics, and the Oppression of Women: Comments on Krell's 'Lucinde's Shame.' " *Cardozo Law Review* 10:5–6 (1989), 1687–93. Reprinted in Patricia J. Mills, ed., *Feminist Interpretations of G.W.F. Hegel*. University Park: Pennsylvania State University Press, 1996, 109–17; Pateman, Carole. *The Sexual Contract*. Stanford, Calif.: Stanford University Press, 1988; Perkins, Robert L. "Three Critiques of Schlegel's *Lucinde*." In David Goicoechea, ed., *The Nature and Pursuit of Love: The Philosophy of Irving Singer*. Amherst, N.Y.: Prometheus, 1995, 149–66; Popper, Karl R. (1945) "Hegel and the New Tribalism." In *The Open Society and Its Enemies*, vol. 2: *The High Tide of Prophecy: Hegel, Marx, and the Aftermath*, 5th ed. Princeton, N.J.: Princeton University Press, 1966, 27–80; Ricoeur, Paul. "Dialectic: A Philosophical Interpretation of Freud." In *Freud and Philosophy: An Essay on Interpretation*. Trans. Denis Savage. New Haven, Conn.: Yale University Press, 1970, 339–551; Singer, Irving. "Benign Romanticism: Kant, Schlegel, Hegel, Shelly, Byron." In *The Nature of Love*, vol. 2: *Courtly and Romantic*. Chicago, Ill.: University of Chicago Press, 1984, 376–431; Singer, Peter. *Hegel*. Oxford, U.K.: Oxford University Press, 1983; Taylor, Charles. *Hegel*. Cambridge: Cambridge University Press, 1975; Taylor, Mark C. *Journeys to Selfhood: Hegel and Kierkegaard*. Berkeley: University of California Press, 1980; Taylor, Mark C. "Love and Forms of Spirit: Kierkegaard vs. Hegel." In Niels Thulstrup, ed., *Kierkegaardiana X*. Copenhagen, Den.: C. A. Reitzels, 1977, 95–116; Waldron, Jeremy. "When Justice Replaces Affection: The Need for Rights." *Harvard Journal of Law and Public Policy* 11:3 (1998), 625–47; Walsh, William Henry. *Hegelian Ethics*. London: Macmillan, 1969.

HEIDEGGER, MARTIN (1889–1976).

Martin Heidegger is considered by many scholars to be one of the most influential thinkers of the twentieth century. Born in Messkirch, Germany, he was educated at the University of Freiburg and held positions at Freiburg and Marburg. Heidegger became the leading figure in the development of **phenomenology**, hermeneutics, and **existentialism**. He also provided the springboard for the emergence of deconstructionism. Among the ninety volumes of Heidegger's collected works (*Gesamtausgabe*), his magnum opus *Being and Time* (1927) stands out as one of the greatest works of Western philosophy.

Despite Heidegger's voluminous writings, he has little to say about sexuality. Given the ontological thrust of his project, he avoids empirical issues associated with sexuality, arguing instead that in its essential constitution human existence, or "Dasein" (being-there), is gender-neutral. (Jean-Paul Sartre [1905–1980] called it "asexual"; *Being and Nothingness*, 383.) Sexuality arises when Dasein's being (*Sein*) is instantiated in various individuals, since it is this potential to be individuated, or the *possibility* of authentic selfhood, that allows for differentiation into female and male sexes. In this way, Heidegger diverges from later feminists, such as Julia Kristeva, who uphold gender (as the Greeks did) as the essential feature of human selfhood (361–65).

In *The Metaphysical Foundations of Logic* (1978), Heidegger provides his most detailed account of sexuality, arguing that sexuality stems from the self's "thrownness" into the world (137). Heidegger gleaned from **Søren Kierkegaard** (1813–1855) that being thrown into the world prompts the unsettling mood of anxiety (see Stack, 136). As thrown, the individual already finds himself or herself bound to a specific set of circumstances, in which the fact of embodiment is fundamental. Embodiment carries with it an implicit differentiation in regard to sex, male or female. By implication, sex is so basic that, like who one's parents are, the individual is powerless over the origination of the sex he or she becomes and must confront the distinctiveness of the desires constitutive of each.

Given the direction of his phenomenological ontology, Heidegger resisted both the psychoanalytic and behaviorist tendencies of his era that portrayed sexuality in terms of drives and urges. Instead, sexuality serves as a "formal indicator," a basic mode of experience that "points to" or "indicates" the more general ontological structures that determine the constitution of human existence as such, or care (*Sorge*) (*Being and Time*, 83–84). Conversely, sexuality is one way the formal constitution of care comes to be instantiated in each individual, in his or her embodied condition. Hence, sexuality provides a definitive avenue by which the self comes to terms with the central issues of life such as human relationships or occupying a world with others (the structure of *Mitsein*, or "being-with"). Insofar as sexuality hinges on the circumstances of embodiment, and the need to pursue sensuous desires arises from the self's thrownness, the variety of sexual practices can be understood only through the fabric of interpersonal relationships comprising our being-in-the-world.

In formally indicating the self's point of origination or thrownness into the world, sexuality also indicates the opposite extreme or limit: the inevitability of death as intrinsic to the constitution of human nature. The reward of a sexual experience is always overshadowed by the transitoriness of its pleasure, and the fleeting ecstasy of the flesh attests to the finitude of the self's temporality. *Eros* is a temporalizing process that in its futurity anticipates the fulfillment of sexual union and in its pastness acknowledges the transience of **love** and relationships (see Dillon). Spatiality also partially defines the phenomenon of human sexuality. Space as the juxtaposition of bodies—not just as a source of physical interaction in terms of seeing, hearing, smelling, touching, and tasting but also as setting limits of what is allowed and what is forbidden—contributes ontologically to determining the origin of sexual attraction. Because these limits can fluctuate, human beings are open to sexual experimentation in ways animals are not. That eroticism involves transgressing limits that are imposed by inhibition and convention becomes a major theme in the writings of Herbert Marcuse ([1898–1979]; *Eros and Civilization*, 208), one of Heidegger's foremost and "brightest students" (Habermas, 6).

Even though Heidegger does not explicitly address the erotic dimension of sexuality, he does provide the phenomenological framework for doing so. Through its embodiment, human existence participates in the dynamic process whereby things come into presence only by retaining an affinity with absence. This negativity entails that hiddenness is necessarily part of the veil through which we encounter ourselves and others. Human existence as care harbors an erotic dimension, since in the movement into disclosedness and unhiddenness the self endures the tension of confronting the retreat back into concealment and hiddenness, the allure of mystery that pervades any appearance of **beauty**. Thus, phenomenologically speaking, the erotic does not lie purely in nakedness but in that dimension of withholding and withdrawal that necessarily accompanies the unveiling of nudity (for example, in the presence of the other). Eroticism, then, thrives by giving play (*Spiel*) to the dynamic of revealing/concealing, in the offering and taking back of nudity that occurs, say, when the curves of a woman's legs momentarily appear while walking in a split skirt. Sexual intimacy consists of a kind of play that invites variation and exalts in the introduction of new possibilities, the hallmark of imagination and fantasy (as in role-playing). For Heidegger, a fetishistic attachment to certain clothing could be explained by a phenomenological appeal to the enactment of play and **fantasy**, rather than by a psychoanalytic reference to infantile desires and fixations.

In his brief allusions to eroticism, Heidegger does not explicitly link sex and love. As his discussions in *Schelling's Treatise on the Essence of Human Freedom* (160) and *Zollikon Seminars* (190) attest, love is an enactment of care, a way of cultivating openness. It is an activity of "letting be," of allowing the uniqueness of beings, including other people, to become unconcealed and stand forth in the singularity of their manifestation. The self's participation in this openness is an essential condition of intimacy or an authentic response to the other, as when one heeds the "voice of [a] friend" (*Being and Time*, 206). One's uniqueness as an individual and potential for intimacy—the exercise of care toward oneself and others—gives way to the diversity of sexual practices. Heidegger thereby allows for the possibility of different sexual orientations, although he does not explicitly address their occurrence. By the same token, Heidegger's tacit acceptance of sexual experimentation would seem to promote an open climate of sexual involvement with multiple partners. (See Frederick Elliston's [1944–1987] Heideggerian defense of promiscuity.) In *Being and Time*, however, we can find textual support for the opposite position, insofar as Heidegger defines freedom as the selection of one possibility to the exclusion of others (331). He thereby implies that monogamy or an intimate relation with only one significant other might be a preferred avenue by which the self can realize its individuality.

Despite the brevity of Heidegger's discussion of sex, his analysis of authentic existence profoundly influenced the treatment of sexuality undertaken by the two most prominent founders of existential psychotherapy, Ludwig Binswanger (1881–1966) and Medard Boss (1903–1990). Both considered more broadly than Heidegger did the spectrum of sexual behavior as it contributes to or detracts from the individual's quest for self-actualization. Heidegger's circumvention of sexuality also provided the opportunity and point of departure for the French thinkers Sartre, Jacques Derrida (1940–2004), and Luce Irigaray to develop philosophies designed to confront the multifaceted character of eroticism. Heidegger's succinct discussion of sexuality, in terms of its insights and omissions, provides an important cornerstone for addressing eroticism from a phenomenological perspective.

See also Existentialism; Feminism, French; Freudian Left, The; Kierkegaard, Søren; Levinas, Emmanuel; Phenomenology; Poststructuralism

REFERENCES

Binswanger, Ludwig. *Being-in-the-World: Selected Papers of Ludwig Binswanger*. New York: Souvenir Press, 1978; Boss, Medard. *Psychoanalysis and Daseinanalysis*. Trans. Ludwig Lefebre. New York: Basic Books, 1963; Derrida, Jacques. (1983) "*Geschlecht*: Sexual Difference and Ontological Difference." In Nancy J. Holland and Patricia Huntington, eds., *Feminist Interpretations of Martin Heidegger*. University Park: Pennsylvania State University Press, 2001, 53–72; Dillon, M. C. "Sex, Time, and Love: Erotic Temporality." *Journal of Phenomenological Psychology* 18:1 (1987), 33–48;

Elliston, Frederick. "In Defense of Promiscuity." In Robert Baker and Frederick Elliston, eds., *Philosophy and Sex*, 1st ed. Buffalo, N.Y.: Prometheus, 1975, 222–43; Habermas, Jürgen. "Psychic Thermidor and the Rebirth of Rebellious Subjectivity." In Robert Pippin, Andrew Feenberg, and Charles P. Webel, eds., *Marcuse: Critical Theory and the Promise of Utopia*. South Hadley, Mass.: Bergin and Garvey, 1988, 3–12; Heidegger, Martin. (1927) *Being and Time [Sein und Zeit]*. Trans. John Macquarrie and Edward Robinson. New York: Harper and Row, 1962; Heidegger, Martin. *Gesamtausgabe*, 90 vols. Frankfurt am Main, Ger.: Vittorio Klostermann, 1975– ; Heidegger, Martin. (1978) *The Metaphysical Foundations of Logic*. Trans. Michael Heim. Bloomington: Indiana University Press, 1984; Heidegger, Martin. (1971) *Schelling's Treatise on the Essence of Human Freedom*. Trans. Joan Stambaugh. Athens: Ohio University Press, 1985; Heidegger, Martin. (1959–1969) *Zollikon Seminars*. Ed. Medard Boss. Trans. Franz Mayr and Richard Askay. Evanston, Ill.: Northwestern University Press, 2001; Irigaray, Luce. *The Forgetting of Air in Martin Heidegger*. Trans. Mary Beth Mader. Austin: University of Texas Press, 1999; Irigaray, Luce. *Sexes and Genealogies*. Trans. Gillian C. Gill. New York: Columbia University Press, 1993; Kristeva, Julia. (1979) "Women's Time." In Kelly Oliver, ed., *The Portable Kristeva*. New York: Columbia University Press, 1997, 349–68; Marcuse, Herbert. (1955) *Eros and Civilization: A Philosophical Inquiry into Freud*. New York: Vintage, 1962; Sartre, Jean-Paul. (1943) *Being and Nothingness: An Essay on Phenomenological Ontology*. Trans. Hazel E. Barnes. New York: Philosophical Library, 1956; Stack, George J. *Kierkegaard's Existential Ethics*. University: University of Alabama Press, 1977.

Frank Schalow

ADDITIONAL READING

Boss, Medard. (1947) *Meaning and Content of Sexual Perversions: A Daseinanalytic Approach to the Psychopathology of the Phenomenon of Love*. Trans. Liese Lewis Abel. New York: Grune and Stratton, 1949; Corazzon, Raul. "Ontology: A Resource Guide for Philosophers." <www.formalontology. it/heidegger_gesamtausgabe.htm> [accessed 24 May 2005]; Derrida, Jacques. (1983) "*Geschlecht*: Sexual Difference and Ontological Difference." In Nancy J. Holland and Patricia Huntington, eds., *Feminist Interpretations of Martin Heidegger*. University Park: Pennsylvania State University Press, 2001, 53–72. Originally published as "*Geschlecht*: Sexual Difference, Ontological Difference." *Research in Phenomenology* 13 (1983), 65–83; Derrida, Jacques. "*Geschlecht* II: Heidegger's Hand." Trans. John P. Leavey, Jr. In John Sallis, ed., *Deconstruction in Philosophy: The Texts of Jacques Derrida*. Chicago, Ill.: University of Chicago Press, 1987, 161–96; Derrida, Jacques. "Heidegger's Ear: Philopolemology (*Geschlecht* IV)." In John Sallis, ed., *Reading Heidegger*. Bloomington: Indiana University Press, 1993, 163–218; Dillon, M. C. "Sex, Time, and Love: Erotic Temporality." *Journal of Phenomenological Psychology* 18:1 (1987), 33–48. Reprinted in SLF (313–25); Elliston, Frederick. "In Defense of Promiscuity." In Robert Baker and Frederick Elliston, eds., *Philosophy and Sex*, 1st ed. Buffalo, N.Y.: Prometheus, 1975, 222–43. Reprinted in P&S3 (73–90); STW (146–58); Ettinger, Elzbieta. *Hannah Arendt/Martin Heidegger*. New Haven, Conn.: Yale University Press, 1997; Gelven, Michael. "Eros and Projection: Plato and Heidegger." *Southwestern Journal of Philosophy* 4 (1973), 125–36; Giorgio, Agamben. "The Passion of Facticity." In Daniel Heller-Roazen, ed., *Potentialities: Collected Essays in Philosophy*. Stanford, Calif.: Stanford University Press, 1999, 185–204; Guignon, Charles, ed. *The Cambridge Companion to Heidegger*. Cambridge: Cambridge University Press, 1993; Heath, Peter L. "Nothing." In Paul Edwards, ed., *The Encyclopedia of Philosophy*, vol. 5. New York: Macmillan, 1967, 524–25; Heidegger, Martin. *Poetry, Language, Thought*. Trans. Albert Hofstader. New York: Harper and Row, 1971; Heiss, Robert. *Hegel, Kierkegaard, Marx: Three Great Philosophers Whose Ideas Changed the Course of Civilization*. New York: Dell, 1975; Holland, Nancy J., and Patricia Huntington, eds. *Feminist Interpretations of Martin Heidegger*. University Park: Pennsylvania State University Press, 2001; Kristeva, Julia. (1979) "Women's Time." In Toril Moi, ed., *The Kristeva Reader*. Trans. Alice Jardine and Harry Blake. New York: Columbia University Press, 1986, 187–213; Leland, Dorothy. "Authenticity, Feminism, and

Radical Psychotherapy." In Linda Fisher and Lester Embree, eds., *Feminist Phenomenology*. Dordrecht, Holland: Kluwer, 2000, 237–48; Michelfelder, Diane P. "*Eros* and Human Finitude." [Reply to M. C. Dillon, "Sex, Time, and Love: Erotic Temporality"] In Alan Soble, ed., *Sex, Love, and Friendship: Studies of the Society for the Philosophy of Sex and Love, 1977–1992*. Amsterdam, Holland: Rodopi, 1997, 327–31; Mulhall, Stephen. *Inheritance and Originality: Wittgenstein, Heidegger, Kierkegaard*. Oxford, U.K.: Clarendon Press, 2001; Schalow, Frank. *Heidegger and the Quest for the Sacred*. Dordrecht, Holland: Kluwer, 2001; Wyschogrod, Michael. *Kierkegaard and Heidegger: The Ontology of Existence*. New York: Humanities Press, 1969; Zimmerman, Michael E. "Ontical Craving versus Ontological Desire." In Babette Babich, ed., *From Phenomenology to Thought, Errancy, and Desire: Essays in Honor of William Richardson, S.J.* Dordrecht, Holland: Kluwer, 1995, 501–23.

HERDT, GILBERT (1949–   ). Gilbert Henry Herdt, one of the most cited of contemporary anthropologists, is perhaps best known for his studies of ritualistic "fellatio insemination" in a Melanesian culture. Born in Oakley, Kansas, he earned an Honors B.A. in anthropology and an M.A. in medical anthropology from California State University, Sacramento, another M.A. and a Ph.C. in anthropology from the University of Washington (Seattle), and a Ph.D. in anthropology from the Australian National University. He also has postdoctoral certification in psychiatry from the University of California at Los Angeles' Neurophysiology Institute. After teaching at Stanford University (1979–1985) and the University of Chicago (1985–1998), he moved on to San Francisco State University, where he has been professor and director of human sexuality studies and professor of anthropology. Herdt also created and directs the National Sexuality Resource Center, which is dedicated to raising sexual literacy in the United States.

Beginning with *Guardians of the Flutes*, Herdt has written eight books about sexuality and has edited fifteen, focusing on the cultural production of sexual meanings and practices (in, especially, the Papua New Guinea tribe he calls the "Sambia") and on adolescent sexuality, gay identity formation, and AIDS (acquired immunodeficiency syndrome). In *Guardians* and other essays and books (see *The Sambia* and *Sambia Sexual Culture*), Herdt described initiation rites that inducted young Sambia males into society, rites that transform young boys into adult men through a practice of regular semen ingestion. After engaging in this fellatio insemination with bachelors for several years, the boys attain adulthood and are expected to marry, procreate, and abandon same-sex sexuality. The Sambia engage in this practice in part because they believe that semen is not produced naturally by the male body so must be ingested for a male to achieve procreative ability (*Sambia Sexual Culture*, 255). Herdt reported that newlywed Sambia men preferred fellatio by their wives to vaginal intercourse, perhaps due to the social ideology that proximity to a vagina, and especially a womb, is dangerous for men.

Aside from alerting scholars to a sensational sexual practice (at least when viewed from the perspective of homophobic Western culture), Herdt's studies challenged certain theories about **sexual orientation**. Most Sambia men successfully negotiate their culturally expected shift from early, exclusively homosexual practice to exclusively heterosexual practice. Theory about sexual orientation from 1950 to 1970 had moved beyond seeing **homosexuality** either as pathology (as in some post-Freudians) or as sinfulness (as in Catholic theology) to postulating distinct homosexual and heterosexual orientations, understood as relatively permanent structures of **sexual desire**. But if most males in a culture can shift from one exclusive practice to another, their sexual orientation (if it makes any sense to use that term) is not a permanent psychological trait—which, of course, does not imply that earlier theorists were right that homosexuality was pathological or sinful.

Herdt's studies were controversial. They supported neither the traditional view that only heterosexuality was biologically normal nor the stance taken by many gay and lesbian activists that same-sex desire was a natural, inescapable, and unchosen aspect of one's individual psychological constitution. Herdt suggested, instead, that most persons in a society develop their type(s) of sexual desire within boundaries established by their particular culture. The shape of desire can be altered and modified, depending on the degree of cultural authorization of such vicissitudes. (See the work of **John Money**, for example.) This, in part, is why Herdt questioned the notion of "orientation" itself. He also thought that speaking of sexual "identity" or "preference" misleadingly implied that an "intentional choice has been made—an idea that opposes much of what we know about the development of sexuality." At the same time, Herdt pointed out that sexual preference could not be understood simply in terms of "learning" one's sexuality from one's culture. If that were true, "we would not expect to find many homosexuals" in the United States, because "antihomosexual imagery is so profound" in our culture (*Same Sex, Different Cultures*, 19–20). The relationship between one's sexuality and the culture one lives in is complex: Our sexuality is not free of culture's influence, but neither is it entirely determined by it.

Many gay and lesbian advocates feared that Herdt's studies of the Sambia would be used by those antagonistic to homosexuality as evidence that American homosexuals *could* change and, as a result, no longer either engage in sinful behavior or manifest mental pathology. But drawing that conclusion from Herdt's studies is unwarranted, since American history and culture differ significantly from Sambian history and culture. After 1980, other investigations have corroborated Herdt's view that the formation of our sexualities is a complex social process.

By virtue of his theoretical perspective, Herdt has made much of the "third sex" or "third gender" phenomenon. In *Same Sex*, he outlined the acceptance of same-sex desires and relations in various cultures from antiquity to contemporary times. Many cultures have not merely tolerated same-gender relations but have created special, elaborate social roles for "third sex" persons, including religious roles, as in Asian shamans and Native American *berdache* (see *Sambia Sexual Culture*, chap. 8; *Third Sex*). As he does in other books, Herdt in *Same Sex* describes how sexual prejudice causes difficulties for adolescents experimenting with their sexuality (see also *Children of Horizons*).

Herdt collaborated with psychoanalyst and psychiatrist Robert Stoller (1924–1991) in one of his return visits to Papua New Guinea. They conducted interviews with Sambia men (and a few women), inquiring in detail about their sexuality. The interviewees were principally selected not because they represented "typical" patterns of male sexuality but because they manifested varied patterns of male sexual behavior. Subjects were asked not only about sexual activities but also about their feelings and desires in connection with those activities. The study provides, then, a sense of the sexual motivations and concerns of these men, including the extent of their awareness of women's desires and pleasure and the men's understanding of the sexual basis of their masculinity. Stoller's participation, by adding a psychological dimension to Herdt's work, introduced new questions about the interaction between culture and individual psychosexuality.

This research yielded the book *Intimate Communications*, which proposed that what becomes understood collectively as the erotic results from noneorotic psychocultural factors. Defending their sexological investigations, Herdt and Stoller argued that studying the erotic was a powerful way to study culture itself:

[G]etting details about sexual life . . . is not a detour from the great issues of anthropology, but is . . . an ideal way to bring the researcher to the center of a culture. Therefore anthropology's lack of such data, especially if it has occurred because the subject is exciting, disturbing, guilt-producing, or repugnant to the ethnographer, puts the lie to anthropologists' claims of being . . . open to understanding the people they study.

Ominously, they perceived "this failure [as] a crime of the mind" (*Intimate Communications*, 200).

Herdt has also studied the importance of cultural systems in shaping sexual practices relevant to HIV (human immunodeficiency virus) transmission and prevention. During the first decade of the epidemic in the 1980s, most social scientists focused on the behavioral correlates of HIV infection among individuals. Even though valuable, their research failed to examine crucial social and cultural factors. Due in large measure to Herdt's enterprising explorations since the early 1990s (see *Sexual Cultures and Migration* and *The Time of AIDS*), an emphasis on cultural analysis took shape alongside growing anthropological research on the political economy of HIV/AIDS and on structural factors, especially social inequality, that shape vulnerability to HIV infection. Similarly, Herdt has investigated sexuality and social policy in the area of sexual health, sexuality education, and rights. He founded a journal in 2004—*Sexuality Research and Social Policy*—to address these issues.

See also Bisexuality; Boswell, John; Diseases, Sexually Transmitted; Homosexuality, Ethics of; Homosexuality and Science; Intersexuality; Mead, Margaret; Money, John; Orientation, Sexual; Perversion, Sexual; Sexology; Social Constructionism

REFERENCES

Herdt, Gilbert. *Guardians of the Flutes: Idioms of Masculinity*. New York: McGraw-Hill, 1981; Herdt, Gilbert. *The Sambia: Ritual and Gender in New Guinea*. New York: Holt, Rinehart and Winston, 1987; Herdt, Gilbert. *Sambia Sexual Culture: Essays from the Field*. Chicago, Ill.: University of Chicago Press, 1999; Herdt, Gilbert. *Same Sex, Different Cultures: Perspectives on Gay and Lesbian Lives*. New York: Westview Press, 1997; Herdt, Gilbert, ed. *Sexual Cultures and Migration in the Era of AIDS*. Oxford, U.K.: Oxford University Press, 1997; Herdt, Gilbert, ed. *Third Sex, Third Gender: Beyond Sexual Dimorphism in Culture and History*. New York: Zone Books, 1994; Herdt, Gilbert, and Andrew Boxer. *Children of Horizons: How Gay and Lesbian Teenagers Are Leading a New Way Out of the Closet*. Boston, Mass.: Beacon Press, 1993; Herdt, Gilbert, and Shirley Lindebaum, eds. *The Time of AIDS: Social Analysis, Theory, and Method*. Newbury Park, Conn.: Sage, 1992; Herdt, Gilbert, and Robert J. Stoller. *Intimate Communications: Erotics and the Study of Culture*. New York: Columbia University Press, 1990; Money, John. *The Adam Principle. Genes, Genitals, Hormones, & Gender: Selected Readings in Sexology*. Buffalo, N.Y.: Prometheus, 1993; National Sexuality Resource Center. (Web site) <nsrc.sfsu.edu/Index.cfm> [accessed 9 June 2005].

Christine E. Gudorf

ADDITIONAL READING

Boulton, Michael J. "Methodological Issues in HIV/AIDS Social Research: Recent Debates, Recent Developments." *AIDS* 7, supp. 1 (1993), S243–S248; Brown, Paula, and Georgeda Buchbinder, eds. *Man and Woman in the New Guinea Highlands*. Washington, D.C.: American Anthropological Association, 1976; Buckley, Peter. "Observing the Other: Reflections on Anthropological Fieldwork." *Journal of the American Psychoanalytic Association* 42:2 (1994), 613–34; Davenport, William. "Sexual Patterns in a Southwest Pacific Society." In Ruth Brecher and Edward Brecher, eds., *An Analysis of Human Sexual Response*. New York: New American Library, 1966, 175–200; Davis,

Dona, and Gilbert Herdt. "Cultural Issues and Sexual Disorders." In Thomas A. Widiger, Allen J. Francis, Harold Alan Pincus, Ruth Ross, Michael B. First, and Wendy Davis, eds., *DSM-IV Sourcebook*, vol. 3. Washington, D.C.: American Psychiatric Association, 1997, 951–57; Draper, Robert. "The Genius Who Loved Boys." *GQ* (November 1999), 313–30; Ewing, Katherine P. Review of *Intimate Communications: Erotics and the Study of Culture*, by Gilbert Herdt and Robert Stoller. *American Ethnologist* 21:3 (1994), 635–36; Giles, James. Review of *Sambia Sexual Culture: Essays from the Field*, by Gilbert Herdt. *Archives of Sexual Behavior* 33:4 (2004), 413–17; Herdt, Gilbert. "Developmental Discontinuities and Sexual Orientation across Cultures." In David P. McWhirter, Stephanie A. Sanders, and June M. Reinisch, eds., *Homosexuality/Heterosexuality: Concepts of Sexual Orientation*. New York: Oxford University Press, 1990, 208–36; Herdt, Gilbert. *Secrecy and Cultural Reality*. Ann Arbor: University of Michigan Press, 2003; Herdt, Gilbert. (1984) "Semen Transactions in Sambia Culture." In David N. Suggs and Andrew W. Miracle, eds., *Culture and Human Sexuality: A Reader*. Pacific Grove, Calif.: Brooks/Cole, 1993, 298–327; Herdt, Gilbert, ed. *Ritualized Homosexuality in Melanesia*. Berkeley: University of California Press, 1984; Herdt, Gilbert, and Bruce Koff. *Something to Tell You: The Road Families Travel When a Child Is Gay*. New York: Columbia University Press, 2000; Kennedy, Elizabeth L. Review of *Children of Horizons: How Gay and Lesbian Teenagers Are Leading a New Way Out of the Closet*, by Gilbert Herdt and Andrew Boxer. *American Anthropologist* 96:3 (1994), 697–700; Knauft, Bruce M. "Foucault Meets South New Guinea: Knowledge, Power, Sexuality." *Ethos* 22:4 (1994), 391–438; Lorber, Judith. "Beyond the Binaries: Depolarizing the Categories of Sex, Sexuality, and Gender." *Social Inquiry* 66:2 (1996): 143–59; Money, John. "Gender-Crossed Boys Grow Up Gay." In *The Adam Principle. Genes, Genitals, Hormones, & Gender: Selected Readings in Sexology*. Buffalo, N.Y.: Prometheus, 1993, 191–202; Money, John. "What Happens to Boys Whose Lovers Were Men?" In *The Adam Principle. Genes, Genitals, Hormones, & Gender: Selected Readings in Sexology*. Buffalo, N.Y.: Prometheus, 1993, 203–19; Piker, Steven. "Contributions of Psychological Anthropology." *Journal of Cross-Cultural Psychology* 29:1 (1998), 9–31; Rivera, Garza C. Review of *Third Sex, Third Gender: Beyond Sexual Dimorphism in Culture and History*, by Gilbert Herdt. *Ethnohistory* 43:1 (1996), 177–80; Robles, Steve. "The Academics of Lust: SF's New Sex Institute." <www.eros-london.com/articles/2003-03-18/institute/> [accessed 9 June 2005]; Scheffler, Harold W. Review of *Intimate Communications: Erotics and the Study of Culture*, by Gilbert Herdt and Robert Stoller. *American Anthropologist* 94:3 (1992), 728–29; Shrage, Laurie. "Should Feminists Oppose Prostitution?" *Ethics* 99:2 (1989), 347–61. Reprinted in HS (275–89); POS3 (323–38); POS4 (435–50); STW (71–80); Soble, Alan. "Fellatio Insemination." In *Sexual Investigations*. New York: New York University Press, 1996, 124–27; Stoller, Robert J. *Observing the Erotic Imagination*. New Haven, Conn.: Yale University Press, 1985; Stoller, Robert J. *Pain and Passion: A Psychoanalyst Explores the World of S&M*. New York: Plenum, 1991; Stoller, Robert J. *Perversion: The Erotic Form of Hatred*. New York: Pantheon, 1975; Stoller, Robert J. *Sex and Gender: On the Development of Masculinity and Femininity*. New York: Science House, 1968; Stoller, Robert J. *Sexual Excitement: Dynamics of Erotic Life*. New York: Pantheon, 1979; Stoller, Robert J. "Theories of Origins of Homosexuality: A Cross-Cultural Look." *Archives of General Psychiatry* 42:4 (1985), 399–404; Stoller, Robert J., and Gilbert Herdt. "Theories of Origins of Male Homosexuality: A Cross-Cultural Look." In Robert J. Stoller, *Observing the Erotic Imagination*. New Haven, Conn.: Yale University Press, 1985, 104–34; Stoller, Robert, Judd Marmor, Irving Bieber, Ronald Gold, Charles W. Socarides, Richard Green, and Robert L. Spitzer. "A Symposium: Should Homosexuality Be in the APA Nomenclature?" *American Journal of Psychiatry* 130:11 (1973), 1207–16.

HETEROSEXISM.

HETEROSEXISM. Heterosexism is the differential treatment of persons on the basis of **sexual orientation** or sexual identity. Both personal and social in scope, these systematic responses to human sexual diversity have developed over the centuries. In any given culture, heterosexism is synergistically constituted by the intersection of civil laws, public policies, religious practices, and domestic arrangements, as well as by individual attitudes and interpersonal behaviors. Heterosexism invariably results in the prejudicial treatment of gay, lesbian, bisexual, and transgendered (GLBT) people and preferential treatment of most heterosexuals. Though heterosexism can take many forms, in all cases its *raison d'être* is a heterocentric sexual ethic. In the last quarter of the twentieth century, debate about whether such differential treatment is morally justifiable became widespread in North Atlantic countries.

Though disagreement about whether heterosexism is defensible reigns, heterosexism is a fairly cogent, intelligible cluster of practices. Distinguishing heterosexism, as largely cognitive, from visceral responses to human sexual diversity is helpful. Though heterosexism is frequently accompanied and reinforced by phobic responses to what is perceived as "queer," heterosexism is not necessarily tied to such fears and hatreds. Homophobia is to heterosexism as misogyny is to sexism and racial bigotry is to racism. Thus the links between homophobia and heterosexism are complex: Hatred and fear of GLBT people may be, but is not always, the driving force behind heterosexism. A person may tolerate diversity on many fronts but be convinced that heterosexist discrimination is morally justified. Indeed, heterosexist policies have been seen as expressions of **love** (albeit "tough love") for GLBT people.

Heterosexism is not only a personal attitude, a private religious conviction, or an academic matter. It pervades many cultures, shapes social institutions, and deeply influences our lives. In the United States, people are treated differently at work, in the military, at home, in religious communities, and in the wider society on the basis of their sexuality. Most North Americans give preferential treatment in a variety of ways to heterosexuals and treat GLBT people prejudicially.

Though there are notable challenges to these policies, generally in North Atlantic nations only males and females are allowed to marry each other. These (presumed) heterosexuals, through civilly licensed marriages, achieve access to social benefits: In the United States, only married people are granted automatic spousal immigration rights, proxy privileges attributed to next of kin in medical decisions and funeral arrangements, economic benefits (direct and transferred) from social security, Medicare, veterans and other pension plans, and spousal benefits associated with life and health insurance policies. One aspect of heterosexism is that same-sex couples cannot legally marry. As a result, they cannot file joint tax returns or acquire joint home, auto, or health insurance policies. Most receive neither the protection nor privileges afforded heterosexual people by laws governing adoption, foster care, custody, domestic abuse, divorce, child support, and estate and/or inheritance claims. Further, discrimination on the basis of sexual identity is widespread in teaching, coaching, the **military**, and many forms of ministry. Leadership and membership in civic clubs (e.g., the Boy Scouts) are privileges enjoyed only by heterosexuals.

One extreme form of heterosexism denies many people the right to safety or a reasonable expectation of physical safety. According to U.S. Department of Justice statistics, GLBT people are the most common victims of hate crimes. Lesbians experience three times, and gay men four times, as much criminal violence as their straight counterparts (Comstock; Gordon, 185–97). If GLBT people want the safety from verbal abuse and violent attack possessed in general by heterosexuals, they must live inauthentic lives by closeting themselves in other-sex relationships or identifying themselves publically as straight. Because they have not disclosed their sexuality to most family members and friends, they cannot celebrate or even acknowledge either those they love or their own sexuality.

Closets make good hiding places, and the protection they offer might ensure survival and social success. But closets isolate as well as shelter, making those inside them vulnerable to twin terrors: both the threat of discovery and, ironically, the threat of never being discovered and hence never really being intimately known by others. Closeting, further, is not merely a personal choice. It is a socially constructed habit generated by heterosexism. GLBT people are trained to keep silent, while most heterosexuals are trained to turn a deaf ear to them. Those GLBT people who insist on "acting up" in public forfeit the physical and emotional safety that heterosexuals have in comparable situations. According to FBI Bias Crimes statistics, hate crimes in the United States against gays and lesbians doubled in the 1990s ("Assault on Gay America"). Many, though not all, heterosexists deplore this "gay bashing." The Roman Catholic Church, which takes a traditional stand on the morality of GLBT sexuality, officially condemns verbal abuse and violence against these persons. Nevertheless, those who perpetrate these crimes often try to excuse their attacks with arguments similar to those advanced to promote less violent forms of heterosexism.

Heterosexism has other consequences. The fear of finding out about themselves that they are "queer" contributes to the confusion many young GLBT people experience about their sexual identity (see Sullivan, 3–9). It fosters in some of them self-loathing and self-destructive behaviors. GLBT teens are at greater risk for substance abuse, depression, and suicide. Indeed, some studies suggest that gay teens are three times more likely than straight teens to attempt suicide (see Gibson). How best to interpret these facts is not self-evident. Some argue that these studies indicate that GLBT people are abnormal (see Jones and Workman). Others claim that heterosexism itself is responsible for these problems, as racism is responsible for some problems among minorities (see Burr; Ruse, 211–13; Thomas and Levin, 30–32, 129–30, 173–74). When GLBT persons "come out" to family and friends, their responses—if forged by heterosexism—may strain psychological and social support structures to the breaking point. After "coming out," many street kids are expelled by parents or choose to run away as a result of the prejudicial treatment they experience. (On the ethics of the closet, coming out, and being outed, see Murphy, 27–146.) Moreover, fear of being mistakenly perceived as GLBT inhibits intimate behavior between heterosexual same-sex friends, especially men. Heterosexism reinforces sexist stereotypes and rigid standards of gender conformity. It also misidentifies GLBT people as more inclined than their straight peers to seduce, attempt to reorient, or harm children sexually. Heterosexism thereby misdirects communal efforts to protect those most vulnerable to sexual predators.

How the consequences of heterosexism are evaluated varies. Some view the noxious consequences as evidence that heterosexism breaks down instead of builds up community and that, therefore, heterosexism is teleologically unjustifiable. Others view the consequences as the sometimes unfortunate price that must be paid for practices and policies that nevertheless, in the long run and overall, serve the common good in important ways. In particular, GLBT people, on the traditional argument, are a threat to heterosexual **marriage**, family life, and children and hence to the commonweal in general. Sexual or gender complementarity is seen by some who commend heterosexism as required for the survival of the institution of marriage. Thus the reenforcement of heterosexual relationships is claimed to be essential to individual flourishing and the common good. Those who challenge these arguments contend that evidence supporting the conclusion that GLBT people pose a threat to the common good in these ways is unconvincing. According to one traditionalist argument, men are domesticated not by marital commitment or promise-making and -keeping but more precisely by the efforts of women. Even men of goodwill are presumed to be wild and dangerous outside marriage, and women—at least the good ones—are believed to be naturally stable and stabilizing, and nurturing of children and men, to the boon of society. (As Schlafly puts it, a man's wife "can motivate him, inspire him, encourage him, teach him, restrain him, reward him"; 17.) Only if marriage is restricted to opposite-sex couples, and the institution thereby sustained, will men, who would otherwise wander and waiver, be induced into long-term companionship with women and hence be tamed and avoid social irresponsibility. Gay men, similarly—unmarried and free of children—have little incentive to contribute to the viability of future society (see **Roger Scruton**). Those who oppose heterosexism find the presumptions about gender or the natural inclinations of the sexes underlying this argument to be highly contestable. Further, many exemplars of single or unmarried heterosexual and homosexual men who lead pacific and socially valuable lives makes the argument dubious.

Consequently, while some advocate that heterosexism be dismantled, as required by justice and the obligation to protect the human and civil rights of all, others object that such dismantling is hazardous and misguided, if not morally outrageous. In this dispute, much depends on whether heterosexist discrimination is justifiable as a matter of principle (see Thomas and Levin). Important to keep in mind when contemplating this issue is that although respect for equality does not require that we always and everywhere treat people identically, it does mean that advocates of differential treatment, whether preferential or prejudicial, bear the burden of proof.

Underlying heterosexist discrimination are philosophical or theological convictions about "good sex." In particular, heterosexism rests on the judgment that ordinary heterosexuality is morally ideal, if not the only normatively acceptable form of human sexuality. According to this heterocentrism, something is wrong with being bisexual, homosexual, or transgendered. These states are imperfect, diseased, or evil. Hence, in addition to considering its many consequences, the moral evaluation of heterosexism requires examining these premises about human sexuality. Heterosexism presupposes that the human sexual design is monochromatically heterosexual. Whatever else might be required, morally good sex must be open to the possibility of procreation and family, which can be satisfied only by opposite-sex couples.

The procreativity requirement is questionable. Fewer people believe today that the use of **contraception**, sterilization, and the choice not to have children are necessarily morally wrong. Nonprocreative sexuality—solitary **masturbation**, mutual masturbation, oral and anal sex—do not seem, to many, unnatural or immoral, at least when done by heterosexuals. **Sexual activity** carried out by infertile heterosexual women (e.g., those who are pregnant or postmenopausal), or men with low sperm counts or erectile or other **sexual dysfunction**, is not usually judged immoral. Since, short of a miracle, these acts cannot generate life, it is apparently inconsistent to judge the sexual activities of GLBT people wrong on the grounds of their nonprocreativity.

Traditionalists defend the procreativity requirement in general by arguing that exceptions to it can be coherently justified without thereby endorsing GLBT sexuality. They argue that a morally significant difference exists between the coital activity of unintentionally infertile heterosexual couples and gay and lesbian couples who, through their choice of a partner, intentionally frustrate their otherwise normal procreative potential (see **G.E.M. Anscombe** [1919–2001]; Finnis, 1066–68; contrast Jung and Smith, 38, 146, 200–201n.4, 218n.10; Koppelman, 46–50). Therapeutic sterilization can be justified on the grounds that it saves lives, and this rationale has no applicability to GLBT sexuality. Further, the sexuality of pregnant women might be interpreted in a way that vividly proves the procreative rule. But the power of these arguments, their ability to withstand the burden of proof, is highly contested.

Those who challenge heterosexism also point out that the moral goodness of the sexuality of older women is difficult to explain within the traditional framework. The changes associated with menopause are not plausibly a disease state or deviation from women's sexual nature. True, for about thirty-five years most women can expect a periodic link between coitus and reproduction. But the next thirty-five years include no such link; this complete absence of reproductive potential is normal for postmenopausal women. Those who oppose heterosexism argue that the **sexual desire**s and relationships of these women may be good even if not procreative. Similarly, the nonprocreative sexual desires and relationships of gays and lesbians may be good. The lesson (see Gudorf, 65) is that when female physiology is taken into account, the purportedly natural connection between sexuality and reproduction is undermined.

See also Anscombe, G.E.M.; Bible, Sex and the; Ethics, Sexual; Homosexuality, Ethics of; Marriage, Same-Sex; Natural Law (New); Orientation, Sexual; Perversion, Sexual; Scruton, Roger; Sex Education; Sherfey, Mary Jane; Violence, Sexual

REFERENCES

Anscombe, G.E.M. "Contraception and Chastity." *The Human World*, no. 7 (1972), 9–30; "Assault on Gay America: The Life and Death of Billy Jack Gaither." *Frontline*, PBS (15 February 2000). <www.pbs.org/wgbh/pages/frontline/shows/assault> [accessed 11 May 2004]; Burr, Chandler. "Homosexuality and Biology." In Jeffrey S. Siker, ed., *Homosexuality in the Church: Both Sides of the Debate*. Louisville, Ky.: Westminster John Knox, 1994, 116–34; Comstock, Gary D. "Empirical Data on Victims." In *Violence against Lesbians and Gay Men*. New York: Columbia University Press, 1991, 31–55; Finnis, John. "Law, Morality, and 'Sexual Orientation.'" *Notre Dame Law Review* 69:5 (1994), 1049–76; Gibson, Paul. "Gay Male and Lesbian Youth Suicide." In Gary Remafedi, ed., *Death by Denial: Studies in Suicide in the Gay and Lesbian Teenager*. Boston, Mass.: Alyson, 1994, 15–68; Gordon, Kevin. *Homosexuality and Social Justice*. San Francisco, Calif.: Consultation on Homosexuality, Social Justice, and Roman Catholic Theology, 1986; Gudorf, Christine E. *Body, Sex, and Pleasure: Reconstructing Christian Sexual Ethics*. Cleveland, Ohio: Pilgrim Press, 1994; Jones, Stanton L., and Don E. Workman. "Homosexuality: The Behavioral Sciences and the Church." In Jeffrey S. Siker, ed., *Homosexuality in the Church: Both Sides of the Debate*. Louisville, Ky.: Westminster John Knox, 1994, 93–115; Jung, Patricia Beattie, and Ralph F. Smith. *Heterosexism: An Ethical Challenge*. Albany: State University of New York Press, 1993; Koppelman, Andrew. "Homosexual Conduct: A Reply to the New Natural Lawyers." In John Corvino, ed., *Same Sex: Debating the Ethics, Science, and Culture of Homosexuality*. Lanham, Md.: Rowman and Littlefield, 1997, 44–57; Murphy, Timothy F., ed. *Gay Ethics: Controversies in Outing, Civil Rights, and Sexual Science*. Binghamton, N.Y.: Harrington Park Press, 1994; Ruse, Michael. *Homosexuality: A Philosophical Inquiry*. New York: Blackwell, 1988; Schlafly, Phyllis. *The Power of the Positive Woman*. New Rochelle, N.Y.: Arlington House, 1977; Scruton, Roger. "Why Heterosexism Is Not a Vice." *The Sunday Telegraph* (24 September 1989), 20; Sullivan, Andrew. *Virtually Normal: An Argument about Homosexuality*. New York: Knopf, 1995; Thomas, Laurence M., and Michael E. Levin. *Sexual Orientation and Human Rights*. Lanham, Md.: Rowman and Littlefield, 1999.

Patricia Beattie Jung

ADDITIONAL READING

Anscombe, G.E.M. "Contraception and Chastity." *The Human World*, no. 7 (1972), 9–30. Reprinted in Michael Bayles, ed., *Ethics and Population*. Cambridge, Mass.: Schenkman, 1976, 134–53; HS

(29–50); Blaney, Robert W. "Homophobia/Heterosexism and Lesbian/Gay Experience: An Annotated Bibliography." *Annual of the Society of Christian Ethics* 7 (1987), 229–52; Calhoun, Cheshire. *Feminism, the Family, and the Politics of the Closet: Lesbian and Gay Displacement.* New York: Oxford University Press, 2002; Condit, Rebecca. "Heterosexism." In Timothy F. Murphy, ed., *Reader's Guide to Lesbian and Gay Studies.* Chicago, Ill.: Fitzroy Dearborn, 2000, 279–80; Corvino, John, ed. *Same Sex: Debating the Ethics, Science, and Culture of Homosexuality.* Lanham, Md.: Rowman and Littlefield, 1997; Finnis, John M. "Law, Morality, and 'Sexual Orientation.'" *Notre Dame Law Review* 69:5 (1994), 1049–76. Reprinted, revised, in *Notre Dame Journal of Law, Ethics, and Public Policy* 9:1 (1995), 11–39. Reprinted, revised, in John Corvino, ed., *Same Sex: Debating the Ethics, Science, and Culture of Homosexuality.* Lanham, Md.: Rowman and Littlefield, 1997, 31–43; Jung, Patricia Beattie. "Heterosexism: An Introduction." Integrity, Washington, D.C. <www.integrityusa.org/downloadablematerials/HeterosexismAnIntroduction.PDF> [accessed 20 April 2004]; Jung, Patricia Beattie. Review of *Body, Sex, and Pleasure: Reconstructing Christian Sexual Ethics*, by Christine E. Gudorf. *Theological Studies* 56:3 (1995), 603–5; Jung, Patricia Beattie, ed. *Sexual Diversity and Catholicism: Toward the Development of Moral Theology.* Collegeville, Minn.: Liturgical Press, 2001; Jung, Patricia Beattie, Mary E. Hunt, and Radhika Balakrishnan, eds. *Good Sex: Feminist Perspectives from the World's Religions.* New Brunswick, N.J.: Rutgers University Press, 2001; Jung, Patricia Beattie, and Shannon Jung, eds. "Heterosexism." In *Moral Issues and Christian Responses*, 7th ed. Belmont, Calif.: Wadsworth, 2003, 274–306; Jung, Patricia Beattie, and Thomas A. Shannon, eds. *Abortion and Catholicism: The American Debate.* New York: Crossroad, 1988; Levin, Michael E. "Homosexuality, Abnormality, and Civil Rights." *Public Affairs Quarterly* 10:1 (1996), 31–48; Murphy, Timothy F., ed. *Gay Ethics: Controversies in Outing, Civil Rights, and Sexual Science.* Binghamton, N.Y.: Harrington Park Press, 1994. Also published as *Journal of Homosexuality* 27:3–4 (1994); Myers, JoAnne. "Preaching to the Choir, and Beyond." [Review of *Heterosexism: An Ethical Challenge*, by Patricia Beattie Jung and Ralph F. Smith] *Journal of Lesbian Studies* 3:4 (1999), 159–61; Nussbaum, Martha C. "Lesbian and Gay Rights: Pro." In Michael Leahy and Dan Cohn-Sherbok, eds., *The Liberation Debate: Rights at Issue.* London: Routledge, 1996, 89–107; Olyan, Saul M., and Martha C. Nussbaum, eds. *Sexual Orientation and Human Rights in American Religious Discourse.* New York: Oxford University Press, 1998; Peddicord, Richard. *Gay and Lesbian Rights: A Question—Sexual Ethics or Social Justice?* Kansas City, Mo.: Sheed and Ward, 1996; Pharr, Suzanne. *Homophobia: A Weapon of Sexism.* Inverness, Calif.: Chardon, 1988; Ratzinger, Joseph (Cardinal). "Considerations Regarding Proposals to Give Legal Recognition to Unions between Homosexual Persons." *Origins* 33:11 (2003), 177, 179–82; Ratzinger, Joseph (Cardinal). "Letter to the Bishops of the Catholic Church on the Pastoral Care of Homosexual Persons." *Origins* 16:22 (1986), 377–81. Reprinted in Jeannine Gramick and Robert Nugent, eds., *The Vatican and Homosexuality: Reactions to the "Letter to the Bishops of the Catholic Church on the Pastoral Care of Homosexual Persons."* New York: Crossroad, 1988, 1–10; and Robert M. Baird and M. Katherine Baird, eds., *Homosexuality: Debating the Issues.* Amherst, N.Y.: Prometheus, 1995, 203–10; Remafedi, Gary, ed. *Death by Denial: Studies in Suicide in the Gay and Lesbian Teenager.* Boston, Mass.: Alyson, 1994; Rich, Adrienne. "Compulsory Heterosexuality and Lesbian Existence." *Signs* 5:4 (1980), 631–60. Reprinted in *Blood, Bread, and Poetry: Selected Prose 1979–1985.* New York: Norton, 1986, 23–75; and Henry Abelove, Michèle Aina Barale, and David M. Halperin, eds., *The Lesbian and Gay Studies Reader.* New York: Routledge, 1993, 227–54; Scruton, Roger. "Gay Reservations." In Michael Leahy and Dan Cohn-Sherbok, eds., *The Liberation Debate: Rights at Issue.* London: Routledge, 1996, 108–24; Scruton, Roger. "Sexual Morality and the Liberal Consensus." In *The Philosopher on Dover Beach—Essays.* Manchester, U.K.: Carcanet, 1990, 262–72; Sears, James T., and Walter L. Williams, eds. *Overcoming Heterosexism and Homophobia: Strategies That Work.* New York: Columbia University Press, 1997; Siker, Jeffrey S., ed. *Homosexuality in the Church: Both Sides of the Debate.* Louisville, Ky.: Westminster John Knox, 1994; Soble, Alan. Review of *Heterosexism: An Ethical Challenge*, by Patricia Beattie Jung and Ralph F. Smith. *Ethics* 105:4 (1995), 975–76; Sullivan, Andrew. *Love Undetectable: Reflections on Friendship, Sex, and Survival.* New York: Knopf, 1998.

HINDUISM. Hinduism is an ancient Indian tradition of thought made up of mythological, religious, and philosophical elements. Whether one takes Hinduism primarily as a repository of myths, a religion, or a philosophical tradition depends on which elements one chooses to emphasize.

The historical background of Hinduism is likewise unclear. One view is that the first records of Hindu thought come from an Indo-European people who seem to have migrated into the Indus valley about 1500 BCE. However, archaeological evidence going back to at least 2000 BCE suggests that elements of Hindu thought were already present in the Indus valley. This evidence partially consists of terra cotta figurines that seem connected to the origins of the Hindu cults of Śiva and Śakti. Further, there are also seals with a figure seated in what might be a yogic posture. Since both the Śiva and Śakti cults along with the practice of yoga and meditation are central features of Hindu religion and philosophy, some basic aspects of Hinduism might have had their roots in the ancient Indus valley civilization. A more recent view, which also suggests that Hinduism might have originated from more ancient traditions, is that the first Hindu texts can be traced to a mixing of two peoples: ruling families from the north of India and poets and seers from the south, whose distant maritime roots go back to South East Asia (Frawley). In addition to this ancient history, Hindu thought has also undergone several periods of distinctive development.

As a result, defining the exact essence of Hinduism is difficult. Clearly, however, Hinduism has something to do with the attempt to overcome suffering by acquiring knowledge, particularly of the self. This is also achieved with *karma*, or self-determination, and the following of one's *dharma*, or responsibility to uphold the cosmic and social orders (here is where the role of caste plays its role in Hindu thinking). This pursuit of knowledge and *dharma* is frequently connected to various forms of yoga or meditative and devotional practices. Following such a path enables one to achieve *mokṣa*, or liberation from the cycle of rebirth. Connected with this system of thought is an orientation to a pantheon of central gods and goddesses who can be understood in mythical, religious, or philosophical ways. These include Indra (the warrior god), Agni (the fire god), Śiva (the destroyer), Viṣṇu (the preserver), Brahmā (the creator), Pārvatī (Śiva's consort), Devī (the mother goddess), Kāma (god of desire), Rati (goddess of passion), and Kṛṣṇa (an incarnation of Viṣṇu).

One striking feature of Hindu thought, an element deeply woven into its mythology, religion, and philosophy, is eroticism. This is of such importance in Hindu thought that a separate branch of Indian scholarship (**Indian erotology**) developed early, at least by 400 CE, that dealt specifically with erotic theory and techniques. Of course, there are Hindu traditions of celibacy and asceticism, as when someone in the student *āśrama* (stage of life) avoids all forms of sexual contact. But even here the awareness of eroticism seems paramount; the celibate focuses on and seeks to control his sexual urges by channeling their energy in various directions. (See Doniger, *Asceticism*, on the close connection between asceticism and eroticism in Hinduism.)

Eroticism makes its first appearance in the earliest Hindu texts. In the *Ṛg Veda* (ca. 1200 BCE), the god Indra chooses his wife for her sensuality, while his wife, the most sexually yearning of women, celebrates the size of Indra's penis and speaks widely of his sexual abilities. Similarly, the god Agni pursues and sexually engages numerous young maidens, including his sister. In the later *Śatapatha-Brāhmaṇa* (ca. 600 BCE), an account is given of how the primal being Prajāpati (identified in later texts with Brahmā) desires and has **incest** with his daughter. This early mythological relation between eroticism and the gods is one that takes on religiophilosophical dimensions in the *Bṛhadāraṇyaka Upaniṣad* (ca.

400 BCE). Here we find Prajāpati creating woman to make a "firm basis" for his semen. Having created her, he places her "below" and worships her. This worshiping takes the form of having sexual intercourse with her. Thus, the *Upaniṣad* tells us "one should worship a woman, placing her below" (370).

Becoming more explicit about this connection between religious worship and sexual intercourse, the *Upaniṣad* then links sexual intercourse and the *Vājapeya* sacrifice (a Vedic rite involving drinking the juice of a hallucinogenic plant, "soma"). Here we are told of woman:

> Her lap is the [sacrificial] alter, her hair the [sacrificial] grass, her skin [within the organ] the lighted fire; the two labia of the vulva are the two stones of the soma-press. . . . He who, knowing this, practices sexual intercourse wins as great a world as is won through the Vājapeya sacrifice; he acquires for himself [the fruit of] the good deeds of the woman. But he who, without knowing this, practices sexual intercourse turns over to the woman his own good deeds. (371)

Thus, already at this early stage in Hindu thought erotic interaction takes on religious and metaphysical significance. Sexual intercourse is explicitly seen as a form of activity in which the man worships the woman. Further, through this worship a man gains special access to the merit of the woman's actions. Although the woman referred to here is not strictly a goddess or religious figure, still the primary sexual features of her body—her lap, pubic hair, vagina, vulva—are said to be the same as elements used in a religious offering. Consequently, sexual intercourse with her is equivalent to a religious rite.

Of course, the ideas here, like the ideas of many other ancient systems of thought, are expressed from a male perspective. This is especially evident when we are told that the man who fails to practice sexual intercourse in this reverential way turns over his own good deeds to the woman. Nevertheless, the important feature in this account, as far as one wants to understand the pervasive eroticism in Hindu thought, is the designation of eroticism as a religious practice imbued with metaphysical significance. Hindu thought is greatly composed of religious and metaphysical elements, and eroticism is, in Hindu eyes, fused with these elements. In this way eroticism pervades Hindu thought.

In the later *Purāṇas* (300 BCE–300 CE), texts of Hindu mythology interwoven with religious and philosophical meanings, various dimensions of eroticism are played out in the interactions of a variety of gods and goddesses. In what is called the "Śiva" cycle of these myths, we encounter the eroticism of Śiva and his consort Pārvatī, a god and goddess who made **love** for a thousand years. In one of these myths Dakṣa, a son of Brahmā, gives to Śiva in **marriage** his daughter Satī, an incarnation of Devī, who is later reborn as Pārvatī. Dakṣa, however, insults Śiva. This so infuriates Satī that she burns herself to death (*Śiva-Purāṇa*, 415–16). In a continuation of this myth, Śiva finds Satī's body and takes her on his shoulders, dancing in great sorrow and shedding many tears. This wild and tearful dance is of such cosmic proportions that it threatens the stability of the universe. Other gods finally intervene, entering Satī's body, cutting it up, and letting the pieces fall to the earth. Śiva then goes to the place where Satī's vulva fell and takes the form of a penis. With this, worldly harmony is reestablished (Doniger, *Hindu Mythology*, 250–51).

In another myth Śiva, naked and with an erection, wanders through the Pine Forest, dancing and begging with a skull. Coming upon the wives of the sages of the Pine Forest, he is overcome with desire and seduces them or, in another version, the wives pursue him. This angers the sages, who curse Śiva's penis, which falls off. The penis, landing on the ground, immediately grows to such an enormous size that it "pervaded the entire earth and enveloped the firmament" (*Skanda-Purāṇa*, 44). Neither Brahmā nor Viṣṇu could discover the top nor the root of the penis, which caused everything to merge in an instant. This awes and frightens the sages, who admit their ignorance and begin to worship Śiva's penis. In a related myth, Śiva leaves the Pine Forest and returns to Pārvatī. Full of burning desire, they immediately make love. Their sexual interaction is so powerful that the gods fear that off-spring conceived in this way would pose great danger to the world. They therefore send Agni (here the god of the erotic fire or the heat of sexual intercourse) to interrupt Śiva and Pārvatī's coitus. Pārvatī is furious and curses the god's wives so that they will be barren, likewise not producing offspring (*Brahma-Vaivarta Purāṇa*, 50–53).

In addition to eroticism, numerous other themes and meanings are contained in these myths, for example, **jealousy**, anger, and conception. Further, Śiva is not only erotic but also, strangely enough, ascetic. Thus, we find him naked, begging, and performing austere *tapas* or forms of asceticism. He is also the destroyer, which is why he carries a skull and, as we are told in other places, frequents cremation grounds, smearing himself with human ashes. Further, he is chaste, rejecting attempts by those who would seduce him. Neverthe-less, eroticism pervades his actions. The eroticism's meaning is revealed in the instability caused by the lack of sexual fulfillment. Thus, Śiva dances wildly with tears while bearing his consort's body. This also, of course, points to the loss of love and the sorrow of death. But the fact that Śiva seeks out Satī's vulva rather than, say, her heart or face, and that he turns himself into a penis rather than something else, suggests that the main point of the myth is the loss of sexual fulfillment. This is further suggested by the fact that peace is es-tablished in the universe only when the penis is again united with the vulva.

This meaning is echoed in the myth in which Śiva seduces the wives of the sages of the Pine Forest. Here, upon losing his penis, a massive upheaval takes place, once again threat-ening the order of the universe. This turmoil, the extent of which not even the gods can dis-cover, can be dealt with only by humans, the sages, worshiping the penis. This worshiping occurs, significantly, after both sexual fulfillment (the **seduction** of the wives of the sages) and after the penis has been cursed and castration occurs. Consequently, the myth suggests that even upon the fulfillment of **sexual desire**, the rejection of such desire (castration and cursing of the penis) leads to cataclysm. This upheaval can be overcome only by worship-ing the sex organs or, as it might also be put, an acceptance and veneration of sexuality as a central feature of human existence.

It is important to note that it is not only the penis that is worshiped in Hindu thought but also the vulva. Thus, the *Bṛhadāraṇyaka Upaniṣad* compares the vulva to the elements of the *Vājapeya* sacrifice. Also, although the places where Satī's tongue, nipples, and vulva are said to have fallen have become seats for holy pilgrimages in Hinduism, the most im-portant of these, Kāmarūpa in Assam, is where her vulva is said to have fallen. Here a cleft stone resembling a vulva is worshiped, and Satī's menstrual cycle is venerated by covering the stone with red powder. This Śaktism, or worship of the goddess, is also a powerful ele-ment in Hinduism. Those who partake of such worship are *Śaktas*, who celebrate *śakti*, the female energies. These energies can be the erotic, ferocious, or fertile aspects of the god-dess. Although there are many goddesses in Hinduism, they are generally considered as avatars of the Great Devī.

Moreover, the upheaval caused by lack of sexual fulfillment is not only an event for the male, for in one myth Pārvatī too becomes furious with the gods' interruption of her sexual pleasure. Although this myth contains the extra feature of conception—insofar as the gods try to prevent conception, and Pārvatī curses their wives with barrenness—her immediate frustration is clearly due to the disruption of her sexual play. This myth is significant also in demonstrating the power of sexual desire itself. Although destruction can result from the frustration of sexual desire, its fulfillment is such that it, too, can shake the world, not only through the power of sexual interaction but also by creating dangerous offspring. In sexual engagement the world as we experience it becomes threatened; we enter a state of deep vulnerability as our sense of time and space, and the distinction between self and other, become scattered in the fury of sexual desire (see Giles, chap. 2).

It might be tempting to see the eroticism in the mythology of Śiva and Pārvatī as merely a feature of this pair's own divine and highly erotic relationship. Such eroticism, however, is prevalent in many other myths and other literary forms. In the *Viṣṇu* and *Bhāgavata Purāṇas* (ca. 400 CE), for example, the youthful Kṛṣṇa, an avatar of Viṣṇu, sexually pursues the *gopīs*, the wives and daughters of the cowherds, through the forest of Vṛndāvana. These women are enraptured with him, melt in his amorous attentions, and make love with him under the moon in the warm autumnal night. The *Bhāgavata Purāṇa* brings the religious element into this myth by seeing the devotion and sexual surrender of the *gopī* to Kṛṣṇa as a model of *bhakti*, or the passionate devotion to god (*Bhāgavata Purāṇa*, 167–70, 359–66).

Moreover, the *Bhāgavata Purāṇa*, which was composed in the south of India, was influenced by the devotional practices and ideas of the indigenous Tamil culture. This culture thrived—having its own language, forms of love poetry, and worship of Murukan, a god of love and war—long before northern Brahmanical ideas arrived. Tamil Cankam poetry, as it came to be called, is distinctive in its focus on the personal and emotional aspects of erotic love. This literary focus on the erotic was easily absorbed by the northern system of thought and helped to pave the way for *bhakti* (see Dehejia; Hart).

The *Purāṇa*'s interpretation of the women's love for Kṛṣṇa as religious devotion is strengthened by the references to Kṛṣṇa in the *Bhagavad Gītā* (ca. 200 BCE) section of the epic poem *Mahābārata* (compiled between 1000 BCE and 100 CE). Here Kṛṣṇa is not merely an avatar of a god, appearing as youthful lover, but rather is the supreme incarnation of the godhead. Thus, Kṛṣṇa declares, "I am the source of everything, and everything proceeds from me; filled with my existence, wise men realizing this are devoted to me" (Miller, 45 [chap. 10]). This devotion, however, contrasts sharply with the devotion extolled in the *Purāṇa*. In the *Bhagavad Gītā*, Kṛṣṇa says of the person who would be dear to him, "He does not rejoice or hate, grieve or feel desire," while in the *Purāṇa* the women are swept away with sexual desire for Kṛṣṇa (Miller, 49 [chap. 12]).

In the *Purāṇa*, then, as in the *Bṛhadāraṇyaka Upaniṣad*, we have a picture of sexual intercourse as a religious rite. In the *Upaniṣad* that rite is worship; in the *Purāṇa* it is devotion, which can also be viewed as worship. The difference is that while in the *Upaniṣad* the man worships the woman through sexual intercourse, in the *Purāṇa* the woman worships the man. Together, these two accounts make a religious rite of sexual intercourse for both the male and the female.

Further, in both accounts eroticism occurs at two levels: One is the metaphysical or divine level (depending on how one interprets the myth); the other is the human level, which has a special relationship to the other level. Thus, in the *Upaniṣad*, the primal being creates a woman and worships her through sexual intercourse. This is the metaphysical or divine level. The *Upaniṣad* then relates this sexual intercourse and human sexual intercourse by proclaiming that men should worship women the same way. This is the human level. Likewise, in the *Purāṇa*, on the metaphysical or divine level the women have sexual intercourse with the god Kṛṣṇa. The human level appears when the *Purāṇa* makes this lovemaking a model of *bhakti*.

The Hindu tendency to see different levels in eroticism enters a new phase in Jayadeva's love poem *Gītagovinda* (1200), a work in the *kāvya* or Sanskrit love poetry tradition. Here Kṛṣṇa again appears as a young lover chasing the *gopī*. In this poem, however, something new enters the story, namely, the female character Rādhā. What is special about Rādhā's relationship to Kṛṣṇa is that not only does she burn with desire for Kṛṣṇa, but also Kṛṣṇa burns with desire for her. Despite Kṛṣṇa's purported divinity, the relationship that unfolds between Kṛṣṇa and Rādhā takes on a deeply human quality. Here Kṛṣṇa is also immersed in human desires. In the closing sections of the poem, when Kṛṣṇa and Rādhā at last have sexual intercourse, Kṛṣṇa becomes overwhelmed in "the battle mixed with love-play." "Held-captive by her arms, pressed by the weight of her breasts, pierced by her finger-nails, the cup of his lower lip bitten by her teeth, crushed by the slope of her hips, bent down by his hand on her hair, crazed by the trickling flow of honey from her lower lip, the lovely beloved somehow obtained delight" (Siegel, 282).

In Jayadeva's reworking of this myth there is little to distinguish a level of eroticism that differs from the human level. The eroticism displayed by Kṛṣṇa and Rādhā is not a divine act that human beings are encouraged to imitate, nor is it obviously a symbol of the devotion human beings should entertain toward a god. Rather, it is simply an account of the unfolding of human erotic desire in all its "heated-pain of love," as Jayadeva puts it. The only religious element remaining in the poem is Kṛṣṇa's identity as a god. Yet this is enough to suggest that something deeper than our immediate awareness of **sexual activity** and erotic pleasure—perhaps an existential need—is taking place in human eroticism (see Giles, chap. 6).

About the time that the *Viṣṇu* and *Bhāgavata Purāṇas* and the idea of *bhakti* were starting to circulate, another development in Hindu thought was taking place: This is the way of **Tantrism**. Tantrism is an esoteric body of thought and practice that finds expression not only in Hinduism but also in other Asian traditions. In its Hindu version, Tantrism is concerned with acquiring various powers and attaining supreme bliss through the practice of yoga and various rituals, including goddess worship and veneration of the goddess in individual females. (Here we see the Śaktism roots of Tantra.) One such practice is *maithuna*, or sexual intercourse. Although the idea of bringing sexual activity into the realm of the religious and metaphysical was not new to Hinduism, Tantric thought was distinct in advocating sexual activity as a way to attain higher states of consciousness. In the Vaiṣṇava Sahajiyā Tantric sect, for example, our original state was seen to be *sahaja*, or cosmic unity and bliss, something that, living in the everyday world of *saṃsāra*, we fail to realize. The Tantric practices of this tradition are designed to enable us to regain an awareness of this primordial unity and bliss.

In the late Vaiṣṇava Sahajiyā Tantric work *Amṛtaratnāvalī* (*The Necklace of Immortality*; ca. 1650), sexual interaction is specifically put forward as a path to this attainment. Here Mukunda-dāsa, the work's author, tells us that "divine love came into being through the churning of the Female Partner during intercourse" and that "continually churning the Female Partner produces the essence of the Female Partner [i.e., the goddess]. Deeply entranced day and night, a state of wonder develops." Referring to the story of Kṛṣṇa, the author says, "the Female Partner and Divine Essence will lead you to the heaven of Goloka and Vṛndāvana [where Kṛṣṇa had sexual intercourse with the *gopī*]. . . . You should carefully realize the Female Partner in the Pond of lust. Through such practices with a Female Partner, you will attain the Primordial Cosmic Substance" (Hayes, 324–25). That Mukunda-dāsa says to *carefully* realize the female partner is important. For this implies that the advocated sexual intercourse is to be done in a specially attuned state of awareness. Grasping at and pursuing sexual intercourse in a careless way (perhaps for nonsexual reasons) will not lead to consciousness of cosmic unity and bliss (what might be called sexual fulfillment). Again, although this particular text focuses on the male, other texts affirm that *maithuna* will lead to the realization of cosmic unity and bliss for both male and female.

Although the Tantric and earlier Hindu approaches to sexuality diverge, nevertheless there is an underlying unity: The basis of the Tantric tradition is already present in the *Bṛhadāraṇyaka Upaniṣad*: Here sexual intercourse is practiced as a religious rite. What the Tantric tradition does is to actively pursue sexual intercourse practiced in this way.

See also Bestiality; Buddhism; Chinese Philosophy; Desire, Sexual; Existentialism; Freud, Sigmund; Freudian Left, The; Gnosticism; Indian Erotology; Jainism; Manichaeism; Plato; Tantrism

REFERENCES

The *Bhāgavata-Purāṇa*, part 1. Trans. Ganesh Vasudeo Tagare. [*Ancient Indian Tradition and Mythology Series*, vol. 7] Delhi, India: Motilal Banarsidass, 1979; *The Brahma-Vaivarta Purāṇa*, part 1. Trans. Rajendra Nath Sen. [*Sacred Books of the Hindus*, vol. 24] Allahabad, India: Panni Office, Bhuvaneshwari Ashram, 1920; Dehejia, Vidya. *Antal and Her Path of Love: Poems of a Woman Saint from South India*. New York: State University of New York Press, 1990; Doniger [O'Flaherty], Wendy. *Asceticism and Eroticism in the Mythology of Śiva*. Oxford, U.K.: Oxford University Press, 1973. Paperback reprint, *Siva: The Erotic Ascetic* (1981); Doniger [O'Flaherty], Wendy. *Hindu Mythology*. Harmondsworth, U.K.: Penguin, 1975; Frawley, David. *The Rig Veda and the History of India* [*Rig Veda Bharata Itihasa*]. New Delhi, India: Aditya Prakashan, 2001; Giles, James. *The Nature of Sexual Desire*. Westport, Conn.: Praeger, 2004; Hart, George. *The Relationship between Tamil and Classical Sanskrit Literature*. Wiesbaden, Ger.: Otto Harrassowitz, 1976; Hayes, Glen A. "The Necklace of Immortality: A Seventeenth-Century Vaiṣnava Sahajiya Text." In David Gordon White, ed., *Tantra in Practice*. Princeton, N.J.: Princeton University Press, 2000, 308–25; Miller, Barbara Stoller, trans. *Bhagavad Gītā*. In John M. Koller and Patricia Koller, eds., *A Sourcebook in Asian Philosophy*. Upper Saddle River, N.J.: Prentice Hall, 1991, 33–50; *Śatapatha-Brāhmaṇa*. Trans. Julius Eggeling. [*Sacred Books of the East*, vol. 12] Delhi, India: Motilal Banarsidass, 1967; Siegel, Lee. *Sacred and Profane Dimensions of Love in Indian Traditions as Exemplified in the Gītagovinda of Jayadeva*. Delhi, India: Oxford University Press, 1978; *The Śiva-Purāṇa*. Trans. Board of Scholars. [*Ancient Indian Tradition and Mythology Series*, vol. 1] Delhi, India: Motilal Banarsidass, 1970; *The Skanda-Purāṇa*, part 1. Trans. G. V. Tagare. [*Ancient Indian Tradition and Mythology Series*, vol. 49] Delhi, India: Motilal Banarsidass, 1992; *The Upanishads*, vol. 3: *Aitareya and Brihadaranyaka*. Trans. Swami Nikhilananda. New York: Bonanza Books, 1956; *Vedic Hymns*, part 1. Trans. Max Muller. [*Sacred Books of the East*, vol. 32] Delhi, India: Motilal Banarsidass, 1967; *Vedic Hymns*, part 2. Trans. Herman Oldenberg. [*Sacred Books of the East*, vol. 46] Delhi, India: Motilal Banarsidass, 1967.

James Giles

ADDITIONAL READING

Baird, Robert D. "Hinduism." In Ruth Chadwick, ed., *Encyclopedia of Applied Ethics*, vol. 2. San Diego, Calif.: Academic Press, 1998, 571–82; Doniger, Wendy. *Splitting the Difference: Gender and Myth in Ancient Greece and India*. Chicago, Ill.: University of Chicago Press, 1999; Dynes, Wayne R., and Stephen Donaldson, eds. *Asian Homosexuality*. New York: Taylor and Francis, 1992; Giles, James. *No Self to Be Found: The Search for Personal Identity*. Lanham, Md.: University Press of America, 1997; Giles, James. "Sartre, Sexual Desire, and Relations with Others." In James Giles, ed., *French Existentialism: Consciousness, Ethics, and Relations with Others*. Amsterdam, Holland: Rodopi, 1999, 155–73; Giles, James. "A Theory of Love and Sexual Desire." *Journal for the Theory of Social Behaviour* 24:4 (1994), 339–57; Goss, Robert E. "Hinduism." In Timothy F. Murphy, ed., *Reader's Guide to Lesbian and Gay Studies*. Chicago, Ill.: Fitzroy Dearborn, 2000, 281–82; Hardy,

Friedhelm. *Viraha Bhakti.* Delhi, India: Oxford University Press, 1983; Klostermaier, Klaus K. (1989) *A Survey of Hinduism,* 2nd ed. New York: State University of New York Press, 1994; Macfie, John Mandeville. *Myths and Legends of India: An Introduction to the Study of Hinduism.* Edinburgh, Scot.: T. and T. Clark, 1924; Miller, Barbara Stoller. *The Bhagavad Gītā.* New York: Bantam Books, 1986; Nanda, Serena. (1990) *Neither Man nor Woman: The Hijras of India,* 2nd ed. Belmont, Calif.: Wadsworth, 1998; Rukmani, T. S. *A Critical Study of the Bhāgavata Purāṇa (with Special Reference to Bhakti).* Varanasi, India: Chowkhamba Sanskrit Series Office, 1970; Sharma, Arvind. "Homosexuality and Hinduism." In Arlene Swidler, ed., *Homosexuality and World Religions.* Valley Forge, Pa.: Trinity Press, 1993, 47–80; Thadani, Giti. "The Politics of Identities and Languages: Lesbian Desire in Ancient and Modern India." In Evelyn Blackwood and Saskia E. Wieringa, eds., *Female Desires: Same-Sex Relations and Transgender Practices across Cultures.* New York: Columbia University Press, 1999, 67–90; Thadani, Giti. *Sakhiyani: Lesbian Desire in Ancient and Modern India.* New York: Cassell, 1996; Thomas, Paul. *Epics, Myths and Legends of India: A Comprehensive Survey of the Sacred Lore of the Hindus, Buddhists and Jains,* 11th ed. Bombay, India: D. B. Taraporevala, n.d.; Vanita, Ruth, ed. *Queering India: Same-Sex Love and Eroticism in Indian Culture and Society.* New York: Routledge, 2002; Vanita, Ruth, and Saleem Kidwai, eds. *Same-Sex Love in India: Readings from Literature and History.* New York: St. Martin's Press, 2000.

HOBBES, THOMAS (1588–1679). One of the most famous passages in Western philosophy, right up there alongside **Ludwig Wittgenstein**'s (1889–1951) *Tractatus Logico-Philosophicus* 7.0, is a description "Of the Natural Condition of Mankind as concerning their Felicity and Misery":

> Whatsoever therefore is consequent to a time of war, where every man is enemy to every man, the same consequent to the time wherein men live without other security than what their own strength and their own invention shall furnish them withal. In such condition there is no place for industry, because the fruit thereof is uncertain: and consequently no culture of the earth; no navigation, nor use of the commodities that may be imported by sea; no commodious building; no instruments of moving and removing such things as require much force; no knowledge of the face of the earth; no account of time; no arts; no letters; no society; [no latté; no pantyhose; no Italian opera;] and which is worst of all, continual fear, and danger of violent death; and the life of man, solitary, poor, nasty, brutish, and short. (Hobbes, *Leviathan,* part 1, chap. 13; 100)

Charlotte Becker once blurted out to His Nibs what she thought **sexual activity** would look like from a Hobbesian perspective. "Of *course,*" she nimbly quipped, "a sexual encounter between a woman and a man"—even in civil society, let alone the State of Nature—"would be nasty, brutish, and short" (unless you were poor, in which case it would certainly be solitary). This picture of Hobbesian sexuality is actually not far from the truth (think about its non-Augustinian implications for Adam and Eve), despite the attempts of recent commentators— Simon Blackburn and Jean Hampton (1954–1996), in particular—to rehabilitate Hobbes as a wholesome philosopher of sex and to make him into a kind of cult hero. When all is said and done, Hobbes might come off looking good (which is not difficult) compared with **Immanuel Kant** (1724–1804), for whom the sexual act was akin to sucking a lemon dry, besides being essentially objectifying (*Lectures,* Ak 27:384–85). But there is, in Hobbes, the notion that sexual interactions are employed by a person to rejoice pleasurably in the expression of his (or her?) power. This idea will get him muffled cheers from some students of **Friedrich Nietzsche** (1844–1900) and **Sigmund Freud** (1856–1939) and reproachful boos from many feminists.

Why is there, in the State of Nature, a war of every person against every other person? Each person desires power; and each person fears death. Such are the basic ingredients of human nature. Moving from the State of Nature into a well-regulated civil society makes life much less "solitary, poor, nasty, brutish, and short" by eliminating random violence, feuds, vigilante justice, and fighting over food, shelter, and a piece of the river from which to drink and in which to bathe and swim. The fear of death remains, even if it no longer screams itself in our consciousness, yet we are able to relax, for the most part, while sleeping in our beds, driving to and from work, shopping at the mall, and hunting wild boar. In addition to the conspicuously reliable police and courts and prisons (the Leviathan), organized religion—one beneficiary of civil society—helps alleviate the fear of death, too. (See Freud's *Future of an Illusion*. And on giving up the full and repeated sexual satisfaction of the State of Nature for the sake of establishing and maintaining civilized society, see his *Civilization and Its Discontents*.) The desire for power remains as well, even if repressed, sublimated, controlled, and transformed into socially useful energy and labor. In that quiescence, it lurks, waiting for the right, propitious, safe time to express itself, knowing by calculation whether *here* and *now* it will be successful and satisfied. There is no reason to suppose that in the arena of sexual interaction the fundamental ingredients of human nature, the fear of death and the desire for power, will be altogether absent, and that there would not be any free-riders.

Frances Ferguson blandly reads "Sadean pornography" (in particular) as affirming that "there would be no sexual pleasure without the demonstration of power" (26). But one need not be even 20 percent of the **Marquis de Sade** (1740–1814) to make that observation. Consider, for example, the Slovenian disciple of **Jacques Lacan** (1901–1981), Slavoj Žižek, who, it must be admitted, does not argue very cogently for his thesis:

> [S]exuality as such (an intersubjective sexual relationship) always involves a relationship of power: there is no neutral symmetrical sexual relationship/exchange, undistorted by power. The ultimate proof is the dismal failure of the "politically correct" endeavour to free sexuality of power: to define the rules of "proper" sexual rapport in which partners should indulge in sex only on account of their mutual, purely sexual, attraction, excluding any "pathological" factor (power, financial coercion, etc.): if we subtract from sexual rapport the element of "asexual" (physical, financial . . .) coercion, which distorts the "pure" sexual attraction, we may lose sexual attraction itself. In other words, the problem is that the very element which seems to bias and corrupt pure sexual rapport . . . may function as the very phantasmic support of sexual attraction— in a way, sex as such is pathological. (72)

"Sex as such is pathological"—a sentiment also held, for their own reasons, by Kant, Freud ("Universal Tendency"), and **Andrea Dworkin** ([1946–2005], 122 ff.). We get the same sort of unsettling message from existentialist philosopher Jean-Paul Sartre (1905–1980):

> [S]adism and masochism are the two reefs on which desire may founder— whether I surpass my troubled disturbance toward an appropriation of the Other's flesh or, intoxicated with my own trouble, pay attention only to my flesh and ask nothing of the Other except that he should be the look which aids

> me in realizing my flesh. It is because of this inconstancy on the part of desire
> and its perpetual oscillation between these two perils that "normal" sexuality is
> commonly designated as "sadistic-masochistic." (*Being and Nothingness*, part 3,
> chap. 3, sec. 2)

But one need not be a Sadean, in whole or in part, nor must one appraise sex as pathological, to insist on the role of power:

> [I]t's the radical inappropriateness that makes lust lust. . . . [I]n sex there is no
> point of absolute stasis. There is no sexual equality and there can be no sexual
> equality, certainly not one where the allotments are equal, the male quotient
> and the female quotient in perfect balance. There's no way to negotiate metri-
> cally this wild thing. It's not fifty-fifty like a business transaction. It's the chaos
> of eros we're talking about, the radical destabilization that is its excitement.
> You're back in the woods with sex. You're back in the bog. What it is is trading
> dominance, perpetual imbalance. You're going to rule out dominance? You're
> going to rule out yielding? The dominating is the flint, it strikes the spark, it
> sets it going. (Philip Roth, 17–18)

It is one of the confusing things about late-twentieth-century and early-twenty-first-century
thought about sexuality that this passage could almost have been written by the "unmodified" feminist **Catharine MacKinnon**: "If there is no inequality, no violation, no dominance, no force, there is no sexual arousal"—for men, she means (211). Power, dominance,
and inequality either corrupt sex or are an erotic blessing and natural to the phenomenon.
Which is it for Hobbes?

Hobbes's account of sexuality does not appear in *Leviathan* but in a shorter and lesser
known work, "Human Nature":

> The appetite which men call *lust*, and the fruition that appertaineth thereunto,
> is a *sensual* pleasure, but *not only* that; there is in it also a delight of the mind:
> for it consisteth of two appetites together, to *please*, and to *be pleased*; and the
> delight men take in delighting, is not sensual, but a pleasure or joy of the mind
> consisting in the imagination of the power they have so much to please. (Chap.
> 9, sec. 15; 47–48)

Lust or, we may presume, the appetite of **sexual desire**, has two components, or is composed of two appetites "together," the appetite or desire "to be pleased" and the appetite or
desire "to please." We can immediately see why it might be thought that Hobbes has hit
upon an especially wholesome account of sexuality. All we have to do is to contrast his
dual appetite view of sexual desire with a common and commonsensical mono-appetite
view, as found, for example, in an essay by Alan Goldman. Sexual desire is, on his account,
the "desire for contact with another person's body and for the pleasure which such contact
produces," *period* (268). What we want, first and foremost, in attempting to satisfy sexual
desire, is our own pleasure, which results from the physical contact we have with another
person's body. There is no component Hobbesian desire "to please" in Goldmanian sexual
desire.

Goldman realizes that something may be thought missing here, but he relegates the possibly missing factor to the realm of the moral. "Giving pleasure" to the other person and
"ensuring that the pleasures of the act are mutual" (283), for Goldman, are that which make
sexual activity morally permissible (from the Kantian perspective he embraces). Goldman,

we might say, "admit[s] the most damaging facts" about sexual desire (Baumrin, 301)—that even if it is not by its nature selfish, it is at least self-centered, self-interested. As a result, sexuality must be redeemed by obligating any person X who wants to satisfy sexual desire to attempt to bring pleasure to the other person Y whose body is the source of sexual pleasure for X. Goldman's account allows logical space for the *bad lover*, the one who cares only about his or her own pleasure and not a whit for the pleasure of the other, and Goldman's version of Kant admonishes us not to *be* this bad lover. Sade, more radically, *encourages* us to be this bad lover and even asserts (which contains some truth) that the other's pleasure is an impediment to our own (343–44). In contrast to both Goldman and Sade, Hobbes, with his dual appetite account of sexual desire, seems to rule out, as logically impossible, this bad lover, the one who desires his or her own pleasure but does not desire to please the other. (Or, on his view, those who do not desire to please the other do not experience sexual desire at all, even if they desire their own pleasure.) Further, Hobbes's account appears to solve straightaway or, better, altogether avoids Goldman's moral issue, for he builds the desire to please the other person right into sexual desire itself, and so sexual desire is naturally, automatically moral. This appearance, however, is deceptive.

Without roaming farther into the details of the passage in which Hobbes provides his account of sexual desire as a dual appetite (doing so will come later), we can already see that neither Goldman, with his mono-appetite account of sexual desire buttressed by the Kantian demand for reciprocity, nor Hobbes, who builds the desire to please the other into sexual desire, escapes or has solved the moral problem. Jean Hampton, too, falls into the trap when she writes (in praising Hobbes), that "when sex is as much about pleasing another as it is about pleasing oneself, it certainly doesn't involve using another as a means and actually incorporates the idea of respect and concern for another's needs" (147). This is not true. Merely pleasing the other does not resolve the moral problem, for much depends on *why* one pleases the other. The mistake is made frequently. Consider David Archard's example:

> If Harry has sex with Sue solely for the purpose of deriving sexual gratification from the encounter and with no concern for what Sue might get out of it, if Harry pursues this end single-mindedly and never allows himself to think of how it might be for Sue, then Harry treats Sue merely as a means. . . . If, by contrast, Harry derives pleasure from his sex with Sue but also strives to attend to Sue's pleasure and conducts the encounter in a way that is sensitive to her needs [as in Goldman], then Harry does not treat Sue merely as a means. (41)

To the contrary, whether X in pleasing Y is acting in a morally permissible way that does not use Y in a manner to which Kant would object depends on the reason X "strives" to provide pleasure for Y. The point is that there is a second type of *bad lover*, one that cuts across both Goldman's and Hobbes's accounts of sexual desire. This is the lover whose motive for producing pleasure for the other is morally suspicious or even wicked.

X's desire that Y experience pleasure may be demonic and manipulative: X wants to *control* the other, by giving pleasure to Y; even worse, X wants to make the other person one's *slave*, by giving pleasure to Y; X wants to make the other *dependent*, by giving pleasure to Y, who comes to require more of the same; X wants to make the other *return pleasure*, even if she would rather not, by giving pleasure to Y (creating a felt obligation to reciprocate); X wants to create desire in the other, by giving pleasure to Y, and then to exert power over the one reduced to *vulnerable* flesh by his or her desire; X wants to relish in the pleasure of Y's *downfall* (Morgan, 382), having seduced Y against Y's better judgment by providing irresistible pleasure. What **Søren Kierkegaard** (1813–1855) did to Regine Olsen (1822–1904) (see "Diary of the Seducer"), or what the devilish female does, flirting with the naive male who is ignorant that he is being teased, is small potatoes compared with what is possible for the morally demented provider of sexual pleasure.

Now, Hobbes *does* say something (as we have seen) about the motive of the X who produces pleasure for Y, and it is not pretty: "[T]he delight men take in delighting, is not sensual, but a pleasure or joy of the mind consisting in the imagination of the power they have so much to please." The human being who, for Hobbes, seeks and exerts power by his or her nature seeks and exerts power in the sexual act as well. That it is a power "to please," to give pleasure, does not entail that it is benevolent. Thus Blackburn inexplicably asserts that the *very same* Hobbes of the "war of all against all . . . *nevertheless*" saw in sexual relations "a joint symphony of pleasure" and "pure mutuality" (87–88; emphasis added), as if Hobbes's psychological egoism disappears between the sheets.

Although *occasionally* a sentimentalist, Robert Nozick (1938–2002) can be counted on to call the Hobbesian spade a spade: "Pleasing another feels best when it is an accomplishment, a surmountable challenge. Consequently, an orgasm is less satisfying to the giving partner when it comes too early or too late" (65). What a burden to put on Y, to attain orgasm at precisely the right time for the X who is trying to produce it!—so as not to damage his poor, solitary, brutish, vulnerable ego. **Irving Singer**, who is *very often* a sentimentalist, also calls the spade a spade: "A man who is pleasuring a woman . . . gives her pleasures in the strict sense of that word, but he himself may experience simply the enjoyment of knowing that his amatory efforts are succeeding" (73). "*I* did it. Me! *I* did it!" declares the triumphant male to himself, exalting in his Hobbesian power to please and hearing in this internal dialogue his partner enthusiastically agree: "Yes you did, *big boy!*" (If he did not really do it, she says it anyway, in the external dialogue.) Singer, probing deeper into the matter than Nozick, proceeds to make a fine point: "[P]eople do not ordinarily enjoy knowing that they are giving pleasure unless their physical gestures—the actual means by which the giving occurs—are enjoyable in themselves" (74). The pleasure of the giving of pleasure is contingent on the getting, which is what we should have expected from a Hobbesian account of sexuality. Where is Blackburn's "pure mutuality"? The Hungarian novelist Stephen Vizinczey also cannot find it: "Paola . . . burst out unexpectedly. 'You men are all vain monkeys. You don't enjoy your own orgasm. The only thing you really want is to make a woman go off with a big bang' " (184).

The motive of the Hobbesian lover X in providing pleasure for Y is to celebrate X's own power. X is on a "nasty, brutish" ego trip—or he is just a silly goose: X wants to be esteemed by Y so that X can esteem himself. X is bursting with **Jean-Jacques Rousseau's** (1712–1778) *amour propre* (see Rapaport, 195–97). Were Y *not* to have an orgasm, X would bemoan X's ineffectual calisthenics sooner than Y's frustration. Thus Hobbes is a champion of the (masculine or feminine) sexual performance principle. Hampton, as Blackburn does, shies away from the self-centered, self-interested nature of Hobbesian sexual desire. The "spin of the last phrase [in Hobbes's account of sexual desire]," she remarks, is "vaguely egoistic" (155n.61). Vaguely? What did she expect from Hobbes—warm compassion and selfless generosity? That otherwise eminently astute philosophers as Hampton and Blackburn would allow (or help) Hobbes to pull the wool over their eyes is as amusing as it is baffling. Maybe they should have consulted the Sunday funnies. Hobbes once said to Calvin that he preferred his meals alive and running—it made eating so much more delightful.

See also Activity, Sexual; Completeness, Sexual; Ethics, Sexual; Existentialism; Feminism, Liberal; Freudian Left, The; Hegel, G.W.F., Hume, David; Kant, Immanuel; Kierkegaard, Søren; MacKinnon, Catharine; Nagel, Thomas; Nietzsche, Friedrich; Rape, Acquaintance and Date; Russell, Bertrand; Sade, Marquis de; Sadomasochism; Schopenhauer, Arthur; Seduction

REFERENCES

Archard, David. *Sexual Consent.* Boulder, Colo.: Westview, 1998; Baumrin, Bernard. (1975) "Sexual Immorality Delineated." In Robert B. Baker and Frederick A. Elliston, eds., *Philosophy and Sex*, 2nd ed. Buffalo, N.Y.: Prometheus, 1984, 300–311; Blackburn, Simon. *Lust: The Seven Deadly Sins.* New York: Oxford University Press and New York Public Library, 2004; Dworkin, Andrea. *Intercourse.* New York: Free Press, 1987; Ferguson, Frances. *Pornography, the Theory: What Utilitarianism Did to Action.* Chicago, Ill.: University of Chicago Press, 2004; Freud, Sigmund. (1930) *Civilization and Its Discontents.* In *The Standard Edition of the Complete Psychological Works of Sigmund Freud*, vol. 21. Trans. James Strachey. London: Hogarth Press, 1953–1974, 57–145; Freud, Sigmund. (1927) *The Future of an Illusion.* In *The Standard Edition of the Complete Psychological Works of Sigmund Freud*, vol. 21. Trans. James Strachey. London: Hogarth Press, 1953–1974, 5–56; Freud, Sigmund. (1912) "On the Universal Tendency to Debasement in the Sphere of Love." In *The Standard Edition of the Complete Psychological Works of Sigmund Freud*, vol. 11. Trans. James Strachey. London: Hogarth Press, 1953–1974, 179–90; Goldman, Alan. "Plain Sex." *Philosophy and Public Affairs* 6:3 (1977), 267–87; Hampton, Jean. "Defining Wrong and Defining Rape." In Keith Burgess-Jackson, ed., *A Most Detestable Crime: New Philosophical Essays on Rape.* New York: Oxford University Press, 1999, 118–56; Hobbes, Thomas. (1640, 1650) "Human Nature, or the Fundamental Elements of Policy." In *The English Works of Thomas Hobbes*, vol. IV. Ed. Sir William Molesworth. Aalen, Ger.: Scientia Verlag Aalen, 1966, 1–76; Hobbes, Thomas. (1651) *Leviathan, Or the Matter, Forme and Power of a Commonwealth Ecclesiastical and Civil.* Ed. Michael Oakeshott. 1962. New York: Touchstone/Simon and Schuster, 1997; Kant, Immanuel. (ca. 1762–1794) *Lectures on Ethics.* Trans. Peter Heath. Ed. Peter Heath and J. B. Schneewind. Cambridge: Cambridge University Press, 1997; Kierkegaard, Søren. (1843) "Diary of the Seducer." In *Either/Or*, vol. 1. Trans. David F. Swenson and Lillian M. Swenson (1944). Rev. Howard A. Johnson. Princeton, N.J.: Princeton University Press, 1959, 297–440; MacKinnon, Catharine A. *Toward a Feminist Theory of the State.* Cambridge, Mass.: Harvard University Press, 1989; Morgan, Seiriol. "Dark Desires." *Ethical Theory and Moral Practice* 6:4 (2003), 377–410; Nozick, Robert. "Sexuality." In *The Examined Life.* New York: Simon and Schuster, 1989, 61–67; Rapaport, Elizabeth. "On the Future of Love: Rousseau and the Radical Feminists." *Philosophical Forum* 5:1–2 (1973–1974), 185–205; Roth, Philip. *The Dying Animal.* Boston, Mass.: Houghton Mifflin, 2001; Sade, The Marquis de. *Justine, Philosophy in the Bedroom, and Other Writings.* Trans. Richard Seaver and Austryn Wainhouse. New York: Grove Press, 1965; Sartre, Jean-Paul. (1943) *Being and Nothingness: An Essay on Phenomenological Ontology.* Trans. Hazel E. Barnes. New York: Philosophical Library, 1956; Singer, Irving. *Sex: A Philosophical Primer.* Lanham, Md.: Rowman and Littlefield, 2001; Vizinczey, Stephen. *In Praise of Older Women: The Amorous Recollections of András Vajda.* New York: Ballantine, 1967; Wittgenstein, Ludwig. (1912) *Tractatus Logico-Philosophicus.* Trans. D. F. Pears and B. F. McGuinness. New York: Routledge, 1961; Žižek, Slavoj. *The Plague of Fantasies.* London: Verso, 1997.

Alan Soble

ADDITIONAL READING

Baumrin, Bernard. "Sexual Immorality Delineated." In Robert B. Baker and Frederick A. Elliston, eds., *Philosophy and Sex*, 1st ed. Buffalo, N.Y.: Prometheus, 1975, 116–28. Reprinted in P&S2 (300–311); Blackburn, Simon. "Sex." In *The Oxford Dictionary of Philosophy.* Oxford, U.K.: Oxford University Press, 1994, 349; Gilbert, Paul. "Power Struggles." In *Human Relationships: A Philosophical Introduction.* Oxford, U.K.: Blackwell, 1991, 32–55; Goldman, Alan. "Plain Sex." *Philosophy and Public Affairs* 6:3 (1977), 267–87. Reprinted in HS (103–23); POS1 (119–38); POS2

(73–92); POS3 (39–55); POS4 (39–55); Hobbes, Thomas. (1640) *The Elements of Law Natural and Politic*. [Part 1: "Human Nature"; Chap. 9: "Of the Passions of the Mind"; sec. 15] <www.ecn.bris.ac.uk/het/hobbes/elelaw> and <cepa.newschool.edu/het/profiles/hobbes.htm> [accessed 2 February 2005]; MacKinnon, Catharine A. "Desire and Power: A Feminist Perspective." In Cary Nelson and Lawrence Grossberg, eds., *Marxism and the Interpretation of Culture*. Urbana: University of Illinois Press, 1988, 105–21; Pateman, Carole. (1989) " 'God Hath Ordained to Man a Helper': Hobbes, Patriarchy, and Conjugal Right." In Mary Lyndon Shanley and Carole Pateman, eds., *Feminist Interpretations and Political Theory*. University Park: Pennsylvania State University Press, 1991, 53–73; Rapaport, Elizabeth. "On the Future of Love: Rousseau and the Radical Feminists." *Philosophical Forum* 5:1–2 (1973–1974), 185–205. Reprinted in POS1 (369–88); Thurman, Judith. "Sentimental Re-education." [Review of *Lust*, by Simon Blackburn] *The New Yorker* (16 and 23 February 2004), 195–97.

HOMOSEXUAL MARRIAGE. *See* Marriage, Same-Sex

HOMOSEXUALITY, ETHICS OF. Homosexuality, like sexuality in general, provides the occasion for many ethical issues to arise: issues regarding, for example, honesty, commitment, fidelity, chastity, and benevolence. While most of these issues arise in both heterosexual and homosexual contexts (as well as in nonsexual contexts), some are more relevant for homosexuality—for example, whether revealing a person's **sexual orientation** to others, thereby "outing" the person, is morally permissible or even morally required (see the essays in Murphy, *Gay Ethics*, 27–146). Yet despite the large variety of ethical issues connected with homosexuality *qua* sexuality, most ethical discussions of homosexuality focus on whether homosexual **sexual activity** is morally permissible. This focus reflects the fact that homosexual conduct has been morally condemned in many societies throughout history and remains controversial. At the same time, moral opposition to homosexuality seems to be losing favor, especially among younger generations in the West.

Those who argue morally in favor of homosexual relationships typically contend that such relationships promote or realize several important and familiar goods, including pleasure, mutual affection, and emotional fulfillment. Although these goods can be achieved nonsexually, sexual relationships seem to realize them in a distinctive or especially powerful way. This approach thus places the burden of proof on anyone who condemns homosexual relationships in which these goods exist. This burden is especially great if the persons are incapable of having satisfying heterosexual relationships, for it seems cruel and unjust to foreclose the possibility of romantic fulfillment to anyone in the absence of strong reasons for doing so (see Vacek). This last point raises the issue of the voluntariness of sexual orientation, which merits a brief discussion.

One might argue that if sexual orientation is involuntary, then homosexual conduct is morally permissible. But this argument conflates sexual orientation (a disposition or set of desires) with sexual conduct, and the voluntariness of the latter is not in question. Further, even if sexual orientation is involuntary, opponents of homosexuality could argue that **sexual desire** for persons of the same sex should be understood as a temptation to wrongful conduct, which is to be avoided despite the (involuntary) temptation. These opponents might draw an analogy with alcoholism: Although alcoholics are unable to change their desire for alcohol, they should nevertheless avoid drinking. While the analogy is imperfect (relatively few people think that drinking alcohol is *always* immoral), it illustrates the importance of distinguishing homosexual orientation from homosexual conduct in certain contexts.

However, the voluntariness of sexual orientation might be relevant to the moral status of homosexual conduct in another way. Suppose that one believes that homosexual conduct is morally inferior to heterosexual conduct but that for some people, namely "constitutional" homosexuals, heterosexual conduct is not a feasible or desirable option. One might then concede that in such cases homosexual conduct is a permissible "second-best" option—morally inferior to heterosexual conduct but morally preferable to having no satisfying sexual relationships at all. One might hold, then, that the voluntariness of sexual orientation is relevant to whether homosexual conduct is morally permissible *for a given individual*, despite the independent judgment that homosexual conduct is objectively inferior. Alternatively, even if one holds that homosexual conduct is *never* morally permissible, one might treat "constitutional" homosexuality as a mitigating factor when evaluating moral culpability for homosexual conduct.

The positions just discussed share the assumption that homosexual conduct is morally inferior to heterosexual conduct. But is this assumption justified? Those who argue morally against homosexual conduct tend to argue either that it is harmful, that it is unnatural, or that it violates divine commands.

Harm. One may argue that homosexual conduct is morally wrong on consequentialist grounds. A common (but naive) consequentialist argument asserts that homosexual conduct is harmful to society because it involves a failure to procreate. But this argument proves too much, since it is equally an argument against **celibacy** (see Bentham). Moreover, it would not apply to homosexuals who procreate through **reproductive technology** or through erstwhile heterosexual relationships.

Somewhat more sophisticated consequentialist arguments invoke correlations between homosexual conduct and **sexually transmitted diseases** or other undesirable things (see Satinover). These arguments suggest several important questions. First, do the alleged correlations hold, or is the evidence for them solid? Second, are they intrinsic to homosexuality, or do they result from contingent factors, including social ostracism of homosexual persons? It seems unfair to condemn a group for characteristics that result from the condemnation itself. Indeed, some gay rights advocates argue that the alleged harms of homosexuality largely result from lack of support for, and even explicit hostility toward, homosexual relationships. Homosexual people, pressured to live in the closet, may find it difficult to sustain long-term relationships and may thus face the emotional and physical risks typical of transient encounters (Corvino, "Why Shouldn't Tommy"). Third, what is the connection between the alleged risks and the morality of homosexual behavior? The fact that one alternative is more risky than another does not automatically make it less moral, even according to consequentialist reasoning. (Driving an automobile is more risky than walking, but consequentialists do not oppose driving.) A consequentialist must also weigh the risks against the expected gains—pleasure, mutual affection, and emotional fulfillment—and take into account the **consent** of the parties involved.

An ingenious consequentialist argument has been advanced by philosopher Michael Levin in two articles and a book coauthored with Laurence Thomas. Levin does not contend that homosexual conduct is immoral. Rather, he holds that it is *abnormal* (in a technical sense; see below) and therefore likely to cause unhappiness. On these grounds, Levin concludes that it is rational to avoid homosexual people and to discourage homosexual conduct.

On Levin's account, homosexual conduct is abnormal insofar as it involves using an organ in a way inconsistent with our evolutionary history. Levin argues that penises are for inserting into vaginas, not for inserting into mouths or other orifices; vulvas are for receiving penises, not for rubbing against other vulvas. For Levin, an organ is *for* some function if and only if that function explains its existence through **evolution**. For example, our teeth are *for* chewing: We have teeth because our (mammalian, primate, human) ancestors who had teeth and used them for chewing tended to have an advantage in surviving and reproducing, creating progeny who also had teeth and used them for chewing. In a similar vein, Levin argues that those among our ancestors who put their penises into vaginas (or put their vaginas around penises) had a reproductive advantage over those that put them elsewhere and passed to later generations this tendency to use penises and vaginas this way. So that is what genitalia are *for*. Any other uses are abnormal.

Levin connects the normal use of an organ with its possessor's happiness by arguing that evolution makes us enjoy (and thereby reinforces) normal behavior. Our ancestors who enjoyed using their teeth for chewing tended to use their teeth this way, lived longer as a result, and left more offspring, who in turn enjoyed using their teeth this way. Conversely, we are likely to be unhappy when we use organs abnormally. Levin offers the example of a person who removes all his teeth and wears them as a necklace. Due to the evolutionary processes of which he is a product, this person is likely to experience dissatisfaction from not being able to chew. (Consider also the likely unhappiness of the person who flagrantly uses his or her teeth to crack butternuts or open beer bottles.) Similarly, for Levin, those who use their genitalia abnormally are likely to experience dissatisfaction. So, he claims, we should expect homosexuals to be less happy than heterosexuals, and he thinks that the evidence, particularly the incidence of homosexual **promiscuity**, confirms this expectation. (Homosexual men engage in promiscuous, **casual sex**, according to Levin, because—unlike heterosexuals—they do not find their sexual relationships sufficiently satisfying.) For these reasons, even though Levin denies that homosexual conduct is immoral, he does think that avoiding homosexuals and discouraging homosexuality is rational. (Note that some consequentialists, such as hedonistic utilitarians, hold that the moral and the prudential are directly related: That something produces unhappiness is a moral strike against it, although not necessarily decisive. So one might try to *transform* Levin's argument into a moral critique of homosexual conduct.)

Levin's argument has been criticized on a number of grounds. Some have argued that he misunderstands evolutionary theory and has not adequately linked abnormality with unhappiness (Koppelman, "Is Marriage"; Murphy, "Homosexuality and Nature"). After all, it is clear that some people are much happier in homosexual relationships than they would be in heterosexual relationships; if they were not, they would be unlikely to pursue homosexual relationships, especially in the face of social ostracism. Yet Levin need not deny that some people are happier in homosexual relationships than they would otherwise be. He just denies that they are, in general, as happy as heterosexuals and on this basis defends the right of other people to avoid them. In this sense Levin's argument is not exactly utilitarian (or not a *good* utilitarian argument): Rather than considering what would promote the *general* happiness (including that of homosexual people), Levin focuses on defending the rights of heterosexuals to do what they believe promotes their *own* happiness.

Any consequentialist view about homosexual conduct will depend on empirical claims about the relative happiness/unhappiness (or other valuable/worthless states) of homosexual persons. Given the large number of apparently happy, open homosexuals, the prospects for a strong consequentialist argument against homosexuality seem dim. Skepticism about such an argument is not new. As utilitarian Jeremy Bentham (1748–1832) wrote over 150 years ago,

I have been tormenting myself for years to find, if possible, a sufficient ground for treating [homosexuals] with the severity with which they are treated at this time of day by all European nations: but upon the principle of utility I can find none. (354)

Nature. Many opponents of homosexuality have opted for a nonconsequentialist approach, usually claiming that homosexual conduct is unnatural in some sense, and hence wrong, regardless of its consequences. This argument suggests two questions: (1) Is homosexual conduct unnatural in a relevant sense? And if so, (2) does that sense carry any moral weight? Opening an umbrella to block the rain interferes with nature and hence is unnatural in *some* sense, but doing so is not therefore immoral. Housing, medicine, computers, and government—to take a random list—involve similar "interferences" with nature. So proponents of the unnaturalness argument must carefully specify what they mean when they claim that homosexuality is unnatural. (See Leiser, 51–57, for a catalog of senses of "unnatural" as applied to homosexuality.)

Some think that genetics are important here. But showing that homosexual orientation has a genetic basis (is due to "nature") does not show that homosexual conduct is morally permissible, any more than showing that alcoholism has a genetic basis shows that excessive drinking is morally permissible (Corvino, "How Not to Argue"; Stein). Conversely, if homosexuality lacks a genetic basis (is due to "nurture"), it does not follow that homosexual conduct is unnatural in any morally relevant sense. That someone speaks English instead of French is not determined genetically, but that does not entail that doing so is unnatural or immoral. The moral status of homosexual conduct cannot be settled merely by investigating its etiology. The more general problem with invoking science to resolve ethical issues is that doing so typically confuses *descriptive* and *normative* senses of "natural." In one sense, what is natural is simply whatever occurs "in nature." In this descriptive sense, homosexuality is undoubtedly natural, as is any other human behavior. But establishing that something *does* occur, whether by genetics or other causes, is not sufficient to establish that it *should* occur. The latter is a normative claim and requires normative premises.

One well-known attempt to develop a normative account of the natural is **Saint Thomas Aquinas**'s (1224/25–1274), though the Natural Law tradition is older and broader than Aquinas (see Finnis, "Law, Morality"). Aquinas held that human nature dictates certain moral constraints on behavior, including sexual behavior. His **sexual ethics** is rich and nuanced, yet a central premise is that sex is for procreation. Sexual acts that preclude procreation (for example, **masturbation**, homosexual acts, heterosexual intercourse with **contraception**, oral and anal sex) are unnatural and therefore wrong, on Aquinas's account. In the late twentieth century, a group of philosophers known as the "New Natural Lawyers" honed and expanded Natural Law philosophy, thereby producing a significant nonconsequentialist argument against homosexuality.

The **New Natural Law** (NNL) holds that there are certain basic goods that are intrinsically worthy of pursuit. The goods are "basic" insofar as they are irreducible to other goods. One of these basic goods is "the marital good," the two-in-one-flesh union of a husband and wife. This union realizes two important values (although it is not reducible to either): procreation and **friendship**. NNL claims that engaging in sexual activity as a *means* to either of these goods is wrong, for doing so treats one's body as an instrument for the satisfaction of desire. Rather, the good realized in (uncontracepted, married, heterosexual) intercourse is the intrinsic good of the marital union itself, where "marital union" is understood in a prepolitical, prelegal sense. NNL criticizes all sexual acts that fall short of pursuing this marital good (the list is the same as Aquinas's, although the reasoning differs somewhat). These acts not only fail to realize the marital good; they also damage it. As John Finnis explains,

> [C]omplete exclusion of the nonmarital acts from the range of acceptable and valuable human options is existentially, if not logically, a precondition for the truly marital character of one's intercourse as and with a spouse. Deliberate approval of nonmarital sex acts is among the states of mind (understanding and willingness) which damage one's capacity to choose and carry out as marital even those actual sex acts which in all other respects are marital in kind. It is a state of mind which, even in those people who are not interested in marrying, is contrary to, and violative of, the good of marriage. ("The Good of Marriage," 123)

The idea seems to be that sexual acts that do not pursue the marital good erroneously treat the marital good merely as an optional feature of sexual activity; for a sexual act to be truly marital, its marital character must be seen as necessary to it. But why sexual acts that do not pursue the marital good *damage* it is not clear. One can grant that chewing sugarless gum is not nourishing but deny that doing so damages the good of nourishment.

NNL has been criticized on other grounds (see Koppelman; Macedo; Moore). The most familiar objection, which plagues any sexual philosophy that designates procreation as a morally essential purpose of sexuality, doubts whether NNL can consistently permit sex for sterile or infertile heterosexual **marriage** partners while prohibiting masturbation, homosexual acts, heterosexual oral and anal sex, and other nonprocreative acts. (Any theory that judges illicit the sexual activity of sterile partners, including married couples where the wife is postmenopausal, is unlikely to capture a wide following.) The fundamental idea behind NNL's argument and, more generally, behind other nonconsequentialist arguments against homosexuality, is that *even if* homosexual relationships realize pleasure, affection, fulfillment, and happiness, there is still something else, some essential moral feature, they lack. The challenge for NNL and other nonconsequentialisms is to articulate that feature in a compelling manner, without ruling out other sexual acts that few people believe are morally wrong. Whether they can meet that challenge remains controversial.

Religion. Religious positions on the morality of homosexuality are as varied as religions themselves. For example, some Protestant denominations are critical of homosexuality; others embrace homosexual persons, perform weddings for them, and even ordain them. The same can be said of Orthodox versus some Reform Jewish congregations. Given this variety, it is useful to detail some questions that must be asked about any religious argument—either for or against homosexuality.

First, one must consider the authority of the sources of religious claims. Quoting scripture (the Hebrew Bible, the Christian Bible, **Islam**'s Qur'an) to justify a claim does not show that claim to be true beyond reasonable doubt, unless scripture is an infallible moral guide. Many scriptures, however, contain questionable and contradictory moral teachings—on slavery, women's roles, stoning adulterers, sex during menstruation, and a variety of other topics (see Vacek). Appeals to religious authorities (bishops, popes, rabbis, mullahs), similarly, are reliable only to the extent that these persons are reliable. To raise these doubts is not in itself to doubt God but only to doubt the human ability to discern God's voice infallibly. Even believers have conceded that history indicates the need for humility and caution regarding religious authority.

Second, even if one grants the authority of the source, one must also accurately interpret or read what the source says. Doing so can be difficult, especially if the source was written in an ancient language, is rich with metaphor and other literary devices, and (like any text) is liable to ambiguity. (See **John Boswell**'s [1947–1994] influential book.) For example, scholars have debated the meaning of the Greek word *arsenokoitai*, which **Saint Paul** (5–64?) uses in 1 Corinthians and 1 Timothy. Translators have rendered the word "abusers of themselves with mankind," "sodomites," "sexual perverts," and "homosexual offenders," which mean different things and, further, are ambiguous. Is anyone who engages in homosexual acts a homosexual "offender," or is some behavior or situation required, beyond mere homosexual conduct, to constitute an offense? The text does not say.

Consider also the story of Sodom and Gomorrah, which is often cited as a condemnation of homosexual conduct (Gen. 19:1–28). Two angels were visiting Lot at Sodom when the men of that town surrounded Lot's house. "Where are the men that came to you tonight? Bring them out to us, so that we may know them," they demanded. Lot refused, even offering his daughters to the townsmen so they would leave his guests alone. But the townsmen would not relent, and the angels struck them blind. God later destroyed Sodom and nearby Gomorrah, raining down "fire and brimstone" upon them.

What was Sodom's crime? Some scholars argue that the city was inhospitable to strangers, while others point to the Sodomites' attempted gang-**rape** of Lot's visitors (if "to know" means "to have sex with"), which would be just as horrifying if it were heterosexual (see Helminiak, 31–54). That homosexuality is the issue is by no means clear. Indeed, scripture itself interprets Sodom's sin differently. "This was the guilt of your sister Sodom: she and her daughters had pride, surfeit of food, and prosperous ease, but did not aid the poor and needy" (Ezek. 16:49).

There are other scriptural texts that appear to condemn homosexual conduct; each must be evaluated on its own merits. At the same time, we should ponder the inconsistency of those who cite religion when condemning homosexuality but ignore similar religious teachings about divorce, contraception, and other common practices. This sort of inconsistency raises moral questions about the use of religion as a weapon rather than as a source of moral illumination.

The focus here on moral arguments against homosexuality should not obscure either the positive case in its favor (see Mohr; Sullivan) or the many other ethical issues surrounding homosexuality and homosexual persons. Indeed, if current trends in the West continue, the arguments against homosexuality, much like the arguments against equality for women and racial minorities, may someday be seen as the shameful relic of a morally insensitive past.

See also Animal Sexuality; Bible, Sex and the; Boswell, John; Chinese Philosophy; Consequentialism; Ethics, Sexual; Ethics, Virtue; Evolution; Feminism, Lesbian; Greek Sexuality and Philosophy, Ancient; Heterosexism; Homosexuality and Science; Judaism, History of; Judaism, Twentieth- and Twenty-First-Century; Kant, Immanuel; Natural Law (New); Queer Theory; Roman Sexuality and Philosophy, Ancient; Social Constructionism

REFERENCES

Bentham, Jeremy. "An Essay on 'Paederasty.'" In Robert B. Baker and Frederick A. Elliston, eds., *Philosophy and Sex*, 2nd ed. Buffalo, N.Y.: Prometheus, 1984, 353–69; Boswell, John. *Christianity, Social Tolerance, and Homosexuality: Gay People in Western Europe from the Beginning of the Christian Era to the Fourteenth Century*. Chicago, Ill.: University of Chicago Press, 1980; Corvino, John. "How Not to Argue for Gay Rights." In Juha Räikkä, ed., *Do We Need Minority Rights? Conceptual Issues*. The Hague, Holland: Martinus Nijhoff, 1996, 215–35; Corvino, John. "Why Shouldn't

Tommy and Jim Have Sex?" In John Corvino, ed., *Same Sex: Debating the Ethics, Science, and Culture of Homosexuality*. Lanham, Md.: Rowman and Littlefield, 1997, 3–16; Finnis, John M. "The Good of Marriage and the Morality of Sexual Relations: Some Philosophical and Historical Observations." *American Journal of Jurisprudence* 42 (1997), 97–134; Finnis, John M. "Law, Morality, and 'Sexual Orientation.'" *Notre Dame Journal of Law, Ethics, and Public Policy* 9:1 (1995), 11–39; Helminiak, Daniel. *What the Bible Really Says about Homosexuality*. San Francisco, Calif.: Alamo Square, 1994; Koppelman, Andrew. *The Gay Rights Question in Contemporary American Law*. Chicago, Ill.: University of Chicago Press, 2002; Koppelman, Andrew. "Is Marriage Inherently Heterosexual?" *American Journal of Jurisprudence* 42 (1997), 51–95; Leiser, Burton. (1973, 1979) *Liberty, Justice, and Morals: Contemporary Value Conflicts*, 3rd ed. New York: Macmillan, 1986; Levin, Michael. "Homosexuality, Abnormality, and Civil Rights." *Public Affairs Quarterly* 10:1 (1996), 31–48; Levin, Michael. "Why Homosexuality Is Abnormal." *The Monist* 67:2 (1984), 251–83; Macedo, Stephen. "Homosexuality and the Conservative Mind." *Georgetown Law Journal* 84:2 (1995), 261–300; Mohr, Richard D. *Gays/Justice: A Study of Ethics, Society, and Law*. New York: Columbia University Press, 1988; Moore, Gareth. *A Question of Truth: Christianity and Homosexuality*. New York: Continuum, 2003; Murphy, Timothy F. "Homosexuality and Nature: Happiness and the Law at Stake." *Journal of Applied Philosophy* 4:2 (1987), 195–204; Murphy, Timothy F., ed. *Gay Ethics: Controversies in Outing, Civil Rights, and Sexual Science*. Binghamton, N.Y.: Harrington Park Press, 1994; Satinover, Jeffrey. *Homosexuality and the Politics of Truth*. Grand Rapids, Mich.: Baker Books, 1996; Stein, Edward. "The Relevance of Scientific Research on Sexual Orientation to Lesbian and Gay Rights." *Journal of Homosexuality* 27:3–4 (1994), 269–308; Sullivan, Andrew. *Virtually Normal: An Argument about Homosexuality*. New York: Knopf, 1995; Thomas, Laurence M., and Michael E. Levin. *Sexual Orientation and Human Rights*. Lanham, Md.: Rowman and Littlefield, 1999; Thomas Aquinas. (1265–1273) *Summa theologiae*, 60 vols. Cambridge, U.K.: Blackfriars, 1964–1976; Vacek, Edward. "A Christian Homosexuality?" *Commonweal* (5 December 1980), 681–84.

John Corvino

ADDITIONAL READING

Arkes, Hadley. "Questions of Principle, Not Predictions: A Reply to Macedo." *Georgetown Law Journal* 84:2 (1995), 321–29; Baird, Robert M., and M. Katherine Baird, eds. *Homosexuality: Debating the Issues*. Amherst, N.Y.: Prometheus, 1995; Batchelor, Edward J., Jr., ed. *Homosexuality and Ethics*. New York: Pilgrim Press, 1980; Bentham, Jeremy. "An Essay on Paederasty." In Robert B. Baker and Frederick A. Elliston, eds., *Philosophy and Sex*, 2nd ed. Buffalo, N.Y.: Prometheus, 1984, 353–69. Reprinted in P&S3 (350–64); Bentham, Jeremy. "Offences against One's Self: Paederasty." *Journal of Homosexuality* 3 (1978), 383–405; continued in *Journal of Homosexuality* 4 (1978), 91–107; Bradshaw, David. "A Reply to Corvino" ["Why Shouldn't Tommy and Jim Have Sex?"]. In John Corvino, ed., *Same Sex: Debating the Ethics, Science, and Culture of Homosexuality*. Lanham, Md.: Rowman and Littlefield, 1997, 17–30; Card, Claudia. *Lesbian Choices*. New York: Columbia University Press, 1995; Corvino, John. "Homosexuality and the Moral Relevance of Experience." In Hugh LaFollette, ed., *Ethics in Practice*, 2nd ed. Malden, Mass.: Blackwell, 2002, 241–50; Corvino, John. "Justice for Glenn and Stacy: On Gender, Morality, and Gay Rights." In James P. Sterba, ed., *Social and Political Philosophy: Contemporary Perspectives*. New York: Routledge, 2001, 300–318; Corvino, John. "Why Shouldn't Tommy and Jim Have Sex?" In John Corvino, ed., *Same Sex: Debating the Ethics, Science, and Culture of Homosexuality*. Lanham, Md.: Rowman and Littlefield, 1997, 3–16. Reprinted in James E. White, ed., *Contemporary Moral Problems*, 7th ed. Belmont, Calif.: Wadsworth, 2002, 308–18. Revised and reprinted as "Homosexuality: The Nature and Harm Arguments," in Terence Ball and Richard Dagger, eds., *Ideals and Ideologies*. New York: Longman, 2002, 373–81; POS3 (137–48); POS4 (135–46). Revised and reprinted in part in Robert C. Solomon, ed., *Introducing Philosophy*, 7th ed. New York: Harcourt College Publishers, 2001, 571–74; and Thomas A. Mappes and Jane S. Zembaty, eds., *Social Ethics: Morality and Social Policy*, 6th ed.

McGraw-Hill, 2002, 189–96; Corvino, John, ed. *Same Sex: Debating the Ethics, Science, and Culture of Homosexuality*. Lanham, Md.: Rowman and Littlefield, 1997; Countryman, William. *Dirt, Greed, and Sex: Sexual Ethics in the New Testament and Their Implications for Today*. Philadelphia, Pa.: Fortress Press, 1988; Finnis, John M. "Law, Morality, and 'Sexual Orientation.'" *Notre Dame Law Review* 69:5 (1994), 1049–76. Reprinted, revised, in *Notre Dame Journal of Law, Ethics, and Public Policy* 9:1 (1995), 11–39. Reprinted, revised, in John Corvino, ed., *Same Sex: Debating the Ethics, Science, and Culture of Homosexuality*. Lanham, Md.: Rowman and Littlefield, 1997, 31–43; Furey, Pat, and Jeannine Gramick, eds. *The Vatican and Homosexuality*. New York: Crossroad, 1988; Greenberg, Rabbi Steven. *Wrestling with God and Men: Homosexuality in the Jewish Tradition*. Madison: University of Wisconsin Press, 2004; Hannigan, James P. *Homosexuality: The Test Case for Christian Sexual Ethics*. New York: Paulist Press, 1988; Hoagland, Sarah Lucia. *Lesbian Ethics: Toward New Value*. Palo Alto, Calif.: Institute of Lesbian Studies, 1988; Jordan, Jeff. "Is It Wrong to Discriminate on the Basis of Homosexuality?" *Journal of Social Philosophy* 25:1 (1995), 39–52. Reprinted in Stephen M. Cahn and Tziporah Kasachkoff, eds., *Morality and Public Policy*. Upper Saddle River, N.J.: Prentice Hall, 2003, 117–29; Jordan, Mark D. *The Invention of Sodomy in Christian Theology*. Chicago, Ill.: Chicago University Press, 1997; Lee, Patrick, and Robert P. George. "What Sex Can Be: Self-Alienation, Illusion, or One-Flesh Union." *American Journal of Jurisprudence* 42 (1997), 135–57; Leiser, Burton. (1973, 1979) "Is Homosexuality Unnatural?" In *Liberty, Justice, and Morals: Contemporary Value Conflicts*, 3rd ed. New York: Macmillan, 1986, 51–57. Reprinted in James Rachels, ed., *The Right Thing to Do: Basic Readings in Moral Philosophy*, 3rd ed. New York: McGraw-Hill, 2003, 144–52; Levin, Michael. "Why Homosexuality Is Abnormal." *The Monist* 67:2 (1984), 251–83. Reprinted in P&S3 (337–49); POS3 (95–127); Macedo, Stephen. "Reply to Critics." *Georgetown Law Journal* 84:2 (1995), 329–37; Mohr, Richard D. "Gay Basics: Some Questions, Facts, and Values." In *Gays/Justice: A Study of Ethics, Society, and Law*. New York: Columbia University Press, 1988, 21–45. Reprinted in James Rachels, ed., *The Right Thing to Do: Basic Readings in Moral Philosophy*, 3rd ed. New York: McGraw-Hill, 2003, 128–43; Mohr, Richard D. *Gay Ideas: Outing and Other Controversies*. Boston, Mass.: Beacon Press, 1992; Mohr, Richard D. *A More Perfect Union: Why Straight America Must Stand Up for Gay Rights*. Boston, Mass.: Beacon Press, 1994; Moon, Dawne. *God, Sex, and Politics: Homosexuality and Everyday Theologies*. Chicago, Ill.: University of Chicago Press, 2004; Moore, Gareth. "Natural Sex: Germain Grisez, Sex, and Natural Law." In Nigel Biggar and Rufus Black, eds., *The Revival of Natural Law: Philosophical, Theological, and Ethical Responses to the Finnis-Grisez School*. Aldershot, U.K.: Ashgate, 2001, 223–41; Nussbaum, Martha C., and Kenneth J. Dover. "Dover and Nussbaum Respond to Finnis." Appendix 4 (1641–51) to Martha C. Nussbaum, "Platonic Love and Colorado Law: The Relevance of Ancient Greek Norms to Modern Sexual Controversies." *Virginia Law Review* 80:7 (1994); Perry, Michael J. "The Morality of Homosexual Conduct: A Response to John Finnis." *Notre Dame Journal of Law, Ethics, and Public Policy* 9:1 (1995), 41–74; Primoratz, Igor. "Homosexuality." In *Ethics and Sex*. London: Routledge, 1999, 110–32; Pronk, Pim. *Against Nature? Types of Moral Argumentation Regarding Homosexuality*. Grand Rapids, Mich.: Eerdmans, 1993; Ramsey Colloquium. "The Homosexual Movement." *First Things*, no. 41 (March 1994), 15–20. Reprinted in John Corvino, ed., *Same Sex: Debating the Ethics, Science, and Culture of Homosexuality*. Lanham, Md.: Rowman and Littlefield, 1997, 58–68; and Robert M. Baird and M. Katherine Baird, eds., *Homosexuality: Debating the Issues*. Amherst, N.Y.: Prometheus, 1995, 31–40; Ruse, Michael. *Homosexuality: A Philosophical Inquiry*. Oxford, U.K.: Blackwell, 1988; Schaff, Kory. "Kant, Political Liberalism, and the Ethics of Same-Sex Relations." *Journal of Social Philosophy* 32:3 (2001), 446–62; Schmidt, Thomas E. *Straight and Narrow? Compassion and Clarity in the Homosexuality Debate*. Downers Grove, Ill.: InterVarsity Press, 1995; Stein, Edward. "The Relevance of Scientific Research on Sexual Orientation to Lesbian and Gay Rights." *Journal of Homosexuality* 27:3–4 (1994), 269–308. Reprinted in HS (191–230); Sullivan, Andrew. *Love Undetectable: Reflections on Friendship, Sex, and Survival*. New York: Knopf, 1998; Vacek, Edward. "A Christian Homosexuality?" *Commonweal* (5 December 1980), 681–84. Reprinted in POS3 (129–35); POS4 (127–33); Weithman, Paul J. "Natural Law, Morality, and Sexual Complementarity." In David M. Estlund and Martha C. Nussbaum, eds., *Sex, Preference, and Family: Essays on Law and Nature*. Oxford, U.K.: Oxford University Press, 1998, 227–46; Williams, Thomas. "A Reply to the Ramsey Colloquium." In John Corvino, ed., *Same Sex: Debating the Ethics, Science, and Culture of Homosexuality*. Lanham, Md.: Rowman and Littlefield, 1997, 69–80; Wolfe, Christopher, ed. *Homosexuality and American Public Life*. Dallas, Tex.: Spence Publishing, 1999; Wolfe, Christopher, ed. *Same-Sex Matters: The Challenge of Homosexuality*. Dallas, Tex.: Spence Publishing, 2000; "Wolfenden Report." Report of the Committee on Homosexual Offences and Prostitution (U.K.). Cmd. 247, 1957.

HOMOSEXUALITY AND SCIENCE. "Homosexuality" refers to sexual attraction and behavior among people of the same sex. The term was coined in 1869 by Károly Mária Benkert (1824–1882; Herzer and Kennedy, 325) and prevailed over other terms such as "Uranism" and "inversion." In his *Symposium*, **Plato** (427–347 BCE) offered a mythical (perhaps comic) explanation of homosexuality. Humans were originally of three kinds, each composed of two bodies. One kind combined a male and female body (including genitals), another two male bodies, and the third two female bodies. Zeus, angered by human ambitions, split them in two. Each half desired (here enters eroticism) to return to its original state: Some men desired women (and vice versa), some women desired women, and some men desired men—depending on from which type they originally came (190e–91e).

Scientific researchers have supplanted mythmakers as the reigning authorities about the origins of **sexual desire**. For the greatest span of history, however, science was not interested in homosexuality. Religion, moral philosophy, and the **law** made influential judgments about homosexuality largely without reference to biology. Only in the nineteenth century did **sexology** begin seriously looking for the origins of homosexuality in psychological or biological causes. This research continues and has itself become the subject of moral debate.

Since the 1800s, biological researchers have looked at many different traits in attempting to distinguish homosexual and heterosexual people: height, fat distribution, hair texture, angles at which people carry their arms, whistling ability, rectal neurology, scrotal folds, the preference for the color green, and many others (Murphy, "Redirecting"; Suppe). Most of these studies—then and now—depend on finding a correlation between a physical trait and **sexual orientation** and then explaining how that trait and homosexual orientation might be causally related.

In 1991, neuroanatomist Simon LeVay reported that homosexual men were more likely to have a smaller neuron structure (INAH-3) than heterosexual men, a size more typical of women. Because this region of the brain is known to influence sexuality, LeVay hypothesized that this structure might influence men's sexual orientation. And in 1994, two researchers reported that homosexual men were more likely than heterosexual men to have more finger skin ridges on their left hands than on their right hands, a trait more common in women. Because prenatal hormones influence skin patterns, the researchers speculated that they might have effects on both skin ridge patterns and sexual orientation (Hall and Kimura). In 2003, another researcher (Lippa) reported that the difference in length between the index and the ring finger was typically greater in homosexual men than heterosexual men, a trait more typical of women (no difference was found in the length ratios of homosexual and heterosexual women). The researcher speculated that prenatal hormone exposure might link this trait to the origin of male homosexual orientation. In 1998, a research team (McFadden and Pasanen) reported that homosexual women's capacity to hear very soft sounds is less pronounced than in heterosexual women. Researchers also found that certain eye blink reflexes in homosexual women are similar to men's (Rahman et al.). These reflexes are involuntary and not influenced by learning. The researchers hypothesized that prenatal hormones might link the two traits.

In the 1970s, Edward O. Wilson proposed that homosexuality might be a heritable trait (genetically transmitted) despite the fact that homosexual sex is not reproductive. Instead of focusing on individual survival, Wilson focused on the survival of the kinship group. Wilson thought that homosexual men and women might contribute to the group's tasks and survival because they had no children of their own and thus would be free to contribute in other and significant ways (142–47). Thus, a group with some homosexuals in its population would have a survival advantage over other groups. Homosexuality might be carried as a recessive trait, guaranteeing that it would appear consistently even if not frequently in a population, passed on by heterosexuals (see Kitcher; Rice and Barbone; Ruse, "Gay Genes").

Direct genetic analysis was not available to early researchers of homosexuality, so most genetic studies proceeded by indirection and circumstantial evidence. In the 1940s, one German researcher examined criminal subjects to study their sibling ratios (Lang). How many brothers, how many sisters, did they have? Homosexual and heterosexual subjects had different sibling ratios, but the ratios would look more alike if the homosexual men were counted as females. It was therefore hypothesized that homosexual men might be genetically female. In the 1950s, another researcher suggested a genetic basis for homosexuality after pointing out that monozygotic twins shared sexual orientation at a high rate (Kallman). Critics pointed out that a genetic influence was not certain here because twins share similar environments (Suppe).

Despite their limitations, twin studies are an interesting way to gauge genetic aspects of homosexuality. One research team reported that siblings' sharing the same sexual orientation varied with the degree of genetic relatedness (Bailey and Pillard). If a male was homosexual, the chance that his monozygotic twin would be homosexual was 52 percent, the chance that a fraternal twin would be homosexual was 22 percent, and the chance that an adopted brother would be homosexual was 11 percent. Similarly, if a female was homosexual, the chance that her monozygotic twin would be homosexual was 48 percent, the chance that her fraternal twin would be homosexual was 16 percent, and the chance that an adopted sister would be homosexual was 6 percent (Bailey et al.). That shared sexual orientation correlates with genetic relatedness is a circumstantial case for a genetic contribution to homosexuality, according to these researchers.

Using a pedigree study, in 1993 Dean Hamer and his colleagues reported a matrilineal pattern of heritability for male homosexuality. They also found that homosexual brothers shared a particular genetic region at a significantly higher rate than did homosexual men and their heterosexual brothers. These researchers did not find a "gay gene." The genetic region in question is capable of containing several hundred genes, and the shared region might involve some other trait that the affected brothers shared. No similar shared genetic region has been found in homosexual women (Hu et al.). In 2003, the National Institutes of Health funded a continuation of this research, providing five years of grant support to Alan Sanders at Northwestern University (NIH Grant 1RO1HD041563-01A2).

Finding genes linked to sexual orientation—if they exist—would be only the first step in devising a causal, explanatory story about the genesis of homosexuality. Researchers would have to describe the pathway through which genes affect sexual orientation: How *exactly* would the genes dispose people toward erotic interest in members of their own sex? One psychologist, Daryl Bem, has suggested in broad outline how this might occur. Genes might influence temperament, and children who experience themselves as unlike others proceed to eroticize those from whom they feel different. This view is speculative (see Peplau et al.) and does not plot a specific pathway from protein production by genes to sexual orientation. Explaining this chain of events challenges all researchers even if genetic aspects to sexual orientation are uncovered.

Some researchers look outside the human species when trying to explain homosexuality. Many animals engage in same-sex erotic activities (Bagemihl). Some behaviors that appear "homosexual" in animals may not be "sexual" but rooted in domination rituals and other species practices. Even so, some animals do seem to seek out erotic and pair-bonding relationships with others of the same sex. This behavior also raises, but does not answer, the question of biological basis or components of animal homosexuality.

Early psychologists like Richard von Krafft-Ebing (1840–1902), **Havelock Ellis** (1859–1939), and **Sigmund Freud** (1856–1939) distinguished between "acquired" and "congenital" homosexuality, between situational homosexuality and homosexuality fated by biology. Krafft-Ebing thought congenital homosexuality was a kind of biological dead-end, the evidence of genetic degeneracy. Thus many psychologists studied homosexuality to find treatments and methods of prevention. Even so, others in the same period were less hostile to homosexuality. Freud did not believe homosexuality was necessarily impairing. To the mother of a homosexual man, Freud wrote in 1935 that it "is nothing to be ashamed of, no vice, no degradation; it cannot be classified as an illness" (*Letters*, 423; see Jones, 195–96). Early homosexual rights advocate Karl Heinrich Ulrichs (1825–1895) believed that homosexuals represented mixed biological types. Because biology grounded homosexuality, homosexual men and women could only have the sexual interests they had. Ulrichs therefore advocated the decriminalization of consensual adult homosexuality and criticized barriers to **same-sex marriage**.

Some writers agree with Ulrichs that a biological basis to homosexuality justifies moral and social acceptance. Unfortunately, showing that homosexuality is biological (in the sense that it emerges as an involuntary sexual orientation) does not advance the cause of homosexual rights as much as advocates like to think. To treat the facts of nature as a moral justification is to commit "the naturalistic fallacy." Murder and **rape** would not be morally acceptable even if people were inclined to do them by biological factors beyond their control. The *morality* of homosexuality depends, instead, on its compatibility with the values and ethical standards that apply in human life generally, and there is no shortage of philosophers, ethicists, and theologians making exactly that case (see, for example, Mohr). Still, the *political* effect of showing homosexuality to be biological seems real: People are more tolerant of traits, including homosexuality, if they believe them to be fixed parts of a person's makeup (Ernulf et al.).

But research about homosexuality can expose factual errors, as the social sciences, in studying populations of homosexual men and women, have done. The pioneering studies of Alfred Kinsey (1894–1956) found a surprising amount of homosexual behavior in the United States in all age and social groups. Evelyn Hooker's (1907–1996) psychological tests showed that homosexual men could not be distinguished from heterosexuals by having distinctive mental functions. The Bell and Weinberg studies (1978) offered detailed perspectives on the lives, sexual practices, and social views of homosexual men and women. In the early 1990s, Edward O. Laumann and his colleagues revisited questions about homosexual behavior in a more sophisticated way than Kinsey. Charlotte Patterson's studies (1992) help to dispel the view that children suffer psychological harm when raised by homosexual parents. All these studies—limited in their sampling methods, sample sizes, and use of sexual categories—have, nonetheless, shed light on the actual lives of men and women with same-sex erotic attractions and identities.

An important philosophical issue shadows sexual orientation research: the possibility that sexual orientations are social artifacts (see Halperin). Some philosophers deny that heterosexuality and homosexuality are natural kinds or "essences" in the way that maple trees or diamonds are fixed entities in nature. Human sexuality is capable of taking many forms, and social forces shape that capacity, making sexual orientations a kind of social role. **Social constructionism**, as this view is called, argues that social dynamics script people into one sexual category or another (see Stein). If so, looking for biological explanations of "homosexuals" would be as mistaken as looking for biological explanations of social categories such as magistrates and teachers. To be sure, the meaning and expression of same-sex eroticism (and other-sex eroticism) depends on cultural mores. But even with all the variability in sexual practices around the globe and even within a given society, some men are only interested in having sex with other men and some women only with women. Even in societies with fluid sexual boundaries, some people drift more or less exclusively toward members of their own sex. Their nuclear sexual fantasies, desires, and behaviors provide enough reason to suggest that biological dispositions and/or psychological events influence this outcome. As the philosopher Michael Ruse has put it (*Homosexuality*, 15–18), homosexuals are facts of nature.

It is undeniable that human sexual interests are always expressed in social contexts. No one's sexual unfolding occurs in a socially unmediated state of nature. The unseen, guiding hand of society influences how people take sexual pleasure in one another. Sometimes people do so through openly accepted rituals. Sometimes people do so in stolen opportunities beyond the gaze of authorities. Nevertheless, saying that "society" mediates sexual development does not explain why particular individuals come to have their specific erotic interests. Schoolmates of the same age can diverge dramatically in their sexual interests despite having similar family structures, social backgrounds, and educational experiences. Some men (women) end up interested in males (females), others end up interested in females (males), some men end up interested in males who appear to be female, and some men and women (a possibility excluded in Plato's myth) end up interested in both males and females. There is no doubt that societies influence the formation of many sexual interests. Still, that biology plays a dispositional role in the determination of one's fundamental orientation should not be ignored.

It has been recognized that what counts as "homosexuality" varies from culture to culture. In some Melanesian societies, as reported by **Gilbert Herdt**, adolescent boys perform fellatio on older males as a rite of passage established by their society. Is this practice "homosexuality"? Would it make sense to look for a biological or genetic cause of this tribal behavior? U.S. history also shows that sexual practices do not cleave neatly into homosexual and heterosexual. In nineteenth-century New York, many men had oral sex with other men for reasons having to do with access to sexual outlets (Chauncey). Would it make sense to look at the biology of *all* these men, as opposed to their social circumstances, to explain their sexual behavior? Similarly, some imprisoned men engage in sex with other inmates; does this count as "homosexuality"? These examples illustrate that the lines about what (and who) counts as "homosexual" are blurry (Brookey). As a result, remaining skeptical about biological explanations of such widely disparate sexual behavior may be wise.

Perhaps we are pursuing the wrong questions: The specifics of sexual development rather than sexual orientation per se should be the focus of research (see Money). This approach does not ask biology to confirm the existence of a class of homosexuals set apart from the class of heterosexuals and then explain how that class comes into existence. Instead, the central question is how any sexual interests emerge in individuals or in people generally. Why do some men prefer hairy men, some men prefer thin blonde females, some women prefer butch women in leather, and others prefer the tall, dark, and handsome male? What accounts for these myriad differences might be a more intriguing and significant question than simply why some people are straight and others are gay.

Another issue is why homosexuality attracts so much attention, from all the possible topics that sex researchers could study. Perhaps scientific investigations of homosexuality are largely a moral residue, an interest shaped under conditions of hostility and misunderstanding (Hubbard and Wald). If all moral stigma were stripped away from homosexuality, maybe little interest would be left in explaining it. Scientific researchers have not been especially interested in the genetics of great writers, painters, philanthropists, or educators. Is moral suspicion the engine that drives the science of homosexuality?

Suspicion about the morality and pathology of homosexuality has, in fact, driven much sexual orientation research. Since the 1800s, psychiatrists and psychologists have looked for the causes of homosexuality to prevent and treat it. Even so, must homosexuality be studied *only* as pathology or *only* as stigmatized behavior? Human beings develop various sexual interests in males, females, or combinations thereof. Why is it not important or interesting to ask how this happens? Freud urged (*Three Essays*, 146, note added in 1915) that the development of "exclusive" heterosexuality is not self-evident but needs as much explanation as homosexuality. What general rules of sexual development are discernible as children mature through adolescence to adult sexual interests, and how do biological traits, history, and social structures influence that development? This is an altogether reasonable question to ask, and not only of homosexuality. It will not always, perhaps never, be easy to sort through the determinants of human behavior, be it novelty-seeking, alcoholism, obesity, or sexual orientation. But we will not know where study in these areas can lead without doing the research. It is overly pessimistic to think that sexual orientation research cannot benefit sex research and other sciences.

Some commentators wonder not whether sexual orientation research can attain plausible results but whether it should be done at all. They worry that the risks of the research outweigh the benefits, so that biological testing for homosexuality, were it possible, would be ethically dubious. Government, the **military**, employers, and even family members might want people tested for sexual orientation, sometimes involuntarily, and "positive" results could be used in harmful ways (Murphy, *Gay Science*, 137–64). A dictator might use the test to wrest sexual secrets from political dissidents. Officials outside a royal household might extort the reigning monarch by threatening to reveal that the crown prince is gay. Military personnel might test soldiers with a view toward discharge. Parents might test teenagers who are concealing, they believe, their real sexual interests. Very little in terms of social benefit would seem to result from testing, at least not enough to offset the possible damage.

These possible effects raise questions that are entirely speculative, because there are no biological tests that disclose people's sexual histories or sexual interests. Nonetheless, what needs to be discussed are protections that will be available if research moves closer toward its goal. The prospect of discriminatory treatment and damage attaches to all genetic and other kinds of biomedical tests (for example, for drug use; for a proclivity for alcoholism). Avoiding the effects of prejudice requires that strong standards of free and informed **consent** guide the use of sexual orientation tests. Yet informed consent might not go very far in protecting individuals from test results. Some people might agree to assume the immediate risks of testing, only to find out later that they have lost social benefits for unforeseeable reasons. Testing makes people vulnerable in multiple ways.

One common speculation about genetic tests for sexual orientation is that parents will use them in reproductive decisions, perhaps to abort children with an unwanted sexual orientation (Murphy, *Gay Science*, 103–35). Some parents *would* want to avoid having homosexual children, though their reasons might not always involve antipathy toward homosexuality. Some object to homosexuality on religious grounds and would want to spare their children the temptations of sin. Others might wish to avoid having homosexual children because homosexuality is alien to them, something removed from their own experience, and they might doubt they could adequately raise homosexual children with the special care and attention they need. Other parents might wish to protect their potential children from the disadvantages in civil rights and social opportunities that accompany being homosexual. For all these reasons, parents might use genetic tests in assisted conception or **abortion** decisions, if such tests were available (Murphy, "Abortion"). Further, it is not clear that embryos and fetuses have rights, either moral or legal, that trump parents' interests in obtaining genetic information important for making reproductive decisions (Botkin; Murphy, *Gay Science*, 125 ff.). Perhaps, absent a compelling reason to the contrary, parents should be entitled to genetic information that helps them reach decisions about the kind of children they will have.

One compelling reason might be that if widely used, genetic tests for sexual orientation would diminish the number of homosexual men and women, and this might well be thought to be harmful to the homosexual community. And if Wilson is right about the kin-selection explanation and benefits of homosexuality, a reduction in their number would be harmful both to the kin-group and to society at large. But, ultimately, the welfare of any minority group rests not on the size of the group but on its access to social advantages and equity in civic matters large and small. The front line for the protection of homosexual men and women should be here, rather than in the genetic counselor's office (see Kaplan). Improving opportunities for homosexual men and women might by itself reduce the worries of potential parents. If they did not believe their children would face social obstacles, some objections to having homosexual children might disappear.

See also Abortion; Animal Sexuality; Bisexuality; Evolution; Herdt, Gilbert; Homosexuality, Ethics of; Intersexuality; Natural Law (New); Orientation, Sexual; Psychology, Twentieth- and Twenty-First-Century; Reproductive Technology; Sexology; Social Constructionism

REFERENCES

Bagemihl, Bruce. *Biological Exuberance: Animal Homosexuality and Natural Diversity.* New York: St. Martin's Press, 1999; Bailey, J. Michael, and Richard C. Pillard. "A Genetic Study of Male Sexual Orientation." *Archives of General Psychiatry* 48:12 (1991), 1089–96; Bailey, J. Michael, Richard C. Pillard, Michael C. Neale, and Yvonne Agyei. "Heritable Factors Influence Sexual Orientation in Women." *Archives of General Psychiatry* 50:3 (1993), 217–23; Bell, Alan P., and Martin S. Weinberg. *Homosexualities: A Study of Diversity among Men and Women.* New York: Simon and Schuster, 1978; Bem, Daryl J. "Exotic Becomes Erotic: A Developmental Theory of Sexual Orientation." *Psychological Review* 103:2 (1996), 320–35; Botkin, Jeffrey R. "Fetal Privacy and Confidentiality." *Hastings Center Report* 25:5 (1995), 32–39; Brookey, Robert Alan. *Reinventing the Male Homosexual.* Bloomington: Indiana University Press, 2002; Chauncey, George. *Gay New York: Gender, Urban Culture, and the Making of the Gay Male World, 1890–1940.* New York: Basic Books, 1994; Ellis, Havelock. (1897–1928) *Studies in the Psychology of Sex.* New York: Random House, 1936; Ernulf,

Kurt E., Sune M. Innala, and Frederick L. Whitam. "Biological Explanation, Psychological Explanation, and Tolerance of Homosexuals: A Cross-National Analysis of Beliefs and Attitudes." *Psychological Reports* 65 (1989): 1003–10; Freud, Sigmund. *Letters of Sigmund Freud*. Ed. Ernst L. Freud. New York: Basic Books, 1960; Freud, Sigmund. (1905) *Three Essays on the Theory of Sexuality*. In *The Standard Edition of the Complete Psychological Works of Sigmund Freud*, vol. 7. Trans. James Strachey. London: Hogarth Press, 1953–1974, 125–245; Hall, J.A.Y., and D. Kimura. "Dermatoglyphic Asymmetry and Sexual Orientation in Men." *Behavioral Neuroscience* 108:6 (1994), 1203–6; Halperin, David. *One Hundred Years of Homosexuality: And Other Essays on Greek Love*. New York: Routledge, 1990; Hamer, Dean H., Stella Hu, Victoria L. Magnuson, Nan Hu, and Angela M. Pattatucci. "A Linkage between DNA Markers on the X Chromosome and Male Sexual Orientation." *Science* 261:5119 (1993), 321–27; Herdt, Gilbert. *Guardians of the Flutes: Idioms of Masculinity*. New York: McGraw-Hill, 1981. 2nd ed., Chicago, Ill.: University of Chicago Press, 1994; Herzer, Manfred, and Hubert Kennedy. "Kertbeny, Karl Maria." In Timothy F. Murphy, ed., *Reader's Guide to Lesbian and Gay Studies*. Chicago, Ill.: Fitzroy Dearborn, 2000, 325–26; Hooker, Evelyn. "The Adjustment of the Male Overt Homosexual." *Journal of Projective Techniques* 21:1 (1957), 18–31; Hooker, Evelyn. "Male Homosexuality in the Rorschach." *Journal of Projective Techniques* 22:1 (1958), 33–54; Hu, Stella, Angela M. L. Pattatucci, Chavis Patterson, Lin Li, David W. Fulker, Stacey S. Cherns, Leonid Kruglyak, and Dean H. Hamer. "Linkage between Sexual Orientation and Chromosome Xq28 in Males, But Not Females." *Nature Genetics* 11:3 (1994), 248–56; Hubbard, Ruth, and Elijah Wald. "The Search for Sexual Identity: False Genetic Markers." *New York Times* (2 August 1993), A11. Jones, Ernest. *The Life and Work of Sigmund Freud*, vol. 3. New York: Basic Books, 1957; Kallman, Franz J. "Studies in the Genetic Determination of Homosexuality." *American Journal of Human Genetics* 4:2 (1952), 136–46; Kaplan, Morris B. *Sexual Justice: Democratic Citizenship and the Politics of Desire*. New York: Routledge, 1997; Kinsey, Alfred, Wardell Pomeroy, and Clyde Martin. *Sexual Behavior in the Human Male*. Philadelphia, Pa.: Saunders, 1948; Kinsey, Alfred, Wardell Pomeroy, Clyde Martin, and Paul Gebhard. *Sexual Behavior in the Human Female*. Philadelphia, Pa.: Saunders, 1953; Kitcher, Philip. "Two Cheers for Homosexuality." In *Vaulting Ambition: Sociobiology and the Quest for Human Nature*. Cambridge, Mass.: MIT Press, 1985, 243–52; Krafft-Ebing, Richard von. (1886) *Psychopathia Sexualis*, 12th ed. Trans. F. J. Rebman. New York: Paperback Library, 1965; Lang, Theo. "Studies in the Genetic Determination of Homosexuality." *Journal of Nervous and Mental Disorders* 92:1 (1940), 55–64; Laumann, Edward O., John H. Gagnon, Robert T. Michael, and Stuart Michaels. *The Social Organization of Sexuality: Sexual Practices in the United States*. Chicago, Ill.: University of Chicago Press, 1994; LeVay, Simon. "A Difference in the Hypothalamic Structure between Heterosexual and Homosexual Men." *Science* 253:5023 (1991), 1034–37; Lippa, Richard A. "Are 2D/4D Finger Length Ratios Related to Sexual Orientation? Yes for Men, No for Women." *Journal of Personality and Social Psychology* 85:1 (2003), 179–88; McFadden, Dennis, and Edward G. Pasanen. "Comparison of the Auditory Systems of Heterosexuals and Homosexuals: Click-Evoked Otoacoustic Emissions." *Proceedings of the National Academy of Sciences* 95:5 (1998), 2709–13; Mohr, Richard D. *Gays/Justice: A Study in Society, Ethics, and Law*. New York: Columbia University Press, 1988; Money, John. *Gay, Straight, and In-Between: The Sexology of Erotic Orientation*. New York: Oxford University Press, 1988; Murphy, Timothy F. "Abortion and the Ethics of Genetic Sexual Orientation Research." *Cambridge Quarterly of Healthcare Ethics* 4:4 (1995), 340–50; Murphy, Timothy F. *Gay Science: The Ethics of Sexual Orientation Research*. New York: Columbia University Press, 1997; Murphy, Timothy F. "Redirecting Sexual Orientation: Techniques and Justifications." *Journal of Sex Research* 29:4 (1992), 501–23; Patterson, Charlotte. "Children of Lesbian and Gay Parents." *Child Development* 63:5 (1992), 1025–42; Peplau, Letitia, Linda Garnets, Leah Spalding, Terri Conley, and Rosemary Veniegas. "A Critique of Bem's 'Exotic Becomes Erotic' Theory of Sexual Orientation." *Psychological Review* 105:2 (1998), 387–94; Plato. (ca. 380 BCE) *Symposium*. Trans. Alexander Nehamas and Paul Woodruff. Indianapolis, Ind.: Hackett, 1989; Rahman, Qazi, Veena Kumari, and Glenn D. Wilson. "Sexual Orientation-Related Differences in Prepulse Inhibition of the Human Startle Response." *Behavioral Neuroscience* 117:5 (2003), 1096–1102; Rice, Lee, and Steven Barbone. "Hatching Your

Genes before They're Counted." In Alan Soble, ed., *Sex, Love, and Friendship*. Amsterdam, Holland: Rodopi, 1997, 89–98; Ruse, Michael. "Are There Gay Genes? Sociobiology Looks at Homosexuality." *Journal of Homosexuality* 4:1 (1981), 5–34; Ruse, Michael. *Homosexuality: A Philosophical Inquiry*. Oxford, U.K.: Blackwell, 1988; Stein, Edward, ed. *Forms of Desire: Sexual Orientation and the Social Constructionist Controversy*, 1st pnt. New York: Garland, 1990. 2nd pnt., New York: Routledge, 1992; Suppe, Frederick. "Explaining Homosexuality: Philosophical Issues, and Who Cares Anyway?" In Timothy F. Murphy, ed., *Gay Ethics: Controversies in Outing, Civil Rights, and Sexual Science*. Binghamton, N.Y.: Haworth Press, 1994, 223–68; Ulrichs, Karl Heinrich. (1864–1880) *The Riddle of "Man-Manly" Love: The Pioneering Work on Male Homosexuality*, 2 vols. Trans. Michael A. Lombardi-Nash. Buffalo, N.Y.: Prometheus, 1994; Wilson, Edward O. *On Human Nature*. Cambridge, Mass.: Harvard University Press, 1978.

Timothy F. Murphy

ADDITIONAL READING

Balch, David L. "Romans 1:24–27, Science, and Homosexuality." *Currents in Theology and Mission* 25:6 (1998), 433–40; Balch, David L., ed. *Homosexuality, Science, and the "Plain Sense" of Scripture*. Grand Rapids, Mich.: Eerdmans, 2000; Bayer, Ronald. (1981) *Homosexuality and American Psychiatry*, 2nd ed. Princeton, N.J.: Princeton University Press, 1987; Bell, Alan P., Martin S. Weinberg, and Sue Kiefer. *Sexual Preference: Its Development in Men and Women*. Bloomington: Indiana University Press, 1981; Bergler, Edmund. (1956) *Homosexuality: Disease or Way of Life?* New York: Hill and Wang, 1957; Cameron, Paul. *The Gay 90s: What the Empirical Evidence Reveals about Homosexuality*. Franklin, Tenn.: Adroit, 1993; Chauncey, George, Jr. (1983) "From Sexual Inversion to Homosexuality: The Changing Medical Conceptualization of Female Deviance." In Kathy Peiss and Christina Simmons, eds., *Passion and Power: Sexuality in History*. Philadelphia, Pa.: Temple University Press, 1989, 87–117; Dahl, Edgar. "Ethical Issues in New Uses of Preimplantation Genetic Diagnosis." *Human Reproduction* 18:7 (2003), 1368–69; Díaz, Jesús A. "Hooker, Evelyn." In Timothy F. Murphy, ed., *Reader's Guide to Lesbian and Gay Studies*. Chicago, Ill.: Fitzroy Dearborn, 2000, 290–92; Gonsiorek, John C. "The Empirical Basis for the Demise of the Illness Model of Homosexuality." In John C. Gonsiorek and James D. Weinrich, eds., *Homosexuality: Research Implications for Public Policy*. Newbury Park, Calif.: Sage, 1991, 115–36; Gouws, Dennis. "Biological Studies of Homosexuality." In Timothy F. Murphy, ed., *Reader's Guide to Lesbian and Gay Studies*. Chicago, Ill.: Fitzroy Dearborn, 2000, 84–86; Hamer, Dean, and Peter Copeland. *The Science of Desire: The Search for the Gay Gene and the Biology of Behavior*. New York: Simon and Schuster, 1994; Henry, William A., III. "The Hamer Study." In Robert Baird and M. Katherine Baird, eds., *Homosexuality: Debating the Issues*. Amherst, N.Y.: Prometheus, 1995, 91–94; Hooker, Evelyn. "The Adjustment of the Male Overt Homosexual." *Journal of Projective Techniques* 21:1 (1957), 18–31. Reprinted in Hendrik Ruitenbeek, ed., *The Problem of Homosexuality in Modern Society*. New York: Dutton, 1963, 141–61; Hooker, Evelyn. "What Is a Criterion?" *Journal of Projective Techniques* 23:2 (1959), 278–81; Lancaster, Roger N. *The Trouble with Nature: Sex in Science and Popular Culture*. Berkeley: University of California Press, 2003; LeVay, Simon. *Queer Science: The Use and Abuse of Research on Homosexuality*. Cambridge, Mass.: MIT Press, 1996; LeVay, Simon. *The Sexual Brain*. Cambridge, Mass.: MIT Press, 1993; LeVay, Simon, and Dean H. Hamer. "Evidence of a Biological Influence in Male Homosexuality." *Scientific American* (May 1994), 44–49; Lewontin, Richard C. "Women versus the Biologists." *New York Review of Books* (7 April 1994), 31–35; Lewontin, Richard C., Steven Rose, and Leon J. Kamin. *Not in Our Genes: Biology, Ideology, and Human Nature*. New York: Pantheon, 1984; Murphy, Timothy F., ed. *Gay Ethics: Controversies in Outing, Civil Rights, and Sexual Science*. Binghamton, N.Y.: Haworth Press, 1994; Pattatucci, Angela M. L., and Dean H. Hamer. "The Genetics of Sexual Orientation: From Fruit Flies to Humans." In Paul R. Abramson and Steven D. Pinkerton, eds., *Sexual Nature Sexual Culture*. Chicago, Ill.: University of Chicago Press, 1995, 154–74; Rosario, Vernon A., II, ed. *Science and Homosexualities*. New York: Routledge, 1997; Ruse, Michael. "Are There Gay Genes? Sociobiology Looks at Homosexuality."

Journal of Homosexuality 4:1 (1981), 5–34. Reprinted as "Are There Gay Genes? Sociobiology and Homosexuality," in SLF (61–86); Schwartz, Mark F., and William H. Masters. "The Masters and Johnson Treatment Program for Dissatisfied Homosexual Men." *American Journal of Psychiatry* 141:2 (1984), 173–81; Stein, Edward. *The Mismeasure of Desire: The Science, Theory, and Ethics of Sexual Orientation.* New York: Oxford University Press, 2001; Stein, Edward. "The Relevance of Scientific Research about Sexual Orientation to Lesbian and Gay Rights." *Journal of Homosexuality* 27:3–4 (1994), 269–308. Reprinted in HS (191–230); Stein, Edward, Jacinta Kevin, and Udo Schüklenk. "Sexual Orientation." In Ruth Chadwick, ed., *Encyclopedia of Applied Ethics*, vol. 4. San Diego, Calif.: Academic Press, 1998, 101–8; Suppe, Frederick. "The Bell and Weinberg Study: Future Priorities for Research on Homosexuality." *Journal of Homosexuality* 6:4 (1981), 69–97.

HUME, DAVID (1711–1776). Scottish philosopher David Hume aspired to lay the foundations of a comprehensive science of humanity. His treatment of sexuality is not integrated but diffused over a number of works. His writings on this topic can be subsumed under two categories: those that deal with the intrinsic nature of "amorous passions" and those that treat the conventions that regulate their indulgence or satisfaction.

Hume's earliest and longest philosophical work, *A Treatise of Human Nature*, includes both. It was originally published in three volumes (1739–1740), titled *Of the Understanding*, *Of the Passions*, and *Of Morals*. Book 2 includes a short section "Of the amorous passion, or love betwixt the sexes," and Book 3 includes "Of chastity and modesty." The first of these is Hume's attempt to incorporate sexual impulses within his more general mechanistic theory of the passions, which is confidently summarized in the final sentence of *A Dissertation on the Passions* (1757; a much abbreviated reworking of Book 2 of the *Treatise*): "[I]n the production and conduct of the passions, there is a certain regular mechanism, which is susceptible of as accurate a disquisition, as the laws of motion, optics, hydrostatics, or any part of natural philosophy" (i.e., physics). The second is an account of some of the social conventions that govern sexual conduct. Both sections constitute in total 4 out of about 400 pages. We may therefore conclude that sexuality was not a subject with which he was greatly preoccupied. Though now regarded as Hume's greatest philosophical work, the *Treatise* was not well received on publication and was not reprinted in his lifetime, nor indeed until 1817. However, much of the material from Books 1 and 3, including his treatment of chastity and modesty, was reworked in *An Enquiry Concerning Human Understanding* (1748) and *An Enquiry Concerning the Principles of Morals* (1751). These were frequently reprinted both during Hume's life and thereafter.

The central tenet of Hume's account of "love betwixt the sexes" is that it incorporates three elements that reinforce one another in a quasi-mechanical way: "the pleasing sensation arising from beauty; the bodily appetite for generation; and a generous kindness or good-will" (*Treatise*, bk. II, ii, 11). Any one of these is likely to be attended by the other two:

> One, who is inflam'd with lust, feels at least a momentary kindness towards the object of it, and at the same time fancies her more beautiful than ordinary; as there are many, who begin with kindness and esteem for the wit and merit of the person, and advance from that to the other passions. But the most common species of love is that which first arises from beauty, and afterwards diffuses itself into kindness and into the bodily appetite.

Hume goes on to highlight the mediating role of an aesthetic appreciation of objects of **sexual desire**: "Kindness or esteem, and the appetite to generation, are too remote to unite easily together. The one is, perhaps, the most refin'd passion of the soul; the other the most gross and vulgar. The love of beauty is plac'd in a just medium betwixt them, and partakes of both their natures: From whence it proceeds, that 'tis so singularly fitted to produce both."

Hume believed that the amorous passion constitutes a striking instance of his unifying theory of the double relation of impressions and ideas, a complex psychological mechanism by which he thought that certain passions were excited and maintained. While this quasi-mechanistic account might not seem very plausible in an age less enthralled by the Newtonian model from which it was derived, and while it has generated far less interest than most of Hume's other doctrines, it nonetheless incorporates certain valuable insights. By including strong benevolent and aesthetic elements it may well have been a conscious reaction against **Bernard Mandeville**'s (1670–1733) almost bestial account of sexual desire (*Fable of the Bees*, Remark N), which seeks to explain sexual passion as little more than a physical appetite. It might be argued, however, that Hume inclined too far in the opposite direction, proffering a theory that was naively optimistic, blurring or even annihilating any practical distinction between **love** and lust (see Lesser; Stafford), and unable to accommodate comfortably sexual desires and activities of a cruel and sadistic type.

While Hume reacted against Mandeville's account of the nature of sexual desire, he wholeheartedly concurred that chastity and modesty are "artificial virtues," inasmuch as they are the product of education and evolving convention rather than inherent in human nature. This claim might now seem obvious, but in the 1720s and 1730s it was innovative and controversial, for many persevered in the belief that the rules governing sexual morality were divinely ordained. Some even avowed that there is in humans an intrinsic natural modesty inhibiting them from **sexual activity**, perhaps as a vestige of that innocence that preceded the fall of Adam and, especially, Eve. Such was the intellectual landscape in which Hume worked and to which he presented his innovative theories. It is therefore surprising that in the *Treatise* he embarks on his psychosocial account of these virtues with a preamble that takes for granted that "such notions arise from education, from the voluntary conventions of men, and from the interest of society" (bk. III, ii, 12). The origin and justification of chastity and its close relation, modesty, is the need to assure men that the children on whom they expend their resources are their own. Since paternity, unlike maternity, is subject to doubt, women must be constrained to fidelity by the most rigorous pressures that social convention can exert. This incentive to chastity must be further reinforced by inculcating from an early age a modesty that "may give the female sex a repugnance to all expressions, and postures, and liberties, that have an immediate relation to [carnal] enjoyment." The obligation to chastity and modesty is extended even to women beyond childbearing age, whose lapse from the prescribed standard would undermine a general rule and set a bad example to younger women.

Hume might have been right in claiming the reason he cites as the primary one why chastity is accounted a virtue, but it is surely not the only one. Just as, according to **Herbert Spencer** (1820–1903), people wish to have exclusive possession of their clothes, ornaments, tools, and weapons, so they develop a proprietary attitude toward their sexual partners, irrespective of whether infidelity has any reproductive potential (*Principles of Sociology*, pt. 2, chap. 5, §292). Sexual **jealousy** is not peculiar to humans but is also experienced by other highly evolved animals (see **Edward Westermarck** [1862–1939], *History*, chap. 9).

While many of Hume's contemporaries were shocked by his assertion that certain virtues are in a significant sense "artificial" (without being arbitrary), some recent commentators (e.g., Immerwahr) are offended by the disparity in the degree of rigor with which chastity is imposed on men and women. Hume seems to have been prepared to acquiesce in the fact that, under pain of greater social disapproval, more self-restraint is required of women than men. He does not quantify this disparity but does point out that it is "contrary to the interest of civil society that men shou'd have an *entire* liberty of indulging their appetites to venereal enjoyment" (*Treatise*, III, ii, 12). It is, moreover, a consequence of his general account of the obligation to practice artificial virtues that men should impose on themselves a high degree of self-restraint in this particular case. That chastity and modesty serve a public good in which men share both directly and by sympathy with the other beneficiaries constitutes a cogent reason for men to conform. The man who indulges himself irresponsibly while requiring his own wife (and other men) to restrain themselves is no better than the man who hopes with impunity to steal the possessions of others but expects them to respect his own property. (Exactly the sort of case **Immanuel Kant** [1724–1804] would later condemn as violating his Categorical Imperative.) The failure to appreciate this corollary (which, admittedly, Hume did not make explicit) would evidence a superficial and selective reading of Hume's text. A gross disparity in the sexual obligations of the sexes would also be inconsistent with the equality that Hume believed should, ideally, exist between them.

Hume also dealt with sexual relations in three of his *Essays*. The most substantial of these, "Of Polygamy and Divorces" (1742), was retained in all subsequent editions of his essays and frequently revised. He begins the essay by striking a deceptively radical note: "As marriage is an engagement entered into by mutual consent, and has for its end the propagation of the species, it is evident, that it must be susceptible of all the variety of conditions, which consent establishes, provided they be not contrary to this end. . . . [I]t is mere superstition to imagine that marriage can be entirely uniform, and will admit only of one mode or form." Hume reviews different kinds of conjugal arrangements, including those found among animals, and proceeds to assess the merits of various systems, including polygamy as practiced in the Middle East, concluding that polygamy "destroys that nearness of rank, not to say equality, which nature has established between the sexes." Being incompatible with true affection, highly productive of jealousy, and a poor environment in which to raise children, polygamy has nothing to commend it. Hume then discusses divorce, finding three "unanswerable objections" to it: first, the adverse effects on children; second, that where divorce is unavailable people will make the best of their situation (successful **marriage** depends on **friendship**, which is more constant than love); and third, permanence of marriage is necessary to guarantee an identity of interest between the parties. Characteristically, and in contrast to the apparent radicalism of the essay's first sentence, Hume concludes with a conservative endorsement of contemporary European practice.

The essay "Of Love and Marriage," published in 1741, was excised from collections of the *Essays* after the 1760 edition. Hume had written to Adam Smith (1723–1790) in September 1752, saying that he would have discarded it from the third edition in 1748 as being "too frivolous . . . and not very agreeable" (*Letters*, no. 78), had he not been dissuaded from doing so by his publisher, Andrew Millar (1707–1768). Writing in a very light vein, he discusses such issues as which sex exercises dominion over the other and whether men provoke resentment in women by abusing their authority. Relations between the sexes would, Hume maintains, be better if founded on equality (without specifying in what this equality might consist). He describes the conflicts between pleasure and responsibility and asserts the need to reconcile them.

"Of Moral Prejudices," published in 1742, was never reprinted during Hume's lifetime. At the end of this essay, under pretext of relating a true story from a Parisian correspondent, he raises the question of whether "a young lady of birth and fortune" should be allowed as a single mother to raise her son, having expressly so contracted with the gentleman who sired him. Without pronouncing on the matter, Hume seems sympathetic to the woman's plight. She must indeed have been "a woman of strong spirit and an uncommon way of thinking," perhaps so uncommon that Hume felt constrained to suppress the piece from subsequent editions of his essays.

Some recent commentators (e.g., Immerwahr), inspired more by their own agendas than by a concern to read an eighteenth-century author sympathetically, have castigated Hume for his sexism and **heterosexism**. But Hume's account of "love betwixt the sexes" might easily be modified so as to apply just as well to homosexual desire, and his attitude toward women, though equivocal, was in many respects modern. Since Hume lived and wrote two and a half centuries ago, it is hardly surprising that some of his opinions do not accord with those now in vogue. What is remarkable is how progressive his ideas were for his time and how influential they have continued to be.

See also Abstinence; Beauty; Desire, Sexual; Jealousy; Kant, Immanuel; Love; Mandeville, Bernard; Marriage; Rousseau, Jean-Jacques; Spencer, Herbert

REFERENCES

Hume, David. (1757) *A Dissertation on the Passions*. In Thomas Hill Green and Thomas Hodge Grose, eds., *Philosophical Works*, vol. 4. London: Longman, Green, 1874–1875; Hume, David. (1748) *An Enquiry Concerning Human Understanding*. Ed. Tom L. Beauchamp. Oxford, U.K.: Clarendon Press, 2000; Hume, David. (1751) *An Enquiry Concerning the Principles of Morals*. Ed. Tom L. Beauchamp. Oxford, U.K.: Oxford University Press, 1998; Hume, David. *Essays Moral, Political, and Literary*. Ed. Eugene F. Miller. Indianapolis, Ind.: Liberty Classics, 1985; Hume, David. *The Letters of David Hume*, 2 vols. Ed. J.Y.T. Greig. Oxford, U.K.: Clarendon Press, 1932; Hume, David. (1739–1740) *A Treatise of Human Nature*. Ed. David Fate Norton and Mary J. Norton. Oxford, U.K.: Oxford University Press, 2000; Immerwahr, John. "David Hume, Sexism, and Sociobiology." *Southern Journal of Philosophy* 21:3 (1983), 359–69; Lesser, A. H. "Love and Lust." *Journal of Value Inquiry* 14:1 (1980), 51–54; Mandeville, Bernard. (1714, 1723) *The Fable of the Bees*, 2 vols. Ed. F. B. Kaye. Oxford, U.K.: Clarendon Press, 1924; Spencer, Herbert. *The Principles of Sociology*, 3rd ed., vol. 1. London: Williams and Norgate; New York: Appleton and Co., 1885; Stafford, J. Martin. "On Distinguishing between Love and Lust." *Journal of Value Inquiry* 11:4 (1977), 292–303; Westermarck, Edward. (1891) *The History of Human Marriage*, 5th ed., 3 vols. London: Macmillan, 1921.

J. Martin Stafford

ADDITIONAL READING

Baier, Annette. "Good Men's Women: Hume on Chastity and Trust." *Hume Studies* 5 (1979), 1–19; Harman, Gilbert. "Explaining Value." *Social Philosophy and Policy* 11:1 (1994), 229–48; Hume, David. *A Treatise of Human Nature*. Ed. L. A. Selby-Bigge. Oxford, U.K.: Clarendon Press, 1968; Lesser, A. H. "Love and Lust." *Journal of Value Inquiry* 14:1 (1980), 51–54. Reprinted in HS (75–78); Mandeville, Bernard. *The Fable of the Bees*. Indianapolis, Ind.: Liberty Classics, 1988; Neu, Jerome. *Emotion, Thought, and Therapy: A Study of Hume and Spinoza and the Relationship of Philosophical Theories of the Emotions to Psychological Theories of Therapy*. London: Routledge and Kegan Paul, 1977; Shalit, Wendy. "Can Modesty Be Natural?" In *A Return to Modesty: Discovering the Lost Virtue*. New York: Free Press, 1999, 118–43; Singer, Irving. *Explorations in Love and Sex*. Lanham, Md.: Rowman and Littlefield, 2001; Stafford, J. Martin. "On Distinguishing between Love and Lust." *Journal of Value Inquiry* 11:4 (1977), 292–303. Reprinted in J. Martin Stafford, ed., *Essays on Sexuality and Ethics*. Solihull, U.K.: Ismeron, 1995, 53–64.

HUMOR. In the 2000 movie *Me, Myself, and Irene,* Hank (the comically aggressive side of Jim Carrey's Jekyll-Hyde character) says to his new acquaintance Irene (Renee Zellweger), *"I hope we can get to know each other better. . . . Do you swallow?"* The question violates norms about personal inquiry but reveals how Hank is thinking about the relationship. It suggests boldness (which we admire), aggression (about which we have reservations), and social ignorance or ineptness (which we can both sympathize with and make fun of). It challenges conventional romanticism: Learning what to expect from potential sexual partners *is* part of getting to know them (though here premature). There is gender asymmetry, since it would have made no sense for Irene to ask the same question, though comebacks were available if she had wanted to encourage mutual disclosure. There is a reductive element to the question, but the joke is not a putdown, nor is it based on hostility or stereotype. The nonsexist sex joke, as Harvey Mindess and his colleagues observe, "reduces love and sex to acrobatics, but no one is demeaned" (52). At least, the joke is nonsexist if we assume that fellatio is a normal and dignified component of sexual encounters. (*Asked by her professor to define "fellatio," the student answers: "Wait, I know that, it's . . . I can't get it out, it's on the tip of my tongue"* [cf. Strean, 65].)

Though no one knows why human beings laugh, philosophers and social scientists have not hesitated to theorize about humor, wit, comedy, jokes, and what is funny. Some theorists—for example, **Immanuel Kant** (1724–1804) and **Arthur Schopenhauer** (1788–1860)—have focused on cognitive features of humor, such as surprise or incongruity (see texts in Morreall, 45–64). Others have focused on affective features, such as feelings of superiority (**Thomas Hobbes** [1588–1679]; Morreall, 19–20), or the sense of release from social and psychological constraints (**Sigmund Freud** [1856–1939]; Morreall, 111–16). There are many theories (for surveys, see Apte; Carroll; Cohen; Davis; Lauter; Mindess et al.; Morreall; Provine). Each explains some forms of humor better than others. (*Q: According to Freud, what comes between fear and sex? A: Fünf* [Cohen, 11].)

One key element of humor is its power to disrupt ordinary expectations and social proceedings in an acceptable way. (When humor becomes conventional, as in after-dinner jokes or sitcoms, it may itself need to be disrupted by a yet more radical humorous shift; cf. Bolle, 92.) Humor licenses temporary suspension of the usual rules, and this possibility creates new levels of social interaction. I can criticize, but I can also *pretend* to criticize. And I can also pretend to pretend, when I really *am* being critical. To say "I'm only kidding" allows me to state things that would be harsh if offered as straightforward criticism. Laughter "takes the edge off " criticism, and so pretending to laugh—invoking the protective cover of the joking relationship—allows us to explore subjects that would otherwise be taboo. Humor allows people to talk without committing themselves and so lets them feel each other out, permitting a process of mutual adjustment. In areas of conflicting interests, divergent viewpoints, and social sensitivity, humor introduces valuable ambiguity.

Humor creates energy by flirting with taboos, which it both questions and affirms. This is seen in the universal myth-figure of the clown, fool, or trickster, whose sexual (and other) pranks disrupt the status quo (Apte, 212–36; cf. Towsen). Through humor, myth breaks the hold of established categories (Bolle, 86–92; Hyde, 271–80). Paradoxically, such humor also supports the status quo, as Towsen notes:

> The clown's humor is also considered to be of therapeutic value when it deals explicitly with sexual and scatological matters. . . . Although many early anthropologists were repulsed by this obscene clowning, it has proved surprisingly

popular among cultures with puritanical standards of morality, for they recognize it as a necessary safety valve. By laughing at taboo subjects, the community confronts the inhibition in an open yet vicarious manner. (15)

Polymath comedian Steve Allen (1921–2000) suggests that

the primary reason that sex jokes—whether specifically "dirty" or not—will almost invariably produce laughter, either hearty or nervous, is that some part of our consciousness knows that material of that sort ought to be repressed, at least in certain social settings. There are even times when nothing more than the mere factor of inappropriateness can make an audience laugh. (52–53)

Consider this joke: *A guy meets a woman in a bar. She is depressed: her husband left her because she's too kinky. Hey, says the guy, small world: my wife left me because she thought I was too kinky! They decide to go back to her place, and she slips into the bedroom to change. She puts on leather skirt and boots, and a rubber bra with the nipples cut out. She grabs a riding crop and handcuffs and returns to the living room, where she sees the guy heading for the door. "Where are you going? I thought we were going to get kinky." The guy looks at her, and says: "Hey, I fucked your dog and I've shit in your purse. . . . I'm gone!"* Comedian Drew Carey insists, "You can tell that joke a hundred different ways, but it's never as funny as when you say 'fucked' and 'shit' in the punch line" (xiv; cf. Joel Feinberg [1926–2004], 244–48). As Karl Kraus (1874–1936) philosophizes, *"The most tragic fate in the whole world must be that of the fetishist who goes after only a woman's shoe, but gets the whole woman"* (Szasz, 153).

While humor is benign in helping us deal with our ambivalent feelings about taboos, it can also serve as a vehicle for venting hostility. Laughter often derives from social anxiety and the hostility that is a response to anxiety. Alan Dundes suggests, "As dreams provide essential outlets for the anxieties of the individual, so joke cycles serve a similar role for the society at large" (95). (*Why are cucumbers better than men? You know how firm it is before you take one home* [84]. *Why are sheep better than women? A sheep will never leave you for a cucumber* [94].) Such humor has a substantial presence in Reinhold Aman's maverick journal *Maledicta: The International Journal of Verbal Aggression*. Gershon Legman (1918–1999), the rather humorless "Diderot of the dirty joke" (Brottman, 42), also saw humor as inspired by aggression. He devoted most of his life, including a brief early stint working for Alfred Kinsey (1894–1956), to studying sexual and scatological humor; the two volumes he published on the "rationale of the dirty joke" consist of more than 1,800 pages of minutely categorized lore and (largely Freudian-inspired) analysis. Legman also devoted extensive time to collecting limericks and other erotic folklore. His work demonstrates the male-centered character of most traditional comedy with a vengeance (Barreca, 154–55).

It is sexual humor's close link with (verbal) aggression that has fueled feminist discussions of humor and sexual inequality (Barreca; Crawford; Tiefer). (*Q: How many radical feminists does it take to change a light bulb? A: That's not funny!* [Barreca, 178].) Comedy's ambiguity has also made sexual humor *non grata* in the workplace. This advice to middle management is typical:

Any sexual remarks, pictures, jokes, or innuendo should be taboo at work. The prevalence of sexual harassment complaints . . . leaves little choice for any other alternative. . . . When you see any type of conduct that could potentially create a sexually hostile work environment, end it, and end it fast, even if you think the conduct is funny or amusing. It may be only a joke to you, but it may be something much more serious to someone else. The point is that you have to ignore your own personal tolerance for the conduct in question. (Orlov and Roumell, 76)

Though the goal of managers is to minimize the risk of legal liability, defenders of the role of robust sexual humor in life (Aristophanes [ca. 450–380 BCE], Rabelais [ca. 1494–1553]) will critique what they see as the "political correctness" of humorless **sexual harassment** law (see Johnson). (*A woman goes into a bank to cash a $100 check. The cashier returns it, saying, "I'm sorry, but this check is no good." "Omygod!" exclaims the woman, "I've been raped"* [cf. Mindess et al., 50].)

Humor and sex may be seen as natural allies in challenging authority, political or religious, that insists on the delay, or denial, of gratification in the service of "serious" ends. V. A. Kolve, writing about medieval drama, notes that

> where each action is scrutinized in terms of its eternal consequence, comedy and delight are impossible. . . . [And] a powerful case was established and reiterated throughout the Middle Ages that laughter and frivolity, the temporary abstention from involvement in all that is serious in the human condition, was an offense against God, a negation of the example of Christ, and a peril to men's souls. (125–26)

Irving Kristol writes similarly about the social preconditions of "Jewish humor":

> The Jews of an earlier day were rich in proverbs (some of them witty), parables, moralistic anecdotes—but not, it seems, in humor. This fact is no occasion for surprise if we cast a glance at the development of humor in the various Western Christian nations of the Middle Ages. There we see that humor could exist only in the interstices of a religious civilization . . . that the religious authorities frowned upon it, and that it won popular affection to the extent that the dominion of religion became questionable, and that, indeed, one of its functions was to challenge this dominion. Humor needs to breathe the air of skepticism, and prior to the modern epoch the Jews were men of faith, piety, and hence sobriety. When one believes that this life on earth is implicated in eternal salvation or eternal damnation, there is little motive for levity. (422)

We may well have reservations about these claims. First, this view obviously does not apply to humor in the broadest sense (note the exception of "witty" proverbs). Kristol is concerned with a very particular kind of humor ("Jewish humor"), a kind of humor that was particularly important in the United States during the twentieth century: the humor of Freud, of Lenny Bruce (1925–1966) and Woody Allen, the humor of an entertainment medium significantly shaped by Jewish sensibilities (see Gabler; for the African American contribution, see Watkins). Second, the view rests on a dubious empirical premise ("not, it seems, in humor"). Unquestionably, religious thinkers have discouraged humor of particular types but rarely humor of every kind. After all, as the medieval translator Notker Labeo (ca. 952–1022) remarked, a human being is rational, mortal, and able to laugh: *homo est animal rationale, mortale, risus capax* (Kolve, 127). Even from the most rigorous religious perspective, we need courage to live virtuously and, as Legman says, "*casting off of fear by rollicking in its details is the one classic function of jokes and humor generally*" (*Second Series*, 302). Or as Barreca puts it, "You have an instinctive desire to render the information funny so that it won't be scary or bizarre" (150).

When I was a boy, I rode once on a ferris wheel, along with my mother and brother. On one of the revolutions, as we rose up, the wheel for some reason stopped, and we hung there in the sky a long time. After a while, it began to rain from the seat right above my head, whose occupant (a girl) was squealing. That it was rain I frankly doubted. A spilled drink? Not likely. Without umbrella, and escape being impossible, there was little for it but to clown in the thin stream. For **Havelock Ellis** (1859–1939), such an experience might have been quintessentially sexual. For me, it was merely a brief, soggy inconvenience, a rinsing off of someone else's fear. Eventually, the wheel began to move again and brought us all back to the ground we had left behind. (*An elderly man calls his young wife to his bedside. "I've made all the arrangements," he says. "All the estate will be yours. But do this one thing for me. When I'm gone, take that thousand-dollar bottle of wine we were saving, and pour it on my grave. Will you do that?" Yes, she will, she says, adding, "Do you mind, darling, if I drink it first?"*)

Why we find some things funny, and not others, and why we desire, or **love**, one individual, and not another, we can hardly say. Mindess and his colleagues suggest that "enjoyment of sexual jokes is part of our human heritage. At puberty we all become the playthings of powerful mating urges, which at once ensure the survival of our species and the absurdity of much of our future behavior" (56). Sex reminds us we cannot always hold on to our rationality or evade our personal mortality, but we can laugh about both.

See also Arts, Sex and the; Ellis, Havelock; Flirting; Freud, Sigmund; Greek Sexuality and Philosophy, Ancient; Harassment, Sexual; Hobbes, Thomas; Lacan, Jacques; Language; Liberalism; Masturbation; Philosophy of Sex, Overview of; Poststructuralism

REFERENCES

Allen, Steve, with Jane Wollman. *How to Be Funny: Discovering the Comic You*. New York: McGraw-Hill, 1987; Aman, Reinhold, ed. *The Best of Maledicta*. Philadelphia, Pa.: Running Press, 1987; Apte, Mahadev L. *Humor and Laughter: An Anthropological Approach*. Ithaca, N.Y.: Cornell University Press, 1985; Barreca, Regina. *They Used to Call Me Snow White . . . But I Drifted: Women's Strategic Use of Humor*. New York: Viking Penguin, 1991; Bolle, Kees W. *The Freedom of Man in Myth*. Nashville, Tenn.: Vanderbilt University Press, 1968; Brottman, Mikita. "Gershon Legman: Lord of the Lewd." In Catherine Johnson, Betsy Stirratt, and John Bancroft, eds., *Sex and Humor: Selections from the Kinsey Institute*. Bloomington: Indiana University Press, 2002, 42–52; Carey, Drew. *Dirty Jokes and Beer: Stories of the Unrefined*. New York: Hyperion, 1997; Carroll, Noël. "On Jokes." *Midwest Studies in Philosophy* 16 (1991), 280–301; Cohen, Ted. *Jokes: Philosophical Thoughts on Joking Matters*. Chicago, Ill.: University of Chicago Press, 1999; Crawford, Mary. "On Conversational Humor." In *Talking Difference: On Gender and Language*. London: Sage, 1995, 129–69; Davis, Murray S. *What's So Funny? The Comic Conception of Culture and Society*. Chicago, Ill.: University of Chicago Press, 1993; Dundes, Alan. *Cracking Jokes: Studies of Sick Humor Cycles and Stereotypes*. Berkeley, Calif.: Ten Speed Press, 1986; Feinberg, Joel. *The Moral Limits of the Criminal Law*, vol. 2: *Offense to Others*. New York: Oxford University Press, 1985; Freud, Sigmund. (1905) *Jokes and Their Relation to the Unconscious*. Trans. James Strachey. New York: Norton, 1960; Gabler, Neal. *An Empire of Their Own: How the Jews Invented Hollywood*. New York: Crown Publishers, 1988; Hobbes, Thomas. *Leviathan, or The Matter, Forme, and Power of a Common-wealth Ecclesiastical and Civill*. London: Andrew Crooke, 1651 (part I, chap. 6); Hyde, Lewis. *Trickster Makes This World: Mischief, Myth, and Art*. New York: Farrar, Straus and Giroux, 1998; Johnson, Edward. "Political Correctness." In Ruth Chadwick, ed., *Encyclopedia of Applied Ethics*, vol. 3. New York: Academic Press, 1997, 565–79; Kant, Immanuel. (1793) *Critique of Judgment*. [§54] Trans. Werner S. Pluhar. Indianapolis, Ind.: Hackett, 1987, 201–7; Kolve, V. A. *The Play Called Corpus Christi*. Stanford, Calif.: Stanford University Press, 1966; Kristol, Irving. (1951) "Is Jewish Humor Dead?" In *Neoconservatism: The Autobiography of an Idea*. New York: Free Press, 1995, 420–28; Lauter, Paul, ed. *Theories of Comedy*. Garden City, N.Y.: Anchor Books, 1964; Legman,

G[ershon]. *No Laughing Matter: An Analysis of Sexual Humor (Second Series)*. New York: Breaking Point, 1975. Reprinted as *Rationale of the Dirty Joke: An Analysis of Sexual Humor (Second Series)*; Legman, G[ershon]. *Rationale of the Dirty Joke: An Analysis of Sexual Humor (First Series)*. New York: Grove Press, 1968; Legman, G[ershon], ed. *The New Limerick*. New York: Crown Publishers, 1977; Mindess, Harvey, Carolyn Miller, Joy Turek, Amanda Bender, and Suzanne Corbin. *The Antioch Humor Test: Making Sense of Humor*. New York: Avon Books, 1985; Morreall, John, ed. *The Philosophy of Laughter and Humor*. Albany: State University of New York Press, 1987; Orlov, Darlene, and Michael T. Roumell. *What Every Manager Needs to Know about Sexual Harassment*. New York: Amacom, 1999; Provine, Robert R. *Laughter: A Scientific Investigation*. New York: Viking Penguin, 2000; Schopenhauer, Arthur. (1818/1844/1859) *The World as Will and Representation*. [Vol. 1, §13; Vol. 2, chap. 8] Trans. E.F.J. Payne. Indian Hills, Colo.: Falcon Wing's Press, 1958. Reprinted, New York: Dover, 1966, 58–61, 91–101; Strean, Herbert. *Jokes: Their Purpose and Meaning*. Northvale, N.J.: Jason Aronson, 1994; Szasz, Thomas. *Karl Kraus and the Soul-Doctors: A Pioneer Critic and His Criticism of Psychiatry and Psychoanalysis*. Baton Rouge: Louisiana State University Press, 1976; Tiefer, Leonore. "The Capacity for Outrage: Feminism, Humor, and Sex." In Catherine Johnson, Betsy Stirratt, and John Bancroft, eds., *Sex and Humor: Selections from the Kinsey Institute*. Bloomington: Indiana University Press, 2002, 22–38; Towsen, John H. *Clowns*. New York: Hawthorn Books, 1976; Watkins, Mel. *On the Real Side: Laughing, Lying, and Signifying— The Underground Tradition of African-American Humor That Transformed American Culture, from Slavery to Richard Pryor*. New York: Simon and Schuster, 1994.

Edward Johnson

ADDITIONAL READING

Allen, Woody. *Getting Even*. New York: Vintage, 1978; Allen, Woody. *Without Feathers*. New York: Ballantine, 1983; Aman, Reinhold, ed. *Maledicta: The International Journal of Verbal Aggression*. Maledicta Press. Published irregularly, 1977–. <www.sonic.net/maledicta/journal.html> [accessed 10 June 2005]; Aman, Reinhold, ed. *Opus Maledictorum: A Book of Bad Words*. New York: Marlowe, 1996; Aman, Reinhold, ed. *Talking Dirty: A Bawdy Compendium of Abusive Language, Outrageous Insults and Wicked Jokes*. London: Robson, 1993; Aristophanes. *The Eleven Comedies*. Anonymous translation. London: Athenian Society, 1912. Reprint, New York: Liveright, 1943; Bakhtin, Mikhail. "Rabelais in the History of Laughter." In *Rabelais and His World*. Trans. Hélène Iswolsky. Cambridge, Mass.: MIT Press, 1968, 59–144; Baring-Gould, W. S. *The Lure of the Limerick: An Uninhibited History*. London: Rupert Hart-Davis, 1968; Barreca, Regina, ed. *The Penguin Book of Women's Humor*. New York: Penguin, 1996; Benatar, David. "Prejudice in Jest: When Racial and Gender Humor Harms." *Public Affairs Quarterly* 13:2 (1999), 191–203; Berger, Peter. *Redeeming Laughter: The Comic Dimension of Human Experience*. Hawthorne, N.Y.: Walter de Gruyter, 1997; Bibby, Cyril. *The Art of the Limerick*. Hamden, Conn.: Archon Books, 1978; Boskin, Joseph. *Rebellious Laughter: People's Humor in American Culture*. Syracuse, N.Y.: Syracuse University Press, 1997; Bruce, Lenny. *The Essential Lenny Bruce*. Ed. John Cohen. New York: Random House, 1967; Caesar, Sid, with Eddy Friedfeld. *Caesar's Hours: My Life in Comedy, with Love and Laughter*. New York: PublicAffairs/Perseus Books, 2003; Chou, Eric. "Sex, Humor, and Imagery." In *The Dragon and the Phoenix*. New York: Arbor House, 1971, 195–206; Christen, Kimberly A. *Clowns and Tricksters: An Encyclopedia of Tradition and Culture*. Denver, Colo.: ABC-CLIO, 1998; Cohen, Ted. "Jokes." In Eva Schaper, ed., *Pleasure, Preference and Value: Studies in Philosophical Aesthetics*. Cambridge: Cambridge University Press, 1983; Conard, Mark T., and Aeon J. Skoble, eds. *Woody Allen and Philosophy: You Mean My Whole Fallacy Is Wrong?* Chicago, Ill.: Open Court, 2004; Davies, Christie. *Ethnic Humor around the World: A Comparative Analysis*. Bloomington: Indiana University Press, 1990; Davis, Murray S. *Smut: Erotic Reality/Obscene Ideology*. Chicago, Ill.: University of Chicago Press, 1983; Douglas, Norman. *Some Limericks*. New York: Grove Press, 1967; Eastman, Max. *Enjoyment of Laughter*. New York: Simon and Schuster, 1936; Esar, Evan. *Humorous English*. New York: Horizon Press, 1961; Feibleman, James. (1939) *In Praise of Comedy:*

A Study in Its Theory and Practice. New York: Russell and Russell, 1962; Flieger, Jerry Aline. *The Purloined Punch Line: Freud's Comic Theory and the Postmodern Text*. Baltimore, Md.: Johns Hopkins University Press, 1991; Gaut, Berys. "Just Joking: The Ethics and Aesthetics of Humor." *Philosophy and Literature* 22:1 (1998), 51–68; Gilliatt, Penelope. *To Wit: Skin and Bones of Comedy*. New York: Charles Scribner's Sons, 1990; Grote, David. *The End of Comedy: The Sit-Com and the Comedic Tradition*. Hamden, Conn.: Archon Books/Shoe String Press, 1983; Hamilton, Marybeth. *"When I'm Bad, I'm Better": Mae West, Sex, and American Entertainment*. Berkeley: University of California Press, 1997; Hanks, Donald. "Self-Deprecating Humor in Relation to Laughter." *Contemporary Philosophy* 23:5–6 (2001), 29–33; Hartogs, Renatus, and Hans Fantel. *Four-Letter Word Games: The Psychology of Obscenity*. New York: M. Evans, 1967; Hazlett, William. *Lectures on the English Comic Writers*. London: Taylor and Hessey, 1819; Hazlitt, W. Carew. *Studies in Jocular Literature: A Popular Subject More Closely Considered*. London: Elliot Stock, 1890; Heimel, Cynthia. *Sex Tips for Girls*. New York: Simon and Schuster, 1983; Hendra, Tony. *Going Too Far*. New York: Doubleday, 1987; Hockett, C. F. "Jokes." In *The View from Language: Selected Essays 1948–1974*. Athens: University of Georgia Press, 1977, 257–89; Isaak, Jo Anna. *Feminism and Contemporary Art: The Revolutionary Power of Women's Laughter*. New York: Routledge, 1996; Johnson, Catherine, Betsy Stirratt, and John Bancroft, eds. *Sex and Humor: Selections from the Kinsey Institute*. Bloomington: Indiana University Press, 2002; Kadushin, Alfred. "The Use of Humor." In *The Social Work Interview: A Guide for Human Service Professionals*, 3rd ed. New York: Columbia University Press, 1990, 234–42; Kierkegaard, Søren. *The Humor of Kierkegaard: An Anthology*. Ed. Thomas C. Oden. Princeton, N.J.: Princeton University Press, 2004; Kinney, Harrison. *James Thurber: His Life and Times*. New York: Holt, 1995; Koestler, Arthur. *The Act of Creation*. New York: Macmillan, 1964; Legman, G[ershon]. *The Horn Book: Studies in Erotic Folklore and Bibliography*. New Hyde Park, N.Y.: University Books, 1964; Legman, G[ershon], ed. *The Limerick: 1700 Examples, with Notes, Variants, and Index*. Paris: Hautes Etudes, 1953. Reprinted, New York: Castle Books, 1978; Lehman, Peter. "Penis-Size Jokes and Their Relation to Hollywood's Unconscious." In Andrew Horton, ed., *Comedy/Cinema/Theory*. Berkeley: University of California Press, 1991, 43–59; Lyman, Peter. (1987) "The Fraternal Bond as a Joking Relationship: A Case Study of the Role of Sexist Jokes in Male Group Bonding." In Michael S. Kimmel and Michael A. Messner, eds., *Men's Lives*, 3rd ed. Boston, Mass.: Allyn and Bacon, 1995, 86–96; Milburn, D. Judson. *The Age of Wit: 1650–1750*. New York: Macmillan, 1966; Mr. "J." *The World's Best Dirty Jokes*. Secaucus, N.J.: Lyle Stuart, 1976; Moore, Thomas. "Priapus the Scarecrow: The Comic and the Vulgar in Sex." In *The Soul of Sex: Cultivating Life as an Act of Love*. New York: HarperCollins, 1998, 115–36; Nachman, Gerald. *Seriously Funny: The Rebel Comedians of the 1950s and 1960s*. New York: Pantheon Books, 2003; Oring, Elliot. *The Jokes of Sigmund Freud: A Study in Humor and Jewish Identity*. Philadelphia: University of Pennsylvania Press, 1984; Otto, Beatrice K. *Fools Are Everywhere: The Court Jester around the World*. Chicago, Ill.: University of Chicago Press, 2001; Parrott, E. O. *The Penguin Book of Limericks*. London: Allen Lane, 1983; Paulos, John Allen. *Mathematics and Humor*. Chicago, Ill.: University of Chicago Press, 1980; Pearsall, Ronald. "Sexual Humor." In *The Worm in the Bud: The World of Victorian Sexuality*. London: Weidenfeld and Nicholson, 1969, 392–407; Phillips, Adam. "Jokes Apart." In *Promises, Promises: Essays on Psychoanalysis and Literature*. New York: Basic Books, 2001, 347–57; Piddington, Ralph. *The Psychology of Laughter: A Study in Social Adaptation*. New York: Gamut Press, 1963; Plessner, Helmuth. *Laughing and Crying: A Study of the Limits of Human Behavior*. Evanston, Ill.: Northwestern University Press, 1970; Rabelais, François. (1532–1564) *Gargantua and Pantagruel*. Trans. Burton Raffel. New York: Norton, 1990; Reich, Annie. "The Structure of the Grotesque-Comic Sublimation." *Bulletin of the Menninger Clinic* 13 (1949), 160–71. Reprinted in *Psychoanalytic Contributions*. New York: International Universities Press, 1973, 99–120; Sacks, Harvey. "An Analysis of the Course of a Joke's Telling in Conversation." In Richard Bauman and Joel Sherzer, eds., *Explorations in the Ethnography of Speaking*. Cambridge: Cambridge University Press, 1974, 337–53; Screech, M. A., and Ruth Calder. "Some Renaissance Attitudes to Laughter." In A.H.T. Levi, ed., *Humanism in France: At the End of the Middle Ages and in the Early Renaissance*. New York: Barnes and Noble, 1970, 216–28; Simon, Richard

Keller. *The Labyrinth of the Comic: Theory and Practice from Fielding to Freud.* Tallahassee: Florida State University Press, 1985; Sorrell, Walter. *Facets of Comedy.* New York: Universal Library/Grosset and Dunlap, 1973; Thurber, James, and E. B. White. (1929) *Is Sex Necessary? Or Why You Feel the Way You Do.* New York: Harper and Row, 1975; Updike, John. "Libido Lite." [Review of *Is Sex Necessary?* by James Thurber and E. B. White] *New York Review of Books* (18 November 2004), 30–31; Wells, Henry W. *Traditional Chinese Humor: A Study in Art and Literature.* Bloomington: Indiana University Press, 1971; Welsford, Enid. *The Fool: His Social and Literary History.* London: Faber and Faber, 1935. Reprinted, Garden City, N.Y.: Anchor Books, 1961; Wilson, Christopher P. *Jokes: Form, Content, Use, and Function.* New York: Academic Press, 1979; Wolfenstein, Martha. *Children's Humor: A Psychological Analysis.* New York: Free Press, 1954. Reprinted, Bloomington: Indiana University Press, 1978.

HUSSERL, EDMUND. *See* Phenomenology

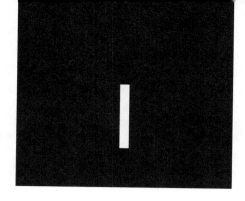

INCEST. Incest, **sexual activity** that occurs between individuals who are closely related by consanguinity or affinity, has not been a central topic in the history of philosophy, although it has been touched on by some of the great theologians and philosophers, for example, **Plato** (427–347 BCE; *Republic*, 457c–462e).

Thomas Aquinas (1224/25–1274) argued that incest was a sexual sin (*Summa theologiae*, IIa-IIae, ques. 154, art. 1, 9, 12; see *Summa contra gentiles*, bk. 3, pt. 2, chap. 125; *De Malo*, ques. 15, art. 3). For Aquinas, some vices of lechery are contrary to nature, and some are not. The unnatural sexual vices, which Aquinas considers the gravest, are acts that cannot be procreative, as in **bestiality**, **masturbation**, and **homosexuality**. Acts that are not unnatural, because from them generation could result—heterosexual **adultery**, **rape**, **seduction**, and incest—are also sexual sins, for Aquinas, but for other reasons (and they are not as morally serious). Thus Aquinas does not condemn incest as always being contrary to nature. Here Aquinas follows **Augustine** (354–430), who acknowledged the necessity, and hence the naturalness, of incest among the children of Adam and Eve (*City of God*, bk. 15, chap. 16). Instead, Aquinas's reasons are that (1) incest and the respect one owes to blood relations are inconsistent; (2) incest would lead to inordinate indulgence in sexual pleasure, thereby weakening the mind and corrupting both prudence and chastity (similarly, for Augustine the incest prohibition "restrains concupiscence within due bounds"); (3) marrying their sisters prevents men from forming intricate interfamilial connections (this is a predominant theme in Augustine; exogamy is the "seed-bed of the city"); and (4) children are naturally subject to parents, which is incompatible with conjugal union between them.

Immanuel Kant's (1724–1804) discussion of incest is limited to a handful of lines spread over two sections of his *Lectures on Ethics*. Kant partially avoids moral questions about incest, because he claims that "nature, by itself" blocks it: "[W]here bonding and familiarity are all too excessive, the impulse produces indifference and disgust. . . . [T]he inclination towards a person one has known from youth upwards is very cold. . . . Thus nature has already by itself set limits to such inclinations between siblings" (Ak 27:389; see **Roger Scruton**, 314). Yet Kant admits that the "original" humans must have engaged in sibling incest. Against parent-child incest Kant provides two moral objections (Ak 27:390). First, it is incompatible with a necessary "respect" that "has to endure throughout life" between parents and children (see Aquinas's reason [1]). Second, sexual union is permissible for Kant only when both parties become subordinate to each other through a mutual surrender of their selves (Ak 27:388). This condition is unsatisfiable between parent and child, because only the child is subordinate in their relationship (see Aquinas's reason [4]). Kant also asks whether incest might be a *crimen carnis contra naturam*, an unnatural crime of the flesh (Ak 27:391). He admits that it seems not to be, because human incest can be heterosexual and procreative and because animals engage in it (see also **David Hume** [1711–1776], *Treatise*, bk. III, pt. 1, sec. 1). But the rest of Kant's discussion is uncertain.

In recent philosophy of sexuality, incest is largely ignored. Even philosophers who have written extensively about sexuality, such as Igor Primoratz (63–65) and Alan Soble (28–29), mention incest only incidentally. More substantial philosophical discussions of incest are found in David Archard (99–103), Raymond Belliotti (242–46), Jerome Neu ("What Is Wrong with Incest?"), **Richard Posner** (199–204; see also Posner and Silbaugh, 129–42), Scruton (311–15), and Ben Spiecker and Jan Steutel. These writings, like those of Augustine, Aquinas, and Kant, address the morality of incest and therefore belong to the field of practical ethics. Incest suggests intriguing philosophical questions, for example, about the authenticity of recovered memories of incest (see Russell, xx–xl). Here the focus will be on its morality.

Arguments about what is morally wrong with incest frequently refer to its harmful effects. One harmful-effects argument is *biological*, which cites inbreeding's detrimental genetic effects (see Arens, 16–24). The basic idea is that the closer the parents of a child are related genetically, the greater the probability that their child will inherit recessive genes that are phenotypically expressed in physical or mental disorders and hence in reduced viability and, perhaps, fertility (or "fitness"). Though based on empirical research, the biological argument is not fully adequate for judging incest wrong (see Archard, 101; Neu, 29). It applies only to incest between biologically related persons, not to another sort of incest, that between genetically unrelated individuals (say, stepfather and stepdaughter). Moreover, pregnancy from incest can be prevented by using reliable contraceptives or by the persons engaging only in noncoital sexual acts (Belliotti, 243).

A second harmful-effects argument is *sociological*, which cites the disruptive social repercussions, were incest widespread (see Arens, 48–60; Wolf). Functionalists in the social sciences, such as Bronislaw Malinowski (1884–1942) and Talcott Parsons (1902–1979), but also scholars not usually associated with functionalism, such as **Sigmund Freud** (1856–1939) and Claude Lévi-Strauss (1908–   ), explain the incest prohibition in terms of its social functions, in particular its contribution to the organization of the nuclear family and, more broadly, to an orderly society. In this argument, if the prohibition of incest were relaxed, the family and, in turn, society would collapse into confusion and chaos. Without the incest prohibition, family members would engage in sexual competition and exchange roles and positions, and the socialization of children would be seriously subverted. (Consider the child of incest in the Jack Nicholson and Faye Dunaway film *Chinatown*, whose mother is also her sister and whose father is also her grandfather.) Further, society would dissolve into small, isolated groups, because (as in Aquinas's reason [3]; see also Neu) family members would not be forced to leave the family to establish the interfamilial structures required for complex social organizations.

The alleged social advantages of the incest prohibition might explain its existence or persistence. But these benefits might also be reasons for morally condemning incest. (Augustine and Aquinas rely on the interference with interfamilial connections as a moral argument against sibling incest.) These reasons would be convincing only if the purported dire effects of lifting the prohibition would actually occur, which may be doubted. Anthropologists and historians have documented the existence of condoned and even mandatory incestuous marriages: sibling unions in royal families of ancient Egypt and in the Egyptian middle class during the Roman era, as well as father-daughter, brother-sister, and mother-son unions among Zoroastrians in ancient Persia (Arens, 9–10). Organized family life and an orderly society seem possible without an incest prohibition.

Further, this functionalist sociology presupposes a view of human sexual nature that may be untenable. It assumes that humans are naturally inclined to incest and that the prohibition is required to counteract this inclination (see Wolf). This view is challenged by evolutionary biology, which argues that inbreeding avoidance mechanisms have been selected that decrease the expression of recessive deleterious genes. One kin-recognition system that adaptively generates incest avoidance among close relatives was suggested by **Edward Westermarck** (1862–1939). In *The History of Human Marriage* (192–218, 236), he claimed (as did Kant) that individuals living closely together from childhood (for example, siblings) are not sexually attracted to each other. Long after Westermarck, empirical research has yielded evidence for this mechanism (Lieberman et al.). Evolutionary biology also predicts cross-generational inbreeding avoidance mechanisms: Men have no genetic interest in engaging in coitus with their biological daughters. Consistently with Westermarck's hypothesis, it has been proposed that the involvement of fathers in the early care of daughters inhibits sexual attraction. This claim has some empirical support (Seto et al., 267–68). A kin-recognition system that generates cross-generational incest avoidance seems to explain salient differences between biological father-daughter incest and stepfather-stepdaughter sexual activity. Incestuous abuse by biological fathers, as compared with abuse by stepfathers, is not only much less prevalent but also less coercive and severe (Beitchman et al., "Short-Term Effects," 550; Finkelhor, 25; Russell, 231–40, 255). In contrast to functionalist interpretations of incest and its prohibition, according to which humans are naturally inclined toward incest and the incest prohibition is a cultural device needed for its *suppression*, evolutionary accounts argue that humans tend to be indifferent sexually to close relatives and the incest prohibition is an *expression* of this tendency. Evolutionary biologists do not share, therefore, the functionalist concern that relaxing the incest prohibition, if conceivable at all, would result in ubiquitous incestuous behavior.

A third harmful-effects arguments is *psychological*, which invokes the detrimental impact of incest on children. Readers of the many publications on child sexual abuse, including incestuous abuse, can easily get the impression that its effects are devastating. There is virtually no domain of symptomatology that has not been associated with child sexual abuse (Kendall-Tackett et al., 173). Much of this research is methodologically questionable. Most empirical studies are confined to clinical samples, to individuals referred to a mental health setting for assessment or treatment of sexual abuse. The findings of these studies might not be generalizable to the wider population, that is, to nonclinical cases of child sexual abuse. Further, few studies include relevant control groups of nonsexually abused individuals. Consequently, it is unclear whether reported symptoms are attributable to sexual abuse or to other factors: physical abuse, family disturbance, parental attitudes, or even actions taken by professionals in response to disclosure. Nevertheless, there is enough evidence to make some warranted claims about the effects of sexual abuse. One short-term effect is that sexually abused children exhibit, more than nonvictims, various sexualized behaviors: putting objects into anuses or vaginas, excessive or public masturbation, seductive or sexually aggressive acts, and compulsive talk, play, and **fantasy** with sexual content (Beitchman et al., "Short-Term Effects," 552; see also Kendall-Tackett et al.). Along with posttraumatic stress disorder, this syndrome appears to be the only consistent short-term effect. Regarding long-term effects, women who report child sexual abuse more commonly exhibit **sexual dysfunction** or disturbance, anxiety and fear, depression, suicidal ideation and attempts, as well as revictimization—for example, being a victim of battering in an adult relationship or being raped (Beitchman et al., "Long-Term Effects," 115).

Psychological arguments therefore provide strong reasons that cross-generational incest is morally wrong. However, even if the psychological harm argument is strong enough to justify a prohibition of adult-child sex, it might not get to the heart of incest's immorality. Perhaps what makes incest wrong is that the child cannot validly **consent** to sexual activity with adults: "[A]t the core of incest's immorality is nonconsensuality" (Belliotti, 246; see Finkelhor, 17–18).

It may very well be admitted that a child does not have the capacity for making competent decisions in matters of sexuality. But it cannot be immediately concluded that adult-child sex is a violation of the principle of mutual consent. The principle of consent is derived from a more basic principle of respect for persons, that is, for individuals who are regarded as competent decision makers. Accordingly, the principle of mutual consent specifies how adult humans should be treated. In particular, having sexual relations with them is morally permissible only if they have freely given consent on the basis of adequate information. This respect is what we owe to agents having the capacities of self-determination. On this interpretation of the principle of consent, incest between adults and children falls outside its scope: By itself the principle does not imply any judgment about the morality of incestuous adult-child sex. Compare the role of consent in other spheres of life, especially health care (and education). In matters of illness, children do not yet have the capacities required for competent decision making. But that children are incapable of consenting does not make health-care intervention morally wrong. On the contrary, because they lack capacities for self-determination, our interventions for their sake for health reasons, from selecting their food to taking them to the dentist, are not just morally permissible but obligatory, whether they "like" it or not (see Shrage, 52–54).

Because children do not have the capacity for making competent decisions in many areas of life, competent adults have the right and responsibility to make decisions for them. The adults who usually have this power are a child's biological parents or their substitutes: stepparents, foster parents, guardians. Adults who function as surrogates or proxies for a child should choose those actions that protect or promote the child's interests or welfare. Their refraining from interventions is inconsistent with their duties to act as a child's surrogate. Parents unwilling to intervene for pressing health-care reasons might be seriously neglecting their children.

In the domain of sexuality, parents also have the authority and responsibility to act as the child's surrogate. But parental interventions out of their own sexual motives cannot be justified in terms of their surrogacy duties. Such behaviors are likely detrimental to the child's welfare or at least are not in the child's best interests. Because parents cannot reasonably claim that engaging in sexual activity with their children is for the good of the children themselves, a parent's having sex with a child violates the surrogacy relationship. (See Belliotti, 246; Scruton, 313. Perhaps this is what Aquinas and Kant had in mind with their "respect" argument.) Indeed, because a parent is expected to protect a child's interests, the harmful effects of parent-child sex might be greater than other forms of (nonincestuous) adult-child sex. The child might experience parental sexual abuse as a breach of trust (Archard, 102), and this often unarticulated feeling of betrayal might have its own independent harmful effects. Incestuous experiences involving a father or stepfather are generally more harmful than abuse by brothers or outsiders. This greater traumatic impact could be explained by the loss of trust involved in parental sexual abuse (see Finkelhor and Browne; Phelan).

Note, however, that both the consent and harm arguments for the moral wrongness of parent-child incest apply fairly well to any adult-child sex, even if not incestuous. Also, neither argument seems to imply that other types of incest are always wrong. On the contrary, cross-generational and intragenerational incest between adults who have given valid consent (but see Archard, 100–101), as well as incest between young siblings (as long as they enjoy it and no detrimental effects are likely) might be permissible. Those who wish to condemn such practices morally probably must resort either to a version of functionalism or to Natural Law arguments.

See also Aristotle; Augustine (Saint); Bible, Sex and the; Consent; Ethics, Sexual; Evolution; Fichte, Johann Gottlieb; Freud, Sigmund; Kant, Immanuel; Natural Law (New); Pedophilia; Perversion, Sexual; Plato; Psychology, Evolutionary; Rape; Tantrism; Thomas Aquinas (Saint); Violence, Sexual; Westermarck, Edward

REFERENCES

Archard, David. *Sexual Consent.* Boulder, Colo.: Westview, 1998; Arens, William. *The Original Sin: Incest and Its Meaning.* New York: Oxford University Press, 1986; Augustine. (413–427) *The City of God.* Trans. Marcus Dods. New York: Modern Library, 1993; Beitchman, Joseph H., Kenneth J. Zucker, Jane E. Hood, Granville A. DaCosta, and Donna Akman. "A Review of the Short-Term Effects of Child Sexual Abuse." *Child Abuse and Neglect* 15:4 (1991), 537–56; Beitchman, Joseph H., Kenneth J. Zucker, Jane E. Hood, Granville A. DaCosta, Donna Akman, and Erika Cassavia. "A Review of the Long-Term Effects of Child Sexual Abuse." *Child Abuse and Neglect* 16:1 (1992), 101–18; Belliotti, Raymond. "Incest." In *Good Sex: Perspectives on Sexual Ethics.* Lawrence: University Press of Kansas, 1993, 242–46; Finkelhor, David. *Child Sexual Abuse: New Theory and Research.* New York: Free Press, 1984; Finkelhor, David, and Angela Browne. "The Traumatic Impact of Child Sexual Abuse: A Conceptualization." *American Journal of Orthopsychiatry* 55:4 (1985), 530–41; Freud, Sigmund. (1913) *Totem and Taboo.* In *The Standard Edition of the Complete Psychological Works of Sigmund Freud,* vol. 13. Trans. James Strachey. London: Hogarth Press, 1953–1974, ix–161; Hume, David. (1739) *A Treatise of Human Nature.* Ed. L. A. Selby-Bigge. Oxford, U.K.: Clarendon Press, 1968; Kant, Immanuel. (ca. 1762–1794) *Lectures on Ethics.* Trans. Peter Heath. Cambridge: Cambridge University Press, 1997; Kendall-Tackett, Kathleen A., Linda M. Williams, and David Finkelhor. "Impact of Sexual Abuse on Children: A Review and Synthesis of Recent Empirical Studies." *Psychological Bulletin* 113:1 (1993), 164–80; Lévi-Strauss, Claude. "The Family." In Harry L. Shapiro, ed., *Man, Culture, and Society.* New York: Oxford University Press, 1960, 261–85; Lieberman, Debra, John Tooby, and Leda Cosmides. "Does Morality Have a Biological Basis? An Empirical Test of the Factors Governing Moral Sentiments Relating to Incest." *Proceedings of the Royal Society (Biological Sciences)* 270:1517 (2003), 819–26; Malinowski, Bronislaw. *Sex and Repression in Savage Society.* London: Routledge and Kegan Paul, 1927; Neu, Jerome. "What Is Wrong with Incest?" *Inquiry* 19:1 (1976), 27–39; Parsons, Talcott. "The Incest Taboo in Relation to Social Structure and the Socialization of the Child." *British Journal of Sociology* 5:2 (1954), 101–17; Phelan, Patricia. "Incest and Its Meaning: The Perspectives of Fathers and Daughters." *Child Abuse and Neglect* 19:1 (1995), 7–24; Plato. (ca. 375–370 BCE) *Republic.* Trans. G.M.A. Grube. Indianapolis, Ind.: Hackett, 1992; Posner, Richard A. *Sex and Reason.* Cambridge, Mass.: Harvard University Press, 1992; Posner, Richard A., and Katharine B. Silbaugh. *A Guide to America's Sex Laws.* Chicago, Ill.: University of Chicago Press, 1996; Primoratz, Igor. *Ethics and Sex.* London: Routledge, 1999; Russell, Diana E. H. (1986) *The Secret Trauma: Incest in the Lives of Girls and Women,* 2nd ed. New York: Basic Books, 1999; Scruton, Roger. *Sexual Desire: A Moral Philosophy of the Erotic.* New York: Free Press, 1986; Seto, Michael C., Martin L. Lalumière, and Michael Kuban. "The Sexual Preferences of Incest Offenders." *Journal of Abnormal Psychology* 108:2 (1999), 267–72; Shrage, Laurie. *Moral Dilemmas of Feminism: Prostitution, Adultery, and Abortion.* New York: Routledge, 1994; Soble, Alan. *Sexual Investigations.* New York: New York University Press, 1996; Spiecker, Ben, and Jan Steutel. "A Moral-Philosophical Perspective on Paedophilia and Incest." *Educational Philosophy and Theory* 32:3 (2000), 283–91; Thomas Aquinas. (1269) *De Malo* [*On Evil*]. Trans. Richard Regan. Oxford, U.K.: Oxford University Press, 2003; Thomas Aquinas. (1258–1264) *On the Truth of the Catholic Faith. Summa contra gentiles. Book Three: Providence. Part II.* Trans. Vernon J. Bourke. Garden City, N.Y.: Image Books, 1956; Thomas

Aquinas. (1265–1273) *Summa theologiae*, 5 vols. Trans. Fathers of the English Dominican Province. London: Burns, Oates, and Washbourne, 1911–1934; Westermarck, Edward. (1891) *The History of Human Marriage*, 5th ed., vol. 2. London: Macmillan, 1921; Wolf, Arthur P. "Incest Prohibition, Origin and Evolution of." In Neil J. Smelser and Paul B. Baltes, eds., *International Encyclopedia of the Social and Behavioral Sciences*, vol. 11. Amsterdam, Holland: Elsevier, 2001, 7259–62.

Jan Steutel and Ben Spiecker

ADDITIONAL READING

Aberle, David F., Urie Bronfenbrenner, Eckhard H. Hess, Daniel R. Miller, David M. Schneider, and James N. Spuhler. "The Incest Taboo and the Mating Patterns of Animals." *American Anthropologist* 65 (April 1963), 253–64; Aldridge, Alfred Owen. "The Meaning of Incest from Hutcheson to Gibbon." *Ethics* 61:4 (1951), 309–13; Appelbaum, Paul S., Charles W. Lidz, and Alan Miesel. *Informed Consent: Legal Theory and Clinical Practice*. New York: Oxford University Press, 1987; Archard, David. "The Limits of Consensuality I: Incest, Prostitution, and Sado-masochism." In *Sexual Consent*. Boulder, Colo.: Westview, 1998, 98–115; Bancroft, John. (1983) "Child Sexual Abuse, Paedophilia and Incest." In *Human Sexuality and Its Problems*. Edinburgh, Scot.: Churchill Livingstone, 1989, 689–708; Bittles, Alan H. "Incest, Inbreeding, and Their Consequences." In Neil J. Smelser and Paul B. Baltes, eds., *International Encyclopedia of the Social and Behavioral Sciences*, vol. 11. Amsterdam, Holland: Elsevier, 2001, 7254–59; Culver, Charles M., and Bernard Gert. "Competence." In Jennifer Radden, ed., *The Philosophy of Psychiatry: A Companion*. New York: Oxford University Press, 2004, 258–70; Denov, Myriam. "The Myth of Innocence: Sexual Scripts and the Recognition of Child Sexual Abuse by Female Perpetrators." *Journal of Sex Research* 40:3 (2003), 303–14; Ehman, Robert. "Adult-Child Sex." In Robert Baker and Frederick Elliston, eds., *Philosophy and Sex*, 2nd ed. Buffalo, N.Y.: Prometheus, 1984, 431–46; Faden, Ruth R., and Tom L. Beauchamp. *A History and Theory of Informed Consent*. New York: Oxford University Press, 1986; Fox, Robin. *The Red Lamp of Incest*. London: Dutton, 1980; Frye, Marilyn. "Critique" [of Robert Ehman]. In Robert Baker and Frederick Elliston, eds., *Philosophy and Sex*, 2nd ed. Buffalo, N.Y.: Prometheus, 1984, 447–55. Revised version, "Not-Knowing about Sex and Power." In *Willful Virgin: Essays in Feminism 1976–1992*. Freedom, Calif.: Crossing Press, 1992, 39–50; Krober, A. L. (1939) *The Nature of Culture*. Chicago, Ill.: University of Chicago Press, 1952; Leventhal, John M. "Epidemiology of Sexual Abuse of Children: Old Problems, New Directions." *Child Abuse and Neglect* 22:6 (1998), 481–91; Levine, Judith. *Harmful to Minors: The Perils of Protecting Children from Sex*. Minneapolis: University of Minnesota Press, 2002; Mitchell, Juliet. *Siblings*. Malden, Mass.: Polity, 2004; Neu, Jerome. "Genetic Explanation in *Totem and Taboo*." In Richard Wollheim, ed., *Freud: A Collection of Critical Essays*. Garden City, N.Y.: Doubleday, 1974, 366–97; Neu, Jerome. "What Is Wrong with Incest?" *Inquiry* 19:1 (1976), 27–39. Reprinted in *A Tear Is an Intellectual Thing: The Meanings of Emotion*. New York: Oxford University Press, 2000, 166–76; Okami, Paul, Richard Olmstead, Paul R. Abramson, and Laura Pendleton. "Early Childhood Exposure to Parental Nudity and Scenes of Parental Sexuality ('Primal Scenes'): An 18-Year Longitudinal Study of Outcome." *Archives of Sexual Behavior* 27:4 (1998), 361–84; Oxenhandler, Noelle. "The Eros of Parenthood." *The New Yorker* (19 February 1996), 47–49; Pollak, Ellen. *Incest and the English Novel, 1684–1814*. Baltimore, Md.: Johns Hopkins University Press, 2003; Posner, Richard A. "Incest." In *Sex and Reason*. Cambridge, Mass.: Harvard University Press, 1992, 199–204; Posner, Richard A. "Sexual Abuse of Children." In *Sex and Reason*. Cambridge, Mass.: Harvard University Press, 1992, 395–402; Posner, Richard A., and Katharine B. Silbaugh. "Abuse of Position of Trust or Authority," "Age of Consent," and "Incest." In *A Guide to America's Sex Laws*. Chicago, Ill.: University of Chicago Press, 1996, 111–28, 44–64, 129–42; Rosen, Stanley. (1968) "A Digression on Incest." In *Plato's Symposium*, 2nd ed. New Haven, Conn.: Yale University Press, 1987, 211–15; Rudd, Jane M., and Sharon D. Herzberger. "Brother-Sister Incest—Father-Daughter Incest: A Comparison of Characteristics and Consequences." *Child Abuse and Neglect* 23:9 (1999), 915–28; Singer, Peter, ed. "Sexual Morality." In *Ethics*. Oxford, U.K.: Oxford University Press, 1994, Part I.B.iii, 93–112;

Smith, Carol. "Challenged by the Text: Two Stories of Incest in the Hebrew Bible." In Athalya Brenner and Carole R. Fontaine, eds., *A Feminist Companion to Reading the Bible: Approaches, Methods and Strategies.* Sheffield, U.K.: Sheffield Academic Press, 1997, 114–35; Smith, Carol. "Stories of Incest in the Hebrew Bible: Scholars Challenging Text or Text Challenging Scholars?" *Henoch* 14 (1992), 227–42; Spain, David H. "The Westermarck-Freud Incest-Theory Debate: An Evaluation and Reformulation." *Current Anthropology* 28:5 (1987), 623–45; Spiecker, Ben, and Jan Steutel. "Paedophilia, Sexual Desire, and Perversity." *Journal of Moral Education* 26:3 (1997), 331–42; Trepper, Terry S., and Mary Jo Barrett. *Systematic Treatment of Incest: A Therapeutic Handbook.* New York: Brunner/Mazel, 1989; Tsai, Mavis, Shirley Feldman-Summers, and Margaret Edgar. "Childhood Molestation: Differential Impacts on Psychosexual Functioning." In Larry L. Constantine and Floyd M. Martinson, eds., *Children and Sex: New Findings, New Perspectives.* Boston, Mass.: Little, Brown, 1981, 201–16; Walter, Alex. "Putting Freud and Westermarck in Their Places: A Critique of Spain." *Ethos* 18:4 (1990), 439–46; Westermarck, Edward. (1934) "The Oedipus Complex." In *Three Essays on Sex and Marriage.* London: Macmillan, 1934, 1–123; Wolf, Arthur P. *Sexual Attraction and Childhood Association: A Chinese Brief for Edward Westermarck.* Stanford, Calif.: Stanford University Press, 1995.

INDIAN EROTOLOGY. Ancient Indian thought divides the principal aims of human existence into *dharma* (religion, morality, social obligations), *artha* (economics, politics, power), and *kāma* (erotic pleasure, sexual interaction, sensual gratification). To this triad (*trivarga*) is sometimes added a fourth, *mokṣa* (liberation or release from rebirth). Around each of these aims a *śāstra* or body of literature has developed that seeks to guide the student in the achievement of the aim. The *kāma-śāstra* is the Indian literature that seeks to aid the student in his or her pursuit of *kāma*. Although the Sanskrit term *kāma* can be used to refer to any pleasure, within the *kāma-śāstra* it refers primarily to erotic pleasure. ("Kāma" is also the name of the Hindu god of **love** and erotic pleasure.) For this reason the content of the *kāma-śāstra* is often referred to as erotology, that is, the study of eroticism.

Indian erotology began in unknown antiquity and has continued to modern times. The central texts include the *Kāma Sūtra* or *Treatise on Erotic Pleasure* by Vātsyāyana (ca. 300–400), *Ratirahasya* or *Secrets of Love* by Kokkoka (ca. 1100–1200), the *Jayamangalā* commentary on the *Kāma Sūtra* by Yaśodhara (ca. 1200–1300), *Smaradīpikā* or "The Light of Love" by Rudra (ca. 1300–1400), *Ratimañjarī* or "The Posy of Love" by Jayadeva (ca. 1300–1500), *Ratiratnapradīpikā* or *Explanation of the Jewels of Love* by Devarāja (ca. 1400–1500), *Anaṅga Ranga* or *Stage of the Love God* by Kalyāṇamalla (ca. 1500–1600), and the modern (1964) *Jaya* commentary on the *Kāma Sūtra* by Devadatta Shāstri (1912–1982). Of these texts, the most important is the *Kāma Sūtra*, the oldest, though only the oldest *extant*, work. Vātsyāyana makes it clear that there were numerous erotological treatises well before his *Kāma Sūtra*, none of which has survived. The *Kāma Sūtra*, he tells us, is only a summary or "condensation" of the earlier works, though his critiques of them reveal that this is not fully true. The erotological importance of the *Kāma Sūtra* is shown by the fact that most later works in this tradition use the *Kāma Sūtra* as their model or are commentaries on it.

Although Indian erotology is one of the oldest traditions to deal explicitly with human sexuality, it has received little attention from scholars of sexuality (or even from Indologists). It has all but been ignored by philosophers of sexuality (but see Giles). Part of the reason for this seems to be that in the popular imagination the *Kāma Sūtra* is little more than a catalog of the different positions for sexual intercourse (along the lines of popular self-help sex manuals). Yet the *Kāma Sūtra* and other erotological works are much more than this: They are treatises on the sexual dimensions of the human condition. The *Kāma Sūtra* discusses the nature of erotic pleasure (in both its male and female manifestations), **sexual desire**, the sexual process, sexual typology, sexual techniques (including positions), ways of increasing pleasure, courtship, **adultery**, and aphrodisiacs. Although most of these discussions are from the male's perspective, the *Kāma Sūtra* contains much that is aimed at women; for example, there is material on being a wife and on living the life of a courtesan. (**Prostitution** was a highly esteemed profession in ancient India.)

Although much of this is advanced as practical advice, alongside it runs a philosophy of human sexuality, a treatment of the fundamental questions of the nature and value of erotic pleasure and sexual desire, issues that have long engaged philosophers in the West. Of course, much in the erotological tradition is culturally bound and might not be especially relevant for other cultures and times. This is true of any intellectual work. To appreciate the philosophical contributions of the *kāma-śāstra* one must not get sidetracked by aspects of these works that hold only for ancient India (e.g., the discussions of auspicious dates for intercourse). Looking at these fundamental philosophical issues provides a sense of the projects underpinning Indian erotology.

In the opening of the *Kāma Sūtra*, Vātsyāyana discusses cultivating the three aims of life, *dharma*, *artha*, and *kāma*, in such a way that they enhance rather than interfere with each other. (Compare this with **Friedrich Nietzsche**'s [1844–1900] discussion, in *The Birth of Tragedy*, of the balance between the Dionysian and Apollonian tendencies.) Vātsyāyana does this by defending the value of each aim against those who reject it. Thus, he defends *dharma* against materialists, *artha* against fatalists, and *kāma* against those who claim that sexual pursuits are an obstacle to religion and to the acquisition of wealth or power. He responds by saying that although the pursuit of pleasure should be moderate, pleasure, like food, sustains the body. Unfulfilled desire, says Vātsyāyana, can lead to madness and even death. One is reminded here of **Havelock Ellis**'s (1859–1939) early modern view of the value of **masturbation** and other sexual activities, which should nevertheless be pursued, at least by men, in moderation (vol. 1, 203; vol. 5, 195).

The position taken by Vātsyāyana is that the quest for erotic pleasure is basically of equal importance to the quest for religious truth or wealth (though there are exceptions). In the works of writers such as Rudra and Kokkoka, however, the pursuit of erotic pleasure is argued to be more important than the pursuit of the other aims. Thus, says Kokkoka, "the enjoyment of love . . . is honoured, even among the gods, before all other studies" (102). The reason is that erotic pleasure is the one substantial good in a fleeting world. This is because no human pleasure can compare to the quality of erotic pleasure. Though here, as with Vātsyāyana, erotic pleasure must be understood broadly as something that occurs throughout the sexual dimensions of human existence (e.g., courtship, love, **marriage**, sexual interaction). For Kokkoka and other erotologists even brief touches between strangers can give rise to erotic pleasure. The significance of erotic pleasure, then, points to the urgency of studying the *kāma-śāstra*, for "where shall a benighted man find such joy, other than in being thoroughly grounded in the principles, arts and techniques proper to the God of Love [Kāma]" (102).

What is the nature of this pleasure that the erotological literature teaches us to pursue? According to Vātsyāyana, erotic pleasure consists of "a direct experience of an object of the senses, which bears fruit and is permeated by the sensual pleasure of erotic arousal that results from the particular sensation of touch" (*Kamasutra*, 8). This compact, unclear definition (typical of Vātsyāyana's sutra form) is developed by Yaśodhara in the *Jayamangalā* commentary. He elaborates the definition by dividing erotic pleasure into two types, primary and secondary. The former occurs when the touch that stimulates erotic pleasure is directed to the genitals (giving rise to the fruit of "bliss" when orgasm ensues), while the latter takes place when touch is directed to other parts of the body.

But, then, what is it, asks Yaśodhara, that makes secondary pleasure a form of erotic pleasure at all? His answer is that touch on places other than the genitals gives rise to erotic pleasure in the recipient so far as the person nevertheless imagines the passion of genital stimulation. Many questions can be asked here. Are genital and nongenital erotic pleasures phenomenologically distinct? During nongenital touching, must one imagine genital stimulation to experience erotic pleasure? What about erotic pleasure that involves no touching at all, as in nocturnal orgasms or **fantasy**-generated erotic pleasure (including orgasm; see Bruijn)? There are also questions about how accurately Yaśodhara's commentary reflects Vātsyāyana's ideas. Shastri, for one, argues that bearing "fruit" in Vātsyāyana's definition refers to offspring and not, as Yaśodhara has it, to orgasm (*The Complete Kāma Sūtra*, 30).

Equally significant in Indian erotology is the nature of sexual desire. Vātsyāyana writes that sexual desire "springs from nature" and is therefore part of our constitution. Further, sexual desire, in its more forceful appearances, has the power to carry us away, beyond our control—though Vātsyāyana and other erotologists allow for individual differences. Kalyānamalla, as part of his sexual typology, refers to the *chanda-vega*, *manda-vega*, and *madhyamā-vega*, or women of high, low, and medium degrees of sexual desire. (Compare this with Kaplan's contemporary account [57–79] of the degrees of sexual desire.)

Because of this power, Indian erotologists stress the need to cultivate control over sexual desire whereby sexual desire can be consciously directed in the use of specific sexual techniques. Such techniques are said to increase erotic pleasure. Yet erotic pleasure is at its highest intensity when we are "intoxicated" with passion and overcome with desire. Therefore, the cultivation of sexual desire is meant to enable us to arrive in a controlled fashion at a point where passion and sexual desire at last sweep our control away. As Vātsyāyana puts it (*Kamasutra*, 42):

> The territory of the text extends
> only so far as men have dull appetites;
> but when the wheel of sexual ecstasy is in full motion,
> then there is no textbook at all, and no order.

See also Activity, Sexual; Buddhism; Chinese Philosophy; Desire, Sexual; Ellis, Havelock; Hinduism; Jainism; Nietzsche, Friedrich; Philosophy of Sex, Overview of; Tantrism

REFERENCES

Bruijn, Gerda de. "From Masturbation to Orgasm with a Partner: How Some Women Bridge the Gap—and Why Others Don't." *Journal of Sex and Marital Therapy* 8:2 (1982), 151–67; Devarāja. *Ratiratnapradīpikā*. Trans. Rangaswami Iyengar. Mysore, India: Royal Press, 1923; Ellis, Havelock. (1897–1927) *Studies in the Psychology of Sex*, 7 vols. Philadelphia, Pa.: F. A. Davis, 1929; Giles, James. *The Nature of Sexual Desire*. Westport, Conn.: Praeger, 2004; Kalyānamalla. *The Ananga Ranga of Kalyānamalla*. Trans. Richard Burton and F. F. Arbuthnot. London: Kimber, 1963; Kaplan, Helen Singer. *The Sexual Desire Disorders: Dysfunctional Regulation of Sexual Motivation*. New York: Brunner/Mazel, 1995; Kokkoka. "The Ratirahasya of Kokkoka." Trans. Alex Comfort. In Alex Comfort, ed., *The Koka Shastra: Being the Ratirahasya of Kokkoka and Other Medieval Indian Writings on Love*. London: Allen and Unwin, 1964, 101–7 (includes the *Ratimañjarī* and extracts from the *Smaradīpika* and other works); Nietzsche, Friedrich. (1872) *The Birth of Tragedy or Hellenism and Pessimism*. Trans. Walter Kaufmann. In Walter Kaufmann, ed., *Basic Writings of Nietzsche*. New

York: Modern Library, 1968, 1–144; Vātsyāyana. *The Complete Kāma Sūtra.* Trans. Alain Daniélou. Rochester, Vt.: Park Street Press, 1994. (Includes the *Jayamangalā* and extracts from *Jaya* commentaries); Vātsyāyana. *Kamasutra.* Trans. Wendy Doniger and Sudhir Kakar. Oxford, U.K.: Oxford University Press, 2002. (Includes extracts from the *Jayamangalā* and *Jaya* commentaries.)

James Giles

ADDITIONAL READING

Bhattacharya, Narendra Nath. *History of Indian Erotic Literature.* New Delhi, India: Munshiram Manoharlal, 1975; Chand, Khazan. *Indian Sexology.* New Delhi, India: S. Chand, n.d.; Comfort, Alex. *The Joy of Sex.* New York: Crown, 1972; Comfort, Alex. *More Joy of Sex.* New York: Simon and Schuster, 1973; Comfort, Alex. *Nature and Human Nature.* London: Weidenfeld and Nicholson, 1966; Comfort, Alex. *The New Joy of Sex.* New York: Crown, 1991; Comfort, Alex, ed. *The Koka Shastra: Being the Ratirahasya of Kokkoka and Other Medieval Indian Writings on Love.* New York: Stein and Day, 1965; De, Sushil Kumar. *Ancient Indian Erotics and Erotic Literature.* Calcutta, India: Firma K. L. Mukhopadhyay, 1959; Ellis, Albert. (1960) *The Art and Science of Love,* rev. ed. New York: Lyle Stuart, 1966; Meyer, Johann Jakob. *Sexual Life in Ancient India: A Study in the Comparative History of Indian Culture,* 2 vols. London: George Routledge and Sons, 1930; Rai, Ram Kumar. *Encyclopedia of Indian Erotics.* Varanasi, India: Prachya Prakashan, 1983; Zysk, Kenneth, G. *Conjugal Love in Ancient India: Ratiśāstra and Ratiramaṇa.* Leiden, Holland: Brill, 2002.

INFIDELITY. *See* Adultery

INTERGENERATIONAL SEX. *See* Pedophilia

INTERNET SEX. *See* Cybersex

INTERSEXUALITY. Two very different kinds of clinical cases have been labeled "intersexuality" or "intersex" conditions. The first involves clinical conditions in which there is doubt neither about the child's genotype—girl, boy—nor about the alignment of phenotype, that is, genital anatomy, with genotypic sex. Problematic cases arise because severe anatomic damage to the genital anatomy has occurred. Such damage results from catastrophic accidents of malformation during gestation, such as cloacal exstrophy (in which the genitalia are largely missing), and from catastrophic iatrogenic damage (for example, penile ablation from circumcision). The problem in the cases of boys with these anomalies or injuries can be that no surgical technique is adequate for correcting the extensive anatomic damage (say, by reconstructing male genitalia). That is, surgical technique is not able to reassign male genital sex to the patient. The celebrated case of John/Joan involved this kind of intersex condition (see Colapinto).

The second kind are the genuine intersex conditions, in which the child's genomic sex, hormonal sex, and anatomic sex do not align and result in sometimes unstable gender identity. Such conditions are usually detected at birth, when the infant is discovered to have abnormal genitalia on initial physical examination. The clinical and social management of both kinds of conditions raises ethical issues.

Before turning to these ethical issues it is necessary to address some important contextual matters that are often overlooked in the literature on the ethics of intersexuality. These concern (1) nomenclature; (2) whether sex and gender should be understood dimorphically (a matter of either/or); (3) the history of scientifically undisciplined innovation in surgery; (4) mind-body dualism in psychoanalytic theory; and (5) the labeling of intersex conditions as social emergencies.

(1) *Sex* refers to the biological categories or classifications into which human beings can be reliably sorted. *Gender* involves the social construction of social roles and personal identity by individuals, families, cultures, and societies—often unwittingly—under the constraints of and in response to sexual differences. Gender *identity* involves a combination of self-discovery and social construction of oneself as male (or a man), female (or a woman), or transsexual. Gender or **sexual orientation** is a matter of the sex(es) or gender(s) of the people to whom one is preferentially sexually attracted and with whom one can attain sexual satisfaction. In clinical discourse it is sometimes said that the main issue with intersex conditions is the surgical assignment of sex, that is, fashioning male or female genital anatomy. However, this discourse is inadequate to the complexity of the issues, for not only can sex be "assigned," but gender and gender identity, to a certain extent, can also be "assigned." At the same time, because gender, gender identity, and gender orientation are *only in part* functions of personal choices, on the one side, and social constructions and expectations, on the other, the ability of surgeons—and parents—to "assign" them is limited. Failing to appreciate that there are such limits, that the biological puts constraints on the "assignment" of gender features, has helped generate ethical controversy over the clinical management of intersex conditions.

(2) Until the advent of modern biology and its concept of biological variability in the late nineteenth century, and its clinical application in the twentieth century in the form of molecular medicine—in which health and disease are understood as functions of the interaction of genes, proteins, and the environment (that is, everything not a gene or a protein)—sex was understood mainly in anatomic terms. There were two main categories, male and female, into which almost everyone could be sorted (dimorphism). Some human beings, hermaphrodites, had both female and male anatomy and thus could not be assigned to either sex; this "intersex" condition was regarded as anomalous or abnormal (see Dreger, *Hermaphrodites*).

This dimorphic picture of sex had enormous implications for gender and gender identity, especially in northern European societies whose influence on American attitudes has been long and deep. Babies were either boys or girls. Children were either boys or girls, too; they used boys' and girls' restrooms and attended boys-only and girls-only gym classes. Schools, especially, can still enforce a rigid gender dimorphism, which reflects the persistence of the older dimorphic picture of sex. One grew up to be a man or a woman; men were sexually oriented toward women as sexual partners and women toward men. In the United States, until the last part of the twentieth century, similarly rigid social attitudes based on dimorphism considered **homosexuality** abnormal, rather than as an expected, unsurprising biopsychosocial variation in our species (see Engel). With the advent of modern biology, and especially the discoveries of molecular medicine, understanding sex dimorphically has been found inadequate to explain the observed variability of sex. Sex is a trait of our species and, like all traits, should be expected to display a wide range of variation (see Fausto-Sterling; McCullough; Sax).

At the chromosomal level, it does appear that there are only two sexes, female (XX) and male (XY). However, recent discoveries have shown that at the level of the genome (the gene sequences that constitute the chromosomes), there is considerable variation; for example, multiple crossovers of gene sequences between the X and Y chromosomes. A dimorphic concept of sex is unable to map this variation or capture its structural and functional significance. At this level of analysis, there are no "intersex" conditions. That term presupposes that there are two and only two sexes into which all normal human beings are sorted, with a third group between male and female, *inter*sex persons, who are abnormal and hence must be assigned to one of them. Ethical issues in the management of intersex conditions came about, in part, because the discredited dimorphic conception of sex persisted.

Exposure to hormones during gestation, infancy, and puberty is a second important aspect of biological sex, because female and male hormones affect developing anatomy, especially the brain. This is an important biological constraint on gender identity. Hormonal sex also displays variability both within itself and with respect to chromosomal and genomic sex. We can expect that genomic, chromosomal, and hormonal sex can align in various patterns, not just two, male and female. This multifaceted biological variation of sex means that we should expect at least the same, if not wider, variation in gender identity and gender roles. The latter are a function of the former, as well as of the complex factors of personal choice, family rearing, cultural influences, social attitudes, and social institutions (for example, schools, churches) that reflect and reinforce those attitudes.

Any attempt to label a variation in sex, gender identity, or gender orientation cannot succeed by invoking the authority of biology, that is, the "natural" categories of male and female, heterosexual boys and men, and heterosexual girls and women. Labeling of this kind should be understood for what it is: a set of value or normative judgments about what sex, gender identity, and gender orientation *ought* to be. To justify the labeling, arguments must be provided for the priority or importance of the values appealed to. Such arguments involve formidable intellectual challenges.

(3) Because intersex conditions involve anomalous anatomy, they are usually managed surgically. Surgery came into academic medicine only in the nineteenth century and has developed throughout most of its history by innovation, notable changes in surgical technique pioneered by individual surgeons. Sometimes these changes were creative extensions of accepted principles and practices of surgery; sometimes these changes broke new ground. If the results look promising after (usually) a small number of attempts, surgeons continue the innovation. At some point, the innovation is publicized through a presentation at a professional meeting, in a publication, or in the lay media, and other surgeons become aware of it. Out of a sincere desire to help patients and an understandable impetus to remain competitive, other surgeons adopt (and even adapt) the new technique, and if it continues to benefit patients, it becomes the standard of care (see Frader and Caniano). But contrast, new drugs and medical devices are not permitted to be introduced and become standard of care in this fashion. Instead, the U.S. Food and Drug Administration requires new drugs and devices to undergo rigorous scientific evaluation that produces evidence of benefit to patients from well-designed, controlled clinical trials.

Much surgical innovation turned out to be successful, in the sense of clinically benefiting patients. But some surgical innovation has been found, when subjected to rigorous scientific evaluation, to be worthless or even dangerous. Honesty requires surgeons to admit that surgical innovation has occurred in a scientifically undisciplined fashion. This process is now changing; evidence-based medical standards are being introduced into surgical practice and research.

This history of scientifically undisciplined surgical innovation has important implications for the surgical management of intersex conditions. First, intersex conditions are relatively rare, and for rare conditions surgeons often have only anecdotal reports of procedures and outcomes (and usually only short-term outcomes). Reports or results may not be inclusive (failures may not be reported) and are therefore biased. Second, in the absence of data about both short-term and long-term outcomes from a large number of case studies, the justification for surgical intervention is only theoretical—the judgment that, however serious the complications of surgery might be, they are not as bad as the consequences of not intervening. This way of thinking is reinforced by anecdotal reports of poor outcomes in the absence of intervention. Third, surgeons who have some success in their cases (anecdotal evidence) can point to them with authority as the basis for intervening. Parents, as laypersons, are not able to sort out the clinical judgments that should be regarded as authoritative (based on scientifically disciplined investigation) from those that should not be. As a consequence, parents may mistakenly accept as authoritative clinical judgments and recommendations that lack scientific authority. The surgeon's authority received reinforcement at a time when the clinical management of intersex conditions did not involve multidisciplinary teams of pediatricians, pediatric endocrinologists, pediatric surgeons and urologists, social workers, nurses, and psychiatrists and psychologists who specialize in early childhood and adolescent development. In such a team setting, it is rare for the perspective of any one member of the team to go unchallenged and achieve controlling authority.

(4) Mind-body dualism is the philosophical view, systematically developed by French philosopher **René Descartes** (1596–1650), that mind and body are distinct, separate entities causally independent of each other. Cartesian dualism had a profound influence on the development of psychoanalytic theory, and that theory had a profound influence on the understanding of intersex conditions in the 1950s and helped to spur innovative surgical interventions (Money et al.).

If mind and body are causally independent, then gender identity and gender orientation are highly plastic, not subject to biological constraints. Gender identity and orientation can therefore be molded by clinical experts when it becomes necessary to do so. Intersex conditions make it necessary to do so. The goal of surgical management is to transform the genital anatomy of an intersexed child to the sex and gender possible given the nature of the anomaly or injury and the limited ability of surgeons to correct it. Gender identity and orientation can then be molded as needed, by consistent parental rearing and reinforcement, for example, the way the child is dressed, the kind of toys the child is given, the sort of sports and other games the child is allowed to play, and which restrooms the child uses at school. Contemporary neuroscience, and clinical practice and research based on it in such medical specialties as psychiatry and neurology, rejects Cartesian dualism, but this recent conceptual shift has not yet succeeded in removing all of the vestiges of the scientifically inadequate dualism that shaped developmental theory of intersex conditions for almost three decades.

(5) Intersex conditions have come to be understood as social emergencies. Parents want to know immediately the sex of their newborn child and are expected by family, friends, neighbors, and coworkers to say immediately after birth, "It's a boy" or "It's a girl." This need to know and inform others creates an atmosphere of urgency, in which clinical decisions must be made quickly and there is not much time or, indeed, any time for gathering information to reach a considered clinical judgment, to take the parents through a detailed informed **consent** process, and to initiate assignment of sex. The ethical logic of pediatric emergencies also shifts authority and control away from parents to physicians.

Strictly speaking, a medical emergency means a condition that is immediately health- or life-threatening, for which clinical intervention must be immediately initiated, making it impossible to start, much less complete, the informed consent process. When a newborn infant's—or any minor child's—life is at stake in an emergency, both medical ethics and law rightly give physicians full authority to initiate life-saving treatment without delay (American Academy of Pediatrics). To be sure, there are life-threatening emergencies associated with congenital adrenal hyperplasia, which can occur with an intersex condition. However, this medical condition can be effectively managed by administration of indicated medication, and surgical assignment of sex is not required to manage this life-threatening condition. No true intersex condition constitutes a surgical emergency. Moreover, the concept of assignment of sex as a social emergency entered clinical thinking and discourse without careful reflection on whether an urgent need—one that, even so, physicians could support parents postponing a decision about—counts as a true medical or surgical emergency.

Cloacal exstrophy and penile ablation are much closer to being surgical emergencies, because they do require prompt medical and surgical intervention. However, these patients are usually stable enough to allow time for the gathering of information, evaluation, and an adequate informed consent process with the parents.

These contextual matters help explain how the clinical and social management of intersex conditions have become ethically controversial (see Chase; Dreger, *Intersex*; Kipnis and Diamond; McCullough; Schober). Consider, first, intersex conditions in which the genomic, chromosomal, and hormonal sex, and previous anatomy (as in penile ablation) or expected anatomy (as in cloacal exstrophy), all align on male or female sex. Gender identity and orientation are not completely plastic; they are subject to biologic constraints. When sex appears univocal, expectations that a discordant gender identity could nonetheless be successfully assigned—where success means that the child will not later experience dysphoria or other more severe psychological sequellae such as chronic depression and suicidal ideations or gestures—face a nearly insurmountable burden of proof. This explains why cases such as the celebrated John/Joan case developed as they did (see Colapinto). There was no doubt that at birth John was a boy, in all the senses of male sex and therefore male gender identity. The problem was that so much of his penis was destroyed that his surgeons believed that they could not restore male anatomy. His case also occurred at a time during which the dualistic views of gender identity remained influential, thus (mistakenly, we would now say) justifying assignment of female gender and its enforcement through rearing. It should come as no surprise that the biological constraints and conceptual confusion about the limitless plasticity of human identity set up this experiment for failure.

By contrast, in true intersex conditions there is variation among the various kinds of sex—genomic, chromosomal, hormonal, anatomic—and so clinicians should expect gender identity and orientation to vary. To think that a sex and therefore a gender could be permanently assigned in all such cases, so that a social "emergency" is solved once and for all (to the great relief of parents, were it the case), is to expect too much from the effects of surgery and rearing on the plasticity of the child's sex and gender.

There is another implication of these contextual matters worth identifying. They call into question the adequacy of postmodern accounts of gender. Postmodernism is, roughly, the view that there is no privileged perspective on reality. Accounts from science, medicine, different cultures and ethnicities, and personal experience compete with each other for intellectual and moral authority (see Komesaroff). It is interesting, and perhaps ironic, that a postmodernist view of intersexuality implicitly endorses the mind-body dualism of psychoanalytic views of the 1950s, because postmodernism shares with those views the commitment notion that gender is essentially plastic, not subject to biological constraints. Modern medicine is just that, modern. It is not postmodern; it takes the view that adherence to scientific method in research and to evidence-based medicine in practice does produce privileged perspectives on health, disease, and injury and how clinical intervention affects them.

Ethically responsible management of intersex conditions begins with the recognition that assignment of sex is more than that, that it also has implications for the assignment of gender. Management also requires recognition of sometimes (nearly) unyielding biological constraints by sex on the assignment of gender. In such cases, assignment of a clearly discordant gender should be assumed to produce clinical harm to the future child and adult. This clinical prognostic judgment requires the moral management of medical uncertainty. In the case of true intersex conditions, the moral management of clinical uncertainty is accomplished on the basis of a well-known medical ethical principle: Physicians should act in ways that avoid or minimize irreversible biopsychosocial harm to patients, both in the short term and in the long term.

In the case of children with aligned genomic, chromosomal, and hormonal sex, clinicians should expect gender identity to conform to male or female sex and should expect the normally observed variation in gender orientation. This analysis is justified by the consistent biological constraint that sex creates for construction of gender in such cases. There is therefore little or no uncertainty about the clinical prognostic judgment of the gender of the patient. A discordant gender should not be assigned, because doing so only sets up the patient for biopsychosocial harm (along with harm for his or her parents). Surgical management should be conservative and not assign a discordant sex.

For true intersex conditions in which there occur medical emergencies, these should be immediately managed with indicated medication. However, this is intervention to manage a life-threatening emergency, not a so-called social emergency to manage assignment of sex and gender. Cases of true intersex conditions are defined by marked variation among genomic, chromosomal, and hormonal sex and, therefore, variable gender. As a consequence, all clinical prognostic judgments about assignment of sex and gender become uncertain. Recommendations about intervention, especially surgical intervention, should be guided by the long-accepted medical ethical principle of avoiding or preventing irreversible short-term and long-term biopsychosocial harm.

One major problem in the ethical controversy about the clinical management of true intersex conditions is that we have only anecdotal reports of success and failure. To make matters worse, there is no consensus about the biopsychosocial criteria for reaching reliable judgments about success or failure. There is, indeed, no agreement about what outcomes should be measured and how. Ethics by anecdote is no better than science or medicine by anecdote.

See also Bisexuality; Ethics, Professional Codes of; Genital Mutilation; Herdt, Gilbert; Homosexuality and Science; Money, John; Orientation, Sexual; Poststructuralism; Social Constructionism

REFERENCES

American Academy of Pediatrics, Committee on Bioethics. "Informed Consent, Parental Permission, and Assent in Pediatric Practice." *Pediatrics* 95:2 (1995), 314–17; Chase, Cheryl. "Surgical Progress Is Not the Answer to Intersexuality." *Journal of Clinical Ethics* 9:4 (1998), 385–92; Colapinto, John. "The True Story of John Joan." *Rolling Stone* (11 December 1997), 54–97; Dreger, Alice Domurat. *Hermaphrodites and the Medical Invention of Sex.* Cambridge, Mass.: Harvard University

Press, 1998; Dreger, Alice Domurat, ed. *Intersex in the Age of Ethics*. Hagerstown, Md.: University Publishing Group, 1999; Engel, George. "The Clinical Application of the Biopsychosocial Model." *American Journal of Psychiatry* 22:4 (1980), 535–44; Fausto-Sterling, Anne. "The Five Sexes." *The Sciences* 33 (March–April 1993), 20–24; Frader, Joel, and Donna Caniano. "Research and Innovation in Surgery." In Laurence B. McCullough, James W. Jones, and Baruch A. Brody, eds., *Surgical Ethics*. New York: Oxford University Press, 1998, 216–41; Kipnis, Kenneth, and Milton Diamond. "Pediatric Ethics and the Surgical Assignment of Sex." *Journal of Clinical Ethics* 9:4 (1998), 398–410; Komesaroff, Paul A. "Introduction: Postmodern Medical Ethics?" In Paul A. Komesaroff, ed., *Troubled Bodies: Critical Perspectives on Postmodernism, Medical Ethics, and the Body*. Durham, N.C.: Duke University Press, 1995, 1–19; McCullough, Laurence B. "A Framework for the Ethically Justified Clinical Management of Intersex Conditions." In Stephen Zderic, ed., *Advances in Experimental Medicine and Biology*, no. 511 (2002), 149–65; discussion, 165–73; Money, John, J. G. Hampson, and J. L. Hampson. "Hermaphroditism: Recommendations Concerning Assignment of Sex, Change of Sex, and Psychologic Management." *Bulletin of the Johns Hopkins Hospital* 97 (1955), 284–300; Sax, Leonard. "How Common Is Intersex? A Response to Anne Fausto-Sterling." *Journal of Sex Research* 39:3 (2002), 174–78; Schober, J. M. "A Surgeon's Response to the Intersex Controversy." *Journal of Clinical Ethics* 9:4 (1998), 393–97.

Laurence B. McCullough

ADDITIONAL READING

American Academy of Pediatrics, Committee on Genetics/Section on Endocrinology/Section on Urology. "Evaluation of the Newborn with Developmental Anomalies of the External Genitalia." *Pediatrics* 106:1 (2000), 138–42; Blizzard, Robert M. "Intersex Issues: A Series of Continuing Conundrums." *Pediatrics* 110:3 (2002), 616–21; Carr, Brian. "Sexual Orientation: Gender Identity Disorders." In Timothy F. Murphy, ed., *Reader's Guide to Lesbian and Gay Studies*. Chicago, Ill.: Fitzroy Dearborn, 2000, 538–39; Colapinto, John. *As Nature Made Him: The Boy Who Was Raised as a Girl*. New York: HarperCollins, 2000; Diamond, Milton, and Keith Sigmundson. "Sex Reassignment at Birth." *Archives of Pediatric and Adolescent Medicine* 151:3 (1997), 298–304; Dreger, Alice Domurat. "A History of Intersexuality: From the Age of Gonads to the Age of Consent." *Journal of Clinical Ethics* 9:4 (1998), 345–55; Epstein, Julia, and Kristin Straub, eds. *Body Guards: The Cultural Politics of Gender Ambiguity*. New York: Routledge, 1991; Fausto-Sterling, Anne. *Myths of Gender: Biological Theories about Women and Men*. New York: Basic Books, 1985; Feder, Ellen K. "Disciplining the Family: The Case of Gender Identity Disorder." *Philosophical Studies* 85:2–3 (1997), 195–211; Feder, Ellen K. " 'Doctors' Orders': Parents and Intersexed Children." In Eva Feder Kittay and Ellen K. Feder, eds., *The Subject of Care: Feminist Perspectives on Dependency*. Lanham, Md.: Rowman and Littlefield, 2002, 294–320. <www.bodieslikeours.org/research-and-studies/feder-docsorders-2.html> and <www.bodieslikeours.org/respdf/Feder2002.pdf> [accessed 16 February 2005]; Foucault, Michel. (1978) *Herculine Barbin: Being the Recently Discovered Memoirs of a Nineteenth Century Hermaphrodite*. Trans. Richard McDougall. New York: Pantheon Books, 1980; Gert, Bernard. "A Sex Caused Inconsistency in DSM-III-R: The Definition of Mental Disorder and the Definition of Paraphilias." *Journal of Medicine and Philosophy* 17 (1992), 155–71; Gudorf, Christine E. "The Erosion of Sexual Dimorphism: Challenges to Religion and Religious Ethics." *Journal of the American Academy of Religion* 69:4 (2001), 863–91; Hale, C. Jacob. "Tracing a Ghostly Memory in My Throat: Reflections on FTM Feminist Voice and Agency." In Tom Digby, ed., *Men Doing Feminism*. New York: Routledge, 1998, 99–129; Hill, Darryl B. "Transvestism." In Timothy F. Murphy, ed., *Reader's Guide to Lesbian and Gay Studies*. Chicago, Ill.: Fitzroy Dearborn, 2000, 592–94; Kessler, Suzanne J. *Lessons from the Intersexed*. New Brunswick, N.J.: Rutgers University Press, 1998; Kessler, Suzanne J. "The Medical Construction of Gender: Case Management of Intersexed Infants." *Signs* 16:1 (1990), 3–26. Reprinted in Barbara Laslett, Sally Gregory Kohlstedt, Helen Longino, and Evelynn Hammonds, eds., *Gender and Scientific Authority*. Chicago, Ill.: University of Chicago Press, 1996, 340–63; Laqueur, Thomas. *Making Sex:*

Body and Gender from the Greeks to Freud. Cambridge, Mass.: Harvard University Press, 1990; Money, John. *The Adam Principle. Genes, Genitals, Hormones, & Gender: Selected Readings in Sexology.* Buffalo, N.Y.: Prometheus, 1993; Morland, Ian. "Is Intersexuality Real?" *Textual Practice* 15:3 (2001), 527–47; Nanda, Serena. *Neither Man nor Woman: The Hijras of India.* Belmont, Calif.: Wadsworth, 1990. 2nd ed., 1998; Olds, Sharon. "Outside the Operating Room of the Sex-Change Doctor." In Carole S. Vance, ed., *Pleasure and Danger: Exploring Female Sexuality.* London: Routledge and Kegan Paul, 1984, 428; Queen, Carol, and Laurence Schimel, eds. *PoMoSexuals: Challenging Assumptions about Gender and Sexuality.* San Francisco, Calif.: Cleis Press, 1997; Simon, William. *Postmodern Sexualities.* New York: Routledge, 1996; Stone, Allucquère Rosanne. *The War of Desire and Technology at the Close of the Mechanical Age.* Cambridge, Mass.: MIT Press, 1995; Stone, Sandy [Stone, Allucquère Rosanne]. "The Empire Strikes Back: A Posttranssexual Manifesto." In Julia Epstein and Kristin Straub, eds., *Body Guards: The Cultural Politics of Gender Ambiguity.* New York: Routledge, 1991, 280–304; Yudkin, Marcia. "Transsexualism and Women: A Critical Perspective." *Feminist Studies* 4:3 (1978), 97–106; Zucker, Kenneth. "Intersexuality and Gender Identity Differentiation." *Annual Review of Sex Research* 10 (1999), 1–69.

IRIGARAY, LUCE. *See* Feminism, French

ISLAM.

ISLAM. For several reasons, the Islamic philosophy of sex is difficult territory. First, because the Qur'an represents the word of *Allah* as revealed to the prophet Mohammed (571–632), some claim that its meaning is accurate only in classic Arabic (Stowasser, 30) and that any translation is inadequate in some way. Second, much research in this area is contentious, either criticizing or defending Islamic practices, particularly in the area of women's rights. Some contemporary Islamic pro-feminine literature seems to be "apologetic," thereby "betraying a belief that there are Western values against which [Islam] must justify itself " (Haddad, 3). Third, "Islam" can refer either to a religion or to a culture. Muslims are connected by their common faith, but there are different interpretations of the Qur'an and varying degrees to which religious and secular principles have merged over the past fourteen centuries. Commentary distinguishes between Qur'anic and culturally influenced *ahadith* laws (Hourani, 6–11; see Lippman, 62–63). We cannot assume there is one unified Islamic culture, nor should we imagine that there is a single Islamic philosophy of sex or that Qur'anic approaches to sexuality are consistent among diverse Islamic populations. Similarly, even though the various denominations of Protestantism, Roman and Orthodox Catholicism, and so forth, are all Christian, there is hardly full agreement among them about sexuality.

In principle, the laws of Islam permeate the lives of Muslims to such an extent that all thoughts and actions are imbued with an awareness of *Allah*. The Qur'an and the *ahadith* contain clearly defined paths to righteousness; this is a major strength of Islam (Smith, 243). The Qur'anic and cultural laws advanced by Islam seek to optimize the conditions under which every Muslim can be devoted to God. If there is a single prevailing principle in Islamic philosophy, it is oneness with *Allah*, "the peace that comes when one's life is surrendered to God" (Smith, 222–23). Islamic philosophical reflection on sexuality emerges from this principle. God commands a life of modesty, demonstrated in the recognition of oneself as His servant. The interpretation of God's word is contingent on divine revelation and the authority of religious leaders; it is immodest to assume one can understand *Allah*'s intentions on one's own. The demand for modesty presents itself also through social norms that remove temptations to sexual impropriety, thus ensuring the chastity of all Muslims:

> Tell the believing men to lower their gaze and guard their sexuality; that is purer for them. . . . God is aware of what they do. And tell the believing women to lower their gaze and guard against their sexuality. (Haneef, 173)

Defenders of Islam note that regulating the relations between the sexes, and regulating the sexual behavior of both sexes, is the direct instruction of *Allah*. However, although restrictions on men's sexuality occur in both the Qur'an and the *ahadith* (for example, regarding divorce and physical appearance), most sexual restrictions are directed toward women, which fuels controversy when Islam is evaluated from the outside.

American Muslim Suzanne Haneef describes the status of women in Islam as commanding respect. Out of honor for women, laws have been established to protect them and ensure their integrity. The most visually noticeable manifestation of this respectful protection is the traditional dress (*hijab*), which Haneef claims "is prescribed by direct order in the Quran" (172). But Leila Ahmed disagrees (55):

> [Veiling] is nowhere explicitly prescribed in the Quran; the only verses dealing with women's clothing . . . instruct women to guard their private parts and throw a scarf over their bosoms. (*Sura* 24:31–34)

Nevertheless, according to contemporary theory a woman's revealing her body, her sexual nature, is a temptation to sin, both for herself and any witnessing men. (There is a similar injunction in the Christianity of **Saint Paul** [5–64?]; see 1 Cor. 11:4–15.) Clothing creates "a curtain . . . between [a woman] and the men with whom she comes in contact" (Haneef, 170, 188). A Muslim woman in public must be clothed in such a way as to reveal only her hands and face, as Mohammed taught his wives (Haneef, 189). In some societies, a woman's face, too, must be covered, only her eyes showing. At Iranian prayer ceremonies women may expose only one eye, "in order to envelope themselves fully from the gaze of unrelated men" (Torab, 241). Further, Islamic institutions commonly encourage the separation of men and women through gender-specific sections of, for example, schools and hospitals. Islam, as do other religions, reserves a woman's sexuality for her husband (Ahmed, 42). She is permitted to adorn herself and accentuate her **beauty** for her husband alone (Haneef, 189–91).

Hijab can be interpreted as advantageous to women, as a mechanism for achieving social status and making social contributions. Haneef explains that

> *hijab* is not an isolated aspect of the Muslim woman's life but . . . reinforces the Islamic social system and . . . concept of womanhood . . . not only to protect society from the disruption produced by uncontrolled expressions of sexual interest and . . . protect a woman's dignity and honor, but also . . . to neutralize her sexuality so that she can be a positive, constructive force in society rather than a harmful one. (170–88)

Critics often wonder, though, what causes or is responsible for the "disruption" that potentially ensues from male arousal by the mere presence of women (Hekmat, 193). A pious male would not be tempted to seduce a woman who is not his wife or, if he were, he would be capable of resisting temptation. Apparently, a woman must clothe herself modestly and avoid being in the presence of men unrelated to her by **marriage** or family because the sex drive, especially in men, is powerful, "animalistic," and must not be provoked (Danner, 131; Haneef, 169). At the same time, however, men—despite their rampant sexual urges— are seen as "stronger, more perfect, more complete, and more beautiful . . . as is the case with the males in all species." In virtue of this sound and superior constitution, the man is the head of the household "in the God-willed natural order of the family, [in which] the man . . . is to the wife as the head is to the body" (Stowasser, 35).

This Islamic view—clothing, as Haneef says, neutralizes a woman's sexuality "so that she can be a positive . . . force in society rather than . . . harmful"—is problematic for Westerners. From the perspective of societies in which women have appreciable sexual freedom (including opportunities for nonmarital sex), it is difficult to understand why women's sexuality should be "neutralized" or how it could be a potentially harmful force. In attempting to prevent women from being seen as sexual objects and thus being victims of **sexual objectification**—by removing visual cues that could be sexually enticing—*hijab* and the segregation of the sexes may ironically convert women into sex objects: Their power of sexual temptation, through their mere presence or the exposure of their skin, is so predominantly constitutive of their nature that this feature threatens to overwhelm and make invisible other aspects of their humanity. Critics also suggest that viewing the woman as a temptress reinforces the lack of men's accountability (Hekmat, 193).

Islam in many ways improved the lives of women, regarding **consent** to marriage, the rights of inheritance, and the elimination of gynocide (Smith, 251). Allowing unwanted female infants to die, often by burying them alive, was an accepted practice in pagan Arabia until it was forbidden by Mohammed (Lippman, 10). Yet there are other elements in Islam that from a Western perspective seem sexist. Hanafi law, for example, punishes sodomy with whipping, but the Qur'an (2:223) permits a man to sodomize his wife even without her consent, since she is "a tilled field" that a man may "enter . . . any way" he chooses (Hekmat, 166). Some interpretations of the Qur'an allow men to beat their wives (lightly) if necessary (Haddad and Smith, 27). The evolving *ahadith* and *de facto* laws of Islam are, according to some commentators, misogynous, while defenders of Islam point out that the Qur'an attempts to promote righteousness in both sexes. Yet **adultery**, fornication, and sexual impropriety (*zina*) have been crimes generally carrying harsh penalties, especially for women. An early injunction against adultery in the Qur'an confined the unfaithful woman "to her house for the rest of her life," but the man involved in the affair was not punished (Hekmat, 156–57). Those who committed *zina* received, supervised by clergy, public whippings, which were sometimes fatal. Unlike many Western legal systems, in which there is accommodation for extenuating circumstances, "no Islamic judge would dare . . . have mercy on the accused. *Allah*'s law is rigid and the sentence inflexible. There is no appeal" (Hekmat, 159).

These early punishments recommended by the Qur'an were later replaced with stoning for adultery involving a married woman, as ordered by Mohammed. (The punishment for adultery in the Hebrew Old Testament was death; Leviticus 20:10.) Men were to have an opportunity to escape by running, while a convicted woman was to be partially buried to prevent movement as each witness, the judge, and bystanders cast stones at her (Hekmat, 161–67). Stoning has been abolished in many contemporary Muslim communities but continues in, for example, Iran (Hekmat, 163). Where imprisonment is the legally mandated punishment, families sometimes kill transgressors for violating their honor (Brand, 108).

Premarital female virginity is respected in many cultures. Islam values virginity so highly that *Allah* promises a wealth of virgins for men who reach paradise after death (Lippman, 62). To ensure virginity and hence the desirability of women to potential husbands, some Islamic cultures have adopted various types of female **genital mutilation**. Circumcision that includes clitoridectomy prevents or reduces sexual pleasure and thereby lessens the motivation for a girl to engage in sex before marriage. Other forms of mutilation impede vaginal penetration and ensure virginity in the manner of medieval European chastity belts. In the more extensive procedures prevalent in North Africa, the *labia majora* are sliced off or sewn together. Infibulation is performed to guarantee a girl will be intact as a bride. Indeed, the smaller the opening that remains, the higher the bride price. A girl in whom a man is interested for marriage is often inspected by his female relatives (see Hosken). Nonetheless, it has been claimed that "Islamic law protects a woman's right to sexual enjoyment [to the extent] that a woman has the right to divorce [if] her husband does not provide sexual satisfaction. It follows that Islamic law prohibits clitoridectomy . . . or infibulation, or any genital mutilation which impairs the woman's ability to enjoy sexual relations" (Ahmad). About this matter the Qur'an is silent, which suggests that female genital mutilation is a cultural custom rather than a theological imperative. Still, there are exceptions to the prohibition of premarital sexual relations. "Temporary marriages," which are not legally permanent, are "justified by the *Shiites* as having been tolerated by the Prophet and occasionally necessary to give mankind a way of satisfying sexual appetites without committing one of the sins condemned in the Koran" (Lippman, 148).

Homosexual relations are forbidden, insofar as they involve **sexual activity** with a person other than one's spouse. Beyond this injunction it is difficult to assess the Islamic treatment of homosexual relations, which until recently has seldom been studied (see Murray and Roscoe). Some classic Arabic poetry alludes to same-sex relationships. Slavery has been prevalent in Islamic history ("Since its endorsement in the Koran, slavery has never been abolished formally by any law"; Hekmat, 132) and brought with it homosexual relations (as also, for example, in ancient Greece). Some of this **homosexuality** was pederastic (Murray, 168). For some males who remained unmarried, homosexual relations were "the only form of personal relations, sexual or emotional, open to them" (Murray and Roscoe, 310–11). Wealthy Muslim women often owned female slaves, and lesbianism was sometimes a means of revolting against patriarchal sexuality (Ahmed, 185). In contemporary Pakistan, "A lesbian orientation is in perfect harmony with family life, so long as the women are good mothers and wives. . . . It is a private matter. . . . However, if she does anything to subvert her gender and social role, she risks retribution" (Khan, 284). It is interesting that **contraception**, too, even though it (like homosexuality) runs counter to the goal of extending the family and the Muslim population, is not expressly forbidden (Haddad and Smith, 28).

Because Islam was the religion of the descendants of Abraham's son Ishmael, there was precedent among the Hebrews for the polygamy and concubinage later endorsed and practiced by Mohammed. Abraham's servant Hagar bore him a child when it was believed his wife Sarah could not (Hekmat, 153; Smith, 223). During Mohammed's time, "plural marriages were common and casual sex with slave-girls was taken for granted" (Lippman, 56). Neighboring aristocrats who were conquered by Muslims became slaves, and the women were forced into harems as concubines (Ahmed, 117). Mohammad's brother-in-law Al-Zubair left 1,000 concubines when he died in 656 (Ahmed, 80). Mohammed had only 1 concubine but as many as eighteen wives. Some "were the widows of companions who had fallen in battle, women who needed care and shelter and were taken into the Prophet's establishment out of kindness" (Lippman, 56). After Mohammed's death some Muslim groups rejected polygamy, concubinage, and the marriage of girls as young as nine (the age of Mohammed's second wife, Aisha). But in general, Islamic authority, "by licensing polygamy, concubinage, and easy divorce for men," sanctioned, both religiously and legally, what today is often considered "abuses of women" (Ahmed, 87). Saudi Arabia, "one of the most orthodox Muslim communities in the world, [continues to practice] polygamy"

(Hekmat, 148). Defenders of polygamy advise that a man should take at most only that number of wives that he can treat with justice and equality. Some argue that it is not possible to treat more than one wife justly (the way that some argue it is not possible to show the concern of **love** to more than one person).

Divorce has been common among Muslims since the beginning of the religion. Mohammed is believed to have threatened mass divorce to all his wives as punishment for their not accepting his policy of female seclusion (Ahmed, 56). But according to some interpretations of the Qur'an, "among all possible things, divorce is the act most hated by God" (Hekmat, 234). The rules of divorce—who may divorce whom and on what grounds—have changed over time and vary from culture to culture. The Arabic word for divorce, *talaq*, originally meant "to release a camel from a tether," as a wife is released from her marriage bond (Hekmat, 227). A three-month waiting period precedes her next marriage, during which time the husband may change his mind (228). The wife may sue for divorce for "the impotency of her husband, nonpayment of maintenance, or his insanity" (230). Once divorced, the dowry is usually returned and the husband is responsible for three months' alimony. A widow must usually wait four months before marrying again (239). Traditionally, "if a husband deserted his wife or was missing for a period, the woman could marry again" within from one to ninety-six years. (Hanafi law considered average life expectancy to be about ninety-six years; the wife could marry again only when her husband could be presumed deceased.)

Critics note that much Islamic philosophy of sexuality and gender relations is based on the fallacious or indefensible assumption that men are superior in many ways to women (Smith, 251). Yet Western philosophy of sex has also adopted these views about male superiority and implied male privilege, and only within the past century has it significantly yielded to the pressure to promote more egalitarian principles.

See also Abstinence; Adultery; African Philosophy; Bible, Sex and the; Genital Mutilation; Greek Sexuality and Philosophy, Ancient; Judaism, History of; Marriage; Paul (Saint)

REFERENCES

Ahmad, Imad-ad-Dean. *Female Genital Mutilation: An Islamic Perspective.* Bethesda, Md.: Minaret of Freedom Institute, Pamphlet no. 1 (2000). <www.minaret.org/fgm-pamphlet.htm> [accessed 8 June 2005]; Ahmed, Leila. *Women and Gender in Islam.* New Haven, Conn.: Yale University Press, 1992; Brand, Laurie A. "Women and the State in Jordan." In Yvonne Yazbeck Haddad and John L. Esposito, eds., *Islam, Gender, and Social Change.* New York: Oxford University Press, 1998, 100–123; Danner, Victor. *The Islamic Tradition.* Amity, N.Y.: Amity House, 1988; Haddad, Yvonne Yazbeck. "Islam and Gender: Dilemmas in the Changing Arab World." In Yvonne Yazbeck Haddad and John L. Esposito, eds., *Islam, Gender, and Social Change.* New York: Oxford University Press, 1998, 3–29; Haddad, Yvonne Yazbeck, and Jane I. Smith. "Islamic Values among American Muslims." In Barbara C. Aswad and Barbara Bilgé, eds., *Family and Gender among American Muslims: Issues Facing Middle Eastern Immigrants and Their Descendants.* Philadelphia, Pa.: Temple University Press, 1996, 19–40; Haneef, Suzanne. (1979) *What Everyone Should Know about Islam and Muslims,* 14th ed. Library of Islam. Chicago, Ill.: Kazi Publications, 1996; Hekmat, Anwar. *Women and the Koran.* Amherst, N.Y.: Prometheus, 1997; Hosken, Fran P. "Female Genital Mutilation: Strategies for Eradication." International Symposium on Circumcision (1–2 March 1989), Anaheim, Calif. <www.nocirc.org/symposia/first/hosken.html> [accessed 29 November 2004]; Hourani, George F. *Reason and Tradition in Islamic Ethics.* Cambridge: Cambridge University Press, 1985; Khan, Badruddin. "Not-So-Gay Life in Pakistan in the 1980s and 1990s." In Stephen O. Murray and Will Roscoe, eds., *Islamic Homosexualities: Culture, History, and Literature.* New York: New York University Press, 1997, 275–96; Lippman, Thomas W. *Understanding Islam: An Introduction to the*

Moslem World. New York: Mentor, 1982; Murray, Stephen O. "Male Homosexuality, Inheritance Rules, and the Status of Women in Medieval Egypt: The Case of the Mamlūks." In Stephen O. Murray and Will Roscoe, eds., *Islamic Homosexualities: Culture, History, and Literature*. New York: New York University Press, 1997, 161–73; Murray, Stephen O., and Will Roscoe, eds. *Islamic Homosexualities: Culture, History, and Literature*. New York: New York University Press, 1997; Smith, Huston. "Islam." In *The World's Religions*. San Francisco, Calif.: HarperCollins, 1991, 221–70; Stowasser, Barbara. "Gender Issues and Contemporary Quran Interpretation." In Yvonne Yazbeck Haddad and John L. Esposito, eds., *Islam, Gender, and Social Change*. New York: Oxford University Press, 1998, 30–44; Torab, Azam. "Piety as Gendered Agency: A Study of Jalasch Ritual Discourse in an Urban Neighborhood in Iran." *Journal of the Royal Anthropological Institute* 2:2 (1996), 235–52.

Elisa Ruhl

ADDITIONAL READING

Ali, A. Yusef. *An English Interpretation of the Holy Quran with Full Arabic Text*. Lahore, India: Muhammad Ashraf, 1995; Anway, Carol L. *Daughters of Another Path: Experiences of American Women Choosing Islam*. Lee's Summit, Mo.: Yawna Publications, 1996; Arkoun, Mohammed, and Robert D. Lee. *Rethinking Islam: Common Questions, Uncommon Answers*. Boulder, Colo.: Westview, 1994; Aswad, Barbara C., and Barbara Bilgé, eds. *Family and Gender among American Muslims: Issues Facing Middle Eastern Immigrants and Their Descendants*. Philadelphia, Pa.: Temple University Press, 1996; Badawi, Jamal [Gemal] A. "The Status of Woman in Islam." *Al-Ittihad* 8:2 (1971), 7–16. Plainfield, Ind.: Muslim Students' Association of the United States and Canada. Reprinted, "The Religion of Islam." *The Islamic Affairs Department at the Royal Embassy of Saudi Arabia*. <www.iad.org/PDF/women.pdf> [accessed 29 November 2004]; Barlas, Asma. *Believing Women in Islam: Unreading Patriarchal Interpretations of the Quran*. Austin: University of Texas Press, 2002; Beck, Lois, and Nikki Keddie, eds. *Women in the Muslim World*. Cambridge, Mass.: Harvard University Press, 1978; Brussat, Frederic, and Mary Ann Brussat. *Spiritual Literacy: Reading the Sacred in the Everyday*. New York: Scribner's, 1996; Cooey, Paula M., William R. Eakin, and J. B. McDaniel, eds. *After Patriarchy: Feminist Transformations of the World Religions*. New York: Orbis Books, 1991; Duran, Khalid. "Homosexuality and Islam." In Arlene Swidler, ed., *Homosexuality and World Religions*. Valley Forge, Pa.: Trinity Press, 1993, 181–97; Farah, Madelain. *Marriage and Sexuality in Islam*. Salt Lake City: University of Utah Press, 1984; Haddad, Yvonne Yazbeck, and John L. Esposito, eds. *Islam, Gender, and Social Change*. New York: Oxford University Press, 1998; Haddad, Yvonne Yazbeck, and Adair T. Lummis. *Islamic Values in the United States: A Comparative Study*. New York: Oxford University Press, 1987; Halwani, Raja. "Islam." In Timothy F. Murphy, ed., *Reader's Guide to Gay and Lesbian Studies*. Chicago, Ill.: Fitzroy Dearborn, 2000, 309–11; Holes, Clive. "The Koran." In Peter France, ed., *The Oxford Guide to Literature in English Translation*. Oxford, U.K.: Oxford University Press, 2001, 141–45; Hunter, Shirley. *Islam, Europe's Second Religion: The New Social, Cultural, and Political Landscape*. Westport, Conn.: Praeger, 2002; Ishaq, Farid. *Islam and Pluralism: An Islamic Perspective on Interreligious Solidarity against Oppression*. Oxford, U.K.: Oneworld, 1997; Khan, Shahnaz. *Aversion and Desire: Negotiating Muslim Female Identity in the Diaspora*. Toronto, Can.: Women's Press, 2002; Lapidus, Ira. *History of Islamic Societies*. Cambridge: Cambridge University Press, 1990; Lewis, Bernard. *The Jews of Islam*. Princeton, N.J.: Princeton University Press, 1987; Mernissi, Fatima. (1975) *Beyond the Veil: Male-Female Dynamics in Modern Muslim Society*, rev. ed. Bloomington: Indiana University Press, 1987; Minaret of Freedom Institute. (Web site) <www.minaret.org/index.html> [accessed 8 June 2005]; Nafisi, Azar. *Reading Lolita in Tehran*. New York: Random House, 2003; Nussbaum, Martha C. "Religion and Women's Human Rights." In Paul Weithman, ed., *Religion and Contemporary Liberalism*. Notre Dame, Ind.: Notre Dame University Press, 1997, 93–137. Reprinted in *Sex and Social Justice*. New York: Oxford University Press, 1999, 81–117; "Polygamy by Light of Life." Polygamy.com. <www.polygamy.com/Islam/Polygamy.htm> [accessed 27 September 2004]; Rahman, Fazlur. "A Survey of Modernization of Muslim Family Law." *International Journal of Middle East Studies* 11:4

(1980), 451–65; Robinson, Francis, ed. *Cambridge Illustrated History of the Islamic World*. Cambridge: Cambridge University Press, 1996; Sahebjam, Freidoune. (1990) *The Stoning of Soraya M.* Trans. Richard Seaver. New York: Arcade Publishing, 1994; Schmitt, Arno, and Jehoeda Sofer, eds. *Sexuality and Eroticism among Males in Moslem Societies*. New York: Haworth, 1991; Seager, Richard Hughes, ed. (1893) *The Dawn of Religious Pluralism: Voices from the World's Parliament of Religions*. LaSalle, Ill.: Open Court, 1993; Shepherd, John J. "Islam." In Ruth Chadwick, ed., *Encyclopedia of Applied Ethics*, vol. 2. San Diego, Calif.: Academic Press, 1998, 733–40; Soble, Alan. "Some Mysteries of Eros: The Sexuality of the Veil." Lecture, Eastern Kentucky University (10 October 2002). <www.uno.edu/~asoble/pages/mystery.htm> [accessed 29 November 2004]. Video. <www.mediaresources.eku.edu/streaming/lectures/chautauqua02-03.htm> and <www.uno.edu:8010/ramgen/philosophy/sobleEKU.rm> [accessed 29 November 2004]; Wadud, Amina. *Qur'an and Woman: Reading the Sacred Text from a Woman's Perspective*. Oxford, U.K.: Oxford University Press, 1999; Walther, Wiebke. *Woman in Islam: From Medieval to Modern Times*. Princeton, N.J.: Marcus Winer, 1981; Warraq, Ibn, ed. *The Origins of the Koran: Classic Essays on Islam's Holy Book*. Amherst, N.Y.: Prometheus, 1998; Warraq, Ibn, ed. and trans. *What the Koran Really Says: Language, Text, and Commentary*. Amherst, N.Y.: Prometheus, 2002; Wolper, Ethel Sara. "Islamic Law and Culture." In Timothy F. Murphy, ed., *Reader's Guide to Lesbian and Gay Studies*. Chicago, Ill.: Fitzroy Dearborn, 2000, 311–12.

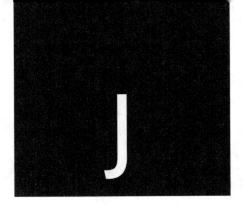

JAINISM. Jainism is one of the three great religious-philosophical traditions of India, the others being **Buddhism** and **Hinduism**. While its last noted *tīrthaṇkara*, Mahāvīra (literally, "Ford-maker," the guide across the "river of ignorance"), lived at the same time as Buddha (sixth century BCE), Jainism's origins are generally regarded as pre-Vedic (early second millennium BCE or before). Jainism is known both for its adherents' stringent observance of *ahiṃsā* (nonviolence) and the extreme asceticism and nudity of its monks. The fundamental Jain doctrine is embodied in the lay followers' *aṇuvrata* or five restraints or vows (*vratas*): nonviolence (*ahiṃsā*), truth-speaking (*satya*), nonstealing (*asteya*), chastity (*brahma*), and nonattachment to worldly things (*aparigraha*). These vows are not simply ethical guidelines but shape the Jain psyche, identity, and way of life. The first vow, *ahiṃsā*, is by far the most important, and all Jain ideas and policies about **love** and **sexual activity** are grounded in it. *Ahiṃsā* can be seen as a noble gesture of love for all creatures. While the emotion love spontaneously arises as a basic human disposition, its further refinement, control, diffusion, and articulation are accomplished though *ahiṃsā*.

The reasons behind the doctrine of *ahiṃsā* are both altruistic and egoistic. First, all living beings desire to live and avoid suffering. Just as each human person seeks life and avoids pain, so one can infer that all life has the same sentiments. One should therefore avoid actions that injure others. Second, all intentional actions that affect other living beings result in the accumulation of karma that adheres to one's soul. This weight of karma-contamination is the root cause of transmigration and suffering (*saṃsāra*). So one must not cause harm to other living beings if one wants to attain release (*mokṣa*) from bondage to this cycle of rebirth.

Jainism, like nearly all Indian philosophical traditions, is classified as *mokṣa-darśana*, a viewpoint that leads to liberation. (Compare Plotinus's [204–270] goal of liberation through ascent back to the One; see Rist.) Jainism recognizes that some actions promote that goal, while others hamper it. Two of the worst impediments are passions and violent acts toward others. Violence leads to the accumulation of karma that is hard to remove from the soul (*jīva*), while passion activates or exhilarates the binding process.

Vibrations (*yoga*) within the soul are caused by body, speech, and mind activity. This causes the influx (*āsrava*) of karmic matter to the soul. However, the actual *binding* (*bandha*) of karmic matter to the soul is caused by passions (*kaṣāyas*). Hence, any advancement toward liberation requires the discontinuation of one's passions. This absence of passions is found during the eleventh, twelfth, and thirteenth stages (*guṇasthāna*) toward enlightenment. Nevertheless, there is still the influx of karmic matter because there is still activity. Yet it does not bind with the soul, because there are no passions. The only type of "bondage" that takes place is momentary bondage of *sātā-vedanīya karma*, and this does not accumulate but produces its effects instantaneously.

Jain authors (like those of other religious traditions, e.g., **Manichaeism**) distinguish the duties/vows of the lay follower (*aṇuvrata*) from the vows of the mendicant (*mahāvrata*).

The monk's regiment of vows is more rigorous than the layperson's vows, although the underlying principles and reasons for the prohibitions are the same. In accordance with *aṇuvrata* restrictions for the layperson (*śrāvaka-pratimā*), the follower must pay particular attention to the fourth vow of chastity (*brahma-vrata*). Unlike mendicants, laypersons are not required to observe strict chastity but are expected to engage in sexual activity only in **marriage** and refrain from illicit extramarital sexual activity. One should create a long-term caring relationship with one's spouse and attempt to engage only in moderate sexual activity, avoiding any overindulgence in carnal pleasure or deviate sexuality (a view found also in some Western religions, for example, the Catholicism of **Thomas Aquinas** [1224/25–1274]). As fathers, men should provide a moral model for their children with respect to sexuality. They should also find suitable mates for them. The layperson, though not prohibited from sexual relations and its accompanying emotions and passions, is expected to mitigate sexual feelings, thoughts, and actions toward women other than his spouse, treating them, as one would treat one's siblings or parents, with respect and sexual indifference. As one progresses along the stages of renunciation (*pratimās*), one's vows of sexual restraint become gradually more pronounced. This begins with engaging in sex only at night and ends with complete continence.

For the mendicant, there is no gradual tapering off of sexuality in stages, for no allowance is made for the expression of this urge in a monk's life. All sexual activity violates the *mahāvrata* vow of chastity. The basis of this prohibition lies in the fact that romantic love and amorous activities bring harm to the aspirant's soul and hence impede the ultimate goal, enlightenment. Not only do romantic love and sexual activity involve passions that function to bind the karmas to the soul, but romantic love, being born of passion, leads to carelessness (*pramāda*), which generally involves harm to others and hence accumulation of more karma.

Jains believe that the sexual act slaughters thousands of minute one- and two-sensed beings that reside in the genitals and in the moist area between a woman's breasts. In addition, millions of sperm meet a violent end when they are helplessly ejaculated. For monks or nuns who have devoted their lives to an intense effort to gain liberation, merely one sexual encounter incurs enough karma to hamper that effort significantly. Even householders are encouraged to curb their sexual acts as much as feasible while still maintaining a fulfilling marriage and producing offspring. Worldly life is necessary for the preservation of humanity and the continuation of the Jain tradition. Still, the social phenomena of marriage and parenthood have negative consequences for householders due to the sexual acts that accompany them. No one, except the near-liberated soul, is free from karmic debt and its future-life consequences.

Despite their sympathy toward procreative sexuality, Jain writers have never portrayed sex in a positive way. Again and again one finds strong warnings against consorting with women and the entrapment of the sexual act. The frequent portrayal of women as sirens obsessed with snaring would-be ascetics underscores the advice to avoid sexuality once the path to enlightenment has begun. As in some Christian interpretations of Eve, women are portrayed as "the deadliest of all poisons . . . blinding men by the intoxication of the wine of lust" (*Sūtrakṛtāṇga*, 273–75). Such misogynistic attitudes were predominant in Indian society at the time (sixth century BCE), fueled in part by the concern that both **flirting** with women and sexuality would distract monks or even laypersons from focusing on the quest for spiritual liberation.

Within the Jain literature a unique and heated debate between two opposing sects, Svetāmbara and Digambara, raged for centuries about whether women could attain liberation.

Both sides agreed that the female-gendered body is inferior to the male-gendered body (due to the female reproductive organs and menstruation, as well as the fact that women lack certain skills, e.g., debating). The Śvetāmbara acknowledged that women can still attain liberation in their lifetime; the Digambara disagreed. The difference arose in part from the Digambara assumption (not shared by Śvetāmbaras) that nudity was a necessary condition for liberation. Women, however, could not fulfill this requirement, since their public nudity would offend prevailing standards of modesty and likely incite **rape**. Further, their bodies could not hold up to the demands of extreme Jain asceticism. And there is the frequent destruction of life that is inherent in the female body form: the higher number of organisms living in her damp groin and breast areas that die as a result of the female layperson's daily activity and sexual activities. Menstruation, too, is destructive.

Nevertheless, Jainism is unique in its acceptance and support of an order of nuns. The Hindu tradition never truly embraced the idea of female renunciation. Buddha only reluctantly agreed to the ordination of women (*bhikṣuni-saṃgha*), and today in the Theravada tradition all lineages of nuns have died out. Compare this gender disparity with the Śvetāmbara text, the *Kalpasūtra*, which notes that during Mahāvīra's lifetime there were more than twice the number of nuns than monks (36,000:14,000) in Jain religious orders; 1,400 women reached *mokṣa*, but only 700 men attained liberation in his presence. The Śvetāmbara also recognize that the nineteenth *tīrthaṅkara*, Malli, was a woman. Within India and the ancient world, Jainism is in the forefront in recognizing that women have just as much right to spiritual advancement as men. Jainism stands apart in legitimating a woman's choice for an alternative lifestyle of intense spiritual commitment and lifelong dedication instead of marriage and child rearing. It is difficult to think of any culture in antiquity (or even today) that openly recognizes and abundantly encourages the value of women choosing to live a life of chastity instead of childbearing.

The pervasive negative attitude toward sexuality in Jainism may account for its refusal to embrace two adaptations of sexuality to spirituality that arose in India. In devotional Hinduism, stories about the female Rādhā's intense passion for Kṛṣṇa served to model how one should approach God. After knowing the intoxicating rapture of romantic love and the ecstasy of sexual union, one is asked to transform them into an analogous ecstatic devotional fervor for Kṛṣṇa. In the West, Heloise (1101–1164) similarly wrote to Peter Abelard (1079–1142) about transforming the passion of their infamous illicit love affair into devotion to God, once their romantic love was squashed and they joined the clergy: "Without changing the ardour of our affections, let us change their object; let us leave our songs, and sing hymns; let us lift up our hearts to God, and have no transports but for his glory" (*Letter II*, 53).

But for Jainism, an analogical connection between sexuality and spirituality is nonsensical. Sexuality, even as a metaphor, is antithetical to spirituality, because the loss of control, the carelessness, the inherent destruction of life, and the passionate fervor of sexuality lead to *saṃsāra* and away from spiritual liberation. A more appropriate analogy, for Jainism, would be between spousal affection (apart from sexuality) and the adherents' love for their spiritual teacher.

Within the Jain community, and particularly among lay followers, ritual activities, such as the *stavas* or *stavans* (hymns of praise), reflect love for the *jinas* (literally, "victors" over transmigration and ignorance) or *tīrthaṅkaras* (principal revealers of the Jain path). Central to the Jain life are the three jewels (*ratnatraya*): true faith (*samyak-darśana*), right knowledge (*samyak-jñāna*), and proper conduct (*samyak-cāritra*). The real path to salvation begins on the fourth step of the fourteen steps (*guṇasthānas*) to liberation, where one has faith in the omniscient teaching of the *tīrthankara* and the validity of the Jain means to salvation. Similarly, the layperson's steps toward becoming a mendicant are found in the eleven steps of *sravaka-pratimā*, which relies heavily on the commitment of the layperson to Jain ideals. This all-embracing love for the tradition that vitalizes the aspirant toward his or her goal is grounded in *ahiṃsā*.

Ahiṃsā guides the activities of the aspirant, gradually building the aspirant's love and compassion (*anukampā*) for all living beings as she or he moves up the fourteen steps toward enlightenment, annihilating the destructive (*ghātiya*) karmas. Indeed, Jains traditionally have valued acts of giving (*dayā*) to monks and nuns as well as compassion (*anukampā*) to living beings as socially beneficially and ethically/spiritually positive; yet such acts do not constitute a path to liberation in and of themselves. Transcendental love or compassion eventually must give way when passion is eradicated from the eleventh step or *guṇasthāna* onward.

Here we see a striking difference between Jain views and their Buddhist and Hindu counterparts. The compassion (*karuṇā*) of the Buddha and fervent devotion (*bhakti*) toward God in medieval Hinduism play a central role in the spiritual development of its aspirants and the character of the central spiritual figure(s) in their tradition. Yet Jainism—with its emphasis on the necessity of extinguishing *all* passions—must view Jinas and spiritually advanced monks as void of such compassion. Even when the *tīrthankara* sends out his *dharma* (spiritual teaching and guidance), it would be a mistake to interpret this as a supreme gesture of compassion, as has often been expressed within the Buddhist view of the teaching of Buddha and the legend of *bodhisattvas* that has followed him. It is intriguing to note that while Buddhist polemicists repeatedly attacked the Jain claims of the Jinas' omniscience (*sarvajñāna* or *kevalajñāna*), Jain authors did not reciprocate by attacking what they must have perceived as the false Buddhist claims of the "compassion" of the Buddha once he reached enlightenment (*nirvāṇa*) or the persistent life of compassion expression by *bodhisattvas* in later Mahayana Buddhism doctrine.

The Jains likewise had a very different attitude toward the influx of Tantra elements in India religion and philosophy when compared with the Buddhist and Hindu schools of thought. Tantric practices began to flourish by the fifth to sixth century in India, and existing religious traditions were compelled to incorporate some of its elements into their own practices. Orthodox Jain leaders integrated elements of Tantra for three reasons: (1) it provided comfort, betterment, and guidance for the here and now life found in samsaric existence; (2) Jain followers, lay and mendicants, already were engaging in Tantric practices that involved passionate and spiritually ignorant (*mithyātva*) deities, so it was important to redirect their spiritual interactions with vegetarian deities sympathetic to Jain principles; and (3) by laying out a "proper" adaptation of Tantra, they could model (and correct) other concurrent, non-Jain traditions' erroneous and dangerous use of Tantra (Chapple, 77; Cort, "Worship," 417; Dundas, "Jain Monk," 231; Qvarnström, 597).

Given that the Jinas are dispassionate (*vītarāga*) and hence removed from life's daily challenges and trauma, they cannot respond to the petitions and worldly needs of the faithful Jain followers. While they offer invaluable guidance for liberating oneself from the world of suffering, little help was provided in excelling or even surviving in the world until that point of departure. Jain Tantric texts and rituals are directed toward the "six actions" (*ṣatkarmāṇi*): pacification of foes (*śānti*); subjugation of others (*vaśī*); immobilization of opponents (*stambhana*); causing one's adversaries to argue with one another (*vidveṣaṇa*); causing foes to retreat (*uccāṭana*); and causing the death of one's enemies (*marana*) (Cort, "Tantra," 121).

Most striking are the goal of killing one's adversaries and the goal to attract and control women, ostensibly in conflict with Jain ideals. No doubt this was instrumental in bringing about reformers such as Buddhisāgarsūri (1847–1925) and Haribhadra (700–770) (Chapple, 75–85; Cort, "Tantra," 125). Given the limited focus and nearly unattainable goals within Jain thought, it is only natural that Jain followers turned to an auxiliary resource in coping with daily life. Accordingly, from approximately the sixth century to the present, the use of magic (*mantras*, *yantras*) has been an integral part of Jain religious life and ritual. There arose a pantheon of otherworldly "heroes" (*vīras*) who served to protect the Jain followers, provide them with worldly needs, and defeat enemies of the Jain community.

Nevertheless, unlike Hinduism and Buddhism, Jainism never employed "left-handed Tantra" practices. These Tantric devices advocate the selective, deliberate breaking down of traditional religious and cultural taboos (for spiritual gain) against eating meat, fornication, sexual deviance, and misuse of rituals. Further, Tantra in Jainism never served as an alternative route to liberation as it did in some Hindu and Buddhist schools of thought; given that the heroes and deities evoked in Tantric rituals and hymns were themselves nonliberated beings, clearly they could not bestow liberation to others (Cort, "Worship," 417; Qvarnström, 597). For Jain thinkers, such misuse of Tantra teachings wrongly steered adherents in a direction that could be devastating to their spiritual progress. Haribhadra in his *Yogadṛṣṭisamuccaya* chastises Tantra-based yoga schools (Kula schools) for employing licentiousness (*advedyasaṃvedya*), which "greatly agitates the aspirant by involvement with objects," while genuine yoga schools employ temperance (*vedyasaṃvedya*), which "destroys obstacles and turns one's thoughts away from woman" (see *Yogadṛṣṭisamuccaya*, passages 72–73, in Chapple, 119–20; see 78–79).

In the *Tattvārtha Sūtra*, Umāsvāti (ca. 135–219) offers some observations about the nature of sexual attraction and physiology. He notes that the sex organs and the accompanying sexual (emotional) dispositions, or preferences, are both determined by karma. Though Umāsvāti does not directly address **homosexuality** or **bisexuality**, he does identify the cause of hermaphroditism as "inauspicious body-making karma." It could be inferred that other "unusual" sexual phenomena such as androgyny, homosexuality, or bisexuality would also be the product of "inauspicious" sexual disposition karma. This sort of karmic analysis, though foreign to contemporary medical science, shares a common feature with it: Both search for the cause of homosexuality. The Jain and the biologists are looking for a mechanical explanation for the phenomena rather than attributing them merely to perverted lifestyle choices.

There is some evidence for Jain intolerance of homosexual behavior, at least among monks. It is not clear, however, if this condemnation centers on the fact that monks would be engaging in sexual activity per se or in homosexual behavior in particular. Given the secluded, male-only monastery, homosexual behavior was the only available means of sexual gratification. Sexuality is something that all monks must be on guard against, since sexual disposition continues to tempt the mendicant all the way until the final stages (tenth to fourteenth steps or *guṇasthāna*) of spiritual development.

See also Buddhism; Catholicism, History of; Chinese Philosophy; Hinduism; Indian Erotology; Judaism, History of; Manichaeism; Tantrism

REFERENCES

Chapple, Christopher Key. *Reconciling Yogas: Haribhadra's Collection of Views on Yoga*. Albany: State University of New York Press, 2003; Cort, John. "Tantra in Jainism: The Cult of Ghaṇṭākarṇ Mahāvir, the Great Hero Bell-Ears." *Bulletin D'études Indiennes* 15. Paris: Association Française Pour Les Études Indiennes, 1997, 115–33; Cort, John. "Worship of Bell-Ears the Great Hero, a Jain

Tantric Deity." In David Gordon White, ed., *Tantra in Practice*. Princeton, N.J.: Princeton University Press, 2000, 417–33; Dundas, Paul. "The Jain Monk Jinapati Sūri Gets the Better of a Nāth Yogī." In David Gordon White, ed., *Tantra in Practice*. Princeton, N.J.: Princeton University Press, 2000, 231–38; Dundas, Paul. *The Jains*. New York: Routledge, 1992; Heloise and Abelard. *Letters* [selections]. In Robert C. Solomon and Kathleen M. Higgins, eds., *The Philosophy of (Erotic) Love*. Lawrence: University Press of Kansas, 1991, 49–55; Jaini, J. L., ed. *The Sacred Books of the Jainas: Original Texts and Commentaries*. New York: AMS Press, 1974; Jaini, Padmanabh S. *The Jaina Path of Purification*. Delhi, India: Motilal Banarsidass, 1979; Qvarnström, Olle. "Jain Tantra: Divinatory and Meditative Practices in the Twelfth-Century Yogaśāstra of Hemacandra." In David Gordon White, ed., *Tantra in Practice*. Princeton, N.J.: Princeton University Press, 2000, 595–604; Rist J. M. "Mysticism." In *Plotinus: The Road to Reality*. New York: Cambridge University Press, 1967, 213–30; *Sūtrakṛtāṅga*. (ca. fourth century BCE) Trans. Hermann Jacobi. In *Jaina Sūtras*, part 2. *The Sacred Books of the East*, vol. 45. Delhi, India: Motilal Banarsidass, 1989, 235–436; Umāsvāti. (ca. 200 CE) *That Which Is = Tattvārtha Sūtra*. [with commentaries] Trans. Nathmal Tatia. San Francisco, Calif.: HarperCollins, 1994.

Kim Skoog

ADDITIONAL READING

Bhadrabahu. *The Kalpa Sūtra*. Trans. Hermann Jacobi. In *Jaina Sūtras*, part 1. *The Sacred Books of the East*, vol. 22. Delhi, India: Motilal Banarsidass, 1989, 217–311; Chapple, Christopher Key. "Religious Dissonance and Reconciliation: The Haribhadra Story." In Tara Sethia, ed., *Ahiṃsā, Anekānta, and Jainism*. Delhi, India: Motilal Banarsidass, 2004, 137–60; Cheng, Hsueh-li. "Jainism." In Lawrence C. Becker and Charlotte B. Becker, eds., *Encyclopedia of Ethics*, 2nd ed., vol. 2. New York: Routledge, 2001, 897–99; Dupuche, John R. *Abhinavagupta: The Kula Ritual, as Elaborated in Chapter 29 of the Tantrāloka*. Delhi, India: Motilal Banarsidass, 2003; Haribhadra. (eighth century) *Yogadṛṣṭisamuccaya*. Trans. Christopher Key Chapple and John Thomas Casey. In Christopher Key Chapple, *Reconciling Yogas: Haribhadra's Collection of Views on Yoga*. Albany: State University of New York Press, 2003, 102–53; Heloise and Abelard. *Letters* [selections]. In Ellen K. Feder, Karmen MacKendrick, and Sybol S. Cook, eds., *A Passion for Wisdom: Readings in Western Philosophy on Love and Desire*. Upper Saddle River, N.J.: Prentice Hall, 2004, 175–87; Jain, Kailash Chand. *Lord Mahāvīra and His Times*, rev. ed. Delhi, India: Motilal Banarsidass, 1991; Jain, Surender K., ed. *Glimpses of Jainism*. Delhi, India: Motilal Banarsidass, 1999; Qvarnström, Olle, ed. *Jainism and Early Buddhism: Essays in Honor of Padmanabh S. Jaini*. Part 1. Fremont, Calif.: Asian Humanities Press, 2003; Roth, Philip. *American Pastoral*. Boston, Mass.: Houghton Mifflin, 1997; Schubring, Walther. *The Doctrines of the Jainas*. Delhi, India: Motilal Banarsidass, 1995; Skoog, Kim. "The Jaina Response to Terrorism." In Tara Sethia, ed., *Ahiṃsā, Anekānta, and Jainism*. Delhi, India: Motilal Banarsidass, 2004, 25–46; Skoog, Kim. "The Morality of *Sallekhanā*: The Jaina Practice of Fasting to Death." In Olle Qvarnström, ed., *Jainism and Early Buddhism: Essays in Honor of Padmanabh S. Jaini*. Part 1. Fremont, Calif.: Asian Humanities Press, 2003, 293–304; Skoog, Kim, ed. "Special Issue: The Philosophy of Jainism." *Philosophy East and West* 50:3 (2000); "Introduction" by Kim Skoog, 321–23; Thomas, Paul. *Epics, Myths and Legends of India: A Comprehensive Survey of the Sacred Lore of the Hindus, Buddhists and Jains*, 11th ed. Bombay, India: D. B. Taraporevala, n.d.; Von Glasenapp, Helmuth. *Jainism: A Religion of Salvation*. Trans. Shridhar B. Shrotri. Delhi, India: Motilal Banarsidass, 1999; White, David Gordon, ed. *Tantra in Practice*. Princeton, N.J.: Princeton University Press, 2000; Wiley, Kristi L. "Views on Ahiṃsā, Compassion, and Samyaktva in Jainism." In Tara Sethia, ed., *Ahiṃsā, Anekānta, and Jainism*. Delhi, India: Motilal Banarsidass, 2004, 15–24.

JEALOUSY. According to one plausible analysis of jealousy, to experience this emotion, or to be jealous, is to be "bothered" by the fact that one is not, as one sees things, "favored" by another person in some way in which one wants to be favored by that other, while someone else is, or so one believes, favored by that other instead (Farrell, "Jealousy and Desire," 166). "Bothered" and "favored" need explanation, but the general idea is clear. In William Shakespeare's (1564–1616) play, Othello wants to be favored by Desdemona's affections, he wants her affection to be directed only at himself, and he is bothered, to put it mildly, by the fact, as he believes, that Cassio is also a recipient of her affection.

Othello is a paradigm example of a *sexually* jealous person. The analysis has the merit, though, of being applicable to other jealousies as well. I might be professionally jealous when I see that a colleague is viewed by our students as a better teacher than I am. (Jealousy "is particularly common among scholars in a given field, for they cannot allow anyone else to surpass them there," says **Immanuel Kant** [1724–1804], Ak 27:438.) I might be "interpersonally" jealous if my children show more interest in what you say to them than in what I say. And Yahweh admits that He is "a jealous God" (Deut. 5:9), wanting the Israelites to "have no other gods before" Him (5:7). In each case there are three parties: *A* wants to be favored in some way by *B*, either over all others or over a specific other, and *A*, believing that *C* is or might be favored by *B* instead, is bothered by that fact. (Cases of apparent jealousy that involve only two people are perhaps better analyzed as envy; see Farrell, "Jealousy," 530–34; "Jealousy and Desire," 170–71; Roberts, 263–64. Note, in this regard, that **Baruch Spinoza** [1632–1677] thought that jealousy was a combination of hate for the beloved and envy of the interloper. See *Ethics* 3, proposition 35.)

This analysis posits three elements in jealousy: a *conative* element (the desire to be favored by another); a *cognitive* element (the belief that one is not, or is at risk of not being, favored); and an *affective* element (being bothered by the fact that one is not favored). Jealousy is not simply the affective state (being bothered). It is the emotion someone has when he is in that state *because* he believes that he is not, or is at risk of not being, favored in some way in which he wants to be favored. The theoretical idea is that emotions are more than and different from phenomenological feelings (see Green).

On this analysis, the affective component in jealousy need not be a particular state that is phenomenologically invariant in all occurrences of the emotion. It might be that some people experience jealousy as something like what they experience when they feel fear, while others experience it as anger, and so on, for any number of ways of being "bothered" by what is believed to be a frustration of the relevant desire. **Saint Augustine** (354–430), for example, gives jealousy a hellish tone: "I was scourged with the red hot rods of jealousy" (*Confessions*, bk. 3, chap. 1). For attributions of jealousy, *any* kind of conscious or unconscious botherment will do, caused by the belief or suspicion that one is not favored in some way one wants to be favored. (On unconscious jealousy, see Greenspan, 26–28.)

This analysis also sets no *a priori* limit on the ways a person might want to be favored by another, thereby becoming vulnerable to jealousy if she believes she is not favored in that way. Indeed, the analysis does not require that the desire is to be favored by another *person*. I might be jealous because my dog appears to be showing you affection. In fact, my awareness of being jealous might make me realize that it is important to me to be favored this way by my dog. Thus, far from assuming that all instances of jealousy involve a desire to be favored in some particular way, this analysis holds only that jealousy involves a desire to be favored in some way or other, the particular way in any given case being revealed by what it is that, in its absence or threatened absence, causes botherment.

Sexual jealousy, then, entails someone's being bothered in some way due to believing that he is not, or is at risk of not being, favored in some way that has to do with sexuality, while someone else, as he believes, is being favored instead. Sexual jealousy is jealousy because it exhibits the belief-desire-affect structure of all jealousy. But what does "has to do with sexuality" involve? One paradigm for a desire's having something to do with sexuality is that it is a desire for sexual exclusivity: *A* might desire that *B* engage in sexual relations only with *A* and would be bothered by the thought that *B* was doing so with *anyone* else. But this scenario does not exhaust sexual jealousy. *A* might desire to be favored by *B* in some way having to do with sexuality without desiring exclusivity: *A* might not care if *B* has sexual relations with *C* or *D* but would be devastated by the thought of *B*'s having sexual relations with the specific person *E* (see Roberts, 259).

It is worthwhile to distinguish sexual jealousy from a broader class, romantic jealousy, of which the former is a subclass. In romantic jealousy, one member of a romantic relationship is bothered because she believes she is not favored in some way she wants to be favored by the other member of the romantic relationship. This distinction enables us to talk about jealousy when there is no concern about sexual behavior as such, but the person's jealousy is still very much about a loved one's attention to others, and her jealousy is related to their relationship's being sexual or romantic. I might be convinced of my partner's sexual fidelity and yet be consumed with jealousy, desperately bothered, because she finds another man more witty, charming, or intelligent than I. My jealousy here need not be based on my believing that my partner's admiration for the other's wit will lead to my losing her or her sexual attention. For I might be certain that I will never lose her and still be bothered by believing that she believes he has more wit than I.

Whether jealousy is largely a natural emotion (see **Edward Westermarck** [1862–1939], 76–78) or to a significant extent social in origin, or conventional, has been disputed. **Bertrand Russell** (1872–1970) seemed to think that while jealousy was in part instinctive, related to the need of males to be assured of paternity, it was more importantly social (*Why I Am Not a Christian*, 170, 174). Recent work in **evolutionary psychology** has proposed that jealousy in men is an adaptive solution to the problem of avoiding cuckoldry (Daly et al.). In women, jealousy is related, instead, to their need to preserve resources. As a result, "Men and women do not differ in either the frequency or the magnitude of their jealousy experience" (Buss, 127).

Regardless of its origin, jealousy, especially but not only sexual jealousy, is often claimed to be bad or to reveal bad things about the jealous person. "With some emotions, like envy and jealousy, we might feel that we should always stifle their expression simply because we find them demeaning and believe that they reveal one to be small-minded" (Lyons, 201; see Primoratz, 85–87). Whether Yahweh's jealousy indicates a divine defect is a fascinating question. But, regarding mere mortals, why is jealousy supposed to be objectionable? One claim is that it involves possessiveness: The jealous person thinks of the other as an object or thing that he owns or with respect to whom he has rights that entitle him to limit the other's freedom of conduct or decision. ("Jealousy always has its source . . . in the attitude of possessiveness towards another person"; Richard Taylor [1919–2003], 143.) Another claim is that jealousy reveals personal insecurity; a psychologically healthy or mature person would not be prone to jealousy. Yet another claim is that jealousy is irrational. It involves irrational beliefs; for example, the belief that **love** is a limited commodity, the allocation of which must be tracked carefully. Or it involves irrational desires; for example, to have someone sexually available only to oneself. (See Farrell, "Jealousy," 546–58; "Jealousy and Desire," 176–84.)

How plausible are these claims? We can agree with Russell that children should not be instructed that "jealousy [involves] a justifiable insistence upon rights" (*On Education*, 120) and admit that the lesson has not always been taught or learned well: Many jealous lovers are possessive and think of their partners as owned objects. But this fact does not go far in establishing that the existence of jealousy, especially sexual jealousy, shows the jealous person to be possessive in an objectionable way. Actually, our analysis of jealousy makes it implausible. Any assertion about what jealousy shows about the jealous person must be an assertion about the *desire* that jealousy requires, about the *belief* it requires, or about the jealous person's being *bothered* by that belief. Thus, if the existence of jealousy shows that the jealous person is objectionably possessive, this would have to be because the desire to be favored (for example, with sexual exclusivity) shows possessiveness, *or* because a belief that one is not favored shows it, *or* because being bothered by that belief shows it.

However, the mere belief that one is not favored cannot itself show that a jealous person is objectionably possessive, because that belief might be true or reasonable apart from whether the jealous person is possessive. So the charge of objectionable possessiveness must rest on either her being bothered by believing that her desire to be favored has been thwarted or her desire to be favored in some way.

But why suppose that a jealous person's being bothered by the fact that she is not favored the way she wants to be favored, while someone else is, is an infallible or even reliable sign that she is objectionably possessive? An especially intense reaction to the frustration of the desire will invite critical scrutiny and might in the end show objectionable possessiveness. But *any* reaction or degree of botherment at all? That is implausible. That the loss of a lover, or its anticipation, is painful does not mean that we view our lover as someone over whom we have "claims of right" (Neu, 444–45). We are often upset when desires of this (or almost any) kind are frustrated, and being upset is possible even if one is not possessive, much less a person who sees others as "things" one has a right to control. As **Roger Scruton** suggests, jealousy "forces . . . into the light of day" the psychic blow that I am not unique, not irreplaceable (164). This distressing self-observation has nothing to do with thinking that I own my (ex-)lover.

Hence, if sexual jealousy shows the person to be possessive, this must be because she has the desire to be favored in the first place. But why suppose that a person's desire to be favored sexually shows that she is objectionably possessive? It might be true that to have this desire is *eo ipso* to convict oneself of various *other* charges, for example, insecurity or irrationality—but possessiveness of an insidious sort? It is difficult to see why this should be so.

What about the claim that jealousy, and especially sexual jealousy, is unhealthy or shows that a person is insecure in ways inconsistent with genuine psychological health? (See McMurtry, 178–79.) Some jealous people probably are insecure to a degree that discredits their psychological health. Their insecurity might cause them to desire to be preferentially favored by another person or to believe (even falsely) that they are not favored the way they want to be. But this does not establish that a person must be insecure, and to such a serious degree, to be susceptible to jealousy. This critic of jealousy must establish that jealousy is impossible without insecurity.

Establishing this claim, however, is difficult, and it seems implausible. Jealousy shows, trivially, that the person believes or suspects he is not favored in the way he wants to be favored, so jealousy might show that he is unsure of his "hold" on the other's affections and hence is *in that sense* insecure. But this insecurity is not the profound psychological defect that the critic of jealousy is, or should be, talking about. (Even without being Cartesian doubters, we are unsure of many things, and this innocuous uncertainty is no sign of mental weakness. Indeed, it can be a sign of mental strength, if it rules out inflexible dogmatism.) For the critic's view of jealousy to be plausible, there must be a kind of insecurity that is independent of any particular belief that one is not favored, a kind of insecurity that explains the desire to be favored, or the belief that one is not favored, or the botherment at not being favored. But there is little reason to suppose that a person whose concern for being favored is sufficient to generate serious botherment, when he believes that he is not so favored, is *by this very fact* shown to be significantly, unhealthily insecure.

Alternatively, the critic of jealousy could argue not that all instances of jealousy show the person to be insecure but only that some instances show this—for example, when the jealousy is unusually intense. Consider Othello's reaction to his belief (perhaps delusional; see Prins, 8–10) that Desdemona has betrayed him. To say that Othello is "bothered" by the fact that, as he believes, this has happened, would be an almost perverse understatement. He kills her! How could someone care that much about sexual fidelity without thereby revealing profound, unhealthy insecurity? On this way of understanding the critic's point, neither Othello's believing that Desdemona has been unfaithful nor the intensity of his reaction is the problem with Othello's jealousy. The belief, though mistaken, could have been correct, yet the critic would still say that Othello's reaction was excessive. Nor is it simply Othello's formidable "feeling," the affective component of his emotion, that is the most plausible object of the critic's doubts. Given the quality of Othello's desire for Desdemona's fidelity, his extreme emotional reaction—the emotional reaction *per se*, not the actions it leads to—is not surprising. Thus, the intensity of Othello's desire for faithfulness is the most plausible object of the critic's concern. That Othello *cares so much* about sexual exclusivity accounts for his excessive reaction, and hence the quality of his desire must show, if anything does, that something is psychologically unhealthy about Othello or his emotion.

What remains, then, is the idea that even though a desire to be favored *simpliciter* is not necessarily a sign of unhealthy insecurity, a desire for sexual exclusivity as intense as Othello's cannot be entirely unobjectionable. Such a strong desire cannot be consistent with a healthy sense of oneself. Intuitively, there *is* something odd (or "pathological"; Neu, 449) about someone who cares so strongly about sexual exclusivity that he is vulnerable to being driven into a murderous rage by the thought that he has been betrayed. (In general, strong desires, including the desire for sexual relations, that cause us, in virtue of their power, to commit risky or harmful acts recklessly, suggest psychological problems.) But that an intense desire for fidelity could be due *only* to profound psychological insecurity is empirically questionable. (For some empirical studies, see White and Mullen.)

The final claim is that an Othello-like desire, given its intensity, is irrational. This might be the most plausible claim to make about Othello, that there is something *crazy* about the intensity of his caring for fidelity. This might be what people mean when they judge jealousy negatively. However, a proponent of this claim will have to defend a view about desire that the history of philosophy suggests will be difficult to defend, namely, the view that desires (or emotions, *qua* entities that involve desires) can, like actions, be appraised as rational or irrational. Scottish philosopher **David Hume** (1711–1776) argued forcefully to the contrary (*Treatise*, bk. II, pt. iii, sec. 3), and subsequent theorists have been inclined to follow him. We shall eventually see how much success critics of Hume (e.g., Charles Taylor) will have.

See also Adultery; Casual Sex; Desire, Sexual; Evolution; Friendship; Hume, David; Judaism, History of; Love; Marriage; Psychology, Evolutionary; Psychology, Twentieth- and Twenty-First-Century; Westermarck, Edward

REFERENCES

Augustine. (397) *Confessions*. Trans. F. J. Sheed. Indianapolis, Ind.: Hackett, 1993; Buss, David M. *The Evolution of Desire: Strategies of Human Mating*. New York: Basic Books, 1994; Daly, Martin,

Margo Wilson, and Suzanne Weghorst. "Male Sexual Jealousy." *Ethology and Sociobiology* 3:1 (1982): 11–27; Farrell, Daniel M. "Jealousy." *Philosophical Review* 89:4 (October 1980), 527–59; Farrell, Daniel M. "Jealousy and Desire." In Roger E. Lamb, ed., *Love Analyzed*. Boulder, Colo.: Westview, 1997, 165–88; Green, O. Harvey. *The Emotions: A Philosophical Theory*. Dordrecht, Holland: Kluwer, 1992; Greenspan, Patricia S. *Emotions and Reasons: An Inquiry into Emotional Justification*. New York: Routledge, 1988; Hume, David. (1739–1740) *A Treatise of Human Nature*. Ed. L. A. Selby-Bigge. Oxford, U.K.: Clarendon Press, 1968; Kant, Immanuel. (ca. 1762–1794) *Lectures on Ethics*. Trans. Peter Heath. Ed. Peter Heath and Jerome B. Schneewind. Cambridge: Cambridge University Press, 1997; Lyons, William. *Emotion*. Cambridge: Cambridge University Press, 1980; McMurtry, John. "Sex, Love, and Friendship." In Alan Soble, ed., *Sex, Love, and Friendship*. Amsterdam, Holland: Rodopi, 1997, 169–83; Neu, Jerome. "Jealous Thoughts." In Amélie Oksenberg Rorty, ed., *Explaining Emotions*. Berkeley: University of California Press, 1980, 425–63; Primoratz, Igor. "Marriage, Adultery, Jealousy." In *Ethics and Sex*. London: Routledge, 1999, 69–87; Prins, Herschel. *Bizarre Behaviours: Boundaries of Psychiatric Disorder*. London: Tavistock/Routledge, 1990; Roberts, Robert C. *Emotions: An Essay in Aid of Moral Psychology*. Cambridge: Cambridge University Press, 2003; Russell, Bertrand. (1926) *On Education, Especially in Early Childhood*. London: Unwin, 1973; Russell, Bertrand. *Why I Am Not a Christian and Other Essays on Religion and Related Subjects*. Ed. Paul Edwards. New York: Simon and Schuster, 1963; Scruton, Roger. "Jealousy." In *Sexual Desire: A Moral Philosophy of the Erotic*. New York: Free Press, 1986, 162–67; Shakespeare, William. (1603–1604) *The Tragedy of Othello, the Moor of Venice*. In Stephen Greenblatt, ed., *The Norton Shakespeare*. New York: Norton, 1997, 2100–2172; Spinoza, Baruch. (1677) *Ethics*. In *The Collected Works of Spinoza*, vol. 1. Trans. E. Curley. Princeton, N.J.: Princeton University Press, 1985, 401–617; Taylor, Charles. *Sources of the Self: The Making of the Modern Identity*. Cambridge, Mass.: Harvard University Press, 1989; Taylor, Richard. *Having Love Affairs*. Buffalo, N.Y.: Prometheus, 1982; Westermarck, Edward. "Adultery and Jealousy." In *The Future of Marriage in Western Civilization*. New York: Macmillan, 1936, 58–79; White, Gregory L., and Paul E. Mullen. *Jealousy: Theory, Research, and Clinical Strategies*. New York: Guilford Press, 1989.

Daniel M. Farrell

ADDITIONAL READING

Bohm, Ewald. "Jealousy." In Albert Ellis and Albert Abarbanel, eds., *The Encyclopedia of Sexual Behavior*. New York: Jason Aronson, 1973, 567–74; Buss, David M. "Evolutionary Psychology: A New Paradigm for Psychological Science." *Psychological Inquiry* 6:1 (1995), 1–30; Daly, Martin, Margo Wilson, and Suzanne Weghorst. "Male Sexual Jealousy." *Ethology and Sociobiology* 3:1 (1982), 11–27; Davis, Kingsley. "Jealousy and Sexual Property." *Social Forces* 14:3 (1936), 395–405; de Sousa, Ronald. *The Rationality of Emotion*. Cambridge, Mass.: MIT Press, 1987; de Sousa, Ronald. "The Rationality of Emotions." In Amélie Oksenberg Rorty, ed., *Explaining Emotions*. Berkeley: University of California Press, 1980, 127–51; de Sousa, Ronald. "Self-Deceptive Emotions." In Amélie Oksenberg Rorty, ed., *Explaining Emotions*. Berkeley: University of California Press, 1980, 283–97; Deigh, John. "Cognitivism in the Theory of Emotions." *Ethics* 104:4 (1994), 824–54; Farber, Leslie. *Lying, Despair, Jealousy, Envy, Sex, Suicide, Drugs, and the Good Life*. New York: Basic Books, 1976; Farrell, Daniel M. "Of Jealousy and Envy." In George Graham and Hugh LaFollette, eds., *Person to Person*. Philadelphia, Pa.: Temple University Press, 1989, 245–68. Reprinted in Christina Sommers and Fred Sommers, eds., *Vice and Virtue in Everyday Life: Introductory Readings in Ethics*, 3rd ed. Fort Worth, Tex.: Harcourt Brace Jovanovich, 1993, 393–419; Freud, Sigmund. (1922) "Some Neurotic Mechanisms in Jealousy, Paranoia, and Homosexuality." In *The Standard Edition of the Complete Psychological Works of Sigmund Freud*, vol. 18. Trans. James Strachey. London: Hogarth Press, 1953–1974, 223–32; Giroud, Françoise, and Bernard-Henri Lévy. (1993) "On Jealousy as Consubstantial with Love." In *Women and Men: A Philosophical Conversation*. Trans. Richard Miller. Boston, Mass.: Little, Brown, 1995, 71–89; Gonzalez-Crussi, Frank. "On Male Jealousy." In *On the Nature of Things Erotic*. San Diego, Calif.: Harcourt Brace Jovanovich, 1988, 25–45; Green, O. Harvey. "Is

Love an Emotion?" In Roger E. Lamb, ed., *Love Analyzed*. Boulder, Colo.: Westview, 1997, 209–24; Hamilton, Christopher. "Sex." In *Living Philosophy: Reflections on Life, Meaning and Morality*. Edinburgh, Scot.: Edinburgh University Press, 2001, 125–41; Konstan, David, and N. Keith Rutter, eds. *Envy, Spite, and Jealousy: The Rivalrous Emotions in Ancient Greece*. Edinburgh, Scot.: Edinburgh University Press, 2003; LaFollette, Hugh. "Sex and Jealousy." In *Human Relationships: Love, Identity, and Morality*. Oxford, U.K.: Blackwell, 1996, 168–81; Lamb, Roger E. "Love and Rationality." In Roger E. Lamb, ed., *Love Analyzed*. Boulder, Colo.: Westview, 1997, 23–45; Lear, Jonathan. "Love's Authority." In Sarah Buss and Lee Overton, eds., *Contours of Agency: Essays on Themes from Harry Frankfurt*. Cambridge, Mass.: MIT Press, 2002, 279–92; Neu, Jerome. "Jealous Afterthoughts." In *A Tear Is an Intellectual Thing: The Meanings of Emotion*. New York: Oxford University Press, 2000, 68–80; Neu, Jerome. "Jealous Thoughts." In Amélie Oksenberg Rorty, ed., *Explaining Emotions*. Berkeley: University of California Press, 1980, 425–63. Reprinted in *A Tear Is an Intellectual Thing: The Meanings of Emotion*. New York: Oxford University Press, 2000, 41–67; Pilardi, Jo-Ann. "Why Should We Exclude Exclusivity?" [Reply to John McMurtry, "Sex, Love, and Friendship"] In Alan Soble, ed., *Sex, Love, and Friendship*. Amsterdam, Holland: Rodopi, 1997, 185–89; Reeve, C.D.C. "Jealousy, Perversity, and Other Liabilities of Love." In *Love's Confusions*. Cambridge, Mass.: Harvard University Press, 2005, 77–91; Rorty, Amélie Oksenberg, ed. *Explaining Emotions*. Berkeley: University of California Press, 1980; Schwartz, Mimi. "Negotiating Monogamy." In *Thoughts from a Queen-Sized Bed*. Lincoln: University of Nebraska Press, 2002, 26–29; Soble, Alan. "A Lakoma." [Reply to John McMurtry, "Sex, Love, and Friendship"] In Alan Soble, ed., *Sex, Love, and Friendship*. Amsterdam, Holland: Rodopi, 1997, 191–97; Solomon, Robert C. *The Passions*. Garden City, N.Y.: Anchor/Doubleday, 1976; Stern, Lawrence. Review of *Having Love Affairs*, by Richard Taylor. *Ethics* 98:1 (1987), 190–92; Taylor, Gabriele. "Envy and Jealousy: Emotions and Vices." In Peter A. French, Theodore E. Uehling, Jr., and Howard K. Wettstein, eds., *Midwest Studies in Philosophy*, vol. 13. *Ethical Theory: Character and Virtue*. Notre Dame, Ind.: University of Notre Dame Press, 1988, 233–49; Taylor, Gabriele. *Pride, Shame and Guilt: Emotions of Self-Assessment*. Oxford, U.K.: Clarendon Press, 1985; Taylor, Richard. *Having Love Affairs*. Buffalo, N.Y.: Prometheus, 1982. Reprinted as *Love Affairs: Marriage and Infidelity*. Amherst, N.Y.: Prometheus, 1997; Tov-Ruach, Leila. "Jealousy, Attention, and Loss." In Amélie Oksenberg Rorty, ed., *Explaining Emotions*. Berkeley: University of California Press, 1980, 465–88.

JOHN PAUL II (POPE). *See* Wojtyła, Karol

JUDAISM, HISTORY OF. Judaism has traditionally assumed that procreative sex and heterosexual **marriage** are essential elements of a fully realized human existence. Although **sexual desire** and pleasure play necessary roles within marriage, they are also fraught with spiritual danger, mainly because they may drive people to commit prohibited sexual acts. These ideas are firmly rooted in the Hebrew Scriptures and Jewish law (*halakhah*) as authoritatively explicated in Talmudic literature, and they have inspired and constrained the attitudes toward sexuality that have been proposed in various times and places throughout Jewish history.

Biblical and Rabbinic Background. The Hebrew Scriptures treat sexuality as an enjoyable element of human life lacking any special religious significance. Although semen is included among the body fluids whose emission results in temporary ritual impurity, sexuality is not incorporated into worship, nor is it viewed as undermining spirituality. The story of the creation of woman expresses the notion that Adam's solo existence was fundamentally defective ("it is not good for man to be alone") without Eve's companionship. The begetting of children is both commanded by God and viewed as one of God's chief blessings to human beings. The desire for children, especially women's, is an important factor in biblical narratives, motivating the actions of many biblical heroes, including Abraham, Sarah, Isaac, Rebecca, Rachel, Leah, Tamar, and Hannah.

While sexual activities are constrained by various ritual rules, so are many other aspects of everyday life, including agriculture, eating, and dressing. The only infractions of sexual mores that receive much attention in the nonlegal sections of the Hebrew Scriptures involve sex between a man and someone else's wife and **rape** (and acts combining the two). These serve as paradigms of gentile depravity in Genesis: Abraham's wife Sarah and Isaac's wife Rebecca are forced to join the harems of gentile kings. The angels visiting Sodom are threatened with gang rape. Dinah is raped by Shechem, son of Hamor, and Potiphar's wife tries to force Joseph into having sex with her.

In later biblical stories one finds that King David's great sin was having sex with Batsheva, a married woman, and later arranging for her husband to be killed in battle. David's unwillingness to punish Amnon for the rape of Tamar sets into motion the tragic course of events described in the Second Book of Kings, whose later plot-turns are largely motivated by different instances of male sexual **jealousy**. Condemnation of sexual relations between a man and another man's wife is also an important theme in the Book of Proverbs. In the prophetic literature, the relationship between God and Israel is often portrayed metaphorically in terms of erotic **love**. As a result, the Israelites' sin of idolatry is frequently compared to female sexual infidelity.

Any treatment of biblical attitudes toward sexuality must mention the Song of Songs. Its male and female protagonists address each other with erotic love poems that are charmingly evocative of the culture and geography of ancient Israel. Although this book may be understood as reflecting something of the notion of love current at the time of its composition, it has had little influence on later rabbinic discussions of love between human beings and has always been interpreted allegorically.

The reconstruction of "biblical" law is a problematic and largely speculative venture. Normative Judaism assumes that when Moses received the written Torah (the first five books of the Bible) from God, he was also taught an Oral Torah, consisting of divinely authorized interpretations and extensions of the written text. This additional material, along with later interpretive debates and legal decrees, was first systematically compiled around 200 by Rabbi Judah the Prince in a work known as the Mishnah. Later legal discussions, many of which deal with the proper interpretation of the Mishnah, were recorded in the Talmud or, to be precise, two different *Talmudim*: the Talmud of the Land of Israel, or Jerusalem Talmud, compiled around 400, and the more authoritative Babylonian Talmud, compiled around 500. Throughout the ages, Jews continued to study and expand their legal tradition, producing a huge and intricately intertextual literature, including *teshuvot* (scholarly letters addressing particular legal questions), *hiddushim* (collections of new interpretations of canonical texts), commentaries, and codifications.

The following account of those aspects of the *halakhah* concerned with sexuality will mix biblical, Talmudic, and medieval materials in a manner that reflects the self-understanding of the normative Jewish legal tradition. It should be noted that while normative Judaism places significant emphasis on the well-being of women, especially within the marital relationship, practically all traditional Jewish religious literature was written by men who were addressing a presumably male readership.

The *Arba'ah Turim*, authored by Rabbi Jacob Ben Asher (1270?–1340), is one of the most authoritative codifications of Jewish law. Its discussion of marital laws begins with a statement of the rabbinical attitude toward marriage:

May the Holy One . . . be blessed, for he sought the welfare of His creations. Knowing that it is not good for man to be alone, He made a fitting helper for him [woman]. Furthermore, since the point of the creation of man was to be fruitful and multiply (this being impossible without the helper), He commanded him to cleave to the helper He had made for him. Thus every man is required to marry a woman in order to be fruitful and multiply, for anyone who does not engage in being fruitful and multiplying is similar to [one who] sheds blood . . . and it is as if he diminishes the image [of God] . . . and he causes the Divine Presence to take leave of Israel. And anyone who remains without a wife remains without well-being, without blessing, without habitation, without Torah, without a [protective] wall, without peace. And Rabbi Eliezer said, "Anyone who does not have a wife is not a man, and upon marrying a woman, his sins are lightened." The commandment [to marry] is of such great importance that one is permitted to sell a Torah scroll only in order to [use the money it brings] to either study Torah or marry a woman. (*Arba'ah Turim*, *Tur Even Ha-Ezer*, chap. 1, para. 1; Samet, vol. 11, 1) [Unless stated otherwise, all translations are by BDL.]

Normative Judaism could never view celibacy as a viable way of life. The High Priest in the Temple, who was bound to the strictest laws of ritual purity, was required to be married, as are those who lead synagogue prayers on the High Holy days. Even today, prominent Orthodox rabbis who become widowers in old age sometimes marry again to avoid the spiritual deficiencies of the unmarried state.

In Jewish tradition, the celebration of a wedding constitutes the ultimate apotheosis of human joy. Dancing and feasting at a wedding are viewed as the fulfillment of a divine command, and helping to finance the wedding of an impoverished couple is an especially profound act of charity. Celebration of a wedding is viewed as the celebration of the power and value of life itself, a notion expressed by ritual laws such as the rule that a funeral procession must yield right of way to a bridal procession. The wedding and its participants might be said to generate a kind of "field" of ritual joy that competes successfully with Judaism's omnipresent motif of mourning for the destruction of the Temple and the exile from the Land of Israel. The *Sheva Brakhot* ("Seven Benedictions") recited at the wedding ceremony and at the festive meals following it explicitly connect the rejoicing of bride and groom with the future joy of the messianic redemption. One benediction strikingly illustrates the rabbinic assumption that the Garden of Eden narrative is not to be read as a condemnation of human sexuality. It asks God to bless the new couple with the erotic bliss enjoyed by Adam and Eve before their expulsion from Paradise: "Verily, grant joy to the beloved friends, as you granted joy to your creation in the Garden of Eden of old. Blessed are you, Lord, who grants joy to groom and bride."

While Judaism approves strongly of marriage, there are certain people with whom a Jew is not allowed to engage in sexual intercourse, and it is simply impossible for a valid marriage with the forbidden partner to take place under Jewish law. The most serious violations belong to the category of *giluy arayot* (the "uncovering of nakedness"). These include sex between a man and another man's wife, various consanguineous relationships, male homosexual intercourse, and **bestiality**. Polygamy is not prohibited by Talmudic law, but monogamy has always been tacitly considered the norm. Polygamy was officially banned for European Jews by Rabbi Gershom ben Yehudah's (960–1028) famous edict, which has gradually been accepted by practically all Jewish communities. Marriages between Jews and non-Jews (who have not converted to Judaism) are not recognized by the *halakhah*.

Jewish law recognizes only the penetration of a living body by a penis as constituting a complete sexual act that can consummate a marriage or constitute a genuine violation of *giluy arayot*. As a result, lesbian acts, while frowned upon, are essentially without legal consequences. Male **masturbation** to ejaculation is an infringement of the rule against "wasting seed" that, while not an offense punishable by human courts, is viewed as a grievous sin by Jewish law. Female masturbation is of practically no interest to the rabbis.

Together with murder and idolatry, *giluy arayot* is one of the three sins that a Jew is expected to refuse to commit, even at the price of certain death. The deliberate and unrepented commission of such an act invites the divine punishment of *karet* ("extirpation"), which is understood to involve an early natural death and/or annihilation of the soul at death, leaving no hope for an afterlife. Some acts of *giluy arayot* are also punishable with various forms of death penalty. The Talmudic interpretation of biblical law restricts the prosecution of capital crimes to historical periods during which the Temple stands in Jerusalem; even then it makes successful prosecution practically impossible by requiring fantastically stringent standards of evidence and criminal intent.

Jewish law views illicit heterosexual acts as a genuine problem in Jewish society, while Jews are presumed to be uninterested in committing male homosexual acts (or bestiality). But gentiles are suspected of such activities, and Jewish men held captive by gentiles are thought to be in danger of homosexual rape. When it is mentioned in rabbinic literature, consensual male homosexual intercourse is thought to be an especially depraved form of *giluy arayot*. Although the *halakhah* grants no legitimacy to the nonheterosexual orientations of anatomically male or female human beings, it does recognize the anatomically intermediate categories of the *androgynos*, who possesses both male and female anatomical characteristics, and the apparently sexless *tumtum*.

Sexual contact is not always allowed within marriage. The *halakhah* includes a great body of laws concerning various degrees of ritual impurity, mostly resulting from the emission of bodily fluids or contact with dead bodies. Since the main repercussions of impurity involve temporary disqualification from participation in rituals associated with the Temple in Jerusalem, they have lost most of their practical significance since its destruction almost 2,000 years ago. However, Scripture plainly prohibits men from having sex with women who are in certain states of ritual impurity, which are usually referred to by the technical term *niddah*. These rules have been interpreted and expanded by the rabbis, resulting in the prohibition of all sexual contact (and intimate behavior that may lead to sexual contact) from the time a woman expects to menstruate until seven days after all flow of blood has stopped, with the assumption that blood flows for a minimum of five days. On completion of the seven "clean days," the woman may immerse herself in a ritual bath, or *mikveh*, and is permitted to engage in sex.

Technically speaking, premarital sex with a permitted partner is not a serious offense under Jewish law. However, by restricting the access of unmarried women to the *mikveh*, the rabbis effectively banned premarital sex by ensuring that unmarried women are in a state of *niddah*. Additional precautionary rules were developed with the hope of limiting the opportunities for illicit sexual conduct and avoiding situations that could lead to the "wasting of seed." In communities where these rules are most stringently applied and interpreted, they impose a rigid separation of the sexes outside of the immediate family circle.

Beyond explicit prohibitions, the rabbis of the Talmud rely on other psychological, legal, theological, and medical principles to work out a coherent view of human, especially *male*, sexuality and its proper expression. On the one hand, sexual desire, often referred to as *yetzer ha-ra* (the "evil inclination"), is viewed as a dangerous force that leads people to perform grievous sins. Even within marriage, excessive sexual indulgence damages a man's health and diverts his attention from spiritual pursuits. On the other hand, the *yetzer ha-ra* is viewed as a profoundly creative psychological drive that not only guarantees the future of the human race but also, in sublimated form, powers the growth of human civilization. An oft-cited rabbinical comment tries to explain why God judges His creation to be "*very* good" (Gen. 1:31) after the creation of humans: "*Very* good" refers to the *yetzer ha-ra*; without the *yetzer ha-ra*, a man would not build a house, or marry a woman, or beget children, or engage in commerce (Genesis Rabbah 9:7).

In the final chapter of his treatise on the laws of sex, *Ba'alei ha-nefesh* (see Cohen), Rabbi Abraham ben David of Posquieres (ca. 1125–1198) summarized the legitimate motives for a husband to engage in intercourse with his wife. These include: sex for procreation; sex during the last two trimesters of pregnancy, which, according to Talmudic medical notions, is beneficial to the fetus (and in the last trimester to the mother as well); sex that satisfies the woman's desire and fulfills her conjugal rights; and sex that preserves a man's health and keeps him from straying into prohibited sexual liaisons. The upshot of this list is that while a man's **sexual activity** should really have an ulterior motive beyond the simple enjoyment of erotic pleasure, he must respect his wife's interest in sex for its own sake. Since it is considered immodest for a woman to make explicit sexual demands of her husband, he is expected to remain vigilant to any erotic hints she might be expressing through dress and behavior. Jewish law takes a woman's conjugal rights seriously, prescribing set quotas for the minimum frequency of intercourse a woman can expect from her husband, depending on his occupation. Scholars are expected to have sex with their wives every Friday night. As a result, Friday night intercourse has become recognized as one of the "delights of the Sabbath" (see Isa. 58:13), joining prayer and feasting as an integral element of the celebration of the Sabbath.

The rabbis accept the physiological thesis that a child's sex follows that of the parent who was last to achieve orgasm in the course of the sexual encounter that led to its inception. Since a premium is placed on the birth of male children, men are expected to try to help their wives reach orgasm first, or to engage twice in intercourse in quick succession with the hope that their wives would reach orgasm before them the second time.

Although the rabbis hardly speak of engaging in sex to express love, they insist that sex must be suffused with love. Great emphasis is placed on the intentions and state of mind of marital partners engaged in sexual intercourse, and the psychological condition of the parents at the moment of conception is thought to influence the well-being and character of the children thereby conceived. Men are expected to help their wives "get into the mood" through ingratiating conversation. Partners must take practical steps (such as avoiding hearing the voices of other people) to ensure that they direct their attention toward each other during intercourse. Intercourse must not be forced or engaged in while angry at one's partner. The rabbis are aware, however, that sex can help restore and maintain the emotional bond between husband and wife. The Babylonian Talmud (Shabbat, 152a) euphemistically refers to the penis as "the bringer of domestic peace."

Rabbinical attitudes toward sex found a fascinating and somewhat extreme crystallization among the thirteenth-century Jewish Pietists living in Germany, known as the *Hassidei Azhkenaz*. The Hassidei Ashkenaz viewed human existence as shot through with constant and powerful sexual attraction. Resistance to elicit sex was seen as a (or perhaps *the*) major spiritual challenge facing Jews. One of the group's prominent leaders, Rabbi Judah He-Hassid

(1150–1217), composed a book, *Sefer Hassidim (Book of the Pious)*, that includes many detailed references to particular adulterous incidents, how they are to be avoided, and how penance should be made for them. In some passages, Judah calls on men to temper their erotic interests in their wives. But sexuality in marriage is not viewed as implicitly sinful. Rather, it may simply distract a man from his devotion to God in the same way that a man's love for his children can interfere with his study of the Torah. While the rabbis of the Talmud were hardly embarrassed to discuss sexual matters openly, Judah goes further, using a vivid description of sexual pleasure in marriage as a rhetorical device to extol the spiritual pleasures of communion with God: "Even when a young man did not visit his wife for many days, and his desire is great, and has pleasure at the moment that he shoots [semen] like an arrow, this is as nothing compared to the great joy of loving God" (sec. 300; Margaliot, 240).

The Hassidei Ashkenaz felt that the maintenance of a high level of erotic attraction within marriage was the only practical safeguard from the ever-present danger of illicit sex. One of their other prominent leaders, Rabbi Eliezer of Worms (eleventh century), instructs husbands:

> He should give her pleasure and embrace her and sanctify himself with sexual intercourse. He should not use foul language and should not see in her anything contemptible, but should rather arouse her with caresses and with all manner of embracing in order to fulfill his desire and hers so that he doesn't think of another, but rather only of her, since she is his intimate partner, he should display love and affection toward her. (Biale, 78)

Medieval Jewish Philosophy. Conventionally philosophical texts were first produced within normative Judaism in the Middle Ages as a result of its encounter with Islamic thinkers who themselves had assimilated much of the Greco-Roman philosophical tradition. The first important figure in medieval Jewish philosophy was Saadia ben Joseph, widely known as Saadia Gaon (882–942). As a scholar, Saadia pioneered many important fields of Jewish learning (biblical translation and exegesis, systematic theology) and as a leader played a crucial role in confronting several of the great challenges facing early medieval Jewry. His philosophical-theological magnum opus, *The Book of Beliefs and Opinions*, was born of the confrontations between Rabbinic Judaism, the antirabbinic Jews known as the Karaites, and early Islamic Kalaam theology.

In the tenth treatise of the *Book*, "Concerning How It Is Most Proper for Man to Conduct Himself in This World," Saadia lists thirteen principal goals that God has implanted in the human psyche to motivate our behavior. He argues that a proper life strikes a balance among all, giving each its due. Four goals involve sexuality: **abstinence**, sexual intercourse, eroticism, and the begetting of children. While Saadia recognizes the spiritual value of abstinence from worldly pleasure, he is concerned that complete sexual abstinence interferes with the crucial goal of human procreation. The spiritual drive for abstinence should be channeled toward the successful avoidance of illicit pleasure. Sexual intercourse could not be inherently reprehensible, since the prophets engaged in it. Factors favoring the pursuit of sexual intercourse include the pleasure and good moods it produces and reproduction. However, excessively frequent intercourse has bad physical and mental effects. Its single-minded pursuit leads to unseemly behavior and illicit and adulterous acts. Eventually one's entire household would adopt such behavior, and the legitimacy of one's children would fall into question.

"Eroticism" refers to a state of intense, all-consuming (perhaps homosexual?) infatuation, allegedly rooted in astrological factors and the Platonic myth of the androgyne. Saadia rejects the astrological and Platonic accounts of "eroticism" and condemns its practice as completely disruptive of both religion and proper human living. However, it is reasonable for a man to experience a restrained version of such emotions toward his wife, inasmuch as it "bind[s] them closely together . . . for the sake of the maintenance of the world" (Saadia, 377). While great biblical heroes take pains to enjoy the blessing of the begetting of children, Saadia points out that a reasonable person will take into account counterbalancing factors such as the dangers of childbirth and the hardships of parenting. In any event, Saadia asks, what is the point of begetting children unless one can make provision for their proper care and education?

Moses Maimonides (1135–1204) is often viewed as the single most influential personality in medieval Judaism. An outstanding physician and leader of the Jewish community, Maimonides's great codification of Jewish law, the Mishneh Torah, revolutionized the study of *halakhah*, and his philosophical masterpiece *The Guide of the Perplexed* set the agenda for the remainder of the classical period of medieval Jewish philosophy. Despite his enormous prestige, Maimonides's writings have always generated vigorous debate. His legal codification has been condemned by some for failing to cite sources and opposing views. His philosophical ideas have been criticized as unduly influenced by **Aristotle** (384–322 BCE). Great controversies still rage regarding the interpretation of Maimonides's philosophical doctrines, largely fueled by what may be deliberate contradictions within and between his various works.

In the section of his *Commentary on the Mishnah* known as the *Eight Chapters*, Maimonides offers a system of ethics that combines elements of Aristotle's **virtue ethics**, the Jewish idea of a divinely legislated Torah, and an idealization of the contemplative life. Following Aristotle, Maimonides claims that the best personality traits may be described as occupying the midpoint of a continuum drawn between traits at opposite extremes. For example, the extreme traits of recklessness and cowardice predispose a person to behave poorly, while a moderate person will display courage or caution in ways appropriate to different situations. Attitudes toward sexual pleasure may be mapped onto such a model, in which the sexual addict is located at one extreme and the celibate at the other. People who relate properly to their sexuality are found at the preferred, middle position. Since it is easier for people to moderate a deficiency of sexual desire than to moderate a surplus, it is wise for them to accustom themselves to be somewhat on the ascetic side of the perfect sexual mean. The Torah's restrictions on sexual activity serve to limit one's opportunities for sexual intercourse, keeping the faithful safely away from excessive sensuality. People of good temperament do not engage in sex merely to enjoy a fleeting pleasure. Rather, they do so to perform the Torah's commandment of reproduction and, as needed, to remain fit and able to pursue the knowledge of God. Their motivations mirror those of the divinely ordained natural order; if sex had been intended to serve principally a source of pleasure, men would have been endowed with the ability to continue enjoying it after performing their reproductive role (ejaculation).

In Maimonides's parallel discussion of ethics in the section of the Mishneh Torah known as *Hilkhot De'ot* ("Laws of Moral Dispositions"), he strays further from Aristotelian theory. He introduces a new religious ideal of saintliness, which can be achieved only by embracing certain extreme character traits. Significantly, while the Maimonidian saint must abandon the middle ground to strive to be completely bereft of pride and anger, he is *not* called on to make a similarly radical rejection of erotic sensuality.

In the *Guide*, Maimonides tends to offer a less balanced approach to sexuality. There sexuality appears as a major impediment to the achievement of the philosophical knowledge and love of God, which constitute Maimonides's ideal human goals. It seems that only the *halakhic* strictures against celibacy hold Maimonides back from suggesting that the spiritual elite should adopt complete cessation of sexual activity. Maimonides scoffs at the philosophically unenlightened reader of the Bible, who finds time for his studies only in those few hours of leisure not devoted to "drinking and copulating" (I:2; Pines, 24); a naturally oversexed man might as well give up on philosophy (I:34; Pines, 77). The prohibitions of *giluy arayot* come not merely to reduce one's opportunities to engage in intercourse; they are also "directed . . . to instilling disgust for it so that it should be sought only very seldom" (III:49; Pines, 606). One purpose of circumcision is to lessen the pleasure of sex. Most important for future philosophical developments, in four different places (II:36, II:40, III:8, III:49; Pines, 371, 384, 432, 608) the *Guide* cites a mistranslation of Aristotle's *Nicomachean Ethics* (bk. III, 10, 1118b2) that was widely accepted by Islamic and Jewish philosophers, to the effect that the sense of touch is intrinsically repugnant. These citations offered Jewish tradition the classical expression of the idea that philosophical reason is opposed to sexuality.

The use of sex as an allegory for the relationship of form to matter is another important Aristotelian idea imported into Judaism by Maimonides. The *Guide* compares matter to a "married harlot" (III:8; Pines, 431). On the one hand, matter never appears without form; it is always "married" to some form or another. On the other hand, matter incessantly takes on different forms. Like a "harlot," matter is unfaithful to any *particular* form. For Maimonides, form, identified with the male, is the spiritual, eternal, and superior element. Matter, equated with the female ("married harlot"), drags down "male" form into imperfect, changing material existence. The form or soul of the individual human being is similarly torn away from spiritual pursuits by the demands and appetites of the material body. Relations with presumably ignorant and irrational women, who are identified with lowly substance, drag men down from their intrinsic spiritual superiority into the morass of bodily pleasure.

Bolstered by Maimonides's great personal authority, misogynistic and antisexual attitudes became trademarks of the mainstream tradition of Greek-inspired medieval Jewish philosophy. Jews who viewed themselves as enlightened, rationalist, and appreciative of the achievements of philosophy and science repressed the Talmud's insistence on the centrality of marriage in Jewish life. While Maimonides addressed his *Guide* to an extremely select audience of the intellectual elite, later Jewish philosophers introduced its sexual outlook to a broader audience. For example, the fourteenth-century circle of Jewish Neo-Platonists viewed sexual asceticism as "a path for all who seek wisdom and religious perfection" (Schwartz, 239). Once again, only the strictures of the *halakhah* keep these Jewish philosophers from advocating complete celibacy.

The rationalists had strayed from several well-established elements of Jewish tradition. Since Scripture plainly refers to women as prophets (Miriam, Deborah, and Huldah), and the rationalists identified biblical prophecy with philosophical enlightenment, it would seem that the philosophers' assumption that women suffer from inherent spiritual and intellectual inferiority explicitly contradicts biblical claims. By rejecting the importance of the heterosexual bond, they not only ran afoul of Talmudic attitudes toward married life, but they also degraded the central metaphor for the relationship between God and the Jewish people. It is hardly surprising that some Jewish writers who were critical of the philosophical tradition took exception to its views on women and sexuality. Joseph Albo (d. 1444) devotes part of his *Sefer Ha-'Ikkarim* (*Book of Principles*) to the nature of God's love for Israel (bk. 3, chap. 37). He discusses his topic in terms largely borrowed from Aristotle's analysis of **friendship**, suggesting that God's love for Israel is, in part, similar in nature to the mutually beneficial yet nonegalitarian relationship between man and wife (inasmuch as their love goes beyond the purely sexual bond required for the preservation of the species). Remarkably, Albo takes his analysis one step further by proposing that God's love for Israel also contains an element of *heshek* ("desire"), the inexplicable erotic infatuation of a particular man for a particular woman. In effect, Albo executes a neat theological rehabilitation of the category of *eroticism* that had troubled Saadia even before the rise of Jewish philosophical asceticism.

Isaac Arama (Spain, 1420–1494), author of the collection of sermons and biblical exegesis known as *Akedat Yitzhak*, was also among the critics of the rationalists. Although hardly a protofeminist, Arama genuinely liked women (see Schwartzmann). In *Akedat Yitzhak* (chap. 45), he openly attacks the misogynistic opinions of the prominent early Neo-Platonic biblical exegete Abraham ibn Ezra (1089–1164) and claims that men, rather than women, are more often the instigators of sinful behavior. While discussing the quasi-marital relationship between God and the Jewish people (chap. 58), Arama lists rules for a successful marriage, the first of which is that "a perfect man will never be satisfied with his wife, to form with her a beneficial union, unless she is of good grace and well educated; Scripture says, 'the wisest of women builds her house . . .' (Proverbs 14:1)." Chapter 8 of *Akedat Yitzhak* contains a philosophical *tour de force*, in which Arama tries to beat the rationalists at their own game by demonstrating the dignity and value of the heterosexual bond through selective quotation of Aristotle. To an extent, Arama may be viewed as correcting the overly antisexual reading of Aristotle popular among Jewish authors. However, he also appears to undermine the genuine Aristotelian doctrine that marriage is a friendship of *inequality*. Arama explains at some length that the biblical story of the creation of woman teaches that men and women could never be so powerfully attracted to each other unless they were essentially similar and equal to each other. The heterosexual bond thus appears to be assigned to the Aristotelian category of friendships based on equality.

The Kabbalistic Tradition. Albo and Arama arrived late enough to have had an appreciation for the Kabbalah, a body of mystical thought and practice that first came to light in the thirteenth century and that would eventually push the rationalist philosophical tradition to the margins of Jewish intellectual concern. The Kabbalah brought about a radical revolution in the role of sexuality in Judaism. If the Talmud views sexuality as an essential part of human life, and the rationalist philosophers fear it as an impediment to spiritual enlightenment, the Kabbalists make sexuality central to the drama of Divine activity. The fundamental theological concern of the Kabbalah is to explain how the Deity, who in the final analysis is identified with the absolutely transcendent *ein sof* (Infinite), creates and interacts with the physical world of human affairs. This theological task is achieved through the production of subtle and complicated accounts of the relationships between different aspects of Divinity (*sefirot*) as it is conceptualized in its manner of relating to the world. The interactions between *sefirot* are described in terms of erotic metaphors. Cosmic harmony, indeed harmony within the Godhead itself, is understood in terms of a perfect act of sexual intercourse between the more transcendent and more immanent aspects of Divinity, "the union of God and His *Shekhinah*" (Divine Presence).

The Kabbalah grants human beings profound spiritual empowerment; the way people think and behave directly affect the nature and quality of the processes taking place in the Godhead. Properly conducted human sexual activity becomes a force encouraging harmony within the Godhead and, as a result, it promotes cosmic redemption:

Here we have a good example of how the kabbalists added a new, mystical layer to the traditional Jewish doctrine that perfection was possible only in the married state. . . . [M]arriage is a state of perfection in which human reality duplicates and thereby promotes the divine perfection which is the union of God-and-his-Shekhinah. This latter unity, disrupted by the fall and human sinfulness, is one that has to be realized. Therefore the sexual act in holy matrimony has an almost sacramental quality, for it is a symbol that mystically promotes the analogous divine union. A man without a wife is mystically a cripple; like a surgeon without hands he cannot perform his most essential twofold duty, to commune with the Shekhinah and unite her with her husband. (Werblowsky, 134)

Unsurprisingly, the Kabbalists quickly found themselves in conflict with the rationalist philosophers. The early Kabbalistic treatise on sex *Iggeret Hakodesh* (*The Holy Letter*; see Cohen) opens with a frontal assault on the sexual asceticism of the philosophical rationalists. It directly attacks Maimonides and suggests that his distaste for sex may be related to Aristotle's heretical claim that the world exists eternally rather than having been created by God at a particular moment in time:

This matter is not as Rabbi Moses [Maimonides] of blessed memory, believed and thought in the *Guide for the Perplexed*. There he praised Aristotle for having said that the sense of touch is a disgrace for us. God forbid, God forbid, the Greek's statement is wrong, for it has a trace of undetected heresy to it. If that worthless Greek had believed that the world was created in time by an act of [divine] will, he would not have said it. But we, the sons of the masters of the holy Torah believe that God created everything in accordance with His wisdom's decree, and created nothing disgraceful or ugly. [Chavel, vol. 2, 323; trans. BDL]

The legacy of the Kabbalistic attitude toward sex is somewhat ambiguous. By endowing sexual intercourse with profound religious significance, the Kabbalah acted against the idealization of celibacy, but it also added a new and powerful source of anxiety regarding sexual activity. For instance, the dominant view in Talmudic law sees nothing wrong with couples enjoying a variety of sexual positions and techniques. But how can one dare stray from the "missionary" position if it alone represents and promotes the ideal union of "God-and-His-*Shekhina*?" Even the author of the *Iggeret Hakodesh* seems to feel that sexual intercourse can be spiritually acceptable only when undertaken in full cognizance of its mystical meaning and performed in accordance with a long list of conditions and instructions. These tensions within the Kabbalah were worked out in a variety of ways, spanning a spectrum that reaches from the holy libertinism of Jacob Frank's (1726–1795) heretical cult to the near endorsement of celibate marriage in some early-nineteenth-century European Hassidic circles.

Hebrew Scripture views sexual pleasure and erotic love as human goods to be enjoyed in heterosexual marriage. Rabbinic tradition builds on the scriptural foundation, positing marriage to be essential for a truly human and Jewish existence, while explicating and extending biblical prohibitions with the hope of helping the avoidance of sexual transgressions. With the rise of Greek-inspired rationalist Jewish philosophy in the Middle Ages, some thinkers writing within the normative Jewish community began to dismiss the importance of the heterosexual bond and rejected sexuality as inimical to philosophical enlightenment and intellectual love of God. Bolstered by the rise of Kabbalistic mysticism, opponents of rationalism eventually reintroduced rabbinical attitudes toward sex into systematic Jewish philosophy. By making sex an important theme for religious theory and practice, the Kabbalah generated various new attitudes toward sexuality that, as always, found themselves restrained by the technical demands of Jewish law.

See also Abstinence; Aristotle; Augustine (Saint); Bestiality; Bible, Sex and the; Buddhism; Catholicism, History of; Ethics, Virtue; Friendship; Gnosticism; Greek Sexuality and Philosophy, Ancient; Hinduism; Islam; Jainism; Judaism, Twentieth- and Twenty-First-Century; Levinas, Emmanuel; Marriage; Paul (Saint); Plato; Protestantism, History of; Roman Sexuality and Philosophy, Ancient; Spinoza, Baruch; Thomas Aquinas (Saint)

REFERENCES

Albo, Joseph. *Sefer Ha-'Ikkarim.* Trans. Isaac Husik. Philadelphia, Pa.: Jewish Publication Society of America, 1946; Aristotle. (ca. 325 BCE?) *Nicomachean Ethics.* Trans. Terence Irwin. Indianapolis, Ind.: Hackett, 1985; Biale, David. *Eros and the Jews: From Biblical Israel to Contemporary America.* New York: Basic Books, 1992. Berkeley: University of California Press, 1997; Chavel, Charles Ber, ed. (1963) *Kitvei Rabbeinu Moshe ben Nahman,* 2 vols. Jerusalem, Israel: Mossad Ha-Rav Kook, 1994; Cohen, Seymour J., trans. *The Holy Letter: A Study in Medieval Jewish Sexual Morality, Ascribed to Nahmanides.* New York: Ktav, 1976; Maimonides, Moses. (1190) *The Guide of the Perplexed.* Trans. Shlomo Pines. Chicago, Ill.: University of Chicago Press, 1963; Margaliot, Reuven, ed. *Sefer Hassidim she-Hiber Rabbeinu Yehudah He-Hassid.* Jerusalem, Israel: Mossad Ha-Rav Kook, 2004; Saadia Gaon. *The Book of Beliefs and Opinions.* Trans. Samuel Rosenblatt. New Haven, Conn.: Yale University Press, 1948; Samet, Aharon, ed. *Arba'ah Turim Ha-Shalem.* Jerusalem, Israel: United Torah Institutions "Shirat Devorah," 1993; Schwartz, Dov. *Yashan BeKankan Hadash (The Philosophy of a Fourteenth Century Neoplatonic Circle).* Jerusalem, Israel: Bialik Institute, 1996; Schwartzmann, Julia. "Isaac Arama and His Theory of Two Matches." *Jewish Studies Quarterly* (2005), forthcoming; information available at <JuliaS@yvc.ac.il>; Werblowsky, R. J. Zwi. *Joseph Karo: Lawyer and Mystic.* Philadelphia, Pa.: Jewish Publication Society of America, 1977.

Berel Dov Lerner

ADDITIONAL READING

Allen, Prudence. *The Concept of Woman: The Aristotelian Revolution.* Grand Rapids, Mich.: Eerdmans, 1997; Anderson, Gary. "The Garden of Eden and Sexuality in Early Judaism." In Howard Eilberg-Schwartz, ed., *People of the Body: Jews and Judaism from an Embodied Perspective.* Albany: State University of New York Press, 1992, 47–68; Baskin, Judith R. "From Separation to Displacement: The Problem of Women in *Sefer Hasidim.*" *Association for Jewish Studies Review* 19:1 (1994), 1–18; Berger, Michael S. "Two Models of Medieval Jewish Marriage: A Preliminary Study." *Journal of Jewish Studies* 52:1 (2001), 59–84; Biale, David. "Ejaculatory Prayer: The Displacement of Sexuality in Chasidism." *Tikkun* 6:4 (1991), 21–25, 87–89; Biale, David. *From Intercourse to Discourse: Control of Sexuality in Rabbinic Literature.* San Anselmo, Calif.: Center for Hermeneutical Studies, 1992; Bos, Gerrit. "Maimonides on the Preservation of Health." *Journal of the Royal Asiatic Society* [series 3] 4:2 (1994), 213–35; Boyarin, Daniel. "Are There Any Jews in 'The History of Sexuality'?" *Journal of the History of Sexuality* 5:3 (1995), 333–55; Boyarin, Daniel. *Carnal Israel: Reading Sex in Talmudic Culture.* Berkeley: University of California Press, 1993; Boyarin, Daniel. *Unheroic Conduct: The Rise of Heterosexuality and the Invention of the Heterosexual Jewish Man.* Berkeley: University of California Press, 1997; Boyarin, Daniel. "Women's Bodies and the Rise of the Rabbis: The Case of Sotah." *Studies in Contemporary Jewry* 16 (2000), 88–100; Bronner, Leila Leah. *From Eve to Esther: Rabbinic Reconstructions of Biblical Women.* Louisville, Ky.: Westminster John Knox Press; Bulka, Reuven P. *Jewish Marriage: A Halakhic Ethic.* New York: Ktav/Yeshiva University Press, 1986; Carr, David M. *The Erotic Word: Sexuality, Spirituality, and the Bible.*

Oxford, U.K.: Oxford University Press, 2003; Cohen, Jeremy. *"Be Fertile and Increase, Fill the Earth and Master It": The Ancient and Medieval Career of a Biblical Text.* Ithaca, N.Y.: Cornell University Press, 1989; Cohen, Jeremy. "Rationales for Conjugal Sex in RaABaD's *Ba'alei ha-nefesh.*" *Jewish History* 6:1–2 (1992), 65–78; Daube, David. *The New Testament and Rabbinic Judaism.* London: Athlone Press, 1956. Reprinted, New York: Arno Press, 1973; Davidson, Herbert A. *Moses Maimonides: The Man and His Works.* New York: Oxford University Press, 2005; Dershowitz, Alan M. "The Talmud as Sexual Harassment." In *The Abuse Excuse and Other Cop-outs, Sob Stories, and Evasions of Responsibility.* Boston, Mass.: Little, Brown, 1994, 251–54; Dorff, Elliot N. *Matters of Life and Death: A Jewish Approach to Modern Medical Ethics.* Philadelphia, Pa.: Jewish Publication Society, 1998; Eilberg-Schwartz, Howard. *God's Phallus and Other Problems for Men and Monotheism.* Boston, Mass.: Beacon Press, 1994; Eilberg-Schwartz, Howard, ed. *People of the Body: Jews and Judaism from an Embodied Perspective.* Albany: State University of New York Press, 1992; Epstein, Louis M. *Sex Laws and Customs in Judaism.* New York: Bloch, 1948. Reprinted, New York: Ktav, 1967; Eron, Lewis John. "Homosexuality and Judaism." In Arlene Swidler, ed., *Homosexuality and the World Religions.* Philadelphia, Pa.: Trinity Press, 1993, 103–34; Feldman, David M. *Birth Control in Jewish Law.* New York: Jason Aronson, 1998; Feldman, David M. (1968) *Marital Relations, Birth Control, and Abortion in Jewish Law.* New York: Schocken Books, 1974; Friedman, Mordechai A. "The Ethics of Medieval Jewish Marriage." In Shlomo D. Goitein, ed., *Religion in a Religious Age.* Cambridge, Mass.: Association for Jewish Studies, 1974, 83–102; Frymer-Kensky, Tikva Simone. *In the Wake of the Goddesses: Women, Culture, and the Biblical Transformation of Pagan Myth.* New York: Free Press, 1992; Green, Arthur. "Bride, Spouse, Daughter: Images of the Feminine in Classical Jewish Sources." In Susannah Heschel, ed., *On Being a Jewish Feminist.* New York: Schocken, 1983, 248–60; Green, Arthur. "The Song of Songs in Early Jewish Mysticism." *Orim: A Jewish Journal at Yale* 2:2 (1987), 49–63; Guberman, Karen. "The Language of Love in Spanish Kabbalah: An Examination of the *Iggeret Ha-Kodesh.*" In David R. Blumenthal, ed., *Approaches to Judaism in Medieval Times.* Chico, Calif.: Scholars Press, 1984, 53–95; Harris, Monford. "The Concept of Love in *Sefer Hasidim.*" *Jewish Quarterly Review* 50:1 (1959), 13–44; Harris, Monford. "Marriage as Metaphysics: A Study of the *Iggereth Hakodesh.*" *Hebrew Union College Annual* 33 (1962), 197–220; Harvey, Steven. "The Meaning of Terms Designating Love in Judaeo-Arabic Thought and Some Remarks on the Judaeo-Arabic Interpretation of Maimonides." In Norman Golb, ed., *Studies in Muslim-Jewish Relations III.* Chur, Switz.: Harwood Academic Publishers, 1997, 175–96; Idel, Moshe. "Erotic Images for the Ecstatic Experience." In *The Mystical Experience in Abraham Abulafia.* Albany: State University of New York Press, 1988, 179–227; Idel, Moshe. *Kabbalah: New Perspectives.* New Haven, Conn.: Yale University Press, 1988; Idel, Moshe. "Sexual Metaphors and Praxis in the Kabbalah." In David Kraemer, ed., *The Jewish Family: Metaphor and Memory.* New York: Oxford University Press, 1989, 197–224; Koltun-Fromm, Naomi. "Sexuality and Holiness: Semitic Christian and Jewish Conceptualizations of Sexual Behavior." *Vigiliae Christianae* 54:4 (2000), 375–95; Lamm, Norman. *A Hedge of Roses: Jewish Insights into Marriage and Married Life.* New York: Philipp Feldheim, 1972; Lerner, Berel Dov. *Rules, Magic, and Instrumental Reason: A Critical Interpretation of Peter Winch's Philosophy of the Social Sciences.* London: Routledge, 2002; Mopsik, Charles. "The Body of Engenderment in the Hebrew Bible, the Rabbinic Tradition, and the Kabbalah." In Michel Feher, Ramona Naddaff, and Nadia Tazi, eds., *Zone 3: Fragments for a History of the Human Body.* New York: Zone Books, 1989, 48–73; Olyan, Saul. " 'And with a Male You Shall Not Lie the Lying Down of a Woman': On the Meaning and Significance of Leviticus 18:22 and 20:13." *Journal of the History of Sexuality* 5:2 (1994), 179–206; Pearson, Birger. *Gnosticism, Judaism, and Egyptian Christianity.* Studies in Antiquity and Christianity, 5. Minneapolis, Minn.: Fortress Press, 1990; Ravven, Heidi M. "The Garden of Eden: Spinoza's Maimonidean Account of the Genealogy of Morals and the Origin of Society." *Philosophy and Theology* 13:1 (2001), 3–47; Rosenfeld, Yiskah. "Taking Back Our Rites: Lighting Candles, Baking Challah, and the Laws of Married Sex." *Lilith* 26:2 (2001), 22–24; Rosenheim, Eliyahu. "Sexual Attitudes and Regulations in Judaism." In John Money and Herman Musaph, eds., *Handbook of Sexology.* Amsterdam, Holland: Excerpta Medica, 1977, 1315–23; Rosner, Fred. *Sex Ethics in the Writings of Moses*

Maimonides. New York: Bloch, 1974; Satlow, Michael L. *Jewish Marriage in Antiquity*. Princeton, N.J.: Princeton University Press, 2001; Satlow, Michael L. " 'One Who Loves His Wife Like Himself': Love in Rabbinic Marriage." *Journal of Jewish Studies* 49:1 (1998), 67–78; Satlow, Michael L. "Rhetoric and Assumptions: Romans and Rabbis on Sex." In Martin Goodman, ed., *Jews in a Graeco-Roman World*. Oxford, U.K.: Clarendon Press, 1999, 135–44; Satlow, Michael L. "Shame and Sex in Late Antique Judaism." In Vincent L. Wimbush and Richard Valantasis, eds., *Asceticism*. New York: Oxford University Press, 1995, 535–43; Satlow, Michael L. *Tasting the Dish: Rabbinic Rhetorics of Sexuality*. Atlanta, Ga.: Scholars Press, 1995; Satlow, Michael L. " 'They Abused Him Like a Woman': Homoeroticism, Gender Blurring, and the Rabbis in Late Antiquity." *Journal of the History of Sexuality* 5:1 (1994), 1–25; Satlow, Michael L. "Try to Be a Man: The Rabbinic Construction of Masculinity." *Harvard Theological Review* 89:1 (1996), 19–40; Satlow, Michael L. " 'Wasted Seed': The History of a Rabbinic Idea." *Hebrew Union College Annual* 65 (1994), 137–69; Scholem, Gershom. "Shekhinah: The Feminine Element in Divinity." In *On the Mystical Shape of the Godhead: Basic Concepts in the Kabbalah*. New York: Schocken, 1991, 140–96; Schwartzmann, Julia. "Gender Concepts of Medieval Jewish Thinkers and the Book of Proverbs." *Jewish Studies Quarterly* 7:3 (2000), 183–202; Sherwin, Byron. "Moses Maimonides on the Perfection of the Body." *Listening* 9 (1974), 28–37; Smith, Carol. "Challenged by the Text: Two Stories of Incest in the Hebrew Bible." In Athalya Brenner and Carole R. Fontaine, eds., *A Feminist Companion to Reading the Bible: Approaches, Methods and Strategies*. Sheffield, U.K.: Sheffield Academic Press, 1997, 114–35; Smith, Carol. "Stories of Incest in the Hebrew Bible: Scholars Challenging Text or Text Challenging Scholars?" *Henoch* 14 (1992), 227–42; Sokol, Moshe Z. "Attitudes towards Pleasure in Jewish Thought: A Typological Perspective." In Jacob J. Schachter, ed., *Reverence, Righteousness, and Rahamanut: Essays in Memory of Rabbi Dr. Leo Jung*. Northvale, N.J.: Jason Aronson, 1992, 293–314; Solomon, Lewis D. *The Jewish Tradition, Sexuality, and Procreation*. Lanham, Md.: University Press of America, 2002; Steinberg, Jonah. "From a 'Pot of Filth' to a 'Hedge of Roses' (and Back): Changing Theorizations of Menstruation in Judaism." *Journal of Feminist Studies in Religion* 13:2 (1997), 5–26; Tishby, Isaiah. "Conjugal Life." In *The Wisdom of the Zohar*. Trans. David Goldstein. Littman Library of Jewish Civilization, vol. 3. London: Littman Library, 1989, 1355–1406; Trible, Phyllis. *God and the Rhetoric of Sexuality*. Philadelphia, Pa.: Fortress Press, 1978; Wasserfall, Rahel R., ed. *Women and Water: Menstruation in Jewish Life and Law*. Hanover, N.H.: Brandeis University Press, 1999; Winston, David. "Philo and the Rabbis on Sex and the Body." *Poetics Today* 19:1 (1998), 41–62; Wolfson, Elliot. *Circle in the Square: Studies in the Use of Gender in Kabbalistic Symbolism*. Albany: State University of New York Press, 1995; Wolfson, Elliot. "Coronation of the Sabbath Bride: Kabbalistic Myth and the Ritual of Androgynisation." *Journal of Jewish Thought and Philosophy* 6:2 (1997), 301–44; Wolfson, Elliot. "Eunuchs Who Keep the Sabbath: Becoming Male and the Ascetic Ideal in Thirteenth-Century Jewish Mysticism." In Jeffrey J. Cohen and Bonnie Wheeler, eds., *Becoming Male in the Middle Ages*. New York: Garland, 1997, 151–85; Wolfson, Elliot. *Through a Speculum That Shines: Vision and Imagination in Medieval Jewish Mysticism*. Princeton, N.J.: Princeton University Press, 1994; Zeidman, Reena. "Marginal Discourse: Lesbianism in Jewish Law." *Women in Judaism* 1:1 (1997). <www.utoronto.ca/wjudaism/journal/vol1n1/v1n1zeid.htm> [accessed 23 August 2004].

JUDAISM, TWENTIETH- AND TWENTY-FIRST-CENTURY.

There are any number of Jewish philosophies of sex, sexuality, and gender. Positions have also shifted over the course of the twentieth century. Although the U.S. Jewish population remains the largest concentration in a single nation-state, to talk about Jews in the United States is not to talk about Jews as a whole. It is impossible, at any rate, to discuss Jewish philosophy on any subject as a whole and certainly so given that a discussion of the diversity of Jewish philosophies in the United States will differ from a similar discussion of Jewish communities in India, Ethiopia, Europe, South America, and Israel. Jews around the world may refer to similar texts and share historical trends, but different communities claim different texts as authoritative, remain tied to particular interpretations, and ground their philosophies and theologies in differing aspects of Jewish history.

The majority of Jews in the United States have roots in Europe and adhere in varying degrees to what in Jewish ethnic terms is "Ashkenazi" culture, which is based in the history of Jews in northern Europe. (The first literary references to the Germanic region called "Ashkenaz" were made in the tenth century.) Central thinkers contributing to Jewish theologies of sex in the twentieth and twenty-first century—Rachel Adler, Rebecca Alpert, David Biale, Martin Buber (1878–1965), Louis Epstein (1887–1949), Robert Gordis (1908–1992), Judith Plaskow—start from and speak within such cultural specificity. Sephardi thought, from the cultures that grew out of the experiences of the Jews of Spain, beginning with the period of Muslim rule (eighth century) and extending into the exile caused by the Inquisition; Mizrachi thought, which was constructed from the lives of Jews in communities in a range of Middle Eastern regions and countries (often thought of as those who never left the area of the ancient origins of the Jewish people); and Ethiopian Jewish thought (and still others) are alive and well amidst the dominant Ashkenazi culture and thought of the United States.

Jewish thought in the United States on matters of sexuality in the twentieth century grew out of the Jewish European experience. The Jewish community in the United States began as a tiny group of Sephardis from Portugal and other areas who were fleeing the Spanish Inquisition. In the late nineteenth century a large migration of German Jews to the United States occurred. Most important for the twentieth century, however, was the migration of millions of Jews from Eastern Europe, which began at the turn of the century and ended, due to new restrictive immigration legislation, in the second quarter. These Eastern European Jews arrived during the most extensive immigration period in U.S. history. The Jewish philosophy and theology of sex of the twentieth century, as in other areas of thought, resulted from the interaction between Jewish thought and that which created (as well as mirrored) much of U.S. thought of the period as well. Jewish thought about sexual and gender matters in the United States in this period can be understood only in this context of a historical encounter that was constituted by altering communal experiences and norms.

All communities, including the religious, embody multiplicity and change. Jewish thinking on sexuality differs, however, from some other groups in that there is no single authority source, such as a church hierarchy. Jewish thought *is* grounded in what is called "Halacha," Jewish law. But although all texts are subject to interpretation, the most authoritative Jewish text, the Talmud, is itself written as a conversation of cross-historical competing arguments on a variety of subjects. Further, and unique to the United States, is the multiplicity of movements generally recognized as Jewishly legitimate by the population—though of course legitimacy is always contested. The four main Jewish religious movements, the Reform, Reconstructionist, Conservative, and Orthodox, each has its own law committees, traditions, and somewhat differing sexual theologies.

In the early 1800s, "Orthodox" began to be used, in the United States, about more traditionally observant Jews. The U.S. Orthodox rabbinical seminary, Yeshiva University, was founded in 1915 on the site of an Orthodox yeshiva that had existed there since 1886. Orthodox Judaism generally understands the Bible as authored by G-d and, *therefore*, *mitzvot* (i.e., commandments) as G-d's word. The Conservative movement began in the United States around 1880. Conservative Judaism may take the Bible to be divinely inspired, but it is open to modern religious, archeological, and historical scholarship regarding the human authorship of such texts. Nevertheless, Conservativism is bound to Ashkenazi interpretations of *Halacha*, which will then be subject to particular readings by those within the movement. The Reform movement began in Germany in the early 1800s, moving to the United States in the 1870s. Traditionally, Reform Judaism has not deemed *Halacha* binding in and of itself; observance of the *mitzvot* is more a (hopefully studied) choice. Much of the movement's energy has been directed toward the social justice trends of the Jewish tradition. Reconstructionism, the newest of the movements, began to develop between the 1920s and the 1940s. It was formalized with the establishment of a rabbinical seminary, the Reconstructionist Rabbinical College, in 1968. Reconstructionist Judaism is grounded in the philosophy of Mordechai Kaplan (1881–1983), a Conservatively trained rabbi who understood Judaism as a civilization, firmly linked to its history yet also needing to adapt to new environs and new eras. It is unique to the U.S. Jewish community that this range beyond the Orthodox matters. Further, there are smaller movements and myriad sects among the ultraorthodox and among Left-leaning Jews, as well as transdenominational seminaries. Though movement differences are significant, most U.S. Jews do not consider themselves explicitly committed to any religiously grounded philosophies at all, but this does not mean that they are not profoundly affected by them.

Each of these religious movements is primarily Ashkenazi in origin and either developed in line with the tremendous twentieth-century changes in the community (Orthodox and Reform) or was created out of this encounter with change (Conservative and Reconstructionist). Understanding the threads of U.S. Jewish sexual theology and philosophy thus requires grasping the experiences of Jews and the Jewish community in the specific time and place in which such thought emerged.

For example, in a frequent pattern of immigration, individuals or family subsets—often, though not exclusively, a young male adult or head of household—came to the United States first, worked, and earned enough money to bring over other family members. This process shattered family structures and generational power dynamics that were long the norm in Jewish life. These immigrant Jews, even those who were married and had a family in the old country, experienced new sexual possibilities. They were confronted with the prospect of premarital and extramarital sex at rates inconceivable previously as well as of cross-religious liaisons and long-term relationships. Many immigrant single persons lived as boarders in Jewish households, which brought these strangers and families into intimate contact in radically new ways. The novel living arrangements contributed to the rise of unprecedented forms of sexual and other relationships between and among the sexes; one result was a change in the conditions in which sexual abuse occurred. The greater necessity of women to work for pay in this urban economy, compared to previous generations, meant that the boundaries for masses of Jewish women were greatly expanded and that men could associate with more women outside the family. Like the new living arrangements, this contact between men and women occasioned a loosening of traditional sexual segregation in ways that many people found liberating, yet it also created vast arenas for the workplace **sexual harassment** of women. The higher level of literacy of Jewish women, compared with that of their old neighbors in Europe and other minority racial or ethnic groups in the United States, also contributed to a different sense of sexual propriety. Through work and domestic duties, Jewish women had connections with many more people and men than they formerly had. Further, the need to take language courses and an emphasis on education meant that after their long workday, many Jewish women attended classes and cultural events designed for the urban poor and immigrant populations. With a small amount of money in their pockets, young men and women, especially in the cities, were out at night, unchaperoned, which would not have been thought proper by earlier generations.

Not only rabbis and theologians but Jewish literature, theater, popular culture, and the media were constantly responding to and working to make sense of these fundamental changes in the familial and sexual norms within the community and providing guidance for people affected by them. For example, ready-to-wear clothing—developed, manufactured, and marketed primarily in small factories owned by Jewish men—became a quintessential symbol of the break from tradition, transforming Jewish women's self-conceptions of independence, the body, and sexual freedom. Heavily infected with progressive to radical politics (also an old-world legacy for these Eastern European Jews) and utopian desires for advancement (a mixture of Jewish messianic individualist and socialist yearnings, fed by American myths), masses of Jews made it through the first half of the twentieth century in this dramatic entanglement between traditions, transformations of gendered and **sexual ethics**, expectations, ideas, and practices.

While some people strengthened the fence around Jewish tradition, others sought to tear it down. Though many individual Jews supported women's suffrage, Jews were more likely to be leaders in other movements—for free speech, for free **love**, for **contraception**, and for changing U.S. divorce laws. The Jewish anarchist Emma Goldman (1869–1940) worked with prostitutes and along with others challenged the tyranny of the institution of **marriage** (see her *Essays*). Fannia Cohen (1885–1962) created educational programs expanding vistas for workers, particularly for women workers, through her position in the International Ladies' Garment Workers' Union. Jews' role in the budding fields of psychology and psychoanalysis greatly influenced theories on sex and gender. Prominent examples are **Sigmund Freud** (1856–1939) and Magnus Hirschfeld (1868–1935). Jews were active in movements for religious freedom and in the intercultural movement, which laid the groundwork for the civil rights movement.

At mid-century, the United States was in the midst of an intense ideological struggle. In the post–World War II environment, the world reeled from news of racial and cultural genocide in Europe; women were being asked again to redefine their identities as men returned home and needed the jobs women had performed in their absence; and economic opportunity became available to some in a partial financial boom. In 1952, Christine Jorgensen (1926–1989) had sex reassignment surgery, and this news was splattered across both the U.S. press and medical literature (see Meyerowitz). In this historical moment, aspects of one's identity presumed to be immutable were suddenly open to change. Whether in the realms of race, class, sex, gender roles, religion, culture, and ethnicity, identities long held to be "facts" were coming undone. Simultaneously, there was a move to shore up such identities, to fix them in more permanent ways. For example, some Jews, long seen in the United States as a race apart from (and below) Anglo-Christians, slowly began to move across an invisible color line to honorary status as "white." This was made possible only by marginalizing elements of Jewish practice and portions of the community that could not or would not assimilate to middle-class expectations of whiteness. As part of this dynamic, as much as new psychological theories on sex and gender were seen as radical and liberating, new pathologies were also invented—which applied not only to Jews but other Americans as well.

By the 1950s Senator Joseph McCarthy (1908–1957) and his followers had succeeded in hindering progressive and radical political activism in the United States while attempting to eliminate communist and other "un-American" activities. Many draconian measures effected during this "Red Scare" directly targeted Jews, sexual liberationists of different stripes, and other minorities. In the post-McCarthy world of the 1960s, the civil rights movement became one of the most viable avenues for historic Jewish work in radical politics with significant implications for new trends in sex/gender politics (see Brettschneider, chap. 2; Singer; Svonkin). Jewish women were among the earliest northerners to go to the southern United States at the beginning of the civil rights movement. Jewish women were often the only women at many of the crucial sites of protest and were usually the only nonblack civil rights workers at the start of the movement (Schultz). In the 1960s, at the moment when interracial friendships and erotic relationships of choice exploded on the U.S. landscape, Jews were more likely to engage in them, entering interreligious and mixed-race marriages, thereby creating the new phenomenon of mixed-race children by choice. In 1963 it was reported that in nearly half of the "Negro-white intermarriages in New York" the "white" spouse was Jewish and most often female (Berger, 122–26; Blustain). These relationships were also fraught with problems. There were a disproportionate number of mixed-race children born out of wedlock and offered for adoption, children created by liaisons between Jewish Euro-heritage women and African American and other minority men (see McKinley).

The phenomenon in the mid-century of the U.S. Jewish community assimilating, and perceived as becoming white, required conforming to certain sex/gender/sexuality norms. But assimilation proceeded only so far. White gender norms can be seen as bourgeois Western and Christian constructions, and these have been anything but static. They have also generally differed from Western Jewish constructions of gender. Due to their "different" gender assignments more broadly, Jews have historically been seen as queer in the Christian West (see Sicular). As Western Christian notions of manhood increasingly included physical prowess and chivalry, Jewish self-identity, by contrast, reinforced its commitment to manhood through learning (Boyarin). Though most Christian women in the West engaged in physical labor, the elite association of white womanhood with chastity and a gendered, quiet etiquette excluded Jewish women not only from "womanhood" but also from being Gentile. An elite Jewish expectation that corresponded to men as scholars was that of the wife or woman as the businessperson who would financially support the household (Hyman). Jewish businesswomen were a far more common occurrence than gentile independent businesswomen, and the Jews were generally respected within the community as conforming to Jewish gender norms. Also, although excluded from formal religious study, Jewish women still tended to have higher literacy rates than women in their surrounding areas. Jewish men stereotyped as being comparatively physically weak, "effeminate," and studious, and women as being strong, savvy, independent agents in the economic sphere, helped to cast Jews as a whole as queer (in sexed/gendered terms).

Part of what made Jews eligible for honorary status as whites in the mid-twentieth-century United States was the entry of select groups of Jews into the economic middle class. Part of the "cost" of that whiteness was the expectation of assimilation to sets of norms related to sex/gender/sexuality. In the United States, the idea of the Jewish man as businessman or a man of the professions emerges as a stereotype. In the West more broadly, as modern European Zionism, starting in the early 1800s, became a mass movement for the liberation of the Jewish people through statehood, Jewish men devoted themselves to overturning the association, which had developed through centuries of diaspora life, of Jewishness with the "weak-muscled," "effeminate," "studious," and "pious" ideals of manhood. With the creation of the state of Israel, Jewish men claimed a stake in military prowess and physical strength as markers of manhood (Cohen; Zerubavel). In the United States, white Christian middle-class ideals found their way into many Jewish communities: Nice Jewish girls were now expected to be quiet, not feisty political activists and bearers of strong opinions. Jewish women were now supposed to be "kept," not working outside the home with an independent income base.

In examining twentieth- and twenty-first-century Jewish philosophies on sexuality, it is important to note the mutually constitutive constructs of heterosexuality, gender/sex, class, and race as they have come to work for Jews in the postwar United States. One of the costs of whiteness that was required of Jews as some moved into the middle class was the quieting of women: unbending the Jewish style of queerish gender-bending. Relying on Jewish daughters to marry up was also important in making it possible for some Jews to be granted honorary status as whites (Brodkin). Complying with Western, Christian, middle-class norms of heterosexuality was necessary for the "whitening" of Jews as a group in the postwar era. But many Jewish women challenged the sexualized gender roles that some Jewish parents were coming to demand of their daughters (Schultz). Some Jewish women activists married up, by marrying men in the professions only newly available to Jewish men; they also tended not simply to class-climb but to use this access in the service of radical and progressive political movements. Other Jewish women partnered with or married nonwhite men and created a generation of not-so-white Jews in ways that some of their class-climbing parents had not exactly expected. Many of these women coupled with other women and became activists as lesbians, bisexuals, and later transgendered Jews (among the most well-known figures, Judith Butler, Leslie Feinberg, and Kate Bornstein are Jewish), fundamentally challenging their potential status as part of the American mainstream. (See also Balka and Rose; Beck; Dickson and Goldmacher's film *Ruthie and Connie*; Kaye/Kantrowitz; and Kaye/Kantrowitz and Klepfisz.)

Jewish experiences in the United States demonstrate that the more open sexual mores of the 1960s, of which Jews made ample use, made possible—as they were made possible by—the involvement of Jewish men and women in the civil rights movement. As Jewish women in particular made use of these openings in traditional heterosexual mores, they were able to take more risks in political work. They thereby continued to classify themselves beyond mainstream Western, Christian, gendered, and heterosexual norms of whiteness that contributed to the ways Jews were often considered "queerly gendered." Jewish men's work in the civil rights movement also continued to cast them as not-quite-white, even as many might have taken the opportunity to get advanced degrees and enter white-collar professions. To the extent that many Jewish men get involved in the service of critical race and other justice politics, they remain beyond traditionally (white) ideals of manhood. Despite their elite academic credentials, most Jewish men in the professions do not meet the narrow standards of U.S. white masculine citizenship.

Jews have been and continue to be highly active in debates on issues of sexuality and gender: the feminist and neo-men's movements, the reproductive rights movement, domestic violence and sexual harassment movements, and the gay, lesbian, bisexual, transgender, and queer movements. We can see the religious grounding for the involvement of Jews in these areas. Jewish law does not simply forbid **abortion**: The health of the woman bearing the fetus takes precedence. Jewish law does not forbid divorce or contraception (particularly for women). Jewish law does acknowledge the function of marriage as creating an opportunity for companionship and sexual pleasure and not only as procreative. Jewish law does recognize women's sexual needs. (For various Jewish theological explorations, see Adler; Dorff; Feldman; Plaskow.)

The modern religious movements continue their exploration of sexual ethics, though they remain somewhat out of touch with the actual practices of U.S. Jews. The rabbinical movements still generally condemn premarital and extramarital sex and interreligious marriage in ways that do not reflect popular Jewish ethics. Jews therefore increasingly write their own *ketubot* (marriage contracts). Transgendered people and same-sex couples have been forming unions officiated by rabbis or employing adaptations of Jewish liturgy. (Jewish law does not require a rabbi to perform a wedding.) Orthodox women have challenged *Halacha* regarding *agunot*—"chained women"—who are denied religious divorces by their husbands. (If they obtain a civil divorce and marry again, their children are branded *mamzer*—bastards—by Orthodoxy; their children's children, *ad infinitum*, are *mamzer* as well. A *mamzer* is permitted to marry only another *mamzer* or a convert to Judaism.) Orthodox women have also established battered women's shelters to cater to the particular needs of Orthodox Jewish women and their children.

The move for recognition of the dignity and needs of queer Jews has grown even within Orthodoxy as well as the three other Jewish movements. Jewish institutions generally support civil rights for women and homosexuals, though this support does not always extend to full and equal participation religiously within Judaism. Women rabbis within the Conservative and Reform movements are still a relatively new phenomenon. All the synagogue movements have for a long time at least distinguished between same-sex acts and homosexual persons, allowing even orthodox congregations to welcome individual gay people into their communities. The Reform and Reconstructionist movements have opened their arms widest, admitting sexual minorities into their rabbinical seminaries and ordaining them as rabbis. The Reconstructionist movement has been exploring issues concerning transgendered Jews, and the Reform movement was the first to admit a transgender-identified student into its rabbinical seminary. Despite much activism, little has been written about transgendered Jews. (See Coleman; Kanegson; Krawitz; Michaels and Cannon.) These movements also allow their rabbis to perform **same-sex marriage** and/or commitment ceremonies. A decision later subject to reconsideration, the rabbinic arm of the Conservative movement in 1992 voted not to ordain gay rabbis or perform same-sex marriages. At the same time, the Conservative movement did not forbid their rabbis from performing ceremonies for same-sex partners, thereby leaving room for individual rabbis to make their own decisions. The Union of Orthodox Rabbis does not ordain queers as rabbis and does not sanction religious same-sex marriage ceremonies. On the other hand, some Orthodox Jewish feminists do forecast that women will be ordained Orthodox rabbis in the twenty-first century (see Greenberg).

See also Bible, Sex and the; Boswell, John; Feminism, Lesbian; Heterosexism; Islam; Judaism, History of; Levinas, Emmanuel; Marriage, Same-Sex; Marxism; Protestantism, Twentieth- and Twenty-First-Century; Psychology, Twentieth- and Twenty-First-Century; Queer Theory; Sexology

REFERENCES

Adler, Rachel. *Engendering Judaism: An Inclusive Theology and Ethics*. Philadelphia, Pa.: Jewish Publication Society, 1998; Alpert, Rebecca T. *Like Bread on the Seder Plate: Jewish Lesbians and the Transformation of Tradition*. New York: Columbia University Press, 1997; Balka, Christie, and Andy Rose, eds. *Twice Blessed: On Being Lesbian, Gay, and Jewish*. Boston, Mass.: Beacon Press, 1989; Beck, Evelyn Torton, ed. *Nice Jewish Girls: A Jewish Lesbian Anthology*. Trumansburg, N.Y.: Crossing Press, 1984; Berger, Graenum. *Black Jews in America: A Documentary with Commentary*. New York: Commission on Synagogue Relations/Federation of Jewish Philanthropies of New York, 1978; Biale, David. *Eros and the Jews: From Biblical Israel to Contemporary America*. New York: Basic Books, 1992. Berkeley: University of California Press, 1997; Blustain, Sarah. "Are You Black or Are You Jewish? The New Identity Challenge." *Lilith: The Independent Jewish Women's Magazine* 21:3 (1996), 21–27; Bornstein, Kate. *Gender Outlaw: On Men, Women, and the Rest of Us*. New York: Vintage, 1995; Boyarin, Daniel. *Unheroic Conduct: The Rise of Heterosexuality and the Invention of the Jewish Man*. Berkeley: University of California Press, 1997; Brettschneider, Marla. *Democratic Theorizing from the Margins*. Philadelphia, Pa.: Temple University Press, 2002; Brodkin,

Karen. *How Jews Became White Folks and What That Says about Race in America.* New Brunswick, N.J.: Rutgers University Press, 1998; Buber, Martin. (1922) *I and Thou [Ich und du].* Trans. Gregor Smith. New York: Collier, 1958; Butler, Judith. (1990) *Gender Trouble: Feminism and the Subversion of Identity,* 10th anniv. ed. New York: Routledge, 2000; Cohen, Rich. *Tough Jews.* New York: Simon and Schuster, 1998; Coleman, Alex. "Variations on a Theme." *Sh'ma* 33, no. 602 (June 2003), 5–6; Dickson, Deborah, dir. *Ruthie and Connie: Every Room in the House.* Produced by Donald Goldmacher. Distributed by Women Make Movies, 2002; Dorff, Elliot N. *Love Your Neighbor and Yourself: A Jewish Approach to Modern Personal Ethics.* Philadelphia, Pa.: Jewish Publication Society, 2003; Epstein, Louis M. (1948) *Sex Laws and Customs in Judaism.* New York: Ktav, 1967; Feinberg, Leslie. *Stone Butch Blues.* Ithaca, N.Y.: Firebrand Books, 1993; Feldman, David M. (1968) *Marital Relations, Birth Control, and Abortion in Jewish Law.* New York: Schocken Books, 1974; Goldman, Emma. (1910) *Anarchism and Other Essays.* New York: Dover, 1969; Gordis, Robert. *Sex and the Family in Judaism.* New York: Burning Book, 1967; Greenberg, Blu. (1981). *On Women and Judaism: A View from Tradition.* Philadelphia, Pa.: Jewish Publication Society of America, 1981; Hyman, Paula. *Gender and Assimilation in Modern Jewish History: The Roles and Representation of Women.* Seattle: University of Washington Press, 1995; Kanegson, Jaron. "A Young Man from Chelm: Or a Nontraditionally Gendered Hebrew School Teacher Tells All." In Caryn Aviv and David Shneer, eds., *Queer Jews.* New York: Routledge, 2002, 55–69; Kaye/Kantrowitz, Melanie. *The Issue Is Power: Essays on Women, Jews, Violence, and Resistance.* San Francisco, Calif.: Aunt Lute Books, 1992; Kaye/Kantrowitz, Melanie, and Irena Klepfisz, eds. *The Tribe of Dina: A Jewish Women's Anthology.* Boston, Mass.: Beacon Press, 1989; Krawitz, Cole. "A Voice from Within: A Challenge for the Conservative Jewish Movement." In Marla Brettschneider, ed., *Symposium:* "Tense Dialogues: Speaking (across) Multicultural Difference in the Jewish Feminist World." *Nashim: A Journal of Jewish Women's Studies and Gender Issues* 8 (Fall 2004), 165–74; McKinley, Catherine E. *The Book of Sarahs: A Family in Parts.* Washington, D.C.: Counterpoint, 2002; Meyerowitz, Joanne. *How Sex Changed: A History of Transsexuality in the United States.* Cambridge, Mass.: Harvard University Press, 2002; Michaels, T. J., and Cannon, Ali. "Which Side Are You On? Transgender at the Western Wall." In Caryn Aviv and David Shneer, eds., *Queer Jews.* New York: Routledge, 2002, 84–99; Plaskow, Judith. *Standing against Sinai: Judaism from a Feminist Perspective.* San Francisco, Calif.: Harper and Row, 1989; Schultz, Debra L. *Going South: Jewish Women in the Civil Rights Movement.* New York: New York University Press, 2001; Sicular, Eve. "Gender Rebellion In Yiddish Film." *Lilith: The Independent Jewish Women's Magazine* 20:4 (1995–1996), 12–17; Singer, Ilana Gerard. "Red-Diaper Daughter." *Lilith: The Independent Jewish Women's Magazine* 17:3 (1992), 7–10; Svonkin, Stuart. *Jews against Prejudice: American Jews and the Fight for Civil Liberties.* New York: Columbia University Press, 1997; Zerubavel, Yael. *Recovered Roots: Collective Memory and the Making of Israeli National Tradition.* Chicago, Ill.: University of Chicago Press, 1995.

Marla Brettschneider

ADDITIONAL READING

Agunot Campaign. (Web site) <www.agunot-campaign.org.uk> [accessed 17 February 2005]; Alpert, Rebecca T. "Guilty Pleasures: When Sex Is Good Because It's Bad." In Patricia Beattie Jung, Mary E. Hunt, and Radhika Balakrishnan, eds., *Good Sex: Feminist Perspectives from the World's Religions.* New Brunswick, N.J.: Rutgers University Press, 2001, 31–43; Alpert, Rebecca T. "Religious Liberty, Same-Sex Marriage, and the Case of Reconstructionist Judaism." In Kathleen M. Sands, ed., *God Forbid: Religion and Sex in American Public Life.* New York: Oxford University Press, 2000, 124–34; Alpert, Rebecca T., Sue Levi Elwell, and Shirley Idelson, eds. *Lesbian Rabbis: The First Generation.* New Brunswick, N.J.: Rutgers University Press, 2001; American-Israeli Cooperative Enterprise. "Theodor (Binyamin Ze'ev) Herzl." *Jewish Virtual Library* (2004). <www.jewishvirtuallibrary.org/jsource/biography/Herzl.html> [accessed 17 February 2005]; Artson, Bradley Shavit. "Judaism and Homosexuality." *Tikkun* 3:2 (1988), 52–54, 92–93; Beck, Evelyn Torton. "Teaching about Jewish Lesbians in Literature: From 'Zeitl and Rickel' to 'The Tree of

Begats.' " In Bonnie Zimmerman and Toni A. H. McNaron, eds., *The New Lesbian Studies: Into the Twenty-First Century*. New York: Feminist Press at CUNY, 1996, 34–40; Biale, Rachel. *Women and Jewish Law: An Exploration of Women's Issues in Halakhic Sources*. New York: Schocken Books, 1984; Biale, Rachel. *Women and Jewish Law: The Essential Texts, Their History, and Their Relevance for Today*. New York: Schocken/Pantheon, 1995; Boteach, Shmuley. *Moses of Oxford: A Jewish Vision of a University and Its Life*, vol. 1. London: André Deutsch, 1994; Boteach, Shmuley. *Kosher Adultery: Seduce and Sin with Your Partner*. Avon, Mass.: Adams Media, 2002; Boteach, Shmuley. *Kosher Sex: A Recipe for Passion and Intimacy*. New York: Doubleday, 1999; Boyarin, Daniel. *Unheroic Conduct: The Rise of Heterosexuality and the Invention of the Jewish Man*. Berkeley: University of California Press, 1997; Boyarin, Daniel, Daniel Itzkov, and Ann Pellegrini, eds. *Queer Theory and the Jewish Question*. New York: Columbia University Press, 2003; Brod, Harry, ed. *A Mensch among Men: Explorations in Jewish Masculinity*. Freedom, Calif.: Crossing Press, 1988; Broyde, Michael J., and John Witte, Jr., eds. *Human Rights in Judaism: Cultural, Religious, and Political Perspectives*. Northvale, N.J.: J. Aronson, 1998; Christ, Carol P., and Judith Plaskow, eds. *Womanspirit Rising: A Feminist Reader in Religion*. San Francisco, Calif.: Harper and Row, 1979; Cohen, Uri C. *Bibliography of Contemporary Orthodox Responses to Homosexuality* (18 December 2002). Academy for Torah Initiatives and Directions. <www.atid.org/resources/ATIDbiblio1.doc> [accessed 1 February 2005]; Diamond, Malcolm Luria. *Martin Buber, Jewish Existentialist*. New York: Oxford University Press, 1960; Eilberg-Schwartz, Howard, ed. *People of the Body: Jews and Judaism from an Embodied Perspective*. Albany: State University of New York Press, 1992; Eron, Lewis John. "Homosexuality and Judaism." In Arlene Swidler, ed., *Homosexuality and World Religions*. Valley Forge, Pa.: Trinity Press, 1993, 103–34; Feldman, David M. *Birth Control in Jewish Law*. New York: Jason Aronson, 1998; Frymer-Kensky, Tikva. "Virginity in the Bible." In Victor H. Matthews, Bernard M. Levinson, and Tikva Frymer-Kensky, eds., *Gender and Law in the Hebrew Bible and the Ancient Near East*. [*Journal for the Study of the Old Testament*; supp. series, no. 262] Sheffield, U.K.: Sheffield Academic Press, 1998, 79–96; Gordis, Robert. *Love and Sex: A Modern Jewish Perspective*. New York: Farrar, Straus and Giroux, 1978; Greenberg, Steven. *Wrestling with God and Men: Homosexuality in the Jewish Tradition*. Madison: University of Wisconsin Press, 2004; Gross, Robert E., and Mona West, eds. *Take Back the Word: A Queer Reading of the Bible*. Cleveland, Ohio: Pilgrim Press, 2000; Katz, Claire Elise. *Levinas, Judaism, and the Feminine: The Silent Footsteps of Rebecca*. Bloomington: Indiana University Press, 2003; Kessel, Barbara. *Suddenly Jewish: Jews Raised as Gentiles Discover Their Jewish Roots*. Hanover, N.H.: University Press of New England, 2000; Kimmel, Michael S. (1987) "Judaism, Masculinity, and Feminism." In Michael S. Kimmel and Michael A. Messner, eds., *Men's Lives*, 3rd ed. Needham Heights, Mass.: Allyn and Bacon, 1995, 42–44; Klepfisz, Irena. *Dreams of an Insomniac: Jewish Feminist Essays, Speeches, and Diatribes*. Portland, Ore.: Eighth Mountain Press, 1990; Koltun, Elizabeth, ed. *The Jewish Woman: New Perspectives*. New York: Schocken Books, 1976; Kornberg, Jacques. *Theodor Herzl: From Assimilation to Zionism*. Bloomington: Indiana University Press, 1993; Lawton, Phillip. "Love and Justice: Levinas' Reading of Buber." *Philosophy Today* 20 (1976), 77–83; Levado, Yaakov, and Reuven Kimelman. [Exchange on Homosexuality and Judaism] In Robert M. Baird and M. Katherine Baird, eds., *Homosexuality: Debating the Issues*. Amherst, N.Y.: Prometheus, 1995, essays 31–33, 254–77; Lewis, Bernard. *The Jews of Islam*. Princeton, N.J.: Princeton University Press, 1987; Magonet, Jonathan, ed. *Jewish Explorations of Sexuality*. Providence, R.I.: Berghahn, 1995; Mandel, Siegfried. *Nietzsche and the Jews*. Amherst, N.Y.: Prometheus, 1998; Nugent, Robert, and Jeannine Gramick. "Homosexuality: Protestant, Catholic, and Jewish Issues: A Fishbone Tale." In Richard Hasbany, ed., *Homosexuality and Religion*. New York: Harrington Park Press, 1989, 4–76; Olyan, Saul M., and Martha C. Nussbaum, eds. *Sexual Orientation and Human Rights in American Religious Discourse*. New York: Oxford University Press, 1998; Oring, Elliot. *The Jokes of Sigmund Freud: A Study in Humor and Jewish Identity*. Philadelphia: University of Pennsylvania Press, 1984; Plaskow, Judith. "Authority, Resistance, and Transformation: Jewish Feminist Reflections on Good Sex." In Patricia Jung, Mary Hunt, and Radhika Balakrishnan, eds., *Good Sex: Feminist Perspectives from the World's Religions*. New Brunswick, N.J.: Rutgers University Press, 2001, 127–39; Podet,

Allen Howard. "Judaism and Sexuality." In Vern L. Bullough and Bonnie Bullough, eds., *Human Sexuality: An Encyclopedia*. New York: Garland, 1994, 325–30; Prager, Dennis. "Homosexuality, the Bible, and Us—A Jewish Perspective." *The Public Interest*, no. 112 (Summer 1993), 60–83; Prell, Riv-Ellen. "Why Jewish Princesses Don't Sweat: Desire and Consumption in Postwar American Jewish Culture." In Howard Eilberg-Schwartz, ed., *People of the Body: Jews and Judaism from an Embodied Perspective*. Albany: State University of New York Press, 1992, 329–59; Raphael, Lev. *Journeys and Arrivals: On Being Gay and Jewish*. Boston, Mass.: Faber, 1996; Robertson, Ritchie. *Theodor Herzl and the Origins of Zionism*. Edinburgh, Scot.: Edinburgh University Press, 1997; Rosenberg, Mila. "Trans/positioning the (Drag?) King of Comedy: Bisexuality and Queer Jewish Space in the Works of Sandra Bernhard." In Jonathan Alexander and Karen Yescavage, eds., *Bisexuality and Transgenderism: InterSEXions of the Others*. New York: Harrington Park Press, 2003, 171–79; Roth, Philip. *Goodbye, Columbus and Five Short Stories*. Boston, Mass.: Houghton Mifflin, 1959; Roth, Philip. (1969) *Portnoy's Complaint*. 25th anniv. ed. New York: Vintage, 1994; Satlow, Michael L. " 'Try to Be a Man': The Rabbinic Construction of Masculinity." *Harvard Theological Review* 89:1 (1996), 19–40; Schimel, Lawrence. "Diaspora, Sweet Diaspora." In Carol Queen and Lawrence Schimel, eds., *PoMoSexuals: Challenging Assumptions about Gender and Sexuality*. San Francisco, Calif.: Cleis Press, 1997, 163–73; Schwartz, Mimi. *Thoughts from a Queen-Sized Bed*. Lincoln: University of Nebraska Press, 2002; Seidman, Naomi. *A Marriage Made in Heaven: The Sexual Politics of Hebrew and Yiddish*. Berkeley: University of California Press, 1997; Smith, Carol. "Challenged by the Text: Two Stories of Incest in the Hebrew Bible." In Athalya Brenner and Carole R. Fontaine, eds., *A Feminist Companion to Reading the Bible: Approaches, Methods and Strategies*. Sheffield, U.K.: Sheffield Academic Press, 1997, 114–35; Smith, Carol. "Stories of Incest in the Hebrew Bible: Scholars Challenging Text or Text Challenging Scholars?" *Henoch* 14 (1992), 227–42; Solomon, Lewis D. *The Jewish Tradition, Sexuality, and Procreation*. Lanham, Md.: University Press of America, 2002; Spiegel, Marcia Cohen. *Bibliography of Sexual and Domestic Violence in the Jewish Community* (2004). <www.mincava.umn.edu/documents/bibs/jewish/jewish.html> [accessed 1 January 2005]; Tessman, Lisa, and Bat-Ami Bar On, eds. *Jewish Locations: Traversing Racialized Landscapes*. Lanham, Md.: Rowman and Littlefield, 2001; Tirosh-Samuelson, Hava, ed. *Women and Gender in Jewish Philosophy*. Bloomington: Indiana University Press, 2004; Waskow, Arthur. *Down-to-Earth Judaism: Food, Money, Sex, and the Rest of Life*. New York: Morrow, 1997.

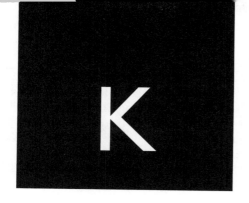

KANT, IMMANUEL (1724–1804).

KANT, IMMANUEL (1724–1804). Born in Königsberg, a center of Prussian political and intellectual life, Immanuel Kant never traveled far from his hometown. He held a series of professorships at the University of Königsberg. His schedule was notoriously regular: Neighbors set their clocks by his evening walk. However, this infamous picture depicts the older Kant (Kuehn, 1–23). The younger Kant was devoted to sartorial elegance and billiards, enjoyed socializing, and decided against **marriage** due to poverty, not from a dislike of female company (George; Kuehn, 117, 169). Kant was reared as a Pietist Protestant but in maturity was skeptical of organized religion (Wood, "Rational Theology," 394–97).

Kant's contributions to philosophy in the areas of metaphysics, epistemology, and ethics are fundamental to modern philosophy. His *Critique of Pure Reason* (1781) addressed, among others, questions about knowledge and freedom. In response to skepticism, the view that we can have no certain knowledge, Kant advanced what may be taken to be a two-world theory: There is the phenomenal world, which we experience through our senses, and the noumenal world, about which we never have direct knowledge. Kant argued that our minds impose categories that order the world of experience. Knowledge of the foundations of science is therefore possible through interrogation of our own reason (Guyer). Similarly, ethical principles are constructions of reason (O'Neill, "Kantian Ethics"). The two-world theory also addresses the problem of free will. Since everything in the physical world is subject to physical laws, human beings must be as well. So our actions are determined, which, for Kant, is incompatible with free will. In two-world theory, we can have freedom in the noumenal realm.

Kant's ethics, expounded primarily in his 1785 *Groundwork of the Metaphysic of Morals*, centers on freedom, rationality, and equality. We must assume that all rational agents possess free will, or autonomy (*Groundwork*, Ak 4:446–48). Autonomous rational agency is the source of our equal moral value (Ak 4:428). It is also the source of moral obligation. Reason prescribes absolute rules for our conduct that, as rational agents, we are committed to follow. These rules are proved through reason alone, not from experience, although human nature plays a role in their application (Ak 4:388–90, 410–12; Wood, *Kant's Ethical Thought*, 8–11). In the *Groundwork*, Kant derives the supreme moral law.

This law, called the Categorical Imperative, is a command we must follow regardless of our desires or inclinations. The "Formula of the Universal Law," the first of Kant's several ways of formulating the Categorical Imperative, enjoins: "Act only on that maxim through which you can at the same time will that it should become a universal law" (*Groundwork*, Ak 4:421). This formula captures the moral importance of universality and impartiality. It also signals Kant's view that an act's intention in part determines its moral status. For Kant, a deontologist in ethics, some actions are inherently wrong. Intending to lie is wrong in itself, no matter what the consequences are. Further, acting morally requires more than simply acting in conformity with duty; an action has moral worth only when done from the motive of duty, as opposed to motives such as self-interest or sympathy (Ak 4:397–99). Although Kant has been criticized for not valuing emotions, he does allow a role for moral emotions such as **love** of one's neighbor (*Metaphysics of Morals*, Ak 6:399–403; for discussion, see Baron, *Kantian Ethics*, 194–226; Velleman).

Kant's second formulation of the Categorical Imperative, the "Formula of Humanity" (FH), commands: "Act in such a way that you always treat humanity, whether in your own person or in the person of any other, never simply as a means, but always at the same time as an end" (*Groundwork*, Ak 4:429). We must respect the autonomy of other people by refraining from using them as mere means or instruments for our own purposes or to achieve our own goals. To respect their autonomy, we must recognize their ability to make their own decisions. We must not treat others, or ourselves, as things or objects, that is, as not being rational and autonomous. Coercion and threats violate this injunction, as do lying to others and manipulating them. Of course, we often do use other people, as when we mail a letter that is handled by post office employees (see Paton, *Categorical Imperative*, 165). We may use other people, however, as long as they **consent**—within important limits. That is, on Kant's view some actions fail to respect humanity even when consent is present and so are morally wrong (O'Neill, "Between"). For example, one may not sell oneself into slavery, engage in unmarried sexual acts, or commit suicide.

Ethical duties are categorized as "perfect duties," which one must follow at all times, and "imperfect duties," which allow some latitude (*Groundwork*, Ak 4:421–24). These two types of duty correspond (roughly) to Kant's later division in *The Metaphysics of Morals* (1797–1798) between the Doctrine of Justice and the Doctrine of Virtue. Justice consists of perfect duties to others and the legal institutions corresponding to these duties (Ak 6:229–40). Kant argues that the state and its legal institutions are morally justified since they are necessary to preserve freedom. Property is fundamental to justice, on his view, and Kant ends up subsuming marriage and family, along with property and contract, under principles of acquisition (*Metaphysics*, Ak 6:276–84). Virtue consists of moral duties that are not coercively enforceable (unlike legal duties) and involve having the ends of one's own perfection and the happiness of others (Ak 6:391–94). In examining Kant's philosophy of sex, the theoretical frameworks provided by both the *Groundwork* and the *Metaphysics* are important.

Kant's views on sex, marriage, procreation, family, and related topics can be found primarily in the *Metaphysics* (Ak 6:276–84, 358–61, 424–26, 469–73); the posthumously published *Lectures on Ethics* (Ak 27:48–52, 384–92); *Observations on the Feeling of the Beautiful and Sublime* (1764; 76–96); "Conjectural Beginning of Human History" (1786); and *Anthropology from a Pragmatic Point of View* (1798; Ak 7:303–11). What emerges is a psychological and anthropological account of sexuality, and an ethics of both **sexual desire** and **sexual activity**, according to which sexuality demeans humanity. From these foundations, Kant concludes that sexual activity is permissible only in marriage. Other expressions of the sexual impulse are, for him, morally wrong as being either contrary to nature (**bestiality, homosexuality, masturbation**) or contrary to reason (**prostitution, adultery**).

In his account of the nature of the sexual, Kant asserts that in sexual activity each person gives himself or herself to the other. A person, however, is a unity. Thus, if one surrenders part of oneself (for example, the genitals), one necessarily surrenders the whole. But— here enters Kant's ethics—such a surrender or giving up of oneself violates the FH: "In this act a human being makes himself into a thing, which conflicts with the Right of humanity in his own person" (*Metaphysics*, Ak 6:278). We have, then, the problem of sex in

Kant: Because all sexual activity seems morally wrong, how can Kant make room for morally permissible sex (only) in marriage? The problem is made even more acute when Kant elaborates his account of the nature of the sexual with respect to desire. Kant thought, dramatically, that sexual desire was inherently immoral:

> In loving from sexual inclination, they make the person into an object of their appetite. As soon as the person is possessed, and the appetite sated, they are thrown away, as one throws away a lemon after sucking the juice from it. The sexual impulse can admittedly be combined with human affection, and then it also carries with it the aims of the latter, but if it is taken in and by itself, it is nothing more than appetite. But, so considered, there lies in this inclination a degradation of man; for as soon as anyone becomes an object of another's appetite, all motives of moral relationship fall away; as object of the other's appetite, that person is in fact a thing, whereby the other's appetite is sated, and can be misused as such a thing by anybody. (*Lectures*, Ak 27:384–85)

Unlike genuine human love, which is benevolent, sexual "love" both objectifies the other and is not concerned about his or her well-being.

Sexual desire, for Kant, violates the FH by making the other an object of appetite. His point is not that sexual desire, *qua* desire, has an "intentional object," in the way one can be the intentional object of respect and other emotions or attitudes (Langton, "Love and Solipsism," 134). Kant's point is that in sexual desire (and only here) another *person* is the "object of another's enjoyment" (*Lectures*, Ak 27:385), so "carnal enjoyment is *cannibalistic* in principle. . . . [E]ach is actually a *consumable* thing . . . to the other" (*Metaphysics*, Ak 6:359–60). Kant's view may be that sexual desire seeks to consume and possess a person as if he or she were merely a thing, which fails to respect the other's humanity (Korsgaard, "Creating the Kingdom," 310). Or Kant's view may be that sexual desire reduces a person to a thing. The sexual "impulse is . . . directed to sex, merely, and not to humanity" (*Lectures*, Ak 27:387). A person is seen, approached, *as* a body to be manipulated, a set of genitals, or an interchangeable representative of his or her sex (Herman; Langton, "Love and Solipsism," "Sexual Solipsism"). If sexual desire causes us to see another person as a mere thing, lack of moral regard for the other naturally follows. Further, if one allows himself or herself to be approached in this way, or welcomes it, one makes oneself into a thing for the other. In this way a person can become an immoral accomplice in the other's objectifying desire—sometimes through the allures of personal adornment (*Lectures*, Ak 27:385). It has been proposed, in light of the FH's prohibition against treating *oneself* as an object, that being an accomplice was perhaps Kant's major worry about sex (Soble, "Sexual Use").

Kant noted that animal instincts, such as the desires for food and sex, can overwhelm duty. While such instincts serve purposes (eating, procreating), Kant adjures that they be disciplined so that sensuality does not overrun intellect (*Lectures*, Ak 27:378–81). He included sexual desire among the passions, which are "appetites directed by men to men, not to things" (*Anthropology*, Ak 267–70; on the passions, compare Wood, *Kant's Ethical Thought*, 256–59, with Baron, *Kantian Ethics*, 199–203). Passions, Kant claims, "do the greatest damage to freedom" (*Anthropology*, Ak 265). Diminishing one's autonomy or rationality through passion or animal instinct, he thinks, violates our duty to pursue moral perfection. (Some of Kant's ideas here—the need to discipline sexuality, the conflict between sex and freedom—were also themes of **Saint Augustine** [354–430]. See *City of God*, bk. 14, *passim*, and Epistle 6*, 102.) But even though Kant understands sexual desire as animalistic, he also identifies purely human elements in sexuality. For example, while interpreting Genesis, he suggests that the leaves concealing the genitals actually served to arouse desire, a sexual technique that marks an important distinction between humans and animals ("Conjectural Beginning," 56–57; see Wood, *Kant's Ethical Thought*, 238, 256–59). Indeed, one might read Kantian sexual desire as a distinctively human passion of domination and competitiveness (see Morgan).

For Kant, a legal institution is required to preserve humanity in the face of these dangers of sexuality. This institution is marriage, which Kant understands as a contract between one man and one woman in which they exchange rights of possession over each other. The marriage right is a "right to a person akin to a right to a thing," so that "if one of the partners in a marriage has left or given itself into someone else's possession, the other partner is justified, always and without question, in bringing its partner back under its control, just as it is justified in retrieving a thing" (*Metaphysics*, Ak 6:278). Each spouse must hold equal rights over the other (as in **Saint Paul** [5–64?], 1 Cor. 7:3–4), which rules out morganatic marriage and polygamy, for these arrangements involve giving oneself totally but receiving in return only half or less of the other person (*Lectures*, Ak 27:389; *Metaphysics*, Ak 6:279).

But how the joint possession of marriage makes sexual activity permissible is unclear. Sex violates the FH because the parties give themselves to each other as things. Kant argues that marriage addresses this by giving the contracting parties equal rights over each other: "[W]hile one person is acquired by the other *as if it were a thing*, the one who is acquired acquires the other in turn; for in this way each reclaims itself and restores its personality" (*Metaphysics*, Ak 6:278). Again, "if I hand over my whole person to the other, and thereby obtain the person of the other in place of it, I get myself back again, and have thereby regained possession of myself. . . . The two persons thus constitute a unity of will. Neither will be subject to happiness or misfortune, joy or displeasure, without the other taking a share in it" (*Lectures*, Ak 27:388). One reading (Ladd's) is that the freedom given up is reciprocally regained. But this reading is complicated by Kant's idea that sexual desire, which compromises freedom, is always directed to sex, not humanity. So the exchange of rights does not seem to rehabilitate desire (see Brake). Further, possession of another person seems to violate the FH, although Kant does distinguish possession from property ownership, which is only of things (*Metaphysics*, Ak 6:359).

Kant's explanation seems to be that marriage *permits* **sexual objectification** rather than *transforms* the objectifying nature of sexuality. Marriage allows spouses "to make direct use of a person *as of* a thing, as a means to my end, but still without infringing upon his personality" (*Metaphysics*, Ak 6:359). A bleak reading of Kant sees this as "a system of mutual exploitation" (Wood, *Kant's Ethical Thought*, 257), and Bertolt Brecht (1898–1956) made Kantian marriage an occasion for satire: "To get those organs duly confiscated," the only recourse is Law (312). **G.W.F. Hegel** (1770–1831) denounced it as "disgraceful," since the ethical content of marriage should not and cannot, *contra* Kant, be represented as a self-interested contract (*Philosophy of Right*, para. 75, 161A; see de Laurentiis; Pateman, 168–88). Kant may be defended against Hegelian dismissals by arguing that marital rights (against abandonment, for example) protect people when the affection of a close relationship begins to fail (see Waldron). In a sympathetic reconstruction, Barbara Herman proposes that Kantian marriage rights "block the transformation of regard that comes with sexual appetite" by "secur[ing] regard for one's partner as a person with a life, which is what the sexual appetite by itself causes one to disregard" (62–63). On this view, marriage does transform, curtail, or diminish the obnoxious nature of sexuality and does not merely make sexual objectification permissible.

Sexual "crimes" are taxonomized by Kant (in a manner reminiscent of **Saint Thomas Aquinas** [1224/25–1274], *Summa theologiae*, 2a2ae, ques. 154, art. 1–12) as those that follow nature but are contrary to reason and those that are contrary to nature (*Lectures*, Ak 27:390–92; *Metaphysics*, Ak 6:424–26). The former category includes unmarried sex and adultery—which is cause, along with "incompatibility," for divorce (*Lectures*, Ak 27:390). Prostitution offends reason and violates the FH: Selling the body treats it as a mere thing, and because we are not our own property, we cannot sell ourselves (Ak 27:386). **Incest** is inherently wrong only between a parent and child, not between siblings, because the subordination that occurs in sexual interactions must be mutual, not one-sided (Ak 27:389–90). (**Plato** [427–347 BCE] reaches the same conclusion about vertical and horizontal incest, but on different grounds; *Republic*, 457c–62e.) Sibling incest, for Kant, is not against nature because it had to occur early in human history.

The sexual crimes contrary to nature discussed by Kant are homosexuality, bestiality, and masturbation, which contravene the natural end of the sexual instinct, procreation:

> [U]nnatural, and even merely unpurposive [nonprocreative], use of one's sexual attribute is inadmissible as being a violation of duty to oneself. . . . [B]y it man surrenders his personality (throwing it away), since he uses himself merely as a means to satisfy an animal impulse. (*Metaphysics*, Ak 6:425)

Kant writes that masturbation makes the agent "an object of enjoyment" and is morally worse than suicide (*Lectures*, Ak 27:391–92; *Metaphysics*, Ak 6:425). Kant's invocation of natural purpose has implications for marital sex; it, too, must not be "unnatural." Yet Kant seems to suggest that nonprocreative sex between spouses might be allowed by "a permissive law of morally practical reason, which in the collision of its determining grounds makes permitted something that is in itself not permitted (indulgently, as it were), to prevent a still greater violation" (*Metaphysics*, Ak 6:426). Perhaps what Kant means here is that sexual intercourse as *remedium ad concupiscentiae* is sometimes permitted—when, for example, the wife cannot become pregnant because she already is.

Regardless, Kant's appeals to nature are controversial, since he does not explain why the unnatural is immoral (Gregor, 133). In *Critique of Judgment* (1790), Kant justifies the attribution of purpose to nature, and he appeals to human nature in other ethical arguments (see Cooke; Williams, 4–10). But these arguments have been criticized as less than rational proofs (Denis, "Kant on the Wrongness"; Gregor, 134, 139–42; Soble, "Kant and Sexual Perversion"). Kant's views on homosexuality have been criticized as inconsistent, and elements of his ethics have even been invoked to defend **same-sex marriage** (Herman, 66n.22; Schaff). Kant does provide other grounds for the immorality of at least masturbation. His comment that "imagination brings forth a desire contrary to nature's end" (*Metaphysics*, Ak 6:425) might condemn the lawlessness of **fantasy** (Kielkopf; see Fortunata, 400; Soble, "Kant and Sexual Perversion," 58–59). And in *Education* (1803), Kant claims that masturbation is self-destructive (117–18).

In reconstructing a happier Kantian view of sex, love, and marriage, some philosophers have turned to his account of **friendship** (Denis, "From Friendship"; Korsgaard, "Creating"; Langton, "Love and Solipsism"). True friendship is an ideal moral relation of mutual benevolence, reciprocity, and self-sharing (*Metaphysics*, Ak 6:469–73; see Paton, "Kant on Friendship"; Wood, *Kant's Ethical Thought*, 275–82), and Kant's description of friendship as a union echoes his view of marriage (Korsgaard, "Creating," 310–11). Notably, he thinks that we have a duty to share ourselves with friends, partly as a release from the "prison" of one's own mind (Langton, "Love and Solipsism," 127–31). Kant conceded that sexuality "can . . . be combined with human affection" and carry with it "the aims" of human love (*Lectures*, Ak 27:384–85). In a letter to a heartbroken young woman who sought his moral advice (Maria von Herbert [1769–1803]), Kant replied that complete communication and mutual esteem are essential to love, "be it for one's spouse or for a friend" (*Correspondence*, Ak 411, Ak 11:331; for the story of this interaction, see Langton, "Duty and Desolation"). Still, on his view, love's tendency to pull people together must always be counterbalanced by the distancing effect of respect (*Metaphysics*, Ak 6:448–49; see Baron, "Love and Respect").

What Kant wrote about women (see *Anthropology*, Ak 7:209, 262–63, 303–11; "On the Common Saying") has been much criticized (Mendus; Schröder). For example, "A woman who has a head full of Greek, like Mme Dacier, or carries on fundamental controversies about mechanics, like the Marquise de Châtelet, might as well even have a beard," so contrary are such activities, Kant thought, to natural feminine "charms" (*Observations*, 78). And in the *Metaphysics* (Ak 6:279) we find his thought that "the natural superiority of the husband to the wife" justifies marriage law that appoints a husband as his wife's "master (he is the party to direct, she to obey)." Perhaps Kant can be defended, in part, as having reported, but not endorsed, the sexist views of his time (Wilson). He did see women as rational agents and aimed to protect their rights in and through marriage (Ladd; Mosser; Wood, *Kant's Ethical Thought*, 395–96n.9): "Scepticism about marriage . . . is bound to have bad consequences for the whole female sex; for woman would be degraded to a mere means for satisfying man's desires. . . . It is by marriage that woman becomes free: man loses his freedom by it" (*Anthropology*, Ak 7:309).

Kant's views on marriage, sex, and friendship reflect diverse influences. His account of friendship draws especially on **Aristotle**'s (384–322 BCE) *Nicomachean Ethics* and Michel Montaigne's (1533–1592) famous essay. His thought about sexuality is indebted in many ways to earlier and continuing debates within Christianity and especially to Paul, Augustine, and Aquinas (although he does not acknowledge these predecessors). Kant's account of the "unity of will" in the marriage contract echoes **Jean-Jacques Rousseau**'s (1712–1778) contract of mutual surrender (*Social Contract*, bk. 1, chap. 6). And Kantian marriage reflects Roman law (Ladd).

Kant's influence in ethical philosophy, as in metaphysics and epistemology, has been extensive. Many contemporary ethicists advance Kantian theories in which rationality and autonomy are key elements (Donagan; Korsgaard; John Rawls [1921–2002]). Not surprisingly, many sexual ethicists draw on Kant, some giving detailed attention to his claims about sexuality, others attending more generally to his ethics. In the latter, the ideals of respecting persons and not using them figure prominently (see O'Neill, "Kantian Ethics"). But the implications of these Kantian notions for sexuality have been contested. Respect for autonomy may be taken to require allowing or adhering to whatever sexual decisions adults make. This reading results in a "liberal Kantian" sexual morality in which consent is not merely necessary (thereby prohibiting coercion and deception) but also sufficient, *ceteris paribus*, for the permissibility of sexual activity (Baumrin; Belliotti; Mappes; Primoratz; for discussion, see Archard; Morgan; Soble, "Sexual Use"; Wertheimer, 131–35). Many contemporary Kantians do not agree that consent is sufficient. For example, it has been argued that the FH prohibits exploitation (Donagan, 107; O'Neill, "Between Consenting Adults"), that even **casual sex** partners must exhibit concern for each other's pleasure (Goldman), that we ought to refrain from mockery or boasting (Klepper), that we ought to attend to others in their particularity (O'Neill, "Between"), and that we should not engage in demeaning, even if consensual, sexual practices such as **sadomasochism**

(Hampton). Further, the value of rational autonomy and the wrongness of using others and the self have also been invoked to generate "conservative Kantian" sexual moralities in which sex ought always to be linked with love, marriage, or procreation (Finnis; **Karol Wojtyła** [1920–2005]).

Respect for persons and Kant's view that sexuality objectifies are important themes in feminist literature. Some feminist philosophers have worked on the analysis of the concept of sexual objectification (Haslanger; LeMoncheck; Nussbaum). **Catharine MacKinnon** has drawn on Kant's moral ideal of respect for free and rational personhood (158), arguing that many contemporary sexual practices fail to respect that personhood by treating women as objects. Feminist discussions of respect and objectification have focused on **sexual harassment**, prostitution, other **sex work**, and **pornography**. Commercial sex, for example, has been regarded as an exchange in which both parties, the prostitute and the client, treat each other merely as means or objects (Anderson and Estes; Estes). Indeed, this may be a case in which, rather than mutual consent morally cleansing their activity, mutual consent is part of the moral problem, since in consenting each makes an object also of himself or herself. (Kant would agree.) Yet more liberal Kantian feminists argue that depending on various factors, including background context and intentions, respect for women may well be compatible with their participation in pornography and prostitution (Garry; Shrage). The philosophical daughters of Kant have stirred up an especially contentious area of ethical, social, and political philosophy. Given the dual influence on Kant's thought—Enlightenment ideals of equal respect, Christian ideals of **sexual ethics**—it is not surprising that his views have been so variously interpreted.

See also Beauty; Casual Sex; Catholicism, Twentieth- and Twenty-First Century; Consequentialism; Descartes, René; Fantasy; Feminism, Liberal; Friendship; Hegel, G.W.F.; Hobbes, Thomas; Liberalism; Marriage; Objectification, Sexual; Personification, Sexual; Prostitution; Rape; Sade, Marquis de; Schopenhauer, Arthur; Scruton, Roger; Wojtyła, Karol (Pope John Paul II)

REFERENCES

Anderson, Clelia Smyth, and Yolanda Estes. "The Myth of the Happy Hooker: Kantian Moral Reflections on a Phenomenology of Prostitution." In Stanley G. French, Wanda Teays, and Laura M. Purdy, eds., *Violence against Women: Philosophical Perspectives.* Ithaca, N.Y.: Cornell University Press, 1998, 152–58; Archard, David. *Sexual Consent.* Boulder, Colo.: Westview, 1998; Aristotle. (ca. 325 BCE?) *Nicomachean Ethics.* Trans. Terence Irwin. Indianapolis, Ind.: Hackett, 1985; Augustine. (413–427) *The City of God.* Trans. Marcus Dods. New York: Modern Library, 1993; Augustine. (421) Epistle 6*. In Elizabeth A. Clark, ed., *St. Augustine on Marriage and Sexuality.* Washington, D.C.: Catholic University of America, 1996, 99–105; Baron, Marcia. *Kantian Ethics Almost without Apology.* Ithaca, N.Y.: Cornell University Press, 1995; Baron, Marcia. "Love and Respect in the *Doctrine of Virtue.*" In Nelson Potter and Mark Timmons, eds., *Kant's Metaphysics of Morals. Southern Journal of Philosophy* 35, supp. (1997), 29–44; Baumrin, Bernard. (1975) "Sexual Immorality Delineated." In Robert B. Baker and Frederick A. Elliston, eds., *Philosophy and Sex*, 2nd ed. Buffalo, N.Y.: Prometheus, 1984, 300–311; Belliotti, Raymond. *Good Sex: Perspectives on Sexual Ethics.* Lawrence: University Press of Kansas, 1993; Brake, Elizabeth. "Justice and Virtue in Kant's Account of Marriage." *Kantian Review* 9 (March 2005), 58–94; Brecht, Bertolt. (1938) "On Kant's Definition of Marriage in *The Metaphysic of Ethics.*" In John Willett and Ralph Manheim (with Erich Fried), eds., *Poems 1913–1956*, rev. ed. Trans. John Willett. New York: Methuen, 1987, 312; Cooke, Vincent M. "Kant, Teleology, and Sexual Ethics." *International Philosophical Quarterly* 31:1 (1991), 3–13; De Laurentiis, Allegra. "Kant's Shameful Proposition: A Hegel-Inspired Criticism of Kant's Theory of Domestic Right." *International Philosophical Quarterly* 40:3 (2000), 297–312; Denis, Lara. "From Friendship to Marriage: Revising Kant." *Philosophy and Phenomenological*

Research 63:1 (2001), 1–28; Denis, Lara. "Kant on the Wrongness of 'Unnatural' Sex." *History of Philosophy Quarterly* 16:2 (1999), 225–48; Donagan, Alan. *The Theory of Morality.* Chicago, Ill.: University of Chicago Press, 1977; Estes, Yolanda. "Moral Reflections on Prostitution." *Essays in Philosophy* 2:2 (2001). <www.humboldt.edu/~essays/estes.html> [accessed 4 January 2005]; Finnis, John M. "Law, Morality, and 'Sexual Orientation.' " *Notre Dame Law Review* 69:5 (1994), 1049–76; Fortunata, Jacqueline. "Masturbation and Women's Sexuality." In Alan Soble, ed., *The Philosophy of Sex: Contemporary Readings*, 1st ed. Totowa, N.J.: Rowman and Littlefield, 1980, 389–408; Garry, Ann. "Pornography and Respect for Women." *Social Theory and Practice* 4:4 (1978), 395–421; George, Rolf. "The Lives of Kant." *Philosophy and Phenomenological Research* 47:3 (1987), 485–500; Goldman, Alan. "Plain Sex." *Philosophy and Public Affairs* 6:3 (1977), 267–87; Gregor, Mary J. *Laws of Freedom: A Study of Kant's Method of Applying the Categorical Imperative in the Metaphysik der Sitten.* Oxford, U.K.: Blackwell, 1963; Guyer, Paul. "Introduction: The Starry Heavens and the Moral Law." In Paul Guyer, ed., *The Cambridge Companion to Kant.* Cambridge: Cambridge University Press, 1992, 1–25; Hampton, Jean. "Defining Wrong and Defining Rape." In Keith Burgess-Jackson, ed., *A Most Detestable Crime: New Philosophical Essays on Rape.* New York: Oxford University Press, 1999, 118–56; Haslanger, Sally. "On Being Objective and Being Objectified." In Louise Antony and Charlotte Witt, eds., *A Mind of One's Own: Feminist Essays on Reason and Objectivity.* Boulder, Colo.: Westview, 1993, 85–125; Hegel, G.W.F. (1821) *Elements of the Philosophy of Right.* Ed. Allen W. Wood. Trans. Hugh Barr Nisbet. Cambridge: Cambridge University Press, 1995; Herman, Barbara. "Could It Be Worth Thinking about Kant on Sex and Marriage?" In Louise Antony and Charlotte Witt, eds., *A Mind of One's Own: Feminist Essays on Reason and Objectivity.* Boulder, Colo.: Westview, 1993, 49–67; Kant, Immanuel. (1798) *Anthropology from a Pragmatic Point of View.* Trans. Mary J. Gregor. The Hague, Holland: Martinus Nijhoff, 1974; Kant, Immanuel. (1786) "Conjectural Beginning of Human History." In Lewis White Beck, ed., *On History.* Indianapolis, Ind.: Bobbs-Merrill, 1963, 53–68; Kant, Immanuel. *Correspondence.* Trans. and ed. Arnulf Zweig. Cambridge: Cambridge University Press, 1999; Kant, Immanuel. (1790) *Critique of Judgment: Including the First Introduction.* Trans. Werner Pluhar. Indianapolis, Ind.: Hackett, 1987; Kant, Immanuel. (1781, 1787) *Critique of Pure Reason.* Trans. Lewis White Beck. Indianapolis, Ind.: Bobbs-Merrill, 1956; Kant, Immanuel. (lectures 1776–1787; published 1803) *Education.* Trans. Annette Churton. London: Kegan Paul, Trench, Trubner, 1899; Kant, Immanuel. (1785) *Groundwork of the Metaphysic of Morals.* Trans. H. J. Paton. New York: Harper Torchbooks, 1964; Kant, Immanuel. (ca. 1762–1794) *Lectures on Ethics.* Trans. Peter Heath. Ed. Peter Heath and J. B. Schneewind. Cambridge: Cambridge University Press, 1997; Kant, Immanuel. (1797–1798) *The Metaphysics of Morals.* Trans. Mary Gregor. Cambridge: Cambridge University Press, 1991, 1996; Kant, Immanuel. (1764) *Observations on the Feeling of the Beautiful and Sublime.* Trans. John T. Goldthwait. Berkeley: University of California Press, 1960; Kant, Immanuel. (1793) "On the Common Saying: That May Be Correct in Theory, But It Is of No Use in Practice." Trans. Mary Gregor. In Mary Gregor, ed., *Practical Philosophy.* Cambridge: Cambridge University Press, 1996, 273–309; Kielkopf, Charles. "Masturbation: A Kantian Condemnation." *Philosophia* 25:1–4 (1997), 223–46; Klepper, Howard. "Sexual Exploitation and the Value of Persons." *Journal of Value Inquiry* 27:3–4 (1993), 479–86; Korsgaard, Christine M. *Creating the Kingdom of Ends.* Cambridge: Cambridge University Press, 1996; Korsgaard, Christine M. "Creating the Kingdom of Ends: Reciprocity and Responsibility in Personal Relations." *Philosophical Perspectives* 6, *Ethics* (1992), 305–32; Kuehn, Manfred. *Kant: A Biography.* Cambridge: Cambridge University Press, 2001; Ladd, John. (1965) "Translator's Introduction." In Immanuel Kant, *Metaphysical Elements of Justice*, 2nd ed. Trans. John Ladd. Indianapolis, Ind.: Hackett, 1999, xv–liv; Langton, Rae. "Duty and Desolation." *Philosophy* 67:262 (1992), 481–505; Langton, Rae. "Love and Solipsism." In Roger E. Lamb, ed., *Love Analyzed.* Boulder, Colo.: Westview, 1997, 123–52; Langton, Rae. "Sexual Solipsism." *Philosophical Topics* 23:2 (1995), 149–87; LeMoncheck, Linda. *Dehumanizing Women: Treating Persons as Sex Objects.* Totowa, N.J.: Rowman and Allanheld, 1984; MacKinnon, Catharine. *Feminism Unmodified: Discourses on Life and Law.* Cambridge, Mass.: Harvard University Press, 1987; Mappes, Thomas A. (1985) "Sexual Morality and the Concept of Using Another Person." In Thomas

A. Mappes and Jane S. Zembaty, eds., *Social Ethics: Morality and Social Policy*, 6th ed. Boston, Mass.: McGraw-Hill, 2002, 170–83; Mendus, Susan. "Kant: 'An Honest But Narrow-Minded Bourgeois'?" In Susan Mendus and Ellen Kennedy, eds., *Women in Western Political Philosophy*. Brighton, U.K.: Wheatsheaf Books, 1987, 24–43; Montaigne, Michel. (1572/1595) "On Affectionate Relationships." In *The Essays of Michel de Montaigne*. Trans. M. A. Screech. New York: Penguin, 1987, 205–19; Morgan, Seiriol. "Dark Desires." *Ethical Theory and Moral Practice* 6:4 (2003), 377–410; Mosser, Kurt. "Kant and Feminism." *Kant-Studien* 90:3 (1999), 322–53; Nussbaum, Martha C. "Objectification." *Philosophy and Public Affairs* 24:4 (1995), 249–91; O'Neill, Onora. "Between Consenting Adults." *Philosophy and Public Affairs* 14:3 (1985), 252–77; O'Neill, Onora. "Kantian Ethics." In Peter Singer, ed., *A Companion to Ethics*. Oxford, U.K.: Blackwell, 1991, 175–85; Pateman, Carole. *The Sexual Contract*. Cambridge, U.K.: Polity Press, 1988; Paton, H. J. *The Categorical Imperative: A Study in Kant's Moral Philosophy*. New York: Harper Torchbooks, 1967; Paton, H. J. (1956) "Kant on Friendship." In Neera K. Badhwar, ed., *Friendship: A Philosophical Reader*. Ithaca, N.Y.: Cornell University Press, 1993, 210–17; Plato. (ca. 375–370 BCE) *Republic*. Trans. G.M.A. Grube. Indianapolis, Ind.: Hackett, 1992; Primoratz, Igor. "Sexual Morality: Is Consent Enough?" *Ethical Theory and Moral Practice* 4:3 (2001), 201–18; Rawls, John. *A Theory of Justice*. Cambridge, Mass.: Harvard University Press, 1971; Rousseau, Jean-Jacques. (1762) *The Social Contract* and *Discourse on the Origin of Inequality*. Trans. Henry J. Tozer and Anonymous (1767). Ed. Lester G. Crocker. New York: Washington Square Press, 1967; Schaff, Kory. "Kant, Political Liberalism, and the Ethics of Same-Sex Relations." *Journal of Social Philosophy* 32:3 (2001), 446–62; Schröder, Hannelore. "Kant's Patriarchal Order." Trans. Rita Gircour. In Robin May Schott, ed., *Feminist Interpretations of Immanuel Kant*. University Park: Pennsylvania State University Press, 1997, 275–96; Shrage, Laurie. "Prostitution and the Case for Decriminalization." *Dissent* (Spring 1996), 41–45; Soble, Alan. "Kant and Sexual Perversion." *The Monist* 86:1 (2003), 57–92; Soble, Alan. "Sexual Use and What to Do about It: Internalist and Externalist Sexual Ethics." *Essays in Philosophy* 2:2 (2001). <www.humboldt.edu/~essays/soble.html> [accessed 4 January 2005]; Thomas Aquinas. (1265–1273) *Summa theologiae*, 60 vols. Cambridge, U.K.: Blackfriars, 1964–1976; Velleman, David J. "Love as a Moral Emotion." *Ethics* 109:2 (1999), 338–74; Waldron, Jeremy. "When Justice Replaces Affection: The Need for Rights." *Harvard Journal of Law and Public Policy* 11:3 (1988), 625–47; Wertheimer, Alan. *Consent to Sexual Relations*. Cambridge: Cambridge University Press, 2003; Williams, Howard. *Kant's Political Philosophy*. New York: St. Martin's Press, 1983; Wilson, Holly L. "Kant's Evolutionary Theory of Marriage." In Jane Kneller, ed., *Autonomy and Community*. Albany: State University of New York Press, 1998, 283–306; Wojtyła, Karol (Pope John Paul II). *Love and Responsibility*. Trans. H. T. Willetts. New York: Farrar, Straus and Giroux, 1981; Wood, Allen W. *Kant's Ethical Thought*. Cambridge: Cambridge University Press, 1999; Wood, Allen W. "Rational Theology, Moral Faith, and Religion." In Paul Guyer, ed., *The Cambridge Companion to Kant*. Cambridge: Cambridge University Press, 1992, 394–416.

Elizabeth Brake

ADDITIONAL READING

Baranzke, Heike. "Does Beast Suffering Count for Kant: A Contextual Examination of §17 in *The Doctrine of Virtue*." *Essays in Philosophy* 5:2 (2004). <www.humboldt.edu/~essays/baranzke.html> [accessed 15 February 2005]; Baron, Marcia. "Love and Respect in the *Doctrine of Virtue*." In Nelson Potter and Mark Timmons, eds., *Kant's Metaphysics of Morals. Southern Journal of Philosophy* 35, supp. (1997), 29–44. Reprinted in Mark Timmons, ed., *Kant's Metaphysics of Morals: Interpretative Essays*. Oxford, U.K.: Oxford University Press, 2002, 391–407; Baumrin, Bernard. "Sexual Immorality Delineated." In Robert B. Baker and Frederick A. Elliston, eds., *Philosophy and Sex*, 1st ed. Buffalo, N.Y.: Prometheus, 1975, 116–28. Reprinted in P&S2 (300–311); Bell, Linda. "Sex as Limited Perspective." *Metaphilosophy* 17 (April–July 1986), 126–34; Belliotti, Raymond. "Immanuel Kant." In *Good Sex: Perspectives on Sexual Ethics*. Lawrence: University Press of Kansas, 1993, 98–103; Belliotti, Raymond. "Sexual Intercourse between Consenting Adults Is Always Permissible."

In Louis P. Pojman, ed., *The Moral Life: An Introductory Reader in Ethics and Literature*. New York: Oxford University Press, 2000, 681–89; Bencivegna, Ermanno. "Kant's Sadism." *Philosophy and Literature* 20:1 (1996), 39–46; Blum, Lawrence. "Kant's and Hegel's Moral Rationalism: A Feminist Perspective." *Canadian Journal of Philosophy* 12 (June 1982), 287–302; Burch, Robert W. "The Commandability of Pathological Love." *Southwestern Journal of Philosophy* [*Philosophical Topics*] 3:3 (1972), 131–40. Reprinted in Alan Soble, ed., *Eros, Agape, and Philia: Readings in the Philosophy of Love*. New York: Paragon House, 1989, 245–53; Cash, Mason. "Distancing Kantian Ethics and Politics from Kant's Views on Women." *Minerva—An Internet Journal of Philosophy* 6 (2002), 103–50. <www.ul.ie/~philos/vol6/kantian.html> [accessed 27 July 2004]; Cohen, G. A. *Self-Ownership, Freedom, and Equality*. Cambridge: Cambridge University Press, 1995; Denis, Lara. *Moral Self-Regard: Duties to Oneself in Kant's Moral Theory*. New York: Garland, 2001; Eaton, Marcia M. "Kant and Contextual Beauty." *Journal of Aesthetics and Art Criticism* 57:1 (1999), 11–15. Reprinted in Peg Zeglin Brand, ed., *Beauty Matters*. Bloomington: Indiana University Press, 2000, 27–36; Finnis, John. "Law, Morality, and 'Sexual Orientation.'" *Notre Dame Law Review* 69:5 (1994), 1049–76. Reprinted, revised, in *Notre Dame Journal of Law, Ethics, and Public Policy* 9:1 (1995), 11–39; and John Corvino, ed., *Same Sex: Debating the Ethics, Science, and Culture of Homosexuality*. Lanham, Md.: Rowman and Littlefield, 1997, 31–43; Garry, Ann. "Pornography and Respect for Women." *Social Theory and Practice* 4:4 (1978), 395–421. Reprinted in Sharon Bishop and Marjorie Weinzweig, eds., *Philosophy and Women*. Belmont, Calif.: Wadsworth, 1979, 128–39; P&S2 (312–26); Garry, Ann. "Sex (and Other) Objects." In Alan Soble, ed., *Sex, Love, and Friendship*. Amsterdam, Holland: Rodopi, 1997, 163–67; Garry, Ann. "Sex, Lies, and Pornography." In Hugh LaFollette, ed., *Ethics in Practice: An Anthology*, 2nd ed. Malden, Mass.: Blackwell, 2002, 344–55; Goldman, Alan. "Plain Sex." *Philosophy and Public Affairs* 6:3 (1977), 267–87. Reprinted in HS (103–23); POS1 (119–38); POS2 (73–92); POS3 (39–55); POS4 (39–55); Green, Ronald M. *Kierkegaard and Kant: The Hidden Debt*. Albany: State University of New York Press, 1992; Guyer, Paul, ed. *The Cambridge Companion to Kant*. Cambridge: Cambridge University Press, 1992; Kant, Immanuel. (1788) *Critique of Practical Reason*. Ed. and trans. Mary Gregor. Cambridge: Cambridge University Press, 1997; Kant, Immanuel. "Duties towards the Body in Respect of Sexual Impulse." In *Lectures on Ethics*. Trans. Louis Infield. New York: Methuen, 1930. Indianapolis, Ind.: Hackett, 1980, 162–71. Reprinted in POS4 (199–205); STW (140–45); Kant, Immanuel. *Education*. Trans. Annette Churton. London: Kegan Paul, Trench, Trubner, 1899. Boston, Mass.: D. C. Heath, 1900. Reprinted, Ann Arbor: University of Michigan Press, 1960; Kant, Immanuel. *Kant's gesammelte Schriften*, 29 vols. Ed. Deutsche Akademie der Wissenschaften. Berlin, Ger.: Walter de Gruyter, 1900–   ; Kant, Immanuel. (ca. 1784–1785) "Lecture on Friendship." In Michael Pakaluk, ed., *Other Selves: Philosophers on Friendship*. Indianapolis, Ind.: Hackett, 1991, 210–17; Kant, Immanuel. (ca. 1788) "On Philosophers' Medicine of the Body." Trans. Mary J. Gregor. In Lewis White Beck, ed., *Kant's Latin Writings: Translations, Commentaries, and Notes*. New York: Peter Lang, 1986, 217–43; Kant, Immanuel. *Philosophical Correspondence: 1759–99*. Trans. Arnulf Zweig. Chicago, Ill.: University of Chicago Press, 1967; Kennedy, Ellen, and Susan Mendus, eds. *Women in Western Political Philosophy: Kant to Nietzsche*. New York: St. Martin's Press, 1987; Kofman, Sarah. "The Economy of Respect: Kant and Respect for Women." Trans. Nicola Fisher. In Robin May Schott, ed., *Feminist Interpretations of Immanuel Kant*. University Park: Pennsylvania State University Press, 1997, 355–72. Reprinted from *Social Research* 49:2 (1982), 383–404; Korsgaard, Christine M. "Creating the Kingdom of Ends: Reciprocity and Responsibility in Personal Relations." *Philosophical Perspectives* 6, *Ethics* (1992), 305–32. Reprinted in *Creating the Kingdom of Ends*. Cambridge: Cambridge University Press, 1996, 188–221; Lacan, Jacques. "Kant avec Sade." In *Écrits*. Paris: Editions du Seuil, 1966, 765–90. "Kant with Sade." Trans. James Swenson. *October*, no. 51 (Winter 1989), 55–75; Madigan, Timothy. "The Discarded Lemon: Kant, Prostitution and Respect for Persons." *Philosophy Now*, no. 21 (Summer–Autumn 1998), 14–16. Reprinted in James E. Elias, Vern L. Bullough, Veronica Elias, and Gwen Brewer, eds., *Prostitution: On Whores, Hustlers, and Johns*. Amherst, N.Y.: Prometheus, 1998, 107–11; Mappes, Thomas A. (1985) "Sexual Morality and the Concept of Using Another Person." In Thomas A. Mappes and Jane S. Zembaty, eds., *Social*

Ethics: Morality and Social Policy, 4th ed. New York: McGraw-Hill, 1992, 203–16. 5th ed., 1997, 163–76. 6th ed., 2002, 170–83. Reprinted in POS4 (207–23); Marshall, John. "Kantian Ethics." In Lawrence C. Becker and Charlotte B. Becker, eds., *Encyclopedia of Ethics*, 2nd ed., vol. 2. New York: Routledge, 2001, 939–43; McEvoy, James. "Friendship within Marriage: A Philosophical Essay." In Luke Gormally, ed., *Moral Truth and Moral Tradition: Essays in Honour of Peter Geach and Elizabeth Anscombe*. Dublin, Ire.: Four Courts Press, 1994, 194–202; Michels, Robert. *Sexual Ethics: A Study of Borderland Questions*. London: Walter Scott, 1914; Millgram, Elijah. "Kantian Crystallization." *Ethics* 114:3 (2004), 511–13; Moscovici, Claudia. *From Sex Objects to Sexual Subjects*. New York: Routledge, 1996; Nussbaum, Martha C. "Objectification." *Philosophy and Public Affairs* 24:4 (1995), 249–91. Reprinted in POS3 (283–321); POS4 (381–419). Reprinted, revised, in *Sex and Social Justice*. New York: Oxford University Press, 1999, 213–39; O'Neill, Onora. "Between Consenting Adults." *Philosophy and Public Affairs* 14:3 (1985), 252–77. Reprinted in *Constructions of Reason: Explorations of Kant's Practical Philosophy*. Cambridge: Cambridge University Press, 1989, 105–25; Paton, H. J. "Kant on Friendship." The Dawes Hicks Lecture on Philosophy, 1956. *Proceedings of the British Academy* 42 (1956), 45–66. Reprinted in Neera K. Badhwar, ed., *Friendship: A Philosophical Reader*. Ithaca, N.Y.: Cornell University Press, 1993, 210–17; Schott, Robin May. *Cognition and Eros: A Critique of the Kantian Paradigm*. University Park: Pennsylvania State University Press, 1993; Schott, Robin May. "Feminism and Kant: Antipathy or Sympathy?" In Jane Kneller, ed., *Autonomy and Community*. Albany: State University of New York Press, 1998, 87–100; Schott, Robin May, ed. *Feminist Interpretations of Immanuel Kant*. University Park: Pennsylvania State University Press, 1997; Schwarzenbach, Sibyl. "On Owning the Body." In James E. Elias, Vern L. Bullough, Veronica Elias, and Gwen Brewer, eds., *Prostitution: On Whores, Hustlers, and Johns*. Amherst, N.Y.: Prometheus, 1998, 345–51; Shell, Susan Meld. *The Embodiment of Reason: Kant on Spirit, Generation, and Community*. Chicago, Ill.: University of Chicago Press, 1996; Shell, Susan Meld. *The Rights of Reason: A Study of Kant's Philosophy and Politics*. Toronto, Can.: University of Toronto Press, 1980; Singer, Irving. "Benign Romanticism: Kant, Schlegel, Hegel, Shelly, Byron." In *The Nature of Love*, vol. 2: *Courtly and Romantic*. Chicago, Ill.: University of Chicago Press, 1984, 376–431; Singer, Irving. "The Morality of Sex: Contra Kant." *Critical Horizons* 1:2 (2000), 175–91. Reprinted in *Explorations in Love and Sex*. Lanham, Md.: Rowman and Littlefield, 2001, 1–20; POS4 (259–72); Singer, Irving. *The Pursuit of Love*. Baltimore, Md.: Johns Hopkins University Press, 1994; Smith, Steven G. (1992) "The Attractions of Gender." In Alan Soble, ed., *Sex, Love, and Friendship*. Amsterdam, Holland: Rodopi, 1997, 547–53; Snow, Nancy E. "Are the Attractions of Gender Really Attractions?" In Alan Soble, ed., *Sex, Love, and Friendship*. Amsterdam, Holland: Rodopi, 1997, 555–57; Soble, Alan. "Sexual Use and What to Do about It: Internalist and Externalist Sexual Ethics." *Essays in Philosophy* 2:2 (2001). <www.humboldt.edu/~essays/soble.html> [accessed 27 July 2004]. Reprinted, revised, in POS4 (225–58); Soble, Alan. "Union, Autonomy, and Concern." In Roger Lamb, ed., *Love Analyzed*. Boulder, Colo.: Westview, 1997, 65–92; Sparshott, Francis. "Kant without Sade." *Philosophy and Literature* 21:1 (1997), 151–54; Spencer, Herbert. "The Ethics of Kant." In *Essays: Scientific, Political and Speculative*, vol. 3. London: Williams and Norgate, 1901, 192–216; Sullivan, Roger J. *Immanuel Kant's Moral Theory*. Cambridge: Cambridge University Press, 1989; Trainor, Brian T. "The State, Marriage, and Divorce." *Journal of Applied Philosophy* 9:2 (1992), 135–48; Ward, Keith. *The Development of Kant's View of Ethics*. Oxford, U.K.: Basil Blackwell, 1972; Wilson, Holly. "Kant's Evolutionary Theory of Marriage." In Jane Kneller, ed., *Autonomy and Community*. Albany: State University of New York Press, 1998, 283–306; Wolff, Robert Paul, ed. *Kant: A Collection of Critical Essays*. Garden City, N.Y.: Anchor Books, 1967; Žižek, Slavoj. "Kant and Sade: The Ideal Couple." *Lacanian Ink* 13 (Fall 1998), 12–25.

KIERKEGAARD, SØREN (1813–1855).

Danish philosopher Søren Aabye Kierkegaard, born in Copenhagen, has had considerable influence and deserved fame. Undergraduates find him perennially fascinating, and much contemporary theology and philosophy has been influenced by his searching and profound investigations. Kierkegaard's literary production, some twenty published volumes and 50,000 pages of journals and papers, is a staggering output for a forty-two-year life.

There are only a few dramatic episodes in his largely literary life, yet they constitute the story line and emotional reservoir for much of his writings. The autobiographical references in Kierkegaard's early aesthetic writings constitute a tantalizing tangle for the interpreter. In particular, his provocative and insightful discussions of sexuality make unavoidable taking his life into cautious consideration. But even though Kierkegaard warns us not to be led astray by a biographical interest, he makes it nearly impossible to pass the Sirens he has established, since he virtually seduces the reader closer to the prohibited shores.

A major sexual event in Kierkegaard's life was breaking his engagement to Regine Olsen (1822–1904). The sixteen-year-old Regine had been close to becoming engaged to another man when, in 1840, Kierkegaard surprisingly asked for her hand. Kierkegaard records immediate doubts about having proposed but did not return the ring until nearly a year later. An engagement in nineteenth-century Denmark was a serious commitment, ushering in a period of ritual family integration. Breaking an engagement was scandalous, a source of gossip, shameful for the families and engaged couple, but mostly the woman. Regine's plea to Kierkegaard not to break with her, her father's equal desperation, and the unbridgeable chasm that resulted from such a rupture must be understood in this context. Regine was a charmingly innocent girl; there is no reason to think that relations between Regine and Kierkegaard were anything but proper by the standards of the day. Indeed, Kierkegaard was shocked and worried about appearances when the jilted Regine despairingly came to his apartment. Kierkegaard sought to appear the cad to the Copenhagen public so as to insulate Regine. (See *Journals and Papers* [*JP*], entry 6472; *Papirer* X⁵, 149 [1849].)

The engagement was the literary inspiration for several works: *Either/Or*, volume 1 (*E/O* 1), including "The Seducer's Diary" and "The Rotation Method of Crops" ("When two people fall in love with each other and sense that they are destined for each other, it is a question of having the courage to break it off, for by continuing there is only everything to lose, nothing to gain" [*E/O* 1, 298]); the prodigious counterargument of "The Aesthetic Validity of Marriage" (*E/O* 2), in which the ethico-religious Judge William argues that eros, **marriage**, and Christianity are compatible; "Guilty?"/"Not Guilty?" (in *Stages on Life's Way*) and *Repetition*, both of which deal with broken engagements; and *Fear and Trembling*, which dwells on the miraculous restoration of an innocent sacrificial victim (Abraham's Isaac). Tinges of regret and a deep sense of loss permeate Kierkegaard's writings, as well as ambivalence about his breaking the engagement. ("Marry, and you will regret it. Do not marry, you will also regret it. Marry or do not marry, you will regret it either way. Whether you marry or do not marry, you will regret it either way" ("Diapsalmata," *E/O* 1, 138). In fact, he gives so many indirect versions of a broken engagement story that one might well see here a classic Freudian repetition compulsion, nowhere more clearly than in the work titled *Repetition* itself (see McCarthy, 274–78).

Kierkegaard felt mild shock when Regine became engaged to Fritz Schlegel (1817–1896), her original intended, at a time when Kierkegaard was still privately indulging thoughts of a reengagement. He remained devoted to Regine, dedicated his authorship to her, had copies of his work specially bound for her, and hoped for some sort of reconciliation, perhaps in their old age. It was not to be.

Why Kierkegaard broke with Regine is fascinating but unanswerable, except by a kind of speculation that Kierkegaard mocked. Since the dawn of the Age of Freud, some have conjectured that Kierkegaard was impotent or homosexual, for which there is no evidence. Was it due to a Freudian, masochistic, self-castration resulting from a sense of guilt? Or—to consider an extreme view—was it the Sadeian culmination of toying with and emotionally torturing an innocent girl (Fenger, 210), as Johannes does to Cordelia in "The Seducer's Diary"? Did he intuit that the marriage of the precocious, intellectual, twenty-seven-year-old son of a wealthy merchant and an innocent girl of sixteen from a good family was a mismatch? Kierkegaard does comment that he did not want to introduce Regine to, and inflict on her, his melancholy and family secrets (*JP*, 5664). Kierkegaard's father, Michael Pedersen Kierkegaard (1756–1838), had impregnated a family servant, Ane Sørensdatter Lund (1768–1834), while his first wife (Kirstine) was ill and married her soon after his wife's death. Ane Lund Kierkegaard was the mother of all seven of the Kierkegaard children, including Søren. When she died (1834), followed quickly by several of his siblings, Kierkegaard sensed that the family was cursed. A journal entry after his father's death (1838) expressed this sense as hopelessness about leading a happy family life, specifically about the continuity of the family line (*JP*, 5431; *Papirer* II, A 806).

In addition to experiencing apprehension about the sexual sins of the father (or parents) being inherited by the son (the Danish term for the "original sin" of Adam and Eve is "inherited sin," *Arvesynden*), Kierkegaard may have been vexed—as was **Saint Augustine** (354–430)—by his youthful dissipation (*JP*, 5403; *Papirer* II, A 520 [28 July 1839]; see Green, 200, 282n.37). Kierkegaard has one of his pseudonyms examine street urchins' faces on Copenhagen boulevards, searching for signs of having fathered one with a prostitute (*Stages*, 283–84). His journals contain a version of this parable that is (only) possibly applicable to Kierkegaard's life:

> Once in his early youth a man allowed himself to be so far carried away in an overwrought irresponsible state as to visit a prostitute. It is all forgotten. Now he wants to get married. Then anxiety stirs. He is tortured day and night with the thought that he might possibly be a father. . . . He cannot share his secret with anyone; he does not have any reliable knowledge of the fact. . . . [T]his very ignorance is the basis of his agitated torment. . . . [H]is misgivings do not really start until he actually falls in love. (*JP*, 5622; *Papirer* IV, A 65 [1843])

In another journal entry, Kierkegaard writes that if he had gone through with the engagement, Regine would have been more his concubine, not a wife, since he could not have been open with her, as demanded by an ethical marriage (*JP*, 5664; *Papirer* IV, A 107 [1843]). And Judge William writes, "[I]f in some way or another you have swallowed a secret that cannot be dragged out of you without costing your life—then never marry" (*E/O* 2, 117; see Watson, 358). As a result, "the curse that hangs over me is that I never dare let any person become deeply and intimately attached to me" (*JP*, 5517; *Papirer* III, A 161 [1841]).

Kierkegaard laments, "I would have had to initiate her into terrible things, my relationship to my father, his melancholy, the eternal brooding night within me, my going astray, my lusts and debauchery, which, however, in the eyes of God are perhaps not so glaring; for it was, after all, anxiety which brought me to go astray, and where was I to seek a safe stronghold when I knew or suspected that the only man [his father] I had admired for his strength was tottering" (*JP*, 5664; *Papirer* IV, A 107 [1843]). Despite his sense of sinfulness, as the Pietism of his time would have emphasized, Kierkegaard apparently knows he is being hard on himself, like the exaggerating Augustine (*Confessions*, bk. 2, chaps. 1–3). Unless guilt and suffering make a sinner, rather than deeds, we witness here only a tortured soul.

Sexuality is most explicitly considered in *Concept of Anxiety* by the pseudonymous Vigilius Haufniensis, a work in which Kierkegaard analyzes anxiety as a summons to self-actualization (in advance of twentieth-century **existentialism**). *Anxiety* takes the form of a theological treatise, focusing on sin as a pressing existential problem to overcome. Comments on sexuality emerge from an exploration of the traditional and medieval theological link between sinfulness and sexuality. But this standpoint eventually reveals itself to have been only a point of departure, and Kierkegaard's understanding of sexuality goes well beyond it. He proposes a higher form of sexuality linked with spiritual striving and provides an account of eros as a dynamism propelling one beyond the merely sensuous (as in Diotima's position presented by Socrates in **Plato**'s [ca. 427–347 BCE] *Symposium*, 210a–12b).

Anxiety considers sexuality narrowly—as a drive to gratify sensuality, combined with a drive to attain immortality through reproduction—to suggest a higher possibility for it. Greek paganism's philosophy of **beauty** is held to be the positive flowering of sensualism, while Judaism is held to represent the other pole of sexuality, self-perpetuation through reproduction, both of which are contrasted with the spirituality held to be introduced by Christianity. Kierkegaard contends that spirituality transcends sensuality and the reproductive urge by subsuming them into the spiritual life enabled by Christianity. Kierkegaard's **language** speaks of Christianity "introducing" spirituality and hence differentiating sensuality from spirituality. His language goes so far as to imply that Christianity suspends the erotic (70) because, in the higher spiritual reality, no difference between man and woman exists. Further, the victory of Christian **love** in a person means that the sexual is overcome and forgotten (80).

Kierkegaard wants to reestablish the preeminence of the spiritual, but he also wants to affirm a positive relationship, beyond ancient Greeks and modern Romantics, between spirituality and sensuality/sexuality (or spirit and flesh). He acknowledges, however, that sexuality, through the traditional biblical interpretation of Adam's original sin, has come to *signify* sinfulness (*Anxiety*, 67). Despite this association, Kierkegaard emphasizes that neither sensuality nor sexuality is the sinful (68, 79–80). But this line of thought is blurred, since *Anxiety*'s pseudonym Haufniensis holds that Adam's sin, while not a sexual sin, is nonetheless the cause of **sexual desire** (49, 79). This asserts traditional Christian theology, but Kierkegaard does so with a gospel freshness that is free of the negative sexual theology of **Saint Paul** (5–64?) and Clement of Alexandria (ca. 150–215). Persons thus have the possibility of becoming, and propagating the species as, spiritually qualified beings. At this higher stage, married parents transmit a well-formed view of life in addition to genes. Kierkegaard cannot resist, however, ironically observing that the maturity required for this parenting emerges only after the years in which sexual desire is strongest (*JP*, 2622; *Papirer* XI², A 250 [1854]).

While establishing spirituality's preeminence, Kierkegaard aims poison-tipped arrows at the formal Christianity of the time that, in his view, had betrayed its core principles in trying to accommodate a reemergent rival philosophy of spiritless sexuality and sensuality. Much of Kierkegaard's early aesthetic authorship is a literary portrayal of this cultural problem. How spiritually indifferent sexuality, tending toward selfishness and frequently resulting in sin, can be elevated to a higher humanity is the task of *E/O 2*, in which Judge William critiques the young aesthete of *E/O 1*, who is lost in sensuality. William argues (and demonstrates in his life) that sexuality finds its proper place in the ethical state of marriage, which he characterizes as open, committed, and charitably loving (*E/O 2*, 116). For William, (Christian) married love leaves room for the eroticism of first love (*E/O 2*, 31) while elevating the lovers to equals before God.

But Kierkegaard elsewhere calls his readers to a life of Christian love that transcends sensuality. "The lover's desire presumably is not selfish in relation to the beloved's, but the desire of both together is absolutely selfish insofar as they in union and in love form one self " (*Stages*, 42–43). Their union eliminates one selfishness, only to replace it with another. "The more securely the two I's come together to become one I" (à la Aristophanes in Plato's *Symposium* [190e–91d]), the more in loving each other the lovers love only themselves. "The beloved [is] therefore called, . . . significantly enough, the other-self, the other-I" (*Works of Love* [*WOL*], 68). Kierkegaard argues, that is, that erotic love, through self-interest and passionate preference, is incompatible with Christian love. (It is water to the fire that is Christian love, *WOL*, 73; see Lindström, 2; Outka, 17–18.) "Confusion," he writes, "develops when the defense amounts to this—that Christianity certainly teaches a higher love but *in addition* praises friendship and erotic love. To talk thus is a double betrayal—inasmuch as the speaker has neither the spirit of the poet nor the spirit of Christianity" (*WOL*, 59; for a similar idea in Augustine, see Schlabach, 133). Kierkegaard also eventually condemns the "superior" married lifestyle that Judge William demonstrates and offers to the young aesthete. Kierkegaard does so not to defend aesthetic sensuality but (as in Paul, 1 Cor. 7:29, 32–33; see Gregory Vlastos [1907–1991] on Plato, 41) to point toward a form of life higher than ethical marriage: "The hearty twaddle of family life constitutes the worst danger for Christianity, and not wild lusts, debauchery, terrible passions and the like. They are not so opposed to Christianity as this flat mediocrity, this stuffy reek, this nearness to one another. . . . There is no greater distance from obedience to the either-or than this flat, hearty family twaddle" (*Papirer* XI², A 152; *The Last Years*, 265). The point seems to be that mere physical "nearness" of the spouses to each other prevents them from focusing on God and thereby leading a fully Christian spiritual life. They "first and foremost belong to God," who should be "the only beloved object" (*WOL*, 118, 124; see Collins, 76; Lindström, 7–8; Watson, 358). This may be why Kierkegaard insists that one's spouse is "first and foremost" one's neighbor (141).

Kierkegaard's authorship is largely concerned about the transformation of individuals from beings in search of satisfying animal needs to beings in whom a religious dimension has suffused all others. This happens when individuals transcend mere aestheticism, including all sensuality, and emerge into the greater sphere of the ethico-religious. Judge William is the symbol and literary instantiation of this view, in contrast to the young aesthete, who functions as the spokesperson and exemplar of the initially fetching but ultimately bankrupt sensual life. Kierkegaard is well known for his doctrine of three stages: the aesthetic, the ethical, and the religious. Here, as elsewhere, his use of a triad is sometimes more formal than substantive and can be frequently viewed as a spoof on the dialectic of **G.W.F. Hegel** (1770–1831).

Kierkegaard's thoughts on sexuality are elaborated in his extended discussions of desire. (The Danish is *Elskov*, the standard term for translating the Greek *eros*.) While Kierkegaard only sparingly mentions "sex" and "sexuality," the erotic and sensuality are major themes in his aesthetic pseudonymous writings of the 1840s. In "The Immediate Stages of the Musical Erotic" (*E/O* 1), the anonymous "A" finds three stages of desire represented in three operas by Wolfgang Amadeus Mozart (1756–1791). Cherubino in *Marriage of Figaro* (1786) is taken to symbolize desire in its first stage, when it is not yet awakened. Desire at this point does not have a clear object, as symbolized by Cherubino's swooning over and chasing woman—virtually any woman and every woman—in bumbling adolescent fashion. In love with love, Cherubino darts wildly in all directions toward the possible gratification of his sexual needs. Any woman will do. As a result he is comical, farcical, even if charmingly so. Papageno of *Magic Flute* (1791) symbolizes awakening desire. The lonely, naive, sweetly melancholic young man is looking for his "other," appropriately named "Papagena," but he does not know what she looks like. Hence his search is blind, but he is convinced he will recognize his "true love" when he finds her. She eventually reveals herself to him in homely disguise, suggesting that any girl who knew the magic word "Papagena" would have had the same success. Desire here is the recognition of a need for a specific, single other to be the possibility of one's emotional and physical satisfaction. (Cf. the discussion of this theme by Walsh, 610–13.) Later, in *Fear and Trembling*, Kierkegaard critiques Papageno's stage:

> Again and again we hear this story in poetry: A man is bound to one girl whom he once loved or perhaps never loved properly, for he has seen another girl who is the ideal. A man makes a mistake in life; it was the right street but the wrong house, for directly across the street on the second floor lives the ideal—this is supposed to be a subject for poetry. A lover has made a mistake, he has seen the beloved by artificial light and thought she had dark hair, but look, on close scrutiny she is a blonde—but her sister is the ideal. This is supposed to be a subject for poetry. In my opinion, any man like that is an impudent young pup who can be unbearable enough in life but ought to be hissed off stage. (91; see Thurber and White's less solemn treatment, 99)

Kierkegaard underscores the point in *Works of Love*: "[T]he task is not: to find—the lovable object; but the task is: to find the object already given or chosen—lovable, and to be able to continue finding him lovable, no matter how he becomes changed" (158; italics omitted). "When it is a duty to love the men we see, then one must first and foremost give up all fanciful and extravagant ideas about a dream-world where the object of love is to be sought and found" (159; italics omitted).

In "The Immediate Stages of the Musical Erotic," genuine desire—the third stage—emerges fully in Mozart's *Don Giovanni* (1787). There is a broad leap from Papageno's innocent desire for his Papagena to the compulsive womanizer Don Giovanni, who desires one woman absolutely—and then for just a moment. His famous list of conquests, including 1,003 in Spain alone, displays the breadth of his interest as well as his unfreedom as the prisoner of sexual compulsion. He is depicted as having a store of seemingly inexhaustible, demonic energy that thrashes about in the thrall of sexual desire. When, at the opera's end, Don Giovanni accepts the challenge of the Commendatore, he tellingly chooses the eternal damnation of hellfire over the seemingly inexhaustible-but-exhausting fires of insatiable sexual desire.

The reader should be wary of Kierkegaard's positing three stages of desire, as it may well be satire on Hegelianism. Indeed, his pseudonym concedes that at least the first stage might not really qualify. Moreover, *E/O* 1 presents a more important and dramatic fourth stage of desire—in Johannes, the psychological seducer of "Diary." In contrast to Don Giovanni, Johannes desires only one woman and desires her in an absolutized moment in which she also desires him. Furthermore, Johannes does not really desire her physically. In this rich thought-experiment, physical conquest is an afterthought. For what Johannes truly desires is *her desire*, that she desire him. In achieving this, he believes that he outdoes Don Giovanni with his 1,003. Johannes's desire, too, might be called demonic, but he appears to be more nearly the master of the demon of desire, as he step-by-step plots the **seduction** of the innocent Cordelia (is she Regine?) and uses those around her for his demonic purposes.

But if this is the culmination of aesthetic desire, Kierkegaard makes sure that his pseudonyms indicate that it is a dead end. The result of this way of life is chronicled in "Diapsalmata," hymns and epigrams of restlessness and self-loathing.

In *Repetition*, the pseudonymous psychologist Constantine Constantius steps backward from desire-run-wild in Don Giovanni and Johannes to consider the paradoxically unsatisfied desire of another Papageno who has found and become engaged to his Papagena. *Repetition*'s nameless Young Man has fallen in love with and become engaged to a nameless young woman. His enduring melancholy (*Melancholi*) is taken as the negative index of desire: He learns by scrutinizing his desire that *it is not she*. In fact, no woman can satisfy the depth of desire that he discovers coursing beneath human desire. Constantius pronounces the young man's melancholy to have a religious depth requiring a religious solution, and Kierkegaard thereby more than hints where this analysis of desire will head. (The degree to which this literary work anticipates **Sigmund Freud**'s [1856–1939] *Beyond the Pleasure Principle*, a study of repetition compulsion and the principle of constancy, is uncanny. See McCarthy.) As if to prevent readers from missing the point, the story line is virtually repeated in *Stages*' "Guilty?"/"Not Guilty?" By way of emphasizing the gravity and depth of a melancholy not satisfied by an earthly beloved, contrary to received romantic wisdom, *Melancholi* is replaced with the darker *Tungsind*, which suggests a melancholy longing about to implode.

Kierkegaard's treatment of these issues is entirely from the male perspective. (See Céline Léon and Sylvia Walsh for discussion.) However, in the manner of his time, he believed that when he wrote of "men" he was achieving a universal analysis applicable to women. By our standards, Kierkegaard is a male chauvinist. But he is not misogynist (in, for example, the manner of **Friedrich Nietzsche** [1844–1900]). Kierkegaard speaks of women as essentially aesthetic, even if equally destined with men for the religious. Women will rightly take offense that Kierkegaard seems to absent them (as did **Arthur Schopenhauer** [1788–1860] and Freud) from the ethical. Feminists will also count against him his indifference to the emerging women's emancipation movement. But when Kierkegaard criticizes women, it is mostly for letting themselves be determined by men, by allowing themselves to become what men want them to be—symbolized above all by fashion— rather than authentically becoming the spiritual equal of men. This theme is advanced in *Stages*' "In Vino Veritas," an imitation of Plato's *Symposium* (ca. 380 BCE) in which various aesthetes gather for a discussion of erotic love but in which the topic shifts to Woman. Throughout, Kierkegaard holds that women are equal to men and that their equality is actualized when, and to the extent that, they are spiritually realized persons.

For Kierkegaard, human sexuality is finally to be understood as part of a deeper, more powerful, more enveloping movement to union and reunion with the One, the Absolute, the Creator God (as in, for example, Tillich, 28). His is the Christian Neo-Platonism of Saint Augustine expressed in the nineteenth-century language of Romanticism and Idealism, even as it seeks to critique and distance itself from those cultural trends. Kierkegaard's philosophy self-consciously updates the classic and medieval journey of the soul to God. In his version of the *Symposium*, he ultimately advocates a view analogous to Diotima's. It would be easy to dismiss Kierkegaard, in Nietzschean-sounding language, as a religious romantic proffering defunct metaphysics. But Kierkegaard has his Augustinian retort: The test of a view about human life lies in existence itself. There it either produces the promised result or it fails. For Kierkegaard, one does not need to argue metaphysics; experience is the arbiter. For him, one needs, above all, to be open to *all* experience, including the pull of a return to the One.

See also Augustine (Saint); Existentialism; Flirting; Hegel, G.W.F.; Hobbes, Thomas; Kant, Immanuel; Love; Paul (Saint); Phenomenology; Plato; Seduction; Wojtyła, Karol (Pope John Paul II)

REFERENCES

Augustine. (397) *Confessions*. Trans. F. J. Sheed. Indianapolis, Ind.: Hackett, 1993; Collins, James D. *The Mind of Kierkegaard*. Chicago, Ill.: H. Regnery, 1965; Fenger, Henning. *Kierkegaard, the Myths and the Origins: Studies in the Kierkegaardian Papers and Letters*. Trans. George C. Schoolfield. New Haven, Conn.: Yale University Press, 1980; Freud, Sigmund. (1920) *Beyond the Pleasure Principle*. Trans. James Strachey. New York: Norton, 1990; Green, Ronald M. *Kierkegaard and Kant: The Hidden Debt*. Albany: State University of New York Press, 1992; Kierkegaard, Søren. (1844) *The Concept of Anxiety*. Trans. Howard V. Hong and Edna H. Hong. Princeton, N.J.: Princeton University Press, 1980; Kierkegaard, Søren. (1843) *Either/Or*, vols. 1 and 2. Trans. Howard V. Hong and Edna H. Hong. Princeton, N.J.: Princeton University Press, 1987; Kierkegaard, Søren. (1843) *Fear and Trembling* and *Repetition*. Trans. Howard V. Hong and Edna H. Hong. Princeton, N.J.: Princeton University Press, 1983; Kierkegaard, Søren. *Journals and Papers*, 7 vols. Ed. and trans. Howard V. Hong and Edna H. Hong. Bloomington: Indiana University Press, 1967–1978; Kierkegaard, Søren. *The Last Years: Journals 1853–1855*. Trans. R. G. Smith. New York: Harper and Row, 1965; Kierkegaard, Søren. *Papirer*, 2nd ed., 16 vols. Ed. Niels Thulstrup. Copenhagen, Den.: Gyldendal, 1968–1978; Kierkegaard, Søren. (1845) *Stages on Life's Way*. Trans. Howard V. Hong and Edna H. Hong. Princeton, N.J.: Princeton University Press, 1988; Kierkegaard, Søren. (1847) *Works of Love: Some Christian Reflections in the Form of Discourses*. Trans. Howard V. Hong and Edna H. Hong. New York: Harper Torchbooks, 1964; Léon, Céline, and Sylvia Walsh, eds. *Feminist Interpretations of Søren Kierkegaard*. University Park: Pennsylvania State University Press, 1997; Lindström, Valter. "A Contribution to the Interpretation of Kierkegaard's book *The Works of Love*." *Studia Theologica* 6:1 (1953), 1–29; McCarthy, Vincent A. "*Repetition*'s Repetitions: Structural and Freudian Repetitions in Kierkegaard's Psychological Novella." In Robert L. Perkins, ed., *International Kierkegaard Commentary: Fear and Trembling and Repetition*. Macon, Ga.: Mercer University Press, 1993, 263–82; Outka, Gene. *Agape: An Ethical Analysis*. New Haven, Conn.: Yale University Press, 1972; Plato. (ca. 380 BCE) *The Symposium*. Trans. Christopher Gill. London: Penguin, 1999; Schlabach, Gerald W. "Friendship as Adultery: Social Reality and Sexual Metaphor in Augustine's Doctrine of Original Sin." *Augustinian Studies* 23 (1992), 125–47; Thurber, James, and E. B. White. *Is Sex Necessary? Or Why You Feel the Way You Do*. New York: Harper and Brothers, 1929; Tillich, Paul. *Love, Power, and Justice*. New York: Oxford University Press, 1960; Vlastos, Gregory. "Sex in Platonic Love." In *Platonic Studies*. Princeton, N.J.: Princeton University Press, 1973, 38–42; Walsh, Sylvia. "Desire and Love in Kierkegaard's *Either/Or*." In Alan Soble, ed., *Sex, Love, and Friendship*. Amsterdam, Holland: Rodopi, 1997, 610–22; Watson, Richard. "The Seducer and the Seduced." *Georgia Review* 39:2 (1985), 353–66.

Vincent A. McCarthy

ADDITIONAL READING

Adorno, Theodor W. "On Kierkegaard's Doctrine of Love." *Studies in Philosophy and Social Science* 8 (1940), 413–29; Allen, Woody. (1971) "My Philosophy." In *Getting Even*. New York: Vintage, 1978, 21–25; Allen, Woody. (1972) "Selections from the Allen Notebooks." In *Without Feathers*. New York: Ballantine, 1983, 7–10; Anderson, Susan Leigh. *On Kierkegaard*. Belmont, Calif.: Wadsworth, 2000; Arbaugh, George E., and George B. Arbaugh. *Kierkegaard's Authorship: A Guide to the Writings of Kierkegaard*. Rock Island, Ill.: Augustana College Library, 1967; Becker-Theye, Betty. *The Seducer as Mythic Figure in Richardson, Laclos, and Kierkegaard*. New York: Garland, 1988; Bourgeois, Patrick. "Kierkegaard: Ethical Marriage or Aesthetic Pleasure?" *The Personalist* 57:4 (1976), 370–75; Cady, Linell E. "Alternative Interpretations of Love in Kierkegaard and Royce." *Journal of Religious Ethics* 10:2 (1982), 238–63; Cappelørn, Neils J., Joakim Garff, and Johnny Kondrup. (1996) *Written Images: Søren Kierkegaard's Journals, Notebooks, Booklets, Sheets,*

Scraps, and Slips of Paper. Trans. Bruce H. Kirmmse. Princeton, N.J.: Princeton University Press, 2003; Cole, J. Preston. *The Problematic Self in Kierkegaard and Freud*. New Haven, Conn.: Yale University Press, 1971; Conant, James. "Nietzsche, Kierkegaard, and Anscombe on Moral Unintelligibility." In D. Z. Phillips, ed., *Religion and Morality*. New York: St. Martin's Press, 1996, 250–98; Dewey, Bradley R. "The Erotic-Demonic in Kierkegaard's 'Diary of the Seducer.'" *Scandinavica* 10 (1971), 1–24; Dunning, Stephen N. *Kierkegaard's Dialectic of Inwardness: A Structural Analysis of the Theory of Stages*. Princeton, N.J.: Princeton University Press, 1985; Emmanuel, Stephen M. "Biography in the Interpretation of Kierkegaard." In Alan Soble, ed., *Sex, Love, and Friendship*. Amsterdam, Holland: Rodopi, 1997, 493–500; Fendt, Gene. "Is *Works of Love* a Work of Love?" In Alan Soble, ed., *Sex, Love, and Friendship*. Amsterdam, Holland: Rodopi, 1997, 473–85; Fendt, Gene. *Works of Love? Reflections on Works of Love*. Potomac, Md.: Scripta Humanistica, 1990; Ferreira, M. Jamie. *Love's Grateful Striving: A Commentary on Kierkegaard's Works of Love*. Oxford, U.K.: Oxford University Press, 2001; Garff, Joakim. (2000) *Søren Kierkegaard: A Biography*. Trans. Bruce H. Kirmmse. Princeton, N.J.: Princeton University Press, 2005; Giles, James, ed. *Kierkegaard and Freedom*. New York: St. Martin's Press, 2001; Hall, Amy Laura. *Kierkegaard and the Treachery of Love*. Cambridge: Cambridge University Press, 2002; Hall, Ronald L. *The Human Embrace: The Love of Philosophy and the Philosophy of Love. Kierkegaard, Cavell, Nussbaum*. University Park: Pennsylvania State University Press, 2000; Hannay, Alastair. *Kierkegaard*. London: Routledge and Kegan Paul, 1982; Hannay, Alastair. *Kierkegaard: A Biography*. Cambridge: Cambridge University Press, 2001; Hannay, Alastair, and Gordon D. Marino, eds. *The Cambridge Companion to Kierkegaard*. Cambridge: Cambridge University Press, 1998; Heiss, Robert. *Hegel, Kierkegaard, Marx: Three Great Philosophers Whose Ideas Changed the Course of Civilization*. New York: Dell, 1975; Hubben, William. *Dostoevsky, Kierkegaard, Nietzsche, and Kafka: Four Prophets of Our Destiny*. New York: Collier, 1962; Kierkegaard, Søren. (1844) *The Concept of Anxiety*. Trans. Howard V. Hong and Edna H. Hong. Princeton, N.J.: Princeton University Press, 1980; Kierkegaard, Søren. (1843) *Either/Or*, vols. 1 and 2. Trans. Howard V. Hong and Edna H. Hong. Princeton, N.J.: Princeton University Press, 1987. Vol. 1: Trans. David F. Swenson and Lillian M. Swenson. Princeton, N.J.: Princeton University Press, 1971. Vol. 2: Trans. Walter Lowrie. Princeton, N.J.: Princeton University Press, 1971; Kimball, Roger. "What Did Kierkegaard Want?" *The New Criterion* 20:1 (2001). <www.newcriterion.com/archive/20/sept01/kierk.htm> [accessed 17 June 2005]; Liehu, Heidi. *Søren Kierkegaard's Theory of Stages and Its Relation to Hegel*. Helsinki: Philosophical Society of Finland, 1990; Lowrie, Walter. *A Short Life of Kierkegaard*. Princeton, N.J.: Princeton University Press, 1951; Mackey, Louis. *Kierkegaard: A Kind of Poet*. Philadelphia: University of Pennsylvania Press, 1971; Martin, Vincent. *Existentialism: Søren Kierkegaard, Jean-Paul Sartre, Albert Camus*. Washington, D.C.: Thomist Press, 1962; Matuštík, Martin J., and Merold Westphal, eds. *Kierkegaard in Post/Modernity*. Bloomington: Indiana University Press, 1995; McCarthy, Vincent A. " 'Melancholy' and 'Religious Melancholy' in Kierkegaard." In Niels Thulstrup, ed., *Kierkegaardiana X*. Copenhagen, Den.: C. A. Reitzels, 1977, 151–65; McCarthy, Vincent A. "Mourning and Melancholia in 'Quidam's Diary.' " In Robert L. Perkins, ed., *International Kierkegaard Commentary: Stages on Life's Way*. Macon, Ga.: Mercer University Press, 2000, 149–71; McCarthy, Vincent A. "Narcissism and Desire in Kierkegaard's *Either/Or*, Part One." In Robert L. Perkins, ed., *International Kierkegaard Commentary: Either/Or, Part 1*. Macon, Ga.: Mercer University Press, 1995, 51–72; McCarthy, Vincent A. *The Phenomenology of Moods in Kierkegaard*. The Hague, Holland: Martinus Nijhoff, 1978; McDonald, William. (1996) "Søren Kierkegaard." In *The Stanford Encyclopedia of Philosophy*. <plato.stanford.edu/entries/kierkegaard> [accessed 30 January 2004]; Morris, T. F. "Kierkegaard on Despair and the Eternal." *Sophia* 28 (1989), 21–30; Morris, T. F. "Kierkegaard on Despair in *Works of Love*." In Alan Soble, ed., *Sex, Love, and Friendship*. Amsterdam, Holland: Rodopi, 1997, 487–91; Mulhall, Stephen. *Inheritance and Originality: Wittgenstein, Heidegger, Kierkegaard*. Oxford, U.K.: Clarendon Press, 2001; Nordentoft, Kresten. "Erotic Love." In Niels Thurstrup and M. Mikulová Thulstrup, eds., *Kierkegaard and Human Values*. Copenhagen, Den.: C. A. Reitzels, 1980, 87–99; Nordentoft, Kresten. *Kierkegaard's Psychology*. Trans. Bruce H. Kirmmse. Pittsburgh, Pa.: Duquesne University Press, 1972; Nygren, Anders. (1953) *Agape and Eros*. Trans.

Philip S. Watson. Chicago, Ill.: University of Chicago Press, 1982; Perkins, Robert L. "Three Critiques of Schlegel's *Lucinde.*" In David Goicoechea, ed., *The Nature and Pursuit of Love: The Philosophy of Irving Singer.* Amherst, N.Y.: Prometheus, 1995, 149–66; Perkins, Robert L. "Woman-Bashing in Kierkegaard's 'In Vino Veritas': A Reinscription of Plato's *Symposium.*" In Céline Léon and Sylvia Walsh, eds., *Feminist Interpretations of Søren Kierkegaard.* University Park: Pennsylvania State University Press, 1997, 83–102; Perkins, Robert L., ed. *International Kierkegaard Commentary: The Concept of Anxiety.* Macon, Ga.: Mercer University Press, 1985; Perkins, Robert L., ed. *International Kierkegaard Commentary: Either/Or, Part 1.* Macon, Ga.: Mercer University Press, 1995; Perkins, Robert L., ed. *International Kierkegaard Commentary: Either/Or, Part 2.* Macon, Ga.: Mercer University Press, 1995; Perkins, Robert L., ed. *International Kierkegaard Commentary: Fear and Trembling and Repetition.* Macon, Ga.: Mercer University Press, 1993; Perkins, Robert L., ed. *International Kierkegaard Commentary: Stages on Life's Way.* Macon, Ga.: Mercer University Press, 2000; Perkins, Robert L., ed. *International Kierkegaard Commentary: Works of Love.* Macon, Ga.: Mercer University Press, 1999; Piety, M. G., and P. A. Bauer. "Not a Seducer" [Letter in reply to Updike]. *New York Review of Books* (25 September 1997), 77; Singer, Irving. "Anti-Romantic Romantics: Kierkegaard, Tolstoy, Nietzsche." In *The Nature of Love,* vol. 3: *The Modern World.* Chicago, Ill.: University of Chicago Press, 1987, 38–94; Smith, Joseph H.M.D., ed. *Kierkegaard's Truth: The Disclosure of the Self.* New Haven, Conn.: Yale University Press, 1981; Smyth, John Vignaux. *A Question of Eros: Irony in Sterne, Kierkegaard, and Barthes.* Tallahassee: Florida State University Press, 1986; Stack, George J. *Kierkegaard's Existential Ethics.* University: University of Alabama Press, 1977; Taylor, Mark C. *Journeys to Selfhood: Hegel and Kierkegaard.* Berkeley: University of California Press, 1980; Taylor, Mark C. "Love and Forms of Spirit: Kierkegaard vs. Hegel." In Niels Thulstrup, ed., *Kierkegaardiana X.* Copenhagen, Den.: C. A. Reitzels, 1977, 95–116; Thompson, Josiah. *Kierkegaard: A Critical Biography.* London: Gollanz, 1974; Updike, John. "On 'The Seducer's Diary.'" *New York Review of Books* (29 May 1997), 27–28; Utterback, Sylvia Walsh. "Don Juan and the Representation of Spiritual Sensuousness." *Journal of the American Academy of Religion* 47:4 (1979), 627–44; Vlastos, Gregory. "Sex in Platonic Love." In *Platonic Studies.* Princeton, N.J.: Princeton University Press, 1973, 38–42. Reprinted in Alan Soble, ed., *Eros, Agape, and Philia: Readings in the Philosophy of Love.* New York: Paragon House, 1989, 124–28; Walsh [Perkins], Sylvia. "Forming the Heart: The Role of Love in Kierkegaard's Thought." In Richard H. Bell, ed., *The Grammar of the Heart: New Essays in Moral Philosophy and Theology.* San Francisco, Calif.: Harper and Row, 1988, 234–56; Walsh [Perkins], Sylvia. "Ironic Love: An Amorist Interpretation of Socratic Eros." In Robert L. Perkins, ed., *International Kierkegaard Commentary: Concept of Irony,* vol. 2. Macon, Ga.: Mercer University Press, 2001, 123–40; Walsh [Perkins], Sylvia. "Issues That Divide: Interpreting Kierkegaard on Woman and Gender." In Niels J. Cappelørn and Jon Stewart, eds., *Kierkegaard Revisited.* New York: Walter de Gruyter, 1997, 191–205; Walsh [Perkins], Sylvia. "Kierkegaard's Philosophy of Love." In David Goicoechea, ed., *The Nature and Pursuit of Love: The Philosophy of Irving Singer.* Amherst, N.Y.: Prometheus, 1995, 167–79; Walsh [Perkins], Sylvia. *Living Poetically: Kierkegaard's Existential Aesthetics.* University Park: Pennsylvania State University Press, 1994; Walsh [Perkins], Sylvia. "Veni, Vidi, Vici: Immediacy and Reflection as Gendered Categories in Kierkegaard's Thought." In Paul Cruysberghs, Johan Taels, and Karl Verstrynge, eds., *Immediacy and Reflection in Kierkegaard's Thought.* Leuven, Den.: Leuven University Press, 2003, 25–39; Wood, Robert E. "Recollection and Two Banquets: Plato's and Kierkegaard's." In Robert L. Perkins, ed., *International Kierkegaard Commentary: Stages on Life's Way.* Macon, Ga.: Mercer University Press, 2000, 49–68; Xie, Wenyu. *The Concept of Freedom: The Platonic-Augustinian-Lutheran-Kierkegaardian Tradition.* Lanham, Md.: University Press of America, 2002; Yang, Chi-ming. *Pseudonymous Authorship and Kierkegaard's* Either/Or: *The Anxiety of the Aesthetic.* Stanford Honors Essay in Humanities Number XLII. Stanford, Calif.: Stanford University Humanities Honors Program, 1998; Zweig, Paul. (1968) "Kierkegaard, the Isolated One." In *The Heresy of Self-Love: A Study of Subversive Individualism.* Princeton, N.J.: Princeton University Press, 1980, 183–203.

KOLNAI, AUREL (1900–1973). When Aurel Thomas Kolnai's 439-page *Sexualethik* (*Sexual Ethics*) appeared in Germany in 1930, the review in *Literarischer Handweiser* called it the "prolegomenon to any future sexual ethics" (Wewel, 263). *Sexualethik* contains untechnical analyses of virtually every aspect of sexuality and is based firmly on the experience of the ordinary moral agent.

Kolnai was born in Budapest, Hungary. For his first twenty years, he enjoyed the bourgeois comfort of home life in the social environment of central European liberal Jewry. After World War I, the collapse of the Habsburg Empire, and the local revolutions that followed, he immigrated to Vienna and began a life of impoverished exile. In 1926 he became a Doctor of Philosophy of Vienna University and a member of the Roman Catholic Church. Partly supported by his family, he wrote several books as well as articles for political, sociological, and philosophical journals. Kolnai left Austria in 1937 to expedite the publication of his anti-Nazi book *The War against the West*, spending the next three years in England, France, and Switzerland. In 1940, between two spells of French internment, he married Elisabeth Gémes (1906–1982). They spent the rest of the war in New York and Boston, largely dependent on charity, before moving to Quebec in 1945, where Kolnai taught at Laval University. In 1955 they moved to London, England, where they lived out their days. They were supported at first by Kolnai's research grants, then by a part-time "visiting" lectureship at the former Bedford College in London University, supplemented by allowances from wealthy relations. (For details, see Dunlop.)

Kolnai's *oeuvre*, centered on ethics and political philosophy and written in five languages, displays a realist version of **phenomenology**. He was never formally trained in this area, but after devouring the ethics of Max Scheler (1874–1928), he could introduce his revised thesis, *Der ethische Wert und die Wirklichkeit*, as a completion of Scheler's phenomenological value-ethics. Kolnai's later talk about "the sovereignty of the object" (allowing the immediate data of experience to "speak for themselves" and refusing to generalize or theorize about them unless the objects clearly required it) is in obvious continuity with Edmund Husserl's (1859–1938) early phenomenological "*zurück zu den Sachen*" ("back to the things themselves"). Thus Kolnai was convinced that moral common sense, the knowledge (often only implicit) that "the plain man" has of human nature and practice, was, despite its imperfections, an indispensable treasury of philosophical truth. As a result, Kolnai's work is hard to encapsulate in summary form; it is always nuanced and qualified and lacks strict definitions and precise boundaries. These facts, in his view, simply reflect the complications of human practice.

Sexualethik was published a few years after what Kolnai called his "psychoanalytic episode." Originally a protégé of Sándor Ferenczi (1873–1933), the Hungarian colleague of **Sigmund Freud** (1856–1939), Kolnai was a member of the Vienna Psychoanalytical Association in the early 1920s. He contributed to the movement a short book, *Psychoanalyse und Soziologie*, and various other philosophical and cultural writings. His contributions became increasingly critical, and eventually he left the Association. His decision to write on **sexual ethics** expressed a deep personal interest in sexuality. He also desired to recall his readers from a concern with theories about sex, based on science or ideology, to the question of how we actually experience sexuality.

In *Sexualethik*'s introduction, Kolnai describes his main philosophical aim: He wants to investigate the "meaning" of sexual conduct and the "logic" of sexual ethical judgments, asking what the ordinary person has in mind when he judges sexual conduct morally. Kolnai appeals to the deliverances of our moral sense or intuitions; the primary objects of these cognitions are moral values and disvalues, felt as their particular "tonalities." In practical, as opposed to contemplative, contexts the conduct's value-tonalities are given to us with a particular "emphasis," a dynamic element felt not as *uniform* moral obligations but as *graduated* nuances of deprecation, warning, or prohibition (on the negative side) and of **consent**, approval, or admiration (on the positive). For the moral agent or spectator to express this complexity linguistically demands sensitivity and conscientious self-scrutiny and probably also dialogue with others and an appeal to what Kolnai later calls "the moral consensus of mankind" ("Moral Consensus," 105). Kolnai's thesis is that the whole edifice of morality is ultimately supported by such immediately apprehended tonalities. It might seem to be possible to elaborate the broad sphere of justice or human welfare by a full-scale ethical theory that only occasionally appeals to immediate experience. But insofar as judgments about lying and stealing are *moral* judgments, they ultimately rest on primordial moral experiences that are inescapably affective and dynamic. Because sexual ethical judgments are a universal feature of human societies, and are yet hard to justify in terms of easily intelligible public criteria, sexual matters are often discussed as though they were simply matters of hygiene or of physical and emotional injury. (Obviously, they may *also* be regarded in this light.) Kolnai's radical claim is that unless we understand the basis of sexual ethics, we will have an imperfect understanding of any other moral sphere.

According to Kolnai, the fundamental experience underlying sexual ethics is the demand to cleanse life from certain "material," from disvalue apprehended as moral "dirt," which threatens personal life in a different way from disvalue apprehended as disturbance, obstruction, or injury. Although other moral disvalues emphasize cleansing (in *Ethischer Wert* Kolnai mentions malice and baseness; 124–28), the sense of moral dirt as attaching primarily to what is actually done, as opposed to the agent's character, makes sexual morality, for Kolnai, *sui generis*. There is in *Sexualethik* much on the positive aspects of sexuality, its connection with spiritual goods and emotional well-being, apart from its function in continuing the species. But there is an urgency about the negative aspects such that, where they are present, positive moral values cannot be realized. Kolnai does not attempt to lay down any detailed moral rules but points to three general principles: limitation of **sexual activity** regarding partner, type of activity, and frequency; each sexual act should be a "normal" coupling; and sexual activity should not conflict with other concerns of life.

This general approach to sex presupposes a "high" conception of the human person. Kolnai admits that his stress on the personal, spiritual, and rational, as opposed to the psychosocial and biological aspects of humans, is religiously inspired, while pointing out that it is shared by secular ethical approaches emphasizing rationality or metaphysical freedom. All such "personalisms" must condemn unrestrained self-abandon or any hedonistic attitude to sex. (*Sexualethik*, though far from constituting a straightforward version of Catholic teaching on sex, generally conforms with the Catholic tradition.) In his analysis of orgasm, Kolnai points to the total surrender of the spiritual personality to overpowering physical pleasure and the shared immersion in a "non-personal, 'material,' stream of life" (*Sexualethik*, 66). There is, he writes, "a fundamental tension, a *germ* of radical incompatibility, between human sexuality and the personal, spiritual, ethically ordered values of human existence" (123). On the other hand, sex can also "lead one to a special kind of self-consciousness, self-awareness, and hence fulfillment *as a person*" (124). "Sexuality is both *evil* 'in itself,' " that is, "in its pure, isolated form as end in itself," and "yet also good in itself" (126), both as the essential means of reproduction and as potentially the basis of a well-ordered life.

There is much in *Sexualethik* on the general nature of human sexuality and its often disruptive presence in the lives of rational beings and much on the nature of the sexes and of what this fundamental biological division means for human life. Kolnai also discusses, among other things, monogamy, fidelity, promiscuity, **prostitution**, and the nature of the **marriage** tie, the sexual ethical significance of the social milieu, the meaning of the (traditional) family, and **sex education**.

Kolnai's treatment of sexual normality emphasizes its "psycho-physical structure," that is, "the internal composition of the sexual experience . . . intimately related to the external movements. . . . The decisive element here is procreation . . . as the point to which the experience naturally leads" (*Sexualethik*, 231). Other essential elements, intelligible in terms of Kolnai's three basic principles of sexual ethics together with "teleology, anatomy and also phenomenology (the essential link between the 'sexes' and sex!)" (239), are " 'union of man and woman,' 'sexual act involving union of the genitals,' and 'continuing up to orgasm' " (232). As for **sexual perversion**, "we can only speak sensibly of [it] . . . when the intentional content of the pleasure is itself made different from the normal one . . . or when the external form of the sex act clearly expresses an altered feeling of pleasure" (231–32). Since there is no possibility of simply "staying put" in sexual matters, perversion "presupposes a counter-movement, a particular obstruction of normality" (239). The key element is perhaps contained here: "[T]he partial withdrawal from the genital zone by the perversions . . . is an expression of withdrawal from the partner, in that pleasure *derived from* a 'part' or 'aspect' of the partner has taken the place of pleasure *in* becoming one with the partner. . . . For the intention to accomplish a genuine 'act' . . . is displaced by the idea of an endless current of 'passive' pleasure" (242). **Homosexuality** implies "a comprehensive alteration of the categorial structure of the world" (266). But Kolnai is never primarily concerned to affirm or condemn. His purpose is always to bring understanding.

See also Catholicism, History of; Catholicism, Twentieth- and Twenty-First-Century; Perversion, Sexual; Phenomenology; Sexuality, Dimensions of

REFERENCES

Dunlop, Francis. *The Life and Thought of Aurel Kolnai.* Aldershot, U.K.: Ashgate, 2002; Kolnai, Aurel. *Der ethische Wert und die Wirklichkeit* [*Ethical Value and Reality*]. Freiburg im Breisgau, Ger.: Herder, 1927; Kolnai, Aurel. "Moral Consensus." *Proceedings of the Aristotelian Society* [n.s.] 70 (1969–1970), 93–118; Kolnai, Aurel. *Psychoanalyse und Soziologie.* Vienna, Austria: Internationaler Psychoanalytischer Verlag, 1920. Trans. Eden Paul and Cedar Paul as *Psycho-Analysis and Sociology.* London: Allen and Unwin, 1921; Kolnai, Aurel. *Sexualethik: Sinn und Grundlagen der Geschlechtsmoral* [*Sexual Ethics: The Meaning and Foundations of Sexual Morality*]. Paderborn, Ger.: Schöningh, 1930. Trans. Francis Dunlop as *Sexual Ethics.* Aldershot, U.K.: Ashgate, 2005 [references are to the original]; Kolnai, Aurel. *The War against the West.* London: Gollancz; New York: Viking, 1938; Wewel, Erich. "Um Ehe und Eros" ["On Mariage and Love"]. *Literarischer Handweiser* 67:5 (February 1931), 261–66.

Francis Dunlop

ADDITIONAL READING

Dunlop, Francis, ed. *Early Ethical Writings of Aurel Kolnai.* Trans. Francis Dunlop. Aldershot, U.K.: Ashgate, 2002; Dunlop, Francis, and Brian Klug, eds. *Ethics, Value, and Reality: Selected Papers of Aurel Kolnai.* London: Athlone, 1977. Indianapolis, Ind.: Hackett, 1978; Kolnai, Aurel. (1962) "Deliberation Is of Ends." In Elijah Millgram, ed., *Varieties of Practical Reasoning.* Cambridge,

Mass.: MIT Press, 2001, 259–78; Kolnai, Aurel. "Der Ekel." In Edmund Husserl, ed., *Jahrbuch für Philosophie und phänomenologische Forschung*, vol. 10. Halle/Saale, Ger.: Max Niemeyer Verlag, 1929, 515–69. *On Disgust*. Carolyn Korsmeyer and Barry Smith, eds., Chicago, Ill.: Open Court, 2003; Kolnai, Aurel. *Der ethische Wert und die Wirklichkeit* [*Ethical Value and Reality*]. Freiburg im Breisgau, Ger.: Herder, 1927. In Francis Dunlop, ed. and trans., *Early Ethical Writings of Aurel Kolnai*. Aldershot, U.K.: Ashgate, 2002, 1–167; Kolnai, Aurel. "Moral Consensus." *Proceedings of the Aristotelian Society* [n.s.] 70 (1969–1970), 93–118. Reprinted in Francis Dunlop and Brian Klug, eds., *Ethics, Value and Reality: Selected Papers of Aurel Kolnai*. London: Athlone, 1977, 144–64; Kolnai, Aurel. *The Utopian Mind and Other Papers: A Critical Study in Moral and Political Philosophy*. Ed. Francis Dunlop. London: Athlone, 1995; Wiggins, David, and Francis Dunlop. "Kolnai, Aurel Thomas." In Brian Harrison, ed., *Oxford Dictionary of National Biography*, vol. 32. Oxford, U.K.: Oxford University Press, 2004, 73–74.

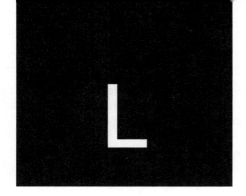

LACAN, JACQUES (1901–1981). The work of Jacques Lacan has come to be associated with a particularly dense style and jargon. Perhaps due in part to his association with literary theory in the United States, Lacan is widely held to be a thinker who had little to say about sexuality and was interested primarily in textuality: how **language** shapes human existence. With his famous claim that the unconscious is structured like a language and his reorientation of the Freudian Oedipus complex around the "name of the father," language seems to be more primary for the psyche than is sexuality. Lacan always considered himself to be a strict Freudian, however, and elements of **Sigmund Freud**'s (1856–1939) theory of sexuality remain present in his theory with some important modifications, especially regarding female sexuality.

Lacan worked in Paris as a doctor and psychiatrist for several years before becoming a psychoanalyst in the 1930s. He began giving weekly theoretical seminars for analysts-in-training with the Société française de psychanalyse (SFP) in 1953. This seminar continued for twenty-seven years. Each year Lacan elaborated on one or several of Freud's works, complying with his injunction that psychoanalysts should "return to Freud" (*Écrits*, 107). In 1963 Lacan was both stripped of his ability to train psychoanalysts with the SFP and banned from the International Psychoanalytic Association (IPA), the global organization founded by Freud. What Lacan referred to as his "excommunication" was partly due to what many of his colleagues perceived to be the personality cult that had developed around him. But the ban was mainly due to his practice of the "variable length session," whereby Lacan reserved the right to end his sessions with patients not after a regular fifty-minute period but at any moment during the session. Leaving open the moment at which the session would end, Lacan held, allowed the end of the session to punctuate what the patient was saying during the session. Thus, the end of the session could act as an obscure interpretation on the part of the psychoanalyst that would avoid suggestion. His excommunication from the SFP and IPA did not keep Lacan from holding his seminar, and with the support of philosopher Louis Althusser (1918–1990) in 1964 the seminar was moved to the École Normale Supérieure. Later the same year Lacan founded his own school, École Freudienne de Paris, and by the early 1970s it had grown to be one of the largest psychoanalytic organizations in Paris. He remained as its head until he dissolved it in 1980, one year before his death. (See Roudinesco's *Jacques Lacan* for more biographical details.)

Lacan's work has received much attention largely because it fused Freudian theory with structuralist influences from linguistics (Ferdinand de Saussure [1857–1913]) and anthropology (Claude Lévi-Strauss [1908–   ]). This fusion allowed Lacan to rethink Freudian psychoanalysis in nonbiological terms. Psychoanalytic symptoms were viewed as linguistic signs whose meaning may be revealed through psychoanalytic interpretation. Using the terms "signifier" (word) and "signified" (meaning) from Saussurian linguistics, Lacan described the symptoms psychoanalysts deal with as "the signifier of a signified that has been repressed from the subject's consciousness. A symbol written in the sand of the flesh" (*Écrits*, 68). The unconscious itself was "structured like a language," and he argued that the unconscious exploits linguistic operations such as metaphor and metonymy for the creation of dreams, symptoms, and slips of the tongue.

Because language is so important in Lacan's work, he has been accused of neglecting the significance of affects, biology, and sexuality. It is true that the primary goal for most of Lacan's career was to illustrate ways in which the structure of language influences everything from desire to psychosis. When he did theorize about sexuality, he saw language and sexuality as antagonistic and claimed that while we are sexual beings as well as speaking beings, these two aspects of our being can never form a harmonious unity. This impossibility results from what Lacan claimed was the fundamentally traumatic nature of sexuality.

A trauma, according to Lacan, is an event that lacks symbolization. Recovery from a trauma occurs by means of symbolization: attaching words and meanings to what has not been symbolized. Something traumatic about sexuality "as such," however, makes it peculiarly resistant to any symbolization ("Kanzer Seminar," 23). Sexuality is traumatic because it is fundamentally "other." Where Freud claimed that childhood sexuality is fundamentally autoerotic, Lacan pointed out that when sexual stirrings first emerge in our lives, we cannot help but feel that we are confronted with something new and alien: Lacan once claimed that no little boy feels that his penis is really his. By modifying Freud's claims about the autoerotic nature of infantile sexuality, Lacan was not saying that sexuality involves a relationship to other people. Rather, his point was that sexuality itself is somehow fundamentally "other" for each of us.

The name for the process by which this traumatic sexuality gets symbolized has been called by some of Lacan's commentators "sexuation," which can be understood to mean becoming "sexed" or what others refer to as "gendered." By means of sexuation an individual not only finds a way to symbolize sexuality (albeit always in a failed manner) but also situates himself or herself within a structure that is either masculine or feminine. For Lacan, masculinity and femininity are structural categories neither anatomically nor biologically determined (*Seminar XX*, 10). Females can be "sexuated" according to feminine structure or masculine structure, and males can be "sexuated" in a feminine or masculine way.

In Lacanian theory the subjective positions of masculine and feminine sexuation are defined in relation to one particular signifier, which Lacan called the phallus. The phallus is a historically contingent, not necessary, way of symbolizing sexuality, yet Lacan maintained that it is pervasive. According to Lacan, children for a time take their mothers to be godlike figures who are capable of fulfilling all the child's needs. Eventually, children learn that their mothers do not have everything. (For one thing, she lacks the phallus attributed to her; see Freud, "Fetishism," 152–53.) She is understood to desire and is thus understood to lack as well (*Écrits*, 252). This realization may occur when the mother delays a satisfaction of the child's needs because she has to pay attention to other things: other children, job, husband, social life. Lacan claims that the awareness that the mother desires beyond the child is very difficult for the child: If its mother desires, the child starts wondering to what extent he or she satisfies that desire and why. When the mother desires beyond the child (as is usually, but not always, the case), the child's status as a desired object is open to question, and the child may wonder, "What does she want from me?" or "Can she afford to lose me?" The question of the mother's desire is raised and insinuates a question about the object of her desire.

Here the phallus as a signifier begins to play a role. In Lacan's structuralist revision of Freud's Oedipus complex, the phallus is the signifier in psychic life for the object toward which the child takes the mother's desire to be directed. Lacan's claim for the centrality of the phallus in psychic life is partly motivated by what he held to be the child's assumptions about the anatomical difference between the sexes (when a child discerns that mother does not have a penis). His claim that the phallus is a signifier is meant to highlight the fact that the phallus is not a real object (a penis) but something produced by an operation much like metaphor. Metaphors put one signifier in place of another, generating thereby an extra meaning-effect that is not reducible to either of the signifiers involved in the metaphor. The two signifiers that produce the phallic signifier are, for Lacan, a signifier for the mother's desire and "the name of the father" (*Écrits*, 140).

This linguistically motivated revision of the Oedipus complex allowed Lacan to argue that even when the father is absent or dead, he is still important in the child's psychic life through what the mother says about the father. Hence Lacan makes the "name" of the father an important factor in the Oedipus complex. When the name of the father is put into a relationship with the mother's desire, the phallus is generated as a signifier for the signified of the mother's desire. So the phallus operates in the psyche as a signifier for what the mother's desire is about, or what it aims at.

Once the phallus becomes a factor for the child, a child either identifies with this signifier (feminine sexuation) or positions himself or herself as one who possesses that signifier (masculine sexuation). In both cases, by "being" or "having" the phallus, the child is able to imagine that he or she is a desirable object. While Freud claimed that only girls take themselves to be castrated, while boys have "castration anxiety," Lacan claimed that both boys and girls see themselves as castrated—in a symbolic, not a literal, sense—because neither really has or is the phallus. For this reason, Lacan claimed that the phallus is also a signifier for lack: a signifier for both the boy and girl of what they are not and do not have (*Écrits*, 278–79).

Another central concept in Lacan's treatment of sexuality and sexuation is "jouissance" (see Evans). He used the term to refer to sexual satisfaction, yet he also frequently used it to refer to enjoyment that went beyond what we normally associate with orgasm or other pleasant and agreeable sexual sensations: Jouissance may be something in which "pleasure *and* pain are presented as a single packet" (*Seminar VII*, 189). An addiction, from a Lacanian perspective, may be the addict's "jouissance"—a fundamental way in which he obtains a type of satisfaction, even despite himself. Similarly, an anorexic's starvation may be her jouissance, or a workaholic's obsession with his job, or an artist's all-consuming productive activity.

Lacan encouraged his students to maintain a sharp distinction between instincts and drives (*VII*, 209), and jouissance "appears not purely and simply as the satisfaction of a need but as the satisfaction of a drive." Instincts are satisfied in a relatively simple manner, by obtaining whatever object is needed. But drives are not satisfied by obtaining their objects; they are satisfied by (so to speak) going "around" their objects. Drives do have objects, but Lacan believed that these objects serve merely as props for a drive's more basic tendency to turn back on the self. This return on the self is the important part of the mechanism of a drive's satisfaction or jouissance. As an image for a drive and its satisfaction, Lacan liked to refer to Freud's evocation of a mouth kissing itself (*The Four Fundamental Concepts*, 179). Like Freud, Lacan held that drives tend to be centered on zones of the body that open up to the outside world, the borders and edges of the body: the mouth, anus, and genitals, as well as the "gaze" and voice. A drive is something that starts out from such body zones, then moves, loops around an object, and turns back to the source from which it originated. A drive can be thought of as a perpetual stimulation of the relevant zone, and the jouissance involved in this "return" movement is entirely divorced from the fulfillment of any biological or instinctual need. So an instinct for eating may be satisfied by food, which object it needs, but an oral drive will want to continue to satisfy itself even after hunger has been satisfied. A need to communicate may be fulfilled by speaking, but a surplus enjoyment arises from continuing to "blah blah blah" after the message has already been communicated. In this way, Lacan emphasizes the excessive, insistent, and repetitive dimension of drives in contrast to the rhythmic coming and going, or rise and decline, of instincts.

Jouissance, then, is the name for a drive-like sexual satisfaction. Generally, it is used by Lacan in a value-neutral way, applicable to socially acceptable as well as self-destructive activities. Lacan later distinguished between two primary types of jouissance, "phallic jouissance" and an "Other" jouissance, which led to some noteworthy revisions in his theory of sexuation. Both sexuations, both masculine and feminine subjects, have access to a phallic jouissance, which Lacan characterizes as a "jouissance of the organ" (*Seminar XX*, 7). However, feminine subjects have access to an "Other" jouissance, also called a "feminine" jouissance, which masculine subjects obtain only with difficulty, if at all. This "Other" jouissance is not typically obtained in genital **sexual activity** (so Lacan calls it a "jouissance beyond the phallus") but in other areas of life: religious ecstasy, meditation, art, and other practices that have a special relationship to language. Lacan, as a Freudian, held that the satisfaction obtained in these practices is still sexual. But since it is neither phallic nor focused on the basic erotogenic zones, the satisfaction is more closely related to Freudian sublimation, in which a drive is satisfied even though it is diverted from its apparent aim. For example, we might want to say that satisfaction from copulation is what a genital drive is aiming at. If this satisfaction is unavailable, some other activity might allow the drive to be satisfied (running around the block, taking a cold shower, writing a poem).

The status of this "Other" jouissance differs in masculine and feminine sexuation. In the masculine, the whole of the person is subject to the phallic function. This means that for masculine subjects nothing beats genital satisfaction. But the masculine subject believes that there is an exception: either a type of jouissance that is unavailable but that would be better than what is available to him, or some person who is not required to position himself with respect to the phallus as a signifier and thus is able to have access to this unhindered "Other" satisfaction. Lacan links this mythical, exceptional "one" to a variety of ideas that play a role in **fantasy** life, most notably to the Freudian myth of the obscene, perverse father of the primal horde (*Totem and Taboo*, 141 ff.), who was not subject to the **incest** taboo and was able to enjoy any woman he wanted. Within the structure of masculine sexuation, the "Other" jouissance and phallic jouissance are in an antagonistic relationship. For masculine subjects, the "Other" jouissance is ruled out as long as there is phallic jouissance, so phallic jouissance is believed to be the only kind going, for better or worse. Yet masculine subjects adamantly, albeit unconsciously, "believe" that this other jouissance must exist somewhere, as desirable, impossible, or abhorrent as they hold it to be.

A feminine subject holds that there is not one person who is not subjected to the phallic function, but she simultaneously holds that the entire person is never subject to that function. Feminine sexuation thus posits an "Other" jouissance not as an impossibility but as an unspeakable, unrepresentable excess. So while there is no individual entirely independent of or free from phallic sexuality, feminine sexuation holds that phallic jouissance is "not-whole." This leaves phallic jouissance and the "Other" jouissance still distinct from each other but perhaps less antagonistic.

Lacan claimed that phallic jouissance and the "Other" jouissance are never able to complement each other. He claimed, in fact, that "there's no such thing as a sexual relationship" (*Seminar XX*, 12; see also Žižek, "There Is No Sexual Relationship"). This was not to deny that men and women have sex but rather to point out that when they do have sex what happens is not what they expect: The sexual act entails a fundamental miscommunication. In sexual acts, the participants are positioned as masculine and feminine with respect to the phallus, and they miss each other or fail to encounter each other as masculine or feminine subjects for this very reason. According to Lacan, only the phallus makes it possible for individuals to identify themselves as masculine or feminine. In any sexual act between two such subjects, we would have a masculine subject identifying himself as such by relating himself to the phallus and a feminine subject identifying herself as such by relating herself to the phallus. But neither is relating to anything proper to the other. This means that for each individual the phallus is a "third party," a *tertium quid* or mediator, to which each individual must first relate to be able to relate to another individual as a sexed being. (This notion is reminiscent of **Søren Kierkegaard**'s [1813–1855] thesis that a man and woman can approach, be with each other, and sustain a successful **marriage** only by each's relating to another *tertium quid*: the Christian God [*Works of Love*, 118, 124]. Indeed, Lacan's "there is no sexual relationship" reminds one of the attempt of another existentialist, and another Frenchman, Jean-Paul Sartre [1905–1980], to argue, on different grounds, that sexual relationships were doomed to impossibility [*Being and Nothingness*, 361–430].)

For Lacan, a masculine subject is able to stage himself as masculine only through the possession of real objects who basically act as stand-ins for the phallus (women). A feminine subject partially identifies with the phallus but, as we have seen, this does not account for the entirety of her subjectivity and enjoyment. She has access not only to the phallic signifier as a signifier but to something beyond the phallus. This "beyond" lacks a signifier, however, and thus remains hidden and silent. While this comes across as a pessimistic account of relations between the sexes, Lacan speculated that some forms of **love** may be able to make up for the failure of the sexual relationship: "[W]hat makes up for the sexual relationship is, quite precisely, love" (*Seminar XX*, 45), and "when one loves, it has nothing to do with sex" (*XX*, 25).

In one of Lacan's more famous passages on the nature of the phallus (*Écrits*, 275), he writes:

> In Freudian doctrine, the phallus is not a fantasy, if we are to view fantasy as an imaginary effect. Nor is it as such an object (part-, internal, good, bad, etc.) inasmuch as "object" tends to gauge the reality involved in a relationship. Still less is it the organ—penis or clitoris—that it symbolizes. . . . For the phallus is a signifier . . . destined to designate meaning effects as a whole, insofar as the signifier conditions them by its presence as signifier.

Many commentators (Luce Irigaray, in particular) accuse Lacan of phallocentrism, charging that there is an overreliance in his work on the male sex organ for understanding sexuality and gender, an overreliance that makes Lacan unable to conceive of feminine sexuality on its own, nonphallic, terms. Aware of Lacan's claim that the phallus is not to be understood as the penis, these critics point out that the phallus is still obviously derived from and closely related to the penis and thus cannot really serve as a neutral term for thinking of both sexes. Others disagree (for example, Fink), claiming that Lacan is not responsible for phallocentrism and that he is describing the way our psyches are structured, without saying this is either good or bad. Yet other critics claim that Lacan really is making normative claims about the function of the phallus in psychic life (Butler). These critics suggest that on Lacan's view anyone who is not sexuated in terms of the phallus is perverse, psychotic, and somehow not capable of becoming a fully socialized subject. On this reading, Lacan is far from being a neutral observer of sexuality and sexuation and is, instead, attempting to perpetuate and legitimize patriarchy and normative heterosexuality.

One of Lacan's most influential and innovative interpreters is Slovenian philosopher and psychoanalyst Slavoj Žižek (b. 1949). While Lacan's works are dense and often unreadable, Žižek's are engaging and remarkably clear. Žižek explains and expands on Lacanian concepts with the help of popular culture and current events. For example, he uses the film *Titanic* (1997) to illustrate Lacan's claim that there is no such thing as a sexual relationship ("The Thing," 222–24). In most disaster films the catastrophic event serves to bring people together despite their social and cultural differences. In the *Titanic*, the sinking of the ship plays a different role: It serves to emphasize class differences, and it also serves to divide the two main characters, Jack and Rose, whose class-crossing romance is central to the film. (Jack dies, Rose lives on.) Žižek argues that the real disaster would have occurred had the ship not sunk and Jack and Rose made it to New York and attempted to live together as a couple. For Žižek, the film uses class difference to cover up this more fundamental, *a priori* impasse of the sexual relationship. This is to say that the film uses class antagonism to suggest that if class differences did not exist, the sexual relationship *would* exist. So the sinking of the ship, according to Žižek, sustains a fantasy according to which any obstacles that exist toward the creation of a sexual relationship are merely artificial. If the disaster did not happen, and/or if class antagonism did not exist, the impossibility of the sexual relationship would dissolve.

Žižek has also made several interventions in **queer theory** and gender theory, generally defending Lacan's views on sexuality and arguing against the idea that **homosexuality** and the perversions are in any way subversive of heterosexual, patriarchal norms. Finding "hysteria" more subversive than **sexual perversion**, he argues that perversion is merely acting out "the secret fantasies that sustain the predominant public discourse, while the hysterical position precisely displays doubt about whether those secret perverse fantasies are 'really *it*' " (*Ticklish Subject*, 248). In other words, Žižek promotes Lacan's idea that perversion is characterized by a certainty that a particular way of obtaining jouissance is the best and superior to other forms. Neurotics, racked by doubt about everything, including whether they are enjoying themselves in the right way, will be inclined to believe that the perversions have enjoyment figured out: This is the fantasmatic role perversion plays for neurotics. Thus, far from contesting the social structures associated with neurosis (patriarchy and heterosexuality, in particular), perversions play an important role for neurotics by sustaining the belief that some people, at least, really know how to enjoy themselves, in a presumably guilt-free way.

Language plays a central role in Lacan's psychoanalytic theory, and its influence on his theory of sexuality is clear. It informs his revision of Freud's account of infantile sexuality, insofar as the phallus is taken to be a signifier for what the infant's mother desires; and it informs his revision of Freud's account of the Oedipus complex, which is structured around "the name of the father." Lacan's structural account of sexuation has been taken by many to be a salubrious step away from the idea, sometimes attributed to Freud, that anatomy is destiny. However, Lacan's account of feminine sexuality still strikes many as being phallocentric, and the debate continues over the extent to which his theory marks a true departure from Freud on this issue.

See also Communication Model; Cybersex; Desire, Sexual; Existentialism; Feminism, French; Firestone, Shulamith; Freud, Sigmund; Language; Masturbation; Perversion, Sexual; Poststructuralism; Psychology, Twentieth- and Twenty-First-Century; Sade, Marquis de; Sherfey, Mary Jane

REFERENCES

Butler, Judith. *Gender Trouble: Feminism and the Subversion of Identity*. New York: Routledge, 1990; Evans, Dylan. "Jouissance." In Dany Nobus, ed., *Key Concepts of Lacanian Psychoanalysis*. New York: Other Press, 1999, 1–28; Fink, Bruce. *The Lacanian Subject: Between Language and Jouissance*. Princeton, N.J.: Princeton University Press, 1995; Freud, Sigmund. (1927) "Fetishism." In *The Standard Edition of the Complete Psychological Works of Sigmund Freud*, vol. 21. Trans. James Strachey. London: Hogarth Press, 1953–1974, 152–57; Freud, Sigmund. (1913) *Totem and Taboo*. In *The Standard Edition of the Complete Psychological Works of Sigmund Freud*, vol. 13. Trans. James Strachey. London: Hogarth Press, 1953–1974, ix–161; Irigaray, Luce. (1977) *This Sex Which Is Not One*. Trans. Catherine Porter, with Carolyn Burke. Ithaca, N.Y.: Cornell University Press, 1985; Kierkegaard, Søren. (1847) *Works of Love: Some Christian Reflections in the Form of Discourses*. Trans. Howard V. Hong and Edna H. Hong. New York: Harper Torchbooks, 1964; Lacan, Jacques. (1966) *Écrits: A Selection*. Trans. Bruce Fink. New York: Norton, 2002; Lacan, Jacques. (1973) *The Four Fundamental Concepts of Psychoanalysis*. Trans. Alan Sheridan. New York: Norton, 1978; Lacan, Jacques. "Kanzer Seminar." *Scilicet*, nos. 6–7 (1975), 7–31; Lacan, Jacques. *The Seminar of Jacques Lacan. Book VII: The Ethics of Psychoanalysis. 1959–1960*. Trans. Dennis Porter. New York: Norton, 1992; Lacan, Jacques. *The Seminar of Jacques Lacan. Book XX: Encore. 1972–1973*. Trans. Bruce Fink. New York: Norton, 1998; Lévi-Strauss, Claude. (1958) *Structural Anthropology*. Trans. Claire Jacobson and Brooke Grundfest Schoepf. New York: Basic Books, 1963; Roudinesco, Elisabeth. *Jacques Lacan*. Trans. Barbara Bray. New York: Columbia University Press, 1997; Sartre, Jean-Paul. (1943) *Being and Nothingness: An Essay on Phenomenological Ontology*. Trans. Hazel E. Barnes. New York: Philosophical Library, 1956; Saussure, Ferdinand de. (1916) *Course in General Linguistics*. Trans. Roy Harris. Ed. Charles Bally and Albert Sechehaye. LaSalle, Ill.: Open Court, 1983; Žižek, Slavoj. (1996) "There Is No Sexual Relationship." In Elizabeth Wright and Edmond Wright, eds., *The Žižek Reader*. Oxford, U.K.: Blackwell, 1999, 174–205; Žižek, Slavoj. "The Thing from Inner Space." In Renata Salecl, ed., *Sexuation*. Durham, N.C.: Duke University Press, 2000, 216–59; Žižek, Slavoj. *The Ticklish Subject*. London: Verso, 1999.

Ed Pluth

ADDITIONAL READING

Althusser, Louis. *Writings on Psychoanalysis: Freud and Lacan*. New York: Columbia University Press, 1996; Barnard, Suzanne, and Bruce Fink, eds. *Reading Seminar XX: Lacan's Major Work on Love, Knowledge, and Feminine Sexuality*. Albany: State University of New York Press, 2002; Boothby, Richard. *Freud as Philosopher: Metapsychology after Lacan*. New York: Routledge, 2000; Borch-Jacobsen, Mikkel. "The Oedipus Problem in Freud and Lacan." In D. Pettigrew and F. Raffoul, eds., *Disseminating Lacan*. Albany: State University of New York Press, 1996, 295–314; Butler, Rex. *Slavoj Žižek: Live Theory*. New York: Continuum, 2005; Clément, Catherine. *The Lives and Legends of Jacques Lacan*. New York: Columbia University Press, 1985; Copjec, Joan. *Read My Desire: Lacan against the Historicists*. Cambridge, Mass.: MIT Press, 1994; Dean, Tim. *Beyond Sexuality*. Chicago, Ill.: University of Chicago Press, 2000; Evans, Dylan. *An Introductory Dictionary of Lacanian Psychoanalysis*. New York: Routledge, 1996; Feldstein, Richard, Bruce Fink, and Maire Jaanus, eds. *Reading Seminars I and II*. Albany: State University of New York Press, 1996; Feldstein, Richard, Bruce Fink, and Maire Jaanus, eds. *Reading Seminar XI*. Albany: State University of New York Press, 1995; Gallop, Jane. *Reading Lacan*. Ithaca, N.Y.: Cornell University Press, 1985; Grosz,

Elizabeth. *Jacques Lacan: A Feminist Introduction*. London: Routledge, 1990; Irigaray, Luce. (1977) *This Sex Which Is Not One*. Trans. Catherine Porter, with Carolyn Burke. Ithaca, N.Y.: Cornell University Press, 1985. Reprinted in Claudia Zanardi, ed., *Essential Papers on the Psychology of Women*. New York: New York University Press, 1990, 344–51; Kay, Sarah. *Žižek: A Critical Introduction*. Cambridge, U.K.: Polity Press, 2003; Lacan, Jacques. (1966) "Guiding Remarks for a Congress on Feminine Sexuality." Trans. Jacqueline Rose. In Juliet Mitchell and Jacqueline Rose, eds., *Feminine Sexuality: Jacques Lacan and the École Freudienne*. New York: Norton, 1985, 86–98; Lacan, Jacques. "Kant avec Sade." In *Écrits*. Paris: Editions du Seuil, 1966, 765–90. "Kant with Sade." Trans. James Swenson. *October*, no. 51 (Winter 1989), 55–75; Leader, Darian. *Lacan for Beginners*. London: Icon Books, 1995; Mead, Rebecca. "The Marx Brother: How a Philosopher from Slovenia Became an International Star." *The New Yorker* (5 May 2003), 38–47; Mitchell, Juliet, and Jacqueline Rose, eds. *Feminine Sexuality: Jacques Lacan and the École Freudienne*. New York: Norton, 1982; Nobus, Dany, ed. *Key Concepts of Lacanian Psychoanalysis*. New York: Other Press, 1998; Ragland-Sullivan, Ellie. *Jacques Lacan and the Philosophy of Psychoanalysis*. Urbana: University of Illinois Press, 1986; Rothenberg, Molly Anne, Dennis Foster, and Slavoj Žižek, eds. *Perversion and the Social Relation*. Durham, N.C.: Duke University Press, 2003; Salecl, Renata, ed. *Sexuation*. Durham, N.C.: Duke University Press, 2000; Sparshott, Francis. "Kant without Sade." *Philosophy and Literature* 21:1 (1997), 151–54; Žižek, Slavoj. *Enjoy Your Symptom! Jacques Lacan in Hollywood and Out*. New York: Routledge, 2001; Žižek, Slavoj. "Kant and Sade: The Ideal Couple." *Lacanian Ink* 13 (Fall 1998), 12–25; Žižek, Slavoj. *The Metastases of Enjoyment: Six Essays on Woman and Causality*. London: Verso, 1994; Žižek, Slavoj. *The Plague of Fantasies*. London: Verso, 1997; Žižek, Slavoj. *The Sublime Object of Ideology*. London: Verso, 1989; Žižek, Slavoj. "There Is No Sexual Relationship." In Renata Salecl and Slavoj Žižek, eds., *Gaze and Voice as Love Objects*. Durham, N.C.: Duke University Press, 1996, 208–49. Reprinted in Elizabeth Wright and Edmond Wright, eds., *The Žižek Reader*. Oxford, U.K.: Blackwell, 1999, 174–205.

LANGUAGE. Human beings do it linguistically. Some theorists have even seen in sexuality the primary origin of language. **Sigmund Freud** (1856–1939) was much taken with a 1912 essay by Hans Sperber (1885–1963), citing it as early as 1913 ("The Interest in Psycho-Analysis," 177) and as late as a footnote added to *The Interpretation of Dreams* in 1925 (*SE*, vol. 5, 352). Freud's fullest account of Sperber's view is found in his 1916 lectures on dreams:

> A philologist, Hans Sperber . . . independently of psycho-analysis, has put forward the argument that sexual needs have played the biggest part in the origin and development of speech. According to him, the original sounds of speech . . . summoned the speaker's sexual partner; the further development of linguistic roots accompanied the working activities of primal man. . . . The words enunciated during work in common thus had two meanings; they denoted sexual acts as well as the working activity equated with them. As time went on, the words became detached from the sexual meaning and fixed to the work. . . . In this way a number of verbal roots would have been formed, all of which were of sexual origin and had subsequently lost their sexual meaning. If the hypothesis I have here sketched out is correct, it would give us a possibility of understanding dream-symbolism. We should understand why dreams . . . have such an extraordinarily large number of sexual symbols. . . . The symbolic relation would be the residue of an ancient verbal identity; things which were once called by the same name as the genitals could now serve as symbols for them in dreams. (*Introductory Lectures*; *SE*, vol. 15, 167)

Important as Sperber's idea seemed to Freud and to Ernest Jones (1879–1958), his chief English disciple (110–11), it is counterintuitive. Otto Rank (1884–1939) criticizes it, suggesting that "what we have to deal with is not a growth of language out of sex-acts or sexual activity, but a comparatively late sexualization of language as a manifestation of the human creative urge which gradually usurps the parenthood of everything by bringing sexual connotations into its nomenclature" (244; cf. 242–52).

Certainly, some kind of sexualization of language occurs. Even ordinary words, such as "do" and "it," take on sexual connotations, and sometimes sexual innuendo crowds out an earlier meaning altogether. The word "intercourse," for example, nowadays virtually unusable except to mean heterosexual coitus, once designated other forms of interaction, which is why coitus was specified as "*sexual* intercourse." Similarly for "making love," which included interactions other than sex, for example, talking.

During the Monica Lewinsky scandal, Bill Clinton took the position that engaging in oral sex was not "having sex." "These encounters," he said, "did not consist of sexual intercourse. They did not constitute sexual relations as I understood that term to be defined at my January seventeenth, 1998, deposition. But they did involve inappropriate intimate contact" (Toobin, 313). The *Journal of the American Medical Association* published, in the middle of Clinton's impeachment trial, a research report according to which 60 percent of 600 college students (surveyed in 1991) did not think oral sex was "having sex" (Sanders and Reinisch). It is easy to understand why the students were divided. In one sense, "having sex" means "going all the way," and stopping short (for example, mutual **masturbation** or oral-genital contact) is specifically *not* having sex. (One can still be "a virgin.") But some would say someone was "having sex" if he or she was engaged in sexually arousing, or being aroused by, another person through manipulation of, or contact with, genital areas. (A prostitute who performs only fellatio may still be said to be "paid to have sex.") Is "foreplay" *having sex* or just a prelude to having sex? In the immortal words (in response to a slightly different question) of the philosophy student who became president, "It depends on what the meaning of the word 'is' is" (Toobin, 314).

Robert Baker proposed in 1975 that "the conception of sexual intercourse that we have in this culture is antithetical to the conception of women as . . . persons rather than objects" (291). He argued, in particular, that the gender-asymmetric character of sexual verbs such as "fuck" points to assumptions about male activity, aggression, or domination, in contrast with female passivity, and that "the metaphor involved would only make sense if we conceive of the female role in intercourse as that of a person being harmed (or being taken advantage of)" (293). Baker presumed that English requires us to say the man *fucks* and the woman *is fucked.* That may not have been true even when Baker wrote his essay (see Moulton, "Reference," 43); it is certainly incorrect now. (See, generally, Sheidlower; Stone. Igor Primoratz suggests that "the usage seems to have changed since [Baker's] article was first published"; 108.) Consider the perfectly grammatical remark, spoken by a man, "She really wanted to fuck (screw) me, but I didn't feel like it." Or the query, girlfriend to girlfriend, "Did you fuck (screw) him?" Of course, the claims of gender asymmetry and of harm are bound to be true for *some* sexual words ("*X* nails *Y*," perhaps; cf. Baker, "Postscript," 303).

Others have also postulated a conceptual connection between being harmed and being a (female) sex object. Ann Garry, for example, in trying to understand how **pornography** can be degrading to women (319; see Shrage, 443), suggests that "the connection between sex and harm helps explain both what is wrong with treating someone as a sex object and why it is worse to treat a woman in this way." But Linda LeMoncheck notes that "conceptually connecting sex with harm that men do to women appears to condemn all heterosexual sex" (129). Of course, there is a sense of "fuck" that implies harm ("we're fucked!"), because fucking *can* be a way of harming someone. But to be fucked is not always to be harmed. Consider the hopeful, "Did you get fucked (laid)?" To be sure, some theorists have found intercourse hostile, violent, or demeaning for women (see **Andrea Dworkin** [1946–2005]), and individuals obviously *can* view their sexual connections in this light.

Because **sexual activity** and language have this double nature, it is also possible for an act or word to express *both* affection and hostility, to suggest both benefit and harm. Few individuals live wholly divorced from such ambivalence, and some may find that it informs the very texture of their sexual experience. Sexual counseling often involves finding the hidden hostility in an ostensibly loving relationship or the disguised affection in an overtly hostile relationship. Identifying attitudes is tricky, in view of multiplicity of meaning (*polysemy*), and sexual language is no easier to interpret than erotic fantasies, dreams, pornography, or art (see Johnson, "Beauty's Punishment"; **Camille Paglia**).

Linguist George Lakoff argues that "lust, or sexual desire" can be understood to embody conceptual metaphors from a variety of source domains that "overlap considerably with the source domains of metaphors for anger" (411). He supports his claim that these metaphors enter into reasoning with an analysis of Timothy Beneke's interviews with rapists, concluding:

> The reason that [such remarks] seem to be so easily understood is that most, if not all, of them are deeply ingrained in American culture. All of the metaphors and folk theories . . . occur again and again in one form or another throughout Beneke's interviews. Moreover, it seems that these metaphors and folk theories are largely held by women as well as men. As Beneke's interviews indicate, women on juries in rape trials regularly view rape victims who were attractively dressed as . . . bringing it upon themselves. . . . The metaphorical expressions that we use to describe lust are not mere words. They are expressions of metaphorical concepts that we use to understand lust and to reason about it. What I find sad is that we appear to have no metaphors for a healthy mutual lust. The domains we use for comprehending lust are HUNGER, ANIMALS, HEAT, INSANITY, MACHINES, GAMES, WAR, and PHYSICAL FORCES. (414–15)

Lakoff's metaphors are hardly exhaustive, however, and his categories are disputable. We could as easily have Body Parts ("I only have *eyes* for you," "you give me a *boner*"), Botany ("My love is like a red, red *rose*"), Magic ("I was *entranced*," "She *cast a spell* on me"), or Religion ("your body is a *temple*," "Oh, *God!*"). Neither is it obvious that such categories as Animals, Heat, Games, or Physical Forces *must* be inconsistent with the idea of "healthy mutual lust."

Sex language is available for expressing love, hate, and ambivalence, so it is hardly surprising that a journal devoted to the study of "verbal aggression" is filled with examples (see Aman) or that "dirty words" should be central to swearing: Excremental functions, blasphemy, and racial epithets figure along with sex (see MacDougald; Montagu). When cultures distinguish acceptable from unacceptable words, part of the point of swearing is to use unacceptable language *because* it is unacceptable. It allows the individual to express passion (understood as involving some loss of control) and to provoke the hearer's passions. One uses impolite speech partially to be impolite. Since one of the ways to be polite is to use (extremely) roundabout language (Brown and Levinson, 132 ff.), one of the ways to be impolite is to be (extremely) direct. For English, this typically involves returning to Anglo-Saxon roots, to "four-letter words." English finds its Latin base useful for euphemism.

The last third of the twentieth century witnessed extensive study of linguistic disparities between men and women, foregrounding concerns about words and metaphors that seem to express, approve, or encourage inegalitarian treatment of women. For example, when American scientists were constructing the atomic bomb in the mid-1940s, they wondered whether it "would be a 'dud' or a success, or, as they said at Los Alamos, a 'girl' or a 'boy'" (Jungk, 197). Such language became politically unthinkable a half century later. Feminist theorists focused attention on differential linguistic treatment in many areas of social life, including compulsive heterosexuality, sexual passivity, wifely deference, reproductive subservience, motherly self-sacrifice, and restrictive domestic dependency. Feminists think "patriarchal" interests have used control of language to bias thought against taking women's choices and voices seriously. They critique derogatory and dismissive language, and violent and degrading images, pointing out that these things, if based on race or religion, would not be tolerated.

The women's movement of the 1970s grew largely from the expectations and disappointments of the civil rights movement of the 1960s. In late 1964, Casey Hayden and Mary King, members of the Student Non-violent Coordinating Committee, wrote a position paper on "women in the movement." (A year later this paper turned into "Sex and Caste: A Kind of Memo," a foundational document of "Second Wave" feminism.) Stokely Carmichael (1941–1998) responded that the proper position of women in the movement was "prone." Though he was apparently joking, and though his comment was later defended by Hayden and others as "really funny" (Hayden, 366; cf. Del Pozzo, 198), for many women the moment encapsulated the problem of their social standing. Wags questioned whether Carmichael meant "supine" rather than "prone" or perhaps was expressing a sexual preference (Brownmiller, 14).

Hayden and King were influenced by Simone de Beauvoir's (1908–1986) *The Second Sex* (Brownmiller, 13). Beauvoir noted "deep similarities between the situation of woman and that of the Negro" (xxiii) and declared, "One is not born, but rather becomes, a woman" (267). Her interpretation of social history in terms of woman's treatment as "the Other" (xvi) shaped much that followed in feminist theory. For many radical feminists, as Valerie Bryson remarks,

> the basis of women's oppression lies not in social organisation or physical domination, but in a male control of culture, religion, language and knowledge that limits the ways in which we can think and causes patriarchal assumptions to be internalised by women as well as by men. . . . [Thus,] feminists have challenged the claims of philosophy and political theory to embody reason and universality, arguing that these are based on a male paradigm that ignores or devalues experiences and ways of thinking associated with women, so that "objectivity" in fact means the subjective perception of men. The whole of cultural and academic life is therefore seen by some feminists as a political arena in which male biases must be exposed and female knowledge asserted. (222)

This project of rescuing language from patriarchal assumptions and asserting female knowledge found weapons in **Friedrich Nietzsche** (1844–1900). "It was Nietzsche, the classical philologist," as Alan Sheridan observes, "who first linked the task of philosophy to a radical reflection on language. For him, it was not a question of knowing what, in themselves, good and evil were, but rather who was speaking and about whom" (77–78). Nietzsche's influence is discernable in **Michel Foucault**'s (1926–1984) concept of "an insurrection of subjugated knowledges," which involves uncovering the power that defines the dominant discourse of objectivity in a given area of life and opening up a space for the assertion of alternatives. The concept of "deconstruction," popularized by Jacques Derrida (1930–2004), suggests that what is most important in a text may be exactly what is missing, occluded, or marginalized. (That can be determined only by further theory, which feminists, queer theorists, and others are happy to provide.)

The work of **Jacques Lacan** (1901–1981) emphasizes the importance of linguistics. "For interpretation is based . . . on the fact that the unconscious is structured in the most radical way like a language, that a material operates in it according to certain laws, which are the same laws as those discovered in the study of actual languages, languages that are or were actually spoken" (234). Some theorists have even drawn a connection between the central Lacanian concept of "desire" and Sperber's theory of the sexual origin of language. Norman Holland remarks:

> Farfetched as [Sperber's] theory sounds, some contemporary analysts have found a core of truth in it. If I think "Jane," I not only bring my mate to mind, I also remind myself of her absence or, even if she were in my study with me, the irreducible difference between Jane and the me who says "Jane." All language— all naming, anyway—by substituting the word for the thing, establishes both a presence and an absence. One could say, therefore, that in all naming "desire speaks," that is, the naming announces both the desire and the absence of what is desired. Following Jacques Lacan, many French analysts of the last decade have drawn just this analogy between unconscious processes and language. (88)

Partly under the influence of Lacan, French feminists such as Hélène Cixous, Catherine Clément, Luce Irigaray, and Julia Kristeva have focused on the theory of language and experimented with forms of writing, suggesting that "the female body can give rise to specifically feminine ways of thinking that defy the logical forms and binary oppositions of 'phallogocentric' thought, and that are based on women's experience of sexual pleasure" (Bryson, 227).

At the same time, Anglo-American feminists were explaining why writers and speakers could, and should, avoid "sexist" language (Miller and Swift, *Handbook*; *Words and Women*). From the 1970s on, a "feminist linguistics" developed. An early landmark was Robin Lakoff's *Language and Woman's Place* (1975), which provoked much discussion, including criticism of her identification of a distinctive "women's style," marked by, for example, tag-questions (Baron, 9; Crawford, 22–48; Smith, 148–50; Spender, 8; Vetterling-Braggin, 34–91). In later work, Lakoff continued to explore the politics of language, questioning the claim that in some cultures men and women speak mutually unintelligible languages but also insisting that in English mutual understanding may be more problematic than people assume:

> In Japanese, there are forms reserved for men, and others for women: to cross over is to invite social disaster. But the forms are nonetheless intelligible to all. So the distinction, to the extent that it exists, is in the *active* use of language; passively, members of these groups understand the forms reserved for the opposite sex. . . . But [in English] there are deep and subtle differences that lead to more serious kinds of misunderstanding: both sexes use the same

words in the same constructions, *but understand them differently.* (*Talking Power*, 201)

The theme of male-female miscommunication was further developed in the 1990s (Cameron; Tannen; cf. Henley).

Janice Moulton offered in 1977 a strong argument against the claim that words such as "man" are gender-neutral labels ("The Myth"). Janet Radcliffe Richards, agreeing, declared that "the use of 'man,' 'he' and the like are not sexually neutral at all" and that "the common use of these male words does influence people's unconscious attitudes to women." Her suggested solution for the "he/she" problem was that "we should get used to using 'they' as a singular word (Jane Austen does it, so it must be stylistically all right)" (293). This advice is sensible, as "they" (with its inflections) has been so used not only by Austen (1775–1817) but by many other distinguished authors and, as Jim Quinn insists, "there is *no* justification for attacking the use of plural pronouns with singular antecedents when the sex is uncertain or mixed" (35). The solution for "man" has been widely adopted: the use of "human" or "person" or, better still, the creation of natural alternatives, such as fire *fighter* and police *officer*. In many contexts, "Miss" has been supplanted by "Ms."

The language reform effort received support, after the Stonewall riots of 1969, from a cohesive gay rights movement (though critics lamented the submergence of the traditional meaning of "gay"). It was also helped by the development of **sexual harassment** law. Suddenly, the feminist critique of differential treatment, linguistic and otherwise, had access to legal teeth. Bosses quickly stopped calling their secretaries "girls," and professors ceased to suggest that "co-eds" were in college to snag husbands. In legal and campus circles, the doctrine of "hate speech" soon developed (see Altman; Walker). One idea of sexual freedom (sexual equality) gradually came into conflict with another idea (sexual openness), as media representations of sex seemed to spark new debate over obscenity and pornography. **Catharine MacKinnon**, the early theorist of sexual harassment law, became one of many "women against pornography." The work of J. L. Austin (1911–1960) on speech acts provided a partial foundation for concern about speech harmful to women (MacKinnon, 121).

But there were also "women against censorship," as American culture entered an era of "political correctness" (see Johnson, "Beauty's Punishment," "Political Correctness"). Even before the shock of a decade of "culture wars" (see LeMoncheck) drawing new energy from post-"9/11" insecurities, some advised greater "reticence" in the face of a culture of overexplicitness in which, as George Steiner lamented, pornographers "do our imagining for us" and the "images of our love-making, the stammerings we resort to in intimacy, come prepackaged" (77). Another critic of overexplicitness, Roger Shattuck, wrote of

> feelings and states of mind so delicate as to be best approached indirectly, by mere hints, by evocation in sound and sense. If I use a word so explicit, so obvious as, for example, *embarrassment* or *anger*, I reduce a complex psychological state to a stereotype, to a convention we think we share, to a caricature of itself. (120)

Though these cautions are salutary, sex has arguably (*pace* Foucault) historically suffered more from repression than from loss of nuance. Looking back to the "Victorian" period in European and American culture, anthropologist Ashley Montagu (1905–1999) reports, "The very word 'sex' is one that could not be freely uttered, especially in mixed company, until after World War I" (300). The period is portrayed bitterly in the autobiography of Viennese writer Stefan Zweig (1881–1942):

> [T]he nineteenth century labored under the illusion that all conflicts could be solved by rationalization, and that the more we hid the natural, the more we could temper our lawless powers. Therefore, if young people were not enlightened about the presence of these forces, they would forget their own sexuality. In this illusion of control through ignoring, all authorities were united in a boycott of hermetic silence. School and church, salon and courts, newspapers and books, modes and manners, in principle avoided every mention of the problem. (69)

Like Steiner (77), Zweig notes that repression can yield an exaggerated interest in sex. But, writing at the beginning of the 1940s, he leaves no doubt about where he thinks the balance lies. What was valuable in reticence may have been lost, along with the excitement of the forbidden. "But all this seems little to me in contrast to the one saving change, that the youth of today is free of fear and depression and enjoys to the full that which was denied us in our time: the feeling of candor and self-confidence" (91).

One could not similarly describe youth at the beginning of the twenty-first century, hemmed in by religious prohibitions, political restrictions, and media vulgarity. To make sense of our feelings and behavior, we must be able to interpret them in terms of familiar cultural references. Boys are confused by the conflicting expectations they are taught (Pollack, 149 ff.), and girls lack coherent emotional models. As Sharon Lamb writes, there are "too few paradigms of women's aggression through which to understand themselves," and the result is psychological self-opacity: "When good girls do bad things, they don't understand it. It seems inexplicable. Instead of saying, I must be more angry than I thought I was, they think, What just happened? Was it me? It doesn't make sense. This is a way of othering the act, seeing it as coming from outside oneself " (168). Can self-opacity be avoided without adequate ways of thinking and talking about one's sexuality?

Language clarifies sexual experience, but often at the cost of imposing prefabricated categories and diminishing its power to reveal and transform. One becomes unable (in Paul Valéry's famous and often misquoted words) "to look, that is, to forget the names of the things one sees" (1240; cf. Shattuck, 120). Sexual mysticism, "one of the least-explored trends in the history of ideas" (Ellenberger, 546), recognizes language's inadequacy as well as its ineluctability (cf. Evola, 273). "Every black drape thrown over the hypnotizing gem of sex with the professed intent of hiding it, becomes the dark backdrop that increases its luster," suggests Frank Gonzalez-Crussi. "And every effort at silencing its language is an effort, conscious or unconscious, at creating new languages that will give it novel and more varied expressions" (114). Perhaps sex is, if not the origin of language, at least its constant source of re-creation.

See also Activity, Sexual; Coercion (by Sexually Aggressive Women); Communication Model; Desire, Sexual; Ellis, Havelock; Existentialism; Feminism, French; Flirting; Foucault, Michel; Freud, Sigmund; Harassment, Sexual; Humor; Lacan, Jacques; Law, Sex and the; MacKinnon, Catharine; Masturbation; Nietzsche, Friedrich; Objectification, Sexual; Personification, Sexual; Pornography; Privacy; Prostitution; Roman Sexuality and Philosophy, Ancient; Seduction; Social Constructionism

REFERENCES

Altman, Andrew. "Liberalism and Campus Hate Speech: A Philosophical Examination." *Ethics* 103 (January 1993), 302–17; Aman, Reinhold, ed. *The Best of Maledicta*. Philadelphia, Pa.: Running Press, 1987; Austin, J. L. *How to Do Things with Words*. Oxford, U.K.: Oxford University Press, 1962; Baker, Robert B. (1975) " 'Pricks' and 'Chicks': A Plea for 'Persons.' " In Robert B. Baker,

Kathleen J. Wininger, and Frederick A. Elliston, eds., *Philosophy and Sex*, 3rd ed. Amherst, N.Y.: Prometheus, 1998, 281–97. Also, " 'Pricks' and 'Chicks': A Postscript after Twenty-Five Years," 297–305; Baron, Dennis. *Grammar and Gender*. New Haven, Conn.: Yale University Press, 1986; Beauvoir, Simone de. (1949) *The Second Sex*. Trans. Howard M. Parshley. New York: Knopf, 1953; Beneke, Timothy. *Men on Rape*. New York: St. Martin's Press, 1982; Brown, Penelope, and Stephen C. Levinson. *Politeness: Some Universals in Language Usage*. Cambridge: Cambridge University Press, 1987; Brownmiller, Susan. *In Our Time: Memoir of a Revolution*. New York: Dial Books, 1999; Bryson, Valerie. *Feminist Political Theory: An Introduction*. New York: Paragon House, 1992; Cameron, Deborah, ed. (1990) *The Feminist Critique of Language*, 2nd ed. London: Routledge, 1998; Crawford, Mary. *Talking Difference: On Gender and Language*. London: Sage, 1995; Del Pozzo, Theresa. "The Feel of a Blue Note." In Constance Curry, Joan C. Browning, Dorothy Dawson Burlage, Penny Patch, Theresa Del Pozzo, Sue Thrasher, Elaine DeLott Baker, Emmie Schrader Adams, and Casey Hayden, *Deep in Our Hearts: Nine White Women in the Freedom Movement*. Athens: University of Georgia Press, 2000, 171–206; Dworkin Andrea. *Intercourse*. New York: Free Press, 1987; Ellenberger, Henri. *The Discovery of the Unconscious: The History and Evolution of Dynamic Psychiatry*. New York: Basic Books, 1970; Evola, Julius. (1969) *Eros and the Mysteries of Love: The Metaphysics of Sex*. Rochester, Vt.: Inner Traditions, 1991; Freud, Sigmund. (1913) "The Interest in Psycho-Analysis." In *The Standard Edition of the Complete Psychological Works of Sigmund Freud*, vol. 13. Trans. James Strachey. London: Hogarth Press, 1953–1974, 163–90; Freud, Sigmund. (1900) *The Interpretation of Dreams*. In *The Standard Edition of the Complete Psychological Works of Sigmund Freud*, vols. 4–5. Trans. James Strachey. London: Hogarth Press, 1953–1974; Freud, Sigmund. (1916) *Introductory Lectures on Psycho-Analysis*. In *The Standard Edition of the Complete Psychological Works of Sigmund Freud*, vols. 15–16. Trans. James Strachey. London: Hogarth Press, 1953–1974; Garry, Ann. "Pornography and Respect for Women." *Social Theory and Practice* 4:4 (1978), 395–421. Reprinted in Sharon Bishop and Marjorie Weinzweig, eds., *Philosophy and Women*. Belmont, Calif.: Wadsworth, 1979, 128–39; P&S2 (312–26); Gonzalez-Crussi, F[rank]. "On Male Genital Anatomy." In *Notes of an Anatomist*. San Diego, Calif.: Harcourt Brace Jovanovich, 1985, 110–29; Hayden, Casey. "Fields of Blue." In Constance Curry, Joan C. Browning, Dorothy Dawson Burlage, Penny Patch, Theresa Del Pozzo, Sue Thrasher, Elaine DeLott Baker, Emmie Schrader Adams, and Casey Hayden, *Deep in Our Hearts: Nine White Women in the Freedom Movement*. Athens: University of Georgia Press, 2000, 333–75; Henley, Nancy M. *Body Politics: Power, Sex, and Nonverbal Communication*. Englewood Cliffs, N.J.: Prentice-Hall, 1977; Holland, Norman N. *The I*. New Haven, Conn.: Yale University Press, 1985; Johnson, Edward. "Beauty's Punishment: How Feminists Look at Pornography." In Dana E. Bushnell, ed., *Nagging Questions: Feminist Ethics in Everyday Life*. Lanham, Md.: Rowman and Littlefield, 1995, 335–60; Johnson, Edward. "Political Correctness." In Ruth Chadwick, ed., *Encyclopedia of Applied Ethics*, vol. 3. New York: Academic Press, 1997, 565–79; Jones, Ernest. (1916) "The Theory of Symbolism." In *Papers on Psycho-Analysis*. Boston, Mass.: Beacon Press, 1961, 87–144; Jungk, Robert. (1956) *Brighter Than a Thousand Suns: A Personal History of the Atomic Scientists*. Trans. James Cleugh. New York: Harcourt Brace, 1958; Lacan, Jacques. (1966) *Écrits: A Selection*. Trans. Alan Sheridan. New York: Norton, 1977; Lakoff, George. *Women, Fire, and Dangerous Things: What Categories Reveal about the Mind*. Chicago, Ill.: University of Chicago Press, 1987; Lakoff, Robin. *Language and Woman's Place*. New York: Harper Colophon, 1975; Lakoff, Robin. *Talking Power: The Politics of Language*. New York: Basic Books, 1990; Lamb, Sharon. *The Secret Lives of Girls: What Good Girls Really Do—Sex Play, Aggression, and Their Guilt*. New York: Free Press, 2001; LeMoncheck, Linda. *Loose Women, Lecherous Men: A Feminist Philosophy of Sex*. New York: Oxford University Press, 1997; MacDougald, Duncan, Jr. "Language and Sex." In Albert Ellis and Albert Abarbanel, eds., *The Encyclopedia of Sexual Behavior*, 2nd ed. New York: Hawthorn, 1967, 585–98; MacKinnon, Catharine A. *Only Words*. Cambridge, Mass.: Harvard University Press, 1993; Miller, Casey, and Kate Swift. *The Handbook of Nonsexist Writing*. New York: Lippincott and Crowell, 1980; Miller, Casey, and Kate Swift. (1976) *Words and Women*. New York: Penguin, 1979; Montagu, Ashley. (1967) *The Anatomy of Swearing*. New York: Collier, 1973; Moulton, Janice. "The Myth of the Neutral 'Man.' " In Mary

Vetterling-Braggin, Frederick A. Elliston, and Jane English, eds., *Feminism and Philosophy*. Totowa, N.J.: Littlefield, Adams, 1977, 124–37; Moulton, Janice. "Sex and Reference." In Robert B. Baker and Frederick A. Elliston, eds., *Philosophy and Sex*, 1st ed. Buffalo, N.Y.: Prometheus Books, 1975, 34–44; Paglia, Camille. "Junk Bonds and Corporate Raiders: Academe in the Hour of the Wolf." In *Sex, Art, and American Culture: Essays*. New York: Vintage, 1992, 170–248; Pollack, William. *Real Boys: Rescuing Our Sons from the Myths of Boyhood*. New York: Random House, 1998; Primoratz, Igor. *Ethics and Sex*. London: Routledge, 1999; Quinn, Jim. *American Tongue and Cheek: A Populist Guide to Our Language*. New York: Pantheon, 1980; Radcliffe Richards, Janet. *The Sceptical Feminist: A Philosophical Enquiry*. Boston, Mass.: Routledge and Kegan Paul, 1980; Rank, Otto. *Art and Artist: Creative Urge and Personality Development*. Trans. Charles Francis Atkinson. New York: Knopf, 1932; Sanders, Stephanie, and June Reinisch. "Would You Say You 'Had Sex' If . . . ?" *Journal of the American Medical Association* 281:3 (10 January 1999), 275–77; Shattuck, Roger. *Forbidden Knowledge: From Prometheus to Pornography*. New York: St. Martin's Press, 1996; Sheidlower, Jesse, ed. *The F Word*, 2nd ed. New York: Random House, 1999; Sheridan, Alan. *Michel Foucault: The Will to Truth*. London: Tavistock, 1980; Shrage, Laurie. "Should Feminists Oppose Prostitution?" In Alan Soble, ed., *The Philosophy of Sex: Contemporary Readings*, 4th ed. Lanham, Md.: Rowman and Littlefield, 2002, 435–50; Smith, Philip M. *Language, the Sexes, and Society*. New York: Blackwell, 1985; Spender, Dale. (1980) *Man Made Language*, 2nd ed. London: Routledge and Kegan Paul, 1985; Sperber, Hans. "Über den Einfluss sexueller Momente auf Entstehung und Entwicklung der Sprache." *Imago: Zeitschrift für Anwendung der Psychoanalyse auf die Geisteswissenschaften* 1 (1912), 405–53; Steiner, George. *Language and Silence: Essays on Language, Literature, and the Inhuman*. New York: Atheneum, 1967; Stone, Leo. "On the Principal Obscene Word of the English Language." *International Journal of Psycho-Analysis* 35 (1954), 30–56; Tannen, Deborah. *Gender and Discourse*. New York: Oxford University Press, 1994; Tannen, Deborah. *You Just Don't Understand: Women and Men in Conversation*. New York: William Morrow, 1990; Toobin, Jeffrey. *A Vast Conspiracy: The Real Story of the Sex Scandal That Nearly Brought Down a President*. New York: Random House, 2000; Valéry, Paul. (1938) "Degas Danse Dessin." In *Oeuvres*, vol. 2. Paris: Gallimard/Bibliothèque de la Pléiade, 1960, 1163–1240; Vetterling-Braggin, Mary, ed. *Sexist Language: A Modern Philosophical Analysis*. Totowa, N.J.: Littlefield, Adams, 1981; Walker, Samuel. *Hate Speech: The History of an American Controversy*. Lincoln: University of Nebraska Press, 1994; Zweig, Stefan. *The World of Yesterday: An Autobiography*. New York: Viking, 1943.

Edward Johnson

ADDITIONAL READING

Adams, Robert M. *Bad Mouth: Fugitive Papers on the Dark Side*. Berkeley: University of California Press, 1977; Baker, Robert B. " 'Pricks' and 'Chicks': A Plea for 'Persons.' " In Robert B. Baker and Frederick A. Elliston, eds., *Philosophy and Sex*, 1st ed. Buffalo, N.Y.: Prometheus, 1975, 45–64. Reprinted in P&S2 (249–67); P&S3 (281–97), with " 'Pricks' and 'Chicks': A Postscript after Twenty-Five Years" (297–305); Boswell, John. " 'What's in a Name?': The Vocabulary of Love and Marriage." In *Same-Sex Unions in Premodern Europe*. New York: Villard, 1994, 3–27; Eakins, Barbara W., and R. Gene Eakins. *Sex Differences in Human Communication*. Boston, Mass.: Houghton Mifflin, 1978; Farmer, J. S., and W. E. Henley. (1890) *Historical Dictionary of Slang*. Ware, U.K.: Wordsworth Editions, 1987; Folb, Edith A. *Runnin' Down Some Lines: The Language and Culture of Black Teenagers*. Cambridge, Mass.: Harvard University Press, 1980; Garry, Ann. "Sex, Lies, and Pornography." In Hugh LaFollette, ed., *Ethics in Practice: An Anthology*, 2nd ed. Malden, Mass.: Blackwell, 2002, 344–55; Goldenson, Robert M., and Kenneth N. Anderson. *The Language of Sex from A to Z*. New York: World Almanac, 1986; Goliard, Roy. *A Scholar's Glossary of Sex*. New York: James H. Heineman, 1968; Henley, Nancy M., and Cheris Kramarae. "Gender, Power, and Miscommunication." In Nikolas Coupland, Howard Giles, and John M. Wiemann, eds., *"Miscommunication" and Problematic Talk*. Newbury Park, Calif.: Sage, 1991, 18–43; Hoey, John, Caralee E. Caplan, Tom Elmslie, Kenneth M. Flegel, K. S. Joseph, Anita Palepu, and Anne Marie Todkill. "Science, Sex and Semantics: The Firing of George Lundberg." *Canadian Medical Association Journal* 160:4 (1999), 507–8; Holmes, Janet. "Women Talk Too Much." In Laurie Bauer and Peter Trudgill, eds., *Language Myths*. London: Penguin, 1998, 41–49; Hughes, Geoffrey. *Swearing: A Social History of Foul Language, Oaths and Profanity in English*. Oxford, U.K.: Blackwell, 1991; Lakoff, Robin. "Language and Woman's Place." *Language in Society* 2 (1973), 45–80; Landau, Sidney I. "*Sexual Intercourse* in American College Dictionaries." *Verbatim: A Language Quarterly* 1:1 (1974). Reprinted in Laurence Urdang, ed., *Verbatim: Volumes I & II*. New York: Stein and Day, 1978, 9–12; Leiber, Justin. "Pornography, Art, and the Origins of Consciousness." In Alan Soble, ed., *Sex, Love, and Friendship*. Amsterdam, Holland: Rodopi, 1997, 601–7; McDonald, James. *A Dictionary of Obscenity, Taboo and Euphemism*. London: Sphere Books, 1988; Michelson, Peter. *Speaking the Unspeakable: A Poetics of Obscenity*. Albany: State University of New York Press, 1993; Moulton, Janice. "The Myth of the Neutral 'Man.' " In Mary Vetterling-Braggin, Frederick A. Elliston, and Jane English, eds., *Feminism and Philosophy*. Totowa, N.J.: Littlefield, Adams, 1977, 124–37. Reprinted in Mary Vetterling-Braggin, ed., *Sexist Language: A Modern Philosophical Analysis*. Totowa, N.J.: Littlefield, Adams, 1981, 100–115; Moulton, Janice. "Sex and Reference." In Robert B. Baker and Frederick A. Elliston, eds., *Philosophy and Sex*, 1st ed. Buffalo, N.Y.: Prometheus, 1975, 34–44. Reprinted in Mary Vetterling-Braggin, ed., *Sexist Language: A Modern Philosophical Analysis*. Totowa, N.J.: Littlefield, Adams, 1981, 183–93; Nabokov, Vladimir. *The Annotated Lolita*. Ed. Alfred Appel, Jr. New York: Vintage Books, 1970. Rev. ed., 1991; Partridge, Eric. (1937) *A Dictionary of Slang and Unconventional English*, 5th ed. New York: Macmillan, 1961; Partridge, Eric. (1948) *Shakespeare's Bawdy*, rev. ed. New York: Dutton, 1969; Primoratz, Igor. "What's Wrong with Prostitution?" *Philosophy* 68:264 (April 1993), 159–82. Reprinted in HS (291–314); POS3 (339–61); POS4 (451–73); Rawson, Hugh. *Wicked Words: A Treasury of Curses, Insults, Put-Downs, and Other Formerly Unprintable Terms from Anglo-Saxon Times to the Present*. New York: Crown, 1989; Reisner, Robert. *Graffiti: Two Thousand Years of Wall Writing*. New York: Cowles, 1971; Richter, Alan. *Dictionary of Sexual Slang*. New York: John Wiley, 1993; Rodgers, Bruce. *The Queen's Vernacular: A Gay Lexicon*. San Francisco, Calif.: Straight Arrow Books, 1972; Ross, Thomas W. *Chaucer's Bawdy*. New York: Dutton, 1972; Sagarin, Edward. *The Anatomy of Dirty Words*. Secaucus, N.J.: Lyle Stuart, 1962; Shoemaker, David W. " 'Dirty Words' and the Offense Principle." *Law and Philosophy* 19 (December 2000), 545–84; Shrage, Laurie. "Should Feminists Oppose Prostitution?" *Ethics* 99:2 (1989), 347–61. Reprinted in HS (275–89); POS3 (323–38); POS4 (435–50); STW (71–80); Soble, Alan. "Beyond the Miserable Vision of 'Vs. Ms.'." In Mary Vetterling-Braggin, ed., *Sexist Language: A Modern Philosophical Analysis*. Totowa, N.J.: Littlefield, Adams, 1981, 229–48; Spears, Richard A. *Forbidden American English*. Lincolnwood, Ill.: Passport Books, 1990; Spears, Richard A. *Slang and Euphemism: A Dictionary of Oaths, Curses, Insults, Sexual Slang and Metaphor, Racial Slurs, Drug Talk, Homosexual Lingo, and Related Matters*. Middle Village, N.Y.: Jonathan David, 1981; Steiner, George. "Night Words: High Pornography and Human Privacy." *Encounter* 25:4 (1965), 14–19. Reprinted in *Language and Silence: Essays on Language, Literature, and the Inhuman*. New York: Atheneum, 1967, 68–77; Stewart, Susan. *Crimes of Writing: Problems in the Containment of Representation*. Oxford, U.K.: Oxford University Press, 1991; Stone, Leo. "On the Principal Obscene Word of the English Language." *International Journal of Psycho-Analysis* 35 (1954), 30–56. Reprinted in *Transference and Its Context*. New York: Jason Aronson, 1984, 323–66; Tannen, Deborah. *That's Not What I Meant! How Conversational Style Makes or Breaks Relationships*. New York: Morrow, 1986; Tisdale, Sallie. "Talk Dirty to Me." *Harper's Magazine* (February 1992), 37–46. Reprinted in POS3 (271–81); POS4 (369–79); Tisdale, Sallie. *Talk Dirty to Me: An Intimate Philosophy of Sex*. New York: Doubleday, 1994; Wilson, Kenneth G. *Van Winkle's Return: Change in American English, 1966–1986*. Hanover, N.H.: University Press of New England, 1987.

LAW, SEX AND THE. Sex is generally thought to be one of the most private, intimate of acts in which one can engage. **Sexual activity**, however, has always been regulated by law. This might seem odd, particularly in liberal democratic societies in which individuals expect the state to protect their freedom, not to interfere with their intimate conduct. This view, clearly articulated by John Stuart Mill (1806–1873) in *On Liberty* (1859), maintains that as long as the individual's behavior, sexual or otherwise, harms neither other people nor society at large, the state should leave the individual alone. Each person is in the best position to determine for themselves what kind of life will be the most meaningful to them and should thus be left alone to construct their own life plans. A happy, prosperous society is one that allows individuals to pursue their own interests when this pursuit does not harm others. If the state, by enacting various laws, were to deny individuals not only the right to make their own choices but the private space to determine what those choices are, individual citizens and society as a whole would suffer. As legal philosopher H.L.A. Hart (1907–1992) suggested, minimizing legal interference "is of particular importance in the case of laws enforcing sexual morality. They may create misery of a quite special degree. . . . [S]uppression of sexual impulses generally is something which affects the development or balances of the individual's emotional life, happiness, and personality" (22). A society composed of miserable, off-balance citizens is not one the law should help create or maintain.

In the United States, the Supreme Court has on occasion, and not without controversy, attempted to limit the power of states whose laws interfered with individuals' sexual freedom, for the very reasons Mill and Hart gave (Burgess-Jackson; for a state-by-state account of the laws that existed in the mid-1990s about various sexual behaviors, see Posner and Silbaugh). In the "privacy" law cases, which have dealt primarily with freedom of reproductive choice, the Court emphasized the fundamental importance to individuals and society of protecting rights to both spatial and decisional **privacy**. As the Court stated in *Planned Parenthood v. Casey* (1992),

> Our law affords constitutional protection to personal decisions relating to marriage, procreation, contraception, family relationships, child rearing, and education. . . . These matters, involving the most intimate and personal choices a person may make in a lifetime, choices central to personal dignity and autonomy, are central to the liberty protected by the Fourteenth Amendment. At the heart of liberty is the right to define one's own concept of existence, of meaning, of the universe, of the mystery of human life.

Though the reasons for protecting sexual and reproductive privacy are eloquently expressed in this opinion, the *Casey* decision is thought by many to interfere (ironically) with a woman's right to an **abortion**. The ruling makes it easier for lawmakers to limit the availability of abortion services, for example, by upholding the constitutionality of laws that require women to make multiple trips to an abortion provider and those laws requiring waiting periods.

Of course, not all sexual choices and actions are harmless, and the liberal view allows state interference in those cases in which harm occurs. There are two classes of sex laws that would be deemed acceptable by even the most liberal position: laws that prohibit sexual activity between an adult and a child, and laws that prohibit sexual assault, **rape**, or nonconsensual sex. But even here there are controversies about who counts as a child and about what counts as assault or the presence/absence of **consent**.

Sex laws exist that specify who counts as a child; these tend to vary from state to state. Age of consent laws specify when a person is old enough to consent to sexual activity and when they are legally able to consent to **marriage**. Ages range from fourteen to eighteen and are frequently different for males and females. In Mississippi, for example, males must be at least seventeen and females fifteen to marry. Statutory rape laws specify the age difference between a minor and an adult, which, if exceeded, makes sexual contact a crime. In Colorado, sexual assault occurs if a child is under fifteen and the other person is at least four years older; it does not matter whether the child consented. For the purpose of protecting children, no one under the age of eighteen may participate in the making of pornographic material; those found in possession of child **pornography** are prosecuted. In 1996, Congress attempted to prohibit not only pornography that employed actual children but also any pornographic visual depiction that appeared to be of a child, including virtual images. This law, the Child Pornography Prevention Act, was struck down by the Supreme Court in 2002 for being overly broad (see *Ashcroft*).

The content of laws prohibiting sexual assault has varied widely, both historically and geographically. In the nineteenth century, for example, in both England and the newly formed United States, sexual assault was defined as sexual intercourse performed by a man on a woman who was not his wife and carried out by force and against her will. This definition entailed that a woman could not be raped by her husband, that men could not be sexually assaulted, and that women could not be sexually assaulted by other women. It also meant that to convict the alleged rapist forcible compulsion had to be established in court by the prosecution. This common-law definition has changed, but many have argued that further reform is needed. Efforts in rape law reform have reexamined the force standard, to shift attention to whether the alleged victim consented, and have questioned what role, if any, the alleged victim's sexual history should play in deciding whether a rape occurred.

Despite the controversies associated with implementing and enforcing sex laws that are designed to prevent harm to others, there is little debate about the appropriateness of legal action in these kinds of cases. Liberty and privacy are important values to be protected up to the point at which an exercise of these freedoms infringes the freedom or well-being of others. When someone is too young to consent, or when an individual of any age clearly does not consent to sexual activity, then that individual is harmed if sex is forced on her or him.

Other types of laws designed to protect public health and well-being may also be justified on liberal grounds. For example, laws that criminalize the sexual transmission of disease and (perhaps) laws prohibiting **prostitution** may be so justified.

In the United States, there is a long history of the law's interfering with individual privacy and freedom to prevent the spread of communicable diseases that are thought harmful to the public health. In the eighteenth century, such laws focused on preventing the spread of smallpox, yellow fever, and plague; in the nineteenth century, the law tried to control cholera and tuberculosis; and in the early twentieth century, legislatures responded to epidemics of polio and certain **sexually transmitted diseases**. In the late twentieth century, various laws were enacted to fight the spread of the HIV (human immunodeficiency virus) virus. How these laws interfere with individual behavior varies by jurisdiction. The Supreme Court established that such legal interventions must have a substantial causal relationship to the public health objective in question, but there is a considerable amount of leeway in this condition. Public health officials can, depending on the type of possible harm, require people to submit to mandatory testing and treatment, to register their health status with local or state authorities, and in certain historical instances to submit to quarantine. In some states, a person can be charged with a criminal offense for exposing another person to a sexually transmitted disease. Although often a misdemeanor, exposing another person to HIV can be a felony if the victim is not informed by the infected person in advance and thus does not consent to the risk of exposure. These laws do not specify that the individual exposed to the sexually transmitted disease actually contracts it and is, as a result, harmed. So one might wonder whether such laws can be justified on traditional liberal grounds. Presumably, the argument would be that even though the law is often a blunt instrument, these laws can be justified insofar as they tend, all things considered, to reduce harm to the public health.

Similar things might be said about laws against prostitution. Several counties in Nevada legally permit prostitution (as do some countries in Europe and elsewhere), although in many jurisdictions it is illegal. Many reasons have been given in defense of the criminalization of prostitution, including safeguarding the public health from the transmission of disease; protecting the public from criminal activities that are commonly associated with prostitution; and protecting women in general from harms that result from the commodification of their sexuality. These are liberal arguments that employ a broad or extended notion of harm, and they may be compelling on their face. But it is not clear that the best way to reduce these and similar harms is by criminalizing prostitution. Some, including prostitutes themselves, have argued that it is precisely the illegality of prostitution that allows for some of these harms, so that a better way to prevent them is to decriminalize prostitution, although some regulation might be necessary. For example, legal prostitution in which providers get regular medical examinations may prevent the transmission of disease better than outlawing prostitution; and many of the criminal activities that go along with prostitution, such as violence, police extortion, and illegal drug dealing, would be reduced if a safe system of providing sexual services were established.

While there is certainly room for disagreement among liberals about the nature or extent of "harm" (see Joel Feinberg [1926–2004], vols. 1–2), the liberal position about the relationship between the state and sexual conduct is clear: Any law that interferes with private, intimate conduct can be justified only by showing that the law prevents harm or is designed to do so. While Mill's philosophical approach is traditionally strong in Anglo-American law and culture, there is another traditionally strong, competing position that is often called "legal moralism." This position, which began as an attack on the Millian view by his countryman James Fitzjames Stephen (1829–1894) in *Liberty, Equality, Fraternity* (1873), attempts to justify laws regulating sexual behavior. According to legal moralists, laws that preserve the sexual mores of a society and promote sexual propriety and decorum and thereby uphold certain standards of appropriate sexual expression are justified. This philosophical approach understands law as an embodiment of social morality and not simply as a tool to prevent harm. Further, legal moralists do not consider the distinction between the public sphere and the private sphere of personal activity to be particularly sharp. Public morality—the foundation of law—is private morality writ large. For legal moralists, right and wrong, moral and immoral, legal and illegal are determined by what every right-minded person sees as right and wrong, moral and immoral, legal and illegal, and these do not change when one leaves one's private home and gets on the public bus.

One of the main features of legal moralism, one that has generated much philosophical controversy (see Dworkin; Feinberg, vol. 4; Gruen and Panichas; Wasserstrom), is the claim that the law may properly be based on "intolerance, indignation, and disgust." As Patrick Devlin says, these reactions

are the forces behind the moral law, and indeed it can be argued that if they or something like them are not present, the feelings of society cannot be weighty enough to deprive the individual of freedom of choice. I suppose that there is hardly anyone nowadays who would not be disgusted by the thought of deliberate cruelty to animals. No one proposes to relegate that or any other form of sadism to the realm of private morality or to allow it to be practiced in public or in private. . . . There is . . . a general abhorrence of homosexuality. We should ask ourselves in the first instance whether, looking at it calmly and dispassionately, we regard it as a vice so abominable that its mere presence is an offence. If that is the genuine feeling of the society in which we live, I do not see how society can be denied the right to eradicate it. (17)

Any sexual activity that elicits this indignation or disgust, even if the activity is not harmful to those who participate in it or to others, violates a common moral code and, according to legal moralism, is therefore rightly criminalized. Hence laws that prohibit, for example, necrophilia, **bestiality**, other activities thought to be **sexual perversion**s, polygamy, and public nudity are perfectly justified. There is a hybrid position, articulated by Robert Bork. He claims, along with Devlin, that "moral outrage is a sufficient ground for prohibitory legislation" (124), but his reason is that "knowledge that an activity is taking place is a harm to those who find it profoundly immoral" (123)—which stretches the Millian principle to justify legal moralism. Hart had already criticized this extended notion of harm on the grounds that mere knowledge cannot be counted as a harm, for doing so would make liberty "nugatory" (47).

Sexual acts between humans and animals, between the living and the dead, and even some sexual acts between consenting adults—such as oral and anal sex—have been considered by the law to be "crimes against nature" that offend common decency and community moral standards. For legal moralists, crimes against nature (sometimes thought of as sins against God, as in **Thomas Aquinas** [1224/25–1274]) are also conceived as social crimes and therefore appropriately prohibited by law. One problem with this justification of the legal denunciation of nonharmful sexual behavior, based on appeals to what is natural or unnatural, pious or impious, virtuous or vicious, is that the specific content of these appeals varies between communities, in any given community, and over time. Legal moralists recognize this variability and urge caution in legislating morals, endorsing legal prohibition and punishment only for those activities that public opinion strenuously condemns. But public opinion is not always or even very often unified or clear.

Consider what occurred in 1992 when voters in Colorado amended the state constitution to deny gay, lesbian, and bisexual individuals redress for discrimination in employment, housing, and public accommodation. "Amendment 2" was approved by 53 percent of the voters. The Supreme Court eventually (in 1996) found Amendment 2 unconstitutional: The majority of justices argued that the Constitution does not permit denying a group equal protection of the law merely on the basis of animosity toward that group (*Romer v. Evans*). Justice Antonin Scalia, a legal moralist, argued in his dissenting opinion that "the seemingly tolerant Coloradans" had properly sought to preserve their traditional sexual mores by passing Amendment 2: The constitution entitled voters "to be hostile toward homosexual conduct" and to express their moral disapproval by singling out this group by enacting laws that deprives its members of certain legal protections.

While interesting questions arise in this case about how to interpret the Constitution, the point relevant here is that it is not obvious how we should identify what "the opinion" of Coloradans is. Scalia apparently believes that a slender 53 percent majority is a condemnation sufficiently strong to justify this legislation, but it can be argued that accurately identifying public opinion is not as simple as recording a majority preference. It may take more sophisticated sociological analysis to determine accurately the depth and breadth of public opinion. For example, does society morally condemn prostitution and find it abhorrent? Evidence can be provided for both sides. There are laws against prostitution, it is routinely denounced by religious spokespersons, many people say that it is immoral, and prostitutes have low social status. Yet prostitution thrives, laws prohibiting it are not rigorously enforced, and those who speak out against it, even religious leaders, have been known to enjoy the services of prostitutes. Further, some would certainly argue that even a vast majority might be wrong in their condemnation or approval of certain activities or practices, as was the case when slavery was legal. Since public morality is the cornerstone of legal moralism, identifying the content of public morality presents difficulties, and public morality can even be wrong, it may seem best to err on the side of the more narrow, harm-based liberal justification for state interference in sexual matters.

See also Abortion; Adultery; Arts, Sex and the; Bestiality; Consent; Consequentialism; Cybersex; Diseases, Sexually Transmitted; Feminism, Liberal; Fichte, Johann Gottlieb; Harassment, Sexual; Incest; Liberalism; Military, Sex and the; Nudism; Objectification, Sexual; Paraphilia; Pedophilia; Pornography; Posner, Richard; Privacy; Prostitution; Rape; Rape, Acquaintance and Date; Sadomasochism; Sex Work; Violence, Sexual

REFERENCES

Ashcroft v. Free Speech Coalition. 122 S.Ct. 1389 (2002); Bonilla, Margaret D. "What Feminists Are Doing to Rape Ought to Be a Crime." *Policy Review* 66 (1993), 22–29; Bork, Robert H. *The Tempting of America: The Political Seduction of the Law.* New York: Free Press, 1990; Burgess-Jackson, Keith. "Our Millian Constitution: The Supreme Court's Repudiation of Immorality as a Ground of Criminal Punishment." *Notre Dame Journal of Law, Ethics, and Public Policy* 18 (2004), 407–17; Devlin, Patrick. *The Enforcement of Morals.* Oxford, U.K.: Oxford University Press, 1965; Dworkin, Gerald, ed. *Morality, Harm, and the Law.* Boulder, Colo.: Westview, 1994; Feinberg, Joel. *The Moral Limits of the Criminal Law.* Vol. 1: *Harm to Others.* New York: Oxford University Press, 1984. Vol. 2: *Offense to Others*, 1985. Vol. 3: *Harm to Self*, 1986. Vol. 4: *Harmless Wrongdoing*, 1988; Gruen, Lori, and George F. Panichas, eds. *Sex, Morality, and the Law.* New York: Routledge, 1997; Hart, H.L.A. (1962) *Law, Liberty and Morality.* Stanford, Calif.: Stanford University Press, 1963; Mill, John Stuart. (1859) *On Liberty.* Ed. Elizabeth Rapaport. Indianapolis, Ind.: Hackett, 1978; *Planned Parenthood v. Casey.* 112 S.Ct. 2791 (1992); Posner, Richard, and Katharine Silbaugh. *A Guide to America's Sex Laws.* Chicago, Ill.: University of Chicago Press, 1996; *Romer v. Evans.* 517 U.S. 620 (1996); Stephen, James Fitzjames. (1873) *Liberty, Equality, Fraternity.* London: Cambridge University Press, 1967; Wasserstrom, Richard A., ed. *Morality and the Law.* Belmont, Calif.: Wadsworth, 1971.

Lori Gruen

ADDITIONAL READING

Altman, Andrew. "Liberalism and Campus Hate Speech: A Philosophical Examination." *Ethics* 103 (January 1993), 302–17; Baird Robert, and M. Katherine Baird, eds. "Part Three: Homosexuality and the Criminal Law." In *Homosexuality: Debating the Issues.* Amherst, N.Y.: Prometheus, 1995, 97–147; Bartlett, Katharine T., and Rosanne Kennedy, eds. *Feminist Legal Theory: Readings in Law and Gender.* Boulder, Colo.: Westview, 1991, 370–403; Bork, Robert H. "After Warren: The Burger and Rhenquist Courts" and "Of Moralism, Moral Relativism, and the Constitution." In *The Tempting of America: The Political Seduction of the Law.* New York: Free Press, 1990, 101–28, 241–50; Brundage, James A. *Law, Sex, and Christian Society in Medieval Europe.* Chicago, Ill.: University of Chicago Press, 1987; Burgess-Jackson, Keith. "Sodomy." In Christopher Berry Gray, ed., *The Philosophy of Law: An Encyclopedia*, vol. 2. New York: Garland, 1999, 819–21; Carmichael, Calum M., ed. *Essays on Law and Religion: The Berkeley and Oxford Symposia in Honour of David Daube.* Berkeley, Calif.: Robbins Collection, 1993; Cohen, David. *Law, Sexuality, and Society: The Enforcement of Morals in Classical Athens.* Cambridge: Cambridge University Press, 1991; Coleman, Jules, and Allen Buchanan, eds. *In Harm's Way: Essays in Honor of Joel Feinberg.* Cambridge: Cambridge University Press, 1994; Edwards, Susan. *Female Sexuality and the Law.* Oxford, U.K.: Martin Robertson, 1981; Ellis, Anthony. "Offense and the Liberal Conception of the Law." *Philosophy and Public Affairs* 13:1 (1984), 3–23; Eskridge, William N., Jr., and Nan D. Hunter, eds. *Sexuality, Gender, and the Law.* Westbury, N.Y.: Foundation Press, 1997. 2nd ed., 2004; Finnis, John. "Law, Morality, and 'Sexual Orientation.' " *Notre Dame Law Review* 69:5 (1994), 1049–76. Reprinted, revised, in *Notre Dame Journal of Law, Ethics, and Public Policy* 9:1 (1995), 11–39; and John Corvino, ed., *Same Sex: Debating the Ethics, Science, and Culture of Homosexuality.* Lanham, Md.: Rowman and Littlefield, 1997, 31–43; Grey, Thomas C. *The Legal Enforcement of Morality.* New York: Knopf, 1983; Gruen, Lori. "Must Utilitarians Be Impartial?" In Dale Jamieson, ed., *Singer and His Critics.* Oxford, U.K.: Blackwell, 1999; Heinze, Eric. "Victimless Crimes." In Ruth Chadwick, ed., *Encyclopedia of Applied Ethics,* vol. 4. San Diego, Calif.: Academic Press, 1998, 463–75; Kipnis, Laura. "Fantasy in America: *The United States v. Daniel Thomas DePew.*" In *Bound and Gagged: Pornography and the Politics of Fantasy in America.* New York: Grove, 1996, 3–63; Lewis, Jacqueline. "Controlling Lap Dancing: Law, Morality, and Sex Work." In Ronald Weitzer, ed., *Sex for Sale: Prostitution, Pornography, and the Sex Industry.* New York: Routledge, 2000, 203–16; MacKinnon, Catharine A. (1983) "Not a Moral Issue." In *Feminism Unmodified: Discourses on Life and Law.* Cambridge, Mass.: Harvard University Press, 1987, 146–62; MacNamara, Donal E. J., and Edward Sagarin. *Sex, Crime, and the Law.* New York: Free Press, 1977; McLaren, Angus. *Sexual Blackmail: A Modern History.* Cambridge, Mass.: Harvard University Press, 2002; Novak, David. "The Clinton Scandal: Law and Morals." In Leonard V. Kaplan and Beverly I. Moran, eds., *Aftermath: The Clinton Impeachment and the Presidency in the Age of Political Spectacle.* New York: New York University Press, 2001, 267–75; Nussbaum, Martha C. *Hiding from Humanity: Disgust, Shame, and the Law.* Princeton, N.J.: Princeton University Press, 2004; Pennock, J. Roland, and J. W. Chapman, eds. *The Limits of Law* [*Nomos XV*]. New York: Lieber-Atherton, 1974; Richards, David A. J. *Sex, Drugs, Death, and the Law: An Essay in Human Rights and Overcriminalization.* Totowa, N.J.: Rowman and Littlefield, 1982; Richter, Duncan J. "Social Integrity and Private 'Immorality': The Hart-Devlin Debate Reconsidered." *Essays in Philosophy* 2:2 (2001). <www.humboldt.edu/~essays/richter.html> [accessed 3 June 2005]; Rivera, Rhonda R. "Sexual Orientation and the Law." In John C. Gonsoriek and James D. Weinrich, eds., *Homosexuality: Research Implications for Public Policy.* Newbury Park, Calif.: Sage, 1991, 81–100; Sartorius, Rolf, ed. *Paternalism.* Minneapolis: University of Minnesota Press, 1983; Tong, Rosemarie. "Women, Pornography, and the Law." *Academe* 73:5 (1987), 14–22. Reprinted in POS2 (301–16); Tong, Rosemarie. *Women, Sex, and the Law.* Totowa, N.J.: Rowman and Littlefield, 1984; Vernon, Richard. "John Stuart Mill and Pornography: Beyond the Harm Principle." *Ethics* 106 (April 1996), 621–32; "Wolfenden Report." Report of the Committee on Homosexual Offences and Prostitution (U.K.). Cmd. 247, 1957.

LEIBNIZ, GOTTFRIED (1646–1716). Gottfried Wilhelm Leibniz, who was born in Leipzig, Germany, began studying philosophy and law at his hometown university at the age of fifteen. After obtaining a doctorate in jurisprudence in 1667, he decided to work for nobility. For the remainder of his life he served various German princes and European courts as an adviser, diplomat, royal historian, and librarian. His services were sought in Austria, Prussia, Russia, and Rome. He also worked as an inventor, mining engineer, and social reformer. In most of these fields, he was a pioneer. For example, he invented new systems of library cataloguing and founded a journal that reviewed newly published books for librarians. In 1700, he founded the Berlin Academy of Sciences, and he initiated similar academies in St. Petersburg and Vienna. He was a member of the Royal Society in London and the Academy of Rome. He also tried to encourage an alliance among the various Christian faiths and, later, among the Christian states.

As an academic, Leibniz was a world-famous philosopher, mathematician, and physicist. In 1676, he discovered differential and integral calculus, a discovery that later caused a controversy with Isaac Newton (1642–1727). Despite the fact that Leibniz was a prolific writer, there is no long, single systematic exposition of his philosophy as a whole. His written works are only short summaries of part of his thought, and he wrote much of his philosophy in letters and notes. His main metaphysical works are *Discourse on Metaphysics* (1686; not published until 1846), *New Essays on Human Understanding* (1704; not published until 1765), *Theodicy* (1710), and *Monadology* (1714).

As a young man, Leibniz was known for his wit and fashionable clothes, but he never married. He became close to the Duchess Sophie (1630–1714) and to her daughter Sophie Charlotte (1668–1705), who was later the queen of Prussia. His intense correspondence and discussions with Sophie Charlotte resulted in his *Theodicy*. Leibniz was an optimistic person, who tried to find the positive in everything. He believed strongly in working for the benefit of humanity and the glorification of God.

Leibniz was a major figure in the rationalist philosophical tradition. There are two major aspects to his thought. First, his main lifelong interest was to devise an alphabet of human thought, a rational **language** that would enable the construction of a reasoning machine. Most of his other projects revolved around this central aim. For example, he invented new systems of formal logic and ways to represent concepts and logical operations numerically. In 1680, he designed a calculating machine that would use binary numbers. He realized that his constructed language would require a huge encyclopedia of organized data, which is why he worked to establish and finance academies throughout Europe. He thought that his alphabet of human thought would help solve Europe's political problems. He believed that the wars of the time, such as the Thirty Years' War, were religious, and these religious differences were based on theological and ultimately philosophical misunderstandings that could be solved rationally.

Second, Leibniz's rationalism led him to metaphysical conclusions that were fundamentally at odds with much of the thinking of the time. His main metaphysical thesis is that the universe consists of an infinite number of mind-like, non-material, independent monads that exist non-spatially. Our ideas of inert matter, mechanical causation, and space are illusions generated by the perceptions of these monads. Leibniz's main thesis rests on three considerations. First, each substance must have a complete concept that distinguishes it from all other possible substances. Consequently, a substance must be identified by all its properties, which means that it is self-contained like a universe unto itself. Second, any substance must be a unity. Because it is infinitely divisible, matter cannot be a unity and must be ideal. In short, reality must consist of substances that are not in space. Third, Leibniz argued that because all propositions can be reduced to those of subject-predicate form, all relations are ideal. Space and time are merely a system of relations rather than absolute entities (as Newton supposed).

According to Leibniz, the universe consists of an infinity of monads, each of which develops independently of all others. At the same time, each monad reflects the universe as a whole. Thus, everything must exist in a preestablished harmony, as chosen by God as being the best of all possibilities. The universe is like a commonwealth of spirits governed by God. Persons can participate in this kingdom of grace through moral growth and **love** (*Discourse on Metaphysics*, sec. 36; *Philosophical Papers*, 640–41).

Leibniz wrote virtually nothing about sexuality, but we may reconstruct his views. Let us start with the metaphysics of sexual identity. According to Leibniz, a person is defined by his or her essence, which includes all his or her properties. An individual's sex is, therefore, part of that person's essence. This is a view that has come to be associated mostly with various traditionalist philosophers. **Roger Scruton**, for example, contrasts his view of the nature of the human being or person with, in particular, one type of Kantian **liberal feminism**, according to which an individual's sex, being male or female, is not part of but is rather incidental to the individual's identity and personhood. Further, on this view, gender, too, is accidental or artificial, and gender differences are not determined by natural sexual differences. It follows from this Kantianism, according to Scruton, that every person, as a fundamentally sex-neutral, gender-neutral moral agent, or as a discrete individual already possessing, without the addition of sex and gender, everything essential to personhood, has exactly the same rights, duties, and freedom as any other person. Further, economic, political, or cultural roles based on sex or gender must be understood as imposed on persons, largely suspiciously, by social arrangements (258–59). Scruton admits that this view is "undeniably appealing" (259), but he rejects it. (One of his arguments is that if gender is artificial, then so too is personhood itself.) Scruton's rejection of this Kantianism, his claim that not only the pure asexual or de-sexed individual, but also the genderless individual, does not exist, not even in some metaphysical sense, amounts to incorporating both sex (our embodiment or "incarnate condition") and gender into personhood or the "self " (260, 274). This move permits the defense of the legitimacy, indeed the desirability, of sex-based social expectations and social roles.

Leibniz denies that the universe is composed of mechanical, inert matter. On the contrary, everything is, to some degree, alive. Even in physics, for Leibniz, the concept of active force is more fundamental than that of matter, and active force is based on the appetites of the relevant monads. Leibniz derived these views from the principle that "nature makes no leaps" (*New Essays*, 307, 324; *Philosophical Papers*, 515), by virtue of which there are no fundamental discontinuities between the inanimate and the animate, so that the inanimate always has something animate about it. Similarly, no fundamental discontinuities exist among plants, animals, and humans (*New Essays*, 306–7). The principle that nature makes no leaps has an interesting application: It suggests that sexual differences are also continuous and that, as a result, there are no sharp basic differences between male and female.

Leibniz also applied his principle of continuity to perception, claiming that one can have ideas of which one is not aware (*New Essays*, 52–54). Even the ideas that we are conscious of are composed of tiny minute ideas of which we are unaware. Leibniz's view of the unconscious, which included the notions of repression and sublimation, has been regarded as an early precursor of the psychoanalytic thought of **Sigmund Freud** (1856–1939; see *Philosophical Papers*, 40).

What appears as the human body really consists of an infinity of non-spatial points of living force. As such, the body is an organized collective, which is expressed by the monad that is the person's soul. In this sense, a person is an organic unity. The purposes and sensations of the monads that form the body are reflected as conscious and self-conscious perceptions and appetites in the person's soul. In Leibniz's metaphysics—unlike the metaphysics of **René Descartes** (1596–1650)—there is no causal relationship between mind and body, because each monad is ultimately self-contained. What *appears* to be a casual relationship between mind and body is really the one (the mind) reflecting spontaneous changes in the other (the body). This metaphysics suggests a Leibnizian account of sexual desires: They are implicit in the appetitive forces of the living body and are (merely) reflected both in the unconscious mind and sometimes in the self-awareness of the soul. Such a view is different from Descartes's, who held that understanding the operation of the passions, including **sexual desire**, provided a way of understanding mind-body interaction.

Leibniz distinguishes three levels of morality. The first relates to the outward conformity of one's actions with the law; the second concerns one's relationships to other people; and the third, one's relationship with God. Intimate personal relationships fall within the second level.

Leibniz says that a true **friendship** must be either the effect of a great and beautiful passion (as, perhaps, in Michel Montaigne's [1533–1592] account of friendship) or of a great virtue found in two people at the same time (as, perhaps, in **Aristotle**'s [384–322 BCE] *Nicomachean Ethics*). Leibniz saw friendship as a sharing of pleasure caused by each person's perceiving and enhancing the other person's perfections, such as feelings of joy and natural capacities (*Philosophical Papers*, 425–27, 630). According to Leibniz, perfections have objective and subjective aspects, which are linked causally. Subjectively, perfections are feelings of pleasure that are caused by the perception of good qualities. Objectively, perfections consist in natural harmony and order, which give rise to feelings of **beauty** and love. Having developed natural capacities would count as an objective aspect of perfection; the subjective counterpart would be a feeling of happiness that someone has well-developed abilities.

In a similar vein, for Leibniz, friendship has a subjective and an objective aspect. The subjective aspect is the feeling of mutual pleasure caused by the perception of perfection, while the objective aspect is the basis of experiencing pleasure in the perfections of others. Now, Leibniz claims that we act, egoistically, only for the sake of our own self-interest, which consists in pleasurable experiences. So Leibniz is a hedonist. Further, our love for other persons is not contrary to this egoism and hedonism, because love requires that we make the other person's happiness and perfection part of our own interests (*Philosophical Papers*, 630). In the history of philosophy, this is a common idea, found in such disparate philosophers as Montaigne ("On Affectionate Relationships"), Robert Nozick (1938–2002; "Love's Bond"), and J.F.M. Hunter (75–76). Finally, it is essential that monads reflect or mirror each other. In the case of persons, this mirroring of monads will consist in part of self-conscious reflections of the other person and, further, reflections of these reflections in the other person (and so on). This implies about sexual relationships that passions will mutually reinforce and strengthen each other, a phenomenon that informs the sexual thought of American philosopher **Thomas Nagel**.

See also Communication Model; Completeness, Sexual; Descartes, René; Friendship; Hobbes, Thomas; Love; Spinoza, Baruch

REFERENCES

Hunter, J.F.M. *Thinking about Sex and Love*. New York: St. Martin's Press, 1980; Leibniz, Gottfried. (1686) *Discourse on Metaphysics and Related Writings*. Trans. and ed. R.N.D. Martin and Stuart Brown. Manchester, U.K.: Manchester University Press, 1988; Leibniz, Gottfried. (1704) *New Essays on Human Understanding*. Trans. and ed. Peter Remnant and Jonathan Bennett. New York: Cambridge University Press, 1981; Leibniz, Gottfried. *Philosophical Papers and Letters*. Trans. and ed. Leroy E. Loemker. Dordrecht, Holland: Reidel, 1969; Leibniz, Gottfried. *Philosophical Writings*. Includes *Monadology* (1714). Trans. Mary Morris and G.H.R. Parkinson. Ed. G.H.R. Parkinson. London: Dent, 1973; Montaigne, Michel. (1572/1595) "On Affectionate Relationships." In *The Essays of Michel de Montaigne*. Trans. and ed. M. A. Screech. London: Penguin, 1991, 205–19; Nozick, Robert. "Love's Bond." In *The Examined Life*. New York: Simon and Schuster, 1989, 68–86; Scruton, Roger. *Sexual Desire: A Moral Philosophy of the Erotic*. New York: Free Press, 1986; Thomson, Garrett. *On Leibniz*. Belmont, Calif.: Wadsworth, 2001.

Garrett Thomson

ADDITIONAL READING

Adams, Robert Merrihew. *Leibniz: Determinist, Theist, Idealist*. New York: Oxford University Press, 1994; Aiton, E. J. *Leibniz: A Biography*. Boston, Mass.: Adam Hilger, 1985; Broad, C. D. *Leibniz: An Introduction*. London: Cambridge University Press, 1975; Brown, Gregory. "Leibniz's Moral Philosophy." In Nicholas Jolley, ed., *The Cambridge Companion to Leibniz*. New York: Cambridge University Press, 1995, 411–41; Brown, Stuart. *Leibniz*. Minneapolis: University of Minnesota Press, 1984; Deleuze, Giles. *The Fold: Leibniz and the Baroque*. Trans. Tom Conley. Minneapolis: University of Minnesota Press, 1993; Frankfurt, Harry G., ed. *Leibniz: A Collection of Critical Essays*. Garden City, N.Y.: Anchor/Doubleday, 1972; Hostler, John. *Leibniz's Moral Theory*. New York: Harper and Row, 1975; Jolley, Nicholas, ed. *The Cambridge Companion to Leibniz*. New York: Cambridge University Press, 1995; Leclerc, Ivor, ed. *The Philosophy of Leibniz and the Modern World*. Nashville, Tenn.: Vanderbilt University Press, 1973; Leibniz, Gottfried. (1716) *Discourse on the Natural Theology of the Chinese*. Trans. and ed. Henry Rosemont, Jr., and Daniel J. Cook. Honolulu: University of Hawai'i Press, 1977; Mates, Benson. *The Philosophy of Leibniz*. New York: Oxford University Press, 1986; Parkinson, G.H.R. *Logic and Reality in Leibniz's Metaphysics*. Oxford, U.K.: Clarendon Press, 1985; Rescher, Nicholas. *Leibniz: An Introduction to His Philosophy*. Totowa, N.J.: Rowman and Littlefield, 1979; Ross, George MacDonald. *Leibniz*. New York: Oxford University Press, 1984.

LESBIAN FEMINISM. *See* Feminism, Lesbian

LEVINAS, EMMANUEL (1906–1995). Emmanuel Levinas was born of Jewish parents in Lithuania and studied Hebrew and German as well as Russian. He became a student in Strasbourg in 1923, where he attended Edmund Husserl's (1859–1938) final lectures and studied **Martin Heidegger**'s (1889–1976) *Being and Time*. His first works, including *Existence and Existents* (1947), showed the influence of Husserl and Heidegger, and he became known for his French translations of their works.

Levinas joined the French army in 1939; an officer, he was taken prisoner of war in 1940. His wife and daughter survived, but the rest of his family was killed. The experience of the war and the treatment of Jews marked his life's work. He spent his life in France and became famous for his ethics based on *alterity* and the *face*. This ethics of responsibility answered the Germans who excused themselves by their lack of knowledge and the SS officers who eliminated knowledge by destroying both concentration camp records and prisoners at the close of the war. Levinas's thought is that I am responsible to the Other, an infinite responsibility that comes from the Other. Who I am I owe to the Other.

Levinas is best known for his view of ethics as "first philosophy," a critical response to Heidegger's ontology in which Levinas perceived the vanishing of the Other into the buzzing (*bourdonnement*) of being.

> Heidegger, with the whole of Western history, takes the relation with the Other as enacted in the destiny of sedentary peoples, the possessors and builders of the earth. Possession is preeminently the form in which the Other becomes the same, by becoming mine. . . . Ontology becomes ontology of nature, impersonal fecundity, faceless generous mother, matrix of particular beings, inexhaustible matter for things. (*Totality*, 46)

Under the heading of Heidegger's ontology, being becomes totality, impersonal, neutral, concerned with knowing and truth. Under the heading of infinity, ethics is relation to the Other; the individual is constituted by and from the Other, whose face signifies infinite alterity. In *Totality and Infinity*, and later more radically in *Otherwise Than Being or Beyond Essence*, Levinas traces alterity through an extraordinary range of notions and in stunning **language**: alterity, beyond, death, metaphysical desire, destitution, excess, exile, exposition (exposure and expression), exteriority, face, grasp, guilt, hither, illeity, interruption, ipseity, luminosity, justice, obligation, Other, other, others, otherwise, outside, overflowing, passivity, persecution, possession, proximity, remoteness, responsibility, restitution, revelation, saying and the said, sensibility, separation, signification, substitution, suffering, surplus, transcendence, vulnerability, wandering, yonder. All these are expressions of alterity and transcendence, understood as beyond being but present as infinity in sensible experience, filled with intimacy, sexuality, and **love**.

This presence of the Other in the face is the condition of ethics and the responsibility that defines my being (for the other).

> The word *I* means *here I am*, answering for everything and for everyone. . . . I am inspired. This inspiration is the psyche. The psyche can signify its alterity in the Same without alienation in the form of incarnation, as being-in-one's-skin, having-the-other-in-one's-skin. ("Substitution," 104)

Who I am comes from the Other, answering beyond limits to the other. In this way, the other as Other, the other's alterity and otherness, are the source of my being as an ethical being, as a subjective, psychic, and inspired being, and as a corporeal, incarnated being in the skin, being oneself by having the Other in one's skin. This relation to the Other does not begin and cannot end but is primordial and infinite: obsessive, traumatic, unrepresentable, immemorial. There is nothing neutral and inert about the face and the idea of the Other in me. The Other is other in the most radical way, an irreducible and exceptional alterity.

Levinas is frequently read as a Jewish philosopher, both in the sense that he practiced **Judaism**, wrote Talmudic studies, drew on Hebrew and other Jewish writings, including Baruch Spinoza (1632–1677), but also in the sense that he introduced Judaic themes into a country that was explicitly Catholic and into a philosophy that claimed to be secular. Many of his commentators have been struck by his Jewish and Hebraic themes. One of these is Levinas's concern with God and God's alterity. Yet he insists that God is neither the source nor efficacy of alterity, which is present in the face of the other. "A face does not function in proximity as a sign of a hidden God who would impose the neighbor on me. It is a trace of itself, a trace in the trace of an abandon, where the equivocation is never dissipated" (*Otherwise*, 94). God is present in alterity, but alterity is not God.

One of Levinas's magical achievements in *Totality*, so eloquent that it influenced many writers on corporeality and desire (for example, Jacques Derrida [1930–2004], Luce Irigaray, Jean-François Lyotard [1924–1998], Jean-Luc Nancy), was to evoke the presence of the infinite in the everyday (another point of difference with Heidegger). The everyday is a site of alterity in enjoyment and corporeality even where it falls short of the infinity and significance of the face. Levinas traces alterity in the everyday through another extraordinary range of notions and again in stunning language, this time of great materiality, desire, and feeling: body, building, caress, contentment, corporeity, desire, domicile, dwelling, earth, eating, ecstasy, emotion, enjoyment, eros, fecundity, feeling, feminine, generosity, gentleness, giving, habitation, happiness, home, hospitality, hunger, indigence, intimacy, joy, *jouissance*, labor, life, living from, living in, love, luxury, mastery, modesty, nakedness, nearness, needs, nourishment, nudity, shame, sojourn, stranger, sweetness, tenderness, virginity, voluptuosity, wants, welcome.

The home here is a site of dwelling, intimacy, and hospitality. Life is lived in intimacy in the home:

> The home that founds possession is not a possession in the same sense as the movable goods it can collect and keep. It is possessed because it already and henceforth is hospitable for its proprietor. This refers us to its essential interiority, and to the inhabitant that inhabits it before every inhabitant, the welcoming one par excellence, welcome in itself—the feminine being. Need one add that there is no question here of defying ridicule by maintaining the empirical truth or countertruth that every home *in fact* presupposes a woman? The feminine has been encountered in this analysis as one of the cardinal points of the horizon in which the inner life takes place . . . as the very welcome of the dwelling. (*Totality*, 157–58)

Levinas welcomes the woman, in the feminine, as a primordial condition of being human, of being able to live in enjoyment, of interiority, of subjectivity. Welcome, hospitality, generosity are states of desire in which an infinite transcendence realizes itself in finite experience (*Totality*, 75–76).

Dwelling is not in relation to myself but in relation to the Other, understood in bodily, affective terms. Intimacy here is alterity.

> [T]he body is not only what is steeped in the element, but what *dwells*, that is, inhabits and possesses. (*Totality*, 137)

> Concretely speaking the dwelling is not situated in the objective world, but the objective world is situated by relation to my dwelling. (153)

It is an alterity experienced in the immediacy of the home and encountered in familiarity and intimacy as gentleness. Affects, feelings, desires, sexual and erotic, spread over the face of things far beyond thought and knowledge, on the one hand, and beyond any sexual organs, on the other (*Totality*, 154–55). Intimacy is the pervasive erotic being of subjectivity.

Much of this writing, well over half of *Totality*, glows with Jewish themes: bread, enjoyment, intimacy, love. The enjoyment of the everyday, the practices that make familiar things and events joyous, belongs historically to Jewish writing. Dwelling in body and home is a biblical theme and can be found in other Jewish writers—in Martin Buber (1878–1965), for example, in the *I-Thou* relation, which takes place in intimacy:

> The woman is the condition for recollection, the interiority of the Home, and inhabitation. . . . The Other who welcomes in intimacy is not the *you* [*vous*] of the face that reveals itself in a dimension of height, but precisely the *thou* [*tu*] of familiarity: a language without teaching, a silent language, an understanding without words, an expression in secret. (*Totality*, 155)

In the home, and in intimacy, sexuality and love are present throughout as primordial conditions of enjoyment, of subjectivity. They are not states of an individual ego but relations with and from an Other, the woman.

Such a view of femininity is not without problems, and Irigaray criticizes Levinas ("Questions") for presenting desire and love for the man from the woman, neglecting women's desire. She does so sharing Levinas's realization that intimacy, love, and desire are manifestations of infinity and transcendence in daily life. In "The Fecundity of the

Caress," Irigaray pursues this critique in so intimate a relation to Levinas himself that his own revelation of the caress as an erotic expression of transcendence comes through intensely: "The caress, like contact, is sensibility. But the caress transcends the sensible. . . . The caress consists in seizing upon nothing, in soliciting what ceaselessly escapes its form toward a future never future enough" ("Fecundity," 257). In the caress, sexuality, nudity, and love come together in transcendence in flesh and skin. Love is from the Other.

The entire final section of Levinas's *Totality*, under the heading "Beyond the Face," can be read as an extended meditation on sexuality across a spectrum of concrete expressions: love, eros, voluptuosity, fecundity. "The metaphysical event of transcendence—the welcome of the Other, hospitality—Desire and language—is not accomplished as love. . . . [I]n love transcendence goes both further and less far than language" (254). Love closes itself around the lovers, separates them from others and from discourse, takes place hidden from society. Sexual intimacy blocks the way to intelligibility:

> The relationship established between lovers in voluptuosity, fundamentally refractory to universalization, is the very contrary of the social relation. It excludes the third party, it remains intimacy, dual solitude, closed society, the supremely non-public. The feminine is the other refractory to society, member of a dual society, an intimate society, a society without language. Its intimacy is to be described. (264–65)

This contrariety to the social relation that is found in love and intimacy—the **privacy** and intimacy of sexuality—is in the end its weakness and its strength. Ethics, justice, and the face all aim toward intelligibility, even as they exceed its possibility. On Levinas's view, the withdrawal of lovers is from transcendence and exceeds transcendence. The alterity of the Other is expressed in **friendship**, not love; in discourse, not sexuality. Erotic pleasure—voluptuosity—closes itself into desire. "In this sense voluptuosity is a pure experience, . . . which remains blindly experience" (*Totality*, 260). Love, sexuality, voluptuosity are a relation with the other that stops short of infinity:

> Love remains a relation with the Other that turns into need, and this need still presupposes the total, transcendent exteriority of the other, of the beloved. But love also goes beyond the beloved. This is why through the face filters the obscure light coming from beyond the face, from what *is not yet*, from a future never future enough, more remote than the possible. (254–55)

> Voluptuosity hence aims not at the Other but at his voluptuosity; it is voluptuosity of voluptuosity, love of the love of the other. Love accordingly does not present a particular case of friendship. Love and friendship are not only felt differently; their correlative differs: friendship goes unto the Other; love seeks what does not have the structure of an existent, the infinitely future, what is to be engendered. I love fully only if the Other loves me. (266)

One may understand these words in terms of signification: Love and **sexual desire** do not aim at understanding, speaking, but at experience and pleasure turned toward themselves, refractory to universalization. One may also understand these words in terms of time. Levinas speaks of *diachronic* as against *synchronic time*, of time as interruption, separation, disruption, as against continuous and successive time—the time of being. Totality and infinity cannot be assembled; the saying and the said cannot occur at the same time.

How, then, does transcendence appear in the succession of time? How does infinity produce in time? Through fecundity: Voluptuosity, sexuality, erotic pleasure, and love issue into paternity in time. The future that is my child, my future in the expression of my pleasure, is the fulfillment of diachronic time.

> [T]he erotic, analysed as fecundity, breaks up reality into relations irreducible to the relations of genus and species, part and whole, action and passion, truth and error; . . . in sexuality the subject enters into relation with what is absolutely other, with an alterity of a type unforeseeable in formal logic, with what remains other in the relation and is never converted into "mine," and that nonetheless this relation has nothing ecstatic about it, for the pathos of voluptuosity is made of duality. (*Totality*, 276)

> Paternity is a relation with a stranger who while being Other . . . *is* me, a relation of the I with a self which yet is not me. . . . In existing itself there is a multiplicity and a transcendence. In this transcendence the I is not swept away, since the son is not me; and yet I am my son. The fecundity of the I is its very transcendence. (277)

Sexuality is a relation to the absolutely Other with an infinite and unmediatable alterity. It is nevertheless a relation, beyond reason, present in everyday life.

See also Existentialism; Feminism, French; Heidegger, Martin; Judaism, History of; Phenomenology; Poststructuralism

REFERENCES

Irigaray, Luce. (1984) "The Fecundity of the Caress: A Reading of Levinas, *Totality and Infinity*, 'Phenomenology of Eros.' " In *An Ethics of Sexual Difference*. Trans. Carolyn Burke and Gillian C. Gill. Ithaca, N.Y.: Cornell University Press, 1993, 85–217; Irigaray, Luce. "Questions to Emmanuel Levinas." Trans. Margaret Whitford. In Margaret Whitford, ed., *The Irigaray Reader*. Oxford, U.K.: Blackwell, 1991, 178–89; Levinas, Emmanuel. (1984) "Ethics as First Philosophy." In Seán Hand, trans. and ed., *The Levinas Reader*. Oxford, U.K.: Blackwell, 1989, 75–87; Levinas, Emmanuel. (1947) *Existence and Existents*. Trans. Alphonso Lingis. The Hague, Holland: Martinus Nijhoff, 1978; Levinas, Emmanuel. (1974) *Otherwise Than Being or Beyond Essence*. Trans. Alphonso Lingis. The Hague, Holland: Martinus Nijhoff, 1978; Levinas, Emmanuel. (1968) "Substitution." In Seán Hand, ed., *The Levinas Reader*. Oxford, U.K.: Blackwell, 1989, 88–125; Levinas, Emmanuel. (1961) *Totality and Infinity*. Trans. Alphonso Lingis. Pittsburgh, Pa.: Duquesne University Press, 1969.

Stephen David Ross

ADDITIONAL READING

Bernasconi, Robert, and David Wood, eds. *The Provocation of Levinas: Rethinking the Other*. New York: Routledge, 1988; Chanter, Tina, ed. *Feminist Interpretations of Emmanuel Levinas*. University Park: Pennsylvania State University Press, 2001; Derrida, Jacques. (1997) *Adieu to Emmanuel Levinas*. Trans. Pascale-Anne Brault and Michael B. Naas. Stanford, Calif.: Stanford University Press, 1999; Derrida, Jacques. (1967) "Violence and Metaphysics: An Essay on the Thought of Emmanuel Levinas." In *Writing and Difference*. Trans. Alan Bass. Chicago, Ill.: University of Chicago Press, 1978, 79–153; Hand, Seán, ed. *The Levinas Reader*. Oxford, U.K.: Blackwell, 1989; Katz, Claire Elise. *Levinas, Judaism, and the Feminine: The Silent Footsteps of Rebecca*. Bloomington: Indiana University Press, 2003; Katz, Claire, and Lara Trout, eds. *Emmanuel Levinas*. New York: Routledge, 2004; Lawton, Phillip. "Love and Justice: Levinas' Reading of Buber." *Philosophy Today* 20 (1976), 77–83; Lechte, John. "Violence, Ethics, and Transcendence: Kristeva and Levinas." In John Lechte and Maria Margaroni, *Julia Kristeva: Live Theory*. New York: Continuum, 2004, 86–115; Levinas, Emmanuel. (1995) *Alterity and Transcendence*. Trans. Michael B. Smith. New York: Columbia University Press, 1999; Levinas, Emmanuel. (1982) *Ethics and Infinity: Conversations with Philippe Nemo*. Trans. Richard A. Cohen. Pittsburgh, Pa.: Duquesne University Press, 1985.

LIBERAL FEMINISM. *See* Feminism, Liberal

LIBERALISM. Three types, or levels, of sexual liberalism may be usefully distinguished. There is liberalism at the level of *policies*; at the level of *principles* underlying those policies; and at the level of *sentiments* concerning sexual tastes and behavior.

Liberal Policies. Sexual liberalism is often conceived in terms of a permissive policy with respect to sexual behavior generally or to behavior of a particular type (one might be a liberal on some sexual matters but not others). The permissive policy might concern what should be allowed by law, or perhaps, following John Stuart Mill (1806–1873), what should be allowed by both law and "public opinion." Mill is interested not so much in the rightful limits of the law as, more generally, in those of "compulsion and control, whether the means used be physical force in the form of legal penalties, or the moral coercion of public opinion" (*On Liberty* [*OL*], chap. 1).

Between the policy of fully tolerating behavior of a given type and the contrary policy of completely prohibiting it, there is the possibility of allowing it in certain restricted circumstances. Many people who consider themselves liberals, and many policies regarded as liberal, take such a middle ground on various matters. A common formula here is "between consenting adults in private." The restriction to consenting parties is intended to protect people from coercion. The restriction to adults aims at protecting minors from subtle forms of involuntariness, consisting in unconsidered or uninformed choices that may later be regretted. While the Australian state of Victoria legally allows **prostitution**, for example, it does not allow either enforced prostitution ("sex slavery") or the presence of anyone under the age of eighteen in a brothel. The **privacy** restriction is meant to protect the sensitivities of nonparticipants, and the notion of privacy may be interpreted more or less broadly. In Victoria, it is not only that commercial sex (like the noncommercial sort) may not be performed in public view; brothels may not have explicit verbal or pictorial external signs, though they seem to be able to identify themselves implicitly by such devices as a red light or a pink-painted facade, together with (interestingly) the *absence* of any explicit indication of the nature of the business.

Liberal Principles. Suppose someone supports a liberal policy with respect to prostitution and explains that while the practice is inherently immoral and its extermination desirable, our limited law enforcement resources are better devoted to tackling even worse things, such as **rape**, robbery, and murder. Despite the liberal policy, there would be some reluctance to describe this person as a true liberal on prostitution. His or her support for legal toleration depends entirely on the contingent fact that the resources for suppression are needed elsewhere, and the implication is that if they were not, there would be no toleration. True liberalism does not rest on such variable contingencies as these; it is a matter of respecting certain *principles* governing the policies we adopt.

A useful perspective from which to view possible principles, and characterize liberalism at this level, is in terms of the following question: While our policies may be subject to various contingencies as noted above, what grounds could *prima facie* justify the prohibition or restriction of any given sexual behavior?

One answer to this question is that no grounds at all could do so. A possible background view here is *moral nihilism*: No behavior is either right or wrong, and this goes for rape and other sexual assaults as well as everything else. An implication of this would seem to be that while the nihilist refuses to condemn the rapist, he cannot condemn those who punish the rapist either, and so his permissiveness is somewhat feeble in practice. A second view is that while some things are right and some are wrong, no *sexual* behavior is in any way wrong, and so none of it ought to be prohibited. A third view is a form of *political anarchism*: We may disapprove of rape and child molesting, but no person or organization has any right to impose such disapproval coercively on anyone else, even if the latter person has imposed *his* values or desires on his victim.

Most people who call themselves liberals, however, and especially those influenced by Mill, do not support such complete tolerance of all sexual behavior. Though not referring directly to sex (or to anything else yet), Mill says that the rightful limits of society's coercive power over the individual are determined by "one very simple principle": "to prevent harm to others. His own good, either physical or moral, is not a sufficient warrant. He cannot rightfully be compelled to do or forbear because it will be better for him to do so, because it will make him happier, because, in the opinions of others, to do so would be wise, or even right" (*OL*, chap. 1). Mill is taking a stand here against what are now known as *paternalism* (see Sartorius), the coercion of people for their own supposed benefit, and *legal moralism* (see Wasserstrom), the enforcement of morality as such.

Mill's "very simple principle" may not, however, be quite as simple as he suggests. There may be clear cases of harm, such as rape, various other forms of sexual assault that cause physical injury or trauma, and infringements on liberty such as sexual enslavement. But there are many problem cases, too, raising questions as to what is to count as harm, or enough of it, and what degree of likelihood of it is required to justify interference (between remote possibility at one end of the scale and virtual certainty at the other). The debate over whether **pornography** is causally connected with harm and, if so, what kinds of pornography and what kinds of harm, and how much of it, and with what degree of probability, illustrates some of these complexities (see Baird and Rosenbaum; Russell; Strossen).

This aside, Mill's liberalism is complicated, or maybe even compromised, by various things he says. We shall consider some of these with respect to sexual conduct.

First, he says that the person's own physical or moral well-being may provide "good reasons for remonstrating with him, or reasoning with him, or persuading him, or entreating him, but not for compelling him, or visiting him with any evil in case he do otherwise" (*OL*, chap. 1). The distinction may be clear in theory but rather fine in practice. Suppose some people think your sexual conduct immoral, though not harmful to others. Mill would seem to allow them to be (constantly?) remonstrating with you, entreating you, and so forth, in ways that you may find intrusive and oppressive. You may in fact think it a lesser evil to be in a social situation where your behavior is merely punishable with, say, a small (even if regular) fine.

Mill later affirms our right not only to condemn someone of whose purely self-regarding conduct we disapprove, and to avoid associating with him ("not to the oppression of his individuality, but in the exercise of ours"), but also to "give others a preference over him in optional good offices, except those that tend to his improvement" (*OL*, chap. 4). He concedes that the consequences for the person may be severe but thinks them acceptable because they are not purposely inflicted as punishment.

Mill gives some examples of "faults" that, he implies, *merit* such treatment. These include the pursuit of "animal pleasures at the expense of those of feeling and intellect." He may well have sexual pleasures in mind, and maybe even *all* sexual pleasures if we go by what he says in *Utilitarianism* (chap. 2) about "higher" and "lower" pleasures, but he does not elaborate.

Second, Mill makes a brief reference to actions that (whether self-harmful or not) "if done publicly, are a violation of good manners, and coming thus within the category of offences against others, may rightly be prohibited. Of this kind are offences against decency; on which it is unnecessary to dwell" (*OL*, chap. 5).

This is a clear departure from the principle that only *harm* to others warrants restrictions on our behavior, given that behavior may be indecent and offensive without being harmful. But is it an illiberal departure? The protection of others from public indecency is not being used as a ground for total prohibition but only for restriction: The conduct may be allowed in private. Many people who consider themselves liberals would be quite comfortable with this stance on behavior such as (1) sexual intercourse, for example. But other things people do might in some places and eras cause offense. Consider these: (2) mutual genital fondling, with or without partial undressing; (3) sensual, prolonged kissing; (4) holding hands; and (5) gazing lovingly at one another. How many people must be offended, and how deeply, to justify prohibiting the public display of each of these, respectively? Do we require some people to be deeply shocked, or most people to be at least embarrassed, or some sort of disjunction or midpoint between these? And are such "quantitative" dimensions the only ones to consider? (See Joel Feinberg [1926–2004], vol. 2.) Suppose that in a certain social milieu many people are very disturbed by witnessing (5). Should it then be prohibited, or would this be pandering to an unhealthy hang-up? If we take the latter view, would the same apply to (4), (3), (2), and (1)? Should a line be drawn, and if so, where and why? Does it matter whether the participants are of different sexes?

Someone wanting to prohibit even heterosexual couples indulging publicly in (5) or (4), on the grounds that it could possibly make some people feel a little uncomfortable, would hardly count as a liberal. On the other hand, someone wanting full tolerance of the public performance of all the above (and perhaps all consensual sexual acts) would be very liberal indeed. Between these poles is a territory in which many liberals would locate themselves, but its borders are hard to specify. Perhaps liberalism should be seen as both a matter of degree and a matter of several dimensions. One liberal might be prepared to ban certain conduct because it may harm others, while another might think that the chance or the amount of harm is insufficient; one liberal might wish to ban a certain public display because it may deeply offend some people, while for another it may be necessary and sufficient that *most* people be affected even if only slightly embarrassed. For these reasons it is difficult to establish a precise formulation of liberal principles concerning harm and offense.

Third, and in the same chapter of *On Liberty*, there is a well-known passage about selling oneself into slavery. Mill supports prohibiting this, on the grounds that in abdicating his liberty, a person would be defeating the very purpose of allowing him to make his own choices: "The principle of freedom cannot require that he should be free not to be free." Adjusting the example for our purposes, what about selling oneself into *sexual* slavery? One would be at the buyer's beck and call for sexual purposes but not for other purposes. There may have to be a contract or law specifying how and where the distinction is to be drawn, but Mill would presumably have none of it and say that his objection to slavery *per se* applies to any particular kind of it such as this.

His words on slavery actually seem to reveal an important tension in his thought: between, on the one hand, the hedonism he occasionally embraces (see, for example, the first two paragraphs of chap. 2 of *Utilitarianism*), which would seem to allow you to sell yourself into slavery if you are going to be more content that way, and, on the other hand, an ideal of rational autonomy that requires you to keep making reflective choices from a range of alternatives harmless to others. Selling yourself into slavery of some kind may increase your net pleasure but at the cost of your continued autonomy, and for Mill here it seems irrelevant that you *do not want* your autonomy and will be more content without it.

His position appears to be interestingly paternalistic. He accepts anyway (as do most people) what is known as *weak* paternalism, where we exercise coercion in the belief that when the coerced party grows up or sobers up or is wised up with relevant knowledge, he or she will be glad of having been coerced. Thus we keep young children away from fires and roads and rivers, and, to take an example of Mill's, we may "seize" a person about to cross an unsafe bridge if there is no time to warn him of the danger. *Strong* paternalism, on the other hand, consists in coercion of someone for the sake of her good not as this is conceived by her or probably will be when she is more mature or rational or informed, but as conceived by the coercer. This is often regarded as illiberal, and Mill's stance on selling oneself into slavery seems to be a case of strong paternalism. "If you were really a liberal," the would-be slave might protest to Mill, "Wouldn't you let me do what I *want* to do, given that I'm not harming others? It's my settled preference; I've actually had a 'trial run' with a potential owner, and I'm quite sure that this is for me!"

Fourth, and again in chapter 5, Mill asks whether society should tolerate brothels and gambling houses. He is uncertain: There are good arguments both ways. On the one hand, he says, it may be argued that since fornication and gambling must be tolerated, so must living or profiting by them, and that society "cannot go beyond dissuasion, and . . . one person should be as free to persuade as another to dissuade." On the other hand, he says, it may be contended that while society should not declare any conduct bad, for the purpose of prohibition, if it affects only the interests of the participants, it may justifiably regard its goodness or badness as being at least "disputable" and try to exclude the influence of those with a personal interest on the side "which the State believes to be wrong." (He presumably means "immoral," at least in the case of brothels.) He tries to resolve the issue by suggesting that although the prohibition of such businesses "is never effectual" and they may always keep operating in some guise, no matter what power is given to the police, yet they will be compelled to do so "with a certain degree of secrecy and mystery, so that nobody knows anything about them but those who seek them; and more than this society ought not to aim at."

Mill implies that he accepts this solution, which looks like a major concession to legal moralism, despite his assurance that the prohibition is "never effectual." This may not much impress those brothel keepers who fail to keep their businesses secret enough and are prosecuted, having facilitated behavior that Mill does not claim to be harmful but at most contrary to the accepted morality.

In 1873, the year of Mill's death, Sir James Fitzjames Stephen (1829–1894) attacked him in *Liberty, Equality, Fraternity*. Criminal law, says Stephen, has not only the function of protecting society from harm; it is also "a persecution of the grosser forms of vice." Persecution of lesser forms may not be practicable, and "it is impossible to legislate directly against unchastity, unless it takes forms that everyone regards as monstrous and horrible. The subject is not one for detailed discussion" (152). He may well be thinking here of **homosexuality**, or at least of sodomy, but, with respect to whatever he does have in mind, Stephen embraces a form of legal moralism.

In 1957, however, the Wolfenden Report in Britain recommended that homosexual behavior between consenting adults in private should no longer be a criminal offense. "There must remain," the Report famously declares in a rallying call for liberals, "a realm of private morality and immorality which in brief and crude terms is not the law's business" (§61).

In 1958 Sir Patrick (later Lord) Devlin published a now famous essay, "Morals and the Criminal Law" (*Enforcement*, 1–25) in which he attacked Wolfenden's thinking and, implicitly, the latter's recommendation as to changing the law. In some places he describes his own position in terms akin to Stephen's, as when he says that with respect to some crimes the function of the criminal law is "simply to enforce a moral principle and nothing else" and that "the law *is* [rightly] concerned with immorality as such" (11). There is a second argument in Devlin, however, which he may not clearly distinguish from the first but for which he is probably more famous. A society depends for its existence, he says, on "community of ideas" as to how its members should govern their lives. Because "a recognized morality is as necessary to society as, say, a recognized government, then society may use the law to preserve morality in the same way as it uses it to safeguard anything else that is essential to its existence" (11). The state may legislate against immorality for the same reason it may legislate against treason and sedition.

Devlin's contemporary critic H.L.A. Hart (1907–1992), in his *Law, Liberty and Morality*, distinguishes Devlin's "extreme" thesis (that the enforcement of morality is a good thing in itself) from his "moderate" thesis (that such enforcement helps to preserve society's "moral cement" and thus its very existence). Mill, as we have seen, comes close to the extreme thesis in connection with brothels. He also has some common ground with the moderate thesis; he says that as well as being prevented from harming other individuals, a person may be rightly compelled "to bear his fair share in the common defense, or in any other joint work necessary to the interest of the society of which he enjoys the protection" (*OL*, chap. 1). Besides **military** service, he may be thinking of such things as taxation. Devlin is suggesting that a further way in which one may be made to serve the interests of society, and indeed to help preserve its very existence, is in being required to conform to the vital shared morality. We may note, however, that his position here differs from the extreme legal moralism advocated by Stephen, and seemingly advocated sometimes by himself, not only in its Millian appeal to the interests of society at large but in its frankly relativist character: What matters is not whether a given act *is* immoral, by some "objective" standard, but whether the society in question *judges* it to be immoral.

Is his moderate view sound? As Hart points out, it may well be true that *some* shared morality is essential to the existence of any society. It does not follow, however, that this morality cannot change without society being destroyed, so that any contravention of its current rules is a threat to society's existence. Even if deviations from the accepted morality become frequent enough to cause it to change, this is nothing like subversion. We should compare such a change, says Hart, "not to the violent overthrow of government but to a peaceful constitutional change in its form, consistent not only with the preservation of a society but with its advance" (52).

In any case, how is the lawmaker to identify the moral judgments of society? Devlin says that unanimity is too much to ask, but a mere majority is not enough. He appeals instead to the traditional English legal standard of the "man in the Clapham omnibus" or the "reasonable man," who, he says, "is not to be confused with the rational man. He is not expected to reason about anything and his judgement may be largely a matter of feeling" (15). It is the strength of this feeling, indeed, that decides when a society may, to protect its own integrity, restrict its members' freedom: "It is not nearly enough to say that a majority dislike a practice; there must be a real feeling of reprobation. . . . No society can do without intolerance, indignation, and disgust; they are the forces behind the moral law. . . . There is, for example, a general abhorrence of homosexuality. [If the genuine feeling of our society is that it is] a vice so abominable that its mere presence is an offence . . . I do not see how society can be denied the right to eradicate it" (17). As Hart observes, such apparent indifference to evidence as to the impact of a practice on society's "moral cement" and reliance instead on the feelings of the ordinary person suggest that Devlin is reverting to, or essentially appealing to, the extreme thesis (50, 55).

Forty years on, the debate in many Western societies is not so much over the legal toleration of homosexual acts (between consenting adults in private) as over such further issues as the legal recognition of homosexual **marriage**. Many conservatives object to the latter on terminological grounds, saying that marriage is by definition a union between a man and a woman. One response to this is that the word is unimportant, and an official same-sex union could easily be called something else. But another response is that the word "marriage" does matter, and we should extend its meaning to acknowledge, in law and in moral thinking, the full equivalence of such unions with heterosexual ones. Besides the terminological issue, however, the main objections raised by conservatives resemble those identified above in Devlin. Some take an extreme legal moralist view, tempered by pragmatism: We may not be able to turn back the clock and recriminalize homosexual acts, but we can at least deny their perpetrators full legal recognition of their relationships. Others embrace a version of the moderate view, claiming that supporters of such unions are "attacking the institution of (heterosexual) marriage," which is vital to the existence of society, at least in any tolerable form. The extent of the institution's importance to society, and to what sort of society, is a matter of debate. But in any case it seems to be no more under attack here than it is by people's choices to live alone or with friends or in a religious community. Presumably not even the most ardent supporter of standard heterosexual marriage will want all these abstentions from it to be prohibited.

Devlin's view of the importance of having and enforcing a shared morality may be regarded as a version of what has recently come to be known as "communitarianism." A common element in communitarian thinking is the idea of *communal goods*. Besides individual goods that you or I may seek and enjoy (goods that in some cases converge, so that we may act jointly to achieve them), there are goods that we see as *ours*, with the sharing of them being an important part of the value. In a "contractarian" picture of society, such as that of **Thomas Hobbes** (1588–1679; *Leviathan*, chaps. 13–18), your need for security converges with mine, and we agree to establish and obey a powerful sovereign to keep the peace; what this fails to recognize, say communitarians, is that there are goods that cannot be reduced to mere convergent ones and that may play important parts in our social and political life. Such goods may include our cultural practices and traditions and our participation at various levels of politics. Might they also include shared **sexual ethics**, based on a shared understanding of the purpose of sexuality?

Some liberals accept a contractarian view of some sort (see, for example, John Rawls [1921–2002]) and the view of human nature on which it is often based: an atomistic conception that sees our identities and interests as formed independently of our social situations and roles, and our need to protect our interests as requiring us to make, or to be understood as having implicitly made, an agreement of some sort with our fellows, an agreement that forms the basis of a sound moral and political system. But liberals are not required to accept any of this. Mill, for example, rejects the atomistic idea in favor of a more Aristotelian one, saying that the social state is "so natural, so necessary, and so habitual" to us that we virtually never conceive ourselves otherwise than as members of a body (*Utilitarianism*, chap. 3; see **Aristotle**'s [384–322 BCE] *Politics*, bk. I, chap. 2). And rather than attempting to base liberal principles and policies on a contract of some sort (a highly problematic notion, as the required contract is hard to discover, and a merely hypothetical contract seems unable to generate real rights and obligations), one may appeal to the value of human autonomy, or happiness, or, as in Ronald Dworkin, to the implications of equality. Mill wavers somewhat between autonomy and happiness and as to their respective natures, but many liberals may appeal to one or more of these goods as justifying their stance on sexual liberty and its limits, rather than to the requirements of any supposedly real or hypothetical contract. Such liberals need not deny the existence of further goods, including communal ones, which may provide rich pleasures and be perfectly acceptable as long as they do not conflict with important individual goods.

Liberal Sentiments. We earlier distinguished liberal policies from liberal principles, noting that one might adopt a liberal policy on some sexual matter for reasons other than liberal principles. But it seems that this distinction is still inadequate to capture an important aspect of what it is to be a truly liberal person. There is a third type of liberalism to be acknowledged, involving a certain *sentiment* toward the behavior in question. Suppose I favor allowing homosexual behavior in private, and do so for the Millian reason that such behavior is purely self-regarding, but am so revolted by the thought of it that I have to force myself to be pleasant and courteous toward people whom I know to be homosexual. As allowed by Mill, perhaps I try to avoid them altogether and give heterosexuals preference in "optional good offices." Should I be regarded as a truly or fully liberal person? To be the latter, it may be said, one must *feel comfortable* with other people's (harmless) sexual tastes and conduct, though they may differ from one's own. This does not mean, of course, that we have to include every such person among our friends, for in a given case there may be other reasons that preclude this, reasons that may indeed involve those sexual tastes in a way: If I am not gay but you are, and you think and talk of nothing but aspects of your gay lifestyle, then it is unlikely that we will have enough common ground to be close friends. On the other hand, if we have common ground on other matters, and both continue to cultivate it, and it is clear to you that I am comfortable with your sexuality and vice versa, there is no reason why we cannot be good or even close friends. This is not merely a theoretical possibility but, for many people of liberal sentiments, a welcome fact of life.

One possible measure of the liberality of our sentiments is **humor**. Consider a common type of joke: The first two sailors or Foreign Legionnaires are "straight," but the third one turns out unexpectedly to be gay. The success of the joke will depend not only on that unexpectedness, and also on some degree of cleverness in the construction of the story, but also on the idea that there is something *wrong* with a sailor or Legionnaire being gay; it would not strike people as funny if the third one were merely *different* from the others in, say, nationality or hair color. If the teller and the hearer of the joke do see something wrong with it, they are not completely comfortable with it, and their sentiments toward it are not (entirely) liberal, even though they may be liberal at the other two levels. Most gay people presumably feel comfortable (in the above way) with others' heterosexuality and find it regrettable when their sentiment is not reciprocated.

An interesting contrast may be drawn between two kinds of reason for which one might not tell or enjoy such a joke (apart from technical matters having to do with how it is composed or told, and social factors such as whether one's prim aunt is listening). On the one hand, someone might reject it simply because it is about sex; such jokes are often called "dirty," like other items with explicit sexual content such as books and pictures. This attitude is hardly a liberal one. On the other hand, it may be because one's sentiments *are* liberal that one does not find it funny: One may be quite comfortable with people being gay, and the third sailor being gay is in itself as unremarkable as his being black or tall or friendly. Those who do enjoy the joke will be liberal enough in their sentiments to find some sexual matters entertaining but not as liberal as they might be when it comes to the particular sexual matters that entertain them.

See also Activity, Sexual; Bestiality; Consent; Consequentialism; Disability; Diseases, Sexually Transmitted; Feminism, Liberal; Feminism, Men's; Humor; Incest; Law, Sex and the; Marriage, Same-Sex; Nudism; Pedophilia; Pornography; Prostitution; Sex Work; Wittgenstein, Ludwig

REFERENCES

Aristotle. (ca. 330 BCE?) *Politics*. Trans. E. Barker. Rev. R. F. Stalley. Oxford, U.K.: Oxford University Press, 1995; Baird, Robert M., and Stuart E. Rosenbaum, eds. (1991) *Pornography: Private Right or Public Menace?* rev. ed. Amherst, N.Y.: Prometheus, 1998; Devlin, Patrick. *The Enforcement of Morals*. Oxford, U.K.: Oxford University Press, 1965; Dworkin, Ronald. *Sovereign Virtue: The Theory and Practice of Equality*. Cambridge, Mass.: Harvard University Press, 2000; Dworkin, Ronald. *Taking Rights Seriously*. London: Duckworth, 1977; Feinberg, Joel. *The Moral Limits of the Criminal Law*. Vol. 1: *Harm to Others*. New York: Oxford University Press, 1984. Vol. 2: *Offense to Others*, 1985. Vol. 3: *Harm to Self*, 1986. Vol. 4: *Harmless Wrongdoing*, 1988; Hart, H.L.A. (1962) *Law, Liberty and Morality*. Stanford, Calif.: Stanford University Press, 1963; Hobbes, Thomas. (1651) *Leviathan*. Ed. C. B. Macpherson. London: Penguin, 1968; Mill, John Stuart. (1859) *On Liberty*. Ed. Elizabeth Rapaport. Indianapolis, Ind.: Hackett, 1978; Mill, John Stuart. (1863) *Utilitarianism*. Indianapolis, Ind.: Bobbs-Merrill, 1957; Rawls, John. *A Theory of Justice*. Cambridge, Mass.: Harvard University Press, 1971; Russell, Diana E. H. *Dangerous Relationships: Pornography, Misogyny, and Rape*. Thousand Oaks, Calif.: Sage, 1998; Sartorius, Rolf, ed. *Paternalism*. Minneapolis: University of Minnesota Press, 1983; Stephen, James Fitzjames. (1873) *Liberty, Equality, Fraternity*. London: Cambridge University Press, 1967; Strossen, Nadine. *Defending Pornography: Free Speech, Sex, and the Fight for Women's Rights*. New York: Scribner's, 1995; Wasserstrom, Richard A., ed. *Morality and the Law*. Belmont, Calif.: Wadsworth, 1971; "Wolfenden Report." Report of the Committee on Homosexual Offences and Prostitution (U.K.). Cmd. 247, 1957.

Douglas Adeney

ADDITIONAL READING

Altman, Andrew. "Liberalism and Campus Hate Speech: A Philosophical Examination." *Ethics* 103 (January 1993), 302–17; Barry, Brian M. *The Liberal Theory of Justice: A Critical Examination of the Principle Doctrines in* A Theory of Justice *by John Rawls*. Oxford, U.K.: Clarendon Press, 1973; Bentham, Jeremy. (1789) *The Principles of Morals and Legislation*. Darien, Conn.: Hafner, 1970; Burley, Justine, ed. *Dworkin and His Critics: With Replies by Dworkin*. Malden, Mass.: Blackwell, 2004; Coleman, Jules, and Allen Buchanan, eds. *In Harm's Way: Essays in Honor of Joel Feinberg*. Cambridge: Cambridge University Press, 1994; Crisp, Roger. "Teachers in an Age of Transition: Peter Singer and J. S. Mill." In Dale Jamieson, ed., *Singer and His Critics*. Oxford, U.K.: Blackwell, 1999, 85–102; Donner, Wendy. "John Stuart Mill's Liberal Feminism." *Philosophical Studies* 69 (1993), 155–66; Dworkin, Gerald, ed. *Morality, Harm, and the Law*. Boulder, Colo.: Westview, 1994; Dworkin, Ronald. *Freedom's Law: The Moral Reading of the American Constitution*. Cambridge, Mass.: Harvard University Press, 1996; Dworkin, Ronald. "Is There a Right to Pornography?" *Oxford Journal of Legal Studies* 1:2 (1981), 177–212. Reprinted in Susan Dwyer, ed., *The Problem of Pornography*. Belmont, Calif.: Wadsworth, 1995, 77–90; Dworkin, Ronald. "Liberty and Pornography." *New York Review of Books* (21 October 1993), 12–15. Reprinted in Susan Dwyer, ed.,

The Problem of Pornography. Belmont, Calif.: Wadsworth, 1995, 113–21; Dworkin, Ronald. *Life's Dominion: An Argument about Abortion, Euthanasia, and Individual Freedom*. New York: Vintage, 1994; Dworkin, Ronald. "Women and Pornography." *New York Review of Books* (21 October 1993), 36–42; [reply to letter] *New York Review of Books* (3 March 1994), 48–49; Dyzenhaus, David. "John Stuart Mill and the Harm of Pornography." *Ethics* 102:3 (1992), 534–51; Ellis, Anthony. "Offense and the Liberal Conception of the Law." *Philosophy and Public Affairs* 13:1 (1984), 3–23; Elshtain, Jean Bethke. "Nineteenth Century Liberal Sons: Jeremy Bentham and John Stuart Mill." In *Public Man, Private Woman: Women in Social and Political Thought*. Princeton, N.J.: Princeton University Press, 1981, 132–46; George, Robert P., and Gerard V. Bradley. "Marriage and the Liberal Imagination." *Georgetown Law Journal* 84:2 (1995), 301–20; Gruen, Lori, and George F. Panichas, eds. *Sex, Morality, and the Law*. New York: Routledge, 1997; Hein, Hilda. "Sadomasochism and the Liberal Tradition." In Robin Ruth Linden, Darlene R. Pagano, Diana E. H. Russell, and Susan Leigh Star, eds., *Against Sadomasochism: A Radical Feminist Analysis*. East Palo Alto, Calif.: Frog in the Well, 1982, 83–89; Hekman, Susan J. "John Stuart Mill's *The Subjection of Women*: The Foundations of Liberal Feminism." *History of European Ideas* 15 (1992), 681–86; Himmelfarb, Gertrude. *On Liberty and Liberalism: The Case of John Stuart Mill*. New York: Knopf, 1974; Laden, Anthony Simon. "Radical Liberals, Reasonable Feminists: Reason, Power, and Objectivity in MacKinnon and Rawls." *Journal of Political Philosophy* 11:2 (2003), 133–52; Langton, Rae. "Whose Right? Ronald Dworkin, Women, and Pornographers." *Philosophy and Public Affairs* 19:4 (1990), 311–59. Reprinted in Susan Dwyer, ed., *The Problem of Pornography*. Belmont, Calif.: Wadsworth, 1995, 91–112; Leidholdt, Dorchen, and Janice C. Raymond, eds. *The Sexual Liberals and the Attack on Feminism*. New York: Teachers College Press, 1990; LeMoncheck, Linda. *Loose Women, Lecherous Men: A Feminist Philosophy of Sex*. New York: Oxford University Press, 1997; Okin, Susan Moller. (1989) "John Rawls: Justice as Fairness—For Whom?" In Mary Lyndon Shanley and Carole Pateman, eds., *Feminist Interpretations and Political Theory*. University Park: Pennsylvania State University Press, 1991, 181–98; Posner, Richard A. *Sex and Reason*. Cambridge, Mass.: Harvard University Press, 1992; Rawls, John. *Political Liberalism*. New York: Columbia University Press, 1993; Reiman, Jeffrey. "Prostitution, Addiction, and the Ideology of Liberalism." *Contemporary Crises* 3 (1979), 53–68; Richards, David A. J. *Sex, Drugs, Death, and the Law: An Essay in Human Rights and Overcriminalization*. Totowa, N.J.: Rowman and Littlefield, 1982; Riley, Jonathan. *Mill on Liberty*. London: Routledge, 1998; Schaeffer, Denise. "Feminism and Liberalism Reconsidered: The Case of Catharine MacKinnon." *American Political Science Review* 95:3 (2001), 699–708; Schaff, Kory. "Kant, Political Liberalism, and the Ethics of Same-Sex Relations." *Journal of Social Philosophy* 32:3 (2001), 446–62; Schulhofer, Stephen. *Unwanted Sex: The Culture of Intimidation and the Failure of Law*. Cambridge, Mass.: Harvard University Press, 1998; Scoccia, Danny. "Can Liberals Support a Ban on Violent Pornography?" *Ethics* 106:4 (1996), 776–99; Scruton, Roger. "Sexual Morality and the Liberal Consensus." In *The Philosopher on Dover Beach—Essays*. Manchester, U.K.: Carcanet, 1990, 262–72; Shrage, Laurie. *Moral Dilemmas of Feminism: Prostitution, Adultery, and Abortion*. New York: Routledge, 1994; Skipper, Robert. "Mill and Pornography." *Ethics* 103:4 (1993), 726–30; Soble, Alan. "Paternalism, Liberal Theory, and Suicide." *Canadian Journal of Philosophy* 12:2 (1982), 335–52; Soble, Alan. *Sexual Investigations*. New York: New York University Press, 1996; Ten, C. L. *Mill on Liberty*. Oxford, U.K.: Clarendon Press, 1980; Vernon, Richard. "John Stuart Mill and Pornography: Beyond the Harm Principle." *Ethics* 106 (April 1996), 621–32; Warburton, Nigel. *Freedom: An Introduction with Readings*. London: Routledge, 2001; Wertheimer, Alan. *Consent to Sexual Relations*. Cambridge: Cambridge University Press, 2003; Wertheimer, Alan. *Exploitation*. Princeton, N.J.: Princeton University Press, 1996; Zerilli, Linda M. G. *Signifying Woman: Culture and Chaos in Rousseau, Burke, and Mill*. Ithaca, N.Y.: Cornell University Press, 1994.

LOVE. "What is love?" may be a question only philosophers would ask. Yet in trying to define love one quickly encounters difficulties. One problem concerns whether love is primarily emotional or volitional. It strikes many as commonsensical that love is an emotion.

Some philosophers, however, argue that the essence of love is not affective but volitional (Frankfurt, *Reasons*, 43, 79). If so, "Concern for the welfare of the loved one [may be] an essential component of all types of love" (Caraway, "Neither Sexist," 361). Some ways of treating the other are good evidence of love or are, perhaps, even constitutive of love, while other ways are incompatible with love. This caring must be exhibited in action and not reside merely in a feeling. While this does not entail that love is not an emotion at all, it does suggest that it is not *only* an emotion.

A popular way of conceiving love's concern claims that love involves a union of interests: When we love each other, your interests become mine and mine become yours. For Neil Delaney, love "includes wanting . . . to take another's needs and interests [as] your own and to wish that she will do the same" (340; see Hunter, 75–76). For **Roger Scruton**, however, there must be more than "wanting" that this happens: Love emerges when "reciprocity becomes community," that is, exactly when "all distinction between my interests and your interests is overcome" (230). As a result of this union, "When something bad happens to one you love . . . something bad also happens *to you*" (Nozick, 68). One advantage of conceiving of concern "in terms of mutual sharing of interests" is that doing so may resolve "the paradoxes of self-interest and altruism" (Fried, 79; see Frankfurt, *Reasons*, 61–62).

The union-of-interests view might not capture everything about love's concern. (For criticism of the view, see Irving SINGER, *Nature*, vol. 3, 406–17; *Pursuit*, 26–29; Soble, "Union.") Even if a better conception of concern—say, **Aristotle**'s (384–322 BCE) in *Nicomachean Ethics* (1156b5–10)—can be found, the emotional aspect of love still requires acknowledgment. Suppose that love is largely an emotion or, better, a passion (for which there are many literary examples, for example, Thomas Mann's [1875–1955] *Death in Venice* [1911]). Which passion is it? **Plato** (427–347 BCE), in *Symposium*, defined love as a desire to possess the good and the beautiful (201a, 202d, 204d, 205e). One's passion for a desirable object (a vase, say) makes her desire to caress it, hold it tightly against her, and put it where she can often gaze on it. A lover might respond precisely the same way to a desirable person, whose **beauty** is overwhelming. But Plato's definition may not adequately illuminate love for persons. Although desire is important in love, it does not exhaust one's feelings for the beloved: Empathy and affection are also involved. And saying that what I desire is "the good" marginalizes the beloved, who is reduced to a mere vehicle for delivering goodness to the lover. Plato's account of love thus looks bleakly impersonal. (For criticisms of Plato, see Gregory Vlastos [1907–1991], "Individual"; Singer, *Nature*, vol. 1, 64–87; contrast Nussbaum, 165–99.)

Love and Value. Suppose we reject these elements of Plato's account. We might still think him to have correctly identified two crucial elements of love: desire and valuation. Presumably, if person *A* loves person *B*, then *A* will have certain desires regarding *B*. In particular, if the love in question is *romantic* love, we may well expect certain *physical* desires to be present. Scruton, for instance, writes that love involves a desire for "that imaginative and immediate acquaintance with the other's mentality, which comes from looking into his face and hearing his voice. Hence, all love shares . . . that emphasis on the other's embodiment which dominates the love that springs from desire" (231). While recognizing the significance of desire, such a conception rejects decisively Plato's occasional approach, which (in some sections of *Symposium* and *Phaedrus*) valorizes purely intellectual or spiritual love (see Vlastos, "Sex in Platonic Love").

What of valuation? Along with Plato, we could view love as the state of responding to an appreciation of the beloved's goodness. The fact that "[a]ll writers on love have agreed that loving something necessarily implies valuing it" might suggest that love is itself a *form* of valuation (Brentlinger, 114). Rather than being a desire for the good, love may be understood as the *judgment* that something or someone *is* good.

While the centrality of valuation to love has been generally recognized, the exact nature of love's relation to value is a matter of dispute. To simplify matters somewhat: There are two views of the relationship between love and value. According to one conceptualization of love, something about the beloved *B* is central in accounting for *A*'s love for *B*. The emphasis is on the perceived merit of the object as grounding *A*'s love. (See Soble, *Structure*, 4–5, who calls this "erosic" love.) By contrast, another view (Soble calls it "agapic" love) sees love as *creating* rather than reflecting antecedent value. The agape tradition in the philosophy of love understands love between persons as akin to God's love for humankind, which is not earned or merited by the objects of God's love but is given freely as a gift. Thus, "God does not love that which is already in itself worthy of love, but on the contrary, that which in itself has no worth acquires worth just by becoming the object of God's love" (Anders Nygren [1890–1978]; 78). While erosic love responds to the independent, preexisting value of the beloved, agapic love is an expression of the loving nature of the lover. Something about the lover *A* rather than about the beloved *B* accounts for *A*'s love. (By the way, it has been argued that not even Plato's account of love is erosic but closer to agapic. He "attempt[s] to capture the notion that our very perception of the beloved as good is dependent on our first seeing with the vision of love"; Osborne, 116.)

Even those who accept that God's love for humanity is *agape* might be skeptical that love between humans, particularly sexual love, can be conceived this way. Erosic love captures more naturally much of the **phenomenology** of (sexual) love. Consider, for example, how we tend to respond to attractive traits when choosing potential partners. Still, some philosophers argue that personal, even sexual, love is (or perhaps should be) largely if not entirely agapic. Irving Singer has claimed that in personal love there is a high degree of "bestowal," as opposed to erosic "appraisal," of value. As if copying God, the lover bestows value on the beloved by loving him (*Nature*, vol. 1, 3–22; vol. 3, 390–406).

One need not be religious to agree with the agapic view. Harry Frankfurt, for example, accepts the agapic model of love within an apparently secular framework. On his view,

> It is true that the beloved invariably *is* . . . valuable to the lover. However, . . . [i]t need not be a perception of value in what he loves that moves the lover to love it. The truly essential relationship between love and the value of the beloved goes in the opposite direction. . . . [W]hat we love necessarily *acquires* value for us *because* we love it. (*Reasons*, 38–39)

Frankfurt then applies this model to parents' love for their children. "Among relationships between humans, the love of parents for their infants or small children is the species of caring that comes closest to offering recognizably pure instances of love" ("On Caring," 166; *Reasons*, 43). Thus "it is not fundamentally because I recognize how important to me my children are that I love them. On the contrary, the relationship between their value to me and my love for them goes essentially the other way. My children are valuable to me in the first place just because I love them" ("Duty and Love," 6). Parents love their children more than they love other children, but they do not believe them to be objectively more valuable. The difference must apparently be explained in agapic, not erosic, terms.

The idea that personal love is agapic, though, raises puzzles (see Wolf on Frankfurt). Should children feel good about their parents' love for them, given that it in no way reflects their value? "A love that does not discriminate forfeit[s] a part of its own value, by doing an injustice to its object," claims **Sigmund Freud** (1856–1939; 49). Perhaps personal love is a complex mixture of both agapic and erosic elements, though we might still wonder, having accepted this reconciliation, whether one tends to dominate in all or any particular case or type of love.

Romanticism and Union. In contemporary Western culture love and sex are most commonly connected through the concept *romantic love*, the major elements of which, according to Carol Caraway, are "concern, admiration, desire for reciprocation, and the passion for union" ("Neither Sexist," 361). Of these, the passion for union (which is something different from "joint interests" discussed earlier) is often taken as a common element of *all* personal love. This passion may be fundamental to romantic love, for even if all four elements are necessary for it, the desire for union may be the only element that is *distinctive* to romantic love (Soble, "Unity," 385–87). After all, concern, admiration, and the desire for reciprocity are present in other relationships, for example, **friendship**.

The idea that a desire for union plays a role in love has a long history. Genesis 2:24 tells us that "a man . . . shall cleave unto his wife: and they shall be one flesh." Aristophanes, in Plato's *Symposium*, relates a myth in which Zeus separates whole human beings into defective halves. As a result, the fundamental desire of a "half-person" is to

> melt together with the one he loves, so that one person emerged from two. Why should this be so? It's because . . . we used to be complete wholes in our original nature, and now "Love" is the name for our pursuit of wholeness, for our desire to be complete. (192e)

Much contemporary thought about romantic love maintains this focus on the passion for union, the desire to form a single entity *we* out of two separate I's (see Delaney, 340–41; Nozick, 82–85; Solomon, 130). "[E]very developed form of sexual desire," Scruton writes, "will tend to reach beyond the present encounter to a project of inner union with its object" (93).

Focusing on the desire for union as the fundamental element of romantic love has the advantage of explaining the link between love and sex, for of all human activities, **sexual activity** (heterosexual or homosexual) most closely approximates a literal union with another—if not a consumption of the other. Robert Nozick (1938–2002), for instance, writes of "the oceanic feeling, the sense of merging, that sometimes occurs with intense sexual experience" (66). Yet the approximation of union provided by sexual intercourse is at best only an approximation (as Plato realized)—and temporary at that. One might wonder whether even the most enjoyable and most satisfying sexual experience could truly satisfy two lovers' desire to unite.

The answer will depend, in part, on how literally union-talk is taken: The more literally we understand it, the more demanding will be the requirements it generates. Vladimir Solovyov (1853–1900), for instance, writes that there must "be a complete and continual interchange, a complete and continual affirmation of oneself in another, a perfect interaction and communion" (26). This sets the bar rather high, for requiring *complete* and *continual* interchanges seems to rule out the occasional, intermittent unions offered by sexual activity. Solovyov, borrowing Aristophanes's "melting" metaphor, claims that the ultimate end of love is that two lovers literally, permanently merge to form one being. Only sexual love "can lead to the effective and indissoluble union of two existences into one; only of it is it also said in the words of Holy Writ: 'Thy twain shall be one flesh,' i.e., shall become one real being" (30). **G.W.F. Hegel** (1770–1831), too, set the bar high: In love, and perhaps during the sexual event, "consciousness of a separate self disappears, and all distinction between the lovers is annulled" (307). Outside the metaphorical, however, it is not clear what Solovyov or Hegel could mean. Perhaps it is that "orgasm, especially simultaneous orgasm, confirms the sexual partners' sense of having merged" (Gregor, 336–37; see Nozick, 65–66). Yet even though intercourse involves intimate contact, including penetration, this is not a real merging of flesh, nor does it result in an "indissoluble union." Nozick suggests that the lovers' genuine union occurs with their first child (85)—an idea Hegel also expresses—which at least suggests how sexuality might yield union: not in the act but as a result of the act.

Perhaps, though, the strict requirement of union through sex means that love is, by its nature, doomed. Aristophanes, in the *Symposium*, hints at this. Even those "half-persons" lucky enough to find their other halves, he says, "finish their lives together and still cannot say what it is they want from one another. No one would think it is the intimacy of sex— that mere sex is the reason each lover takes so great and deep a joy in being with the other. It's obvious that the soul of every lover longs for something else" (192c–d). What each soul wants, on Aristophanes's view, is to merge in the most complete and literal sense. For Aristophanes, then, sexuality contains an unavoidable element of sadness (hence his myth is often seen as tragicomic): "This sadness comes from the reminder that we have not succeeded absolutely in losing our separateness; and the infantile hope that we can recover the womb never becomes a reality" (May, 314).

Some philosophers have wanted to acknowledge the significance of the passion for union while at the same time maintaining a certain skeptical distance from it. For Robert Solomon, the search for a "shared identity" is an essential feature of love, yet he judges the quest hopeless:

> Love is a process, a dialectic, a movement—toward what? Toward a shared identity, the creation of a shared self. But . . . this goal is impossible, unachievable, even incomprehensible. . . . The paradox of love is this, that it presupposes a strong sense of individual autonomy and independence, and then seeks to cancel this by creating a shared identity. (268–69)

Literal merging is, indeed, difficult to understand. But is it really the goal of love? Singer, who is skeptical about romantic lovers' desiring literally to merge, writes that Solomon "seems to confuse the sharing of self with an actual merging. . . . The sharing of self does not mean that lovers are no longer separate selves or that they have given up *all* their independence. There is no reason why either lover should want to lose his or her individual autonomy" (*Nature*, vol. 3, 410). Love is less paradoxical, presumably, for those who reject total merging in favor of a "two overlapping circles" model of shared identity (Nozick, 66) or "republican nation" (Delaney, 341) model.

The desire for union also plays a fundamental role in Erich Fromm's (1900–1980) *The Art of Loving*. In Fromm, however, union is not desired for its own sake but as a means, as an escape from the existential *Angst* that is otherwise humanity's fate. "The experience of separateness arouses anxiety," Fromm writes; "it is, indeed, the source of all anxiety. Being separate means being cut off, without any capacity to use my human powers. Hence to be separate means to be helpless" (8). Mere sex, unaccompanied by love, provides only a temporary escape: "The sexual orgasm can produce a state similar to the one produced by a trance, or to the effects of certain drugs. . . . [But] the sexual act without love never bridges the gap between two human beings, except momentarily" (12). Love, on the other hand, provides a permanent solution, a union in which both participants retain their individual identities. "In love the paradox occurs that two beings become one and yet remain two" (17).

This ideal love, "the union under the condition of preserving one's integrity," Fromm calls "mature love" (20). Fromm contrasts this love with "symbiotic" union, in which one partner submerges his or her identity and submits to the will of the other (as in the relationships, for example, between mother and fetus or between masochist and sadist). As Fromm writes, "If I am attached to another person because I cannot stand on my own feet, he or she may be a lifesaver, but the relationship is not one of love" (94). Yet "mature love" runs the risk of isolating the lovers from the wider community. Fromm claims that love is not genuine unless it extends beyond the beloved and takes in *everybody*, and indeed every*thing*. "If I truly love one person I love all persons, I love the world, I love life. If I can say to somebody else, 'I love you,' I must be able to say 'I love in you everybody, I love through you the world, I love in you also myself ' " (55). In transcending individual lovers and casting a wider net, Fromm's "mature love" comes close to *agape*. At any rate, it is clearly not in any substantial sense romantic or erotic.

Love and Sex. One of C. S. Lewis's (1898–1963) books on love, *The Four Loves*, usefully distinguishes between "Venus," or pure animalistic desire, and "Eros," an especially human type of sexuality:

> Sexual desire, without Eros, wants . . . a sensory pleasure; that is, an event occurring in one's body. We use a most unfortunate idiom when we say, of a lustful man prowling the streets, that he "wants a woman." Strictly speaking, a woman is just what he does not want. He wants a pleasure for which a woman happens to be a necessary piece of apparatus. How much he cares about the woman as such may be gauged by his attitude to her five minutes after fruition (one does not keep the carton after one has smoked the cigarettes). Now Eros makes a man really want, not a woman, but one particular woman. (134–35)

Lewis's distinction between Eros and mere Venus has, for him, an interesting implication. A man who is ruled by Eros "really hasn't leisure to think of sex. He is too busy thinking of a person. . . . If you asked him what he wanted, the true reply would often be, 'To go on thinking of her' " (133), in the same way that mere sex would not satisfy Aristophanic lovers. In Lewis, as in many other writers (e.g., Frankfurt, "On Caring," 170), there is a crucial dimension to love, even genuine sexual or erotic love, that is absent from mere **sexual desire**: its particularity. Unlike hunger (or horniness), which might be satisfied by *any* dish of roast beef (or *any* accommodating person), Eros attaches to one particular person, for whom there can be no substitute.

Suppose that romantic love necessarily includes a desire for union. Must romantic love, as a result, lead to sexual desire for one's beloved? Perhaps. "One might imagine romantic love without full-blown sex, without intercourse and heavy petting, . . . but one cannot imagine romantic love without some form of caress, if only with eyes and the touch of two fingers and an occasional kiss" (Solomon, 259). Others agree: "Central to any plausible contemporary romantic ideal are mutual longings for sexual intimacy together with more sweeping delight in each other's physicality" (Delaney, 347). One argument for this view, offered by Dana Bushnell (1958–2003), is that sexual desire is the only feature that separates romantic love from other attachments, such as friendship and parental love for a child. But there are possible counterexamples. Caraway, for instance, endorses Rolf

Johnson's suggestion that Dante's (1265–1321) love, at age nine, for Beatrice is an example of nonsexual romantic love ("Patchwork," 86). Sexuality may typically play a role in romantic love, but whether it is necessary is controversial.

Some philosophers have assumed that the union must be not only sexual but, specifically, heterosexual. If we picture two people who long for union as in some sense complements to one another (each other's missing half, say), it may seem obligatory to conceive of union in terms of a female-male pair. For such philosophers, "the differences between men and women do not prevent love, but make it possible, because in virtue of these differences men and women are yin-yang complements" (Soble, *Structure*, 251). We find Fromm worrying, "The polarity of the sexes is disappearing, and with it erotic love, which is based on this polarity" (15). Both **Jean-Jacques Rousseau** (1712–1778) and **Arthur Schopenhauer** (1788–1860) held that "romantic love requires [a person] to see in the other the perfections of the opposite sex that [he or she] necessarily lack[s]" (Caraway, "Neither Sexist," 363). Yet Plato's Aristophanes, who might be viewed as the originator of the view that sexual desire is the longing of complements to unite into a whole, did not privilege heterosexuality. To the contrary, Aristophanes's highest praise was reserved for homosexual males who "are bold and brave and masculine. . . . [T]his sort of man grows up as a lover of young men and a lover of Love, always rejoicing in his own kind" (*Symposium*, 191a-b).

In the history of the philosophy of sex, there are views that might be called cynical. For example, Schopenhauer is notorious for reducing love to sexual desire (in a manner that might have anticipated Freud; see Young and Brook): "All amorousness is rooted in the sexual impulse alone, is in fact only a more closely determined, specialized, and, indeed, in the strictest sense, individualized sexual impulse" (*World as Will*, vol. 2, 533). Of course, one need not be a cynic to unite sex and love this way; indeed, such views may express a positive assessment of both sex and love and may thus contribute to the justification and celebration of extensive human sexual freedom. On the other side, there is a long tradition of thinking of love and "lust"—a sentiment closely connected to sex—not only as distinct but as opposed to each other. This might be thought the very opposite of cynicism, since it allows love to achieve a beautiful and glorious autonomy. But the incompatibility of love and lust tends to suggest a hierarchy in which the flesh, the body, is conceived as inferior, perhaps even inherently corrupt. Indeed, this separation of love and lust is combined, in much Christian thinking on the subject, with a profoundly negative evaluation of sexuality (and hence of lust as well) as notorious as anything found in Schopenhauer. "It is better to marry than to burn," said **Saint Paul** (5–64?), in 1 Corinthians 7:9. Yet he also said that it was even better to remain in a state of **abstinence**, unmarried or celibate.

Marriage. While sexual activity made legitimate (or pardoned) by **marriage** may not damn those who engage in it, it is, for **Saint Augustine** (354–430), nonetheless shameful:

> Lawful and respectable though it [marital intercourse] is, does it not seek a chamber secluded from witnesses? . . . [W]ho does not know what goes on between husband and wife for the procreation of children? Indeed, it is for the achievement of this purpose that wives are married with such ceremony. And yet, when the act for the birth of children is being consummated, not even the children that may already have been born from the union are allowed to witness it. . . . What is the reason for this if not that something by nature fitting and proper is carried out in such a way as to be accompanied also by something of shame as punishment? (*City of God*, bk. 14, chap. 8)

The idea that procreation is the only proper function of sexual intercourse suggests that limiting intercourse to married partners is not itself sufficient to reconcile this inherently shameful activity with morality. It is further necessary that every act of intercourse be performed in such a way as to aim at procreation or, as Catholics sometimes say, an act of intercourse must at least be *open* to procreation. This idea emerges strongly in the writings of **Saint Thomas Aquinas** (1224/25–1274):

> [E]very emission of semen, in such a way that generation cannot follow, is contrary to the good for man. And if this be done deliberately, it must be a sin. . . . Likewise, it must also be contrary to the good for man if the semen be emitted under conditions such that generation could result but the proper upbringing would be prevented. . . . [T]he needs of human life demand many things which cannot be provided by one person alone. Therefore, it is appropriate to human nature that a man remain together with a woman after the generative act, and not leave her immediately to have such relations with another woman, as is the practice with fornicators. (*Summa contra gentiles*, 3.122)

It would seem to follow that love cannot make sexual activity ethical, even between married partners. Even so, from the claim that intercourse is permissible only in the bounds of matrimony, it is not difficult to conclude that love is also required. Not romantic love, of course (that notion likely postdates these thinkers), nor sexual love, which would not have been considered genuine love at all. Rather, Aquinas puts his claims in terms of friendship: "[T]he union of male and female in the human species must be not only lasting, but also unbroken [and] the greater that friendship is, the more solid and long-lasting it will be" (3.122).

Immanuel Kant (1724–1804) advances a similar distinction. His starting point is the claim that love, conceived as agapic, rather than erosic, and sexual desire form two poles:

> [T]rue human love . . . admits of no distinction between types of persons, or between young and old. But a love that springs merely from sexual impulse cannot be love at all, but only appetite. Human love is goodwill, affection, promoting the happiness of others and finding joy in their happiness. But it is clear that, when a person loves another purely from sexual desire, none of these factors enter into the love. Far from there being any concern for the happiness of the loved one, the lover, in order to satisfy his desire and still his appetite, may even plunge the loved one into the depths of misery. (163)

Jacques Lacan (1901–1981), too, opines with legions of other philosophers that "when one loves, it has nothing to do with sex" (25). Still, Kant follows Augustine and Aquinas in believing that, somehow, lust can be made moral in marriage: "Matrimony is the only condition in which use can be made of one's sexuality. If one devotes one's person to another, one devotes not only sex but the whole person; the two cannot be separated. . . . In this way the two persons become a unity of will" (167). So, as in the union of interests view, "Whatever good or ill, joy or sorrow befall either of them, the other will share in it." The so-called commonsense morality of our era sometimes seems to follow Augustine, Aquinas, and Kant to some degree, accepting marriage, and procreation within marriage, as the natural ends of human life. But more recent views depart from these predecessors in placing more emphasis on the importance of love, both passionately romantic and simply affectionate, between the partners.

Loveless Sex. A host of Christians and non-Christians hold that sex with love is morally preferable to sex without love. Others have argued that loving sex is preferable in part because loving sex is better *as sex.* Gregor, for one, claims that "in the context of the loving relationship, the pleasure of the sexual act is intensified" (334). While this view is not uncommon, it is far from universal. Russell Vannoy is perhaps the most prominent defender of the view that sex without love is as valuable, as rewarding, as sex between lovers; indeed, sex without love may even be better. "[T]hat sex with love is a rich, complex phenomenon and sex without involvement is a mere sensation in the groin is a fallacious dualism" (*Sex without Love*, 26). Vannoy proceeds to suggest:

> Could it be that the preference for sex with love over sex without love is merely one of taste—tenderness versus raunchiness, predictability and security versus adventure and novelty, attachment versus independence? I am reminded of those who prefer their coffee straight and those who must have it mixed with cream and sugar. In each case something is gained and something is lost. (29)

The claim that sex without love has *some* value, even potentially significant value, is no longer thought wrong by very many (though some within certain religious traditions still reject it). The more controversial and interesting claim is that we should expect loveless sex to be *better* as sex than loving sex. Loving relationships not only require us to sacrifice "raunchiness," "adventure and novelty," and "independence"; they also risk various "emotional entanglements" including "mutual possessiveness" (19). Of course, Vannoy's proposal that the issue is one of mere taste weighs heavily against the notion that loveless sex is *objectively* or *inherently* superior to loving sex (and vice versa). At most we can ask, perhaps counterfactually, what most people, if sufficiently informed, autonomous, and so forth, would prefer.

Vannoy, however, also presses a deeper point (in backhanded agreement with those, like Kant, who sense that love and sex are strictly incompatible), that there really is *no such thing* as loving sex. Loving sex is presumably sex that *expresses* love, and Vannoy is critical of the idea that an animalistic physical act could (or should) be used to express an extremely civilized, if not rather *effete*, emotion. "[J]ust how does a penis that is vigorously thrusting up and down in a vagina express anything at all?" he asks (11).

> Sex is complicated enough without worrying about what or whether one's bodily language is actually communicating. Indeed, a penis thrusting up and down in a vagina may actually "communicate" dominance and aggression more than it does love. . . . finally, there is the possibility that sex used primarily as a tool for communicating emotion would come to devalue the purely sensual aspects of sex. (*Sex without Love*, 22)

In another place Vannoy provides an additional argument: "The only thing that expresses love is the totality of the experiences two persons share through whatever time their love endures. No part of sex can possibly express all or even a major part of what is implied by the phrase *being in love*" ("Express Love," 247–48).

It should come as no surprise that not everyone is convinced. Edward Johnson objects to Vannoy's "totality of experience" argument on the grounds that the view "demands too much from the notion of expression. Many ordinary things are taken to be expressions of love: a poem, a gesture, a look, and so forth. To say that no poem ever expressed love . . . would be hard to defend" (259). And Vannoy's claim that a thrusting penis could not possibly express "anything at all" ignores the impact of social convention. This is exactly how and why, for example, an extended middle finger can and does express hostility.

See also Abstinence; Adultery; Bestiality; Casual Sex; Catholicism, History of; Communication Model; Descartes, René; Existentialism; Fichte, Johann Gottlieb; Friendship; Hegel, G.W.F.; Heterosexism; Hume, David; Kant, Immanuel; Leibniz, Gottfried; Marriage; Nagel, Thomas; Paglia, Camille; Paul (Saint); Personification, Sexual; Philosophy of Sex, Overview of; Rousseau, Jean-Jacques; Scruton, Roger; Thomas Aquinas (Saint)

REFERENCES

Aristotle. (ca. 325 BCE?) *Nicomachean Ethics*. Trans. Terence Irwin. Indianapolis, Ind.: Hackett, 1985; Augustine. (413–427) *City of God* (*De civitate Dei*). Trans. Marcus Dods. New York: Modern Library, 1950; Brentlinger, John. "The Nature of Love." In *Symposium*. Trans. Suzy Q Groden. Amherst: University of Massachusetts Press, 1970, 113–29; Bushnell, Dana E. "Love without Sex: A Commentary on Caraway." *Philosophy and Theology* 1:4 (1987), 369–73; Caraway, Carol. "Romantic Love: A Patchwork." *Philosophy and Theology* 2:1 (1987), 76–96; Caraway, Carol. "Romantic Love: Neither Sexist Nor Heterosexist." *Philosophy and Theology* 1:4 (1987), 361–68; Delaney, Neil. "Romantic Love and Loving Commitment: Articulating a Modern Ideal." *American Philosophical Quarterly* 33:4 (1996), 339–56; Frankfurt, Harry G. "Duty and Love." *Philosophical Explorations* 1:1 (1998), 4–9; Frankfurt, Harry G. (1997) "On Caring." In *Necessity, Volition, and Love*. Cambridge: Cambridge University Press, 1999, 155–80; Frankfurt, Harry G. *The Reasons of Love*. Princeton, N.J.: Princeton University Press, 2004; Freud, Sigmund. (1930) *Civilization and Its Discontents*. Trans. and ed. James Strachey. New York: Norton, 1961; Fried, Charles. *An Anatomy of Values*. Cambridge, Mass.: Harvard University Press, 1970; Fromm, Erich. (1956) *The Art of Loving*. New York: Harper and Row, 1974; Gregor, Thomas. "Sexuality and the Experience of Love." In Paul R. Abramson and Steven D. Pinkerton, eds., *Sexual Nature Sexual Culture*. Chicago, Ill.: University of Chicago Press, 1995, 330–50; Hegel, G.W.F. (1797–1798) "On Love." In *On Christianity: Early Theological Writings*. Trans. Thomas Knox. New York: Harper and Bros., 1948, 302–8; Hunter, J.F.M. *Thinking about Sex and Love*. New York: St. Martin's Press, 1980; Johnson, Edward. "Lovesexpressed." In Alan Soble, ed., *Sex, Love, and Friendship*. Amsterdam, Holland: Rodopi, 1997, 259–63; Johnson, Rolf M. "Love, Passion, and the Need to Be Loved." Paper presented to the Society for the Philosophy of Sex and Love (28 December 1981), Philadelphia, Pa.; Kant, Immanuel. (ca. 1780) *Lectures on Ethics*. Trans. Louis Infield. London: Methuen, 1930; Lacan, Jacques. *The Seminar of Jacques Lacan. Book XX: Encore. 1972–1973*. Trans. Bruce Fink. New York: Norton, 1998; Lewis, C. S. *The Four Loves*. New York: Harcourt, Brace, Jovanovich, 1960; May, Rollo. *Love and Will*. New York: Norton, 1969; Nozick, Robert. *The Examined Life*. New York: Simon and Schuster, 1989; Nussbaum, Martha C. *The Fragility of Goodness: Luck and Ethics in Greek Tragedy and Philosophy*. Cambridge: Cambridge University Press, 1986; Nygren, Anders. (1930, 1936) *Agape and Eros*. Trans. Philip S. Watson. Chicago, Ill.: University of Chicago Press, 1982; Osborne, Catherine. *Eros Unveiled: Plato and the God of Love*. Oxford, U.K.: Clarendon Press, 1994; Plato. (ca. 365 BCE) *Phaedrus*. Trans. Alexander Nehamas and Paul Woodruff. Indianapolis, Ind.: Hackett, 1995; Plato. (ca. 380 BCE) *Symposium*. Trans. Alexander Nehamas and Paul Woodruff. Indianapolis, Ind.: Hackett, 1989; Schopenhauer, Arthur. (1818, 1844, 1859) *The World as Will and Representation*, 2 vols. Trans. E.F.J. Payne. New York: Dover, 1966; Scruton, Roger. *Sexual Desire: A Moral Philosophy of the Erotic*. New York: Free Press, 1986; Singer, Irving. *The Nature of Love*. Vol. 1: *Plato to Luther*, 2nd ed. Chicago, Ill.: University of Chicago Press, 1984. Vol. 2: *Courtly and Romantic*, 1984. Vol. 3: *The Modern World*, 1987; Singer, Irving. *The Pursuit of Love*. Baltimore, Md.: Johns Hopkins University Press, 1994; Soble, Alan. *The Structure of Love*. New Haven, Conn.: Yale University Press, 1990; Soble, Alan. "Union, Autonomy, and Concern." In Roger Lamb, ed., *Love Analyzed*. Boulder, Colo.: Westview, 1997, 65–92; Soble, Alan. "The Unity of Romantic Love." *Philosophy and Theology* 1:4 (1987), 374–97; Solomon, Robert. *Love: Emotion, Myth, and Metaphor*. Garden City, N.Y.: Anchor Press, 1981; Solovyov, Vladimir Sergeyevich. *The Meaning of Love*. Trans.

Jane Marshall. New York: International Universities Press, 1947; Thomas Aquinas. (1258–1264) *On the Truth of the Catholic Faith* [*Summa contra gentiles*]. *Book Three: Providence. Part II*. Trans. Vernon J. Bourke. Garden City, N.Y.: Image Books, 1956; Vannoy, Russell. "Can Sex Express Love?" In Alan Soble, ed., *Sex, Love, and Friendship*. Amsterdam, Holland: Rodopi, 1997, 247–57; Vannoy, Russell. *Sex without Love: A Philosophical Exploration*. Buffalo, N.Y.: Prometheus, 1980; Vlastos, Gregory. "The Individual as an Object of Love in Plato." In *Platonic Studies*. Princeton, N.J.: Princeton University Press, 1973, 3–34; Vlastos, Gregory. "Sex in Platonic Love." In *Platonic Studies*. Princeton, N.J.: Princeton University Press, 1973, 38–42. [Appendix 2 of "The Individual as an Object of Love in Plato"]; Wolf, Susan. "The True, the Good, and the Lovable: Frankfurt's Avoidance of Objectivity." In Sarah Buss and Lee Overton, eds., *Contours of Agency: Essays on Themes from Harry Frankfurt*. Cambridge, Mass.: MIT Press, 2002, 227–44; Young, Christopher, and Andrew Brook. "Schopenhauer and Freud." *International Journal of Psychoanalysis* 75 (1994), 101–18. <www.carleton.ca/~abrook/SCHOPENY.htm> [accessed 18 October 2004].

Troy Jollimore

ADDITIONAL READING

Adams, Robert M. "Pure Love." *Journal of Religious Ethics* 8:1 (1980), 88–99. Reprinted in Charles Taliaferro and Paul J. Griffiths, eds., *Philosophy of Religion: An Anthology*. Malden, Mass.: Blackwell, 2003, 493–503; Babcock, William S. "Cupiditas and Caritas: The Early Augustine on Love and Human Fulfillment." In William S. Babcock, ed., *The Ethics of St. Augustine*. Atlanta, Ga.: Scholars Press, 1991, 39–66; Badhwar, Neera. "Friends as Ends in Themselves." *Philosophy and Phenomenological Research* 48:1 (1987), 1–23. Reprinted, revised, in Alan Soble, ed., *Eros, Agape, and Philia: Readings in the Philosophy of Love*. New York: Paragon House, 1989, 165–86; SLF (333–52); Baier, Annette. "Caring about Caring: A Reply to Frankfurt." *Synthese* 53:2 (1982), 273–90; Barthes, Roland. *A Lover's Discourse: Fragments*. Trans. Richard Howard. New York: Hill and Wang, 1978; Bayles, Michael D. "Marriage, Love, and Procreation." In Robert B. Baker and Frederick A. Elliston, eds., *Philosophy and Sex*, 1st ed. Buffalo, N.Y.: Prometheus, 1975, 190–206. Reprinted in P&S2 (130–45); P&S3 (116–29); Belliotti, Raymond. "The Primacy of Emotion: Love and Intimacy." In *Good Sex: Perspectives on Sexual Ethics*. Lawrence: University Press of Kansas, 1993, 56–85; Benjamin, Jessica. *The Bonds of Love: Psychoanalysis, Feminism, and the Problem of Domination*. New York: Pantheon, 1988; Ben-Ze'ev, Aaron. *Love Online: Emotions on the Internet*. Cambridge: Cambridge University Press, 2004; Berger, Fred R. "Gratitude." *Ethics* 85:4 (1975), 298–309; Bergmann, Martin S. *The Anatomy of Loving: The Story of Man's Quest to Know What Love Is*. New York: Columbia University Press, 1987; Bernstein, Mark. "Love, Particularity, and Selfhood." *Southern Journal of Philosophy* 23 (1986), 287–93; Bertocci, Peter. *Sex, Love, and the Person*. New York: Sheed and Ward, 1967; Betz, Joseph. "The Relation between Love and Justice: A Survey of the Five Possible Positions." *Journal of Value Inquiry* 4 (1970), 191–203; Bloom, Allan. *Love and Friendship*. New York: Simon and Schuster, 1993; Bornoff, Nicholas. *Pink Samurai: Love, Marriage, and Sex in Contemporary Japan*. New York: Pocket Books, 1991; Brake, Elizabeth. "Love's Paradox: Making Sense of Hegel on Marriage." In Stella Stanford and Alison Stone, eds., *Hegel and Feminism*, *Women's Philosophy Review*, Special Issue no. 22 (Autumn 1999), 80–104; Breggin, Peter Robert. "Sex and Love: Sexual Dysfunction as a Spiritual Disorder." In Earl E. Shelp, ed., *Sexuality and Medicine*, vol. 1: *Conceptual Roots*. Dordrecht, Holland: Reidel, 1987, 243–66; Brentlinger, John. "The Nature of Love." In *Symposium*. Trans. Suzy Q Groden. Amherst: University of Massachusetts Press, 1970, 113–29. Reprinted in Alan Soble, ed., *Eros, Agape, and Philia: Readings in the Philosophy of Love*. New York: Paragon House, 1989, 136–48; Brown, Robert. *Analyzing Love*. Cambridge: Cambridge University Press, 1987; Brown, Ursula M. "Love and Color." In *The Interracial Experience: Growing Up Black/White Racially Mixed in the United States*. Westport, Conn.: Praeger, 2001, 97–108; Burch, Robert W. "The Commandability of Pathological Love." *Southwestern Journal of Philosophy* [*Philosophical Topics*] 3:3 (1972), 131–40. Reprinted in Alan Soble, ed., *Eros, Agape, and Philia: Readings in the Philosophy of Love*. New York: Paragon House, 1989, 245–53; Bushnell,

Dana. "Love without Sex: A Commentary on Caraway." *Philosophy and Theology* 1:4 (1987), 369–73. Reprinted as "Love without Sex" in SLF (381–83); Calhoun, Cheshire. "Making Up Emotional People: The Case of Romantic Love." In Susan A. Bandes, ed., *The Passions of Law*. New York: New York University Press, 1999, 217–40; Capellanus, Andreas. (ca. 1174–1186) *The Art of Courtly Love*. Trans. John Jay Parry. New York: Columbia University Press, 1990; Caraway, Carol. "Romantic Love: A Patchwork." *Philosophy and Theology* 2:1 (1987), 76–96. Reprinted in SLF (403–19); Caraway, Carol. "Romantic Love: Neither Sexist Nor Heterosexist." *Philosophy and Theology* 1:4 (1987), 361–68. Reprinted in SLF (375–79); Cicovacki, Predrag. "Can Love Resolve the Problem of Marriage?" In Thomas Magnell, ed., *Explorations of Value*. Amsterdam, Holland: Rodopi, 1997, 221–33; Coleman, Julie. *Love, Sex, and Marriage: A Historical Thesaurus*. Amsterdam, Holland: Rodopi, 1999; De Lauretis, Teresa. *The Practice of Love: Lesbian Sexuality and Perverse Desire*. Bloomington: Indiana University Press, 1994; De Rougemont, Denis. (1939) *Love in the Western World*. Rev. ed. Trans. Montgomery Belgion. New York: Pantheon, 1956; Diorio, Joseph A. "Sex, Love, and Justice: A Problem in Moral Education." *Educational Theory* 31:3–4 (1982), 225–35. Reprinted in Alan Soble, ed., *Eros, Agape, and Philia: Readings in the Philosophy of Love*. New York: Paragon House, 1989, 273–88; Ehman, Robert R. "Personal Love." *The Personalist* 49 (1968), 116–41. Reprinted in Alan Soble, ed., *Eros, Agape, and Philia: Readings in the Philosophy of Love*. New York: Paragon House, 1989, 254–71; Ehman, Robert R. "Personal Love and Individual Value." *Journal of Value Inquiry* 10:2 (1976), 91–105; Ellis, Albert. "The Justification of Sex without Love." In *Sex without Guilt*. New York: Lyle Stuart, 1958, 66–86; Evans, C. Stephen. *Kierkegaard's Ethic of Love*. New York: Oxford University Press, 2004; Feder, Ellen K., Karmen MacKendrick, and Sybol S. Cook, eds. *A Passion for Wisdom: Readings in Western Philosophy on Love and Desire*. Upper Saddle River, N.J.: Prentice Hall, 2004; Ferrari, G.R.F. "Platonic Love." In Richard Kraut, ed., *The Cambridge Companion to Plato*. Cambridge: Cambridge University Press, 1992, 248–76; Fisher, Helen E. *Why We Love: The Nature and Chemistry of Romantic Love*. New York: Holt, 2004; Fisher, Mark. *Personal Love*. London: Duckworth, 1990; Fisher, Mark. "Reason, Emotion, and Love." *Inquiry* 20 (1977), 189–203; Frankfurt, Harry G. (1994) "Autonomy, Necessity, and Love." In *Necessity, Volition, and Love*. Cambridge: Cambridge University Press, 1999, 129–41; Frankfurt, Harry G. "Freedom of the Will and the Concept of a Person." *Journal of Philosophy* 68 (1971), 5–20; Frankfurt, Harry G. "The Importance of What We Care About." *Synthese* 53:2 (1982), 257–72. Reprinted in *The Importance of What We Care About: Philosophical Essays*. Cambridge: Cambridge University Press, 1988, 80–94; Freud, Sigmund. *Sexuality and the Psychology of Love*. Ed. Philip Rieff. New York: Collier, 1963; Fuchs, Eric. (1979) *Sexual Desire and Love: Origins and History of the Christian Ethic of Sexuality and Marriage*. Trans. Marsha Daigle. New York: Seabury Press, 1983; Gaylin, Willard. *Rediscovering Love*. New York: Viking Penguin, 1985; Gilbert, Paul. "Love and Sex." In *Human Relationships: A Philosophical Introduction*. Oxford, U.K.: Blackwell, 1991, 9–31; Giles, James. "A Theory of Love and Sexual Desire." *Journal for the Theory of Social Behaviour* 24:4 (1994), 339–57; Goicoechea, David, ed. *The Nature and Pursuit of Love: The Philosophy of Irving Singer*. Amherst, N.Y.: Prometheus, 1995; Goldman, Alan. "Plain Sex." *Philosophy and Public Affairs* 6:3 (1977), 267–87. Reprinted in HS (103–23); POS1 (119–38); POS2 (73–92); POS3 (39–55); POS4 (39–55); Goode, William J. "The Theoretical Importance of Love." *American Sociological Review* 24:1 (1959), 38–47. Reprinted in Ashley Montagu, ed., *The Practice of Love*. Englewood Cliffs, N.J.: Prentice-Hall, 1975, 120–35; Gould, Thomas. *Platonic Love*. London: Routledge and Kegan Paul, 1963; Green, O. Harvey. "Is Love an Emotion?" In Roger E. Lamb, ed., *Love Analyzed*. Boulder, Colo.: Westview, 1997, 209–24; Gregory, Paul. "Eroticism and Love." *American Philosophical Quarterly* 25:4 (1988), 339–44; Hall, Ronald L. *The Human Embrace: The Love of Philosophy and the Philosophy of Love. Kierkegaard, Cavell, Nussbaum*. University Park: Pennsylvania State University Press, 2000; Halwani, Raja. "Love." In Timothy F. Murphy, ed., *Reader's Guide to Gay and Lesbian Studies*. Chicago, Ill.: Fitzroy Dearborn, 2000, 365–67; Hamlyn, D. W. "The Phenomena of Love and Hate." *Philosophy* 53 (1978), 5–20. Reprinted in Alan Soble, ed., *Eros, Agape, and Philia: Readings in the Philosophy of Love*. New York: Paragon House, 1989, 218–34; Hutcheon, Pat Duffy. "Through a Glass Darkly: Freud's Concept of Love." In David Goicoechea, ed., *The Nature and Pursuit of Love: The Philosophy of Irving Singer*. Amherst, N.Y.: Prometheus, 1995, 183–95; John Paul II (Pope). "Authentic Concept of Conjugal Love." *Origins* 28:37 (1999), 654–56; Johnson, Rolf M. *Three Faces of Love*. DeKalb: Northern Illinois University Press, 2001; Kant, Immanuel. (ca. 1762–1794) *Lectures on Ethics*. Trans. Peter Heath. Cambridge: Cambridge University Press, 1997; Kant, Immanuel. (1797) *The Metaphysics of Morals*. Trans. Mary Gregor. Cambridge: Cambridge University Press, 1996; Kierkegaard, Søren. (1845) *Stages on Life's Way*. Trans. Walter Lowrie. Princeton, N.J.: Princeton University Press, 1945; Kierkegaard, Søren. (1847) *Works of Love: Some Christian Reflections in the Form of Discourses*. Trans. Howard Hong and Edna Hong. New York: Harper and Row, 1962; Kipnis, Laura. *Against Love: A Polemic*. New York: Pantheon, 2003; Kosman, L. A. "Platonic Love." In W. H. Werkmeister, ed., *Facets of Plato's Philosophy*. Amsterdam, Holland: Van Gorcum, 1976, 53–69. Reprinted in Alan Soble, ed., *Eros, Agape, and Philia: Readings in the Philosophy of Love*. New York: Paragon House, 1989, 149–63; Kraut, Robert. "Love *De Re*." In Peter French, Theodore Uehling, and Howard Wettstein, eds., *Midwest Studies in Philosophy*, vol. 10: *Studies in the Philosophy of Mind*. Minneapolis: University of Minnesota Press, 1986, 413–30; Kupfer, Joseph. "Romantic Love." *Journal of Social Philosophy* 24:3 (1993), 112–20. Reprinted, revised, in Alan Soble, ed., *Sex, Love, and Friendship*. Amsterdam, Holland: Rodopi, 1997, 579–85; Lamb, Roger E. "Love and Rationality." In Roger Lamb, ed., *Love Analyzed*. Boulder, Colo.: Westview, 1997, 23–47; Lamb, Roger E., ed. *Love Analyzed*. Boulder, Colo.: Westview, 1997; Langton, Rae. "Love and Solipsism." In Roger E. Lamb, ed., *Love Analyzed*. Boulder, Colo.: Westview, 1997, 123–52; Lawrence, D. H. (1918) "Love." In *Sex, Literature, and Censorship*. Ed. Harry T. Moore. New York: Twayne, 1953, 33–39; Lawton, Phillip. "Love and Justice: Levinas' Reading of Buber." *Philosophy Today* 20 (1976), 77–83; Lear, Jonathan. *Love and Its Place in Nature*. New York: HarperCollins, 1990; Lear, Jonathan. "Love's Authority." In Sarah Buss and Lee Overton, eds., *Contours of Agency: Essays on Themes from Harry Frankfurt*. Cambridge, Mass.: MIT Press, 2002, 279–92; Lesser, A. H. "Love and Lust." *Journal of Value Inquiry* 14:1 (1980), 51–54. Reprinted in HS (75–78); Lessing, Doris. "How I Finally Lost My Heart." In *A Man and Two Women*. New York: Popular Library, 1963, 83–95; Letwin, Shirley Robin. "Romantic Love and Christianity." *Philosophy* 52 (April 1977), 131–45; Levine, Michael P. "Loving Individuals for Their Properties: Or, What Was the Colour of Yeats's Mother's Hair?" *Iyyun: Jerusalem Philosophical Quarterly* 48 (July 1999), 251–67; Levine, Michael P. "Lucky in Love: Love and Emotion." In Michael P. Levine, ed., *The Analytic Freud: Philosophy and Psychoanalysis*. London: Routledge, 2000, 231–58; Levine, Michael P. "Rational Emotion, Emotional Holism, True Love, and Charlie Chaplin." *Journal of Philosophical Research* 24 (January 1999), 489–506; Levine, Michael P. "Why Is Love So Bizarre?" *dotlit: The Online Journal of Creative Writing* 3:2 (2002). <www.dotlit.qut.edu.au/200202/bizarre.htm> [accessed 20 September 2004]; Lewis, C. S. *The Allegory of Love: A Study in Medieval Tradition*. Oxford, U.K.: Oxford University Press, 1936; Mann, Thomas. (1911) *Death in Venice [and Seven Other Stories]*. Trans. H. T. Lowe-Porter. New York: Vintage, 1936; Martin, Mike. *Love's Virtues*. Lawrence: University Press of Kansas, 1996; Martin, Mike. (1989, 2001) "Sex and Love." In *Everyday Morality: An Introduction to Applied Ethics*, 2nd ed. Belmont, Calif.: Wadsworth, 1995, 217–29; Meilaender, Gilbert. *The Limits of Love: Some Theological Explorations*. University Park: Pennsylvania State University Press, 1987; Merino, Noël. "The Problem with 'We': Rethinking Joint Identity in Romantic Love." *Journal of Social Philosophy* 35:1 (2004), 123–32; Millgram, Elijah. "Aristotle on Making Other Selves." *Canadian Journal of Philosophy* 17:2 (1987), 361–76; Millgram, Elijah. "Kantian Crystallization." *Ethics* 114:3 (2004), 511–13; Millgram, Elijah. *Practical Induction*. Cambridge, Mass.: Harvard University Press, 1997; Mirandola, Giovanni Pico Della. (1651) *A Platonick Discourse upon Love*. Ed. Edmund G. Gardner. Boston, Mass.: Merrymount Press, 1914; Montagu, Ashley, ed. *The Practice of Love*. Englewood Cliffs, N.J.: Prentice-Hall, 1975; Montaigne, Michel de. (1572/1595) "On Affectionate Relationships." In M. A. Screech, ed. and trans., *The Essays of Michel de Montaigne*. London: Penguin, 1991, 205–19; Morgan, Douglas. *Love: Plato, the Bible, and Freud*. Englewood Cliffs, N.J.: Prentice-Hall, 1964; Moseley, Alex. (2001) "Philosophy of Love." In James Fieser, ed., *The Internet Encyclopedia of Philosophy*. <www/iep.utm.edu/l/love.htm> [accessed 18 January 2005]; Newton-Smith, W. "A Conceptual

Investigation of Love." In A. Montefiore, ed., *Philosophy and Personal Relations*. Montreal, Can.: McGill-Queens University Press, 1973, 113–36. Reprinted in Alan Soble, ed., *Eros, Agape, and Philia: Readings in the Philosophy of Love*. New York: Paragon House, 1989, 199–217; Nozick, Robert. "Love's Bond." In *The Examined Life*. New York: Simon and Schuster, 1989, 68–86. Reprinted in STW (231–40); Nozick, Robert. "Sexuality." In *The Examined Life*. New York: Simon and Schuster, 1989, 61–67; Nussbaum, Martha C. *Love's Knowledge: Essays on Philosophy and Literature*. New York: Oxford University Press, 1990; Nussbaum, Martha C. "The Speech of Alcibiades: A Reading of the *Symposium*." In *The Fragility of Goodness: Luck and Ethics in Greek Tragedy and Philosophy*. Cambridge: Cambridge University Press, 1986, 165–99. Revised from "The Speech of Alcibiades: A Reading of Plato's *Symposium*." *Philosophy and Literature* 3:2 (1979), 131–72; Nygren, Anders. *Den kristna kärlekstanken genom tiderna* (Part I, 1930; Part II, 1936). *Agape and Eros*. London: S.P.C.K. House, 1932, 1938. Philadelphia, Pa.: Westminster Press, 1953. Trans. Philip S. Watson. Chicago, Ill.: University of Chicago Press, 1982; Ortega y Gasset, José. (1940) *On Love: Aspects of a Single Theme*. Trans. Toby Talbot. New York: Meridian Books, 1957; Outka, Gene. *Agape: An Ethical Analysis*. New Haven, Conn.: Yale University Press, 1972; Phillips, Adam. "On Love." In *On Flirtation*. Cambridge, Mass.: Harvard University Press, 1994, 39–41; Polhemus, Robert M. *Erotic Faith: Being in Love from Jane Austen to D. H. Lawrence*. Chicago, Ill.: University of Chicago Press, 1990; Price, A. W. *Love and Friendship in Plato and Aristotle*. Oxford, U.K.: Clarendon Press, 1989; Price, A. W. "Martha Nussbaum's *Symposium*." *Ancient Philosophy* 11 (1991), 285–99; Primoratz, Igor. "Sex and Love." In *Ethics and Sex*. London: Routledge, 1999, 21–33; Reeve, C.D.C. *Love's Confusions*. Cambridge, Mass.: Harvard University Press, 2005; Reik, Theodor. *A Psychologist Looks at Love*. Oxford, U.K.: Farrar and Rinehart, 1944; Robinson, Jenefer. "Emotion, Judgment, and Desire." *Journal of Philosophy* 80 (1983), 731–41; Rorty, Amélie. "The Historicity of Psychological Attitudes: Love Is Not Love Which Alters Not When It Alteration Finds." In Peter French, Theodore Uehling, and Howard Wettstein, eds., *Midwest Studies in Philosophy*, vol. 10: *Studies in the Philosophy of Mind*. Minneapolis: University of Minnesota Press, 1986, 399–412; Santas, Gerasimos. *Plato and Freud: Two Theories of Love*. Oxford, U.K.: Blackwell, 1988; Scruton, Roger. "Attitudes, Beliefs and Reasons." In John Casey, ed., *Morality and Moral Reasoning*. London: Methuen, 1971, 25–100; Singer, Irving. *Explorations in Love and Sex*. Lanham, Md.: Rowman and Littlefield, 2001; Sircello, Guy. "Love and Sex." In *Love and Beauty*. Princeton, N.J.: Princeton University Press, 1989, 172–79; Small, Meredith F. *What's Love Got to Do with It? The Evolution of Human Mating*. New York: Anchor Books, 1995; Soble, Alan. "Analyzing Love" [Review essay of *Analyzing Love*, by Robert Brown]. *Philosophy of the Social Sciences* 19:4 (1989), 493–500; Soble, Alan. "Irreplaceability." In Alan Soble, ed., *Sex, Love, and Friendship*. Amsterdam, Holland: Rodopi, 1997, 355–57; Soble, Alan. "Love." In *Sexual Investigations*. New York: New York University Press, 1996, 17–20; Soble, Alan. "Love and Value, Yet *Again*." [Review essay of *The Reasons of Love*, by Harry G. Frankfurt] *Essays in Philosophy* 6:1 (2005). <www.humboldt.edu/~essays/soble2rev.html> [accessed 26 December 2004]; Soble, Alan. *The Philosophy of Sex and Love: An Introduction*. St. Paul, Minn.: Paragon House, 1998; Soble, Alan. Review of *Personal Love*, by Mark Fisher. *Canadian Philosophical Reviews* 12:1 (1992), 24–25; Soble, Alan. Review of *The Nature of Love*, vol. 3: *The Modern World*, by Irving Singer. *Canadian Philosophical Reviews* 8:2 (1988), 74–76; Soble, Alan. "The Unity of Romantic Love." *Philosophy and Theology* 1:4 (1987), 374–97. Reprinted in SLF (385–401); Soble, Alan, ed. *Eros, Agape, and Philia: Readings in the Philosophy of Love*. New York: Paragon House, 1989. Corrected reprint, 1999; Soble, Alan, ed. *Sex, Love, and Friendship: Studies of the Society for the Philosophy of Sex and Love, 1977–1992*. Amsterdam, Holland: Rodopi, 1997; Solomon, Robert C. *About Love: Reinventing Romance for Our Times*. New York: Simon and Schuster, 1988; Solomon, Robert C. "The Virtue of (Erotic) Love." In Peter A. French, Theodore E. Uehling, Jr., and Howard K. Wettstein, eds., *Ethical Theory: Character and Virtue. Midwest Studies in Philosophy* 13 (1988), 12–31. Reprinted in Robert C. Solomon and Kathleen Higgins, eds., *The Philosophy of (Erotic) Love*. Lawrence: University Press of Kansas, 1991, 492–518; STW (241–55); Solomon, Robert C., and Kathleen Higgins, eds. *The Philosophy of (Erotic) Love*. Lawrence: University Press of Kansas, 1991; Stafford, J. Martin. "Love and Lust

Revisited: Intentionality, Homosexuality and Moral Education." *Journal of Applied Philosophy* 5:1 (1988) 87–100. Reprinted in *Essays on Sexuality and Ethics*. Solihull, U.K.: Ismeron, 1995, 65–78; HS (177–90); Stafford, J. Martin. "On Distinguishing between Love and Lust." *Journal of Value Inquiry* 11:4 (1977), 292–303. Reprinted in *Essays on Sexuality and Ethics*. Solihull, U.K.: Ismeron, 1995, 53–64; Sternberg, Robert. *The Triangular Theory of Love: Intimacy, Passion, and Commitment*. New York: Basic Books, 1988; Sternberg, Robert, and Michael Barnes, eds. *The Psychology of Love*. New Haven, Conn.: Yale University Press, 1988; Stewart, Robert M., ed. *Philosophical Perspectives on Sex and Love*. New York: Oxford University Press, 1995; Sullivan, Andrew. *Love Undetectable: Reflections on Friendship, Sex, and Survival*. New York: Knopf, 1998; Taylor, Gabrielle. "Love." *Proceedings of the Aristotelian Society* 76 (1976), 147–64; Taylor, Richard. *Love Affairs: Marriage and Infidelity*. Amherst, N.Y.: Prometheus, 1997. Previously published as *Having Love Affairs*. Buffalo, N.Y.: Prometheus, 1982, 1990; Thurber, James, and E. B. White. (1929) "How to Tell Love from Passion." In *Is Sex Necessary? Or Why You Feel the Way You Do*. New York: Harper and Row, 1975, 62–78; Tillich, Paul. *Love, Power, and Justice*: *Ontological Analyses and Ethical Applications*. New York: Oxford University Press, 1954; Trevas, Robert, Arthur Zucker, and Donald Borchert, eds. *Philosophy of Sex and Love: A Reader*. Upper Saddle River, N.J.: Prentice-Hall, 1997; Vacek, Edward Collins. *Love, Human and Divine: The Heart of Christian Ethics*. Washington, D.C.: Georgetown University Press, 1994; Velleman, J. David. "Love as a Moral Emotion." *Ethics* 109:2 (1999), 338–74; Verene, Donald P., ed. *Sexual Love and Western Morality*, 1st ed. New York: Harper and Row, 1972. 2nd ed., Boston, Mass.: Jones and Bartlett, 1995; Vlastos, Gregory. "The Individual as an Object of Love in Plato." In *Platonic Studies*. Princeton, N.J.: Princeton University Press, 1973, 3–34. Reprinted in Alan Soble, ed., *Eros, Agape, and Philia: Readings in the Philosophy of Love*. New York: Paragon House, 1989, 96–124. Also: "Appendix II: Sex in Platonic Love," 38–42; reprinted in Soble, 124–28; Walsh, Anthony. "Love and Sex." In Vern Bullough and Bonnie Bullough, eds., *Human Sexuality: An Encyclopedia*. New York: Garland, 1994, 369–73; Williams, Clifford, ed. *On Love and Friendship*. Boston, Mass.: Jones and Bartlett, 1995; Wilson, John. *Love between Equals: A Philosophical Study of Love and Sexual Relationships*. New York: St. Martin's Press, 1995; Wojtyła, Karol (Pope John Paul II). *Love and Responsibility*. New York: Farrar, Straus and Giroux, 1981.

LUTHER, MARTIN. *See* Protestantism, History of